(continued from front page)

" I am writing to congratulate you on preparing an exceptional study guide. In five years of teaching this course, I have never encountered a more thorough, comprehensive, concise and realistic preparation for this examination. "
Teacher, Davie, FL

" I have found your publications, *The Best Test Preparation...*, to be exactly that. "
Teacher, Aptos, CA

" I used your book to prepare for the test and found that the advice and the sample tests were highly relevant... Without using any other material, I earned very high scores and will be going to the graduate school of my choice. "
Student, New Orleans, LA

" I used your *CLEP Introductory Sociology* book and rank it 99% — thank you! "
Student, Jerusalem, Israel

" Your *GMAT* book greatly helped me on the test. Thank you. "
Student, Oxford, OH

" I recently got the *French SAT II* Exam book from REA. I congratulate you on first-rate French practice tests."
Instructor, Los Angeles, CA

" Your *AP English Literature and Composition* book is most impressive."
Student, Montgomery, AL

" The REA *LSAT* Test Preparation guide is a winner! "
Instructor, Spartanburg, SC

The Best Test Preparation and Review Course for the

MCAT

Medical College Admission Test

**with CD-ROM for both Windows & Macintosh
REA's Interactive MCAT TESTware®**

Joseph A. Alvarez, M.A.
Professor of English
Central Piedmont Community College, Charlotte, NC

Pauline Beard, Ph.D.
Assistant Professor of English
Portland State University, Portland, OR

Robert Chasnov, Ph.D.
Associate Professor of Physics
Liberty University, Lynchburg, VA

Anita P. Davis, Ed.D.
Chairperson, Education Department
Converse College, Spartanburg, SC

Larry A. Giesmann, Ph.D.
Associate Professor of Biology
Northern Kentucky University, Highland Heights, KY

Gary F. Greif, Ph.D.
Chairperson, Philosophy Department
University of Wisconsin-Green Bay, Green Bay, WI

Timothy M. Hagle, J.D., Ph.D.
Assistant Professor of Political Science
The University of Iowa, Iowa City, IA

Marie Hankins, Ph.D.
Chairperson, Chemistry Department
University of Southern Indiana, Evansville, IN

Thomas C. Kennedy, Ph.D.
Professor of English
Washburn University, Topeka, KS

James S. Malek, Ph.D.
Dean of the College of Liberal Arts
University of Nevada, Las Vegas, NV

Mary Rengo Murnik, Ph.D.
Chairperson, Biological Sciences Department
Ferris State University, Big Rapids, MI

Jack C. Norman, Ph.D.
Professor of Chemistry
University of Wisconsin-Green Bay, Green Bay, WI

William R. Oliver, Ph.D.
Associate Professor of Chemistry
Northern Kentucky University, Highland Heights, KY

John G. Robison, Ph.D.
Chairperson, Philosophy Department
University of Massachusetts at Amherst, Amherst, MA

Garrett Ward Sheldon, Ph.D.
Associate Professor of Political Science
Clinch Valley College of University of Virginia, Wise, VA

William L. Stone, Ph.D.
Associate Professor of Pediatrics
James H. Quillen College of Medicine
East Tennessee State University, Johnson City, TN

Barbara A. D. Swyhart, Ph.D.
Professor of Philosophy
California University of Pennsylvania, California, PA

Gail D. Thomas, M.S.
Doctoral Candidate
Program in Physiology and Neurobiology
Rutgers University, New Brunswick, NJ

William C. Uhland, M.S.
Research Scientist
Cooper and Robert Wood Johnson Hospitals, Camden, NJ

William F. Wacholtz, Ph.D.
Assistant Professor of Chemistry
University of Wisconsin-Oshkosh, Oshkosh, WI

Charles M. Wynn, Ph.D.
Professor of Chemistry
Eastern Connecticut State University, Willimantic, CT

Research & Education Association
61 Ethel Road West • Piscataway, New Jersey 08854

The Best Test Preparation and Review Course for the
MEDICAL COLLEGE ADMISSION TEST (MCAT)
with CD-ROM for both Windows & Macintosh
REA's Interactive MCAT TEST*ware*®

Library of Congress Control Number 00-134279

International Standard Book Number 0-87891-350-5

TEST*ware*® is a trademark of
Research & Education Association, Piscataway, NJ 08854.

Windows® is a trademark of Microsoft® Corporation.
Macintosh® is a trademark of Apple Computer, Inc.

Research & Education Association
61 Ethel Road West
Piscataway, New Jersey 08854

 REA supports the effort to conserve and
protect environmental resources by
printing on recycled papers.

CONTENTS

About Research & Education Association

Research & Education Association (REA) is an organization of educators, scientists, and engineers specializing in various academic fields. Founded in 1959 with the purpose of disseminating the most recently developed scientific information to groups in industry, government, high schools, and universities, REA has since become a successful and highly respected publisher of study aids, test preps, handbooks, and reference works.

REA's Test Preparation series includes study guides for all academic levels in almost all disciplines. Research & Education Association publishes test preps for students who have not yet completed high school, as well as high school students preparing to enter college. Students from countries around the world seeking to attend college in the United States will find the assistance they need in REA's publications. For college students seeking advanced degrees, REA publishes test preps for many major graduate school admission examinations in a wide variety of disciplines, including engineering, law, and medicine. Students at every level, in every field, with every ambition can find what they are looking for among REA's publications.

Unlike most test preparation books—which present only a few practice tests that bear little resemblance to the actual exams—REA's series presents tests that accurately depict the official exams in both degree of difficulty and types of questions. REA's practice tests are always based upon the most recently administered exams, and include every type of question that can be expected on the actual exams.

REA's publications and educational materials are highly regarded and continually receive an unprecedented amount of praise from professionals, instructors, librarians, parents, and students. Our authors are as diverse as the subjects represented in the books we publish. They are well known in their respective fields and serve on the faculties of prestigious high schools, colleges, and universities throughout the United States.

About the MCAT Authors

In order to meet our objective of providing exams that reflect the MCAT in both content and degree of difficulty, every practice exam section has been carefully prepared by test experts in each field. Our authors have examined and researched the mechanics of the MCAT in order to develop practice questions that accurately depict the exam and test the knowledge required to do well on it. Our experts are highly regarded in the educational community—they have taught in their respective fields at competitive colleges and universities throughout the United States. Their extensive knowledge of the MCAT has enabled them to create practice questions and detailed explanations of the answers that will help you achieve a top score.

Acknowledgments

In addition to our authors, we wish to thank Dr. Max Fogiel, President, for his overall guidance, which brought this publication to completion, and the following for their significant editorial contributions: Susan Arvay, Jason Biegel, Aaron Bram, Chad Holland, Eric Hollekim, Andrew McIntosh, Paul Olson, Nicholas Paraskevopoulos, Kimberly Parke, Andrew Parks, Muhammad Qureshi, Alexandra Sonshine, Cindy Coe Taylor, Ph.D., Jeanine Todaro, John Tsinetakes, and Albert Zaretskie. Gratitude is also extended to Marty Perzan for composition of type and artwork.

Chapter 1

Preparing for the MCAT

About Our Book and MCAT TESTware®

You Can Achieve a Top MCAT Score

By reviewing and studying the material in this book and accompanying software (MCAT TESTware®), you can achieve a top score on the Medical College Admission Test (MCAT). The book and software have been designed to effectively prepare you for the MCAT Assessment by providing you with six full-length exams that accurately reflect the MCAT in both the level of difficulty and nature of the questions. The exams provided are based on the new format of the MCAT and include every type of question you may encounter during the actual examination. This book's practice exams 5 and 6 are also on CD-ROM as part of our exclusive interactive MCAT TESTware®. By taking the exams on the computer you will have the additional study features and benefits of enforced timed conditions, individual diagnostic analysis of what subjects need extra study, and instant scoring. For your convenience, our interactive MCAT TESTware® has been provided for you in both Windows and Macintosh formats. Many features are included which you will find helpful as you prepare for the MCAT. For instructions on how to install and use our software, please refer to the appendix at the back of this book.

Following each exam in the book you will find an answer key, complete with detailed explanations and solutions designed to clarify the material. Our objective is not only to provide you with the answers, but also to explain to you why one answer is more acceptable than another, and at the same time, review the material most likely to be encountered on the actual MCAT. By completing all six practice exams, and studying the explanations which follow, you can discover your strengths and weaknesses. This will then allow you to concentrate on the sections of the exam which give you the most difficulty. Also included are reviews of each topic covered in the test: chemistry, biology, physics, and mathematics, as well as tips on writing the essay. These reviews also present drills which can help prepare you for the model tests.

About the MCAT

The MCAT is required by virtually all American medical schools and is a very important criterion for admission. Every year, about 40,000 applicants to American and Canadian medical schools submit MCAT results, along with other undergraduate records, as part of the highly competitive medical school admission process.

Every medical school will have its own formula for evaluating your application and will attach a different weight to your MCAT scores. As a general rule, the scores you achieve on the MCAT are equally as important as your overall grade-point average and interviewing performance. For all intents and purposes, you must score well to have a reasonable chance for admission. This is even more important if you are applying to a highly competitive medical school.

The MCAT is administered by the AAMC twice a year—once in the spring and once in the late summer. Medical school admissions advisors generally suggest that you take the MCAT in the spring prior to the year you plan to begin your studies. Spring test dates are most preferable because your test results will be ready in time for early processing of your medical school application. In addition, if you should perform poorly during the spring administration of the MCAT, you will have an opportunity to retake the MCAT during the late summer.

MCAT registration materials, for both the spring and late summer administrations of each year, become available each February. For more information, you should contact your academic advisor, or contact:

MCAT Registration
MCAT Program Office
P.O. Box 4056
Iowa City, IA 52243
Phone: (319) 337-1357
TDD: (319) 337-1701

Association of American Medical Colleges
2450 N St., N.W.
Washington, DC 20037
Phone: (202) 828-0600
Website: www.aamc.org
E-mail: amcas@aamc.org

Format of the MCAT

In addition to testing your basic scientific knowledge in the fields of biology, chemistry, and physics, the MCAT will test your problem solving, critical thinking, and writing skills. The exam is composed of four basic sections, each containing brief passages which outline a situation. Following the passages are multiple-choice questions, which are designed to test your knowledge and various skills.

Verbal Reasoning (85 minutes)

This section consists of 65 reading comprehension questions based on several passages.

Physical Sciences (100 minutes)

This section consists of 77 physics and general chemistry questions. Approximately 10 or 11 passages will be the basis for 62 of the questions and the remaining 15 will be independent.

Writing Sample (30 minutes each essay)

This section consists of two separate essays on assigned topics.

Biological Sciences (100 minutes)

This section consists of 77 general biology and organic chemistry questions. Approximately 10 or 11 passages will be the basis for 62 of the questions; the remaining 15 will be independent.

Total Testing Time: 5 hours and 45 minutes

Test Section	Number of Questions	Minutes Per Section	Minutes Per Break Period
Verbal Reasoning	65	85	10
Physical Sciences	77	100	60 (lunch)
Writing Sample	2 essays	60	10
Biological Sciences	77	100	—

The Review Sections

- The **Biology Review** provides a comprehensive summary of the main areas tested in the Biological Sciences Test Section. It discusses topics in both general biology and organic chemistry.

- The **Chemistry Review** presents all of the topics that constitute the general chemistry half of the Physical Sciences Test Section.

- The **Physics Review** covers all of the topics that constitute the general physics half of the Physical Sciences Test Section.

- The **Mathematics Review** helps sharpen the necessary skills required for the science sections of the MCAT by reviewing the key areas of math you'll need to master before taking the exam.

- The **Writing Sample Review** provides some pointers on answering the Writing Sample section of the MCAT. It also discusses ways to gear your writing skills for this test section and organize your thoughts in a limited amount of time.

The Test Sections

As discussed earlier, the MCAT contains four separate sections: Verbal Reasoning, Physical Sciences, the Writing Samples, and Biological Sciences. The following outline explains these sections in detail and suggests helpful hints for selecting the correct answer.

VERBAL REASONING

The Verbal Reasoning section will ask interpretive, applicative, and inferential questions that refer to several reading passages. Each passage will be approximately 500 to 600 words in length. The questions will not ask about detailed facts from the passage but will include material that will call for the following:

- Understanding the theme of a passage

- Determining and evaluating the important points of an argument

- Drawing inferences from facts and reaching conclusions

All questions will be answerable solely on the basis of information provided in the passages and will not require any medical or special knowledge.

The passages for this section will be drawn from many disciplines, including the social sciences, the humanities, and philosophy. Thus, no particular academic background will afford an advantage.

Suggested Techniques for Answering Verbal Reasoning Questions

- Read the passage for content. Be sure you understand the words and statements in it.

- Skim some of the questions first before reading the passage. This may help you focus on the important points in the passage.

- Try not to spend too much time deciphering the meaning of words and statements upon first reading of the passage. It will be helpful to go over specific parts of the passage later, after reading each question.

- While reading the passage, you should look specifically for inferences, along with the mood or tone of the passage. Such things may hint at the type of questions that might be asked.

- Passages usually have their main idea or theme in the first and/or last sentences.

- Opinion pieces are the core of the MCAT Verbal Reasoning section. You should observe how the author's opinion differs from the general opinion surrounding the issue.

- You should remember that correct choices will usually paraphrase the information from the passages. This is especially true of inferential questions.

- Choices that repeat the material from a passage word-for-word are usually used as a lure to steer you into choosing the wrong answer.

PHYSICAL SCIENCES

The Physical Sciences section is based on several mini-passages that outline a situation. You will be required to interpret, analyze, and apply the information provided as you answer the questions. This section will require you to:

- Understand and apply basic concepts

- Balance simple chemical equations

- Solve general physics problems

All of the questions asked will be at the level of first-year college material. You will not need advanced or special knowledge to answer these questions.

Suggested Techniques for Answering Physical Sciences Questions

- Read each mini-passage thoroughly.

- Be sure you understand what each question is asking.

- Take notes in the margins of your test booklet.

- Do not try to work out the problems in your head.

- If you do not know the answer to a question, try to make an educated guess.

THE WRITING SAMPLE

The Writing Sample will ask you to write two essays on assigned topics. You will be given a short statement or quote to analyze. You must then write a logical and concise essay, addressing all of the required writing tasks in the time allotted. You will not be required to have prior knowledge of medicine in order to write your essays, as topics on medicine will not be assigned. You will, however, be expected to:

- Review and understand the topic statement or quotation

- Formulate a clear position

- Support your position eloquently and effectively

- Use correct grammar and vocabulary

(For suggested techniques on writing the essay, see Chapter 6, WRITING SAMPLE REVIEW, page 352)

BIOLOGICAL SCIENCES

The Biological Sciences section is based on several mini-passages that outline a situation. You must be able to interpret, analyze, and apply the information provided. In this section you will be required to:

- Understand and apply basic concepts

- Balance simple chemical equations

- Solve general biology and organic chemistry problems

All questions will be at the level of first-year college material. You will not be required to possess prior or advanced knowledge to answer these questions.

Suggested Techniques for Answering Biological Sciences Questions

- Read each mini-passage thoroughly.

- Be sure you understand what each question is asking.

- Skim some of the questions before reading each mini-passage.

Scoring the MCAT

Your MCAT test score will be composed of four individual scores—one for each section of the test. All of the multiple-choice sections of your MCAT will first be given a raw score. Your raw score for a particular section is determined by totaling the number of correct answers for that section. Your raw score will then be converted into a scaled score, with 1 being the lowest and 15 being the highest. The conversion of raw scores into scaled scores varies from year to year due to differing levels of question difficulty. The MCAT writing samples are scored by two or three readers.

Computing Your Score

1. Use the answer key after each test to check your answers.

2. Use the space below to mark your raw score.

3. Use the Score Conversion Chart to convert your raw scores into scaled scores.

**Total Number of
Correct Answers
(Raw Score)**

Verbal Reasoning Section _____

Physical Sciences Section _____

Biological Sciences Section _____

Use the following table to convert your raw score to a scaled score. Remember that the conversion value of raw scores to scaled scores will vary slightly from year to year to compensate for different levels of question difficulty.

MCAT Scoring Table

Verbal Reasoning			Physical Sciences			Biological Sciences		
Scaled Scores	Raw Scores	Estimated Percentile Ranks	Scaled Scores	Raw Scores	Estimated Percentile Ranks	Scaled Scores	Raw Scores	Estimated Percentile Ranks
15	61-65	93-99	15	66-77	96-99	15	71-77	98-99
14	56-60	78-90	14	61-65	90-95	14	66-70	92-97
13	51-55	63-75	13	56-60	82-89	13	61-65	83-90
12	46-50	48-60	12	51-55	73-81	12	56-60	73-81
11	41-45	36-46	11	46-50	62-71	11	51-55	61-71
10	36-40	25-33	10	41-45	50-59	10	46-50	49-59
9	31-35	16-23	9	36-40	39-47	9	41-45	37-47
8	26-30	9-14	8	31-35	25-35	8	36-40	26-35
7	21-25	4-7	7	26-30	14-23	7	31-35	16-24
6	17-20	3-4	6	21-25	5-12	6	26-30	7-14
5	13-16	2-3	5	17-20	4-5	5	21-25	2-6
4	10-12	2	4	13-16	3-4	4	16-20	2
3	7-9	1	3	9-12	2-3	3	11-15	1
2	4-6	1	2	5-8	1-2	2	6-10	1
1	0-3	1	1	0-4	1	1	0-5	1

Your estimated percentile rank indicates your rank in comparison to other students who have taken the exam. For example, if your Verbal Reasoning raw score is 59 (correct answers), then, according to the table, your percentile rank would fall between 78 and 90, indicating that you scored better than 78% to 90% of all MCAT examinees.

Scoring the Writing Samples

Your MCAT writing samples will be graded on a scale of 1 to 6, with 1 being "poor" and 6 "excellent." Each writing sample will be graded independently, by two readers. The raw score assigned to your essays will be a combination of four evaluations—two for your first essay and two for your second essay. If there is a discrepancy of more than one point between the two readers, a third reader will evaluate your essay and assign a final score.

After the initial scoring, the evaluations for both of your essays will be added together and assigned a letter grade on a scale from J to T, with J being the lowest and T being the highest. Your scores for the writing samples will also be reported to the medical schools to which you are applying. Each medical school will receive a written explanation describing the meaning of each letter grade, your percentile ranking, and score distributions.

Here are the scoring criteria for evaluating your MCAT writing samples:

POINT VALUE

1. The essay shows very poor spelling and punctuation. The essay may not answer the assigned topic. The structure and writing of the essay may make it difficult to understand.

2. The essay contains major structural and/or grammatical errors. The analysis of the essay topic may be incorrect or incomplete. One or more of the required writing assignments may be executed incompletely or incorrectly.

3. The essay indicates that the writer's basic skills are adequate, but that there are noticeable errors. The essay may be disorganized or poorly planned. One or more of the required writing assignments may be addressed only on a superficial level.

4. The essay is well-organized with only minor digressions from the topic. Points are logical and clearly written, but must be developed in greater depth. All required writing assignments have been addressed, but one or more may need more development.

5. The essay addresses all required writing assignments clearly and thoroughly. The essay's points are concise and well-organized. Grammar and punctuation in the essay are correct.

6. The essay thoroughly addresses the required writing assignments in depth. The essay's points are very clear and well-organized. The grammar and punctuation of the essay are excellent.

MCAT Test-Taking Strategies

HOW TO BEAT THE CLOCK

Every second counts when you are taking the MCAT, so you will want to use your test time in the most efficient manner possible. Since the MCAT is composed of questions which vary in degree of difficulty, you should answer first the questions which you feel are easy, saving the difficult ones for last. Also, you should not spend a great deal of time working out a single difficult question when you could be solving the questions which are easier to answer. Although you should work quickly, do not rush through the exam as this will cause you to answer the questions with less accuracy. Pace yourself and work steadily.

Make every effort to maintain your concentration during the test. Do not waste time watching the proctor or looking around the room. This will waste valuable minutes that will become very important as you approach the end of the exam.

GUESSING STRATEGY

If you are uncertain of a question, guess at the answer rather than not answer it at all. You will not be penalized for answering incorrectly, since wrong answers are not counted. This means that you should never leave a space on your answer sheet blank. Even if you do not have time to guess at an answer, be sure to fill in every space on the answer sheet. Since you will not be assessed a penalty for a wrong answer, you will receive credit for any questions you answer correctly by luck. Remember, your chances of filling in the correct circle are automatically bettered if you do not leave the question blank.

Try to make an educated guess if you do not know the answer. However, if time is short and you cannot make educated guesses, do not simply guess at random. Use one letter and fill in all your guesses with that letter. This has been statistically proven to be one-and-a-half times as effective as blind guessing.

OTHER MUST-DO STRATEGIES

As you work on the test, make sure your answers correspond with the numbers and letters on the answer sheet. You do not want to be marked incorrect simply because you filled in the wrong circle.

Don't hesitate to write in this book, as you are allowed to write in the test booklet of the actual exam. Do not try to solve difficult problems or questions in your head. You will be under a great deal of pressure when taking the actual exam and you may become confused. Work the problem out in your test booklet instead, as the problem is easier to solve when you can see your work on paper.

If you are completely uncertain of a question, skip it at first. Mark the question in your test booklet so that you can go back to it later. This will allow you to go on to questions about which you are certain. Then, if time allows, go back and try to make educated guesses for the questions you skipped.

Good luck on the MCAT!

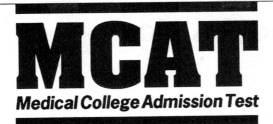

Chapter 2
Biology Review

Chapter 2

I. Molecular Biology

1. Enzymes and Cellular Metabolism

A. ENZYME STRUCTURE AND FUNCTION

An enzyme is a protein that performs a metabolic function. Enzymes are catalysts and affect the rate but not the overall change in free energy of a chemical reaction. Most enzymes have molecular weights over 10,000 daltons.

All enzymes are complex proteins. Some proteins, for example, play only a structural role and have no metabolic function. Proteins are polypeptides, i.e., linear polymers with amino acids serving as the repeating units. Proteins are composed of one or more polypeptide chains and often contain a nonprotein moiety such as carbohydrate (as in glycoproteins), lipid (as in lipoproteins), or a metal ion (as in metalloproteins). Both noncovalent and covalent interactions can be important in stabilizing the structure of a polypeptide. Hydrogen bonds, ionic bonds, and hydrophobic interactions are important noncovalent factors. Disulfide bonds formed by cysteine side chains are a major form of covalent interaction. Each amino acid unit in a polypeptide can be any one of the twenty different naturally occurring amino acids. The sequence of amino acids in a polypeptide can, therefore, be very variable. This great variability enables proteins to assume many different structures and thereby perform many different and specific functions. The function of an enzyme is determined by its structure.

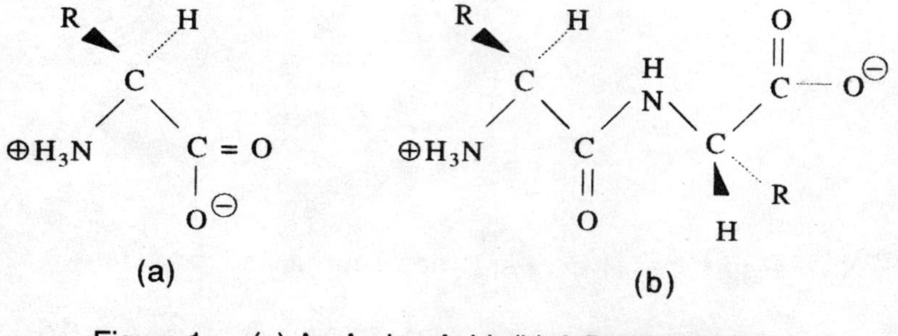

Figure 1 — (a) An Amino Acid; (b) A Peptide Bond

Individual amino acids (see Figure 1a) all possess an alpha-carbon that bonds to a carboxyl group ($-COO^-$), an alpha-amino group ($-NH_3^+$), a side group (R), and a hydrogen atom (H). At physiological pH the carboxyl group is negatively charged and the alpha-amino group is positively charged. With the exception of glycine (where R = H), the alpha-carbon of all amino acid is asymmetric (or chiral). All naturally occurring amino acids have L-stereochemistry.

In humans, not all the amino acids required for protein synthesis are made by the body. Eight amino acids are essential for man, i.e., valine (Val), leucine (Leu), isoleucine (Ile), lysine (Lys), phenylalanine (Phe), tryptophan (Try), threonine (Thr) and methionine (Met). Histidine (His) is required in infants but not in adults. The essential amino acids must come from dietary sources.

In a polypeptide chain the amino acid units are linked together by peptide bonds. The peptide bond is formed between the carboxyl group of one amino acid and the amino group of the next amino acid. As shown in Figure 2, the peptide bond has a partial double-bond character which restricts rotation about the C—N peptide bond. This restricted rotation limits the number of possible conformations obtainable by a polypeptide.

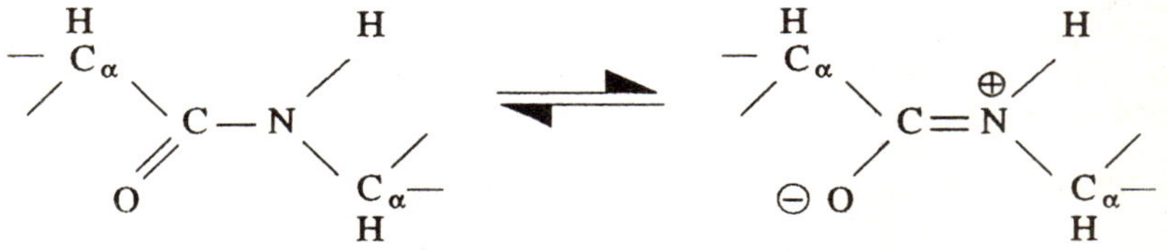

Figure 2 — Partial Double-Bond Character of Peptide Bond.

Proteins (and enzymes) can have four levels of structure. The primary structure is totally determined by the sequence of amino acids. The secondary structure is due to the formation of alpha-helices or beta-sheets. Both alpha-helices and beta-sheets arise from the periodic hydrogen bonding between peptides (see Figure 3).

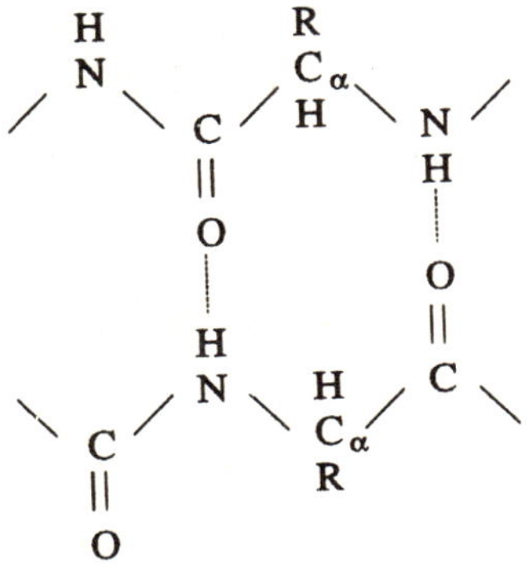

Figure 3 — Hydrogen Bonds Between Polypeptides

The tertiary structure of a protein is the complete three dimensional description of each atom in the protein. Tertiary structure is built from units of secondary structure linked together by turns in the polypeptide backbone. Quaternary structure results when protein subunits combine to form a larger structure. Hemoglobin is an example of a protein with quarternary structure since it contains two alpha-subunits (α) and two beta-subunits (β), i.e., $\alpha_2\beta_2$.

Proteins can be either water-soluble or bound to biological membranes. For water-soluble proteins, the hydrophilic amino acid side chains are generally found near the outer surface of the protein. The hydrophobic amino acid side chains are found in the interior of the protein where they are out of contact with water. Hydrophobic amino acid side chains (Cys, Val, Ile, Leu, Met, Trp, and Phe) are relatively nonpolar and do not interact with water molecules. Hydrophilic amino acid residues (Lys, Arg, His, Asp, Glu, Asn, and Gln) are polar and interact favorably with water.

Membrane proteins are associated with the lipid bilayer of biological membranes. There are two general categories of membrane proteins, i.e., intrinsic membrane proteins and extrinsic membrane proteins. Intrinsic membrane proteins are strongly associated with the biological membrane and can only be removed with a denaturing detergent such as sodium dodecylsulfate (SDS). Intrinsic membrane proteins often have a sequence containing numerous hydrophobic amino acid side chains that are strongly associated with the hydrophobic domain of the lipid bilayer. Extrinsic membrane proteins are only loosely associated with biological membranes and can be removed by alterations in the ionic strength or by a chelator such as EDTA.

PROBLEM

Enzymes are

a)   proteins.   b)   catalysts.

c)   carbohydrates.   d)   Both a) and b).

Solution

d)   Enzymes are proteins that act as catalysts. Carbohydrates are not proteins, and therefore cannot be enzymes.

B. CONTROL OF ENZYME ACTIVITY

For the proper regulation of metabolism it is necessary for all organisms to exert considerable control over the location, amount and activity of enzymes. An enzyme (E) forms a complex with its substrate (S) at a well defined region called the active site. Subsequently, the enzyme-substrate complex (ES) is converted into a product (P) and the enzyme (E) is released.

$$E + S \rightleftharpoons ES \longrightarrow E + P$$

The activity of an enzyme can be regulated by changing or blocking the active site. A competitive inhibitor is one that reversibly binds to the active site and com-

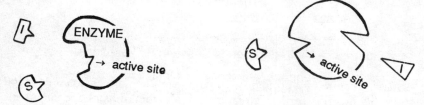

(a) Competitive inhibition
Both substrate (S) and inhibitor (I) compete for the same active site.

(b) Non-competitive inhibition.
The inhibitor (I) binds at a site different from the active site and does not prevent binding of the substrate. The inhibitor does decrease enzymatic activity.

Figure 4 — (a) Competitive Inhibition; (b) Noncompetitive Inhibition petes with the substrate for binding at this same locus (see Figure 4(a)). For competitive inhibition the activity of the enzymatically catalyzed reaction depends upon the concentration of both substrate and inhibitor.

Many enzymes have two (or more) alternative conformations, and the binding of ligands (substrates or other molecules) can influence which conformation the enzyme assumes. For allosteric proteins one conformation is enzymatically active and the other conformation is inactive. Allosteric enzymes are very important in the regulation of metabolic reactions (see below).

PROBLEM

> Organisms can control all of the following EXCEPT
>
> a)   location of enzymes.   b)   type of enzymes.
>
> c)   amount of enzymes.   d)   activity of enzymes.

Solution

b)   Organisms control the activity of enzymes by changing or blocking active sites. Location and amount of enzymes may be controlled through feedback. Types of enzymes are determined genetically and cannot be altered.

C. FEEDBACK INHIBITION

Cells are required to synthesize an enormous number of essential compounds for their survival. Bacteria, although structurally simple, can use glucose to provide for their energy needs and to synthesize necessary organic components. The synthesis of these organic compounds is accomplished by specific metabolic pathways in which a precursor molecule is converted to a product by a series of enzyme-catalyzed reactions. The flow of metabolites in a metabolic pathway is often regulated by controlling the activity of key enzymes in the pathway. Usually, the first enzyme in a metabolic pathway is controlled by the end product of the pathway. This type of regulation is called feedback inhibition. In negative feedback inhibition (see Figure 5) the end product of a pathway inhibits the first enzyme in the pathway.

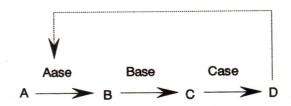

Figure 5 — Feedback Inhibition of a Metabolic Pathway.
Metabolite D inhibits Aase.

The first enzyme in a metabolic pathway is usually an allosteric enzyme. The end product of the pathway binds to a regulatory site on the enzyme, causing it to assume an inactive conformation. The regulatory site is different from the active site. In the case of negative feedback inhibition the pathway end product is usually a noncompetitive inhibitor. A noncompetitive inhibitor binds to the enzyme at a locus different from the active site (see Figure 4(b)). Furthermore, for noncompetitive inhibition the rate of the enzymatically catalyzed reaction depends only on the concentration of the inhibitor and not on the concentration of substrate. In summary, feedback regulation:

(a)   usually involves an allosteric enzyme,

(b)   is very rapid, and

(c)   can involve enzymatic inhibition or enzymatic activators (positive feedback inhibition).

Feedback regulation also provides an efficient method of conserving cellular energy and preventing the build-up of metabolic intermediates which, at high levels, could be toxic.

PROBLEM

In feedback inhibition of metabolic pathways, which are controlled directly?

a)   End products   b)   Metabolites

c)   Enzymes   d)   Precursor molecules

Solution

c)   In feedback inhibition the flow of metabolites is often regulated by controlling the activity of key enzymes in a pathway. Usually, the first enzyme in a metabolic pathway is controlled by the end product of the pathway.

D. GLYCOLYSIS

The sequence of energy producing catabolic reactions called glycolysis takes place in all living cells. Glycolysis results in the production of adenosine triphosphate (ATP), which provides cells with an efficient source of chemical energy. Catabolism is the chemical breakdown of food molecules to provide energy and building blocks for the synthesis of macromolecules. The first step in catabolism is the breakdown of macromolecular polymers to their monomeric units. Polysaccharides are broken down into sugars such as glucose. Glucose is further catabolized by the process of glycolysis.

ANAEROBIC

Glycolysis does not require the presence of oxygen. This metabolic pathway is very ancient, having evolved when the earth's atmosphere contained very little oxygen. In eukaryotes and many prokaryotes, glycolysis results in the net production of two molecules of ATP, two molecules of NADPH, and two molecules of pyruvate per molecule of glucose:

$$\text{D-glucose} + 2HPO_4^{2-} + 2ADP + 2NAD \longrightarrow$$

$$2CH_3C\!\!-\!\!CO_2 + 2ATP + 2\ NADPH + 2H^+.$$

The ten steps in the glycolytic pathway are detailed below (see Figure 6). The first steps of glycolysis (steps 1-3) convert glucose to fructose 1,6-diphosphate (FDP) at the cost of two ATPs. Fructose and glucose are both six-carbon sugars (hexoses). The second stage results in the splitting (by aldolase) of fructose 1,6-diphosphate into two three carbon sugars (trioses), i.e., dihydroxyacetone phosphate (DHAP) and D-glyceraldehyde 3-phosphate. DHAP is converted to D-glyceraldehyde 3-phosphate by triose phosphate isomerase. The third phase of glycolysis produces ATP by converting D-glyceraldehyde 3-phosphate into metabolites that can transfer phosphoryl groups to ADP. The pyruvate produced by glycolysis is a key branch-point metabolite. Under anaerobic conditions yeast converts pyruvate to ethanol and carbon dioxide and animals convert pyruvate to lactic acid. Some prokaryotes utilize different pathways than the one described above. All function to generate ATP, $NADH_2^+$, and pyruvate, but some are less efficient than glycolysis.

AEROBIC

The key regulatory enzyme in glycolysis is phosphofructokinase. Its activity is inhibited by ATP, citrate and fatty acids and activated by ADP, AMP, cyclic AMP, and FDP. When cells that are undergoing anaerobic glycolysis are switched to aerobic conditions the rate of glycolysis rapidly drops. This is called the Pasteur effect. The effect is explained by the fact that under aerobic conditions the pyruvate produced by glycolysis can undergo further oxidation, via the citric acid cycle (see below). This results in the production of 18 ATP molecules per pyruvate. Thus, the energy needs of the cell are met with a considerably reduced rate of glycolysis. The decreased rate of glycolysis with higher levels of ATP is consistent with the fact that phosphofructokinase is inhibited by ATP.

PROBLEM

Glycolysis does not			
a)	occur in the cytoplasm.	b)	require oxygen.
c)	produce ATP.	d)	break down glucose.

Solution

b) Glycolysis is the series of metabolic reactions by which glucose is converted to pyruvate (a 3-carbon sugar) with the concurrent formation of ATP. Glycolysis occurs in the cytoplasm of the cell and for this process the presence of oxygen is unnecessary.

E. KREBS (CITRIC ACID) CYCLE

For most eukaryotic cells and aerobic bacteria the pyruvic acid produced by glycolysis is completely oxidized to CO_2 and H_2O. This process, called cellular respiration, produces reducing power in the form of NADH and $FADH_2$. NADH and $FADH_2$ are then utilized by the electron transport system to produce ATP. Electron transport occurs in the mitochondria of eukaryotic cells and in the membrane of aerobic bacteria.

In eukaryotic cells, the pyruvate produced by anaerobic glycolysis enters the mitochondrion and is decarboxylated. This leaves behind an acetate residue. NAD^+ accepts one hydrogen from pyruvic acid and one from coenzyme A(CoA). This allows the CoA and the acetate to condense, forming acetyl CoA. The primary function of the citric acid pathway is to oxidize acetyl groups to CO_2 and H_2O. The overall reaction is:

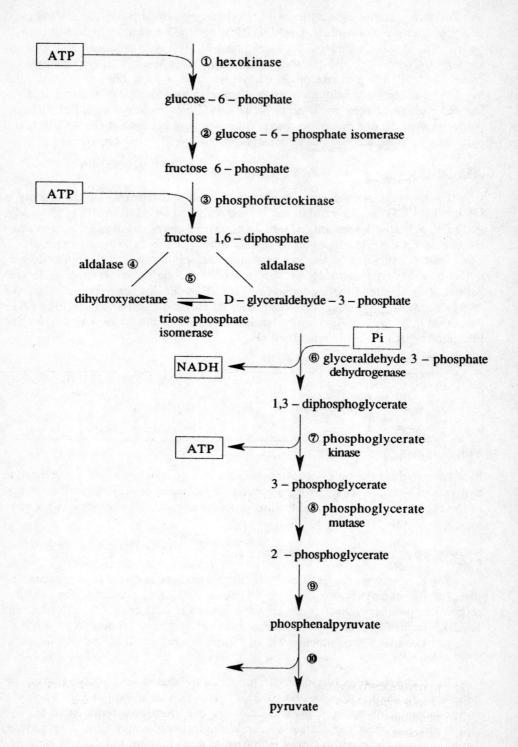

Figure 6 — Glycolysis

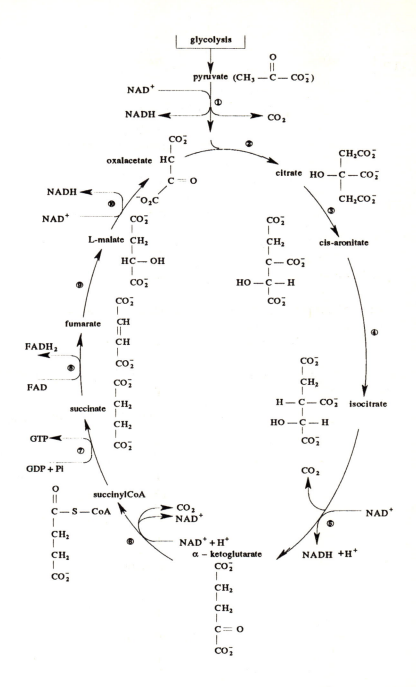

(1) pyruvate carboxylase
(2) citrate synthetase
(3) aconitase
(4) aconitase
(5) isocitrate dehydrogenase
(6) alpha-ketoglutarate dehydrogenase
(7) succinyl CoA synthetase
(8) succinate dehydrogenase
(9) fumarase
(10) malate dehydrogenase

Figure 7 — The Krebs Cycle

$$\text{acetyl CoA} + 2H_2O + 3NAD^+ + FAD + GDP + HPO_4^- \longrightarrow$$

$$2CO_2 + 3NADH + FADH_2 + GTP + 8H^+ + CoA$$

and the enzymatically catalyzed steps shown in Figure 7. The citric acid (or Krebs) cycle occurs in the mitochondrial matrix (see Figure 10).

It is noteworthy that molecular oxygen (O_2) does not enter the citric acid cycle. The additional oxygen atoms required for CO_2 production come from H_2O. The one GTP produced by step 7 is easily converted to ATP (GTP + ADP = GDP + ATP). The oxidation of one NADH molecule by the electron transport system produces three ATPs and, similarly, the oxidation of one $FADH_2$ produces two ATPs. The complete oxidation of glucose yields 38 ATPs.

PROBLEM

In the Krebs Cycle, all of the following occur EXCEPT

a) oxidation of succinate.

b) formation of $FADH_2$.

c) formation of NADH.

d) transformation of NADH to NAD.

Solution

d) NADH is converted to NAD during oxidative phosphorylation, which yields 3 ATP.

F. ELECTRON TRANSPORT CHAIN AND OXIDATIVE PHOSPHORYLATION

The last steps in catabolism, called oxidative phosphorylation, result in the efficient production of ATP. In these steps, electrons (e^-) are ultimately transferred to oxygen (see Figure 8) with the generation of ATP. Oxidative phosphorylation is dependent upon the structure of mitochondria.

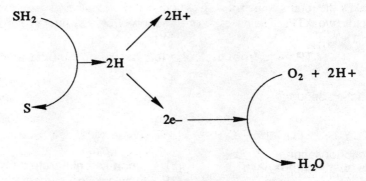

Figure 8 — Electron Transport.
Substrates (SH_2) contain H-atoms consisting of a proton (H^+) and an electron (e^-). The energy locked in H^+ and e^- is harnessed during oxidative phosphorylation to produce ATP.

Oxidative phosphorylation generates ATP by harnessing the energy of the electron transport chain to efficiently phosphorylate ADP. The enzyme catalyzing this reaction is a proton (H^+) driven ATP synthetase (H^+-ATP synthetase). H^+-ATP synthetase is a transmembrane protein embedded in the inner mitochondrial membrane. The energy to drive ATP formation by H^+-ATP synthetase comes from a proton gradient across the inner mitochondrial membrane. This proton gradient is generated by the movement of electrons down the respiratory chain. The respiratory chain is a series of membrane bound redox carriers with cytochrome oxidase being the terminal electron acceptor (see Figure 9).

The electrons that ultimately reach O_2 (and form H_2O) are initially carried by the hydrogen atoms of NADH and $FADH_2$ (from glycolysis and the citric acid cycle). These hydrogen atoms can be dissociated into an electron (e^-) and a proton (H^+). The electrons are transported by the respiratory chain and the protons are released into the aqueous medium. The released H^+ ions are translocated from the matrix space to the intermembrane space, and a pH gradient is established. The energy created by this gradient is trapped by the H^+-ATP synthetase when the H^+ flow back into the matrix (see Figure 10). This process is known as chemiosmosis.

The process of oxidative phosphorylation illustrates a milestone in biochemistry, because it is an example of factorial metabolism — the coupling of metabolism with transport across a membrane.

PROBLEM

The ratio of ATP produced aerobically to anaerobically by the oxidation of one molecule of glucose is

a)   2:1.   b)   1:2.

c)   1:18.   d)   18:1.

Solution

d)   The aerobic production of ATP involves the Krebs (citric acid) cycle and the oxidation of glucose. The anaerobic production of ATP takes place during glycolysis. The citric acid cycle produces 34 ATPs and the oxidation of glucose produces two. This makes the total number of ATPs produced during aerobic processes 36. Glycolysis yields two ATPs. The net ratio of aerobic ATP to anerobic ATP is 36:2 which is equal to 18:1.

ATP yield from the complete oxidation of glucose

Reaction sequence	ATP yield per glucose
GLYCOLYSIS: GLUCOSE TO PYRUVATE (in the cytoplasm)	
Phosphorylation of glucose	− 1
Phosphorylation of fructose 6-phosphate	− 1
Dephosphorylation of 2 molecules of 1, 3-DPG	+ 2
Dephosphorylation of 2 molecules of phosphoenolpyruvate	+ 2

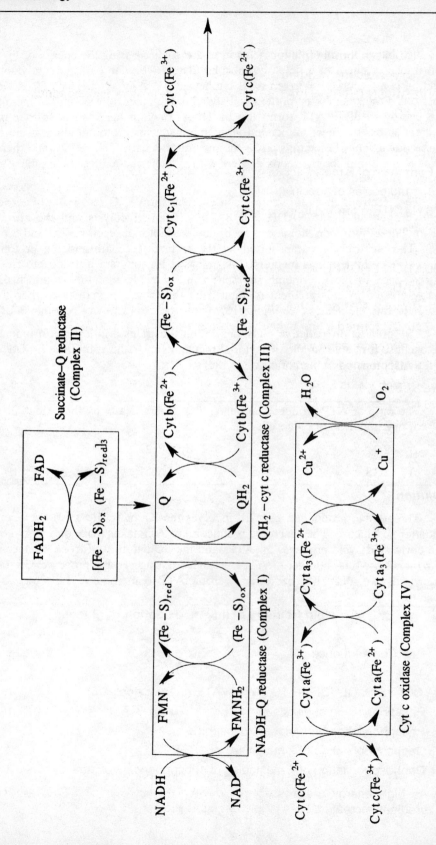

Figure 9 — Respiratory Chain

2 NADH are formed in the oxidation of 2 molecules of
glyceraldehyde 3-phosphate

CONVERSION OF PYRUVATE TO ACETYL CoA (inside mitochondria)
2 NADH are formed

CITRIC ACID CYCLE (inside mitochondria)
**Formation of 2 molecules of guanosine triphosphate from 2
molecules of succinyl CoA**   **+2**
6 NADH are formed in the oxidation of 2 molecules of
succinate

OXIDATION PHOSPHORYLATION (inside mitochondria)
2 NADH formed in glycolysis; each yields 2 ATP
(not 3 ATP each, because of the cost of the shuttle)   **+ 4**
2 NADH formed in the oxidative decarboxylation of
pyruvate; each yields 3 ATP   **+ 6**
2 FADH formed in the citric acid cycle;
each yields 2 ATP   **+ 4**
6 NADH formed in the citric acid cycle;
each yields 3 ATP

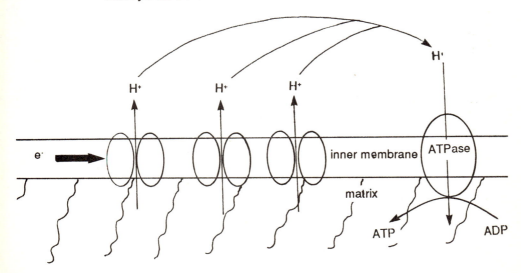

Figure 10 — Oxidative Phosphorylation.
As high energy electrons move down the respiratory chain, a proton
gradient is created. H+-ATPase uses this gradient to make ATP.

2. DNA and Protein Synthesis

A. DNA STRUCTURE AND FUNCTION

The information determining the sequence of amino acids in a polypeptide resides in another linear polymer called deoxyribonucleic acid (DNA). DNA, and nucleic acids in general, are polynucleotides in which the repeating units are nucleotides. DNA contains the cell's genetic information. DNA has been called an "aperiodic crystal." Aperiodicity is a requirement for coding information and the "crystalline" structure of DNA provides considerable thermodynamic stability.

Nucleotides contain either a purine or a pyrimidine base that is attached to a five-carbon sugar-phosphate (see Figure 11). In DNA the sugar is 2-deoxyribose (dRib) and in ribonucleic acids (RNA) the sugar is ribose (Rib). Four bases are found in both DNA and RNA. Adenine and guanine are the two purine bases present in DNA. Thymidine and cytosine are the two pyrimidines. RNA also contains adenine, guanine, and cytosine, but uracil substitutes for thymine. Nucleotides are linked to each other by phosphodiester bonds between the 3′ hydroxyl group of one nucleotide and the 5′ end of the next (see Figure 11).

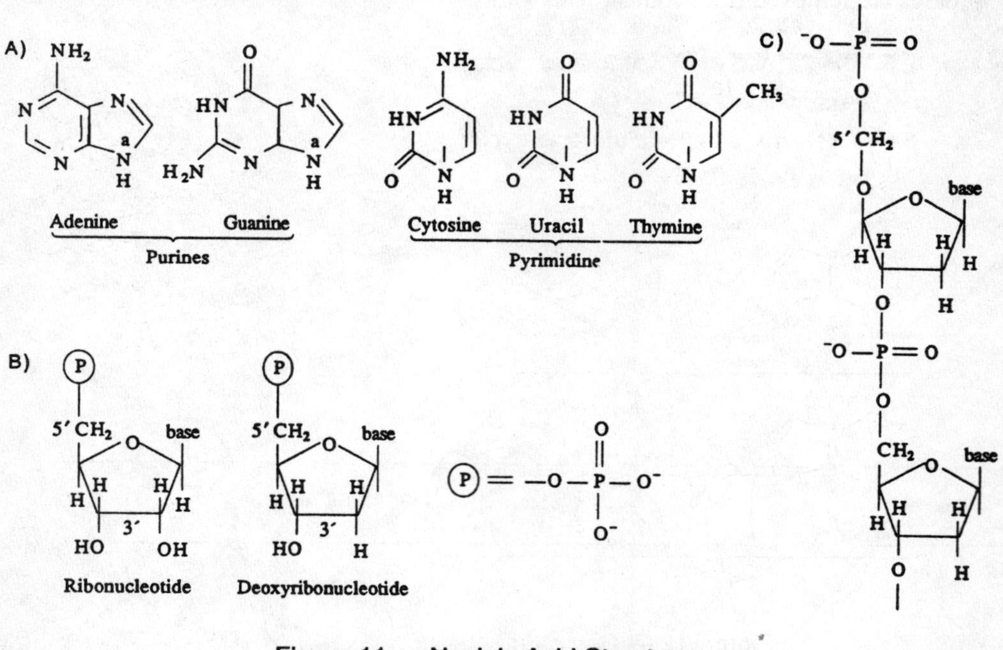

Figure 11 — Nucleic Acid Structure.
(a) Structure of bases in nucleic acids. Purines attach to ribose (or deoxyribose) at the 9-position and pyrimidines at the 1-position. (b) Structure of a ribonucleotide and deoxyribonucleotide. (c) Structure of single chain deoxyribonucleic acid.

The composition of DNA provides important clues with regard to both its function and structure. Chargaff found that:

(1)   the base composition of DNA in different tissues from the same species was identical,

(2) the base composition of DNA from similar species was similar and the base composition of DNA from widely divergent species was dissimilar,

(3) in DNA from all species the number of adenine bases equalled the number of thymine (A = T) bases and the number of guanine bases equalled the number of cytosine bases (G = C).

The Watson-Crick model of DNA provides an immediate and simple explanation for the fact that A = T and G = C. The Watson-Crick model proposes that DNA is a double stranded helix with the two strands running in opposite directions, i.e., antiparallel. The purines and pyrimidine bases are stacked on top of each other forming the inside of the double helix. The planes of the bases are essentially parallel to one another and perpendicular to the long axis of the DNA molecule. Adenine, on one strand, forms a specific base pair with thymine on the other, antiparallel strand. The AT base pair is stabilized by two hydrogen bonds. Guanine and cytosine also form a specific base pair (GC), but it is stabilized by three hydrogen bonds. The complementary base pairing for double stranded DNA is illustrated in Figure 12. In addition to hydrogen bonding and charge separation between phosphates along the helix, the structure of DNA is stabilized by hydrophobic interactions. The stacked bases are removed from contact with water.

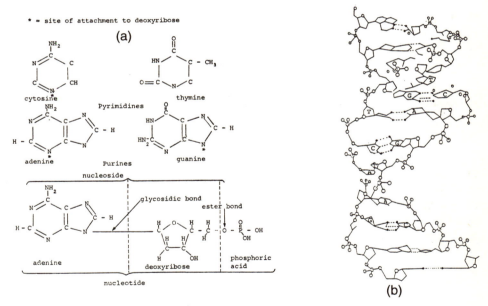

Figure 12 — Complementary Base Pairing in DNA.
(a) Four base pairs; (b) DNA double helix, showing complementary base pairing.

B. DNA AS TRANSMITTER OF GENETIC INFORMATION

The unique structure of DNA enables it to serve two template functions. One function is to serve as a template for its own replication. The other is to provide a template for the synthesis of RNA (transcription).

DNA replication involves:

(1)   strand separation, and

(2)   the synthesis, via DNA polymerase, of a complementary daughter strand from each parent strand.

The biochemical details of this process are complex, involving numerous proteins. DNA replication involves a replication form in which both nascent strands are synthesized in a 5′ to 3′ direction. This results in continuous synthesis for the leading strand but discontinuous synthesis for the lagging strand (see Figure 13). Discontinuous synthesis results in Okazaki fragments, which are later joined to form a continuous strand.

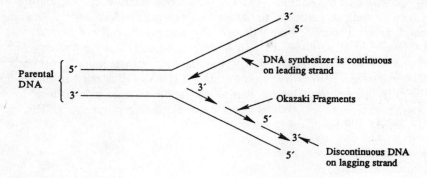

Figure 13 — DNA replication fork with Okazaki fragments.

C. PROTEIN SYNTHESIS: TRANSCRIPTION AND TRANSLATION

Transcription

A second function of DNA is to provide a template for the synthesis of messenger RNA (mRNA), ribosomal RNA (rRNA) and transfer RNA (tRNA), all of which are single stranded ribonucleic acid polymers. Messenger RNA is the intermediary polymer used to transmit information about the sequence of amino acids in protein from DNA. The synthesis of RNA from a DNA template is called transcription. In most cells the flow of genetic information is:

$$DNA \xrightarrow{\text{transcription}} mRNA \xrightarrow{\text{translation}} protein$$

In eukaryotic cells DNA is found almost exclusively in the cell nucleus, and most of the RNA is found in the cytoplasm where protein synthesis occurs. Both rRNA and tRNA are involved in the biosynthesis of proteins (translation) but do not carry any information coding for the sequence of amino acids in a protein. For RNA synthesis the bases on one strand of DNA (the "sense strand") are matched with complementary ribonucleotide triphosphates and polymerized into an RNA molecule.

In prokaryotes a multi-subunit RNA polymerase is responsible for the synthesis of mRNA, tRNA and rRNA from the DNA template. RNA polymerase cannot, however, utilize an RNA template (double stranded or single stranded) or an RNA/DNA hybrid. Transcription involves three steps:

(1) initiation,

(2) elongation, and

(3) termination.

Initiation starts at specific sites on the DNA termed promoters. One subunit of RNA polymerase, the sigma subunit, recognizes these promoters. RNA chain elongation proceeds in a 5′ $\longrightarrow$ 3′ direction until a termination signal is encountered on the DNA template. Some termination signals require a protein called Rho and are referred to as Rho-dependent. After the polymerase encounters the signal, Rho disengages it from the template, or, more specifically, promotes the dissociation of RNA polymerase from the template. Other termination signals are Rho-independent.

Transcription in eukaryotic cells is mechanistically very similar to prokaryotic transcription but more complex. Eukaryotic cells contain three different polymerases, denoted RNA polymerase I, II, and III. Each transcribes a different set of genes. RNA polymerase I transcribes most of the ribosomal RNA. RNA polymerase II transcribes mRNA and most of the snRNP RNAs. RNA polymerase III transcribes small RNAs such as tRNA and the 5S ribosomal RNA. Each polymerase is comprised of ten or more subunits — considerably more complex than *E. coli* RNA polymerases. The three polymerases share common subunits, although each also has private subunits. Unlike *E. coli* RNA polymerase, eukaryotic polymerases cannot bind to promoter sequences. They require that other protein factors first bind the DNA.

The base sequence of an mRNA molecule (or of the DNA gene itself) encodes the information for the amino acid sequence of a protein. Since proteins vary greatly in molecular weight, it follows that mRNAs must be heterologous in length. Each amino acid in a polypeptide is determined by a three base codon. Three bases allow for 64 different codons. However, proteins are comprised of only twenty different amino acids. Therefore, either some codons are not used or more than one codon can code for an amino acid (i.e., the code is degenerate). In fact only three codons (UAA, UAG and UGA) do not code for amino acids. They provide the termination signal for translation and are referred to as "stop codons." The genetic code used in a wide variety of organisms is identical with only minor exceptions.

In prokaryotic cells, the sequence of bases coding for a given polypeptide (the gene or cistron) are continuous. In marked contrast, the coding regions for polypeptides in eukaryotic cells can be discontinuous. The newly synthesized mRNA (the primary transcript) in eukaryotic cells contains regions called introns that are not expressed in the synthesized protein product. These intron regions are removed and the regions that are expressed (exons) are spliced together to form the final functional mRNA molecule.

Translation

The process for translating an mRNA molecule into a polypeptide is very complex. Ribosomes and tRNA are of primary importance, but numerous other proteins are also required. Polypeptides are synthesized by sequentially adding amino acids to the carboxyl end of the growing polypeptide chain. The mRNA contains the codons specifying the sequence of amino acids but cannot itself associate with them. An intermediary RNA molecule called tRNA performs this task. At least one unique tRNA exists for each amino acid. The amino acid is activated and attached to its specific tRNA by an ATP driven process utilizing the enzyme aminoacyl tRNA synthetase. A tRNA carrying its cognate amino acid is said to be "charged."

$$\text{amino acid} + ATP + tRNA + H_2O \longrightarrow \text{aminoacyl-tRNA} + AMP + 2Pi$$

Aminoacyl-tRNA synthetase enzymes are very selective in attaching each amino acid to its cognate tRNA. Without this strict selectivity, the process of polypeptide synthesis would be compromised.

Each tRNA molecule has an anticodon consisting of three bases complementary to the bases of a codon on an mRNA molecule. The process of assembling a polypeptide from aminoacyl-tRNAs and an mRNA takes place on ribosomes. A ribosome is composed of both RNA and protein. It has two binding sites for charged tRNA: a P or peptidyl site and an A or aminoacyl site. Polypeptide synthesis involves initiation, elongation, and termination.

Prokaryote Translation

Initiation results when the mRNA and the initiator tRNA (formylmethionyl-tRNA) bind to 30S ribosome subunit in either order. The charged initiator tRNA

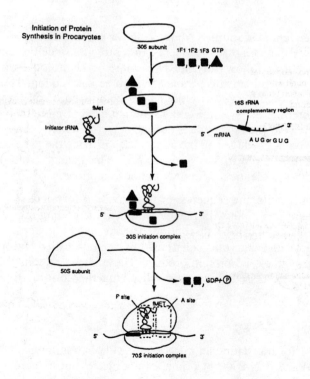

Figure 14 (a) — Protein Synthesis and Role of mRNA, ribosomes and tRNA

binds to the P site. (See Figure 14(a).) mRNA has a purine-rich sequence called the ribosome binding site (RBS) followed by the AUG codon. The RBS promotes the binding of the mRNA to RNA of the 30S ribosomal subunit. The 50S ribosomal subunit then binds to the 30S subunit giving the 70S initiation complex. One GTP is spent to form the 70S initiatition complex. Many non-ribosomal proteins, termed initiation factors; are involved in establishing the 70S unit complex.

Elongation proceeds by binding of a aminoacyl-tRNA to the A site. Formation of a peptide bond between the amino group of incoming aminoacyl-tRNA and the carboxyl group of the adjacent fmet-tRNA costs one GTP and causes the release of uncharged fmet-tRNA. The translocation of the peptidyl-tRNA from the A site to the P side moves the ribosome to the next codon and expends a second GTP. Each elongation step requires the hydrolysis of two GTPs.

Termination of polypeptide synthesis occurs when a stop codon is encountered. The stop codon is read by one of two protein release factors which cause release of the polypeptide chain from the ribosome.

As with transcription, eukaryotic and prokaryotic translation are similar but have several differences. For one, eukaryotic ribosomes are relatively large. Both the small subunit (40S) and the large subunit (60S) are larger than their prokaryotic equivalents. Together they form an 80S ribosome. Also, eukaryotic initiation is nota-

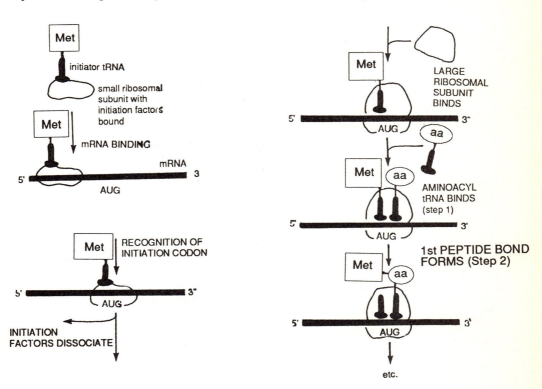

Figure 14 (b) — Initiation of Eukaryotic Protein Synthesis

bly more complex (see Figure 14(b)). It involves more initiation factors, many of which are themselves multi-subunited. The initiator tRNA is a special methoinine tRNA (termed Met-tRNA^Met), but it is not formylated. Also, the initiator tRNA always binds to the 40S subunit before the mRNA does, rather than in either order (as in prokaryotes). Furthermore, binding of the mRNA to the 40S subunit requires the hydrolysis of one ATP. With the exception of the mRNA of a few viruses, eukaryotic mRNA does not possess a ribosome binding site but instead requires a 5′ cap for efficient initiation (see Figure 14(c)). This cap is a 7-methylguanosine linked at its 5′ end to the 5′end of the mRNA via a triphosphate bridge. Finally, one release factor (RF) recognizes all three stop codons.

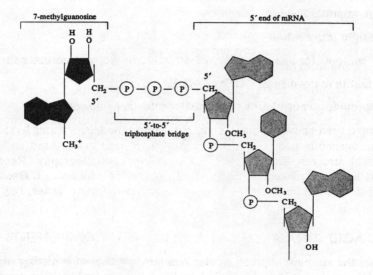

Figure 14 (c) — Structure of Eukaryotic mRNA Cap

PROBLEM

Nitrous acid converts cytosine to uracil by deamination. This type of conversion in one DNA strand would lead to a change in the complementary base in the other strand to

a) adenine.

b) cytosine.

c) thymine.

d) guanine.

Solution

a) Cytosine normally binds to guanine and uracil normally binds to adenine. A conversion of cytosine to uracil would lead to a conversion of guanine to adenine in the complementary strand. Thus a CG to AU (or AT) event has occurred.

II. Microbiology

Knowledge of the properties and characteristics of viruses and bacteria and fungi is essential to understanding the cause of many diseases as well as the therapeutic approaches used to alleviate these diseases. Modern molecular approaches are proving to be particularly useful in this regard.

1. Viral Structure and Life History

Viruses are important because they:

(1) provide insight into evolution,

(2) are important tools for understanding the molecular biology of normal cells,

(3) are important in many diseases such as AIDS,

(4) they may provide powerful molecular tools for the many diseases.

Some viruses have been shown to cause cancer in animal models. Viruses have been obtained in homogeneous state and some viruses have been crystallized and their three dimensional structure fully determined by x-ray crystallography. Recently, much emphasis has been placed on the possibility of using viruses to transmit selected genetic information into eukaryotic cells to correct defective genes, i.e., gene therapy.

A. NUCLEIC ACID (DNA AND RNA) AND PROTEIN COMPONENTS

Viruses are the simplest supramolecular complex capable of initiating replication. They contain nucleic acids (either DNA or RNA but not both) with a surrounding protein coat called the capsid that protects the encapsulated nucleic acid from damage. Some animal viruses also have an envelope of lipid and glycoprotein surrounding the capsid. An extracellular viral particle (or virion) cannot independently reproduce itself and requires a host cell for this function. It accomplishes this task by diverting the biosynthetic machinery of the host cell to synthesize its own components. In some RNA viruses the viral mRNA preferentially bind to the host ribosomes. Hence, synthesis of viral proteins is favored over synthesis of host proteins.

There are four classes of RNA eukaryotic viruses that are distinguishable by the relationship of their viral RNA to their mRNA (see Table 1). mRNA is designated as (+) RNA and, its complementary RNA, as (-) RNA. Class I viruses contain (+) RNA which, in turn, is the template (+) mRNA. The parental RNA also functions as mRNA since it is capable of polymerizing ribonucleotides from an RNA template. For class I, as well as class II and class III viruses, this is accomplished by a viral RNA-directed-RNA polymerase (or RNA replicase).

Class II viruses contain (-) RNA which is transcribed into monocistronic mRNAs by a viral RNA transcriptase contained in the virion. One of these mRNAs codes for an RNA replicase which generates double stranded RNA from the parental (-) RNA. The RNA replicase also synthesizes progeny (-) RNA strands from the double stranded RNA.

Class III viruses contain double-stranded RNA, and the (-) strand provides the template for (+) mRNA. Class IV viruses are particularly important because the flow of genetic information is from (+) RNA to DNA and then back to RNA (see Table 1). Class IV viruses are called retroviruses and they code for an RNA-directed DNA polymerase (or reverse transcriptase). The HIV virus, which causes AIDS, is a retrovirus.

An important property of some RNA retroviruses (class IV RNA viruses) is their ability to induce tumors in animal models. Some DNA viruses (i.e., Simian virus 40 and polyoma virus) can also cause tumors. Cancer-causing viruses (i.e., oncogenic viruses) transform their host cells by inserting their viral specific genes into the host chromosome. Normal cells stop multiplying when in close contact with one another, i.e., contact inhibition. Transformed cells no longer exhibit contact inhibition and, therefore, grow continuously.

Class	Viral RNA	Flow of Genetic Information
I	(+) RNA $\longrightarrow$	(-) RNA $\longrightarrow$ (+) mRNA
II	(-) RNA $\longrightarrow$ ($\pm$) RNA $\longrightarrow$ RNA	(+) mRNA
III	($\pm$) RNA $\longrightarrow$	(+) mRNA
IV	(+) RNA $\longrightarrow$	(-) DNA $\longrightarrow$ ($\pm$) DNA $\longrightarrow$ (+) mRNA

Table 1 — Classes of RNA Viruses

In the DNA or RNA viruses the DNA provides the template for the synthesis of mRNA molecules which preferentially use the host ribosomes to synthesize viral specific proteins and the enzymes necessary for viral DNA synthesis.

Viruses contain very few genes (between 3 and 240) and, therefore, construct much of their molecular machinery from identical protein subunits. For example, the protein coat of the TMV (Tobacco mosaic virus), which contains only 6 genes, is made up of 2,130 identical protein subunits. Coat protein subunits usually arrange themselves into either rods or spheres, or a combination of these shapes.

PROBLEM

> Viruses differ from other living organisms because
>
> a)   viruses possess no bounding membrane.
>
> b)   viruses lack all metabolic machinery.
>
> c)   viruses lack all reproductive machinery.
>
> d)   All of the above.

Solution

d)   Viruses differ from living things in many ways. They do not have any membranes because they have no need to take in or expel material. Viruses lack all metabolic machinery and do not produce ATP because they do not perform energy-requiring processes. Viruses do possess either DNA or RNA, but cannot independently reproduce. They must rely on host cells for reproductive machinery and components.

B. BACTERIOPHAGE: STRUCTURE, FUNCTION AND LIFE CYCLE

Bacteriophages (or phages) are bacterial viruses that have either RNA or DNA genomes. Figure 15 illustrates the structure of a typical bacteriophage which has a head, tail and tail fibers. Infection of a bacterium (1 to 10 µm in length) begins when a phage (100-300 nm) attaches its tail fibers to a surface receptor on the bacterium. The DNA, which is tightly packed in the phage head, is subsequently injected through the cell wall and the cell membrane into the bacterium (see Figure 16). In only a few minutes all the metabolism of the infected bacterium is directed towards the synthesis of a new phage particles. About 30 minutes after infection the bacterium undergoes lysis and hundreds of completed bacteriophages are released.

The complex coordination of phage life cycle is a result of different phage genes being expressed at different times. The early phage genes are expressed before phage DNA synthesis begins. For many phages some of these gene products shut down the biosynthetic capacity of the bacterium. One of early phage gene products that helps to shut down the metabolism of the host cell is a nuclease specific for bacterial DNA but not the phage DNA.

The late gene products are associated with the synthesis of viral DNA, capsid formation, packaging of the viral DNA into preformed heads, and the synthesis of lysozyme to degrade the bacterial cell wall thus causing lysis. Not all phages cause immediate lysis of the infected bacterium. In some cases the phage DNA incorporates itself into the bacterial chromosome and is only replicated when the host chro-

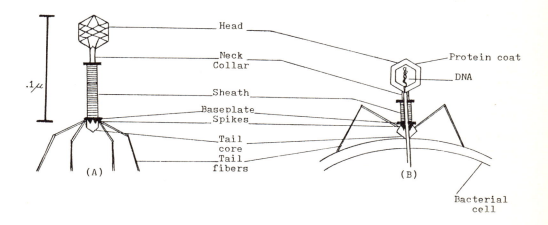

Figure 15 — The Structure of a Typical Bacteriophage

mosome is replicated. This process is called lysogeny. Viruses that exhibit this state are called temperate or moderate viruses.

The viral DNA incorporated into the host chromosome is called a provirus, or prophage. In the case of bacteriophages this prophage can be induced to become virulent and lyse its host bacterium. The resulting infectious phage often carry small amounts of bacterial chromosome which can be transferred to newly infected bacteria. The process whereby DNA is transferred from one bacteria to another by a phage is called transduction.

PROBLEM

> Moderate viruses may
>
> a)   replace DNA only when the host replicates.
>
> b)   induce tumors.
>
> c)   cause immediate lysis of infected bacteria.
>
> d)   have both DNA and RNA.

Solution

a)   In moderate viruses the phage DNA is incorporated directly into the host chromosome, and thus replicates only when the host does. RNA retroviruses may induce tumors. Most viruses, with the exception of moderate ones, cause immediate lysis of infected bacteria. Viruses may contain either DNA or RNA, not both.

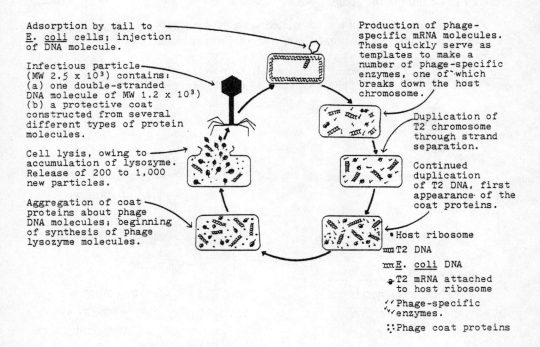

Adsorption by tail to E. coli cells; injection of DNA molecule.

Infectious particle (MW 2.5 x 10³) contains: (a) one double-stranded DNA molecule of MW 1.2 x 10³) (b) a protective coat constructed from several different types of protein molecules.

Cell lysis, owing to accumulation of lysozyme. Release of 200 to 1,000 new particles.

Aggregation of coat proteins about phage DNA molecules; beginning of synthesis of phage lysozyme molecules.

Production of phage-specific mRNA molecules. These quickly serve as templates to make a number of phage-specific enzymes, one of which breaks down the host chromosome.

Duplication of T2 chromosome through strand separation.

Continued duplication of T2 DNA, first appearance of the coat proteins.

Host ribosome
T2 DNA
E. coli DNA
T2 mRNA attached to host ribosome
Phage-specific enzymes.
Phage coat proteins

Figure 16 — The Life Cycle of a Bacteriophage

2. Prokaryotic Cells

A. CELL STRUCTURE AND FUNCTION

All living organisms have a cell structure that can be classified as either eukaryotic or prokaryotic. The prokaryotic cell is distinguished by the absence of a membrane bound nucleus. Prokaryotic cells (1-10 μm in length) are much smaller than eukaryotic cells (10-100 μm in length). Both types of cells can have flagella for motility but these structures are relatively simple in prokaryotic cells. Prokaryotic cells include eubacteria, archaebacteria, blue-green algae, spirochetes, rickettsia, and mycoplasma.

In prokaryotic cells such as bacteria (see Figure 17(a)) the single chromosome is a large single circular double stranded DNA molecule that is not separated from the cytoplasm by a nuclear membrane. The prokaryotic chromosome lies in the nuclear zone. Prokaryotic cells contain less DNA than more advanced eukaryotic cells. Furthermore, in prokaryotic cells the processes of transcription and translation occur simultaneously.

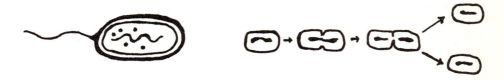

Figure 17 — (a) The Structure of a Bacterium; (b) Bacterial Reproduction

The only two membraneous structures in prokaryotic cells are the plasma membrane and the other membrane which are lipid bilayers with associated intrinsic and

Typical Bacterial Cell

	Prokaryotic	Eukaryotic
DNA		
	No nuclear membrane	DNA contained in nucleus with surrounding nuclear membrane
	No histones	DNA associated with histones
membranes		
	plasma membrane	plasma membrane and other
	outer membrane	membranous organelles such as mitochondria, endoplasmic reticulum, Golgi complex, peroxisomes, and lysosomes

Table 2 — Differences Between Prokaryotic and Eukaryotic Cell

extrinsic membrane proteins. In contrast, eukaryotic cells contain membraneous organelles such a mitochondria and a membrane bound nucleus (see Table 2). Ribosomes and cytosol are present in both cell types. The cytosol contains water soluble enzymes, metabolic intermediates and inorganic ions.

PROBLEM

Which of the following structures is found in a bacterial cell?

a) Golgi apparatus

b) Nuclear membrane

c) Ribosomes

d) Mitochondrion

Solution

c)   Unlike eukaryotes, bacterial cells lack Golgi apparatus, endoplasmic reticulum, mitochondria and a nuclear membrane. The lack of an endoplasmic reticulum means that the ribosomes are free (not bound to rough endoplasmic reticulum).

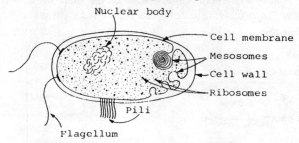

Figure 17 (c) — Typical bacterial cell

B. BACTERIAL LIFE HISTORY AND PHYSIOLOGICAL CHARACTERISTICS

Bacterial growth is the result of cellular division. For bacteria the process of cell division is straightforward, i.e., the cell doubles in size and then divides in two. This type of growth is exponential. The time it takes for a doubling of a number of bacteria is called the mean generation time, which is typically less than one hour. During cellular division, the nuclear body first replicates (see Figure 17(b)), the resulting homologous chromosomes separate, a cross wall forms between the chromosomes, the cell divides and separates.

A considerable store of fundamental information about molecular biology has come from microbiological studies. Strong evidence for DNA being the genetic material comes from studies in which DNA from one bacterial strain is transferred to another. The transfer of the donor DNA is accompanied by the transfer of some donor phenotype(s) (such as virulence) to the recipient strain. DNA can be transferred from one bacterium to another by transformation, conjugation, and transduction.

Transduction is the transfer of a fragment of the bacterial genome from a donor strain to a recipient strain of bacteria using a bacteriophage as the vector. In transformation, a DNA fragment isolated from a donor strain is directly taken up by the recipient strain. In bacterial conjugation the male and female cells adhere, chromosome or episome replication occurs in the male cell and one copy is injected into the female cell. No transfer of DNA occurs from the female to the male bacterium.

Bacterial cells are noted for their metabolic versatility and their highly efficient regulation of metabolic and catabolic activities.

Under adverse conditions some bacteria shift from their normal vegetative state to a dormant state, i.e., they undergo sporogenesis. Sporogenesis is a form of cellular differentiation resulting in a metabolically dormant structure such as an endospore which are formed by the Gram-positive bacteria of the genera Bacillus and Clostridium. Under favorable conditions the spore can undergo germination to return the cells to a vegetative state.

PROBLEM

In transduction, a

a) male chromosome is injected into a female cell.

b) female chromosome is injected into a male cell.

c) bacteriophage transfers genetic material between bacteria.

d) DNA fragment from a donor strain is directly taken up by a recipient strain of bacteria.

Solution

c) a) refers to bacterial conjugation. b) is an impossibility. d) refers to transformation.

3. Fungi

A. MAJOR STRUCTURAL TYPES

All fungi are eukaryotic organisms having at least one nucleus with a nuclear membrane, an endoplasmic reticulum and mitochondria. They lack chloroplasts and chlorophyll. Fungi are spore-bearing organisms with absorptive nutrition. They reproduce sexually and asexually. The primitive plant body formed by fungi is called a thallus but it has no true roots, leaves, stems, or vascular tissue. Although there are over 100,000 species of fungi, only about 100 are important in human diseases. Ringworm (dermatophytoses) is, however, a very common infectious disease caused by a fungus. Fungi are further divided into yeasts and molds.

B. GENERAL LIFE HISTORY AND PHYSIOLOGY

Yeasts are unicellular forms of fungi with a spherical shape (3 - 15 μm in diameter). Yeast reproduce by budding or by binary fission. Molds grow in multicellular tubular colonies called hyphae. During growth these hyphae bunch together to form a mycelium.

Fungi and myxobacterium have the ability to form "fruiting bodies" which are an effective adaptation to a land environment. The fruiting bodies serve to disperse spores or cysts. Asexual spores formed from the body (or thallus) of a fungus are called thallospores and asexual spores formed from specialized structures are called conidia.

Fungi are also capable of sexual reproduction. In all sexual reproduction there is an alteration in chromosome number. At fertilization two haploid nuclei join to form a diploid nucleus. The diploid cells eventually give rise to haploid cells by meiosis. In lower fungi the visible organism often exists primarily in the haploid state (haplophase) and only transiently in the diploid state (diplophase). Sexual reproduction in fungi follows this sequence:

(1)   compatible haploid nuclei are brought together in the same cell of the thallus;

(2)   two genetically different nuclei fuse to form a diploid nucleus;

(3)   meiosis occurs to form haploid nuclei which develop into sexual spores.

PROBLEM

All of the following are true of fungi EXCEPT they do not

a)   reproduce sexually.   b)   reproduce asexually.

c)   produce spores.   d)   produce seeds.

Solution

d)   Fungi may produce spores sexually or asexually. Seeds are produced by plants, not fungi.

III. Generalized Eukaryotic Cell

1. Plasma Membrane: Structure and Function

A. COMPOSITION, STRUCTURE, AND MOVEMENT OF PROTEINS AND LIPIDS

The plasma membrane surrounds the cell and separates the inside (intercellular) from the outside (extracellular) of the cell. Structurally, the plasma membrane is composed of a lipid bilayer and membrane bound proteins (see Figure 18(a)). Lipid bilayers are also present in other organelles of eukaryotic cells, e.g., mitochondria and endoplasmic reticulum. Phospholipid (PL) molecules are the primary lipid constituents of most lipid bilayers (see Figure 18(b)). Cholesterol and glycolipids are also present in many biological membranes. PL molecules are amphipathic molecules, i.e., they have a polar head group and two nonpolar hydrocarbon "tails." PL molecules self aggregate to form a lipid bilayer because in this molecular arrangement their head groups remain in contact with water and their tails are removed from contact with water. The lipid bilayer structure has two important properties:

(1) It is a permeability barrier for charged molecules. Charged, hydrophilic molecules, cannot move through the lipid bilayer because they would have to give up thermodynamically favorable interactions with polar water molecules. Water molecules, although permeable to the bilayer, have an extremely low concentration in the hydrophobic domain of the bilayer. For charged molecules to pass through the bilayer specific transport proteins must be present. Hydrophobic molecules such as O_2 as well as small uncharged polar molecules (H_2O, CO_2 and urea) are, however, membrane permeable.

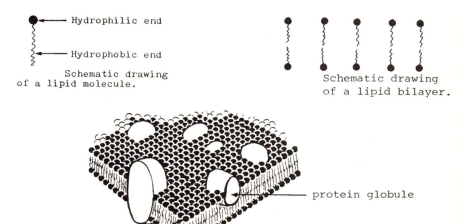

Hydrophilic end

Hydrophobic end

Schematic drawing of a lipid molecule.

Schematic drawing of a lipid bilayer.

protein globule

hydrophilic ends

hydrophobic center

Figure 18 (a) — The Lipid Bilayer

(2)   The individual PL molecules move rapidly in the plane of the lipid bilayer. Proteins associated with the lipid bilayer also can have rapid lateral motion. The bilayer, therefore, acts as two-dimensional fluid and this fluidity is necessary for diffusion of membrane bound enzymes and receptor molecules.

The plasma membrane and the membranes of other subcellular organelles are asymmetric with respect to the head groups found on the inner and outer monolayers. In addition, the proteins associated with biological membranes are also embedded in the bilayer in an asymmetric manner. For example, glycoproteins (as well as glycolipids) in the plasma membrane usually have their carbohydrate moities facing the extracellular space.

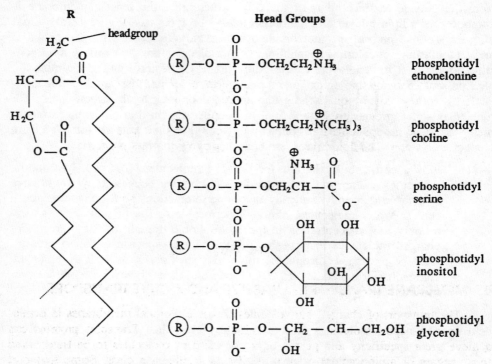

Figure 18 (b) — The Structure of PL Molecules

PROBLEM

Cell membranes are generally composed of a

a)   double layer of phospholipids with proteins dispersed throughout the membrane.

b)   double layer of phosphoproteins with glucose dispersed throughout the membrane.

c)   double layer of nucleic acids.

d)   double layer of proteins with phospholipids dispersed throughout the membrane.

Solution

a)   The plasma membrane contains about 40 percent lipid and 60 percent protein by weight although there is considerable variation between different cell types. The lipid molecules of the plasma membrane are polar. One end is hydrophobic, the other end is hydrophilic. The lipid molecules are arranged in two layers so that the hydrophobic ends are near each other and the hydrophilic ends face outside. The individual lipid molecules can move laterally, so the bilayer is actually fluid and flexible. Protein molecules of the plasma membrane may be arranged at various sites and imbedded to different degrees. The highly selective permeability of the plasma membrane is dependent upon the specific types and amounts of proteins and lipids present.

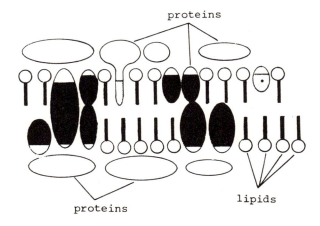

Figure 18 (c)

B. MEMBRANE TRANSPORT — PASSIVE AND ACTIVE TRANSPORT

The transport of charged biomolecules across biological membranes is dependent upon transport molecules most of which are proteins. Transport proteins can achieve great specificity and permit only one class of molecules to be transported (e.g., sugars or amino acids) or one specific molecule in a class. Some transport molecules simply permit a solute to reversibly diffuse from one side of the membrane to the other. This process is called passive transport. The direction of transport for a solute will be influenced by a concentration gradient across the membrane (i.e., from high to low concentration), as well as the electric charge across the membrane, i.e., the membrane potential.

The combination of the chemical and electrical gradient is called the electrochemical gradient. Plasma membranes are more negatively charged on the cytoplasmic side than the extracellular side and this hinders the passive transport of positively charged ions. In some cases, the passive transport of a solute is through an aqueous pore created by the transport protein. This type of transport protein is called a channel protein or porin. Transport of a solute through a channel protein is not saturable (see Figure 19). In other cases, the solute molecule binds to a transport protein which then facilitates its translocation to the other side of the membrane. This process, called facilitated diffusion, is similar to a substrate binding to the active site of an enzyme, which is a saturable process.

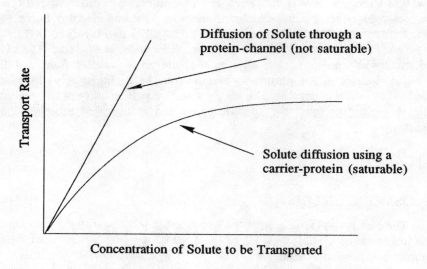

Figure 19 — Passive Transport

In order to transport a solute against an unfavorable electrochemical gradient it is necessary to expend energy, usually ATP. This type of transport is called active transport.

PROBLEM

Porins are important in		
a) facilitated diffusion.	b)	substrate binding.
c) saturable processes only.	d)	passive transport.

Solution

d)   Passive transport may occur when a solute passes through an aqueous pore created by a channel protein, or porin. Transport of a solute through a porin is not saturable. Facilitated diffusion occurs when a substrate binds to the active site of an enzyme.

C. THE Na⁺ - K⁺ PUMP AND MEMBRANE POTENTIAL

The membrane potential of plasma membranes is generated by two important transport proteins: the Na^+, K^+-ATPase and the K^+-channel. Na^+,K^+-ATPase uses ATP to pump Na^+ ions out of the cell and K^+ ions into the cell (see Figure 20). This is an example of active transport because the concentration of Na^+ outside the cell is higher than inside. The reverse is true for K^+ ions.

The K^+-channel permits K^+ ions to diffuse out of the cell and this loss of positive ions causes the inside of the cell to become more negative than the outside. Eventually increasing negative charge inside the cell retards the outflow of K^+ ions (i.e., the negative charge inside the cell attracts the positively charged K^+ ions) and equilibrium is achieved when the inflow of K⁺ ions equals the outflow. The end result is a plasma membrane potential between - 20 and - 70 mV depending on the cell type.

PROBLEM

In most cells, the concentration of Na⁺ is _____ in the cell than outside it, because of _____.

a) higher ... active transport

b) higher ... passive transport

c) lower ... active transport

d) lower ... passive transport

Solution

c) The Na⁺ – K⁺ pump is a form of active transport where energy is used to pump Na⁺ ions out of the cell and K⁺ ions into the cell.

D. OSMOTIC EFFECTS AND CELL VOLUME

The Na⁺,K⁺–ATPase along with the K⁺-channel primarily controls the level of ions inside the cell. Thus, these elements are also the main controllers of intracellular osmotic pressure and cellular volume. The charged macromolecules inside the cell require counterbalancing ions like Na⁺, K⁺ and Cl⁻. This creates an osmotic pressure, causing cellular swelling from the influx of water. Counterbalancing this intracellular osmotic pressure is the osmotic pressure caused by the ions in the extracellular fluid—primarily Na⁺ and Cl⁻. These ions tend to move down their concentration gradient and into the cell. Were it not for the Na⁺, K⁺-ATPase pumping Na⁺ out and consequently preventing Cl⁻ from leaking in (by maintaining a negative membrane potential), the cell would swell and burst.

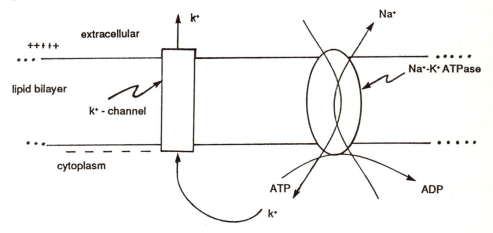

Figure 20 — Membrane Potential and Active Transport

PROBLEM

Which ions must be transported out of the cell to prevent its rupture?

a) Na⁺

b) K⁺

c) Cl⁻

d) All of the above.

Solution

d)   The macromolecules inside the cell require counterbalancing ions outside the cell, such as Na^+, K^+, and Cl^-. These counterbalancing ions create an osmotic balance that prevents the influx of water into the cell, thus preventing cell rupture.

E. MEMBRANE RECEPTORS

The plasma membrane contains a wide variety of protein receptors to which ligands can bind. A major function of these receptors is to receive signals from the extracellular environment. Neurotransmitters and hormones are examples of ligands that bind to protein receptors on target cells and influence the behavior of the cell.

Receptor proteins (see Figure 21) are usually transmembrane proteins that have an extracellular domain where signals are received, a hydrophobic domain going through the lipid bilayer, and a cytoplasmic signal transducing domain. The initial binding of the signal molecule (i.e., the first message) alters the conformation of protein receptor and this activates an intracellular signal pathway. The intracellular signal is often transmitted by a second class of small and rapidly diffusible molecules called second messengers. Calcium and cyclic AMP (see Figure 22) are two important second messengers. Alternately, the cytoplasmic domain of the receptor may have protein kinase activity which is activated upon ligand binding. Thus, the receptor molecule itself can activate or inactivate certain intracellular substrates via phosphorylation.

The second messengers can then regulate a wide variety of biochemical and physiological processes. For example, the release of fatty acids from adipocytes (fat cells) is regulated by catecholamines. When catecholamines (the first message) bind to a surface receptor on the adipocyte plasma membrane, this causes the receptor molecule to activate an adenylate cyclase enzyme, which catalyzes the production of intracellular cAMP from ATP (see Figure 21). The increased cAMP (the second messenger) activates a protein kinase which, in turn, phosphorylates the hormone

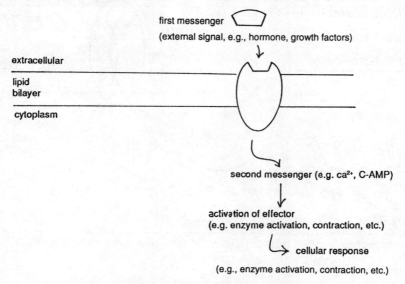

Figure 21 — Cell Receptors and Signals

sensitive lipase enzyme. The phosphorylation activates hormone sensitive lipase, and it then hydrolyzes triglyceride into fatty acids (see Figure 23).

Some receptors serve to bind very large molecules that are brought into the cell as a source of nutrients. Most cells, for example, have receptors for low density lipoprotein (LDL) which is a very large lipid-protein complex. The LDL receptor is called the apoB,E receptor and it recognizes the apoB protein moiety of LDL. After binding to the apoB,E receptor, LDL is internalized by endocytosis (see Figure 24) and provides the cell with an external source of cholesterol and other lipids.

PROBLEM

Ligands bind to		
a) target cells.	b)	neurotransmitters.
c) protein receptors.	d)	hormones.

Solution

c)   Neurotransmitters and hormones are examples of ligands that bind to protein receptors on target cells.

F. EXOCYTOSIS AND ENDOCYTOSIS

Macromolecules are too large to be transported through the plasma membrane by specific transport proteins. The transport of these macromolecules is accomplished by the processes of exocytosis and endocytosis. In exocytosis an intracellular vesicle is transported to the plasma membrane where it fuses with the plasma membrane. The fusion process releases the contents of the vesicle to the extracellular space. Endocytosis is essentially the reverse of this process (see Figure 24 on page 47).

PROBLEM

Which is most likely to be transported by exocytosis?		
a) Urea	b)	Lipoprotein
c) Na+	d)	Hormones

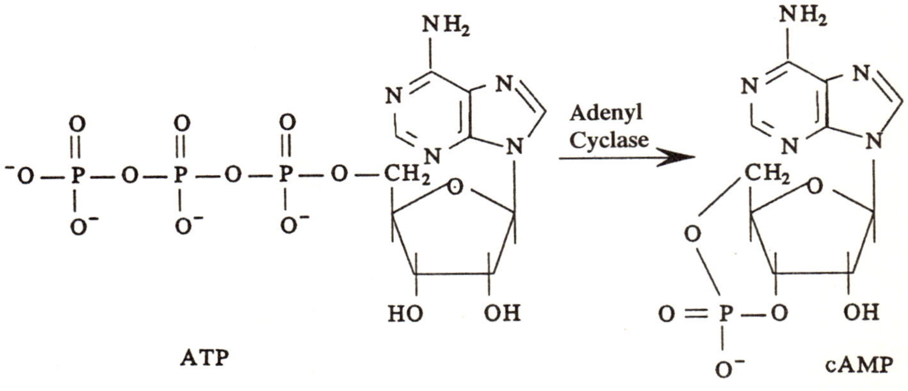

Figure 22 — Structure of cyclic AMP

Solution

b)   Exocytosis is used for the transport of the largest molecules, macromolecules. Lipoproteins have larger molecules than any of the other materials listed.

G. CELLULAR ADHESION

Cells in a tissue are in contact with a network of molecules called the extracellular matrix. This matrix plays a major role in promoting cell-cell adhesion. In addition, cells that are in direct contact with each other can form cell junctions between specialized regions of their plasma membranes.

2.   Membrane-Bound Organelles

A. MITOCHONDRIA

The structure and function of this membrane organelle has been discussed on pages 17 through 21 (see also Figure 10). Mitochondria are the primary site for the production of ATP. Mitochondria appear to be associated with the microtubules of the cytoskeleton. Mitochondria contain their own genome. Proteins from both the

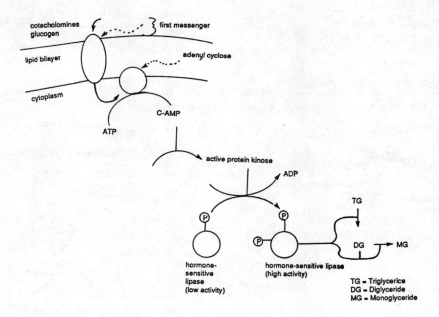

Figure 23 — Hormone Sensitive Lipase

mitochondrial genome and the nuclear DNA are required for mitochondrial replication. In mammals, mitochondrial genes are maternally inherited.

PROBLEM

> Which of the following is responsible for the majority of cellular ATP production?
>
> a)   Endoplasmic reticulum   b)   Lysosomes
>
> c)   Golgi apparatus   d)   Mitochondria

Solution

d)   The mitochondria are responsible for 95 percent of all ATP produced in the cell. For this reason the mitochondria are commonly referred to as the "powerhouse" of the cell. Mitochondria are membrane-bound organelles that are distributed throughout the cell. Mitochondria tend to be most concentrated in regions which require large amounts of energy, such as muscle.

B. ENDOPLASMIC RETICULUM

Eukaryotic cells contain an endoplasmic reticulum (ER) which represents about one-half of all the cellular membrane (see Figure 25 on page 49). Prokaryotic cells do not contain an ER. The ER is a primary site for lipid biosynthesis. It also serves as a delivery site for proteins that are to be excreted from the cell or to be delivered to other intracellular organelles. Structurally, the ER is thought to be a single, highly convoluted, membrane sheet enclosing a single space called the ER lumen. The cytoplasm is separated from the ER lumen by a single membrane (the ER membrane). The ER membrane is continuous with the outer nuclear membrane.

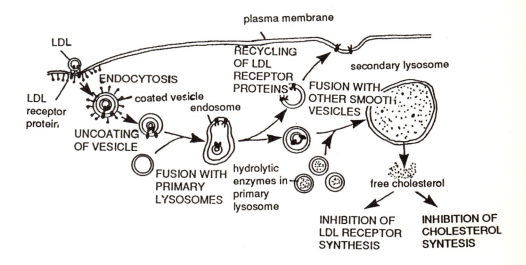

Figure 24 — LDL Uptake by Receptor Mediated Endocytosis

Proteins that are to be secreted by the cell or sent to other intracellular organelles are delivered to the lumen of the rough ER. Rough ER has attached ribosomes. The polypeptides being translated on these ribosomes are transported from the cytoplasmic side of the ER membrane into the ER lumen. The ribosomes attached to the rough ER are identical to ribosomes that are not attached to the rough ER. Attachment of some ribosomes to the ER is directed by small sequence of amino acids at the amino end of the polypeptide being translated (i.e., the signal sequence). The signal sequence is removed once the polypeptide has been delivered to the ER lumen. Many polypeptides undergo "core glycosylation" in the ER. Smooth ER has no attached ribosomes.Transport vesicles carrying newly synthesized lipids and proteins bud off the smooth ER for transport to the Golgi apparatus. Many important detoxification and lipid metabolism reactions take place on the smooth ER.

PROBLEM

Prokaryotic cells contain

a)   an endoplasmic reticulum.

b)   ribosomes.

c)   a nuclear membrane.

d)   both an endoplasmic reticulum and ribosomes.

Solution

b)   Prokaryotic cells contain ribosomes, but they do not have an endoplasmic reticulum or nuclear membrane.

C. GOLGI APPARATUS

The Golgi apparatus is composed of flattened membrane-bound sacs surrounded by a swarm of smaller membrane-bound vesicles called "coated vesicles." Proteins associated with the ER are transported to the Golgi apparatus by these small vesicles which are coated with a protein called clathrin. Glycoproteins are received by the convex side of Golgi apparatus and undergo "terminal glycosylation" in the Golgi apparatus. The sugar moieties of glycoproteins are extensively modified by enzymes in the Golgi apparatus and the modified glycoproteins are sorted and delivered to either other organelles or to the plasma membrane where they can be secreted into the extracellular fluid. It should be noted that the luminal side of both the ER and the Golgi apparatus correspond to the extracellular side of the plasma membrane. Furthermore, two membranes separate the lumen of the ER from the lumen of the Golgi apparatus.

PROBLEM

The Golgi apparatus primarily functions in

a)   packaging protein for secretion.

b)   synthesizing protein for secretion.

c)   packaging protein for hydrolysis.

d)   synthesizing protein for hydrolysis.

Solution

a)   The Golgi apparatus is an organelle that is responsible only for the packaging of protein for secretion.

D. LYSOSOMES

Lysosomes (250 - 750 nm in diameter) are membrane-bound vesicles found in the cytoplasm. These organelles are responsible for the intracellular digestion of macromolecules. A primary lysosome is a newly synthesized vesicle and contains a wide variety of hydrolytic enzymes (all are acid hydrolases) such as proteases phospholipases, and nucleases. These hydrolytic enzymes are almost all glycoproteins and have optimal enzymatic activities at pH 5.0, the pH inside the lysosomes. The primary lysosome arises from budding of specialized regions of the Golgi apparatus. A secondary lysosome is a lysosome that is actively digesting a substrate (see Figure 24). The substrate can be a foreign pathogen such as a bacterium or an endogenous macromolecule such as LDL.

PROBLEM

Lysosomes contain			
a)	glycogen stores.	b)	lipids.
c)	acid hydrolases.	d)	ATP.

Solution

c)   Lysosomes are cell organelles found in the cytoplasm. They are vesicles surrounded by a single membrane and contain enzymes, mostly acid hydrolases. These hydrolases are released when the membrane bursts, permitted the digestion of cellu-

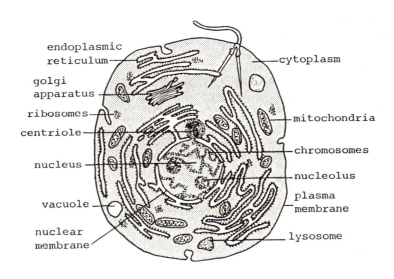

Figure 25 — The Generalized Eukaryotic Cell

lar structures and macromolecules. During the normal metabolism of the cell, enzyme release is carefully controlled by mechanisms which are still very poorly understood.

3. Cytoskeleton

A. MICROFILAMENTS, MICROTUBULES AND INTERMEDIATE FILAMENTS

The cytoskeleton of eukaryotic cells plays a key role in maintaining the cellular structure and cellular motility. Microfilaments and microtubules are composed of cytoskeletal filaments. These filaments are polymers of soluble subunits and can rapidly assemble and dissemble. The assembly process is energy dependent and requires ATP or GTP. A third type of filament is designated as intermediate filament because it has a diameter in between that of microfilaments and microtubules. Intermediate filaments are found in most animal cells. They are of a more permanent nature than either microfilaments or microtubules. The molecular mechanisms involved in the contraction actin and myosin filaments are discussed in the section on muscle tissue.

PROBLEM

Intermediate filaments are

a)   found in animal cells.

b)   more permanent than microfilaments.

c)   intermediate in diameter between microfilaments and microtubules.

d)   All of the above.

Solution

d)   Intermediate filaments, found in animal cells, are more permanent than, and intermediate in diameter between, microfilaments and microtubules.

B. CILIA, FLAGELLA AND CENTRIOLES

Cilia are hair-like projections (0.25 µm) that extend from the surface of many animal cells. These structures are used for cell movement (as in protozoa) or to move fluid (such as mucus) at the surface of the cell. Ciliated epithelial cells are found in the respiratory tract. Ciliary movement is dependent upon movement of the axoneme which is primarily composed of microtubules. It is a relatively permanent structure. The soluble subunit used to construct a microtubule is called tubulin. Ciliary motion requires ATP hydrolysis which generates a sliding movement of microtubules.

In order for microtubules to perform their functions they must be attached to other parts of the cell. Cilia end in a structural unit, the basal body, located at the base of the ciliary axoneme. The cytoplasmic microtubules observed in interphase cells (period between mitoses) are attached to centrioles. Basal bodies and centrioles have very similar structures each having a nine fold array of triplet microtubules.

The centrosome, which is present in most animal cells, has a centriole pair at its center. Higher plants do not have centrosomes. The centrosome, also called the cell center, is adjacent to the cell nucleus. It serves to organize microtubules and plays a major role in cell division.

Flagella in eukaryotic cells have a structure very similar to cilia and generate movement using the same principle detailed for cilia. Sperm cells and protozoa are examples of flagellated eukaryotic cells. The flagella of bacteria differ markedly from those of eukaryotic cells.

4. Nucleus: Structure and Function

The nucleus of the cell contains the nuclear DNA encoding the genetic information required for cellular replication, differentiation and functions. DNA replication and RNA synthesis occur in the nucleus. The RNA in the nucleus can be processed (e.g., RNA splicing) before being transported to the cytoplasm.

Nuclear DNA associates with histone proteins to form nucleosomes, the unit particles of chromatin. Chromatin, in turn, is packaged to form very compact structures called chromosomes. Other proteins, called nonhistone proteins, are also associated with nuclear DNA. Most of the DNA in the nucleus does not code for protein.

A. NUCLEAR ENVELOPE AND NUCLEAR PORES

The nucleus is bound by an envelope that is made up of two membranes, i.e., an inner and an outer nuclear membrane. The inner and outer nuclear membranes are fused at points called nuclear pores. The nuclear pores contain a nuclear pore complex thought to permit the selective transport (in and out) of macromolecules. For example, DNA and RNA polymerases which are synthesized in the cytoplasm must be transported into the nucleus through nuclear pore complexes.

PROBLEM

Nuclear pore complexes
a) transport micromolecules.
b) transport the nucleus.
c) fuse the nuclear and cell membranes.
d) fuse the inner and outer nuclear membrane.

Solution

d) Nuclear pore complexes fuse the inner and outer nuclear membrane to permit the transport of macromolecules to and from the nucleus.

B. NUCLEOLUS

The nucleolus is a highly ordered structure specially designed to produce the rRNA required for ribosomes. The synthesized rRNA immediately combines with ribosomal proteins to form subunits. These subunits join to form functional ribosomes only after they have been transported from the nucleus through nuclear pores to the cytoplasm.

PROBLEM

rRNA is made in the

a) endoplasmic reticulum.   b) nucleolus.

c) ribosomes.   d) cytoplasm.

Solution

b) rRNA is synthesized in the nucleolus and combined with ribosomal proteins.

5. Mitosis

A. MITOTIC PROCESS, PHASES OF THE CELL CYCLE

Cells are continuously subjected to various kinds of stress that can result in cell death. For an organism to grow and survive, cells must reproduce themselves. For cellular division to occur a cell must first double its contents, divide its nucleus and then divide its cytoplasm. The process of nuclear division is called mitosis. A cell that is not undergoing active division is said to be in interphase. The interphase period had been further delineated on the basis of when DNA synthesis occurs (see Figure 26). The period of active DNA synthesis and replication is called S-phase. The gap period before S-phase is called G1 phase, and the gap period after S-phase is called G2 phase. The mitotic phase, designated M-phase, begins after the G2 phase.

PROBLEM

A mitotic cell produces

a) two cells with half of the chromosomes of the first cell.

b) two cells each with the full chromosome complement of the original cell.

c) four cells with half of the chromosome complement of the original cell.

d) four cells with the full chromosome complement of the first cell.

Solution

b) Mitosis refers to the process by which a cell divides to form two daughter cells, each with exactly the same number and kind of chromosomes as the parent cell.

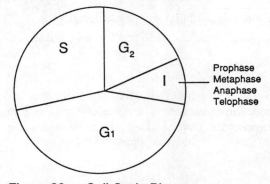

Figure 26 — Cell Cycle Phase

B. MITOTIC STRUCTURES

CHROMATIDS AND CENTROMERE

Most of the synthetic events necessary for cell division occur during interphase. In animal cells the initiation of DNA replication (i.e., the start of S-phase) is closely associated with the replication of the cell's pair of centrioles. The centrioles are the microtubule organizing center of the cell. Each centriole pair forms the spindle pole during mitosis. Once DNA synthesis is initiated, it continues until all the DNA is replicated. As the DNA replicates, new histones are attached and chromatin is formed. Each chromosome is duplicated in S-phase forming two sister chromatids joined by a centromere.

CENTRIOLES, ASTERS, SPINDLES

G2-phase begins at the end of the S-phase. During G2-phase cells prepare for mitosis by constructing much of the macromolecular machinery used in the mitotic spindle (see below). M-phase begins at the end of G2-phase. The M-phase has been further divided into prophase, prometaphase, metaphase, anaphase and telophase (see below). During prophase, chromatin condenses into chromosomes. In addition the mitotic spindle is formed. The mitotic apparatus consists of the two centrioles, a set of microtubules and two pair of centrioles. The microtubules form a radial array called the aster around each pair of centrioles. Some of the microtubules eventually connect each pair of centrioles. These microtubules comprise the spindle. The microtubules are responsible for the movement of chromosomes during mitosis.

KINETOCHORE

Prometaphase starts with the dissolution of the nuclear envelope. Microtubules subsequently become attached to chromosomes at a locus called the kinetochore. During metaphase the chromosomes become aligned at a plate halfway between the spindle poles. At anaphase the chromosomes are broken apart by the microtubules attached to the kinetochores. During telophase the daughter chromosomes arrive at opposite spindle poles, and the kinetochore microtubules dissociated. Furthermore, a nuclear envelope appears around each set of new chromosomes and nucleoli reappear. This completes the process of mitosis. The subsequent division of the cytoplasm is called cytokinesis.

PROBLEM

Kinetochore microtubules dissociate during			
a)	prophase.	b)	metaphase.
c)	telophase.	d)	anaphase.

Solution

c)   Kinetochore microtubules attach during prometaphase. An anaphase they break apart the chromosomes. During telophase the kinetochore microtubules dissociate.

IV. Specialized Eukaryotic Cells and Tissues

1. Neural Cells and Tissues

A. STRUCTURES (CELL BODY, AXON, DENDRITES, MYELIN SHEATH, SCHWANN CELLS, AND NODES OF RANVIER).

The neuron is the key cell type in the brain and the peripheral nervous system. A neuron receives information from other neurons or from sensory receptors and transmits the information to either other neurons or to muscles. The structure of typical nerve cell is shown in Figure 27.

Information is transmitted by neurons either by an action potential or by synaptic transmission. The action potential is an all-or-none response and it is a time dependent change in the transmembrane potential of the neuronal plasma membrane. The action potential is carried (see below for details) away from the cell body by the axon which usually branches and has many termini. When the action potential comes to an axon terminal it contacts the synapse which is a knob-like structure. The synapse is the junction between the end of the axon and the dendrites of an adjacent neuron.

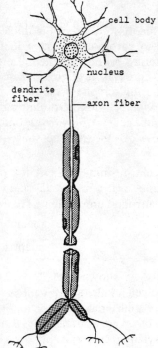

Figure 27 — The Structure of a Typical Vertebrate Neuron

In vertebrates many axons are insulated by layers of myelin that serve to increase the speed at which an action potential is transmitted along the axon. The myelin sheath (in peripheral neurons) is formed by glial cells called Schwann cells (see Figure 28). Between one Schwann cell and the next there is a small region where the axon has no sheathing. This region, called the node of Ranvier, is very rich in Na^+-channels.

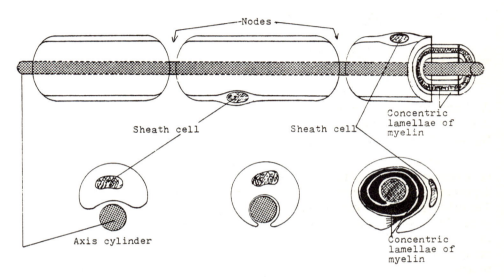

Figure 28 — The Structure of Schwann Cells and the Nodes of Ranvier

PROBLEM

The myelin sheath of many axons is produced by the	
a) node of Ranvier.	b) nerve cell body.
c) Schwann cell.	d) astrocytes.

Solution

c) Schwann cells are the myelin-forming cells of the peripheral nervous system. Each Schwann cell forms a single myelin internodal segment around a portion of an axon. Schwann cells may also surround unmyleinated axons, without producing myelin.

B. SYNAPSE

The structure of a synapse is shown in Figure 29. The presynaptic cell is separated from the postsynaptic cell by the synaptic cleft. The electrical signal from the axon triggers the release of neurotransmitter substances from storage vesicles (synaptic vesicles). The release of the neurotransmitter causes an electrical change in the postsynaptic cell. The postsynaptic cell sums up electrical signals induced by the release of the neurotransmitter and, when a critical total signal level is reached, an action potential is generated by the postsynaptic cell.

PROBLEM

The correct sequence for signal transmission in a synapse is

a)   presynaptic cell, postsynaptic cell, synaptic cleft.

b)   presynaptic cell, synaptic cleft, postsynaptic cell.

c)   synaptic cleft, presynaptic cell, postsynaptic cell.

d)   None of the above.

Solution

b)   Electrical signals in the presynaptic cell cause release of neurotransmitter substances which flow through the synaptic cleft to the postsynaptic cell. The postsynaptic cell creates an electrical signal in response to the received neurotransmitter.

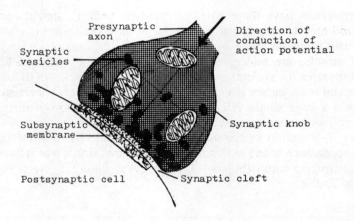

Figure 29 — The Structure of a Typical Synapse

C. RESTING POTENTIAL AND ACTION POTENTIAL

The resting potential of a neuron is established by the Na^+,K^+-ATPase and the K^+-channel as described above (see pg 42 and Figure 20). The action potential is generated by a voltage gated Na^+-channel. A voltage gated channel is one whose permeability can increase or decrease depending upon the level of the membrane potential. The resting membrane potential of a neuron is about -70mV. When the axon receives a nerve impulse this electrical signal reduces the membrane potential to about 0 mV (see top panel of Figure 30). This initial increase is called membrane depolarization. Concomitant with the membrane depolarization there is an opening of a voltage gated N^+-channel which permits Na^+ to flow into the cell (recall that Na^+ is high outside the cell and low inside the cell). This influx of positive charge causes the membrane potential to become even more positive and this is accompanied by a closing of the Na^+-channel and a subsequent drop in membrane potential until the resting potential is reestablished (see lower panel of Figure 30)

PROBLEM

Referring to Figure 30, membrane polarization occurs

a)   before 0 ms.   b)   at 0 ms.

c)   at 1 ms.   d)   at 4 ms.

Solution

b)   The resulting neuron potential of a neuron is about – 70 mV. When the axon receives a nerve impulse the potential reduces to about 0 mV, resulting in a membrane depolarization.

2.   Contractile Cells and Tissues

A. STRIATED, SMOOTH, AND CARDIAC MUSCLE

Vertebrates have three types of muscles: striated, smooth, and cardiac. The specialized muscle cells in muscle tissues all have the ability to contract using actin and myosin filaments. ATP hydrolysis provides the energy for muscle contraction. Striated muscles are under voluntary control and they connect bones in a limb. Striated muscles (or skeletal muscles) are used for complex activities such as walking. Skeletal muscles are made of long muscle fibers (myofibers) and each fiber is considered a large single cell that is formed by the fusion of many separate cells. Each myofiber has many nuclei and bundles of myofibrils. As shown in Figure 31, a myofiber (1-40 mm in length and 10-50 μm in width) has a striated appearance. The striated appearance is due to bundles of aligned myofibrils which have dark bands (A bands) alternating with light bands (I bands). A narrow line bisects each I band and is called the Z-disc.

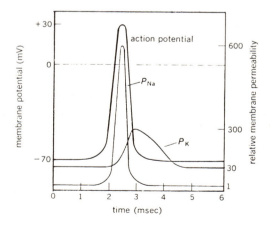

Figure 30 — Action potential

Smooth muscles are under involuntary control by the central nervous system. Smooth muscles are involved with movements of the small and large intestine, the bladder, and they also control the diameter of blood vessels. Smooth muscle cells are not striated and have one nucleus per cell. Cardiac muscle, or heart muscle, is very similar to striated muscle but is under involuntary control. Cardiac muscles produce the synchronous contraction of the heart (i.e., the heartbeat).

PROBLEM

Which of the following statements is false?

a)   Cardiac muscle is uninucleate, striated and controlled by the autonomic nervous system.

b)   Skeletal muscle is multinucleate, striated and controlled by the somatic nervous system.

c)   Smooth muscle is uninucleate, non-striated and controlled by the autonomic nervous system.

d)   None of the above.

Solution

d)   All of the statements regarding muscle types are true. Skeletal muscle is responsible for most voluntary movements, and it is controlled by the somatic nervous system. It contains striations due to the ordered arrangement of thick and thin filaments and has many nuclei. Smooth muscle lines the stomach, intestinal tracts and blood vessels whose involuntary movements are controlled by the autonomic nervous system. Smooth muscle is uninucleate and does not have striations. Cardiac muscle contains features of both types of muscle. It is striated, uninucleate, and is not under voluntary control.

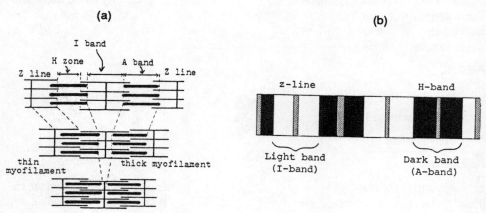

Figure 31 — (a) The Structure of Two Adjacent Myofibrils, and (b) Diagrammatic Structure of a Sarcomere.

B. SARCOMERE

The sarcomere (see Figure 31(b)) is the basic unit of contraction in striated muscles and it is the region between one Z-disk and the next. Myofibrils are made up of repeating sarcomere units. The sarcomere has thick myosin filaments as well as thin actin filaments. The thin filaments are attached to the Z-disk. The movement of thick and thin filaments between each sarcomere leads to muscle contraction.

PROBLEM

During muscular contraction,

a) sarcomeres move between myofibrils.

b) myofibrils move between Z-disks.

c) myosin and actin filaments move between sarcomeres.

d) Z-disks are made of myofibrils.

Solution

c) The sarcomere has myosin and actin filaments. The movement of these filaments between each sarcomere leads to muscular contraction. Actin filaments attach to the Z-disk. Myofibrils are made of sarcomeres.

C. CALCIUM REGULATION OF CONTRACTION

The movement of striated muscles is under voluntary control and muscle contraction is initiated by an electrical impulse from a neuron. The electrical impulse from the neuron triggers an action potential in the plasma membrane of the myofiber and is rapidly spread by transverse (or T) tubules (from the plasma membrane) to the Z-disk of the myofibrils. The signal is then transmitted to the sarcoplasmic reticulum. The sarcoplasmic reticulum surrounds each myofibril; when activated by the electrical impulse, it releases Ca^{+2} ions, causing all the myofibrils in the myofiber to simultaneously contract.

PROBLEM

Which is required for muscular contraction?

a) Electrical impulse

b) Ca^{+2} ions

c) Na^+ ions

d) Both a) and b)

Solution

d) Muscular contraction is initiated by electrical impulse from a neuron. The impulse makes the sarcoplasmic reticulum release Ca^{+2} ions, which cause myofibrils to contract.

3. Epithelial Cells and Tissues

A. Simple Epithelium and Stratified Epithelium

Epithelial cells line the inner and outer surfaces of the body. These cells have many specialized shapes and functions. Epithelial cells adhere to each other and to the basal lamina. Simple squamous epithelium cells (see Figure 32(a)) form a thin layer of cells that cover the inner lining of most blood vessels. Simple cuboidal epithelium (Figure 32(b)) also consist of a single layer of tightly fitting cells but they have a cube-like shape. Cuboidal epithelium cells line the ducts of many glands. A layer of elongated simple columnar epithelial cells form the lining of the stomach, the cervix and the small intestine (Figure 32(c)). Goblet cells are found in simple columnar epithelium and they secrete mucus. Stratified epithelium are several cell layers thick and they form the surface of the mouth, the esophagus, and the vagina. Skin is also formed from stratified squamous epithelial cells that have undergone a process of keratinization. Intestinal epithelial cells are very specialized and the cell surface facing the lumen of the small intestine has many microvilli that are important in the absorption of nutrients. The microvilli contain actin filaments which help maintain their rigidity.

A major function of all epithelial cells is to provide a boundary between different cell types. The basal lamina provides a distinct boundary between the epithelial cells and the cells that underlay the basal lamina.

PROBLEM

Epithelial tissues perform many functions. Which of the following is a function of this tissue?

a) Absorption

b) Protection

c) Secretion

d) All of the above.

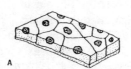
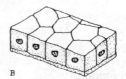
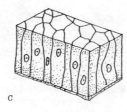

Figure 32 — Types of Epithelial Cells
(a) Simple squamous epithelium; (b) Simple cuboidal epithelium,
and (c) Simple columnar epithelium

Solution

d)   Epithelium exhibits a multiplicity of structural forms, all with the common role of covering the outer surface and lining the inner surfaces of the body. In some cases, such as skin, the function is mainly protective. In many other instances, however, epithelial tissue carries out functions such as surface and transepithelial transport, absorption, and secretion.

4.   Connective Cells and Fiber Types

A. MAJOR CELL AND FIBER TYPES

Connective tissues are characterized by the presence of relatively few cells with a large complement of extracellular matrix. The extracellular matrix is primarily composed of collagen fibers which are secreted by fibroblasts. Cartilage is formed by chondroblast and bone is formed by osteoblasts.

At least four distinct types of collagen fibers have been identified. Type IV is found exclusively in the basal lamina. Types I and III are found in skin whereas bone contains only type I. The extracellular matrix also has polysaccharides which are primarily glycosaminoglycans. These polysaccharides are often cross-linked with protein to form proteoglycans. Bone and teeth are composed of extracellular matrix with a secondary deposition of calcium phosphate crystals.

PROBLEM

Collagen fibers are found in		
a) skin.	b) blood.	
c) bones.	d) Both a) and c)	

Solution

d)   Collagen is found primarily in connective tissue, such as skin and bones. Blood is not a connective tissue.

B. LOOSE VS. STRONG CONNECTIVE TISSUE

Connective tissue is classified as either "loose" or "strong." Loose connective tissue forms the bed for epithelial cells and many glands. Blood vessels are found in loose connective tissues. Strong connective tissue is found in bone, cartilage and tendons.

PROBLEM

Which of the following is not a connective tissue?		
a) Bone	b) Tendons	
c) Cartilage	d) Muscle	

Solution

d)   Connective tissues function to support and hold together structures of the body. Bone, cartilage, tendons, ligaments, and fibrous connective tissues are all different types of connective tissue. The cells of these tissues characteristically secrete a large amount of noncellular material, called matrix. The nature and function of each kind of connective tissue is determined primarily by its matrix. Most of the connective tissue volume is made up of matrix.

C. CARTILAGE

Cartilage is a component of rigid connective tissue and it provides support, framework and protection. There are three types of cartilage, i.e., hyaline, elastic and fibrocartilage. Each contains a different kind of extracellular matrix. Hyaline cartilage is the most abundant and it occurs in many joints and bone ends. During embryonic development skeletal components are first formed from hyaline cartilage which is subsequently replaced by bone. Elastic cartilage is more flexible than hyaline cartilage and it forms the external structure of the ears. Fibrocartilage is mechanically very strong and it serves a protective role by functioning as a cushion between bones in the knees and the pelvic girdle. Cartilage cells are found in small chambers called lacunae which are surrounded by extracellular matrix.

PROBLEM

Elastic cartilage is found

a)   on bone ends.

b)   in ears.

c)   in the pelvis and knees.

d)   Both a) and c)

Solution

b)   Elastic cartilage is found in ears. Hyaline cartilage coats bone ends. The pelvis and knees contain fibrocartilage.

D. EXTRACELLULAR MATRIX

The extracellular matrix is primarily composed of collagen and tropocollagen is the basic structural unit from which collagen is constructed. Collagen fibers are extremely strong. Tropocollagen has a unique triple helix structure and each polypeptide strand is called an alpha-chain. Intramolecular hydrogen bonds link each alpha-chain to the other two alpha-chains. The amino acid sequence of each alpha-strand is given by:

(gly-pro-X)n

where every third residue is glycine and X can be any amino acid. Pro is proline. In collagen fibers, the tropocollagen molecules are aligned along their long axis but are displaced by about 64 nm. The adjacent tropocollagen molecules are also cross linked to one another. This cross-linking greatly enhanced the mechanical strength of the collagen fibers.

PROBLEM

The extracellular fibers found in all connective tissues are composed mainly of

a)   collagen.

b)   calcium.

c)   elastin.

d)   glycans.

Solution

a)   The connective tissues are defined as the complex of cells and extracellular materials which provide the supporting and connecting framework for all other body tissues. The connective tissues consist of extracellular fibers, amorphous ground substance, and connective tissue cells. The fibers are composed mainly of the protein collagen. The ground substance occupies the spaces between the cells and fibers and contains proteoglycans, glycoproteins, and other molecules secreted from the cells.

V. Nervous and Endocrine Systems

1. Nervous System Structure and Function

Neurons are the fundamental cell type of the nervous system. Neurons can transmit information from inside and outside the body to processing centers in the brain and spinal column. The processed signals can evoke responses, also transmitted by neurons, by muscles and glands. The coordination and integration of these events leads to behavioral adaptation to environmental changes and helps maintain a stable internal environment.

A. ORGANIZATION OF THE VERTEBRATE NERVOUS SYSTEM

The structure of the neuron, action potentials and synaptic transmission has already been discussed (see pg 71). The organs of the brain and spinal column form the central nervous system. The nerves that connect the central nervous system to other body parts are called the peripheral nervous system.

PROBLEM

The central nervous system is composed of the

a)   brain and spinal column.

b)   spinal column and nerves.

c)   neurons, synapses, and spinal column.

d)   sense organs, spinal column, and brain.

Solution

a)   The organs of the brain and spinal column form the central nervous system. The nerves that connect the central nervous system to other body parts are called the peripheral nervous system.

B. SENSOR AND EFFECTOR NEURONS

The sensory function of the nervous system is achieved by sensors at the ends of peripheral nerves. Neurons with a sensory function are called afferent or sensory neurons. The dendrites of these neurons have either sensors at their terminals or their dendrites are in close association with specialized sensor cells. Most sensor neurons have a unipolar structure (see Figure 33(a)).

The information from sensory neurons is transmitted, in the form of a nerve impulse, over peripheral nerves to the central nervous system. After integration of the sensory information a response can be transmitted by the peripheral nerves to effectors, i.e., muscles and/or glands. Interneurons form linkages between neurons within the brain (or spinal cord) and are involved with processing and integration. The interneurons are multipolar (see Figure 33(b)).

Motor neurons, also called efferent neurons, transmit nerve impulses from the brain or spinal column to effectors. Motor neurons are usually multipolar.

Neurons are bundled together to form nerve fibers. Some nerve fibers contain only motor neurons (motor nerves), some only sensory neurons (sensory nerves). Most nerve fibers have, however, both motor and sensory neurons (mixed nerves).

PROBLEM

Bundles of neurons are known as

a)   interneurons.   b)   association areas.

c)   nerve fibers.   d)   effectors.

Solution

c)   Neurons are bundled together to make nerve fibers. Interneurons link neurons to the brain. Effectors are muscles or glands that respond to stimuli.

C.   SYMPATHETIC AND PARASYMPATHETIC NERVOUS SYSTEM

The autonomic nervous system is not under voluntary control and functions independently. The contraction of smooth muscles, blood pressure regulation, temperature regulation, and the secretory function of most glands are under the control of

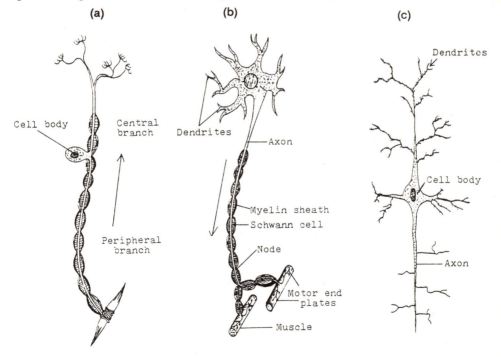

Figure 33 — Neuronal Structures: (a) Unipolar Neuron;
(b) Multipolar Neuron, and (c) Bipolar neuron.

the autonomic nervous system. The autonomic nervous system has been further divided into the sympathetic and parasympathetic nervous systems.

In general, the sympathetic subdivision serves to prepare an organism for energy expenditure while the parasympathetic system restores and maintains an organism in a resting state. Organs are innervated with nerve fibers from both the sympathetic and parasympathetic divisions. The sympathetic nervous system, for example, increases heart rate, and decreases intestinal secretions. These physiological adaptations are restored by the parasympathetic nervous system.

Most of the nerve fibers in the autonomic system are composed of motor neurons and two neurons are used to connect the brain or spinal cord to the effector. The preganglionic axon comes from a neuron in the brain or spinal cord and forms a synapse with a ganglion outside the brain and spinal cord. The postganglionic axon comes from this second neuron and it goes to the effector.

Sympathetic nerves are adrenergic and secrete the neurotransmitter called norepinephrine at the end of their postganglionic fibers. Parasympathetic nerves are cholinergic and secrete acetylcholine at the ends of their postganglionic fibers.

PROBLEM

> Which of the following is characteristic of stimulation of the sympathetic nervous system?
>
> a) Elevated heartbeat
>
> b) Increased saliva excretion
>
> c) Elevated gastric secretion
>
> d) All of the above.

Solution

a) In general, the sympathetic nervous system produces the effects which prepare an animal for emergency situations, such as quickening of the heart and breathing rates and dilation of pupils.

2. Sensory Reception and Processing

A. SOMATIC SENSORS

Somatic sensors transmit information from the nonspecialized parts of the body. The specialized senses refer to smell, taste, hearing, equilibrium and sight. The somatic sensors can be further divided into exteroreceptive, proprioceptive, visceral, and deep sensations. The exteroreceptive sensations arise from the surface of the body. The proprioceptive sensations arise from muscles and tendons as well as body position, the visceral sensations from the internal organs, the deep sensations from "deep" tissues (e.g., bones).

The somatic sensors can be:

(1) mechanoreceptors, which respond to mechanical movement.

(2) thermoreceptors, which respond to hot and cold.

(3)   pain (or nociceptors) receptors which signal tissue damage.

A wide variety of mechanoreceptors exist. These include:

(1)   free ends of sensory nerve fibers which are found predominantly in epithelial cells which respond to touch and pressure.

(2)   Meissner's corpuscles which respond to light touch.

(3)   Pacinian corpuscles which respond to deep pressure and tissue vibrations.

PROBLEM

Somatic sensors could not detect a	
a) bright light.	b) hot stove.
c) stomachache.	d) sunburn.

Solution

a)   Somatic sensors transmit information from non-specialized parts of the body. They do not transmit smell, taste, hearing, equilibrium, or sight.

B.   OLFACTION TASTE

The specialized sensation of smell (olfaction) and taste rely on chemoreceptors. Chemoreceptors are also present on internal tissues where they can detect changes in oxygen levels, glucose levels and pH. In general, chemoreceptors require a threshold level of stimulation in order to generate a receptor potential.

The neurons in the superior part of the nasal cavity that detect odors are called olfactory receptors. These bipolar (see Figure 33(c)) neurons lie in a surrounding matrix of columnar epithelial cells. Bowman's glands, which secrete the mucous necessary for receptor functioning, are also embedded in the columnar epithelial cells. The mucosal ends of the olfactory neurons have many cilia which are the primary receptor sites for gaseous molecules dissolved in the mucosal fluid.

The precise mechanism whereby different gaseous molecules are distinguished is not yet clearly known. When the cilia are stimulated a receptor potential is generated which triggers a nerve impulse in the olfactory nerve fibers. This signal is transmitted to the central nervous system. The olfactory receptors undergo a progressive adaptation; with time that diminishes their response to a stimulus. The taste cells undergo a similar adaptation.

The sense of taste is generated by taste buds located in the tongue, and to a lesser extent, on the roof of the mouth. It is thought that taste consists of different combinations of four primary tastes, i.e., sour, salty, sweet and bitter. The taste receptors are microvilli that protrude from taste cells that are specialized epithelial cells. The outer surface of the taste bud is covered with stratified squamous epithelial cells and the microvilli from the taste cells protrude from a pore on this surface. The taste cells are replaced about every ten days. After stimulation the taste cells generate a receptor potential that, in turn, triggers a nerve impulse that is transmitted to the central nervous system.

PROBLEM

Following exposure to a strong odor over a long period of time, olfactory receptors exhibit a diminished response. This is due to

a) receptor stress.

b) progressive adaptation.

c) receptor death.

d) lack of mucosal fluid.

Solution

b) Progressive adaptation to strong stimuli reduces the response of taste and olfactory receptors.

C. HEARING

EAR STRUCTURE

The ear, which functions in both hearing and balance, has external, middle and internal components. The external ear consists of the auricle, which is funnel shaped, and the auditory meatus, which is tube shaped (see Figure 34). These structures serve to funnel sound waves into the ear where they produce pressure oscillations on the eardrum. The middle ear is in the tympanic of the temporal bone. The eardrum or tympanic membrane separates the external and middle ear.

Three small bones in the tympanic cavity transmit the vibration of the eardrum to the inner ear (see Figure 35). The malleus or hammer is attached to the eardrum.

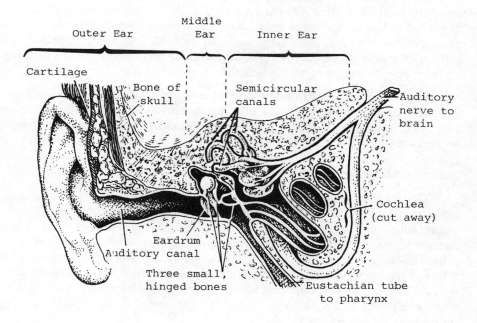

Figure 34 — The Structure of the Ear

The malleus causes the incus (or anvil) to vibrate and this movement is then transmitted to the stapes (or stirrup). It is the movement of the stapes that causes movement of fluid in the inner ear. The stapes is connected to an opening in the middle ear called the oval window.

The inner ear contains the labyrinth (see Figure 36), a complex set of interconnecting and coiled tubes. The labyrinth includes the cochlea and three semicircular canals. The cochlea contains a fluid that is moved by the impact of the stapes. The surface of the basilar membrane inside the cochlea contain the organ of Corti. The organ of Corti has the hair cells that function as the receptors for sound oscillations.

The eustachian tube connects the middle ear to the throat and permits pressure equilibration between the ear and the outside of the body.

MECHANISM OF HEARING

The organ of Corti generates a receptor potential when stimulated by the vibrations of the basilar membrane. The hearing receptor cells have cilia or hair-like structures that project into the endolymph of the cochlear duct. The sensitivity of the

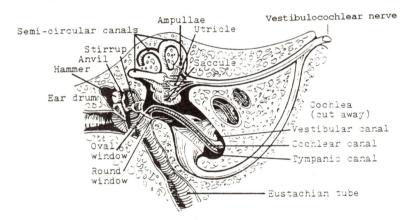

Figure 35 — Structures of the Middle Ear

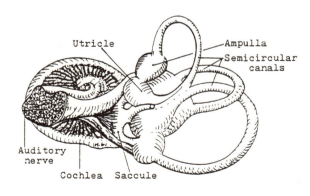

Figure 36 — The Labyrinth of the Inner Ear

ear to different sound frequencies depends upon the differential sensitivity of the hair cells. The movement of the hairs causes a receptor potential to be generated which is transmitted to the cochlear nerve fibers. Some of the nerve impulses from each ear reach both sides of the brain.

PROBLEM

Which of the following items is not part of the human ear?

a) Malleus

b) Cochlea

c) Hyoid

d) Oval window

Solution

c)   Only the hyoid, which is a very small bone near the base of the tongue, is not a part of the human ear. The tectorial membrane is part of the cochlea which is in the inner ear. The oval window is a membrane which separates the middle ear and the inner ear. The malleus is one of the small bones in the middle ear which conducts sound.

D.   VISION

EYE STRUCTURE

The light receptors in the eye are extremely sensitive. A retinal rod cell can detect a single photon. The structure of the human eye is shown in Figure 37. The cornea is transparent and helps focus light and provides mechanical protection to the other underlying tissues. The anterior chamber contains aqueous humor and it lies between the cornea and the lens. The lens focuses light on the retina. The iris controls the diameter of the pupil and helps control the intensity of the light impinging on the retina. The vitreous humor in the eye cup helps control the internal pressure of the eye.

The retina contains the photoreceptor cells which are either specialized for color vision (i.e., the cones) or for night vision (i.e., the rods). In the human retina there is a specialized region called the fovea which has a high density of cone cells. Before

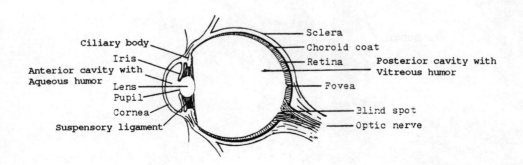

Figure 37 — The Structure of the Human Eye

light reaches the photoreceptor cells it must pass through a number of other retinal layers. The rod photoreceptor cells (see Figure 38) are adjacent to the retinal pigment epithelium. The rod cells shed their tips each day and these tips are phagocytized by the retinal pigmented epithelium. Blood supply to the retina is by way of the choroid or by retinal blood vessels. The choroid is posterior to the retinal pigment epithelium.

The outer segment of the rod photoreceptor cell has numerous disc membranes that are not in direct contact with the plasma membrane. The photosensitive pigment, rhodopsin, is an intrinsic membrane protein found in the disc membranes.

LIGHT RECEPTORS

The rhodopsin molecules in the disc membranes are covalently linked with 11-cis-retinal. Retinal is a aldehyde form of vitamin A. Light causes an isomerization of the cis-retinal to the all-trans-retinal form. This isomerization triggers a change in the conformation of rhodopsin. The light induced conformational change in rhodopsin causes Na^+-channels on the photoreceptor plasma membrane to close. In the dark, the photoreceptor cells are depolarized. This depolarization is due to open Na^+-channels that permit a constant influx of Na^+-ions. The result of a light stimulus is to close the Na^+-channels and thereby cause the receptor cell to become hyperpolarized. This action potential causes a decreased release of inhibitory neurotransmitter.

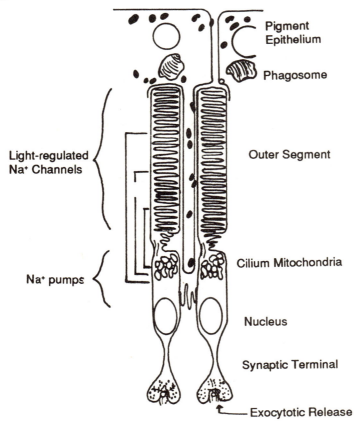

Figure 38 — Structure of the Rod Photoreceptor Cell

> The part of the eye which regulates the amount of incoming light is the
>
> a) retina.   b) lens.
>
> c) iris.   d) cornea.

Solution

c)   Light entering the eye passes through the cornea and enters the lens via a small opening called the pupil. The size of the pupil can be changed by a diaphragm-like muscular structure, the iris, so that the amount of incoming light can be regulated. The iris may contain various colored pigments. The light then falls on a light-sensitive region, the retina, which is located at the rear of the eye.

3.   Endocrine System: Hormones and their Sources

A.   FUNCTION OF ENDOCRINE SYSTEM

Bodily functions are controlled by both the nervous system and the endocrine system as well as the interaction between these two systems. The nervous system, as detailed above, relies on electrical signals. The endocrine system utilizes chemical signals and the signal molecules are called hormones. The endocrine system refers to the set of glands, tissues and cells that secrete hormones directly into bodily fluids.

Hormones regulate a wide variety of metabolic functions and transport functions, as well as development, growth, and reproduction. Hormones are structurally diverse and can exert physiological effects on their target tissues at very low concentrations. Hormones can be peptides, proteins, glycoproteins, biological amines, or steroids.

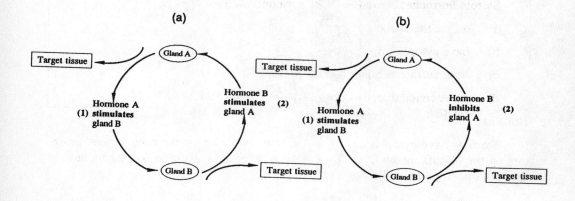

Figure 39 — (a) Positive and (b) Negative Feedback Regulation.

PROBLEM

Hormones do not regulate	
a) growth.	b) reproduction.
c) digestion.	d) temperature.

Solution

d)   Temperature regulation is controlled by the autonomic nervous system. Growth, reproduction, and digestion are controlled, in part, by hormones.

B.   CELLULAR MECHANISMS OF HORMONE ACTION

Many hormones exert their action by first binding to specific receptors on the cell surface. Some of the overall molecular characteristic of this type of signalling process has been discussed above (see the section on the eukaryotic plasma membrane).

Many hormones activate a cyclic AMP system. The first event is the binding of a hormone to a surface receptor on the plasma membrane of the target cell. The receptor-hormone complex then activates adenyl cyclase which produces cAMP from ATP in the cytoplasm. The cAMP is a "second messenger" which relays the initial extracellular signal from the hormone (the first messenger) to an intracellular signal (increased levels of cAMP). The increased cAMP then, in turn, can activate a wide variety of physiological responses. Often a protein kinase is activated which can phosphorylate specific enzymes and thereby regulate their enzymatic activity.

Steroid hormones do not utilize a cAMP system. The steroid hormones are freely permeable to the plasma membrane and do have surface receptors. Instead, they bind to cytoplasmic receptors and the receptor-hormone complex then initiates a series of events leading to the activation of specific genes in the cells' nucleus.

PROBLEM

Steroid hormones are unlike other hormones because they
a)   utilize the cyclic AMP system.
b)   have cytoplasmic receptors.
c)   have surface receptors on the plasma membrane.
d)   are secreted directly into bodily fluids.

Solution

b)   Steroids have cytoplasmic receptors. Most other hormones have surface receptors on the plasma membrane and utilize the cyclic AMP system. All hormones are secreted directly into bodily fluids.

C.   CONTROL OF HORMONE SECRETION

The secretion of hormones into circulating blood is a very regulated process. Both negative and positive feedback loops help regulate this process (see Figure 39). In a negative feedback loop gland A secrets hormone A which stimulates gland B to produce hormone B which then can inhibit the secretion of hormone A by gland A. In a positive feedback loop gland A produces hormone A which stimulates gland B to produce hormone B which further stimulates gland A to secret hormone A.

Hormonal secretions can also be controlled by the nervous system. For example, the adrenal medulla (see below) secretes catecholamines in response to nerve impulses and not by the influence of other hormones or any other stimulus.

PROBLEM

> Hormone secretion is controlled by
>
> a) negative and positive feedback.
>
> b) the nervous system.
>
> c) negative feedback only.
>
> d) Both a) and b).

Solution

d) Hormone secretion can be controlled by positive feedback, negative feedback, or the nervous system.

D. MAJOR ENDOCRINE GLANDS, THEIR HORMONES, SPECIFICITY, AND TARGET ISSUES.

The major endocrine glands, their hormone products, their target tissues and their functions are detailed below.

PITUITARY GLAND

Pituitary Gland — lies at the base of the brain and is connected to the hypothalamus. The pituitary gland is divided into the anterior and posterior pituitary gland.

ANTERIOR PITUITARY GLAND

Anterior pituitary gland — all the major hormones produced by the anterior pituitary gland influence other glands.

Adrenocorticotropic hormone (ACTH) — a protein hormone whose target tissue is the adrenal cortex. ACTH controls the secretion of some adrenocortical hormones and thereby influences the metabolism of glucose, fats, and proteins.

Follicle stimulating hormone (FSH) — a protein hormone whose target tissue is the ovary. FSH stimulates the growth and reproductive activities of the gonads.

Growth hormone (GH) — a protein hormone that promotes body growth and has a major impact upon formation of body protein. It increases:

(1) the transport of amino acids through cell membranes and,

(2) the synthesis of proteins by ribosomes.

It also decreases the rate of protein catabolism.

Luteinizing hormone (LH) — a protein hormone whose target tissue is the ovary. LH stimulates the growth and reproductive activities of the gonads.

Prolactin (PRL) — a protein hormone that stimulates growth of the mammary gland and production of milk.

Thyroid stimulating hormone (TSH) — a protein hormone whose target tissue is the thyroid gland. TSH controls the synthesis of thyroxine in the thyroid gland. Thyroxine, in turn, controls many metabolic reactions.

POSTERIOR PITUITARY GLAND

Antidiuretic hormone (ADH) — this peptide hormone, also called vasopressin, causes a decreased secretion of water by the kidneys, i.e., antidiuresis.

Oxytocin — a peptide hormone whose target tissues include the uterus and the mammary gland. Oxytocin is thought to play a key role in the birthing process, causing contraction of the uterus. Oxytocin also stimulates the expression of milk from the mammary gland in response to suckling.

THYROID GLAND

Thyroid gland — this gland is located below the larynx and on both sides of the trachea.

Thyroxine (T4) — an iodinated amino acid derivative that increases the overall metabolic rate and, in children, promotes growth. In particular, T4 increases protein synthesis, it increases the number and size of mitochondria, and stimulates both carbohydrate and fat metabolism. Secretion of T4 is controlled by TSH from the anterior pituitary gland.

Triiodothyronine (T3) — an iodinated amino acid derivative whose functions are similar to those detailed for thyroxine.

PARATHYROID GLANDS

Parathyroid glands — these glands are located on the posterior surface of the thyroid gland. The parathyroid hormone is the only hormone secreted by the parathyroid gland.

Parathyroid hormone (PTH) — this protein hormone causes an absorption of calcium and phosphate from bone. Moreover, the PTH causes a dramatic increase in the secretion of phosphate by the kidney. The overall result of increased levels of PTH in plasma is an increase in calcium, but a decrease in phosphate levels. PTH promotes the conversion of vitamin D into 1,25-dihydroxycholecalciferol which, in turn, helps promote calcium transport through cell membranes. 1,25-Dihydroxycholecalciferol is the active form of vitamin D. High levels of plasma calcium decrease the secretion of PTH.

ADRENAL GLANDS

The adrenal glands lie at the top of the kidney. The adrenal consists of two distinct glands that secrete different hormones. The exterior part of the adrenal is called the cortex and the central region the medulla. The cells of the medulla are modified postganglionic cells. The cells of the adrenal medulla are in contact with the sympathetic division of the autonomic nervous system.

Adrenal medulla — Nerve impulses from the sympathetic nerve fibers are the stimulus for the secretion of epinephrine and norepinephrine.

Epinephrine — this hormone, also called adrenalin, is a biological amine. Both epinephrine and norepinephrine are catecholamines. Epinephrine prepares the body for a "fight or flight" response, i.e., heart rate, metabolic rate, and systemic blood pressure increases. The liver converts glycogen into glucose, the airways dilate and the force of cardiac muscle contraction increases.

Norepinephrine — this biological amine has a structure similar to that of epinephrine and its biological effects are very similar.

ADRENAL CORTEX

Adrenal cortex — this gland secretes a group of hormones called corticosteroids that are all synthesized from cholesterol. Corticosteroids are further divided into glucocorticoids, mineralocorticoids and androgenic hormones. The glucocorticoids increase blood glucose, the mineralocorticoids affect electrolytes. The androgenic hormones are similar to testosterone.

Aldosterone — is the primary mineralocorticoid and causes sodium ions to be retained and potassium ions to be excreted. This hormone also reduces urinary output, promotes water retention, and increases extracellular fluid volume. Aldosterone exerts its effects on the tubules of the kidney. The secretion of aldosterone is controlled by many factors such as the potassium concentration in extracellular fluid, the renin-angiotensin system, body sodium and adrenocorticotropic hormone.

Cortisol is the primary glucocorticoid and this hormone has the liver as its primary target. Cortisol influences carbohydrate, protein and fat metabolism. One effect of cortisol is to stimulate gluconeogenesis, i.e., the synthesis of glucose from noncarbohydrates, particularly from amino acids. Increased gluconeogenesis, in turn, causes an increased formation of glycogen in the liver. In addition, cortisol causes an increased release of fatty acids from fat cells (adipocytes). The secretion of cortisol is first stimulated by the hypothalamus (of the brain) which secretes *corticotropin-releasing hormone* (CRH). CRH causes the anterior pituitary to secrete ACTH and ACTH causes the adrenal cortex to release cortisol. Stress of almost any kind will cause the release of ACTH which is rapidly followed by secretion of cortisol. Cortisol also exerts an anti-inflammatory effect on tissues damaged by injury.

THE PANCREAS

The *pancreas* lies behind the stomach and is connected to the duodenum. The secretory cells of the pancreas play a role in both the endocrine and exocrine system. The exocrine part of the pancreas secretes digestive enzymes into the small intestine (duodenum). The role of the pancreas in digestion will be discussed below. The endocrine part of the pancreas is due to the islets of Langerhans which contain alpha-, beta-, and delta-cells. These cells secrete their products directly into the blood stream. The alpha-cells secrete glucagon, the beta-cells insulin, and the delta-cells somatostatin. Humans with diabetes have beta-cells that are incapable of secreting insulin. Insulin and glucagon work in concert to control many metabolic activities.

Insulin — a protein hormone that influences carbohydrate, fat, and amino acid metabolism. Insulin decreases the release of fatty acids and fat cells and promotes the utilization of glucose. High levels of blood glucose (e.g., after a meal) stimulate the secretion of insulin. Insulin promotes the uptake and storage of glucose by almost all tissues in the body, particularly those of the liver and muscles. In liver and muscle tissue, glucose is stored as glycogen. The glycogen in the liver is used to supply the blood with glucose when the dietary supply of glucose decreases. Insulin also causes the liver to convert glucose into fatty acids which are subsequently stored in fat cells as triglycerides. Insulin also promotes the transport of amino acids into many tissues. Low levels of insulin causes fatty acids and glycerol to be released from adipocytes into plasma. The increased plasma levels of nonesterified fatty acids stimulate the liver to synthesize triglycerides, cholesterol esters, phospholipids and cholesterol. These lipids are secreted by the liver in the form of very low density lipoprotein. In addition, high levels of plasma fatty acids also stimulate liver mitochondrial fatty acid oxidation producing ketone bodies (i.e., betahydroxybutyrate and acetoacetate). Humans with the inability to secrete insulin often have very high levels of very low density lipoprotein and also develop premature atherosclerosis.

Glucagon — this protein hormone counteracts many of the metabolic effects of insulin. In particular, glucagon promotes an increase in blood glucose levels by causing a breakdown in glycogen, i.e., glycogenolysis. The secretion of glucagon is regulated by blood glucose levels, i.e., low levels of blood glucose stimulate glucagon secretion.

OVARY

See the Section on Reproductive System and Development.

THE TESTES

See the Section on Reproductive System and Development.

PROBLEM

> The adrenal medulla is most closely associated with
>
> a)   insulin.   b)   epinephrine.
>
> c)   chorionic gonadotropin.   d)   vasopressin.

Solution

b)   Epinephrine is a secretory product of the adrenal medulla. It causes a breakdown of glycogen to glucose in the liver and skeletal muscle with a consequent rise in blood glucose levels. Epinephrine elevates the blood pressure and heart rate. It also constricts cutaneous blood vessels and dilates skeletal muscle vessels. In addition, it causes the organs of the digestive tract to experience vasoconstriction.

VI. Circulatory System, Lymphatic, and Immune Systems

1. Circulatory System

A. MULTIPLE FUNCTIONS, INCLUDING ROLE IN THERMOREGULATION

The circulatory system has a major role in maintaining the stability of the body's internal environment, i.e., homeostasis. The fluid in the body can be divided into intracellular fluid and extracellular fluid which have different compositions. The extracellular fluid can be further divided into interstitial fluid and the fluid of the circulatory system, i.e., plasma. The circulatory system is responsible for the movement and mixing of the extracellular fluid.

Some major roles of the circulatory system are:

(a)   the delivery of oxygen and required nutrients,

(b)   the removal of metabolic waste products,

(c)   the transport of regulatory molecules such as hormones,

(d)   the transport of protective chemicals and enzymes. Vitamin E is an example of a protective chemical which inhibits free radical damage to cell membranes and macromolecules,

(e)   the transport of molecules and cells essential to the immune system.

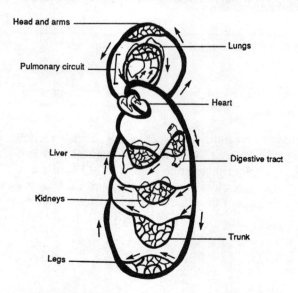

Figure 40 — The Circulatory System

PROBLEM

The circulatory system does all the following EXCEPT

a)   deliver oxygen.

b)   regulate blood pressure.

c)   transport enzymes.

d)   remove waste products.

Solution

b)   The circulatory system transports materials to and from tissues, it does NOT regulate blood pressure. Blood pressure is controlled, in part, chemically.

B.   FOUR-CHAMBERED HEART, PULMONARY, AND SYSTEMIC CIRCULATION.

The overall organization of the circulatory system is shown in Figure 40. In essence, the four-chamber heart is two pumps: one pumps blood to the lungs and the other to the systemic circulation.

The four-chambered heart (see Figure 41) is composed of two atria and two ventricles. The atria are filling chambers and pump blood to the ventricles which provide the main contractile force needed to move blood through the circulatory system.

Deoxygenated venous blood from the venae cavae continuously flows into the right atrium and then directly into the right ventricle (before contraction). Atrial contraction then fills the right ventricle. The contraction of the right ventricle (and the closing of the tricuspid valve) pumps the blood into the pulmonary circulation where the blood is oxygenated and carbon dioxide is lost to the atmosphere. The oxygenated blood is returned to the heart via the pulmonary veins and enters the left atrium. With the contraction of the left atrium the blood enters the left ventricle. The contraction of the left ventricle closes the bicuspid valve and blood is pumped into the systemic circulatory system.

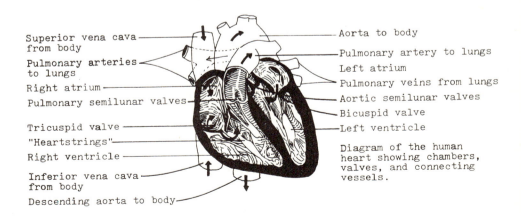

Figure 41 — The Heart

The heart is supplied with oxygenated blood by two branches of the aorta, i.e., the right and left coronary arteries. A major cause of cardiovascular disease is the accumulation of atherosclerotic plaques in the coronary arteries. This severely narrows the lumen of these arteries and a small blood clot can clog these arteries resulting in a cut-off of oxygenated blood to the heart. This results in a coronary heart attack.

The cardiac cycle is the period from the end of contraction and the end of the next contraction. The period of relaxation is called the diastole and the period of contraction is the systole.

PROBLEM

Which of the following is not a true statement?

a)   Blood enters the heart through the superior (anterior) vena cava or through the inferior (posterior) vena cava.

b)   The pulmonary artery carries oxygenated blood.

c)   Oxygenated blood first enters the left atrium of the heart.

d)   The systemic circulation contains oxygenated blood.

Solution

b)   Blood enters the right atrium of the heart through the superior or inferior vena cava. When this chamber is filled, the blood is forced through the tricuspid valve and into the right ventricle. From there, this deoxygenated blood travels through the pulmonary artery to the lungs where it exchanges carbon dioxide for oxygen. Once oxygenated, the blood travels to the left atrium through the pulmonary veins. It travels through the bicuspid valve to the left ventricle, out through the aorta, and is then distributed throughout the body.

C.   ARTERIAL AND VENOUS SYSTEMS, CAPILLARY BEDS, SYSTEMIC AND DIASTOLIC PRESSURE

Arteries carry oxygenated blood away from the heart under high pressure. Arteries have strong vascular walls which pulsate in synchrony with heart pulsations. The maximum pressure reached during the arterial pulse is called the systolic pressure and the lowest pressure is called the diastolic pressure. The arteries end in arterioles which effectively control the flow of blood into the capillary beds. The capillaries have a very permeable membrane which permits the exchange of nutrients, hormones, electrolytes, and other substances between blood and the interstitial spaces between cells. The deoxygenated blood from the capillary beds collects in the venous system and returns to the heart. The venous system is under low pressure and is thin walled.

The arterial pulse pressure is influenced primarily by the stroke volume output of the heart and by the compliance of the arterial vasculature. The stroke volume of the heart is the amount of blood pumped out of the heart with each heartbeat. The greater the stroke volume output, the greater the arterial pulse pressure. The compliance of the arterial vasculature refers to the distendability of the arteries to a pressure load. The greater the arterial compliance, the lower the arterial pulse pressure.

PROBLEM

> The only artery in the human body which carries deoxygenated blood is the
>
> a) pulmonary artery. b) right coronary artery.
>
> c) left coronary artery. d) carotid artery.

Solution

a)   The pulmonary artery carries blood to the lungs to be cleaned of its carbon dioxide. All other arteries carry oxygenated blood.

D.   COMPOSITION OF BLOOD

Whole blood can be separated by low speed centrifugation into a cell free fluid called serum (or plasma if a blood anticoagulant is present) and a pellet containing cells and platelets. Plasma is about 92% water and contains electrolytes, lipoproteins, proteins, hormones, other nutrients and vitamins. The lipoproteins are lipid-protein complexes. Lipoproteins are the primary transport molecules for lipids and also transport vitamin E and beta-carotene (provitamin A). Lipoproteins are further divided into very low density lipoprotein, low density lipoprotein and high density lipoprotein. High plasma levels of low density lipoprotein are associated with atherosclerosis and cardiovascular disease. In contrast, high plasma levels of high density lipoprotein are thought to protect against atherosclerosis.

The primary proteins found in plasma are albumin, globulins, and fibrinogen. Albumin is the most abundant plasma protein (about 60%) and is a carrier molecule for nonesterified fatty acids. Albumin also plays a role in maintaining the osmotic pressure of blood. The globulins are further divided into alpha-, beta-, and gamma-globulins. The gamma-globulin fraction contains molecules that function as antibodies in the humoral immune system (see below). Fibrinogen functions in clot formation.

The red blood cell (or erythrocyte) is the primary cell found in blood. This unique cell has a plasma membrane but no other membranous organelles and does not have a cell nucleus. The primary function of red blood cells is oxygen transport to tissues and the removal of carbon dioxide. The oxygen carrying molecule in the red blood cell is hemoglobin (see below). The red blood cell has a biconcave shape and is extremely deformable and able to move through very small capillaries. In anemia the number of red blood cells in a given volume of blood is low resulting in a decreased ability to deliver oxygen to tissues. Nutritional and/or genetic factors can contribute to anemia.

Blood also contains white blood cells and platelets. White blood cells (or leukocytes) include monocytes, lymphocytes, neutrophils, eosinophils, and basophils. Neutrophils, eosinophiles, and basophils (all three are also called granulocytes) as well as monocytes are phagocytic cells. The role of these phagocytic cells in the immune system will be discussed below. Lymphocytes also play a key role in the immune system (see below). Platelets function in clot formation.

E. ROLE OF HEMOGLOBIN IN OXYGEN TRANSPORT

Hemoglobin is the primary molecule found in red blood cells and its primary function is in the transport of oxygen. The three dimensional structure of hemoglobin is known in detail from X-ray crystallographic studies. Hemoglobin is a tetramer (alpha$_2$beta$_2$) with two identical alpha subunits and two identical beta subunits. Both the alpha and beta subunits have a structure similar to myoglobin. Myoglobin is the monomeric oxygen binding protein of muscle. Each of the hemoglobin subunits has a heme group containing iron in the ferrous (Fe^{+2}) state. Each heme group can bind a single oxygen molecule. Oxygen binding does not change the oxidation state of the heme iron.

Hemoglobin is an allosteric protein. The binding of oxygen to hemoglobin is regulated by other molecules such as protons (H^+), carbon dioxide (CO_2) and 2,3-diphosphoglycerate (DPG). These molecules exert their influence on oxygen binding by binding to sites that are distinct from the oxygen binding sites. A key feature of oxygen binding to hemoglobin is the cooperative nature of this binding (see Figure 42). Cooperative binding occurs when the binding of each oxygen molecule facilitates the binding of the next oxygen molecule. This cooperative binding results in a characteristic sigmoidal dissociation curve as shown in Figure 42. In contrast, the binding of oxygen to myoglobin is not cooperative (and the dissociation curve is a hyperbola) but myoglobin does have a stronger affinity for oxygen than does hemoglobin.

The cooperative binding of oxygen to hemoglobin plays an important physiological role in the delivery of oxygen to tissues. Hemoglobin is almost fully saturated with oxygen at the partial pressure of oxygen found in the lung (pO_2 = 100 mm Hg). Oxygen is readily dissociated from hemoglobin and delivered to myoglobin which has a stronger affinity for the oxygen. As more oxygen is dissociated from hemoglobin the affinity of the remaining oxygen is less. This follows since dissociation is just the reverse of binding. Thus, hemoglobin is able to deliver oxygen to tissues even at the low pO_2 levels found in capillaries (pO_2 = 20-26 mm Hg).

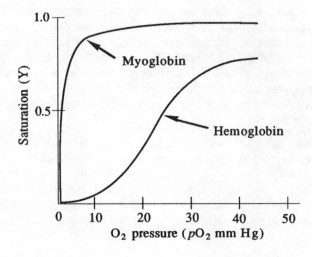

Figure 42 — Oxygen Binding to Hemoglobin and Myoglobin

CO_2, DPG and H^+ shift the oxygen dissociation curve to the right, i.e., the affinity of hemoglobin for oxygen is decreased. Tissues with a high metabolic activity, such as contracting muscle, generate large amounts of H^+ and CO_2. High H^+ and CO_2 lower the affinity of hemoglobin for oxygen and thereby increase the delivery of oxygen to these metabolically active tissues. This is called the Bohr effect.

PROBLEM

In muscles, oxygen leaves hemoglobin to bind with myoglobin because

a)   the presence of H^+ and CO_2 in muscles increases the affinity of hemoglobin for oxygen.

b)   the removal of oxygen from hemoglobin increases hemoglobin's affinity for the remaining oxygen.

c)   myoglobin has a stronger oxygen affinity than hemoglobin.

d)   the bonding of oxygen to myoglobin is cooperative.

Solution

c)   Myoglobin has a stronger oxygen affinity than hemoglobin. Myoglobin does not have the cooperative oxygen binding. The presence of H^+ and CO_2, as well as the removal of oxygen from hemoglobin, decreases the affinity of hemoglobin for oxygen.

2.   Lymphatic System

The lymphatic system provides an important link with the cardiovascular system and the immune system. It consists of lymph fluid, lymphatic vessels (see Figure 43), lymph nodes, the spleen and the thymus gland. The thymus gland plays a key role is the processing of T-lymphocytes (see below).

Almost all tissues in the body have lymphatic capillaries and these merge to form lymphatic vessels. The lymph from the upper and lower portion of the body

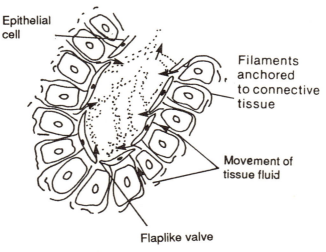

Figure 43 — A Lymphatic capillary

flows into veins in the thorax. A vital role of the lymphatic system is to provide an alternative route for the fluid in between cells (interstitial fluid) to flow back into blood. Interstitial fluid that enters the lymph capillaries is called lymph. In addition, the lymphatic system aids in the removal of proteins and large particles from the interstitial spaces.

Lymph capillaries have many "flaps" or valves that permit the inflow of fluid and particulate matter but prevent their "back flow" into the interstitial spaces. Edema, which is the accumulation of fluid in tissues, can result if fluid flow through the lymphatic system is blocked.

Bacteria and viruses that have entered tissues cannot be directly absorbed via the blood capillaries. These pathogens enter lymph and are subsequently transported into lymph nodes which contain large numbers of lymphocytes and macrophages which defend against these microorganisms. The role of macrophages and lymphocytes in the immune system is detailed below.

PROBLEM

The lymphatic system transports all the following EXCEPT

a) plasma.

b) interstitial fluid.

c) pathogens.

d) macrophages.

Solution

a) Plasma travels in the circulatory system. Interstitial fluid (lymph), pathogens, and macrophages may be transported in the lymphatic system.

3. Immune System

The primary function of the immune system is to provide resistance from attack by infectious agents such as bacteria and viruses. Most immune responses in higher organisms involve the production of antibodies (i.e., acquired immunity) but other innate mechanisms for killing infectious agents also exist. Macrophages, for example, can kill invading bacteria by phagocytosis (engulfing and digesting) and this process can occur in the absence of antibodies. The acidic digestive juice of the stomach is also effective in killing infectious agents introduced by swallowing.

A. ANTIGENS, ANTIBODIES AND ANTIGEN-ANTIBODY REACTIONS

Acquired immunity depends upon the production of recognition molecules that can distinguish "self" from "nonself." The two forms of acquired immunity are:

(1) humoral immunity and,

(2) cellular immunity.

Cellular immunity refers to the formation of lymphocytes that are sensitized against the invading agent. Humoral immunity refers to the binding of circulating antibodies to the invading agent. Antibodies (or immunoglobulins) are remarkably specific recognition molecules.

A typical antibody consists of four polypeptide chains. There are two identical "light chains" and two identical "heavy chains" and the four chains are held together by disulfide bonds as shown in Figure 44a to form a Y-shaped molecule. As shown in Figure 44b, both the heavy and light chains of an antibody are built up from a structurally similar "domain" or polypeptide subunit of about 220 amino acids. Each light chain has two such domains: a "constant" domain and "variable" domain. Similarly, each heavy chain has three (sometimes two) constant domains and one variable domain. The variable domains are at the amino-terminal ends (see Figure 44) of both heavy and light chains and the amino acid sequence in this region is very variable. The variable regions provide the specificity which enables an antibody to bind to a very specific region of another molecule, i.e., the antigen. The constant regions of antibodies provide a mechanism for the binding of the antibody to other cells (such as macrophages) or binding to elements of the complement system (see below).

When antibodies bind to an antigen on an invading organism they mark it for destruction by either the complement system or by macrophages. The proteins of the complement system destroy an invading organism by perforating its cell membrane. Antibodies can also inactivate an invading organism by agglutination (multiple antigenic sites are bound together to form a clump), precipitation (the water soluble antigen complexes with the antibody and the complex is insoluble), or by neutralization (the antibody binds to and covers a toxic site).

PROBLEM

The complement system of immune response does NOT

a) agglutinate antigens.

b) precipitate antigens.

c) ingest antigens.

d) neutralize toxic sites.

Solution

c) The complement system may agglutinate, precipitate, or neutralize antigens. Macrophages ingest antigens.

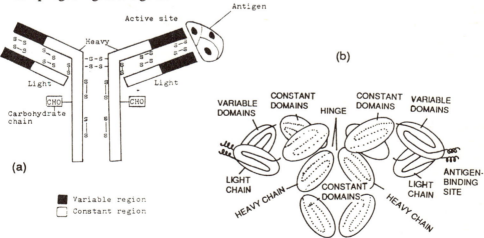

Figure 44 — The Structure of Typical IgG Antibody showing the constant and variable polypeptide segments. (a) shows position of disulfide bonds and (b) shows arrangement of domains.

B.   TISSUES AND CELLS OF THE IMMUNE SYSTEM

T-LYMPHOCYTES, B-LYMPHOCYTES, BONE MARROW, SPLEEN, THYMUS, AND LYMPH NODES).

Lymphoid tissues form the "organ system" responsible for acquired immunity. Acquired immunity does not develop until after contact is made with an invading agent. Lymphoid tissues are widely distributed throughout the body and are particularly concentrated in lymph nodes, the thymus, the bone marrow and the spleen. The white cells or lymphocytes of blood are also lymphoid cells.

T-LYMPOCYTES AND B-LYMPHOCYTES.

Lymphoid tissues contains two types of lymphocytes called T-lymphocytes and B-lymphocytes. The T-lymphocytes form the sensitized cells of the cellular immune system and the B-cells play a key role in the production of antibodies that provide for humoral immunity. T-cells have another class of recognition molecules called T-cell receptors which will only recognize cells that bear both "self" and "nonself" markers.

Both T- and B-lymphocytes arise from embryonic stem cells but before becoming part of lymphoid tissues they require a maturation process. For T-cells this maturation occurs in the thymus gland and for B-cells the exact site is not known but is thought to be in the bone marrow. After the maturation process the T- and B-cells migrate to and become imbedded in the lymphoid tissues.

The immunological events following an infection by an infectious agent such as a virus are as follows:

(1)   Macrophages ingest a number of viruses and display some specific viral "markers" or antigens on their surface. Some helper T-cells in circulation have the proper T-cell receptors to recognize the processed viral antigens on the macrophage surface and these T-cells become activated.

(2)   The activated helper T-cells multiply and also stimulate the multiplication of killer T-cells and activated B-cells that can also recognize the same processed viral antigens. The activated B-cells multiply and differentiate into plasma cells that produce antibodies to the viral antigen. Some of the activated B-cells become memory cells which permit a rapid response to any future infection by the virus.

(3)   The killer T-cells will destroy host cells that have become infected with the virus and thereby inhibit viral replication. The antibodies produced by the B-cells will also bind to the virus and prevent them from infecting additional host cells.

(4)   When the infection is contained, suppressor T-cells halt the immune responses and memory T-cells and memory B-cells remain in the blood and lymphatic system.

The AIDS virus is particularly damaging to the immune system because it invades and kills helper T-cells.

PROBLEM

> The functional difference between B-cells and T-cells is that
>
> a)   B-cells differentiate from stem cells and T-cells differentiate from lymphocytes.
>
> b)   T-cells differentiate from stem cells and B-cells differentiate from lymphocytes.
>
> c)   T-cells secrete antibodies in response to introduced antigens and B-cells direct the cell-mediated response.
>
> d)   B-cells secrete antibodies in response to introduced antigens and T-cells direct the cell-mediated response.

Solution

d)   T-cells and B cells are the cells involved in the immune responses of the body. Both cell types differentiate from stem cells of the bone marrow. The stem cells that migrate to the thymus become T-cells and are responsible for cell-mediated immunity. Those stem cells that migrate to the bursa or analogous structure become B-cells and are the cells of the humoral immune system.

VII. Digestive and Excretory Systems

1. Digestive System

The primary role of the digestive system is to convert food into substances that are capable of being absorbed into the body. Moreover, those substances that are incapable of absorption must be excreted. The digestive system consists of the alimentary canal and the exocrine organs that secrete digestive juices into the alimentary canal. The alimentary canal starts at the mouth and includes the pharynx, esophagus, stomach, small intestine, large intestine and the anus (see Figure 45). The salivary gland, pancreas, liver and gallbladder are organs that secrete substances into the alimentary canal.

A. INGESTION: STRUCTURES AND THEIR FUNCTIONS

The first component of the alimentary canal is the mouth which mechanically reduces the size of food materials and mixes the masticated particles with saliva. The teeth are specialized structures for breaking up food particles and increasing the surface area of the food particles. The incisors cut large food sections, the cuspids serve to grasp and tear food, and the bicuspids and molars are effective in grinding food particles.

Saliva is secreted into the mouth by the salivary glands and it increases the moisture content of the food particles and also initiates the digestion of carbohydrate. Amylase is the digestive enzyme in saliva and it splits starch and glycogen into disaccharides. In plants, glucose is stored as starch granules and in animals, glucose

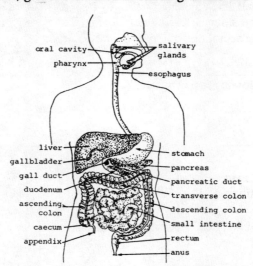

Figure 45 — The Digestive System

is stored as glycogen granules. Starch is a very heterogenous material and its two principal components are amylose and amylopectic polysaccharides.

PROBLEM

> Which of the following organs is not a part of the human digestive system?
>
> a)   Esophagus   b)   Thymus
>
> c)   Gall bladder   e)   Pancreas

Solution

b)   All the choices are a part of the digestive system except for the thymus. The thymus is a gland that does most of its work during childhood and is almost completely inactive by puberty.

B.   STOMACH

The food mass from the mouth passes through the pharynx and the esophagus by a peristaltic wave and enters the stomach. In the stomach the food mass is mixed with gastric secretions and the digestion of protein is initiated. The gastric glands secrete pepsinogen, mucus, hydrochloric acid and intrinsic factor. Intrinsic factor is important in promoting the absorption of vitamin B12. Pepsinogen is the inactive form of pepsin.

The inactive form of an enzyme is called a zymogen. Pepsinogen is activated to pepsin by cleavage of a 44-residue peptide (from the amino terminal end) and this activation occurs spontaneously at pH 2 and is also catalyzed by pepsin. Pepsin is an acid-protease and has maximal enzymatic activity at pH 2 to 3. The hydrochloric acid in the stomach functions to maintain an acidic pH (of l) and also denatures dietary protein to make it more susceptible to protease attack. Pepsin primarily catalyzes the hydrolysis of peptide bonds with an aromatic amino acid residue such as phenylalanine, tryptophane and tyrosine. The polypeptides produced by pepsin digestion are transported to the small intestine for further hydrolysis. The mixture of food mass and gastric juices in the stomach constitutes chyme. Chyme enters the small intestine which also receives the secretions of the liver and pancreas.

PROBLEM

> Which of the following is a zymogen?
>
> a)   Protease   b)   Tyrosine
>
> c)   Chyme   d)   Pepsinogen

Solution

d)   Pepsinogen is a zymogen, an inactive form of an enzyme. Protease is an enzyme, tyrosine is an amino acid, and chyme is the mixture found in the stomach.

C.   DIGESTIVE GLANDS, INCLUDING LIVER AND PANCREAS, BILE PRODUCTION

The pancreas, in addition to it role in the endocrine system (see the Endocrine Section, pg. 72), also functions in the exocrine system. The acinar cells, which form most of the pancreatic mass, secrete pancreatic juice which travels through the pancreatic duct to the duodenum. The bile duct from the liver and gallbladder enter the duodenum at the same site. Pancreatic juice aids the digestion of carbohydrate, fat, and protein. The pH of pancreatic juice is alkaline and it neutralizes the acidic chyme from the stomach. Carbohydrate digestion is assisted by pancreatic amylase which breaks down starch and glycogen into disaccharides (see above). Triglycerides are hydrolyzed into glycerol and free fatty acids by the action of pancreatic lipase.

A mixture of zymogens are released into the small intestine. These zymogens include trypsinogen, chymotrypsinogen and procarboxypeptidase and they are converted into their active forms (trypsin, chymotrypsin and carboxypeptidase, respectively). Trypsin hydrolyzes the carboxyl side of peptide bonds with argine and lysine residues while chymotrypsin acts on the carboxyl side of peptide bonds with aromatic residues (phenylalanine, tryptophane and tyrosine) as well as methionine. Carboxypeptidase A releases the carboxyl-terminal amino acids and carboxypeptidase B is restricted to peptides with an arginine or lysine carboxyl-terminal. The pancreas also secretes nucleases to breakdown nucleic acids into nucleotides.

The liver functions in the process of digestion by secreting bile salts which act like a detergent and emulsifies fat. This emulsification increases the surface area of the fat droplets. Lipases can efficiently utilize triglycerides (fat droplets) that have been emulsified by bile salts. Bile salts are synthesized by hepatic cells from cholesterol and are secreted into the common bile duct. The common bile exits to the duodenum via a sphincter muscle (the sphincter of Oddi). Between meals the sphincter of Oddi is closed and bile is stored in the gallbladder.

PROBLEM

Bile is secreted by the

a)	stomach.	b)	liver.
c)	duodenum.	d)	gallbladder.

Solution

b)   Bile is an aqueous solution which contains various organic and inorganic solutes. Among the major organic solutes are bile salts, phospholipids, cholesterol, and bile pigments. The adult human liver produces about 15 ml of bile per kilogram body weight. The rate of synthesis and secretion is dependent mainly upon blood flow to the liver.

D.   SMALL INTESTINE, LARGE INTESTINE

The small intestine receives chyme from the stomach as well as pancreatic juice and bile from the liver. It starts at the pyloric sphincter and ends at the large intestine. The three segments of the small intestine are the duodenum, the jejunum and the ileum. The small intestine has numerous villi that project into the intestinal lumen. These villi serve to mix chyme with intestinal juices and aid in the absorption of digested nutrients. The small intestine is the primary absorbing organ of the alimentary canal. The epithelial cells of the intestinal mucosa have a variety of digestive enzymes. These include peptidases (which break polypeptides into amino acids), and enzymes that convert disaccharides into monosaccharides.

The large intestine plays almost no role in the digestion of food but does reabsorb water and electrolytes. In addition, it stores feces until defecation of undigestible food components, such as fiber.

PROBLEM

Villi are finger-like protrusions of the

a)   small intestine.   b)   outer ear.

c)   bronchioles.   d)   capillaries.

Solution

a)   Villi line the lumen of the small intestine and thereby increase the intestinal surface area. Most of the nutrient absorption during digestion occurs through the villi.

E.   MUSCULAR CONTROL OF DIGESTION

The smooth muscles of the alimentary canal promote both the mixing of food with gastric juices and the rhythmic wave-like (peristaltic) movements that propel food through the lumen of the digestive tract. The regulation of this muscular contraction is primarily controlled by an "intrinsic nervous system." This intrinsic system also regulates much of the secretory functions required for digestion. In addition, nerve fibers from the parasympathetic and sympathetic branches of the autonomic system also interact with the intrinsic nervous system of the gut. In general, the parasympathetic system increases the activity of the gut and the sympathetic system decreases this activity.

The vagus nerve, which is part of the parasympathetic system arises from the brain, innervates the esophagus, stomach, pancreas and the proximal half of the large intestine. Parasympathetic nerve fibers also originate from the sacral segments of the spinal cord and innervate the distal segment of the large intestine. The sympathetic innervation also regulates the gastrointestinal tract. The preganglionic fibers originate in the spinal cord and the postganglionic fibers innervate all parts of the gut. The norepinephrine secreted by the ends of the sympathetic nerves inhibits the contractions of smooth muscles in the gut and also inhibits the intrinsic nervous system.

PROBLEM

Norepinephrine inhibits all the following EXCEPT

a)   smooth muscle contraction.

b)   peristalsis.

c)   the intrinsic nervous system.

d)   the parasympathetic nervous system.

Solution

d)   Norepinephrine inhibits the intrinsic nervous system and smooth muscles in the gut (which produce peristalsis). Norepinephrine does not affect the parasympathetic nervous system.

2. Excretory System

A. ROLE OF EXCRETORY SYSTEM IN BODY HOMEOSTASIS

Metabolic waste products are often toxic and must be removed from the body to prevent tissue damage. Blood and lymph are the fluids that initially receive metabolic wastes. Gaseous waste products such a CO_2 are removed from blood by the respiratory system. Salts and nitrogenous wastes are removed from the circulatory system by the urinary system. The urinary system also plays a key role in body homeostatsis by helping to regulate the volume and composition of extracellular fluid, the production of red blood cells and blood pressure. The urinary system is composed of a pair of kidneys, a pair of ureters, a urinary bladder and a urethra (see Figure 45).

PROBLEM

Wastes are removed from the blood by the

a) respiratory system. b) urinary system.

c) digestive system. d) both a) and b).

Solution

d) The respiratory and urinary systems both remove wastes. The respiratory system removes gases from the blood and the urinary system removes liquid and dissolved materials from the blood. The digestive system breaks down food, but does not remove wastes.

B. KIDNEY: STRUCTURE AND FUNCTION

The kidneys (see Figure 46) are located on both sides of the spinal column and are behind the parietal peritoneum. The surface of the kidney facing the spinal column (the medial surface) is concave and contains a deep sinus through which the

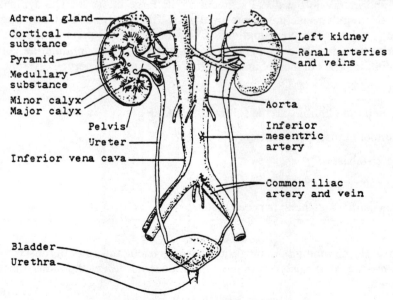

Figure 46 — The Kidneys

renal artery (from the aorta) and the renal vein (from the inferior vena cava) enter. The ureter, which transports urine away from the kidney, also exits from the renal sinus. The extrarenal ureter is expanded into a funnel-shapped sac (the renal pelvis) at its junction with the renal sinus. The intrarenal tubes of the ureter branch to form two major calyces each of which further divides into minor calyces. Urine is delivered into the minor calyces by the renal papillae and then flows through the ureter into the bladder.

The interior of the kidney is divided into an inner renal medulla and an outer renal cortex. The renal medulla forms pyramidal structures whose apexes form the renal papillae. The renal cortex has a granular appearance due to the many small tubules of the nephrons (see below).

In addition to its role of removing metabolic wastes the kidney also secretes erythropoietin which stimulates the production of red blood cells. Renin is also secreted by the kidney and it helps regulate blood pressure. The inactive form of vitamin D (25-hydroxyl-vitamin D) is converted to the active form of vitamin D (1,25-dihydroxyvitamin D) in the kidney. The active form of vitamin D promotes Ca^{+2} absorption.

PROBLEM

The kidney can do all the following EXCEPT

a) remove metabolic wastes.

b) help activate vitamin C.

c) help regulate blood pressure.

d) help stimulate production of red blood cells.

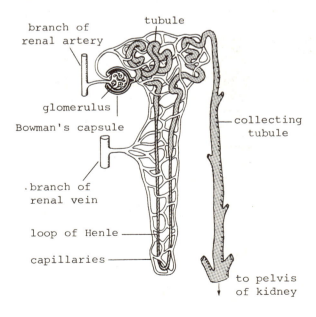

Figure 47 — A Nephron

Solution

b)   The kidney does everything listed above but help in the activation of vitamin C. The kidney helps in the activation of vitamin D.

C.   NEPHRON: STRUCTURE AND FUNCTION

Urine is formed in the nephron which is the functional unit of the kidney. About a million nephrons are present in each kidney. The two major sections of a nephron are the corpuscle and the tubule (see Figure 47)

The corpuscle is a network of intertwined capillaries that surround a capsule (Bowman's capsule) containing the glomerulus. The end of the proximal tubule forms Bowman's capsule. The convoluted proximal tubule from Bowman's capsule forms the loop of Henle followed by the distal convoluted tubule.

PROBLEM

Which of the following is not part of the nephron in the human kidney?

a)   Proximal convoluted tubule   b)   Loop of Henle

c)   Distal convoluted tubule   d)   Major calyx

Solution

d)   The nephron is the structural and functional unit of the kidney consisting of a renal corpuscle (a Glomerulus enclosed within Bowman's capsule), and its attached tubule. The tubule consists of the proximal convoluted portion, the loop of Henle, and the distol convoluted portion. These connect by arched collecting tubules. There are approximately one million nephrons in each kidney.

The major calyx is not part of the nephron, but is, rather, a part of the intrarenal collecting system.

D.   FORMATION OF URINE

Blood enters the glomerulus through the afferent arteriole and exits through the efferent arteriole. The blood in the glomerulus is under pressure (60 mm Hg) and this pressure forces fluid into Bowman's capsule. The fluid in the Bowman's capsule flows into:

(1)   the proximal renal tubule (in the cortex of the kidney),

(2)   the loop of Henle,

(3)   the distal tubule and,

(4)   a collecting duct which, in turn, flows into the renal pelvis.

The end result of this fluid movement is the creation of urine. The solute composition of urine is, however, partly dependent upon environmental and nutritional parameters. The loops of Henle and the vasa recta provide mechanisms for regulating the osmolarity and volume of urine produced by the kidney.

The concentration of electrolytes and other substances in the fluid contained in Bowman's capsule (i.e., the glomerular filtrate) is very similar to that found in interstitial fluid. Most of the water and some of the solutes in the glomerular filtrate (under a pressure of about 18 mm Hg) is reabsorbed into peritubular capillaries which are under about 13 mm Hg of pressure, (i.e., lower than that of the loop of Henle). The solutes that are reabsorbed into circulation are nontoxic and their loss as urine would be wasteful. For example, glucose, amino acids and many electrolytes are reabsorbed. Toxic, unwanted or "excess" solutes are not reabsorbed and appear in urine. In addition to this filtration mechanism, some wastes are directly secreted, from the peritubular capillaries, into the renal tubules.

E.   STORAGE AND ELIMINATION OF WASTES

Urea is a byproduct of amino acid metabolism and it is a main constituent of urine. Uric acid which is formed from the catabolism of purines is also eliminated in urine. Urine, from the renal pelvis, flows through the ureter to the urinary bladder. The flow of urine through the ureter is promoted by peristaltic contraction of the muscular lining of the ureter. The process by which the urinary bladder empties is called micturition. Micturation occurs when the tension in the walls of the bladder reaches a threshold level caused by the increasing volume of urine. This can trigger a reflex that results in the emptying of the bladder. The micturation reflex can also be influenced by both inhibitory and stimulatory signals from the brain. In particular, the relaxation of the urethral sphincter is necessary before urination can proceed.

PROBLEM

Micturation is controlled by			
a)	reflex.	b)	signals from the brain.
c)	hormones.	d)	Both a) and b).

Solution

d)   Micturation is controlled by reflex and signals from the brain, not hormones.

VIII. Muscle and Skeletal Systems

1. Muscle System

A. FUNCTIONS

The primary function of all muscle tissue is contraction during which chemical energy is converted to mechanical energy. The contraction of muscle fibers causes tension on the body parts to which they are attached. Skeletal muscles function by applying tension to their attachment points on bones. Bones and muscles form lever systems which control body movements and help maintain posture. Muscles also function to control the movement of fluids in circulatory and excretory system and help maintain body temperature.

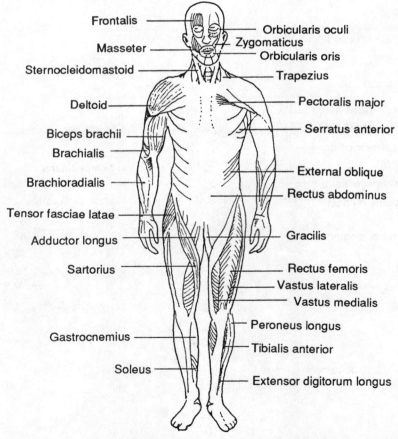

Frontalis — Orbicularis oculi
Zygomaticus
Masseter — Orbicularis oris
Sternocleidomastoid — Trapezius
Deltoid — Pectoralis major
Serratus anterior
Biceps brachii
Brachialis
Brachioradialis — External oblique
Rectus abdominus
Tensor fasciae latae
Adductor longus — Gracilis
Sartorius — Rectus femoris
Vastus lateralis
Vastus medialis
Peroneus longus
Gastrocnemius — Tibialis anterior
Soleus — Extensor digitorum longus

Figure 48 (a) — Anterior View of Superficial Skeletal Muscles

B.   BASIC MUSCLE TYPES AND LOCATIONS

Almost half the body is muscle mass with the vast majority being skeletal muscle. Smooth muscle and cardiac muscle account for about 5-10% of body mass. The structure of various contractile cells and the molecular mechanisms responsible for muscle contraction have been discussed in the section IV. (Specialized eukaryotic cells and tissues, B. Contractile cells and tissues, pp. 57-79).

SKELETAL MUSCLES

Skeletal muscle fibers are about 10-80 microns in diameter and extend the entire length of a muscle. The multinucleated cells of skeletal muscles are striated. Individual skeletal muscles are separated from each other by a surrounding fascia which can also extend beyond the muscle to become part of a tendon. The tendon functions to connect the muscle to bone.

Some major skeletal muscles are described below:

Biceps brachii — this muscle in the upper arm has two heads (immovable origins) that originate on the scapula. The muscle follows the humerus and is connected to the radius by a tendon. Contraction causes the arm to bend at the elbow.

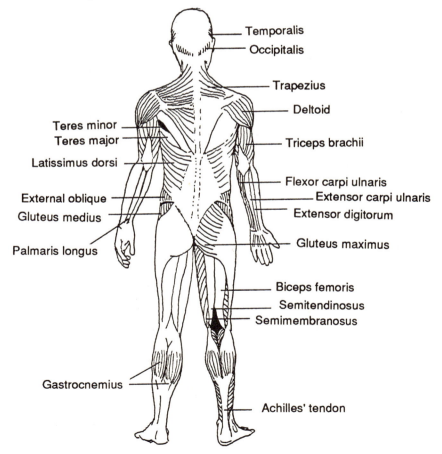

Figure 48 (b) — Posterior View of Superficial Skeletal Muscles

pectoralis major — this large muscle of the chest connects the humerus (in the upper arm) to the bones of the thorax.

deltoid — this triangular muscle is located on the shoulder and is active in all shoulder movements.

extensor digitorum — extensor muscles act to straighten body parts away from the main body. Extensor digitorum muscles extend either the fingers or toes.

sternomastoid — these muscles connect the sternum and mastoid.

Figure 48 shows many of the major skeletal muscles.

SMOOTH MUSCLES

Smooth muscles cells form fibers that are smaller (i.e., 2-5 microns in diameter and 50-200 microns in length) than skeletal fibers and they have only a single nucleus. Smooth muscles contract and relax more slowly than skeletal muscles.

Visceral and multiunit are the two major types of smooth muscles. Visceral smooth muscles are in contact with each other (at points called gap junctions). Stimulation of one portion of a smooth muscle causes the action potential to be conducted to the surrounding fibers. Visceral smooth muscles are found in the intestines, the bile ducts, the ureters, and the uterus. Visceral smooth muscles are responsible for the peristaltic movement of the intestinal tract.

In contrast, each multiunit smooth muscle fiber acts independently and is usually innervated by a single nerve which controls its contraction. Multiunit smooth muscles are found in the walls of blood vessels and in the iris of the eye.

CARDIAC MUSCLES

The primary function of cardiac muscles is the rhythmic pumping action of the heart. The ventricles provide the primary force for pumping blood through the lungs

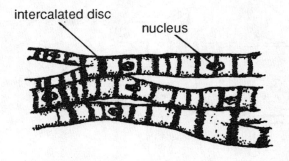

Figure 49 — The Intercalated Disc of Cardiac Muscle

and the peripheral circulatory system. Cardiac muscles exist only in the heart. Cardiac muscle cells are striated and have a single nucleus. Cardiac muscle fibers contain angular intercalated discs (see Figure 49) which are cell membranes that separate one cardiac muscle cell from the next. The three major muscle types present in the heart are: (1) ventricular muscle; (2) atrial muscle and; (3) specialized excitatory and conductive muscle fibers. The atrial and ventricular muscles contract in a manner similar to that of skeletal muscles but the specialized excitatory and conductive fibers contract only very weakly. These specialized muscles fibers do, however, provide a mechanism for the rapid transmission of excitatory impulses throughout the heart.

The intercalated discs of cardiac muscle fibers provide a very low resistance pathway for the rapid transmission of action potentials. Cardiac muscle is, therefore, a syncytium in which the action potentials rapidly propagate throughout the lattice of interconnected fibers. There are, in fact, two separate syncytium systems in the heart, i.e, the atrial syncytium and the ventricular syncytium. Although separated by fibrous tissue, an impulse can be conducted from the atrial to the ventricular syncytium via the A-V bundle.

C. NERVOUS CONTROL OF MUSCLES

MOTOR AND SENSORY CONTROL

Motor (or efferent) neurons carry nerve impulses out from the brain or spinal cord. Each skeletal muscle fiber is connected to a myelinated motor neuron at a region called the neuromuscular junction. The specialized region of the muscle fiber membrane that forms a junction with the axon of the motor neuron is called a motor end plate (see Figure 50)

A nerve impulse reaching the neuromuscular junction will cause the release of acetylcholine which, in turn, triggers the generation of action potential in the muscle fiber. The acetylcholine released into the synaptic cleft between an axon terminal and

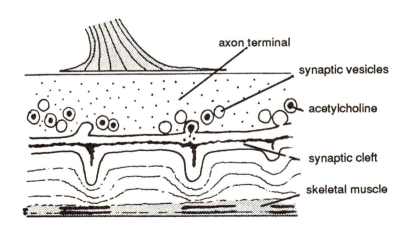

Figure 50 — The Motor End-Plate

the plasma membrane of the muscle fiber is rapidly destroyed by acetylcholinesterase.

THE MOTOR UNIT

Each motor neuron branches to form contacts with many muscle fibers. The neuron and the muscle fibers attached to it form a motor unit. When an impulse is transmitted through the motor neuron it will cause the simultaneous contraction of all muscle fibers to which it is attached. Very fine movements. require the number of connections a motor neuron makes with muscle fibers to be small (e.g., about 10).

THE REFLEX ARC

Motor neurons and sensory (or afferent) neurons usually occur in the same "mixed" nerve. The simplest manner in which sensory and motor neurons are integrated to evoke behavior is in a reflex arc (see Figure 51). For example, the knee-jerk response when striking the patella stimulates a stretch receptor neuron which sends an impulse to the spinal cord. Within the gray matter of the spinal cord the axon of the sensory neuron forms a synapse with a dendrite of an anterior motor neuron. The impulse travels via the anterior motor neuron to the quadriceps femoris muscle which responds by contracting and causing an extension of the leg.

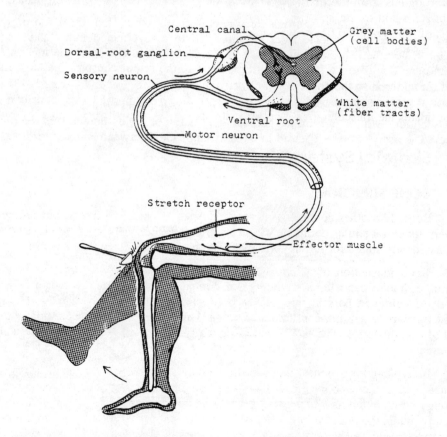

Figure 51 — A Simple Reflex Arc that Elicits a Knee-Jerk Response

Most of the sensory neurons that enter the spinal cord do not terminate on anterior neurons but rather on interneurons. Interneurons are more numerous (by a factor of about 30) than anterior motor neurons and they have numerous connections to each other and also to anterior motor neurons. These interconnections provide the basis for complex reflex responses such as the withdrawal reflex.

VOLUNTARY AND INVOLUNTARY CONTROL

Reflex behavior is unconscious and automatic but plays a critical role in homeostasis. Changes in vascular tone in response to hot or cold, sweating and some motor functions of the gut are all examples of autonomic reflexes that occur in the spinal cord.

The brain stem, which connects the cerebrum to the spinal cord, has numerous nerve pathways that help regulate the involuntary functions involved with equilibrium, respiration, cardiovascular function, eye movements, and support of the body against gravity.

"Voluntary" control of motor functions is primarily under the control of the frontal lobes of the cerebral cortex and the cerebellum of the brain. The cerebral cortex contains a "pyramidal area" that contains very large pyramid shaped cells. Motor signals from the brain originate in the pyramidal cells and travel through the brain stem and to the spinal column via the pyramidal or corticospinal nerve tract. Most of the pyramidal fibers terminate on interneurons in the cord gray matter. These interneurons, in turn, form synapses with motor neurons controlling various voluntary muscles.

In addition to the corticospinal tracts there are "extrapyramidal tracts" that also transmit motor signals from the brain. A specialized region of the frontal lobe that coordinates the muscular area involved with speech is called "Broca's area."

2. Skeletal System

A. BONE STRUCTURE

Bone, like other connective tissues, consists of cells and fibers, but unlike the others its extracellular components are calcified, making it a hard, unyielding substance ideally suited for its supportive and protective function in the skeleton.

Upon inspection of a long bone with the naked eye, two forms of bone are distinguishable: cancellous (spongy) and compact. Spongy bone consists of a network of hardened bars having spaces between them filled with marrow. Compact bone appears as a solid, continuous mass, in which spaces can be seen only with the aid of a microscope. The two forms of bone grade into one another without a sharp boundary.

In typical long bones, such as the femur or humerus, the shaft (diaphysis) consists of compact bone surrounding a large central marrow cavity composed of spongy bone. In adults, the marrow in the long bones is primarily of the yellow, fatty variety, while the marrow in the flat bones of the ribs and at the ends of long bones is primarily of the red variety and is active in the production of red blood cells. Even this red marrow contains about 70 percent fat.

The ends (epiphyses) of long bones consist mainly of spongy bone covered by a thin layer of compact bone. This region of the long bones contains a cartilaginous region known as an epiphyseal plate. The epiphyseal cartilage and the adjacent spongy bone constitute a growth zone, in which all growth in length of the bone occurs. The surfaces at the ends of long bones, where one bone articulates with another are covered by a layer of cartilage, called the articular cartilage. It is this cartilage which allows for easy movement of the bones over each other at a joint.

Compact bone is composed of structural units called Haversian systems. Each system is irregularly cylindrical and is composed of concentrically arranged layers of hard, inorganic matrix surrounding a microscopic central Haversian canal. Blood vessels and nerves pass through this canal, supplying and controlling the metabolism of the bone cells. The bone matrix itself is laid down by bone cells called osteoblasts. Osteoblasts produce a substance, osteoid, which is hardened by calcium, causing

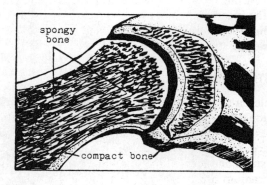

Figure 52 — Longitudinal section of the end of a long bone.

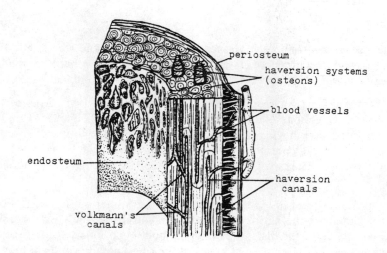

Figure 53 — Cross-section of a long bone showing internal structures

calcification. Some osteoblasts are trapped in the hardening osteoid and are converted into osteocytes which continue to live within the bone. These osteocytes lie in small cavities called lacunae, located along the interfaces between adjoining concentric layers of the hard matrix. Exchange of materials between the bone cells and the blood vessels in the Haversian canals is by way of radiating canals. Other canals, known as Volkmann's canals, penetrate and cross the layers of hard matrix, connecting the different Haversian canals to one another. (See Figure 52.)

With few exceptions, bones are invested by the periosteum, a layer of specialized connective tissue. The periosteum has the ability to form bone, and contributes to the healing of fractures. Periosteum is lacking on those ends of long bones surrounded by articular cartilage. The marrow cavity of the diaphysis and the cavities of spongy bone are lined by the endosteum, a thin cellular layer which also has the ability to form bone (osteogenic potencies).

Haversian type systems are present in most compact bone. However, certain compact flat bones of the skull, such as the frontal, parietal, occipital, and temporal bones, and part of the mandible, do not have Haversian systems. These bones, termed membrane bones, have a different architecture and are formed differently than bones with Haversian systems.

B.   SKELETAL STRUCTURE

The axial skeleton consists of the skull, vertebral column, ribs, and the sternum. The primary function of the vertebrate skull is the protection of the brain. The part of the skull that serves this function is the cranium. The rest of the skull is made up of the bones of the face. In all, the human skull is composed of twenty-eight bones, six of which are very small and located in the middle ear. At the time of birth, several of the bones of the cranium are not completely formed, leaving five membranous regions called fontanelles. These regions are somewhat flexible and can undergo changes in shape as necessary for safe passage of the infant through the birth canal.

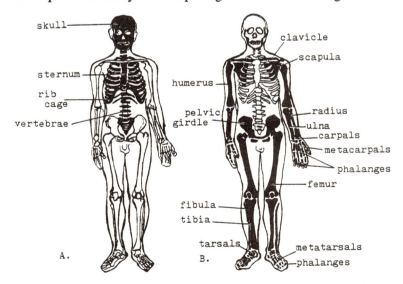

Figure 54 — Diagrams of human body showing, A, the bones of the axial skeleton and B, the bones of the appendicular skeleton.

The human vertebral column, or spine, is made up of 33 separate bones known as vertebrae, which differ in size and shape in different regions of the spine. In the neck region there are 7 cervical vertebrae; in the thorax there are 12 thoracic vertebrae; in the lower back region there are 5 lumbar vertebrae, in the sacral or hip region, 5 fused vertebrae form the sacrum to which the pelvic girdle is attached; and at the end of the vertebral column is the coccyx or tailbone, which consists of four, or possibly five, small fused vertebrae. The vertebrae forming the sacrum and coccyx are separate in childhood, with fusion occurring by adulthood. The coccyx is man's vestige of a tail.

A typical vertebra consists of a basal portion, the centrum, and a dorsal ring of bone, the neural arch, which surrounds and protects the delicate spinal cord which runs through it. Each vertebra has projections for the attachment of ribs or muscles or both, and for articulating (joining) with neighboring vertebrae. The first vertebra, the atlas, has rounded depressions on its upper surface into which fit two projections from the base of the skull. This articulation allows for up and down movements of the head. The second vertebra, called the axis, has a pointed projection which fits into the atlas. This type of articulation allows for the rotation of the head.

In man there are 12 pairs of ribs, one pair articulating with each of the thoracic vertebrae. These ribs support the chest wall and keep it from collapsing as the diaphragm contracts. Of the twelve pairs of ribs, the first seven are attached ventrally to the breastbone, the next three are attached indirectly by cartilage, and the last two, called "floating ribs", have no attachments to the breastbone.

The bones of the appendages and the girdles, which attach the appendages to the rest of the body, make up the appendicular skeleton. In the shoulder region the pectoral girdle, which is generally larger in males than in females, serves for the attachment of the forelimbs; in the hip region, the pelvic girdle serves for the attachment of the hindlimbs. The pelvic girdle, which is wider in females so as to allow room for fetal development, consists of three fused hipbones, called the ilium, ischium and pubis, which are attached to the sacrum. The pectoral girdle consists of two collarbones, or clavicles, and two shoulder blades, or scapulas. Articulating with

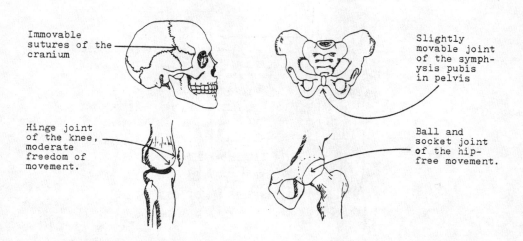

Immovable sutures of the cranium

Slightly movable joint of the symphysis pubis in pelvis

Hinge joint of the knee, moderate freedom of movement.

Ball and socket joint of the hip-free movement.

Figure 55 — Diagrams illustrating the types of joints found in the human body.

the scapula is the single bone of the upper arm, called the humerus. Articulating with the other end of the humerus are the two bones of the forearm called the radius, and the ulna. The radius and ulna permit the twisting movements of the forearm. The ulna has on its end next to the humerus a process often referred to as the "funny bone." The wrist is composed of eight small bones called the carpals. The arrangement of these bones permits the rotating movements of the wrist. The palm of the hand consists of 5 bones, known as the metacarpals, each of which articulates with a bone of the finger, called a phalanx. Each finger has three phalanges, with the exception of the thumb, which has two.

The pattern of bones in the leg and foot is similar to that in the arm and hand. The upper leg bone, called the femur, articulates with the pelvic girdle. The two lower leg bones are the tibia (shinbone) and fibula, corresponding to the radius and ulna of the arm, respectively. These two bones are responsible for rotation of the lower leg. Ventral to the joint between the upper and lower leg bones is another bone, the patella or knee cap, which serves as a point of muscle attachment for upper and lower leg muscles. This bone has no counter part in the arm. The ankle contains seven irregularly shaped bones, the tarsals, corresponding to the carpals of the wrist. The foot proper contains five metatarsals, corresponding to the metacarpals of the hand, and the bones in the toes are the phalanges, two in the big toe and three in each of the others.

The point of junction between two bones is called a joint. Some joints, such as those between the bones of the skull, are immovable and extremely strong, owing to an intricate intermeshing of the edges of the bones. The truly movable joints of the skeleton are those that give the skeleton its importance in the total effector mechanism of locomotion. Some are ball and socket joints, such as the joint where the femur joins the pelvis, or where the humerus joins the pectoral girdle. These joints allow free movement in several directions. Both the pelvis and the pectoral girdle contain rounded, concave depressions to accommodate the rounded convex heads of the femur and humerus, respectively. Hinge joints, such as that of the human knee, permit movement in one place only. The pivot joints at the wrists and ankles allow freedom of movement intermediate between that of the hinge and the ball and socket types. (Refer to Figure 55.)

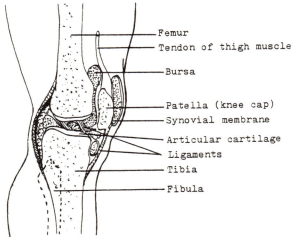

Figure 56 — The structure of a knee joint

The different bones of a joint are held together by connective tissue strands called ligaments. Skeletal muscles, attached to the bones by means of another type of connective tissue strand known as a tendon, produce their effects by bending the skeleton at the movable joints. The ends of each bone at a movable joint are covered with a layer of smooth cartilage. These bearing surfaces are completely enclosed in a liquid-tight capsule, called the bursa.

The joint cavity is filled with a liquid lubricant, called the synovial fluid, which is secreted by the membrane lining the (refer to Figure 56) cavity. During youth and early maturity the lubricant is replaced as needed, but in middle and old age the supply is often decreased, resulting in joint stiffness and difficulty of movement. A common disability known as bursitis is due to the inflammation of cells lining the bursa, and also results in restrained movement.

IX. Respiratory and Skin Systems

1. Respiratory System

A. FUNCTION

Oxygen and carbon dioxide are the important respiratory gases. While a small amount of oxygen is carried dissolved in the blood, most of the oxygen is carried by hemoglobin, an important protein found in red blood cells. Carbon dioxide (CO_2) is also dissolved in the blood and carried by hemoglobin, but most carbon dioxide is carried in the blood as bicarbonate ion (HCO_3).

There are chemoreceptors which are sensitive to changes in the chemical composition of the blood. Central chemoreceptors in the medulla oblongata are quite sensitive to levels of hydrogen ion (H^+) or CO_2. When H^+ or CO_2 increase, the receptors are excited and they in turn send signals to the breathing centers in the medulla oblongata, stimulating breathing. In addition, there are peripherally located chemoreceptors located in the aortic arch and carotid arteries. They too can stimulate the medullary breathing centers when there is an increase in H^+ ($\emptyset$ ph) or CO_2, as well as when there is a decrease in oxygen in the blood. The increase in breathing will function to increase the oxygen and/or decrease the carbon dioxide levels in the blood.

The lungs are the site of gas exchange in the pulmonary circulation. The alveoli or air sacs of the lungs are thin-walled, as are the pulmonary capillaries which supply them. Hence, the respiratory gases can easily diffuse through these walls. Gases diffuse from a region of high partial pressure to one of lower partial pressure. When one inhales, there is an increase in oxygen in the alveoli; when one exhales, there is a decrease in carbon dioxide in the alveoli. Since the blood entering the pulmonary capillaries has a low level of oxygen and a high level of carbon dioxide, oxygen will diffuse from the alveoli into the pulmonary capillaries and carbon dioxide will diffuse from the pulmonary capillaries into the alveoli. Hence the blood returning to the heart from the lungs will be replenished with oxygen, and the body tissues will be ridded of carbon dioxide, the major waste product of cellular metabolism.

B. BREATHING STRUCTURES AND MECHANISMS

The respiratory system in man and other air-breathing vertebrates includes the lungs and the tubes by which air reaches them. Normally, air enters the human respiratory system by way of the external nares or nostrils, but it may also enter by way of the mouth. The nostrils, which contain small hairs to filter incoming air, lead into the nasal cavities, which are separated from the mouth below by the palate. The nasal cavities contain the sense organs of smell, and are lined with mucus secreting epithelium which moistens the incoming air. Air passes from the nasal cavities via the internal nares into the pharynx, then through the glottis and into the larynx. The larynx is often called the "Adam's apple," and is more prominent in men than women. Stretched across the larynx are the vocal cords.

The opening to the larynx, called the glottis, is always open except in swallowing, when a flap-like structure (the epiglottis) covers it. Leading from the larynx to the chest region is a long cylindrical tube called the trachea, or windpipe. In a dissection, the trachea can be distinguished from the esophagus by its cartilaginous C-shaped rings which serve to hold the tracheal tube open. In the middle of the chest, the trachea bifurcates into bronchi which lead to the lungs. In the lungs, each bronchus branches, forming smaller and smaller tubes called bronchioles. The smaller bronchioles terminate in clusters of cup-shaped cavities, the air sacs. In the walls of the smaller bronchioles and the air sacs are the alveoli, which are moist structures supplied with a rich network of capillaries. Molecules of oxygen and carbon dioxide diffuse readily through the thin, moist walls of the alveoli. The total alveolar surface area across which gases may diffuse has been estimated to be greater than 100 square meters.

Each lung, as well as the cavity of the chest in which the lung rests, is covered by a thin sheet of smooth epithelium, the pleura. The pleura is kept moist, enabling the lungs to move without much friction during breathing. The pleura actually consists of two layers of membranes which are continuous with each other at the point at which the bronchus enters the lung, called the hilus (roof). Thus, the pleura is more correctly a sac than a single sheet covering the lungs.

The chest cavity is closed and has no communication with the outside. It is bounded by the chest wall, which contains the ribs on its top, sides and back, and the sternum anteriorly. The bottom of the chest wall is covered by a strong, dome-shaped sheet of skeletal muscle, the diaphragm. The diaphragm separates the chest region

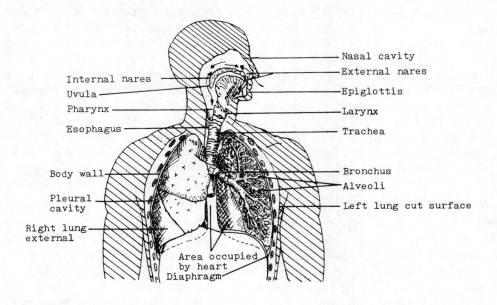

Figure 57 — Diagram of the human respiratory system

(thorax) from the abdominal region, and plays a crucial role in breathing by contracting and relaxing, changing the intrathoracic pressure.

2. Skin System

A. COMPOSITION

Human skin is composed of a comparatively thin outer layer, the epidermis, which is free of blood vessels, and an inner, thick layer, the dermis, which is packed with blood vessels and nerve endings. The epidermis is a stratified epithelium whose thickness varies in different parts of the body. It is thickest on the soles of the feet and the palms of the hands. The epidermis of the palms and fingers has numerous ridges, forming whorls and loops in very specific patterns. These unique fingerprints and palmprints are determined genetically, and result primarily from the orientation of the underlying fibers in the dermis. The outermost layers of the epidermis are composed of dead cells which are constantly being sloughed off and replaced by cells from beneath. As each cell is pushed outward by active cell division in the deeper layers of the epidermis, it is compressed into a flat (squamous), scalelike epithelial cell. Such cells synthesize large amounts of the fibrous protein keratin, which serves to toughen the epidermis and make it more durable.

Scattered at the juncture between the deeper layers of the epidermis and the dermis are melanocytes, cells that produce the pigment melanin. Melanin serves as a

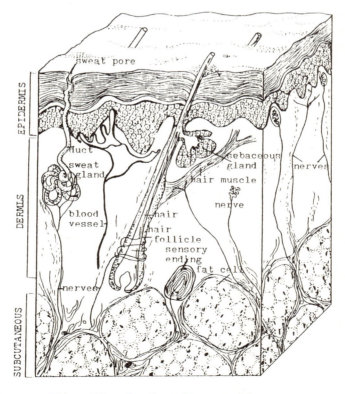

Figure 58 — Section of human skin

protective device for the body by absorbing ultraviolet rays from the sun. Tanning results from an increase in melanin production as a result of exposure to ultraviolet radiation. All humans have about the same number of melanocytes in their skin. The difference between light and dark races is under genetic control and is due to the fact that melanocytes of dark races produce more melanin.

The juncture of the dermis with the epidermis is uneven. The dermis throws projections called papillae into the epidermis. The dermis is much thicker than the epidermis, and is composed largely of connective tissue. The lower level of the dermis, called the subcutaneous layer, is connected with the underlying muscle and is composed of many fat cells and a more loosely woven network of fibers. This part of the dermis is one of the principle sites of body fat deposits, which help preserve body heat. The subcutaneous layer also determines the amount of possible skin movement.

The hair and nails are derivatives of skin, and develop from inpocketings of cells from the inner layer of the epidermis. Hair follicles are found throughout the entire dermal layer, except on the palms, soles, and a few other regions. Individual hairs are formed in the hair follicles, which have their roots deep within the dermis. At the bottom of each follicle, a papilla of connective tissue projects into the follicle. The epithelial cells above this papilla constitute the hair root and, by cell division form the shaft of the hair, which ultimately extends beyond the surface of the skin. The hair cells of the shaft secrete keratin, then die and form a compact mass that becomes the hair. Growth occurs at the bottom of the follicle only. Associated with each hair follicle is one or more sebaceous glands, the secretions of which make the surface of the skin and hair more pliable. Like the sweat glands, the sebaceous glands are derived from the embryonic epidermis but are located in the dermis. To each hair follicle is attached smooth muscle called arrector pili, which pulls the hair erect upon contraction.

B.   PROTECTION AND THERMOREGULATION

Perhaps the most vital function of the skin is to protect the body against a variety of external agents and to maintain a constant internal environment. The layers of the skin form a protective shield against blows, friction, and many injurious chemicals. These layers are essentially germproof, and as long as they are not broken, keep bacteria and other microorganisms from entering the body. The skin is water-repellent and therefore protects the body from excessive loss of moisture. In addition, the pigment in the outer layers protects the underlying layers from the ultraviolet rays of the sun.

In addition to its role in protection, the skin is involved in thermoregulation. Heat is constantly being produced by the metabolic processes of the body cells and distributed by the bloodstream. Heat may be lost from the body in expired breath, feces, and urine, but approximately 90 per cent of the total heat loss occurs through the skin. This is accomplished by changes in the blood supply to the capillaries in the skin. When the air temperature is high, the skin capillaries dilate, and the increased flow of blood results in increased heat loss. Due to the increased blood supply, the skin appears flushed. When the temperature is low, the arterioles of the skin are constricted, thereby decreasing the flow of blood through the skin and decreasing the rate of heat loss. Temperature-sensitive nerve endings in the skin reflexively control the arteriole diameters.

At high temperatures, the sweat glands are stimulated to secrete sweat. The evaporation of sweat from the surface of the skin lowers the body temperature by removing from the body the heat necessary to convert the liquid sweat into water vapor. In addition to their function in heat loss, the sweat glands also serve an excretory function. Five to ten per cent of all metabolic wastes are excreted by the sweat glands. Sweat contains similar substances as urine but is much more dilute.

X. Reproductive System and Development

1. Male and Female Gonads and Genitalia

The successful production of offspring in higher organisms is complex and reserved for mature, fully developed organisms. The organs related to the reproductive process are called genitalia. The specific organs responsible for producing the sex cells (i.e., sperm cells in males and ova in females) are called gonads; in females this organ is the ovary and in males this organ is the testis.

A. THE MALE REPRODUCTIVE SYSTEM

In males (see Figure 59) the reproductive organs include two testes as well as accessory internal organs (i.e., the epididymides, the ductus or vasa deferentia, the seminal vesicles, ejaculatory ducts, the prostate gland, the urethra, and the bulbourethral glands) and accessory external organs (i.e., the scrotum, penis). These accessory organs primarily serve to store and deliver the sperm (or spermatozoa) to the female genitalia. Various glands secrete fluids to aide in this process.

The testes respond to hormones secreted by the anterior pituitary gland (i.e., gonadotropins). The anterior pituitary, in turn, is stimulated by the hypothalamus (see section on the Endocrine system, page 72). The testes also secrete hormones such as testosterone. During puberty testosterone stimulates testicular growth as well as the growth of the accessory male reproductive organs. Testosterone also helps to maintain secondary masculine sex characteristics.

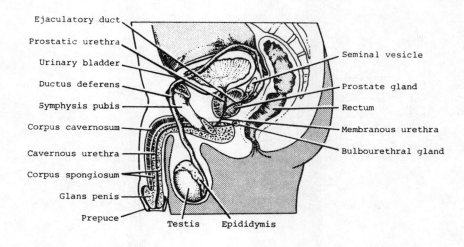

Figure 59 — The Male Reproductive System

B.   THE FEMALE REPRODUCTIVE SYSTEM

The female reproductive system produces, transports and temporarily stores ovum. Ovum are produced in the ovaries which are the primary reproductive organ. Furthermore, the female reproductive system is specialized to accept sperm, to aide in the process of fertilization, to provide a highly controlled environment for long term fetal development, and to deliver the new born from an intrauterine to an extrauterine environment. Hormones are also secreted by the ovaries. Figure 60 illustrates the basic structural features of the female reproductive system. The accessory internal organs of the female reproductive tract include the fallopian tubes and the vagina. The external female accessory organs include the labia majora, the labia minora, the clitoris and the vestibule.

2.   Gametogenesis by Meiosis

A.   SPERMATOGENESIS (SPERM PRODUCTION)

Spermatogenesis occurs in the coiled seminiferous tubules of the testes. The seminiferous tubules have supporting columnar epithelial cells called Sertoli cells as well as spermatogenic cells. The spermatogenic cells form sperm cells. Sperm cells taken directly from the testes are neither functional nor motile. The sperm in the testes pass through ducts into the epididymis where they become motile but still lack the ability to fertilize an ovum. To be fully functional the sperm must incubate in the tubal fluid of the female.

After passing through the epididymis, sperm moves through the vas deferens which is a long muscular tube that ascends to the ejaculatory duct. The ejaculatory duct empties into the urethra.

B.   OOGENESIS (PRODUCTION OF EGG CELLS OR OOCYTES)

The ovaries lie on each side of the pelvic cavity and each ovary has an exterior

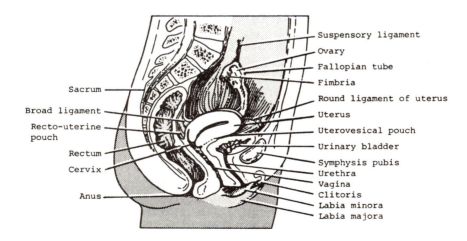

Figure 60 — The Female Reproductive System

monolayer of germinal epithelial cells that give rise to the ovum. At birth these germinal epithelial cells have already differentiated into millions of primordial follicles each of which contains an egg cell (or primary oocyte) and a surrounding single layer of follicle cells. At puberty some of the egg cells in the follicles undergo meiosis to form a secondary oocyte which contains a haploid number of chromosomes. Furthermore the primordial follicles undergo a maturation process at puberty: the oocytes enlarges and the follicular cells proliferate and form a cavity containing the oocyte and a follicular fluid. A mature follicle has an inner layer of granulosa cells and an outer layer of cells formed by ovarian stroma (the theca). The ovum is embedded in a mass of granulosa cells. During ovulation the oocyte is discharged from the mature follicle and then travels to the opening of the uterine tube. If fertilization of the egg cell does not take place the cell will die in a short period of time.

3. Reproductive Sequence

A. MALES

The reproductive sequence in males is: (a) psychic stimulation; (b) erection of the penis; (c) lubrication; (d) emission and ejaculation (orgasm). Erection is primarily a vascular event caused by dilation of arteries and constriction of veins in response to parasympathetic impulses from the sacral portion of the spinal column. The resulting high arterial blood pressure fills the erectile tissues of the penis. There are three cylindrical masses of erectile tissues (venous sinusoids) in the penis, i.e., two corpus cavernosum and one corpus spongiosum.

The parasympathetic impulses that promote erection also stimulate the secretion of a lubricating fluid from the bulbourethral gland. This fluid lubricates the end of the penis facilitating coitus (intercourse).

Emission is the movement of sperm cells (from the testes) and secretions (from the prostate and seminal vesicles) to the internal urethra to form seminal fluid. Emission is a reflex that occurs in response to sympathetic impulses from the spinal cord that results in peristaltic contractions of the smooth muscles of the epididymis, the vas deferens and the ampulla. Sympathetic impulses also trigger the contraction of smooth muscles in the prostate glands and the seminal vesicles which force the sperm down the urethra. Ejaculation is the expulsion of seminal fluid from the urethra by a reflexive contraction of the bulbocavernosus muscle (a skeletal muscle).

B. FEMALES

The reproductive sequence in females involves, in parts, a monthly (28 days is normal) sexual cycle that is under hormonal regulation. Follicle-stimulating hormone (FSH) and lutenizing hormone (LH) are secreted by the anterior pituitary at the beginning of the sexual cycle and these hormones stimulate the process of ovulation. Both FSH and LH bind to cellular receptors that, in turn, activate adenyl cyclase.

About 2 days before ovulation there is a marked increase in the secretion of LH which causes the mature follicle to rupture and release an oocyte which enters the uterine tube (at about day 14). Following ovulation, the follicular cells turn into the corpus luteum which releases increased amounts of estrogen and progesterone. The increased estrogen causes a thickening of the uterine endometrium in preparation for the potential implanting of a fertilized ovum. Similarly, progesterone causes an increased vascularization, swelling and secretory activity of the endometrium which is the innermost layer of tissue forming the uterine wall. Both estrogen and progesterone also inhibit the production of LH and FSH by the anterior pituitary gland. If fertilization does not occur, then the corpus luteum stops secreting estrogen and progesterone causing the disintegration of the uterine lining (i.e., menstrual flow). If fertilization does occur, then the placenta will secret chorionic gonadotropin which extends the life of the corpus luteum to the first 3-4 months of pregnancy.

Coitus in the female also evolves psychic stimulation, erection, lubrication, and orgasm. The clitoris (see Figure 60) contains two columns of erectile tissue called the corpus cavernosa that respond to parasympathetic impulses just as the penis does, i.e., the clitoris becomes erect. Concurrently, the Bartholin's glands located beneath the labia minor secrete a lubricating mucus.

4. Embryogenesis

A. EMBRYONIC DEVELOPMENT

Embryonic development begins when an ovum is fertilized by a sperm and ends at parturition (birth). It is a process of change and growth which transforms a single cell zygote, into a multicellular organism.

The earliest stage of embryonic development is the one-celled, diploid zygote which results from the fertilization of an ovum by a sperm. Next is a period called cleavage, in which mitotic division of the zygote results in the formation of daughter cells called blastomeres. At each succeeding division, the blastomeres become smaller and smaller. When 16 or so blastomeres have formed, the solid ball of cells is called a morula. As the morula divides further, a fluid-filled cavity is formed in the center of the sphere, converting the morula into a hollow ball of cells called a blastula. When cells of the blastula differentiate into two, and later three, embryonic

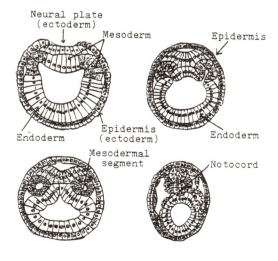

Figure 61 — Early Germ Layer Development

germ layers, the blastula is called a gastrula. The gastrular period generally extends until the early forms of all major structures (for example, the heart) are laid down. After this period, the developing organism is called a fetus. During the fetal period (the duration of which varies with different species), the various systems develop further. Though developmental changes in the fetal period are not so dramatic as those occurring during the earlier embryonic periods, they are extremely important.

Congenital defects may result from abnormal development during this period.

B. GERM LAYERS

Early forms of all major structure are laid down during the gastrula period. These forms, called primary germ layers begin to differentiate rapidly during the fetal stage. There are three primary germ layers: ectoderm, mesoderm and endoderm.

Ectoderm gives rise to the epidermis of the skin, including the skin glands, hair, nails, and enamel of teeth. In addition, the epithelial lining of the mouth, nasal cavity, sinuses, sense organs, and the anal canal are ectodermal in origin. Nervous tissue, including the brain, spinal cord, and nerves, are all derived from embryonic ectoderm. Mesoderm gives rise to muscle tissue, cartilage, bone, and the notochord, which in man is replaced in the embryo by vertebrae.

XI. Genetics and Evolution

1. Genetics

A. GENOTYPE AND PHENOTYPE

Genes are the units of heredity and are located on chromosomes. Genes occur in various forms, or alleles, the combinations of which code for the specific expression of traits. Each individual inherits one allele of each gene from his mother and one from his father. If an individual inherits two identical alleles of a gene, he is said to be homozygous for that trait. If the alleles are different, the individual is heterozygous for that trait.

The genotype is the actual genetic constitution of the individual, but the phenotype is the expression of the genotype. For instance, there are two alleles which determine eye color. Let B represent the dominant allele, dictating brown eyes, and b represent the recessive allele dictating blue eyes. From these two alleles, there are three possible genotypes coding for eye color: BB — homozygous dominant, Bb — heterozygous, and bb — homozygous recessive. There are only two phenotypes: BB and Bb, both coding for brown eye color since B is dominant over b. Blue eyes are possible only with the genotype bb. Note that green eyes are considered as blue, both genotypically and phenotypically. The phenotype includes not only physical characteristics apparent to an observer, but all characteristics that are the result of the genotype. For instance, one's blood type is part of one's phenotype.

B. DOMINANT/RECESSIVE INHERITANCE

There are many different types of genetic inheritance patterns. The simplest is that of dominant and recessive inheritance, as exemplified by the inheritance of eye color above. Suppose two people, heterozygous for brown eyes, have children. The best way to examine the probabilities of eye color in the offspring is to use a Punnett square, where the alleles of each parent form the axes of the square. The Punnett square below shows the cross between the two heterozygotes.

Bb× Bb

	B	b
B	BB	Bb
b	Bb	bb

Phenotypically, 75% of the offspring will have brown eyes (BB and Bb), and 25% (bb) will have blue eyes. The genotypes are 25% BB (homozygous dominant), 50% Bb (heterozygous), and 25% bb (homozygous recessive). The genotypic ratio is

1BB : 2Bb : 1bb.

The Punnett square below shows the cross between a blue-eyed woman and a heterozygous brown-eyed man.

bb × Bb

	b	b
B	Bb	Bb
b	bb	bb

The proportions of the offspring are 50% heterozygous (Bb) and thus brown eyed, and 50% homozygous recessive (bb), and thus blue-eyed.

C.   INCOMPLETE DOMINANCE

Some traits show incomplete dominance in which a dominant allele cannot fully mask the expression of the recessive allele. This is best exemplified in certain flowers, where color is inherited as such. Let R be the dominant allele for red flower color, and r be the recessive allele for white flower color. When a red flower (RR) is crossed with a white one (rr), the first generation will be 100% pink (Rr) as shown in the Punnett square below.

RR × rr

	R	R
r	Rr	Rr
r	Rr	Rr

If the allele for red color were fully dominant, the heterozygotes would all be red, not pink. While the result of this one cross may appear to be a blended trait, in future generations, the dominant and recessive allele can each be independently expressed again (i.e., the original traits will remerge); hence no blending has occurred. The subsequent cross between the pink flowers is shown below:

Rr × Rr

	R	r
R	RR	Rr
r	Rr	rr

The expected probabilities of phenotypic expression are 25% red (RR), 50% pink (Rr) and 25% white (rr).

D. CODOMINANCE

In codominance, a heterozygote has two dominant alleles which are equally expressed. Codominance is best exemplified by the inheritance of blood antigens. There are multiple alleles, IA, IB, and i, possible at the locus that codes for ABO blood type. Of course, any one individual inherits only two alleles. I^A and I^B are dominant to i, but are codominant with each other.

Type A blood is expressed by the genotypes I^AI^A and I^Ai. The person has only A antigens on his red blood cells. A phenotypically type B person has the genotype I^BI^B or I^Bi. This person has only B antigens on his red blood cells. The AB phenotype is expressed by the single genotype I^AI^B. These alleles are codominant and the person has both A *and* B antigens on his red blood cells. The homozygous recessive genotype ii is expressed phenotypically by Type O blood. This person has neither A nor B antigens on his red blood cells.

Punnett squares can be used here as well to determine blood type probabilities for offspring. Suppose a heterozygous type A man mates with a heterozygous type B female. The Punnett square below shows that there will be an equal probability (25%) of each blood type in the offspring.

$$I^Ai \times I^Bi$$

	I^A	i
I^B	I^AI^B	I^Bi
i	I^Ai	ii

There is a 25% probability of type AB(I^AI^B), type B(I^Bi), type A(I^Ai) and type O(ii)

E. SEX-LINKED INHERITANCE

Sex-linked inheritance is a little more complex. There are two sex chromosomes, called X and Y. A female has two X chromosomes, one inherited from each parent. A male has an X chromosome inherited from his mother, and a Y chromosome inherited from his father. The X chromosome is much larger than the Y chromosome and the X chromosome contains genes for color blindness and hemophilia on it, both of which are recessive traits.

When a male inherits an X chromosome with the recessive allele, he will fully express the trait (hemophilia or colorblindness), since his Y chromosome has no dominant allele to mask it. In contrast, when a female inherits an X chromosome with the recessive allele, she most likely will have the normal dominant allele on her other X chromosome, which will mask the recessive trait. Hence, she will merely carry the trait, but will not express it. In order for a female to be afflicted and express the trait, she must inherit two recessive alleles, one on each of her X chromosomes. That means that her father must express the trait, while her mother must either by a carrier or express the trait as well. The likelihood of a mate between two individuals each with this recessive sex-linked allele is low, unless there is mating between relatives.

Thus, the usual transmission of sex-linked traits is from a carrier mother to her son. The father cannot transmit the disease to his son since a male offspring has only one X chromosome which must have come from his mother. The carrier mother has an equal chance of passing the gene on to either a son or a daughter; however the trait is expressed more often in the son, who lacks the dominant allele to mask it. The daughter will not express the disease unless she has also acquired the recessive gene from an afflicted father.

If h represents the recessive allele for hemophilia, then a male can be represented on of two ways: an afflicted male will have the genotype X^hY, and a normal male will have the genotype X^HY. There are three possible genotypes for a female: a normal females is X^HX^H; a carrier female is X^HX^h, and an afflicted female is X^hX^h.

Suppose that C is the dominant allele for normal color vision and c is the allele for color blindness. A male is either normal (X^CY) or color blind (X^cY); a female is either normal (X^CX^C), a carrier (X^CX^c), or colorblind (X^cX^c). As in hemophilia, the carrier genotype in a female means simply that she can transmit the condition, although she does not express the trait.

A cross between a carrier mother and a normal father is shown below:

$$X^CX^c \times X^CY$$

	X^C	X^c
X^C	X^CX^C	X^CX^c
Y	X^CY	X^cY

Note that the offspring are 25% of each of the following: normal female, carrier female, normal male, and colorblind male.

The following cross shows how a female can become afflicted. A carrier women mates with an afflicted man.

$$X^CX^c \times X^cY$$

	X^C	X^c
X^c	X^CX^c	X^cX^c
Y	X^CY	X^cY

Hence the four possible outcomes, occurring with equal probability, are carrier female, colorblind female, normal male, colorblind male.

QUESTIONS

Let squares represent males; circles represent females; shaded are afflicted, white are not. The following questions refer to the pedigree shown in Figure 62.

PROBLEM

> All of the following statements concerning the disease in question are true EXCEPT
>
> a)   it is sex-linked.
>
> b)   it is caused by a recessive gene.
>
> c)   it may be hemophilia.
>
> d)   the afflicted boys must have received two alleles for this disease, since it is recessive.

Solution

   d).

PROBLEM

> If the disease were colorblindness, the genotype of P1 must be
>
> a) X^CX^c. | b) X^CX^C.
>
> c) X^cX^c. | d) X^CY.

Solution

   d).

PROBLEM

> If F_{2-5} were to marry a woman homozygous dominant for the trait in question, the probability that they would have a a child afflicted with the disease is
>
> a)   0%. | b)   25%.
>
> c)   50%. | d)   100%.

Solution

   a).

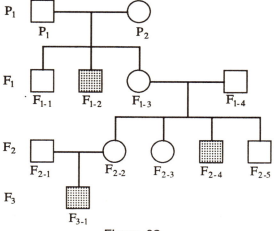

Figure 62

Different traits are characterized by certain patterns of inheritance. Which of the following are incorrectly paired?

a) Eye color — dominance/recessive inheritance

b) Red, pink, white color in plants — incomplete dominance

c) ABO blood typing — incomplete dominance

d) Hemophilia — sex-linked inheritance

Solution

c).

2. Evolution

A. DARWIN'S THEORY — NATURAL SELECTION

In the 1800s, two major theories of evolution were proposed. In 1800, Jean Baptiste Lamarck proposed a theory based on the inheritance of acquired characteristics. In other words, organs, and therefore animals, evolve through use. His classic example was his explanation for why the giraffe had such a long neck: he said that giraffes stretch their necks to reach the leaves high in trees. He assumed that an animal that stretched its neck could pass a stretched and hence lengthened neck on to its offspring,

Lamarck's theory was incorrect, since characteristics acquired in life cannot be passed on to the next generation, since the information is not in the genes. For instance, if a man develops his muscles by lifting weights, his offspring would not necessarily be muscular as well.

Charles Darwin proposed a theory of evolution, largely based on his observations made during the voyage of *the Beagle*. While traveling about the Galapagos Islands off the west coast of Ecuador, Darwin observed that each of the islands had similar birds, all finches. However, these finches were of different species. The most obvious anatomical distinction among the finches was the beak. Since structure often dictates function, Darwin realized that the differences in beak structure were an adaptation to the available food sources (i.e., insects, fruit, seeds) on the various islands. The finches all were of a common ancestor, and through many generations, differentiated into distinct species particularly suited to the environment of their island. While the phrase was not coined at that time, this is a classic example of adaptive radiation, which refers to the emergence of several species from one species due to the segregation of habitats.

According to Darwin's theory, a giraffe would have a long neck because those giraffes that by chance had the selective advantage (long necks) could eat food in the trees and hence survive and reproduce. The offspring, like the parent, would have long necks. Giraffes with short necks would be selected against, and thus not be able to survive to reproduce other short-necked giraffes.

The basic premise of Darwin's theory is that individuals have differing capacities to cope with their environment. Some individuals have characteristics which are advantageous in the environment and hence, those individuals will tend to survive and reproduce. The postulates of his theory came together in his book *On the Origin of Species by Means of Natural Selection* in 1859, and are recapitulated below.

All organisms overproduce gametes. Not all gametes form offspring and of the offspring formed, not all survive. Those organisms that are most competitive (in various different aspects) will have a greater likelihood of survival. These survival traits vary from individual to individual but are passed on to the next generation, and thus over time, the best adaptations for survival are maintained. The environment determines which traits will be selected for or against, but these traits may change in time. A selected trait at one time may later be disadvantageous.

Despite all of Darwin's insight, he never could explain the mechanism whereby traits were passed on. This was the key drawback to his theory. At about the same time, unbeknownst to Darwin, Gregor Mendel was experimenting with garden peas. Mendel was the first to introduce the concept of genes (heritable factors), although he did not use the term.

B.   EVIDENCE FOR EVOLUTION

Evidence for evolution comes from many scientific disciplines. Evidence from comparative biochemistry and molecular biology is based on the analysis of enzymes, proteins, nucleic acids, etc., to determine similarities in nucleotide sequences, and hence amino acid sequences. A similar molecular structure suggests a recent (by evolutionary standards) bifurcation of the original ancestral stock.

COMPARATIVE ANATOMY

Comparative anatomy distinguishes between homologous structures and analogous structures. Homologous structures are those structures that share an anatomical similarity due to a common evolutionary origin; this is exemplified by the basic bone structure in the forelimb of all vertebrates such as the flipper of a whale and the arm of a human. Analogous structures are those that subserve similar functions despite differences in their anatomy, and thus have no common ancestry. The wing of an insect and the wing of a bird exemplify analogous structures.

FOSSIL RECORD

The fossil record is an important clue to evolutionary origins. While fossils can actually be the preserved remnants of life (shells, skeletons), they also include imprints and molds, such as the imprint of an animal footprint. Fossil age can be estimated by the use of carbon dating. The ratio of radioactive carbon (^{14}C) to nonradioactive carbon (^{12}C) is determined. The half life of a radioactive element is the time span in which half the atoms in a sample will have decayed. The half life of ^{14}C (to decay to ^{12}C) is 5730 years. This spontaneous rate of decay is a constant.

C.   FACTORS RESPONSIBLE FOR EVOLUTIONARY CHANGE

There are four factors which bring about evolutionary change—mutation, gene flow, genetic drift and natural selection.

Genetic *mutations* are changes in the base sequence in DNA and hence genes, and as such are passed on to future generations. There are many different types of mutations. A point mutation is a substitution of a single nucleotide by another. This single base substitution changes the codon to another of the 64 possible codons. Because of the degeneracy of the genetic code and because of wobble at the third position of the codon, substitution may or may not change the amino acid encoded. If the codon does call for the incorporation of a different amino acid, there still may not be a deleterious effect, especially if an amino acid is replaced by one with similar chemical characteristics, such as replacing one nonpolar amino acid with another nonpolar one. However, if the base substitution calls for an amino acid with distinct chemical characteristics, such as a difference in the charge on the amino acid, it is more likely to be deleterious. The site of the mutation is also important. For instance if the new amino acid occurs at the functional site of a protein, such as the active site of an enzyme, this is more likely to adversely affect protein function.

Deletion or addition of a multiple of three bases results in the deletion or insertion of several amino acids, which may or may not affect protein function. Deletion or addition of one or two bases (or any other non-multiple of three) causes a reading-frame shift. All the codons beyond the mutation will be incorrectly read, and the wrong amino acids will be incorporated. Furthermore, an amino acid encoding codon may be converted to a stop codon, leading to a truncated version of the protein.

GENE FLOW

Gene flow refers to the change in allele frequency due to migration. Migration can be immigration (entrance) or emigration (exit) of individuals (and their genes) to or from a population.

GENETIC DRIFT

Genetic drift refers to a shift in allele frequency due to random fluctuation. This chance event is of special concern in small populations.

NATURAL SELECTION

Natural selection and differential reproduction are basically synonymous. This differential ability to survive and reproduce is the key factor in evolutionary change. Each individual of the population has a unique genotype (except identical twins, who have a common genotype) responsible for determining its phenotype. The environmental conditions at the time dictate which phenotypes are advantageous for survival. Those individuals with the phenotypes that can cope best in the environment will differentially reproduce and their genes will increase in frequency in the next generations.

D. HARDY-WEINBERG EQUILIBRIUM

The Hardy-Weinberg equilibrium refers to an artificial state in which the proportion of alleles at a given locus remain constant. The four factors required to maintain the equilibrium are: (1) no mutations, (2) isolation (and hence no migration and no gene flow), (3) large population size (and hence no genetic drift), and (4) equal viability and fertility of all genotypes, i.e., random reproduction (and hence no natural selection). In real populations, these factors are not usually all met and changes in allele frequency can occur.

The Hardy-Weinberg rule states that allele frequencies and genotype frequencies will be infinitely stable. For a trait which has only two alleles, p and q, the frequencies are expressed by the equation:

$p + q = 1$

where p is the frequency of one allele at the given locus and q is the frequency of the alternative allele. The sum of the frequencies must equal one.

Another mathematical equation holds true under a Hardy-Weinberg equilibrium:

$(p + q)^2 = p^2 + 2pq + q^2$

If p is the frequency of the dominant allele, then p^2 is the frequency of homozygous dominants in the population. If q is the frequency of the recessive allele, then q^2 is the frequency of homozygous recessives in the population. Thus $2pq$ is the frequency of heterozygotes in the population. Note also that

$p^2 + 2pq + q^2 = 1.$

Suppose a teacher does a statistical analysis of the eye color in students in a junior high school. The analysis shows that of the 1000 students, 910 have brown eyes, while only 90 have blue eyes (or green eyes). Five years later, the analysis is repeated, as the students in the first survey have graduated, and other teenagers are now in the junior high school.

The results now show that of the 1000 students, 840 have brown eyes and 160 have blue eyes. The table below summarizes the data:

Year	Brown eyes	Blue eyes	Total
1986	910	90	1000
1991	840	160	1000

In the original sample, 91% of the students have brown eyes and 9% have blue eyes. Since 9% (0.09) is equal to q^2, q must equal 0.3. Therefore p must equal 0.7 (i.e., $p = 1 - 0.3$). The 910 brown-eyed students consist of those that are homozygous and those that are heterozygous for the dominant allele. The homozygous dominant population represents 49% of the total population ($p^2 = 0.7^2$), while the heterozygous make up 42% of the total population ($2pq = 2 \times 0.7 \times 0.3$). Thus 490 students are homozygous dominant and 420 are heterozygous, giving a total of 910 brown-eyed students.

The data for 1991 is significantly different. The change in allele frequencies can be accounted for by migration (immigration and emigration). In this sample, blue eyes account for 16% of the population (160/1000). Thus $q^2 = 0.16$ and q equals 0.4. To verify this, note that p must equal 0.6 (i.e., $p = 1 - 0.4$). Thus, the homozygous dominant population would account for 36% ($p^2 = 0.6 \times 0.6$) or 360 students, and the heterozygous population would account for 48% ($2pq = 2 \times 0.6 \times 0.4$) or 480 students. Indeed, there are 840 (360 + 480) brown-eyed students in the 1991 population.

PROBLEM

Analysis of the protein insulin shows that there is only one amino acid difference between porcine and human insulin. The scientific discipline which would make these evolutionary conclusions is

a) comparative anatomy. b) the fossil record.

c) ^{14}C dating. d) molecular biology.

Solution

d).

PROBLEM

Gene flow is a factor which brings about evolutionary change due to

a) natural selection. b) migration.

c) chance events. d) point mutations.

Solution

b).

PROBLEM

An equation which correctly describes a Hardy-Weinberg equilibrium is

a) $p^2 + q^2 = 1$. b) $2p + 2pq + 2q = 1$.

c) $p^2 + 2pq^2 + q^1 = 1$. d) $p^2 + 2pq + q^2 = 1$.

Solution

d).

PROBLEM

If the dominant allele p has a frequency of 0.2, what is the percentage of heterozygous in a population under a Hardy-Weinberg equilibrium?

a) 16% b) 4%

c) 64% d) 32%

Solution

d).

XII. Biological Molecules

1. Amino Acids and Proteins

Amino acids, as the name implies, have properties of both amines and carboxylic acids. The general formula for an amino acid is

$$^+H_3N - CHR - COO^-,$$

where R can be any side chain. As can be seen from the structure, amino acids are *zwitterions*, meaning that they have both negative and positive charges at neutral pH. Under acidic conditions they will react as:

$$^+H_3N - CHR - COO^- + H_3O^+ \longrightarrow {}^+H_3N - CHR - COOH + H_2O.$$

Under basic conditions they will react by:

$$^+H_3N - CHR - COO^- + OH^- \longrightarrow {}^+H_2N - CHR - COO^- + H_2O.$$

The simplest amino acid, glycine, has a single hydrogen for its R group. Others, such as alanine and valine, have long aliphatic chains for their R group. Lysine, arginine, and histidine all have an additional amino group, and hence are basic. Serine and threonine have aliphatic hydroxyl side chains. Phenylalanine, tyrosine, and tryptophan have aromatic side chains. Aspartate and glutamate have an additional carboxylic acid group, and hence are acidic. Asparagine and glutamine have amide side chains. Cysteine and methionine contain sulfur in their side chain. Often, a one letter symbol is used to identify these amino acids. Amino acids that cannot be

Amino Acid	Three Letter Abbreviation	One Letter Symbol	Formula
Aliphatic Amino Acids			
Glycine	Gly	G	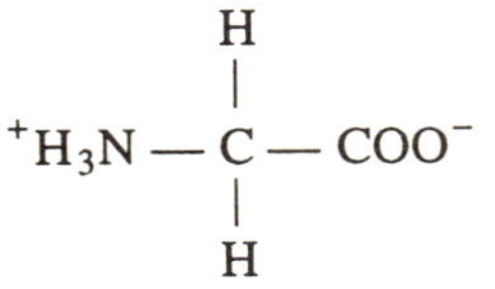 $^+H_3N - C - COO^-$ (H above, H below)
Alanine	Ala	A	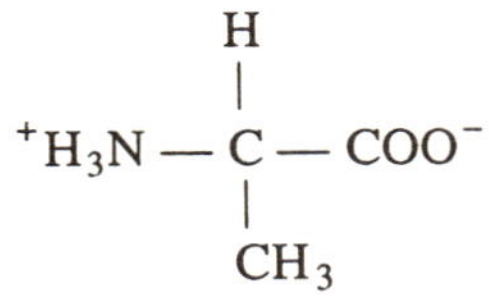 $^+H_3N - C - COO^-$ (H above, CH_3 below)
Valine*	Val	V	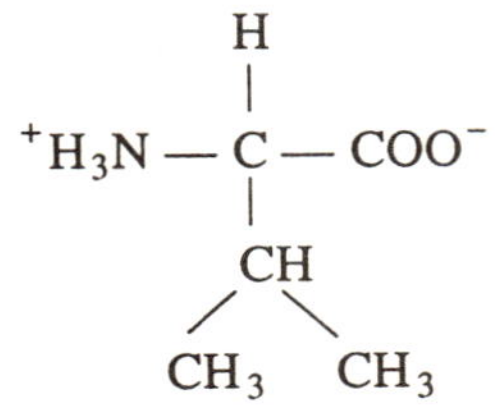 $^+H_3N - C - COO^-$ (H above, CH below with CH_3 and CH_3)

Amino Acid	Three Letter Abbreviation	One Letter Symbol	Formula

Leucine* — Leu — L

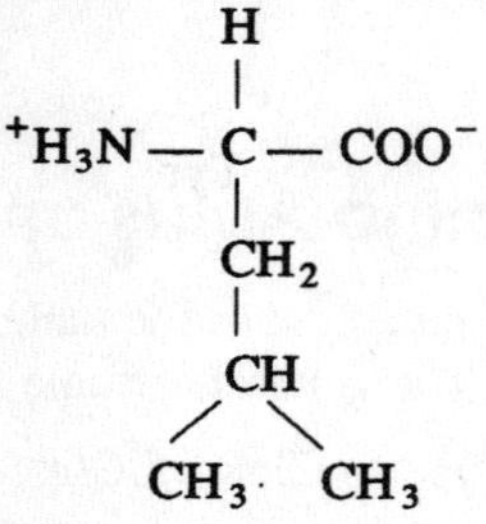

$$^+H_3N - \underset{\underset{\underset{\underset{CH_3 \quad CH_3}{\diagup \diagdown}}{CH}}{\overset{\overset{\overset{H}{|}}{|}}{C}}}{} - COO^-$$

Isoleucine* — Ile — I

$$^+H_3N - \underset{\underset{\underset{CH_3}{|}}{\underset{\underset{CH_2}{|}}{H - C - CH_3}}}{\overset{\overset{H}{|}}{C}} - COO^-$$

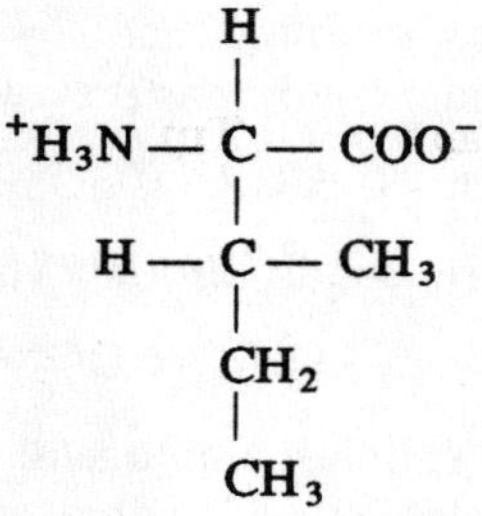

Aliphatic Hydroxyl Side Chains

Serine — Ser — S

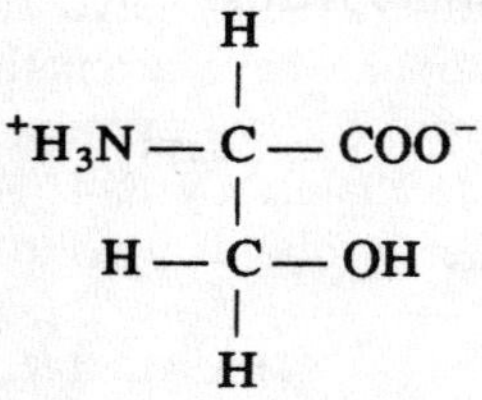

$$^+H_3N - \underset{\underset{\underset{H}{|}}{H - C - OH}}{\overset{\overset{H}{|}}{C}} - COO^-$$

Threonine* — Thr — T

$$^+H_3N - \underset{\underset{\underset{CH_3}{|}}{\underset{\underset{CH_2}{|}}{H - C - OH}}}{\overset{\overset{H}{|}}{C}} - COO^-$$

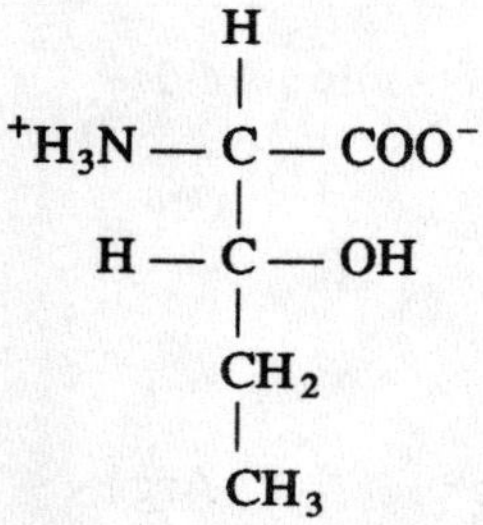

Aromatic Side Chains

Phenylalanine* — Phe — F

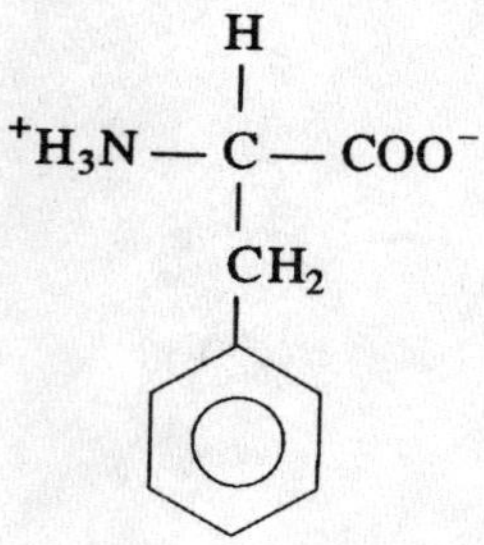

$$^+H_3N - \underset{\underset{CH_2}{|}}{\overset{\overset{H}{|}}{C}} - COO^-$$

Amino Acid	Three Letter Abbreviation	One Letter Symbol	Formula
Tyrosine	Tyr	Y	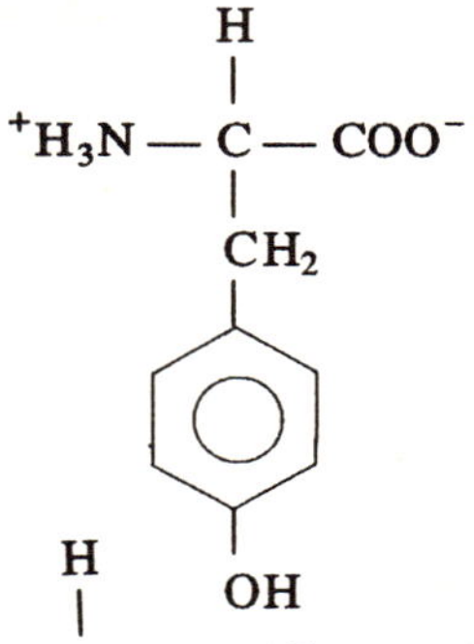 $^+H_3N-\overset{\displaystyle H}{\underset{\displaystyle CH_2}{C}}-COO^-$ with para-hydroxyphenyl ring (OH)
Tryptophan*	Trp	W	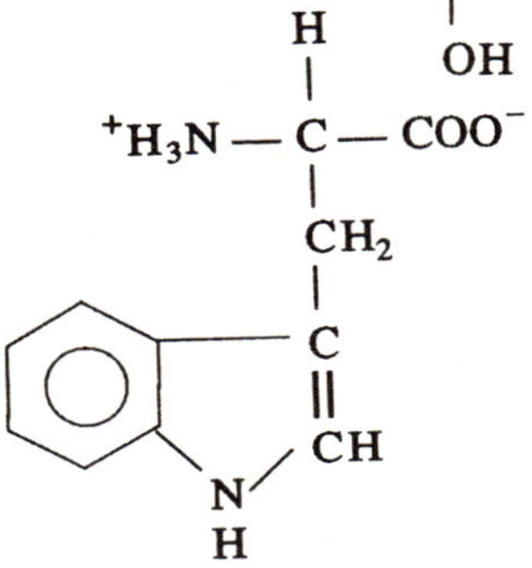 $^+H_3N-\overset{\displaystyle H}{\underset{\displaystyle CH_2}{C}}-COO^-$ with indole ring

Basic Amino Acids

Amino Acid	Three Letter Abbreviation	One Letter Symbol	Formula
Lysine*	Lys	K	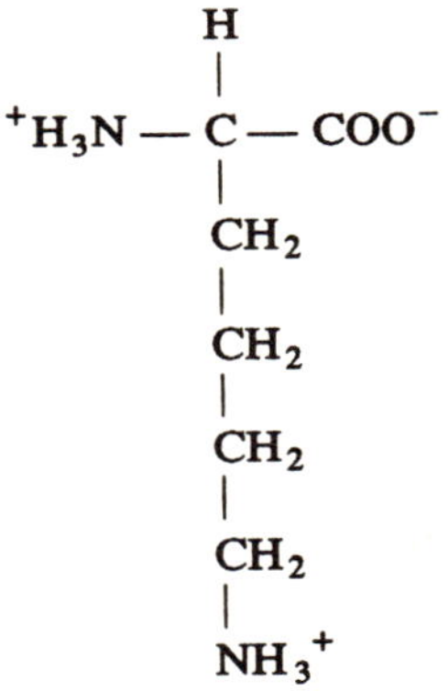 $^+H_3N-\overset{\displaystyle H}{C}-COO^-$, CH_2, CH_2, CH_2, CH_2, NH_3^+
Arginine*	Arg	R	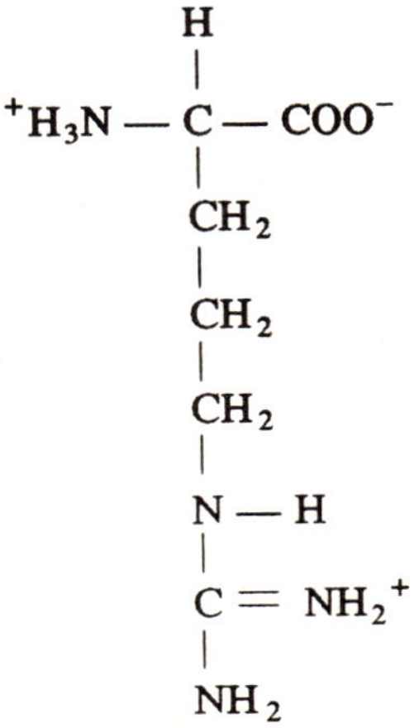 $^+H_3N-\overset{\displaystyle H}{C}-COO^-$, CH_2, CH_2, CH_2, $N-H$, $C=NH_2^+$, NH_2

Amino Acid	Three Letter Abbreviation	One Letter Symbol	Formula
Histadine*	His	H	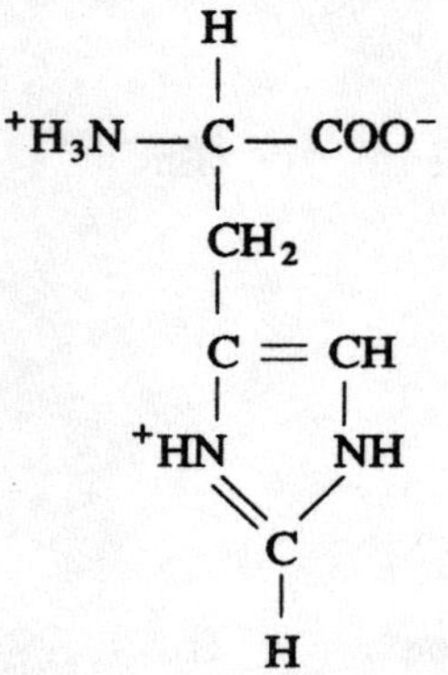
Acidic Amino Acids			
Aspartate (or Aspartic Acid)	Asp	D	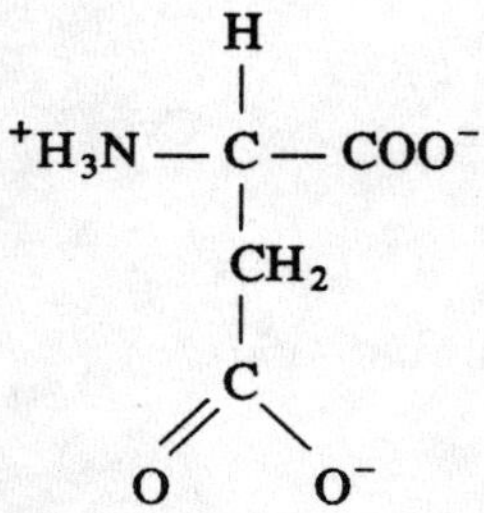
Glutamate (or glutamic acid)	Glu	E	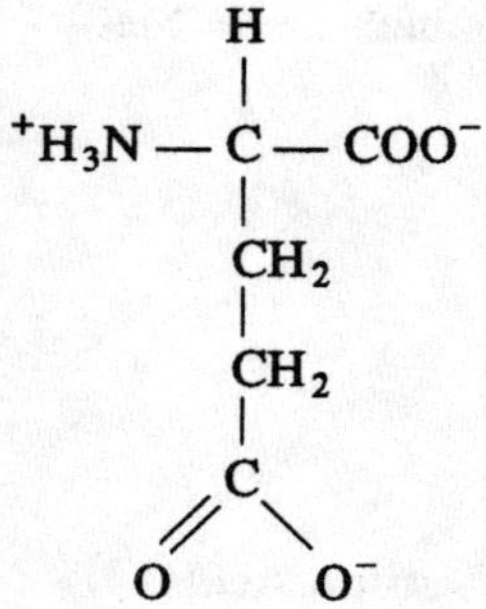
Amide Containing Amino Acids			
Asparagine	Asn	N	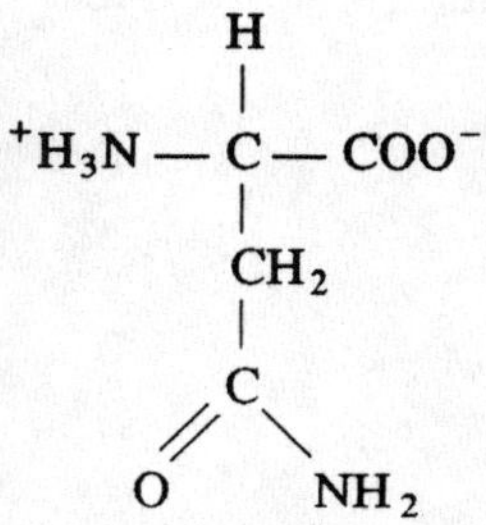

Histadine* His H

$$^+H_3N - \underset{\underset{\underset{\underset{C}{\overset{\displaystyle H}{|}}}{\underset{\underset{\displaystyle C = CH}{}}{}}}{\overset{\displaystyle H}{\underset{|}{C}}} - COO^-$$

Acidic Amino Acids

Aspartate (or Aspartic Acid) Asp D

Glutamate (or glutamic acid) Glu E

Amide Containing Amino Acids

Asparagine Asn N

Amino Acid	Three Letter Abbreviation	One Letter Symbol	Formula
Glutamine	Gln	Q	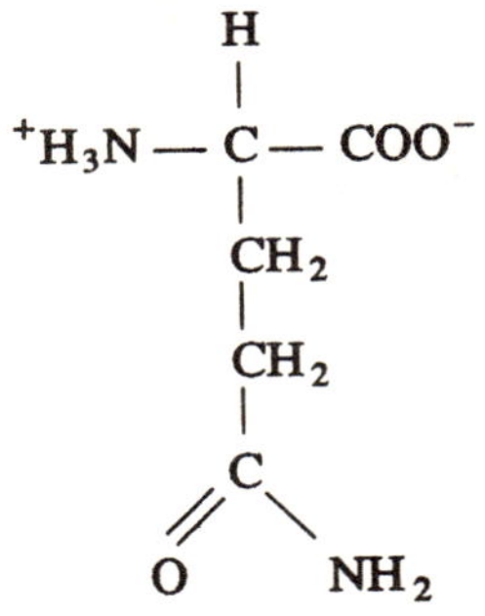 $^+H_3N - C - COO^-$ with H above, CH_2, CH_2, C double bonded to O and NH_2 below

Sulfur Containing Amino Acids

Cysteine	Cys	C	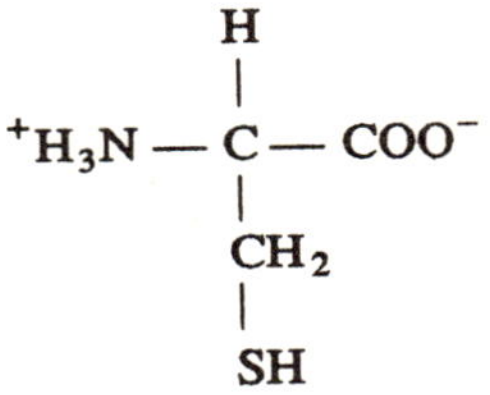 $^+H_3N - C - COO^-$ with H above, CH_2, SH below
Methionine*	Met	M	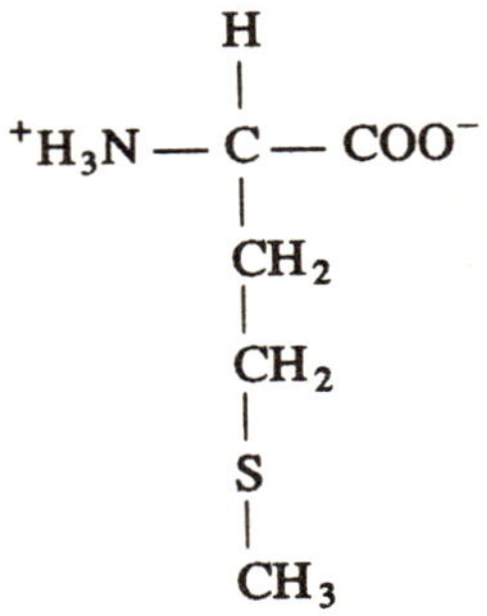 $^+H_3N - C - COO^-$ with H above, CH_2, CH_2, S, CH_3 below

Other Amino Acids

Proline	Pro	P	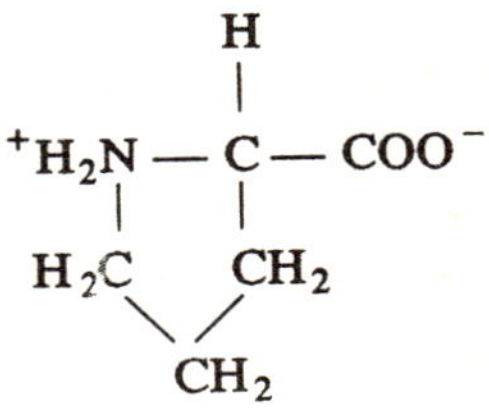 $^+H_2N - C - COO^-$ with H above, ring H_2C and CH_2 joined by CH_2

produced by the organism in question, and must be supplied by an external source, are called "essential amino acids." The table on pp. 127–131 lists the abbreviations, symbols, and R groups for amino acids. Those marked with an asterisk are essential acids for *homo sapiens*.

The primary method of linking amino acids together to form peptides is by a peptide bond. The amino end of one amino acid is attracted to the carboxylic acid end of another amino acid. This bonding results in a dipeptide and water, as can be seen:

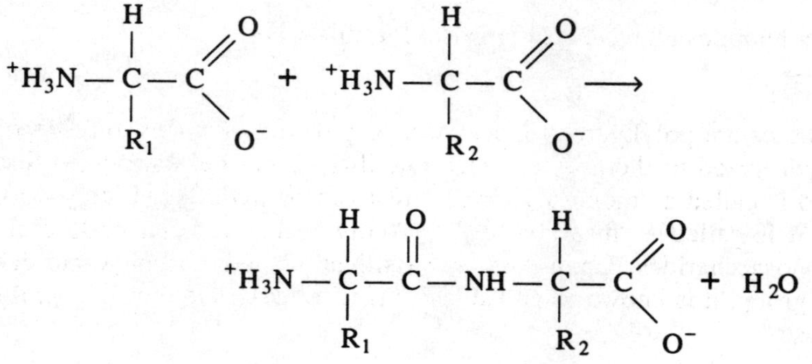

$$^+H_3N - \overset{\overset{\displaystyle H}{|}}{\underset{\underset{\displaystyle R_1}{|}}{C}} - \overset{\displaystyle O}{\underset{\underset{\displaystyle O^-}{}}{C}} \quad + \quad ^+H_3N - \overset{\overset{\displaystyle H}{|}}{\underset{\underset{\displaystyle R_2}{|}}{C}} - \overset{\displaystyle O}{\underset{\underset{\displaystyle O^-}{}}{C}} \longrightarrow$$

$$^+H_3N - \overset{\overset{\displaystyle H}{|}}{\underset{\underset{\displaystyle R_1}{|}}{C}} - \overset{\overset{\displaystyle O}{||}}{C} - NH - \overset{\overset{\displaystyle H}{|}}{\underset{\underset{\displaystyle R_2}{|}}{C}} - \overset{\displaystyle O}{\underset{\underset{\displaystyle O^-}{}}{C}} \quad + \quad H_2O$$

Breaking such a bond requires water; hence, it is known as hydrolysis. The sulfur containing amino acids can also bond with one another by sulfide bonds. This is important because an amino acid in one peptide chain can bond with an amino acid in another by sulfide bonds, as is illustrated below.

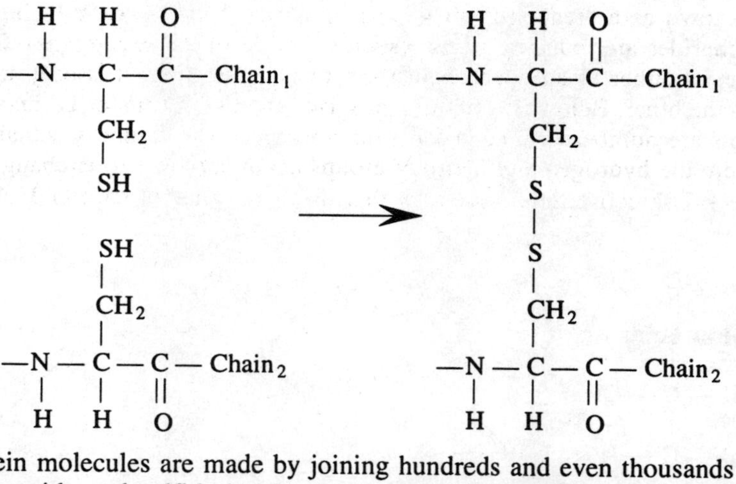

Protein molecules are made by joining hundreds and even thousands of amino acids by peptide and sulfide bonds. Each protein has a unique sequence of amino acids. This sequence of amino acids, along with the location of sulfide bonds, is known as the "primary structure" of the protein. The "second structure" refers to the steric relationship of amino acids that are close to one another in the linear sequence.

"Tertiary structure" refers to the steric relationships of amino acids that are far apart in the linear sequence. (Remember, proteins are not straight chains, but these chains are folded, making a three-dimensional structure.) The dividing line between secondary and tertiary structure is somewhat arbitrary.

"Quaternary structure" of a protein refers to the way the various peptide chains are packed together. Each chain is referred to as a "subunit." The "isoelectric point" is the pH at which there is no net electrical charge on a protein. This is a different value for various proteins. Proteins are important to living things, as they constitute the vast majority of an organism's structure (fibrous proteins) and enzymes involved in the metabolism (globular proteins).

2. Carbohydrates

Carbohydrates all have the empirical formula

CH_2O.

Carbohydrates are polyhydroxy aldehydes, polyhydroxy ketones, or compounds that can be hydrolyzed to them. A carbohydrate that cannot be hydrolyzed to a simpler compound is called a "monosaccharide." If it can be hydrolyzed into two monosaccharides, it is called a "disaccharide." A "polysaccharide" can be hydrolyzed into many monosaccharides. Upon further classification, if a carbohydrate contains an aldehyde group, it is known as an "aldose"; if it contains a ketone group, it is known as a "ketose."

Monosaccharides are also classified by the number of carbon atoms they contain. A triose, tetrose, and pentose carbohydrate would have three, four, and five carbon atoms, respectively. An aldopentose would be a five carbon monosaccharide with an aldehyde group. A ketohexose would be a six carbon monosaccharide containing a ketone group. A ketohexose would be a six carbon monosaccharide containing a ketone group. A carbohydrate that reduces Fehling's, Benedict's, or Tollen's reagent is known as a "reducing sugar." All monosaccharides are reducing sugars. Most disaccharides are reducing sugars (sucrose is one of the exceptions). Carbohydrates can exist either in an open chain form or a closed ring. It is easy to change from one to the other. Below is a figure that shows the two forms for D-glucose. The carbon atoms are numbered in each form for reference. The figure is actually α–D-glucose. Were the hydrogen and hydroxy groups about carbon 1 to exchange places, it would be β-D-glucose. Diastereomers that differ only about carbon 1 are called "anomers."

Among the aldoses, any diastereomers that differ only about the configuration of carbon 2 are called "epimers." Note that any carbohydrate can have an anomer, but only an aldose can have an epimer. Aldoses can be oxidized by Fehling's or Tollen's reagent, bromine water, nitric acid, and periodic acid. Ketoses can also be oxidized by Fehling's or Tollen's reagent, but not any of the other listed oxidants. The oxidation of aldoses are shown by bromine water and nitric acid in the figure below.

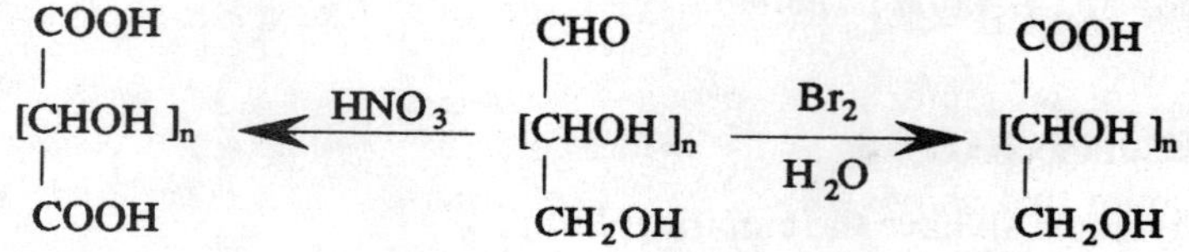

$$
\begin{array}{ccc}
\text{COOH} & \text{CHO} & \text{COOH} \\
| & | & | \\
[\text{CHOH}]_n \xleftarrow{\text{HNO}_3} & [\text{CHOH}]_n \xrightarrow[\text{H}_2\text{O}]{\text{Br}_2} & [\text{CHOH}]_n \\
| & | & | \\
\text{COOH} & \text{CH}_2\text{OH} & \text{CH}_2\text{OH} \\
\text{Aldaric Acid} & \text{Aldose} & \text{Aldonic Acid}
\end{array}
$$

A glycoside linkage connects monosaccharides to form di- or polysaccharides. The breakage of such a linkage is shown below, changing the disaccharide, maltose, to two glucose molecules. Note that since water is involved, it is a type of hydrolysis.

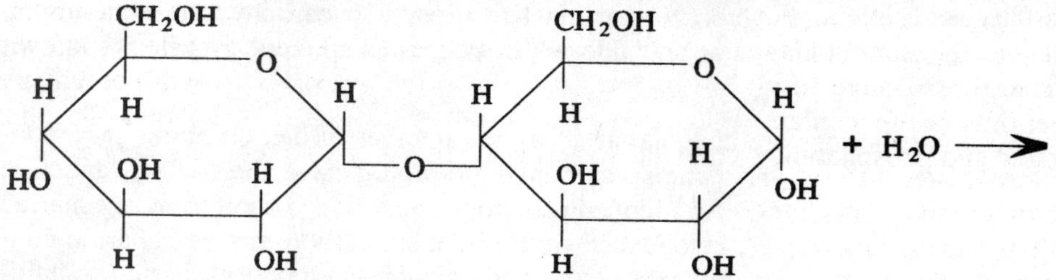

Maltose

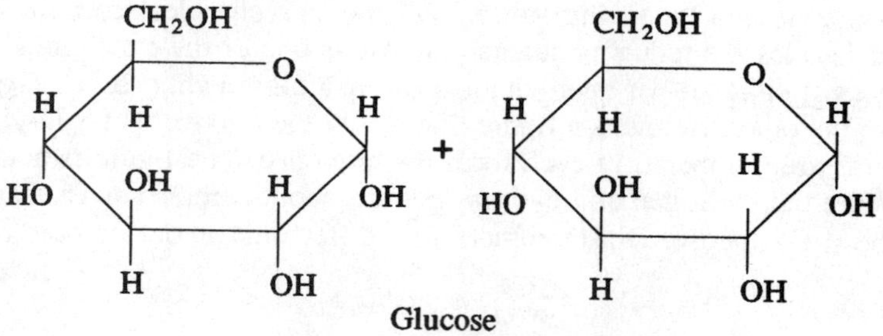

Glucose

3. Lipids

Chemically, fats are carboxylic esters derived from glycerol, and are known as glycerides. The general formula for a triglyceride is shown below, where R can be

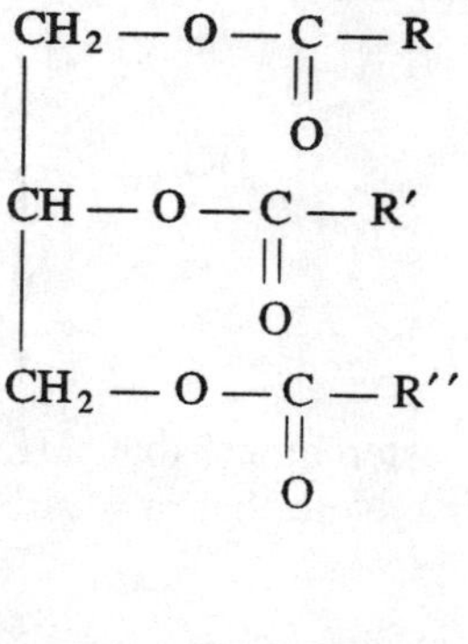

$$
\begin{array}{l}
\text{CH}_2 - \text{O} - \overset{\text{O}}{\underset{\|}{\text{C}}} - \text{R} \\
| \\
\text{CH} - \text{O} - \overset{\text{O}}{\underset{\|}{\text{C}}} - \text{R}' \\
| \\
\text{CH}_2 - \text{O} - \overset{\text{O}}{\underset{\|}{\text{C}}} - \text{R}''
\end{array}
$$

any fatty acid. Fatty acids are generally straight chained compounds from three to eighteen carbons long. As a rule, living organisms tend to produce fatty acids containing an even number of carbons. Were these fatty acids not associated with trigylcerols, they would be considered carboxylic acids. An example of a fatty acid would be linoleic acid,

$$CH_3(CH_2)_4CH=CHCH_2CH=CH(CH_2)_7COOH \text{ (cis, cis-isomer)}.$$

Cholesterol is a precursor to the five major classes of steroid hormones; progestagens, glucocorticoids, mineralocorticoids, androgens, and estrogens. Following is a diagram that shows cholesterol, and some of the steroids that are derived from it.

4. Phosphorus Compounds

The previous section mentions triglycerides with ester linkages to fatty acid chains. There are a group of compounds known as "phospholipids" where there are two fatty acids and a phosphate group attached to the triglycerides. These are important since phospholipids make up cell membranes, adenosine triphosphate is involved in energy exchange in all known life forms, and nucleic acids, which contain the blueprints of life, contain organic phosphates. Below is a figure that shows phosphoric acid and phosphatidic acid, a phosphoglyceride. R and R´ can be any fatty acid.

Phosphoric Acid   Phosphatidic Acid   Various phospate esters

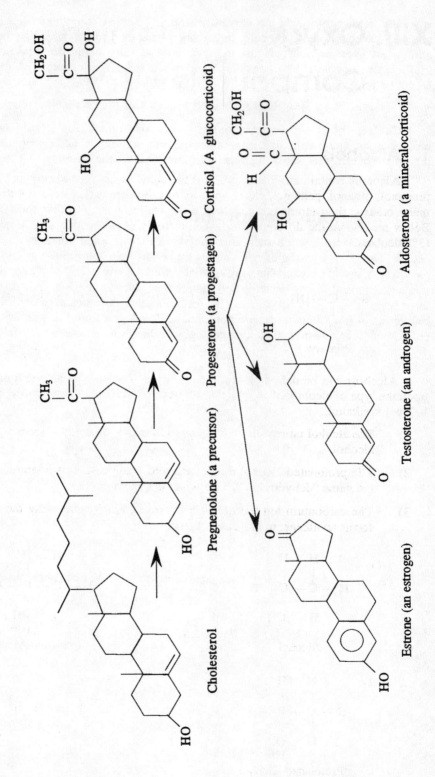

XIII. Oxygen Containing Compounds

1. Alcohols

Alcohols contain an -OH group, and the name of an alcohol ends in "-ol" (e.g., propanol, butanol, pentanol, etc.). An alcohol is further classified according to how many other carbon atoms are attached to the carbon atom that has the -OH group. Below are shown the differences between primary (1°), secondary (2°), and tertiary (3°) alcohols.

$$
\begin{array}{ccc}
\overset{\displaystyle H}{\underset{\displaystyle H}{R - C - OH}} & \overset{\displaystyle H}{\underset{\displaystyle R}{R - C - OH}} & \overset{\displaystyle R}{\underset{\displaystyle R}{R - C - OH}} \\
\text{Primary} & \text{Secondary} & \text{Tertiary}
\end{array}
$$

Alcohols can be dehydrated using hot acids. The ease of dehydration depends upon the type of alcohol: 3° > 2° > 1°. The steps of an alcohol dehydration are shown below for ethanol.

1) The alcohol unites with a hydrogen ion (from the acid) to form a protonated alcohol.

2) The protonated alcohol dissociates into water and a carbonium ion (hence the name "dehydration," since water is removed).

3) The carbonium ion then loses a hydrogen ion (regenerating the acid), and forms an alkene, in this case, ethene.

1)

$$
\underset{\text{Alcohol}}{H - \overset{H}{\underset{H}{C}} - \overset{H}{\underset{OH}{C}} - H} + \underset{\substack{\text{Hydrogen} \\ \text{ion}}}{H^+} \rightleftharpoons \underset{\text{Protonated Alcohol}}{H - \overset{H}{\underset{H}{C}} - \overset{H}{\underset{\substack{OH \\ H\oplus}}{C}} - H}
$$

2)

$$
\underset{\text{Protonated Alcohol}}{H - \overset{H}{\underset{H}{C}} - \overset{H}{\underset{\substack{OH \\ H\oplus}}{C}} - H} \rightleftharpoons \underset{\text{Carbonium ion}}{H - \overset{H}{\underset{H}{C}} - \overset{H}{\underset{\oplus}{C}} - H} + \underset{\text{Water}}{H \diagdown \underset{O}{} \diagup H}
$$

3)

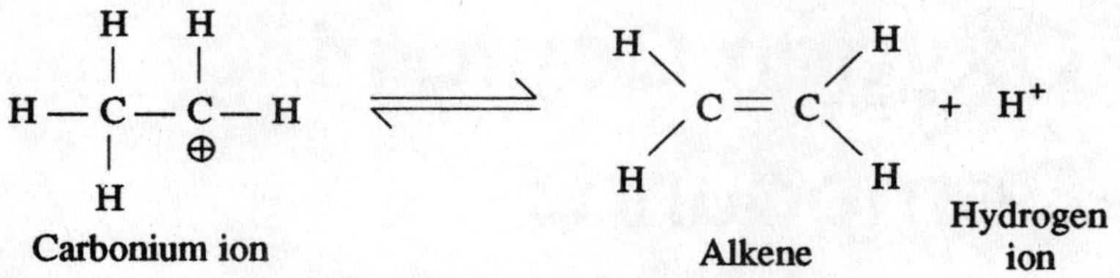

$$H-\overset{\overset{\displaystyle H}{|}}{C}-\overset{\overset{\displaystyle H}{|}}{\underset{\oplus}{C}}-H \quad \rightleftharpoons \quad \overset{H}{\underset{H}{>}}C=C\overset{H}{\underset{H}{<}} \quad + \quad H^+$$

Carbonium ion \qquad Alkene \qquad Hydrogen ion

Alcohols will also react with hydrogen halides to yield alkyl halides and water. The order of reactivity of alcohols toward hydrogen halides is $3° > 2° > 1° >$ methanol. All alcohols except methanol and most $1°$ alcohols will react by what is termed an "S_N1" (substitution-1) reaction, whereby the halide substitutes for the -OH group in its exact location, as is shown in the example below.

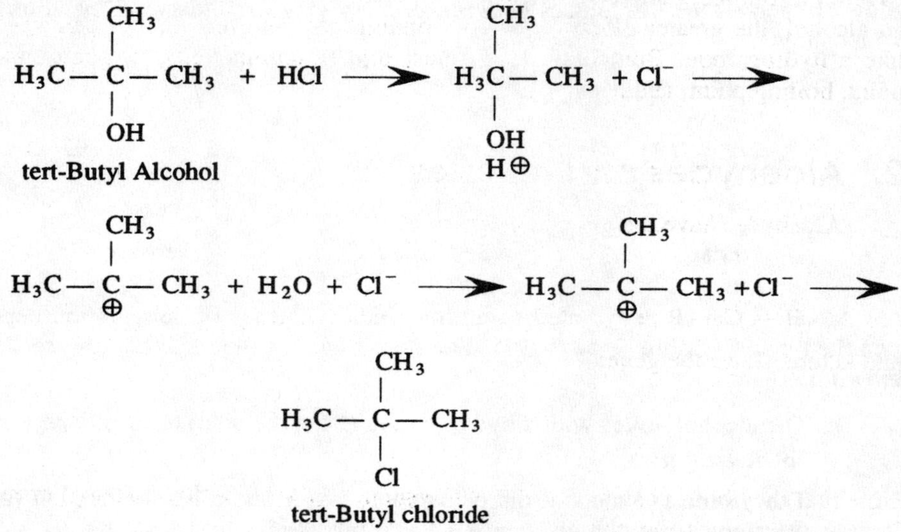

$$H_3C-\overset{\overset{\displaystyle CH_3}{|}}{\underset{\underset{\displaystyle OH}{|}}{C}}-CH_3 \quad + \quad HCl \quad \longrightarrow \quad H_3C-\overset{\overset{\displaystyle CH_3}{|}}{\underset{\underset{\displaystyle OH}{|}}{CH_3}} \quad + Cl^- \quad \longrightarrow$$

tert-Butyl Alcohol \qquad\qquad $H \oplus$

$$H_3C-\overset{\overset{\displaystyle CH_3}{|}}{\underset{\oplus}{C}}-CH_3 \quad + H_2O + Cl^- \quad \longrightarrow \quad H_3C-\overset{\overset{\displaystyle CH_3}{|}}{\underset{\oplus}{C}}-CH_3 \quad +Cl^- \quad \longrightarrow$$

$$H_3C-\overset{\overset{\displaystyle CH_3}{|}}{\underset{\underset{\displaystyle Cl}{|}}{C}}-CH_3$$

tert-Butyl chloride

Most $1°$ alcohols and methanol will react by what is known as an "S_N2" (substitution-2) mechanism. This yields an alkyl halide and water, but there is a rearrangement of the ions formed, and hence the halide is on a different carbon than the -OH group was. This is shown below.

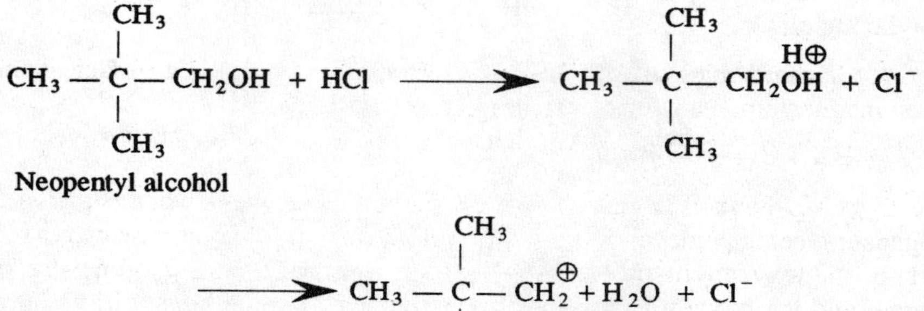

$$CH_3-\overset{\overset{\displaystyle CH_3}{|}}{\underset{\underset{\displaystyle CH_3}{|}}{C}}-CH_2OH \quad + HCl \quad \longrightarrow \quad CH_3-\overset{\overset{\displaystyle CH_3}{|}}{\underset{\underset{\displaystyle CH_3}{|}}{C}}-CH_2OH \quad \overset{H\oplus}{} + Cl^-$$

Neopentyl alcohol

$$\longrightarrow \quad CH_3-\overset{\overset{\displaystyle CH_3}{|}}{\underset{\underset{\displaystyle CH_3}{|}}{C}}-\overset{\oplus}{CH_2} +H_2O + Cl^-$$

$$CH_3 - \overset{\overset{\displaystyle CH_3}{|}}{\underset{\underset{\displaystyle CH_3}{|}}{C}} - \overset{\oplus}{CH_2} + Cl^- \longrightarrow CH_3 - \overset{\overset{\displaystyle CH_3}{|}}{\underset{\oplus}{C}} - CH_2 - CH_3 + Cl^-$$

$$\longrightarrow CH_3 - \overset{\overset{\displaystyle CH_3}{|}}{\underset{\underset{\displaystyle Cl}{|}}{C}} - CH_2 - CH_3$$

tert-pentyl chloride

Hydrogen bonding affects the physical properties of alcohols. This subject is covered in the inorganic chemistry section. Generally speaking, the more carbons in an alcohol, the greater effect hydrogen bonding has, and the alcohol behaves more like a hydrocarbon. Branching, as in most organic compounds, decreases melting point, boiling point, and density.

2. Aldehydes and Ketones

Aldehydes have the general formula

$$\overset{\overset{\displaystyle O}{||}}{H - C - R},$$

and ketones have the general formula

$$\overset{\overset{\displaystyle O}{||}}{R - C - R'}.$$

Note that they both possess the carbonyl group. $C = O$. It is this carbonyl group that largely determines the chemistry of these compounds, hence they are collectively known as "carbonyl compounds." The names of aldehydes end in "-al" (e.g., propanal, butanal, pentanal, etc.). The names of ketones end in "-one" (e.g., 3-pentanone, 3-methyl-2-butanone, propanone, etc.). These carbonyl compounds react typically by nucleophilic addition. Aldehydes will undergo nucleophilic addition even more readily than ketones, due to electronic and steric factors. One such example of this electrophilic addition is the Grignard synthesis of alcohols from carbonyl compounds.

A Grignard reagent is prepared by mixing an appropriate organic halide with metal magnesium, using dry ether as a solvent, such that

$$RX + Mg \longrightarrow RMgX.$$

The C – Mg bond is highly polar, the carbon being somewhat negative and the magnesium being somewhat positive. Due to differences in electronegativity between carbon and oxygen in the carbonyl group, the carbon has a somewhat positive charge, and the oxygen is somewhat negative. The two carbons will be attracted to one another, as will the magnesium and oxygen atoms, the result being the magnesium salt of an alcohol, which upon the addition of water, becomes the alcohol itself. The Grignard synthesis with formaldehyde (methanal) yields a 1° alcohol, higher

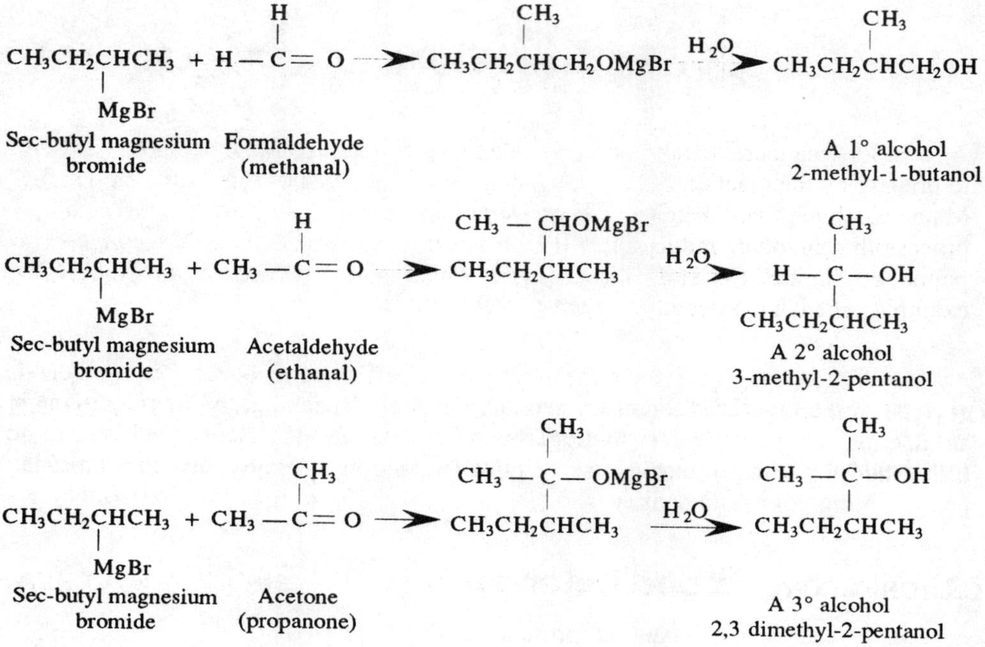

$$CH_3CH_2CHCH_3 + H-C=O \longrightarrow CH_3CH_2CHCH_2OMgBr \xrightarrow{H_2O} CH_3CH_2CHCH_2OH$$

(with H above the C=O; with MgBr below the first structure; with CH₃ above the reactant and product)

Sec-butyl magnesium Formaldehyde   A 1° alcohol
bromide   (methanal)   2-methyl-1-butanol

$$CH_3CH_2CHCH_3 + CH_3-C=O \longrightarrow CH_3CH_2CHCH_3 \xrightarrow{H_2O} H-C-OH$$

(with MgBr below first; with H above the C=O; product CH₃—CHOMgBr above and CH₃ above; final H—C—OH with CH₃ above and CH₃CH₂CHCH₃ below)

Sec-butyl magnesium Acetaldehyde   A 2° alcohol
bromide   (ethanal)   3-methyl-2-pentanol

$$CH_3CH_2CHCH_3 + CH_3-C=O \longrightarrow CH_3CH_2CHCH_3 \xrightarrow{H_2O} CH_3CH_2CHCH_3$$

(with CH₃ above the C=O; MgBr below first; product CH₃—C—OMgBr with CH₃ above; final CH₃—C—OH with CH₃ above)

Sec-butyl magnesium Acetone   A 3° alcohol
bromide   (propanone)   2,3 dimethyl-2-pentanol

aldehydes yield secondary alcohols, and ketones yield 3° alcohols. These reactions are shown above.

Dry alcohols, in the presence of anhydrous acids, can add to the carbonyl group of aldehydes and yield an acetal. For example:

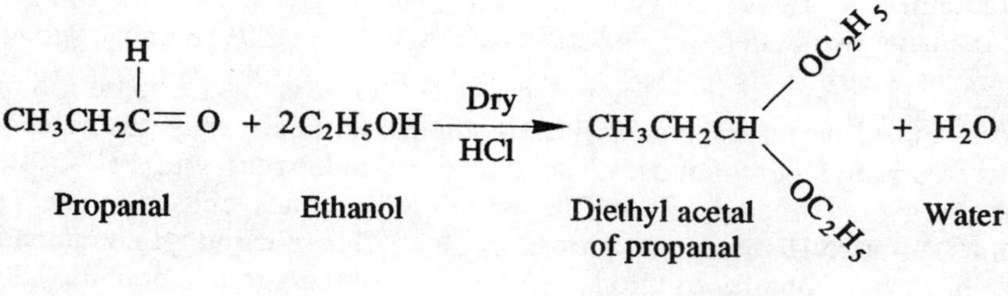

$$CH_3CH_2C=O + 2C_2H_5OH \xrightarrow[\text{HCl}]{\text{Dry}} CH_3CH_2CH\begin{smallmatrix}OC_2H_5\\OC_2H_5\end{smallmatrix} + H_2O$$

(with H above the C=O)

Propanal   Ethanol   Diethyl acetal   Water
                                                of propanal

In an alcoholic solution, there is strong evidence that an aldehyde exists in equilibrium with a compound known as a "hemiacetal." A hemiacetal is formed by the addition of the nucleophilic alcohol to the carbonyl group. Hemiacetals are usually too unstable to be isolated. Below shows such a reaction:

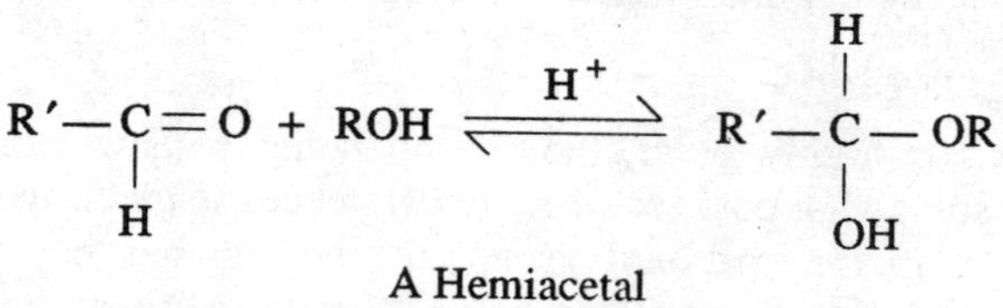

$$R'-C=O + ROH \underset{}{\overset{H^+}{\rightleftharpoons}} R'-C-OR$$

(with H below first C; with H above the product C and OH below)

A Hemiacetal

The basis of acetal chemistry is the "carbonium ion," whose resonating structure is as follows:

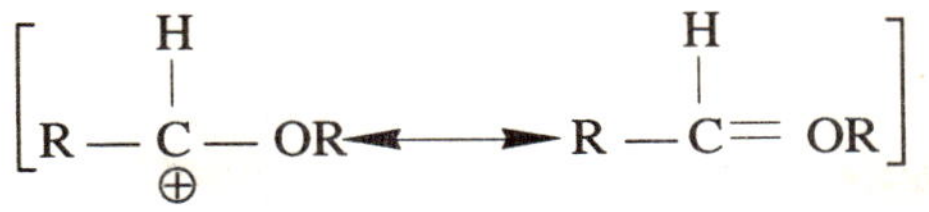

$$\left[R - \overset{\overset{\text{H}}{|}}{\underset{\oplus}{C}} - OR \longleftrightarrow R - \overset{\overset{\text{H}}{|}}{C} = OR \right]$$

In like manner, "ketals" can be made using ketones. (Simple ketals are difficult to prepare by the reaction of ketones and alcohols.) The same is true of "hemiketals." Many aldehydes and ketones are converted to amines by reductive amination, a process that involves reduction in the presence of ammonia. An intermediate compound, an "imine" (RCH=NH), is formed, which is then reduced to an amine. Two examples of such a procedure are shown here.

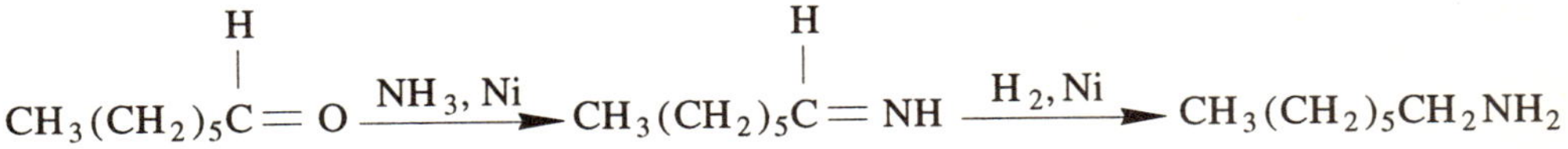

$$CH_3(CH_2)_5\overset{\overset{\text{H}}{|}}{C} = O \xrightarrow{NH_3,\ Ni} CH_3(CH_2)_5\overset{\overset{\text{H}}{|}}{C} = NH \xrightarrow{H_2,\ Ni} CH_3(CH_2)_5CH_2NH_2$$

| n-Heptanal | An Imine | 1-aminoheptane a1° Amine |

$$CH_3(CH_2)_2\overset{\overset{\text{O}}{||}}{C}CH_3 \xrightarrow{NH_3,\ Ni} CH_3(CH_2)_2\underset{\underset{\text{H}}{|}}{\overset{\overset{\text{N}}{||}}{C}}CH_3 \xrightarrow{H_2,\ Ni} CH_3(CH_2)_2\underset{\underset{\text{NH}_2}{|}}{CH}CH_3$$

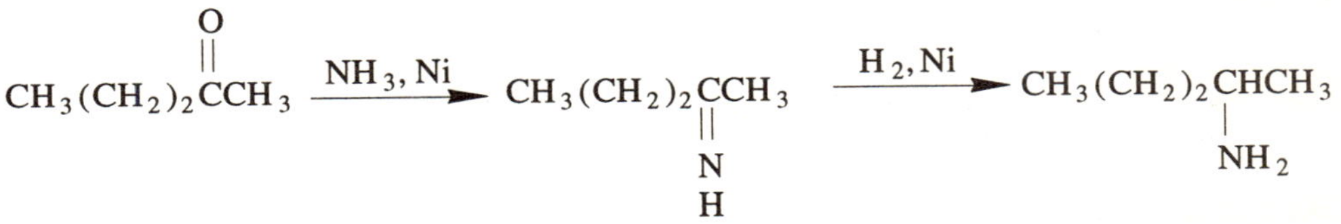

| 2-Pentanone | An Imine | 2-aminopentane a 2° Amine |

Imines can exist in tautomerization with "enamines." Compounds whose structures differ markedly in arrangement of atoms, but which exist in equilibrium, are called "tautomers." "Tautomerism" is the term that describes this equilibrium. An enamine contains two double-bonded carbons, single bonded to an amine group. An imine contains a carbon double-bonded to a nitrogen. An example of such tautomerism is shown below.

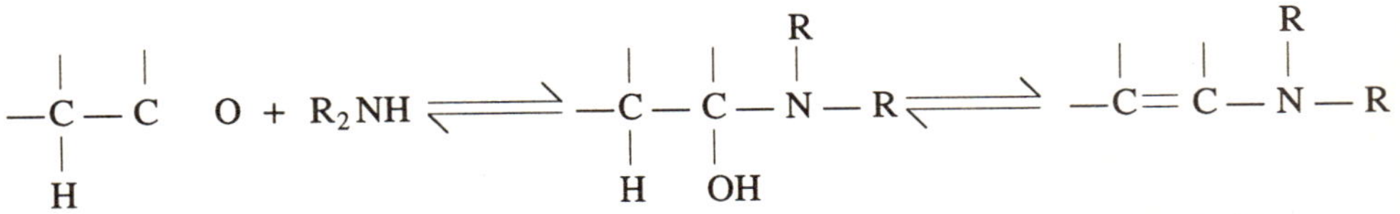

$$-\underset{\underset{\text{H}}{|}}{C} - \overset{|}{C}\ \ O + R_2NH \rightleftharpoons -\overset{|}{\underset{\underset{\text{H}}{|}}{C}} - \overset{\overset{|}{}}{\underset{\underset{\text{OH}}{|}}{C}} - \overset{\overset{\text{R}}{|}}{N} - R \rightleftharpoons -\overset{|}{C} = \overset{|}{C} - \overset{\overset{\text{R}}{|}}{N} - R$$

Two moles of an aldehyde or two moles of a ketone can combine with one another in the presence of a dilute base. This is known as an "aldol condensation," and the product, having the combined properties of a carbonyl (-al) and an alcohol (-ol), is called an "aldo." An aldo can react with a weak base to form a carbonyl compound that was larger than the starting material. A couple of examples follow.

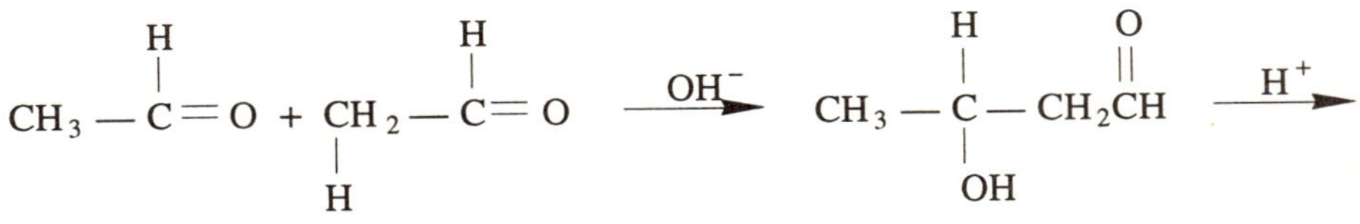

$$CH_3 - \overset{\overset{\text{H}}{|}}{C} = O + \overset{\overset{\text{H}}{|}}{\underset{\underset{\text{H}}{|}}{C}}H_2 - \overset{}{C} = O \xrightarrow{OH^-} CH_3 - \overset{\overset{\text{H}}{|}}{\underset{\underset{\text{OH}}{|}}{C}} - CH_2\overset{\overset{\text{O}}{||}}{C}H \xrightarrow{H^+}$$

| Ethanol (2 moles) | 3-Hydroxybutanal |

$$CH_3 - \overset{\overset{\displaystyle H}{|}}{C} = \overset{\overset{\displaystyle H}{|}}{C} - \overset{\overset{\displaystyle H}{|}}{C} = O \ + \ H_2O$$

2-Butenal

$$CH_3 - \overset{\overset{\displaystyle CH_3}{|}}{C} = O \ + \ CH_3 - \overset{\overset{\displaystyle CH_3}{|}}{C} = O \ \xrightarrow{OH^-} \ CH_3\underset{\underset{\displaystyle OH}{|}}{\overset{\overset{\displaystyle CH_3}{|}}{C}} - CH_2\underset{\underset{\displaystyle O}{||}}{C}CH_3 \ \xrightarrow{H^+}$$

Acetone (2 moles)
(propanone)

Diacetone alcohol

$$CH_3 - \underset{\underset{\displaystyle O}{||}}{\overset{\overset{\displaystyle CH_3}{|}}{C}} = CHCCH_3 \ + \ H_2O$$

4-Methyl-3-penten-2-one

An enol is a compound that contains two doubly bonded carbons (-ene), and an alcohol group (-ol). These will exist in tautomerism with ketones, with the ketone structure the most stable, and hence the most preferred. An example follows:

$$-\underset{\underset{\displaystyle H}{|}}{\overset{\overset{\displaystyle |}{}}{C}} - \overset{\overset{\displaystyle |}{}}{C} = O \ \rightleftharpoons \ -\overset{\overset{\displaystyle |}{}}{C} = \overset{\overset{\displaystyle |}{}}{C} - OH$$

Ketone   enol

Aldehydes will reduce Tollen's reagent. Methyl ketones are oxidized by hypohalite. An aldol condensation will not occur if an aldehyde or ketone lack an alpha hydrogen. This is a hydrogen on the carbon next to the carbonyl group. It is the acidity of this hydrogen that causes the reaction to proceed. These are chemical tests that can be used to identify the various types of carbonyl compounds present.

A compound that not only has a carbonyl group, but also a carbon-carbon double bond, has properties that are characteristic of both functional groups. In α, β-unsaturated (containing carbon-carbon multiple bonds) carbonyl compounds, the carbon-carbon double bond and the carbon-oxygen double bond are separated by just one carbon-carbon single bond.

$$\overset{\displaystyle \beta \quad \alpha}{-\overset{\overset{\displaystyle |}{}}{C} = \overset{\overset{\displaystyle |}{}}{C} - \overset{\overset{\displaystyle |}{}}{C} = O}$$

Because of this conjugation, these compounds have properties of both the double carbon-carbon bond and the carbonyl group, and some special properties as well. The presence of the carbonyl group lowers the reactivity of the carbon-carbon double bond toward electrophilic addition, and also controls the orientation of the addition.

3. Carboxylic Acids

Carboxylic acids possess both a carbonyl and a hydroxide group,

$$R - \overset{\displaystyle O}{\overset{\|}{C}} - OH .$$

It is the -OH group that undergoes change in nearly every reaction, but does so in a way that is only due to the effect of the C=O. These acids are named ending with "-oic acid" (e.g., methanoic acid, ethanoic acid, propanoic acid, etc.), common names also abound, such as formic acid, acetic acid, etc.

When an alcohol is mixed with a carboxylic acid, the result is an ester. The type of alcohol used determines the degree of the reaction, methanol being the most reactive; methanol $> 1° > 2° > 3°$. Below is such a reaction:

$$CH_3\overset{\displaystyle O}{\overset{\|}{C}} - OH + CH_3OH \longrightarrow CH_3\overset{\displaystyle O}{\overset{\|}{C}} - OCH_3$$

Lithium aluminum hydride can decarboxylate an acid to an alcohol. A typical reaction might be the conversion of pentanoic acid to pentanol:

$$CH_3(CH_2)_3COOH \xrightarrow{\ LiAlH_4\ } CH_3(CH_2)_3CH_2OH .$$

Hydrogen bonding, as would be expected, plays an important role in intermolecular forces in carboxylic acids. Intramolecular forces include the inductive effect of substituents on the acid chain. The inductive effect is an effect that is caused by a highly electronegative or electropositive group or atom located on the chain. This effect is felt throughout the whole molecule, although it does decrease with the distance from the group. Electron withdrawing groups (e.g., NO_2, halogens, etc.) increase the stability of the carboxylate ion, and hence strengthen the acid. Again the farther away this group is from the carboxylic acid functional group, the less effect it will have. An electron releasing group, such as an amine, will destablize the ion, and weaken the acid; again, the distance rule also comes into play. The carboxylate ion is further stabilized by resonance. It really has one and one-half bonds from the carbon to each oxygen:

$$\left[R - \overset{\displaystyle O}{\underset{\displaystyle O^-}{C}} \longleftrightarrow R - \overset{\displaystyle O^-}{\underset{\displaystyle O}{C}} \right]$$

4. Common Acid Derivatives

Fats, glycerides, and esters can be "saponificated," literally, made into soap, by using excess base of a known concentration. This is analogous to an acid-base titration. The amount of base needed to convert these materials into soap is known as the "saponification equivalent," and can be used to determine their equivalent weight. The saponification reaction of an ester and a base are shown below:

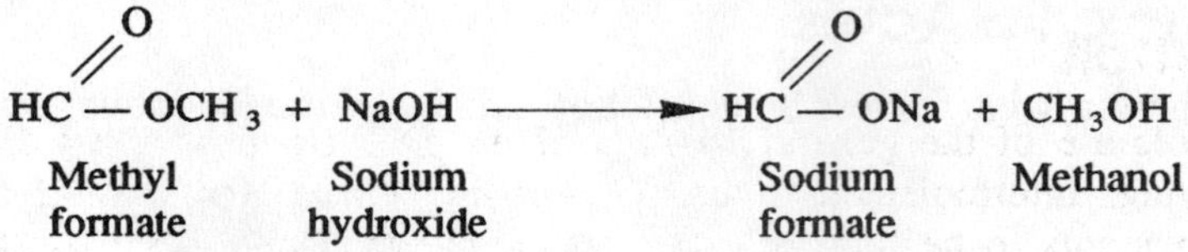

$$HC\overset{O}{\overset{\|}{-}}OCH_3 \ + \ NaOH \longrightarrow HC\overset{O}{\overset{\|}{-}}ONa \ + \ CH_3OH$$

Methyl	Sodium	Sodium	Methanol
formate	hydroxide	formate	

Amides have the general formula

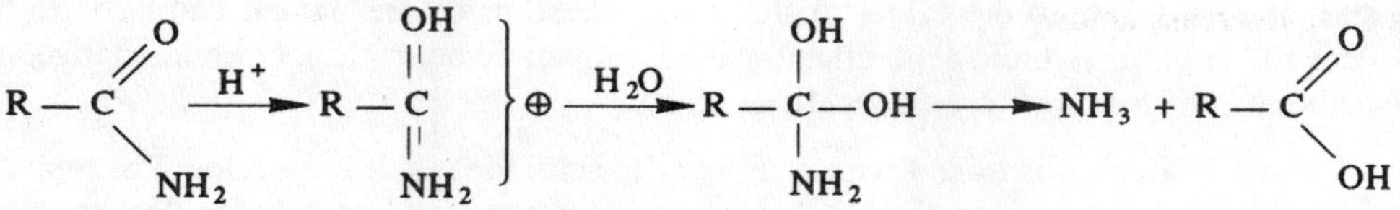

$$R-C\overset{O}{\underset{NH_2}{\diagup}} \xrightarrow{H^+} R\overset{OH}{\underset{\underset{NH_2}{|}}{-}C} \Biggr\} \oplus \xrightarrow{H_2O} R\overset{OH}{\underset{\underset{NH_2}{|}}{-}C}-OH \longrightarrow NH_3 + R-C\overset{O}{\underset{OH}{\diagup}}$$

and can be hydrolized to carboxylic acids. Under acid conditions, hydrolysis involves attack by the hydroxide ion on the amide itself:

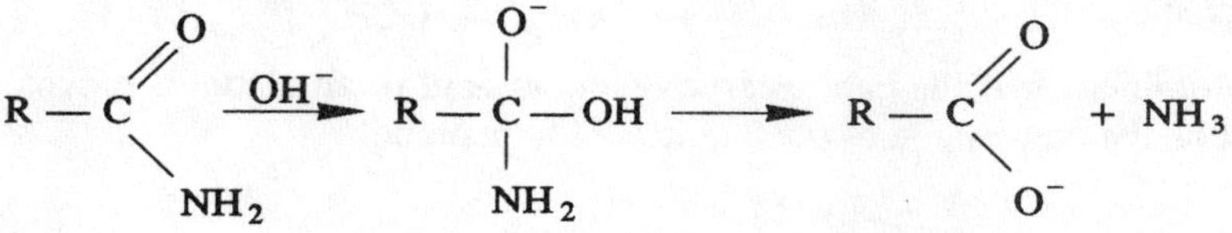

$$R-C\overset{O}{\underset{NH_2}{\diagup}} \xrightarrow{OH^-} R\overset{O^-}{\underset{\underset{NH_2}{|}}{-}C}-OH \longrightarrow R-C\overset{O}{\underset{O^-}{\diagup}} + NH_3$$

As a rule, carboxylic acid derivatives are more reactive toward nucleophilic substitution than are their non-carboxylic acid counterparts. In other words, for nucleophilic substitution, an acid chloride (R-COOCl) is more reactive than a comparable alkyl chloride (R-Cl), an amide (R-COONH$_2$) is more reactive than an amine (R-NH$_2$), and an ester (R-COOR′) is more reactive than an ether (R-OR′). Steric effects must also be taken into account for these reactions. These are the repulsive forces of the positive hydrogen nuclei on the carbons. Carbon atoms are free to swing about single bonds, and it is the repulsion of hydrogens from one carbon atom to another that keep them from getting too close.

5. Ethers

Ethers are of the general formula R-O-R′, and are named by the two groups attached to the oxygen, followed by the word "ether." (e.g., di-ethyl ether, methyl ethyl ether, butyl propyl ether, ect.) Ethers are generally very unreactive since the oxygen bond is quite stable. However, under extreme conditions (high temperatures and concentrations) ethers can be cleaved acids to yield alkyl halides and alcohols. HI is the most reactive acid used for this, followed by HBr, followed by HCl. Cleavage includes a nucleophilic attack by a halid ion on a protonated ether. (Since the ether accepts this proton, it is weakly basic.) The result is the displacement of the weakly basic alcohol molecule. This is shown below:

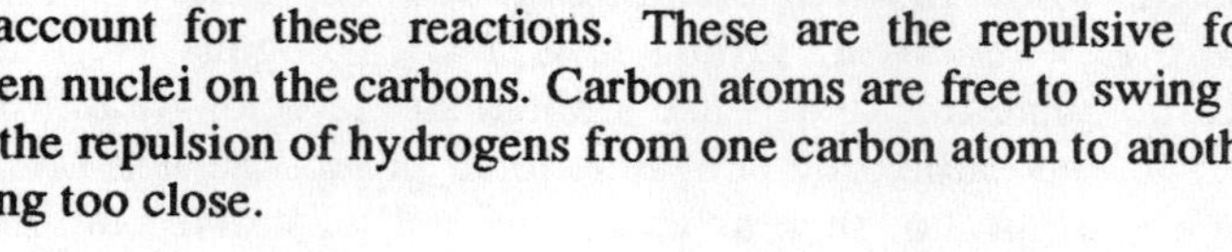

$$H_3-O-CH_3 + HI \rightleftharpoons CH_3-\underset{\underset{H\oplus}{|}}{O}-CH_3 + I^-$$

$$\xrightarrow{S_N1 \ or \ S_N2} CH_3I + CH_3OH$$

6. Phenols

Phenols are of the general formula of an -OH group attached directly to an aromatic ring. Intermolecular hydrogen bonding causes the boiling and melting points of phenols to be high. Phenols are much stronger acids than are alcohols, which is due to the influence of the aromatic ring. Electron attracting groups, such as halides, or NO_2, increase the acidity of phenols, while electron releasing groups, such as CH_3, decrease acidity.

XIV. Amines

An amine has the general formula

RNH_2, R_2NH, and R_3N,

for primary (1°), secondary (2°), and tertiary (3°) amines. Amines are quite basic, strong enough to turn litmus blue. Amines are named by naming the group to which they are attached, and adding the word "-amine" at the end. Stereoisomers of amines do exist, but the energy barrier between two possible arrangements about the nitrogen atom is so low that optical isomers are rapidly interconverted before they can be isolated. Primary and secondary amines can be converted to amides by reaction with acyl chlorides; tertiary amines will not react in this manner. This is shown below.

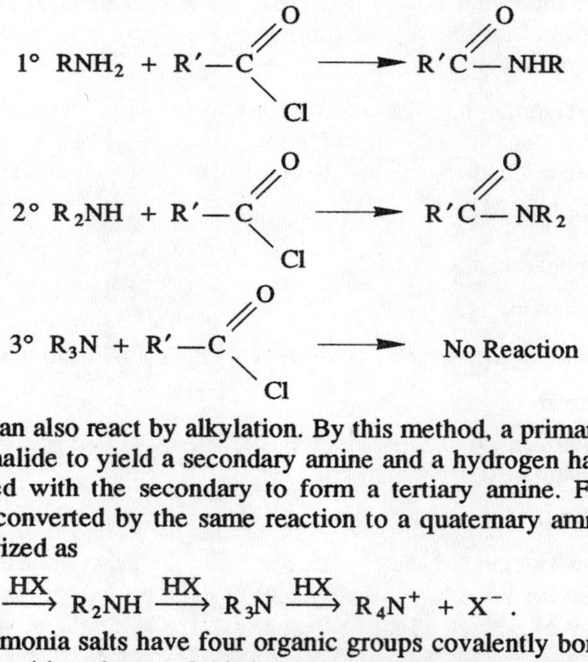

$$1° \quad RNH_2 + R'-C\overset{O}{\underset{Cl}{<}} \longrightarrow R'C\overset{O}{-}NHR$$

$$2° \quad R_2NH + R'-C\overset{O}{\underset{Cl}{<}} \longrightarrow R'C\overset{O}{-}NR_2$$

$$3° \quad R_3N + R'-C\overset{O}{\underset{Cl}{<}} \longrightarrow \text{No Reaction}$$

Amines can also react by alkylation. By this method, a primary amine can react with an alkyl halide to yield a secondary amine and a hydrogen halide. This process can be repeated with the secondary to form a tertiary amine. Finally the tertiary amine can be converted by the same reaction to a quaternary ammonium salt. This can be summarized as

$$RNH_2 \xrightarrow{HX} R_2NH \xrightarrow{HX} R_3N \xrightarrow{HX} R_4N^+ + X^-.$$

Quaternary ammonia salts have four organic groups covalently bonded to a nitrogen atom, and the positive charge of this ion is balanced by some negative ion. When the salt of a 1°, 2°, or 3° amine is treated with hydroxide ion, the nitrogen gives a hydrogen ion and the free amine is liberated. The quaternary ammonium ion has no proton to give up, and hence it is not affected by hydroxide ion. The quaternary ammonium salt does react with silver oxide to form a quarternary ammonium hydroxide and a precipitate of silver halide:

$$R_4N^+ + X + Ag_2O \longrightarrow P_4N^+OH^- + AgX.$$

Amines are more basic than water, and less basic than hydroxide ions. Aliphatic amines have k_b's that are from 10^{-3} to 10^{-4}, stronger than that of ammonia. Aromatic amines have lower k_b's, 10^{-9} or less, far lower than ammonia. Electron releasing groups on the aromatic rings, such as CH_3, stabilize the cation, and increase the basicity. Electron withdrawing groups. on the aromatic ring, such as COOH, halogens, etc. destabilize the cation, and decrease the basicity.

XV. Hydrocarbons

1. Saturated

Compounds made up only of hydrogen and carbon are appropriately called "hydrocarbons." If they contain all of the hydrogen atoms the carbons will allow (i.e., no double or triple bonds), they are referred to as "saturated." These saturated hydrocarbons are known properly as "alkanes." The alkanes are named according to the number of carbon atoms present. Methane has one carbon, ethane has two, propane has three, butane has four, and from there Greek roots are used (e.g., pentane for five, hexane, for six, heptane for seven, etc.). If the alkane is in a ring structure, rather than a chain, the name is prefixed with "cyclo-." The higher the molecular weight of an alkane, and the more branching and side chains, the higher the melting and boiling points are.

Alkanes are generally very unreactive; however, they can be combusted to carbon dioxide and water (this is covered in the inorganic section), and they can be halogenated by a free radical reaction. A free radical chain reaction consist of

1)   A chain initiating step,

2)   Chain propagating steps, and

3)   Chain terminating steps.

The overall reaction for the halogenation of alkanes can be shown as

$$RH + X_2 \longrightarrow RX + HX.$$

The ease of the halogenation decreases as the molecular weight of the halogen increases. In decreasing order of reactivity,

$$F > Cl > Br > I.$$

If ethane is mixed with chlorine gas, nothing will occur. However, if the mixture is heated, or light is shone upon it, the halogenation reaction will begin, and continue even after the source of heat or light has been removed. The light or heat is involved in the chain initiating step. In this instance it is the dissociation of a chlorine molecule into two chlorine radicals:

$$Cl_2 + light/heat \longrightarrow 2Cl\cdot.$$

The chlorine radicals can then react with the ethane to form hydrogen chloride and an ethane radical:

$$Cl\cdot + CH_3CH_3 \longrightarrow HCl + CH_3CH_2\cdot.$$

The ethane radical can react with a molecule of chlorine to produce chloroethane and a chlorine radical:

$$CH_3CH_2\cdot\ Cl_2 \longrightarrow CH_3CH_2Cl + Cl\cdot.$$

The last two reactions presented are chain propagation steps. So long as they continue, so does the chain reaction. Chain terminating steps halt the reaction. One such example is a chlorine radical reacting with an ethane radical. The result is still chloroethane, but no free radicals are generated to continue the reaction:

$$CH_3CH_2{}^{\cdot} + Cl^{\cdot} \longrightarrow CH_3CH_2Cl.$$

Other chain terminating reactions will not only stop the chain reaction, but will not produce any product. Such an example would be two chlorine radicals coming together to form a chlorine molecule. The chain is broken, but no product is formed:

$$Cl^{\cdot} + Cl^{\cdot} \longrightarrow Cl_2{}^{\cdot}.$$

Sometimes a chain terminating step will actually produce a contaminant. Such an example would be two ethane radicals coming together to produce a molecule of butane;

$$2CH_3CH_2{}^{\cdot} \longrightarrow CH_3CH_2CH_2CH_3.$$

Inhibitors can also absorb these radicals and terminate the chain reaction. An example of such would be oxygen. Were oxygen to get into the system, it would react with the ethane radical as shown:

$$CH_3CH_2{}^{\cdot} + O_2 \longrightarrow CH_3CH_2 - O - O^{\cdot}.$$

The radical formed can do very little to continue the chain reaction.

Small cyclic hydrocarbons undergo a great deal of bond strain. Cyclopropane has bond angles of 60°, and cyclobutane 90°. Both rapidly undergo ring opening reactions to relieve this strain. Cyclopentane has carbon bond angles of 108°, and hence is fairly stable. Ring structures over five carbons are quite stable, as the three-dimensional shape of the molecule allows the ring to pucker, and all carbon bonds are at the 109.5° angle of the tetrahedron bond.

2. Unsaturated

Alkenes possess a double carbon-carbon bond, and as a result possess two less hydrogens than their alkane counterparts. The general formula for an alkene is C_nH_{2n}, where n is the number of hydrogen bonds. Geometric isomers can exist for alkenes, due to their double bonds. If two identical functional groups are on the same side of the double-bond, the molecule is referred to as a "cis" isomer. If they are on different sides, it is a "trans" isomer. If there are more than two different groups around the double bond, a different system is used. The atoms on each carbon are ranked according to their atomic weight. If the two higher weight atoms are on the same side of the double bond, it is the Z isomer, and if they are on the opposite sides, it is the E isomer. The illustrations below give examples of how this nomenclature is used.

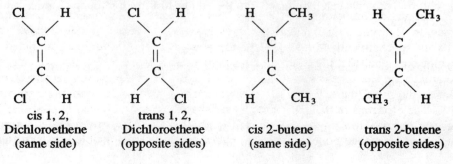

| cis 1, 2,
Dichloroethene
(same side) | trans 1, 2,
Dichloroethene
(opposite sides) | cis 2-butene
(same side) | trans 2-butene
(opposite sides) |

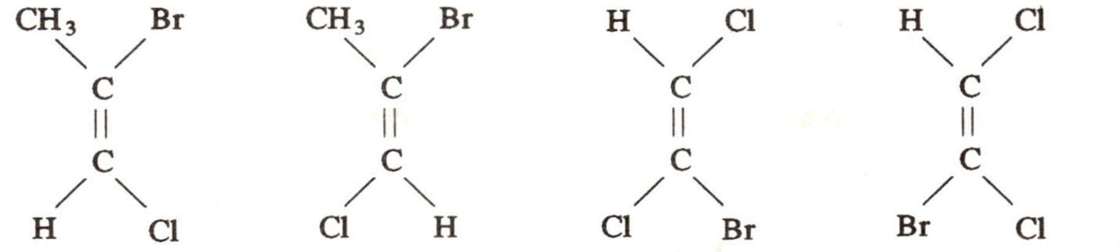

Z 2 Bromo 1 chloropropene	E 2 Bromo-1 chloropropene	Z 1 Bromo 1,2, Dichloroethene	E 1 Bromo 1, 2 Dichloroethene
Br > CH$_3$		Cl > H	
Cl > H		Br > Cl	

Alkenes are named using the same system for alkanes, but the "-ane" ending is replaced with "-ene." (e.g., ethene, propene, hexane, etc.) The boiling and melting points of alkenes are relatively similar to their alkane counterparts.

A notable difference between alkanes and alkenes involves the reaction of alkenes with hydrogen halides and with water. The addition of hydrogen halides destroys the double bond, and the hydrogen and halide will add to the two carbons that were once double bonded. The hydrogen will go to the carbon atom attached to the fewest carbons. This is shown in the following example.

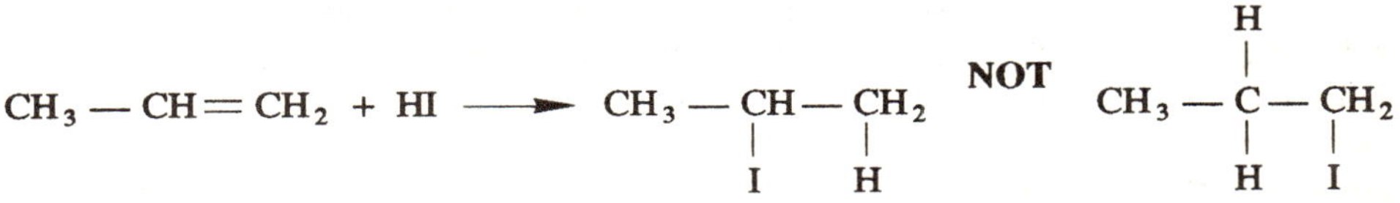

Alkenes will also react with water in the presence of acids to form alcohols. The water is split into H and OH groups, and these groups add at the site of the double bond, destroying it. Again, if there is a difference among the two carbons, the hydrogen will add to the one attached to the fewest other carbons. This is shown below.

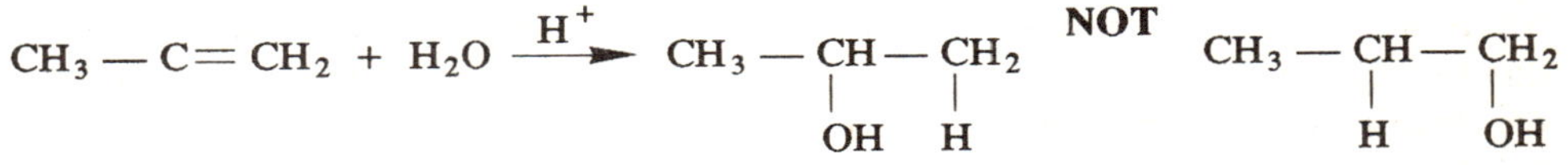

3. Aromatic

Aromatic compounds are benzene and compounds that resemble benzene in behavior. Benzene is a molecule of cyclohexane with three double bonds, but it behaves so chemically different than the properties that would be predicted for "cyclohexatriene" that it has not only been given its own name, but its own category, the aromatics. Benzene is a very flat molecule with all of the hydrogens and carbons lying in the same plane. It is also very symmetrical, with every bond angle equalling 120°. The electrons in the carbon atoms are shared in several bonds in benzene; it is this delocalization of these electrons that make the molecule so stable. Cyclohexadene, (one double-bond) and cyclohexadiene (two double bonds) differ as predicted from cyclohexane. Benzene, with the three double bonds, differs greatly from its predicted properties due to this delocalization of electrons and resonance stability. Below is a diagram of the resonance hybrid to represent benzene, and the symbol that is commonly used to represent benzene, or an aromatic ring.

XVI. Molecular Structure of Organic Compounds

1. σ AND π BONDS

All double and single bonds consist of what is called a sigma (σ) bond. In addition to the sigma bond, double bonds also possess a pi (π) bond. Triple bonds are made of two pi's and a sigma. For example, in a molecule of ethene, $CH_2=CH_2$, there is only one pi bond and five sigmas (don't forget to count the single bonds going to the hydrogens!). Hybrid orbitals and the determination of molecular structure are covered in the inorganic section. The delocalization of electrons in resonating structures are covered in the above section on aromatics.

2. Multiple Bonding

The length of a carbon-carbon single bond is 0.153 nm, a double carbon-carbon bond is 0.134 nm, and a carbon-hydrogen bond is 0.110 nm. Generally speaking, the shorter a bond is, the less energetic it is, hence the *easier it is to break*. Atoms are free to rotate about single bonds, hence we speak of rotational energy and rotational isomers. The more single bonds (carbon-carbon) a molecule has, the more rotational configurations are possible. Double and triple bonds do not permit this type of rotation. For each double bond in a compound, a number of rotational isomers are eliminated. but the possibility of cis, trans, Z, and E isomers are introduced.

3. Stereochemistry

General isomerism is covered in the inorganic chemistry section. Isomers that differ only in the way their atoms are oriented in space are called "stereoisomers." Stereoisomers that are mirror images of one another are called "enantiomers." If they are not mirror images of one another, they are called "diastereomers." The rotational isomers mentioned in the section above are also known as "conformational isomers." Many organic substances possess the ability to rotate a beam of polarized light when in solution. This phenomenon is known as "optical activity." The symbols + and - are used to denote materials that rotate polarized light to the right and to the left, respectively. Enantiomers of the same substance will have identical physical properties, and can only be distinguished by measuring the direction they bend polarized light. Their biological properties, however, can be markedly different. A "racemic mixture" is one that contains equal amounts of both enantiomers, and hence, does not bend polarized light at all. A racemic mixture is designed by ±. Optically active molecules can be classified as R or S. Holding the central atom of such a molecule, with the lowest molecular weight group pointing away, the sequence of the remaining three groups is noted. If they decrease in molecular weight in a clockwise direction, the isomer is denoted R, and if they decrease in a counter-clockwise direction, they are denoted as S. It must be stressed that one cannot tell simply from the R or S nomenclature whether or not they are + or -.

XVII. Separations and Purification

1. Extraction

A material can be transferred from one solvent to another in which it is even more soluble. The only requirement is that the two solvents used must not be miscible in one another. It is standard procedure for the solvent used in the extraction to be volatile so it can be evaporated and the solute recovered. In practice the extraction solvent is added to the solution and the container agitated. The container is then left to stand so the two phases of the immiscible solvents are completely separated. The phase containing the solute is then drained off. In practice, it is more efficient to perform several extractions using a small amount of solvent each time, rather than one extraction using a large amount of solvent.

2. Chromatography

Chromatography uses the differences in polarity and molecular weight to separate compounds. Any chromatography system consists of a mobile phase, such as a gas, which moves with the sample(s), and a stationary phase, which is a type of support that the samples and mobile phase move along.

In gas chromatography, the stationary phase is a liquid that is absorbed onto an inert solid. The two most commonly used solid "support phases" are crushed firebrick, and a similar material, kieselguhr. A variety of liquid stationary phases are used depending upon the nature of the material that is being analyzed. Materials such as squalene, n-hexadecane, polyethylene glycol, and silicone oils and gums are commonly used. The choice depends upon the polarities of the substances being separated, and the maximum temperature that is being used for the separation.

The mobile phase is a gas that will not react with the stationary phase nor the materials being separated. Helium, nitrogen, and hydrogen are commonly used, with helium by far being the most common. The stationary phases are packed into a column, usually stainless steel or glass, connected to a source of gas, and placed into an oven. A small amount of sample (liquid or gas) is injected into one end of the column in the direction of the gas flow. Depending upon the oven temperature and differences in polarity between the stationary phase and the materials being separated, the different components of the sample will have a "retention time," which is the time it takes them to pass through the column under the given conditions.

The two most common detectors at the end of these columns to detect the species as they leave the column are the thermal conductivity detector (TCD, or "hot-wire") and the flame ionization detector (FID). The TCD consists of a simple platinum glow-wire which emits infrared radiation (heat) that passes through the end of the column. A detector on the other side of the column records any changes in the

I.R. radiation passing through the column. Since the most commonly used carrier gas, helium, has such a vastly different thermoconductivity than anything else (except possibly hydrogen), any material that passes through the column other than the carrier gas will absorb the I.R. radiation differently, which will be registered by the detector, and converted into an electronic signal.

An FID consists of a hydrogen-oxygen flame. This flame is hot enough to volatilize and ionize most substances. An ion detector above the flame registers the ions thus produced. This type of detector is about two orders of magnitude more sensitive than the TCD. It has the disadvantage that it cannot detect water, since water is a product of the hydrogen-oxygen flame.

Thin-layer chromatography is technically simpler, but no less useful of a technique. The stationary phase is coated in a thin layer onto some rigid sheet, which is usually a glass plate. Common stationary phases include starch, silica gel, cellulose, and aluminum oxide. These are applied by dissolving them in a solvent (usually water) to make a slurry, and spreading a thin film on a glass plate, which is then baked in an oven to remove the solvent. The sample, in liquid form, or dissolved in the mobile phase, is spotted at the bottom of the plate by a pipet and allowed to dry. The plate is then placed in a jar with a small amount of the mobile phase in the bottom. The jar is covered so the vapor pressure of the mobile phase is in equilibrium with the liquid.

Mobile phases are usually organic solvents such as benzene, chloroform, ethanol, butanol, acetone, and many more, as well as combinations of these. Differences between the polarity of the mobile phase and the substances of analysis cause the mobile phase to carry these to different heights on the plate. Once the solvent has run all of the way to the top of the plate, the plate is removed from the chamber and dried. Unless the materials of interest are naturally colored, they must be stained before they can be detected. Commonly used stains include ninhydrin, pH indicators, iodine, and potassium permanganate. Sometimes, ultraviolet light is used if the material fluoresces.

3. Distillation

A mixture of two substances, only one of which is volatile, can be separated by distillation. A very common example is the removal of salt from water. The water will boil and vaporize at a far lower termperature than the salt. The water boils away, leaving the salt behind. The water vapor can then be condensed, and pure water recovered. This is known as simple distillation, and is a technique that has been used for centuries.

If both components in a mixture have boiling points that are fairly close, such as benzene (b.p. = 85°) and pentane (b.p. = 36°), simple distillation will not do a good job of separating them. In the above example, analysis would show that after distillation, there would be a slight enrichment of pentane (the lower boiling material) in the distillate (that which was vaporized and recondensed), and a slight enrichment of benzene, (the higher boiling component) in the residue (the material that remains in the distillation flask), but not enough of an enrichment in either to be of any use. In such instances "fractional distillation" is used. A column filled with glass beads, or any other inert material offering a larger surface area, is placed between the distillation apparatus and the condenser. The less volatile vapors (in this case, benzene) will condense onto the surface of the beads, and fall back into the distillation flask, directly below. In such a manner a good separation of the above mixture can be realized.

4. Recrystallization

Recrystallization is commonly used to prepare high purity chemicals. The original batch of impure crystals are dissolved in a "good" solvent, one in which they are readily soluble. A second "bad" solvent is then added. The material of interest is insoluble in this, but the impurities present are. The substance of interest will then precipitate out of the solution. Another method involves the use of only one solvent. The impure crystals are dissolved in a minimum amount of hot solvent. The solution is then cooled. If the solubility of the material of interest is minimal in the cold solvent, but the impurities are still soluble, the material of interest will crystallize out. To do this, one must know the solubilities of the material of interest, as well as the impurities that are present, at a variety of temperatures in the solvent used.

XVIII. Use of Spectroscopy in Structural Identification

1. Infrared Spectroscopy

Infrared radiation consists of wavelengths from 0.78 to 1,000 um. The wavelengths from 2.5 to 15 um are most commonly used in spectroscopy, which corresponds to a frequency range of 1.2×10^{14} to 2.0×10^{13} Hz. In spectroscopy, wavenumber (δ), which is the reciprocal of the wavelength in centimeters, is commonly used. This would correspond to a wavenumber of 4,000 to 670 cm^{-1}. Recall from organic chemistry that atoms attached to a carbon atom can rotate about a single bond. The bonds can also vibrate and stretch. The energy needed to excite these molecules in such a manner is present in the I.R. band. For example, I.R. radiation from 3700 to 3100 cm^{-1} (2.7 to 3.2 um) will be absorbed by O-H and N-H bonds and cause them to vibrate. Hence, if I.R. radiation is sent through an organic sample, and the detector finds that the above region has been absorbed by the sample, then it is likely that the sample contains O-H and/or N-H bonds. In a like manner, triple bonds absorb between 2700 to 1850 cm^{-1}, and carbon-carbon double bonds absorb between 1950 to 1550 cm^{-1}. Tables are available that list various organic functional groups, and the I.R. regions that they absorb. Books are available that show the I.R. spectrum of known compounds.

2. NMR Spectroscopy

A strong magnetic field can cause the nuclei of certain atoms to be split into two or more quantisized energy levels. Absorption of electromagnetic energy in the range of 0.1 to 100 MHz (3,000 to 3 m) will cause transitions in the magnetically induced energy levels of the nuclei. This process is known as nuclear magnetic resonance (NMR). The sample is placed in a strong magnetic field and spun. Radio frequencies of the above wavelengths are then introduced to the sample. The nucleus in question must have a quantum spin of $^1/_2$ to be of any use with this procedure. Ordinary hydrogen, H^1, is the most commonly observed nuclei in this procedure; however, none of the solvent used to dissolve the sample can contain H^1. Hence, ordinary water would not be suitable, nor would ordinary pentane. (However, heavy water, or deuterated pentane, where the ordinary H^1 has been replaced by H^2 (deuterium) will work find, provided the sample is soluble in one of them.)

C^{13} is the next most commonly used atom for NMR studies. However, its natural abundance is only 1% (H^1 is 99.99% abundant in nature, by comparison), which limits its use. Other nuclei used in NMR are F^{19} and P^{31}. The frequency of the radiation absorbed (usually calibrated in ppm) gives a clue to the surroundings of the atom of interest (e.g., for a proton, whether it is on a methyl or ethyl group, or a benzene ring.) The number of splits in the absorption peak indicate how many other atoms of the same element are adjacent. The ratio of area of the peaks in the total NMR spectra show the relative ratios of the different types of atoms present.

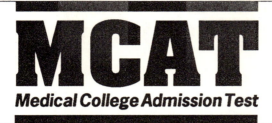

Medical College Admission Test

Chapter 3
Chemistry Review

Chapter 3

I. STOICHIOMETRY

1. Atomic Weight

Atomic weights (or more properly, Atomic Masses) have units of Daltons or a.m.u.'s (atomic mass units) and tell how the weight, in grams, of the average atom of an element compares with the weight of an atom of carbon-12. A mole of a substance contains 6.02 EE+23 atoms. More about this will be covered later. Since the atomic weight of iodine is 127, one mole of iodine atoms will have a mass of 127 grams. The atomic weight of cobalt is 59, therefore 59 grams of cobalt will have one mole of cobalt atoms. Sometimes different atoms of the same elements can have different atomic weights, these are known as isotopes. For example, thallium exists in nature as two isotopes, of atomic weights 205 and 203. The atomic weight listed on the periodic table is an average, based upon both the atomic weights of the element found in nature and upon their natural abundance. For example, in nature lead consists of the following four isotopes in the following natural abundances:

Pb-204	1.42%	abundant
Pb-206	24.1%	
Pb-207	22.1%	
Pb-208	52.4%	

Using this data we can calculate the average atomic weight of lead as:

$$(0.0142)(204) + (0.241)(206) + (0.221)(207) + (0.524)(208) = 207.2$$

The value, 207.2, is the one reported in the periodic table.

2. Molecular Weight

The molecular weight of a compound is determined by simply adding up the atomic weights of **all** of the atoms present. Oxygen gas has the formula O_2; therefore, the molecular weight of one oxygen molecule is 32 (2×16). Molecular weights are usually given in Daltons or a.m.u. [atomic mass units], so it would be properly said that oxygen gas has a molecular weight of 32 Daltons, or 32 a.m.u. The molecular weight of water, H_2O, where H = 1 a.m.u. and O = 16 a.m.u., would be

$$(2 \times 1) + (1 \times 16) = 18 \text{ Daltons.}$$

A table of atomic weights (sometimes called atomic masses) must be available to do such calculations (see page 993). For instance, to find the molecular weight of copper (II) sulfate, we know that the formula is $CuSO_4$, and looking up the proper atomic weights, we get

$(1 \times 63.5) + (1 \times 32) + (4 \times 16) = 159.5$ a.m.u.

PROBLEM

a)	What is the molecular weight of nitrogen gas, N_2? (nitrogen at. wt. = 14)
b)	What is the molecular weight of cobalt chloride, $CoCL_2$? (at.wt Co = 58.9, Cl = 35.4).
c)	What is the molecular weight of benzene, C_6H_6? (C = 12, H = 1)

Solution

a)   28

b)   129.7

c)   78   All units either Daltons, or a.m.u.

For salts such as cobalt chloride, copper sulfate, etc., the term "Formula Weight" is used, since they do not exist in molecular form. Do not let such a term confuse you; for the purposes of the MCAT, formula weight and molecular weight can be used interchangeably.

3. Empirical Formulas vs. Molecular Formulas

The empirical formula is the simplest ratio of atoms present in a compound. The molecular formula shows the actual number of atoms present. From a molecular formula, a molecular weight can be determined, and conversely, if given an empirical formula and molecular weight, a molecular formula can be determined. Sometimes the empirical formula and molecular formula for a compound are the same. Water has an empirical formula of H_2O (the simplest ratio), and a molecular formula of H_2O (the actual numbers present).

Hydrogen peroxide has an empirical formula of HO, and a molecular formula of H_2O_2. If benzene has an empirical formula of CH and a molecular weight of 78, what is its molecular formula? (at. wt. C = 12, H = 1)

$12 + 1 = 13.$

$78/13 = 6$

$\therefore$ multiply all of the subscripts in the empirical formula by 6. The answer is C_6H_6.

PROBLEM

a)	Acetylene, like benzene, has an empirical formula CH, and a molecular weight of 26, what is its molecular formula?
b)	Vitamin C has an empirical formula of $C_3H_4O_3$ and a molecular weight of 176 Daltons, what is its molecular formula?

Solution

a) C_2H_2

b) $C_6H_8O_6$

4. Metric Units

Listed below are the metric units relevant to the MCAT.

SI Prefixes

Fraction	Prefix	Symbol	Multiple	Prefix	Symbol
10^{-1}	deci	d	10	deka	da
10^{-2}	centi	c	10^2	hecto	h
10^{-3}	milli	m	10^3	kilo	k
10^{-6}	micro	μ	10^6	mega	M
10^{-9}	nano	n	10^9	giga	G
10^{-12}	pico	p	10^{12}	tetra	T
10^{-15}	femto	f			

Units and Conversion Factors

Quantity	SI Unit	Symbol	Conversion Factors
length	meter	m	$1 \text{ cm} = 10^{-2}$ m
			$1 \text{ nm} = 10^{-9}$ m
			$1 \text{ A}° = 10^{-10}$ m
			$1 \text{ inch} = 2.54 \times 10^{-2}$ m
mass	kilogram	kg	$1 \text{ g} = 10^{-3}$ kg
			$1 \text{ mg} = 10^{-6}$ kg
			$1 \text{ lb} = 0.454$ kg
time	second	s	$1 \text{ day} = 8.6 \times 10^4$ s
temperature	kelvin	K	$0° \text{ C} = 273.15$ K
volume	cubic meter	m^3	$1L = 10^{-3} \text{ m}^3$
			$= 1000 \text{ cm}^3$
			$1ml = 1cm^3$

PROBLEM

a) How many meters in 5.2 kilometers? How many centimeters? How many millimeters?

b) What is the mass in kilograms of 75.8 cubic centimeters of pure water at 4°C.? $1 \text{ g } H_2O = 1 \text{ cm}^3$ at 4°C

Solution

a) 5,200 meters, 520,000 centimeters, 5,200,000 millimeters.

b) 0.0758 kilograms

5. Description of Composition by % Mass

If a substance consists of 4 grams of material A, 16 grams of material B, and 80 grams of material C, its percent composition by mass is easy to determine. It can readily be seen that the composition by mass is:

4% A, 16% B, and 80% C

More often one does not have the luxury of the sum of all of the masses equalling 100. In such instances, one must divide the mass of each component by the sum of the masses of all components, and multiply this quotient by 100 to obtain the mass percent. For example, if analysis of a sample of baking soda showed it to consist of 35.0 grams of sodium, 1.5 grams of hydrogen, 18.3 grams of carbon, and 73.1 grams of oxygen, what is the percent composition of this baking soda? First, the mass of all of the components must be summed:

35.0 + 1.5 + 18.3 + 73.1 = 127.9 grams

of sample. To find the percentage of each component, simply divide the mass of each component by the total mass, and multiply by 100:

% of sodium = (35.0/127.9) × 100 = 27.4%

% of hydrogen = (1.5/127.9) × 100 = 1.2%

% of carbon = (18.3/127.9) × 100 = 14.3%

% of oxygen = (73.1/127.9) × 100 = 57.1%

PROBLEM

a) A sample of calcium chloride showed upon analysis to consist of 93.0 grams of calcium and 165 grams of chlorine. What is its weight percent composition?

b) A sample of penicillin showed it to consist of 8.62 grams of carbon, 0.808 grams of hydrogen, 2.87 grams of oxygen, 1.26 grams of nitrogen, and 1.44 grams of sulfur. What is its percent composition?

Solution

a) 36.0% calcium, 64.0 chlorine

b) 57.5% carbon, 5.39% hydrogen, 19.1% oxygen, 8.40% nitrogen, 9.60% sulfur.

6. Mole Concept, Avogadro's Number

A mole specifies a definite quantity. Just as a dozen of anything is 12, a gross is 144, a mole is 6.02×10^{23}. This is such a large number that it is usually only used in chemistry where large numbers of atoms and molecules are encountered. One mole of benzene would contain 6.02×10^{23} molecules of benzene. How many molecules would there be in 0.001 moles of benzene? A simple multiplication reveals the answer to be

$0.001 \times 6.02 \times 10^{23} = 6.02 \times 10^{20}$ molecules of benzene.

If there are 7.525×10^{22} atoms of neon present, how many moles are there? Knowing that there are **ALWAYS** 6.02×10^{23} in a mole, the calculations would be:

$$(7.525 \times 10^{22}) / (6.02 \times 10^{23}) = 0.125 \text{ moles}$$

or 1/8 mole of neon. 6.02×10^{23} is known as Avogadro's number, and is defined as the number of atoms in one gram of hydrogen, H. Using this definition, one can see that if one measures out the atomic or molecular weight of a substance in grams, there will be one mole of atoms or molecules present. For example, one mole of helium (At.Wt. = 4) will have a mass of four grams, half a mole 2 grams, ten moles 40 grams, etc. How many molecules (or rather, formula units) of indium chloride are there in 1105.0 grams of $InCl_3$ (M.W. = 221.0 Daltons)?

$$1105.0/221.0 = 5.000 \text{ moles}, 5.000 \times 6.02 \times 10^{23} = 3.01 \times 10^{24} \text{ molecules}$$

(or formula units) of $InCl_3$.

What would the mass of 1.30×10^{22} molecules of carbon dioxide (M.W. = 44) be? First, the number of moles must be found:

$$1.30 \times 10^{22}/6.02 \times 10^{23} = 0.0216 \text{ moles of } CO_2.$$

This is multiplied by the molecular weight to find the mass:

$$0.0216 \times 44 = 0.950 \text{ grams of } CO_2.$$

PROBLEM

a) If one has 6.02×10^{23} of toothpicks, how many moles of toothpicks are present?

b) How many molecules are present in 0.002 moles of napthalene?

c) How much mass will 25 moles of xenon (At.Wt. = 131.3) have?

d) Determine the mass of 7.88×10^{25} atoms of iron (At.Wt. = 55.8).

e) How much mass, and how many molecules in 3.45 moles of water (M.W. = 18)?

Solution

a) 1 mole of toothpicks

b) 1.20×10^{21} molecules of napthalene

c) 3282 grams of xenon

d) 7304 grams of iron

e) 62.1 grams and 2.08×10^{24} molecules of water.

7. Definition of Density

Density is the mass of a substance divided by its volume. For example, 34.8 ml of isobutyl iodide has a mass of 56.1 grams. What is its density? Simple division tells us the answer is

$$56.1 / 34.8 = 1.61 \text{ grams / ml}$$

Sometimes the volume needs to be calculated, as in the following example: If a rectangular block of pure cobalt metal measures 5.23 cm long, 10.3 cm high, and 2.01 cm wide, and has a mass of 944 grams, what is the density of cobalt? First, to find the volume of a rectangular solid the formula $V = lwh$ is recalled,

$$V = 5.23 \times 2.01 \times 10.3 = 108 \text{ cm}^3.$$

With a volume calculated, we proceed as before,

$$944 / 108 = 8.72 \text{ gm} / \text{cm}^3.$$

Sometimes, given the density, one can work backwards to calculate dimensions. What is the radius of a sphere of sulfur with a mass of 26.4 grams? The density of sulfur is 2.05 gm / cm^3. To find the volume,

$$26.4 / 2.05 = 12.9 \text{ cm}^3.$$

To determine the radius, recall that the volume of a sphere = $4/3 \, \pi \, r^3$. Solving for the radius gives a value of 1.45 cm.

PROBLEM

> a) A rectangular block of pure camphor ($C_{10}H_{15}BrO$) measures 10.0 centimeters in width, 50.0 centimeters in length, and 2.00 meters in height. It contains 3.74×10^{26} molecules of camphor. What is the density of camphor?
>
> b) How many moles of hydrogen are there in 20.0 grams of ($C_{17}H_{21}O_4N$)? What is the weight percent of hydrogen?
>
> c) If analysis of pyrene shows it to be composed of 95.0% carbon and 5.00% hydrogen, what is its empirical formula? If the molecular weight is found to be 202 Daltons, what is its molecular formula?

Solution

a) Calculate the volume of the box. (Remember, 2.00 meters = 200 centimeters!)

$$200 \text{ cm} \times 50\text{cm} \times 10\text{cm} = 100,000 \text{ cm}^3. \tag{1}$$

Calculate the number of moles of camphor.

$$3.74 \times 10^{26} / 6.02 \times 10^{23} = 6.21 \times 10^2 \text{ moles.} \tag{2}$$

Calculate the molecular weight of camphor.

$$(10 \times 12) + (15 \times 1) + (1 \times 79.9) + (1 \times 16) = 231 \text{ Daltons.} \tag{3}$$

Calculate the mass of camphor.

$$621 \text{ moles} \times 231 \text{ grams} / \text{mole} = 1.43 \times 10^5 \text{ grams.} \tag{4}$$

Calculate the density of camphor.

$$1.43 \times 10^5 \text{ grams} / 10^{5 \text{ cm3}} = 1.43 \text{ gm} / \text{cm}^3. \tag{5}$$

b) Calculate the molecular weight.

$$(17 \times 12) + (21 \times 1) + (4 \times 16) + (1 \times 14) = 303 \text{ Daltons.} \tag{1}$$

Calculate the number of moles in 20 grams.

$$20 / 303 = 0.0660 \text{ moles.} \tag{2}$$

Note from the formula that every mole has 21 moles of hydrogen in it.

$$21 \times 0.0660 = 1.38 \text{ moles of hydrogen.} \tag{3}$$

This solves the first part. The second part can be solved in two ways.

Calculate the mass of hydrogen.

$$1.38 \times 1 = 1.38 \text{ grams of hydrogen.} \tag{1a}$$

Find the weight percent hydrogen.

$$(1.38 / 20) \times 100 = 6.93\% \text{ hydrogen.} \tag{2a}$$

OR

Calculate the weight of hydrogen in 1 mole.

$$1 \times 21 = 21. \tag{1b}$$

Divide this into the weight of 1 mole.

$$21 / 303 = 0.0693 = 6.93\%. \tag{2b}$$

c)   Assume you have 100 grams of pyrene, in which case there will be 95.0 grams of carbon and 5.00 grams of hydrogen. (Any mass will work, but obviously, when dealing with percentages, 100 is the easiest.)

Calculate the number of moles present of each.

$$95 / 12 = 7.92 \text{ moles of carbon, } 5 / 1 = 5 \text{ moles of hydrogen.} \tag{1}$$

Divide the smallest number of moles into all of the moles present, including itself.

$$7.92 / 5 = 1.58, 5 / 5 = 1. \tag{2}$$

This gives a ratio of 1.58:1 (C:H).

Multiply the ratio by a common factor to eliminate decimals.

$$5 \times (1.58{:}1) = 7.9{:}5, \tag{3}$$

which can be rounded off to 8:5, which means the empirical formula is C_8H_5. The weight of the empirical formula is calculated.

$$(8 \times 12) + (5 \times 1) = 101. \tag{4}$$

Divide this value into the molecular weight.

$$202 / 101 = 2. \tag{5}$$

Multiply the subscripts in the empirical formula by the value obtained in step (5).

$$2 \times (C_8H_5) = C_{16}H_{10}, \tag{6}$$

which is the molecular formula.

8. Oxidation Number

When an atom loses electrons, it is said to be oxidized. The opposite of this process is called reduction. To show the oxidation state of a particular element in a compound, or reaction, chemists have invented oxidation numbers. For example, the oxidation number for aluminum in the metallic state is 0, but in the salt, aluminum chloride, it is +3. There are a few simple rules for assigning oxidation numbers. (Remember, although these numbers are useful, they do not really exist in the molecules; they are artificial aids to help understand certain chemical reactions).

Rule #1: The oxidation number of any element uncombined, or combined with itself, is always zero, e.g., the oxidation numbers for He, Ne, Ar, Xe, and Rn are all 0. O_2, O_3, N_2, Gl_2, Br_2, etc. all have oxidation numbers of 0. Cu, Fe, Au, Pg, etc. all have oxidation numbers of 0. Sometimes metals are written with a zero superscript to their right to show that they are uncombined (zero oxidation number), $Fe°$, $Ag°$, $V°$, etc.

Rule #2: The oxidation number of an ion is equal to the charge of an ion: e.g., the oxidation number of Fe^{++} is +2, that of Fe^{+++} is +3. The oxidation number of Cl^- is -1, of $S^=$ is -2.

Rule #3: in all compounds, the sum of the oxidation is zero. Elements at the edges of the periodic table always have the same oxidation number in the combined state. For example, lithium will always be +1 and flourine will always be -1.

As one moves into the table, the numbers begin to vary. Oxygen is usually -2, but it can be -1 (as in the case of peroxides). Deep in the interior of the table, oxidation numbers can vary greatly, and can only be determined by deduction, using the known oxidation numbers of the atoms in the compound with them. The following examples should clarify this passage: In the compound NaCl, we can tell from the periodic table that Na will form a +1 ion and Cl a -1, hence these are the oxidation numbers for these respective atoms in this compound. It can be written as Na+1 Cl-1. Note that the sum is zero, (+1) + (-1) = 0. We can do the same thing for K_2S. K forms a +1 ion, and S usually forms a -2 ion. Since there are two K's, there is a total charge of +2, and again the sum of the oxidation numbers is zero, 2(+1) + (-2) = 0. This can be written K_2S +1 -2. If we look at PbS_2, Pb is so far into the interior of the table that we cannot tell immediately what its oxidation number is in this compound. We know that S is usually a -2, and since there are two of them, that gives us a total charge of 2 × (-2), or -4. Since the sum of all of the oxidation numbers in a compound must be zero, Pb must have an oxidation number of +4 in this case and it would be written PbS^{+4} -2.

For a final example, consider the compound Fe_2S_3. S is usually -2, and since there are three of them present, 3 ×(-2) = -6. If the total charge on the sulfur is -6, and the sum of the oxidation numbers must equal zero for a compound, then the total charge on the iron must be +6. The total charge must be divided by the total number of iron atoms present ((+6) / 2 = (+3)) to obtain an oxidation number of +3 for iron in this compound.

Rule #4: The sum of oxidation numbers in a polyatomic ion will equal the charge of the ion. For example in NH^+_4, hydrogen has a charge of +1, and since there are four of them, 4 × (+1) = (+4). Since the total charge of the ion equals +1, the oxidation number for nitrogen in this compound is (+1) - (+4) = (-3). If we look at the oxidation number of nitrogen in NO^-_3, it will have a different value. Oxygen is usually -2, and since there are three of them the total charge is 3 ×(-2) = (-6). Since the sum of the oxidation numbers must equal the charge of the ion, the oxidation number for nitrogen in this case is (-1) - (-6) = (-1) + 6 = +5.

PROBLEM

What are the oxidation numbers of the atoms in the following?							
a)	S_8	b)	H_2O	c)	MnO_2	d)	Fe^{++}
e)	CrO	f)	Sn	g)	ClO^-_4	h)	$Mn_2(SO_4)_3$

Solution

a)   0   b)   +1, -2   c)   +4, -2   d)   +2

e)   +2, -2   f)   0   g)   +7, -2   h)   +3, +6, -2

Commonly used oxidizing agents include potassium permanaganate [$KMnO_4$], potassium dichromate [$K_2Cr_2O_7$], and cerium (IV) bisulfate [$Ce(HSO_4)_4$]. Common reducing agents include tin (II) chloride [$SnCl_2$] and sodium thiosulfate [$Na_2S_2O_3$]. Oxidation and reduction are collectively termed "redox." A redox titration is one in which the amount of oxidizing and reducing agents are brought to an equal concentration. Such an example would be the reaction of copper (II) ions reacting with metallic iron,

$$Cu^{++} + Fe^{\circ} \longrightarrow Cu^{\circ} + Fe^{++}.$$

This will be covered in greater detail later.

9. Description of Reactions by Chemical Equations

Chemical equations are written much like a mathematical equation. An arrow replaces the equal sign. To the left of the arrow are the reactants, or starting materials, and to the right are the products, or final materials. The number of atoms shown on the left side of the arrow must equal the number shown on the right side. If we wanted to write "hydrogen and oxygen can combine to form water," the chemical equation would start with

$$H_2 + O_2 \longrightarrow H_2O.$$

This would be a good start, as we are showing hydrogen and oxygen as reactants, and water as a product. However, closer inspection shows two atoms of oxygen on the left of the arrow and only one on the right. Since an atom of oxygen simply cannot disappear from the universe, something is wrong. If one places a coefficient of "2" before the H_2O, this now gives two atoms of oxygen on the right side of the arrow. However, this causes another problem, as now there are four hydrogen atoms to the right of the equation, and only two on the left. This can be remedied by placing a "2" before the hydrogen on the left hand side. At this point the number of atoms on both sides of the arrow are equal. Such an equation is said to be balanced. A balanced equation has an advantage over the English statement, as it also shows the ratios in which the atoms (or moles of atoms) combine and form products. In the example above, the final, balanced equation would be

$$2H_2 + O_2 \longrightarrow 2H_2O,$$

and shows that two moles of hydrogen will combine with one mole of oxygen to produce two moles of water. This will always be the ratio. Four moles of hydrogen will react with two moles of oxygen to produce four moles of water, etc. When working with grams of material, you must first convert to moles to use the ratios in the chemical equation. $2 \times 2 = 4$ grams of hydrogen and $1 \times 32 = 32$ grams of oxygen react to form $2 \times 18 = 36$ grams of water. Note that mass is still conserved when working in grams rather than moles. Let us next look at the reaction of zinc percarbonate with perchloric acid:

$$ZnCO_3 + HClO_4 \longrightarrow Zn(ClO_4)_2 + H_2O + CO_2$$

It can be seen at once that there is only one atom of Cl on the left, and two on the right. Further inspection indicates that the ClO_4 reacts as a group. Hence, putting a coefficient of "2" in front of the perchloric acid gives:

$$ZnCO_3 + 2HClO_4 \longrightarrow Zn(ClO_4)_2 + H_2O + CO_2$$

which balances the equation, and establishes the molar ratios for this reaction. If we have 2.00 kilograms of $ZnCO_3$ and 100 grams of $HClO_4$, how many grams of $Zn(ClO_4)_2$ can be made? First we must calculate molecular weight, and number of moles present.

M.W. for $ZnCO_3$ $(1 \times 65.37) + (1 \times 12) + (3 \times 16) = 125.4$ Daltons,

for $HClO_4$: $(1 \times 1) + (1 \times 35.4) + (4 \times 16) = 100.4$ Daltons,

for $Zn(ClO_4)_2$: $(1 \times 65.37) + (2 \times 35.4) + (8 \times 16) = 264.2$ Daltons.

# of moles of $ZnCO_3$: (2.00 Kg = 2,000 gm) 2,000 / 125.4 = 15.95,

# of moles of $HClO_4$: 100 / 100.4 = 1.00.

By looking at the molar ratios it can be seen that for every mole of $ZnCO_3$ consumed, two moles of $HClO_4$ will be needed, and one mole of $Zn(ClO_4)_2$ will be produced. In this instance, the $HClO_4$ is the **limiting reagent,** since it will be used up, and the other reactant will still have some material left over. Consuming all of the 1.00 mole of $HClO_4$, will require 0.500 moles of the $ZnCO_3$ (using the ratio established in the equation), leaving the remaining 15.45 moles unreacted. By the same ratio, it can be seen that 0.500 moles of $Zn(ClO_4)_2$ will be produced. Converting this into grams gives $0.500 \times 264.2 = 132.1$ grams of $Zn(ClO_4)_2$ produced. So far all of the equations we have written show all of the atoms involved, and are called "gross molecular equations." Some species will exist in ionic form in aqueous solutions (e.g., in water). Consider the gross molecular equation.

$$Na_2CO_3 + CaCl_2 \longrightarrow 2NaCl + CaCO_3$$

The only species that exists in molecular form is the $CaCO_3$; the rest will be present as ions. A "gross ionic equation" will show this as:

$$2Na^+ + CO_3^= + Ca^{++} + 2Cl^- \longrightarrow 2Na^+ + 2Cl^- + CaCO_3$$

Since the sodium and chloride ions do not get involved in the reaction, they are called "spectator ions." Since they are unchanged from one side of the arrow to the other, they can be eliminated. Such an equation is referred to as "net ionic," and would be written as:

$$Ca^{++} + CO_3^= \longrightarrow CaCO_3$$

Below is a list of common types of reactions, and methods to balance the equations for them.

A.   DIRECT COMBINATION REACTIONS OF ELEMENTS

This can be the easiest of the reaction types. Keep in mind the types of ions that the atoms in question prefer to form, and deduce the formula for the product from that. For example, the reaction of zinc with sulfur can be written as:

$$Zn^\circ + S \longrightarrow ?$$

From the periodic table it can be seen that Zn tends to form + 2 ions, and S forms -2 ions. The resulting neutral compound would then be zinc sulfide, ZnS, and the reaction would be written

$$Zn° + S \longrightarrow ZnS.$$

Notice that this equation is already balanced. The reaction of potassium with bromine would be stated $K + Br_2 \longrightarrow$? Since K and Br both form ions with a charge of one, and opposite in signs, the formula for potassium bromide can be deduced as KBr. We can now write the equation as:

$$K + Br_2 \longrightarrow KBr.$$

However, there are twice as many Br's on the left side of the equation as the right. Placing a "2" in front of the product gives the proper number of Br's, but also doubles the number of K's on that side. Placing a "2" in front of the K on the left-hand side balances the equation. The final equation is

$$2K + Br_2 \longrightarrow 2KBr.$$

For a final example, note the combination of aluminum and oxygen. We would start with

$$Al° + O_2 \longrightarrow ? .$$

Since Al forms +3 ion, and oxygen a -2, the formula for aluminum oxide is Al_2O_3, which would give

$$Al° + O_2 \longrightarrow Al_2O_3.$$

In this case we can actually multiply the oxygen on the right hand side by a fraction ($1\frac{1}{2}$) to get it to equal the value on the right side. It can be easily seen that a "2" in front of the Al on the left side will put things in balance:

$$2Al° + 1\frac{1}{2}O_2 \longrightarrow Al_2O_3.$$

However, fractions are not generally tolerated in chemical equations. Multiplying through by 2 will clear this fraction and give:

$$4Al° + 3O_2 \longrightarrow 2Al_2O_3.$$

PROBLEM

Write a balanced reaction for the direct combination of

a) barium and oxygen   b) lithium and oxygen

c) aluminum and sulfur

Solution

a) $2Ba + O_2 \longrightarrow 2BaO$

b) $4Li + O_2 \longrightarrow 2Li_2O$

c) $2Al + 3S \longrightarrow Al_2S_3$

B.   COMBUSTION REACTIONS

In a combustion reaction, an organic (carbon containing) compound combines with oxygen (usually unlimited) to ultimately form carbon dioxide and water. Balancing is done as before. For example, the complete combustion of octane (C_8H_{18}) (a major component in gasoline) would start with

$$C_8H_{18} + O_2 \longrightarrow CO_2 + H_2O.$$

The 8 carbons and 18 hydrogens are easy to account for on the right-hand side:

$$C_8H_{18} + O_2 \longrightarrow 8CO_2 + 9H_2O.$$

This leaves 25 oxygens to be accounted for on the left-hand side, correcting for this gives:

$$C_8H_{18} + 12\frac{1}{2}O_2 \longrightarrow 8CO_2 + 9H_2O.$$

Multiplying through by two to remove the fraction yields the final equation:

$$2C_8H_{18} + 25O_2 \longrightarrow 16CO_2 + 18H_2O.$$

For the complete combustion of acetone $[(CH_3COCH_3)]$, the beginning would be the same as before:

$$CH_3COCH_3 + O_2 \longrightarrow CO_2 + H_2O.$$

Again, the number of carbons and hydrogens are set equal:

$$CH_3COCH_3 + O_2 \longrightarrow 3CO_2 + 3H_2O.$$

All that remains to be done is to balance the oxygen atoms (remember that one oxygen is in acetone):

$$CH_3COCH_3 + 4O_2 \longrightarrow 3CO_2 + 3H_2O,$$

which is the final equation.

PROBLEM

Write a balanced equation for the complete combustion of:

a)   Xylene $[C_6H_4(CH_3)_2]$

b)   Ethanol $[CH_3CH_2OH]$

Solution

a) $2C_6H_4(CH_3)_2 + 21O_2 \longrightarrow 16CO_2 + 10H_2O$

b) $CH_3CH_2OH + 3O_2 \longrightarrow 2CO_2 + 3H_2O$

C.   NEUTRALIZATION REACTIONS

According to classical acid-base theory, an acid forms H^+ ions [or more properly H_3O^+ ions] when dissolved in water, and a base yields OH^- ions when in water. When such an acid and base are mixed in equivalent quantities, a neutralization reaction occurs, and the products are water and a salt (i.e., the combination of a metal and non-metal). For the complete neutralization of sulfuric acid and sodium hydroxide, we would start with

$$H_2SO_4 + NaOH \longrightarrow ?$$

A look at the ions present show

$$H^+, SO_4^=, Na^+, \text{ and } OH^-.$$

Obviously the Na^+ and H^+ would not want to combine, nor would the $SO_4^=$ and OH^-.

Due to the (-2) charge on the sulfate ion, two sodium ions would be needed to electrically balance the charges, resulting in sodium sulfate, Na_2SO_4. The H^+ and the OH^- will combine to form H_2O. The equation can now be written as:

$$H_2SO_4 + NaOH \longrightarrow H_2O + Na_2SO_4$$

To start balancing the equation, it is first noted that two sodiums are needed on the left-hand side:

$$H_2SO_4 + 2NaOH \longrightarrow H_2O + Na_2SO_4$$

Balancing for the hydrogen and oxygen now give us the final equation:

$$H_2SO_4 + 2NaOH \longrightarrow 2H_2O + Na_2SO_4$$

Consider the neutralization of nitric acid with magnesium hydroxide. Of course the start will be,

$$HNO_3 + Mg(OH)_2 \longrightarrow ?$$

From this it can be seen that the salt will be magnesium nitrate, $Mg(NO_3)_2$, and of course, water will still be formed. This gives:

$$HNO_3 + Mg(OH)_2 \longrightarrow H_2O + Mg(NO_3)_2$$

To balance this equation two nitrates are placed on the left-hand side:

$$2HNO_3 + Mg(OH)_2 \longrightarrow H_2O + Mg(NO_3)_2$$

Balancing the oxygen and hydrogen gives us the final, correct equation:

$$2HNO_3 + Mg(NO_3)_2 \longrightarrow 2H_2O + Mg(NO_3)_2$$

PROBLEM

Write a balanced equation for the following neutralization reactions:

a) Orthophosphoric acid and sodium hydroxide, $H_3PO_4 + NaOH$

b) Radium hydroxide and hydrochloric acid, $Ra(OH)_2 + HCl$

c) Hydrogen sulfide and silver hydroxide, $H_2S + AgOH$

Solution

a) $H_3PO_4 + 3NaOH \longrightarrow Na_3PO_4 + 3H_2O$

b) $Ra(OH)_2 + 2HCl \longrightarrow RaCl_2 + 2H_2O$

c) $H_2S + 2AgOH \longrightarrow Ag_2S + 2H_2O$

D.   OXIDATION AND REDUCTION REACTIONS

Oxidation and reduction are known collectively as "redox." In any chemical system, an oxidation cannot occur unless a reduction also occurs, and vice versa. Recall from a previous section that oxidation is loss of electrons, and gaining electrons is reduction. A reducing agent causes another atom to be reduced, and in the process, the reducing agent is oxidized. In like manner, an oxidizing agent causes another atom to be oxidized, while it itself is reduced. There are two main methods used to balance redox equations. The first method is to use oxidation numbers, which were previously introduced. Oxidation numbers have been assigned to the reactants and products of the following unbalanced equations:

$$\overset{+1\ -1}{NaCl} + \overset{+4\ -2}{MnO_2} + \overset{+1\ +6\ -2}{H_2SO_4} \longrightarrow \overset{0}{Cl_2} + \overset{+2\ +6\ -2}{MnSO_4} + \overset{+1\ +6\ -2}{Na_2SO_4} + \overset{+1\ -2}{H_2O}.$$

From these numbers, it can be seen that Mn changes from a +4 to a +2; i.e., it has been reduced. Cl has changed from -1 to 0, i.e., it has been oxidized. Short, partial equations can be written to show these changes:

$$\overset{+4}{Mn} \longrightarrow \overset{+2}{Mn}, \text{ and } \overset{-1}{Cl} \longrightarrow \overset{0}{\tfrac{1}{2}Cl_2} \text{ (or } 2Cl^- \longrightarrow \overset{0}{Cl_2})$$

From this it can be seen that Mn changes by -2, and Cl by +1. A multiplier must be found for each change in oxidation number so that the two products will have the same absolute value. For example, if -2 (Mn) were multipled by 1, and +1 (Cl) multiplied by 2, the absolute value of both products would be "2." Hence, the compound containing Mn will have a "1" placed in front of it, and the compound containing Cl will have a "2" in front of it, as follows:

$$2NaCl + (1)MnO_2 + H_2SO_4 \longrightarrow Cl_2 + MnSO_4 + Na_2SO_4 + H_2O$$

(Note that the "1" really isn't necessary before the MnO_2). This balances the Na, Cl and Mn. Balancing now is done as for previous problems. Placing a "2" in front of the H_2SO_4 balances the sulfur, but causes problems with hydrogen and oxygen. Placing a "2" in front of the H_2O alleviates the problem, resulting in the final equation:

$$2NaCl + MnO_2 + 2H_2SO_4 \longrightarrow Cl_2 + MnSO_4 + Na_2SO_4 + 2H_2O$$

An alternative method is to solve this using half reactions, one to describe the oxidation reaction, and the other to describe the reduction. These two reactions are then summed together to get the correct balanced equation. First, a half-reaction is written for the oxidation of chlorine:

$$2Cl^- \longrightarrow Cl_2 + 2e\text{-}$$

(Note that we are not concerned with the fate of the electrons). Another half-reaction is written for the reduction of manganese. This presents a slight problem at first. On the left-hand side, we have MnO_2, a precipitate in molecular form, on the right-hand side, we have $MnSO_4$, which is ionic. We can start by eliminating the spectator ions:

$$MnO_2 \longrightarrow Mn^{++}$$

Obviously this is not the final form. Looking at the overall reaction, it can be seen that the oxygen ends up as water. This can only be accomplished by having it bond to the hydrogen ions from the acid. We now have:

$$MnO_2 + H^+ \longrightarrow Mn^{++} + H_2O$$

We can now add the two electrons that the Mn gains, and balance the elements:

$$MnO_2 + 4H^+ + 2e^- \longrightarrow Mn^{++} + 2H_2O$$

Note that one equation involves the loss of two electrons, and the other a gain of two. Had they not dealt with the same number, a multiplier would have to have been found for each equation, so the number of electrons dealt with in each would be equal. The two equations are now added:

$$2Cl^- + MnO_2\ 4H^+ + 2e^- \longrightarrow 2e^- + Cl_2 + Mn^{++} + 2H_2O$$

The two electrons can be eliminated since they are on both sides of the arrow, and the spectator ions can be added to give the form:

$$2NaCl + MnO_2 + 2H_2SO_4 \longrightarrow Cl_2 + MnSO_4 + Na_2SO_4 + 2H_2O$$

which is the same result as before. For some equations one method is easier than the other. Sometimes redox equations will deal with ions. In such instances, in the final form, not only do the elements have to balance, but so do the charges (i.e., the net charge on the left must equal the net charge on the right). These equations can still be balanced by either of the two previously described methods. For example, the net ionic form of the previous equation is

$$2Cl^- + MnO_2 + 4H^+ \longrightarrow Cl_2 + 2Na^+ + 2H_2O$$

As was stated, the net charge of the left-hand side

$$[(-2) + (+4)] = +2$$

equals the net charge of the right-hand side [+2]. For a final example the equation

$$Cr_2O^=_7 + H^+ + Fe^{++} \longrightarrow Cr^{+++} + Fe^{+++} + H_2O$$

Solving this by oxidation numbers we start with:

$$\overset{+6 \ -2}{Cr_2O_7^=} + \overset{+1}{H^+} + \overset{+2}{Fe^{++}} \longrightarrow \overset{+3}{Cr^{+++}} + \overset{+3}{Fe^{+-+}} + \overset{+1 \ -2}{H_2O}.$$

It can be seen that chromium is reduced from a +6 to a +3 state and iron is oxidized from a +2 to a +3. Multiplying the chromium equation by "1" and the iron equation by "3" gives a common change in oxidation number of "3" for both species. Putting these coefficients into the equation yields:

$$(1) \ Cr_2O^=_7 + H^+ + 3Fe^{++} \longrightarrow Cr^{+++} + 3Fe^{+-+} + H_2O$$

It can be seen that a "2" is needed in front of the Cr on the right-hand side. The 7 oxygens on the left-hand side can be accounted for in the water on the right-hand side, which would then require 14 hydrogen ions on the left. The supposed final balanced equation is:

$$Cr_2O^=_7 + 14H^+ + 3Fe^{++} \longrightarrow 2Cr^{+++} + 3Fe^{+++} + 7H_2O$$

Note that the net charge on the left-hand side

$$[(-2) + (+14) + (3 \times (+2))] = +18$$

should equal the net charge on the right

$$[(2 \times (+3)) + (3 \times (+3))] = +15$$

when an equation is properly balanced. This shows that an error was made here, since 15 and 18 are not equal. First the calculations are checked, and found in order. What was overlooked? Closer inspection shows that two Cr atoms have a charge of -3 in their oxidation numbers, for a total change of -6. Multiplying the iron equation by this factor yields a new equation:

$$Cr_2O^=_7 + 14H^+ + 6Fe^{++} \longrightarrow 2Cr^{+++} + 6Fe^{+++} + 7H_2O$$

Checking the net charges again gives

$$[(-2) + (14 \times (+1)) + (6 \times +1))] = +24$$

for the left-side, and

$$[(2 \times (+3)) + (6 \times (+3))] = +24$$

for the right-side. It is now balanced. The half-reaction method would be as follows: The oxidation equation is easy to write:

$$Fe^{++} \longrightarrow Fe^{+++} + e^-$$

The reducing equation is a little more difficult. We can start with

$$Cr_2O^=_7 \longrightarrow Cr^{+++}$$

Right away we can see see that two Cr's are needed on the right-hand side. Two Cr's will yield a total of six e⁻'s (the change in oxidation number is "3", 2 × 3 = 6). The 7 oxygens present can react with hydrogen to give water, which would require 14 hydrogen ions on the left. This gives:

$$Cr_2O^=_7 + 14H^+ + 6e^- \longrightarrow 2Cr^{+++} + 7H_2O$$

Since the reduction requires 6 electrons, and the oxidation only gives one, we need six times more of the oxidant (sometimes we need to multiply both half-reactions by a different number to obtain a common number of electrons) Multiplying the iron equation by "6," and adding it to the chromium equation yields:

$$Cr_2O^=_7 + 14H^+ + 6e^- + 6Fe^{++} \longrightarrow 2CR^{+++} + 7H_2O + 6e^- + 6Fe^{+++}$$

Once the six electrons are cancelled, we have the same solution as before.

PROBLEM

Balance the following equations:

a) $H_2O_2 + H^+ + Fe^{++} \longrightarrow H_2O + Fe^{+++}$

b) $Cl^- + Cr_2O^=_7 + H^+ \longrightarrow Cl_2 + Cr^{+++} + H_2O$

c) $I_2 + OCl^- + OH^- \longrightarrow IO^-_3 + Cl^- + H_2O$

Solution

a) $H_2O_2 + 2H^+ + 2Fe^{++} \longrightarrow 2H_2O + 2Fe^{+++}$

b) $6Cl^- + Cr_2O_7^= + 14H^+ \longrightarrow 3Cl_2 + 2Cr^{+++} + 7H_2O$

c) $I_2 + 5OCl^- + 2OH^- \longrightarrow 2IO^-_3 + 5Cl^- + H_2O$

PROBLEM

a) The German airships used to condense the water out of their engines' exhaust to use as ballast. Otherwise, the ship would drift higher as the fuel was consumed. A good rule of thumb was that for every gallon of gasoline burned, a gallon of water was produced. Find out how accurate this is on a mass basis. Assume gasoline to be 100% octane [C_8H_{18}], combustion to be 100%, and the recovery of the water to be 100%, the density of octane is 0.706 gm/ml. How many grams of water are produced for each gram of octane consumed?

b) A sample of (at. wt. Fe = 55.8) iron has a mass of 156 gm. The iron is 95.1% pure and is reacted with hydrochloric acid by the unbalanced reaction,

$$Fe^\circ + HCl \longrightarrow FeCl_3 + H_2.$$

The impurities do not react with HCl, all of the iron is consumed, and all of the hydrogen is recovered. How many grams of hydrogen are produced? If the hydrogen is produced in one, large spherical bubble what is its diameter (H_2 has a density of 0.0898 gm/l under these conditions)?

c)   A lump of solid sodium hydroxide (NaOH) has a mass of 15.3 grams. 19.9 grams of pure nitric acid (HNO_3) are needed to just neutralize it. What is the weight percent purity of the NaOH sample?

Solution

a)   Write a balanced equation for the combustion of octane: 8 carbons and 18 hydrogens would give us:

$$C_8H_{18} + O_2 \longrightarrow 8CO_2 + 9H_2O.$$

This would require a total of $12^1/_2$ O_2's. Multiplying the entire equation by "2" to eliminate the fraction yields

$$2C_8H_{18} + 25O_2 \longrightarrow 16CO_2 + 18H_2O.$$

Find the molecular weights of octane and water:

$$(12 \times 8) + (18 \times 1) = 114, (1 \times 2) + (16 \times 1) = 18.$$

Convert 1 gm of octane into moles of octane: $1/114 = 0.00877$ moles of octane.

Use the balanced equation to go from moles of octane to moles of water:

$$(0.00877 / 2) \times 18 = 0.0789 \text{ moles of water.}$$

Convert moles of water to grams of water:

$$0.0789 \times 18 = 1.42 \text{ grams of water}$$

Note that the density of octane was never used in these calculations. The final answer is 1.42 grams of water are produced for every 1.00 gram of octane consumed.

b)   Calculate the total mass of iron.

$$156 \times 0.951 = 148 \text{ grams pure iron.}$$

Calculate the number of moles of iron.

$$148 / 55.8 = 2.65 \text{ moles of iron.}$$

Balance the equation by either method:

$$\overset{0}{Fe^\circ} + \overset{+1\ -1}{HCl} \longrightarrow \overset{+3\ -1}{FeCl_3} + \overset{0}{H_2}. \quad \overset{0}{Fe} \longrightarrow \overset{+3}{Fe^{+++}},$$

a change of +3.

$$\overset{+1}{2H^+} \longrightarrow \overset{0}{H_2},$$

a change of -2 (2 atoms involved).

To obtain a common change in oxidation number (absolute value), multiply the Fe by 2 and the H by 6. This gives

$$2Fe° + 6HCl \longrightarrow 2FeCl_3 + 3H_2 .$$

OR

$$Fe° \longrightarrow Fe^{+++} + 3e^-, \text{ and } 2H^+ + 2e^- \longrightarrow H_2 .$$

Note that 3 electrons are supplied by the iron, and 2 are consumed by the hydrogen. Multiplying the Fe by 2, and the H by 3 results in a total of 6 e⁻'s swapping atoms.

$$2Fe° \longrightarrow 2Fe^{+++} + 6e^-, \text{ and } 6H^+ + 6e^- \longrightarrow 3H2.$$

Adding these equations, including spectator ions, and cancelling electrons yield:

$$2Fe° + 6HCl \longrightarrow 2FeCl_3 + 3H_2.$$

Calculate moles of H_2 produced per mole of Fe consumed,

$$(2.65/2) \times 3 = 3.98 \text{ moles of } H_2.$$

Convert to grams of H_2, $3.98 \times 2.00 = 7.96$ grams of hydrogen. This answers the first part.

Calculate the volume of hydrogen,

$$7.96/0.0898 = 88.6 \text{ liters of } H_2.$$

Convert to cm^3,

$$88.6 \text{ liters} = 88,600 \text{ cm}_3.$$

The volume of a sphere is $V = 4/3\pi r^3$, and solving for "r," we get 27.6 cm.

The question asked for diameter, which is twice the radius, so

$$2 \times 27.6 = 55.2 \text{ cm}.$$

c)   Determine molecular weights for NaOH & HNO_3,

$$(1 \times 23) + (1 \times 16) + (1 \times 2) = 40.0 \text{ Daltons,}$$

$$\text{and } (1 \times 1) + (1 \times 14) + (3 \times 16) = 63.0 \text{ Daltons, respectively.}$$

Write a balanced equation,

$$HNO_3 + NaOH \longrightarrow \text{water} + \text{salt,}$$

The salt in this case must be sodium nitrate,

$$HNO_3 + NaOH \longrightarrow H_2O + NaNO_3,$$

Looking at the elements on both sides of the arrow, one can see that by luck the equation is already balanced. Calculate the moles of HNO_3 used,

$$19.9/63.0 = 0.316 \text{ moles.}$$

Calculate the number of moles of NaOH present,

$$(0.316/1) \times 1 = 0.316 \text{ moles.}$$

Calculate grams of NaOH present,

$$0.316 \times 40.0 = 12.6 \text{ grams.}$$

Calculate the weight percentage of NaOH of the sample's mass,

$$(12.6/15.3) \times 100\% = 82.4\% \text{ purity.}$$

II. ELECTRONIC STRUCTURE AND THE PERIODIC TABLE

1. Electronic Structure

The model of the hydrogen atom that Niels Bohr introduced early in the twenti-eth century, showing an electron orbiting a central nucleus in a manner analogous to a planet-sun system, is quite outdated and inaccurate. The exact location of a particu-lar electron about a nucleus at any given moment in time cannot be accurately known. Instead, predictions can be made as to the most *likely* location of an electron about a nucleus. These predictions can be made because the electrons do occupy definite energy levels about the nucleus. Within these definite energy levels are regions where there are high probabilities of finding an electron. These areas are often thought of in terms of a cloud of negative charge, called an "electron cloud." This cloud is more dense in areas of high probability, and more diffuse in the areas of lower probability. These electron clouds are referred to as "atomic orbitals." The definite energy levels that contain these atomic orbitals are often referred to as shells. These shells surround the nucleus much like the layers of an onion. The shells are numbered, with the one closest to the nucleus as "1," and also designated by letters of the alphabet, starting with K, for the shell closest to the nucleus. The maximum number of electrons that each energy level can hold is determined by the formula,

$$N = 2n^2.$$

where N is the maximum number of electrons for the given energy level, and n is the shell's number. Below is a table that summarizes this data for the first seven shells. These energy shells can be subdivided into different *subshells*. Electron transitions between different subshells is possible. These subshells are further subdivided into *orbitals*. The maximum number of electrons

ELECTRON ENERGY LEVELS

letter designation	numeric value (n)	maximum number of electrons ($2n^2$)
K	1	2
L	2	8
M	3	18
N	4	32
O	5	50*
P	6	72*
Q	7	98*

* The number given is hypothetical, it should be confirmed when atoms of large enough atomic number to fill these shells are produced.

that can occupy any orbital at one time is two. To help predict the most probable location of these electrons, the following four quantum numbers are used. The "Principal Quantum Number," n, is used to designate the volume of space in which the electron moves and the energy of the electron. The n number refers to the energy shell in which the electron is residing. The n number is always an integer, and can vary in theory from 1 to infinity. In all known atoms, it is never above 7. As was mentioned previously, sometimes the letters K,L,M, ... etc. are used in place of the n numbers 1,2,3, ... etc. The "Subsidiary Quantum Number," ℓ designates the shape of the region that the electron is most likely to occupy. The ℓ number is equal to n-l, and in theory can vary from 0 to infinity. In all known atoms, it is never more than 3. Just as letters are sometimes used for the n number, so they are used for the ℓ. s,p,d, f,g,h,i ... are used in place of 0,1,2,3,4,5,6 ... etc.

The "Magnetic Quantum Number," m, is used to designate the vector, or a general way of orientation of the region of high electron probability in space. m can vary in value from -1 to +1, and every integral value in between (meaning zero can be m). The "Spin Quantum Number," s, specifies the direction of the electron spin about a nucleus. An electron orbiting a nucleus is limited to only two possible spins:

$$+\tfrac{1}{2}h/2\pi, \text{ and } -\tfrac{1}{2}h/2\pi,$$

where "h" is a term known as Planck's constant. Usually the spin term is simply shortened to $+\tfrac{1}{2}$ and $-\tfrac{1}{2}$. No two electrons in a particular atom can have the same four quantum numbers. This means that for two electrons to occupy the same orbital, they must have opposite spin. This concept is known as the *Pauli exclusion principle*.

A. GROUND VS. EXCITED STATES

When all of the electrons in an atom are in the orbitals of lowest possible energy, the atom is said to be in the "ground state." If energy is somehow imparted to these electrons, they are boosted up to higher energy orbitals. Such an atom is said to be in an "excited state." When the electrons return to the ground state, this energy is given off in the form of electromagnetic radiation.

B. CONVENTIONAL NOTATION FOR ELECTRONIC STRUCTURE

The electronic notation involves the use of the first two quantum numbers. For example, hydrogen has only one electron. It is in the first energy level (n = 1), and of subshell s. To designate this, it is written $1s^1$; the superscript 1 meaning there is one electron in this orbital. Helium has a total of two electrons, in the same orbital. The electronic notation for helium would be $1s^2$, where 1 represents the first energy level, s denotes the subshell (s subshells are spherical in shape), and the superscript 2 denotes two electrons occupying this shell. According to the Pauli exclusion principle, these two electrons must have opposite quantum spin numbers. To represent this, sometimes boxes with arrows are used. Each box represents a different subshell, and the arrows represent electrons. Arrows of different direction represent electrons of different spin. Hence, hydrogen would be represented as:

1s

↑

The electronic structure of helium would be:

1s

↑↓

Note that the arrows are going in opposite directions to denote the opposite spins of the electrons. The first energy level contains only the single s subshell. Proceeding to the next element, lithium, a structure of

$1s^2 2s^1$

is obtained. This denotes that the 1s orbital is filled, as in helium, and the 2s subshell has one electron in it. This would be shown as:

1s   2s

↑↓	↑

Note that beryllium has 4 total electrons, as

$1s^2 2s^2$,

and would be shown as

1s   2s

↑↓	↑↓

Note the paired electrons of opposite spin, and a total of 4 electrons, but only 2 valence electrons. Starting with the next element, boron, another subshell of the second energy level begins to fill. The p subshell is shaped like a dumbbell. There are actually three p's, each lying in a plane at right angles from the other two. Using the conventional terminology of Cartesian coordinates, these are known as p_x, p_y and p_z, the subscript denoting which plane they are lying in. All three of the p's are of equal value, the x, y, and z terms being arbitrary. Note that these orientation factors are determined by the m number. [Since $\ell = 1$, and m = all integers between -1 and +1, we get m values of -1, 0, and +1. That shows three subdivisions of the p, and that is what is observed.] The notation for boron would be

$1s^2 2s^2 2p^1$,

and would be shown as:

1s   2s $2p_x$ $2p_y$ $2p_z$

↑↓	↑↓	↑		

Note the unoccupied p orbitals. As can be predicted, carbon would be

$1s^2 2s^2 2p^2$,

and would be shown as

1s   2s $2p_x$ $2p_y$ $2p_z$

↑↓	↑↓	↑	↑	

Note that the p subshell will fill each orbital with a single electron before it will pair an orbital with two electrons of opposite spin. This is true of any subshell; the electrons enter each orbital of a given type singly and with identical spins before any pairing of electrons of opposite spin occurs within those orbitals. This is known as Hund's Rule. Nitrogen will follow this as

$1s^2 2s^2 2p^3$

(for review, note that nitrogen will have a total of 7 electrons, 5 of them valence electrons.), and be depicted as

1s	2s	2p$_x$	2p$_y$	2p$_z$
↑↓	↑↓	↑	↑	↑

With oxygen, the p orbitals begin to pair up

$1s^2 2s^2 2p^4$

1s	2s	2p$_x$	2p$_y$	2p$_z$
↑↓	↑↓	↑↓	↑	↑

Fluorine adds another electron to pair up, and with neon the second energy level is filled, giving

$1s^2 2s^2 2p^6$

[10 total electrons, 8 of which are valence],

1s	2s	2p$_x$	2p$_y$	2p$_z$
↑↓	↑↓	↑↓	↑↓	↑↓

Note all of the elements in the same vertical row in the periodic table will have the same *outer* electron configuration. For example, sodium will have the same outer configuration as lithium, it will just be one energy level higher, with the inner electron configuration matching that of neon;

$1s^2 2s^2 2p^6 3s^1$

1s	2s	2p$_x$	2p$_y$	2p$_z$	3s
↑↓	↑↓	↑↓	↑↓	↑↓	↑

Silicone's outer electrons will match those of carbon,

$1s^2 2s^2 2p^6 3s^2 3p^2$

1s	2s	2p$_x$	2p$_y$	2p$_z$	3s	3p$_x$	3p$_y$	3p$_z$
↑↓	↑↓	↑↓	↑↓	↑↓	↑↓	↑	↑	

Argon will match that of neon,

$1s^2 2s^2 2p^6 3s^2 3p^6$

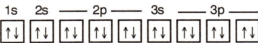

As one begins to fill the fourth energy level, the electron notation follows the predictable rule mentioned above for potassium ($...4s^1$) and calcium ($...4s^2$). However, at scandium, a new rule needs to be introduced. Recall that the ℓ quantum number is equal to n-1. For n = 3, that gives ℓ = 2, or a "d" orbital. Note that although we are in the fourth row of the table, it is the third row that is filling with electrons in these *transition metals,* hence the number of valence electrons will not change. Also, recall that the m quantum number can have any integral value from -1 to +1, for ℓ = 2, this gives m = -2, -1, 0, 1, 2, which gives five sub-levels (orbitals)

for the d subshell. These five orbitals are all of equal value, and follow Hund's Rule for pairing up. The nomenclature for scandium is

$$1s^2 2s^2 2p^6 3s^2 3p^6 3d^1 4s^2,$$

which shows 21 total electrons, but only two valence electrons, just as magnesium has. This would be represented as

1s	2s	—— 2p ——	3s	—— 3p ——	———— 3d ————	4s
↑↓	↑↓	↑↓ ↑↓ ↑↓	↑↓	↑↓ ↑↓ ↑↓	↑ ☐ ☐ ☐ ☐	↑↓

Using the rule as introduced, the electron configuration of titanium would be

$$1s^2 2s^2 2p^6 3s^2 3p^6 3d^2 4s^2,$$

1s	2s	—— 2p ——	3s	—— 3p ——	———— 3d ————	4s
↑↓	↑↓	↑↓ ↑↓ ↑↓	↑↓	↑↓ ↑↓ ↑↓	↑ ↑ ☐ ☐ ☐	↑↓

The same rule can be used for vanadium. At chromium, another aspect of electron behavior must be revealed. The predicted configuration would be:

1s	2s	—— 2p ——	3s	—— 3p ——	———— 3d ————	4s
↑↓	↑↓	↑↓ ↑↓ ↑↓	↑↓	↑↓ ↑↓ ↑↓	↑ ↑ ↑ ↑ ☐	↑↓

However, the attraction of four electrons in the 3d is strong enough to pull in an electron from the 4s, so the proper configuration would be:

1s	2s	—— 2p ——	3s	—— 3p ——	———— 3d ————	4s
↑↓	↑↓	↑↓ ↑↓ ↑↓	↑↓	↑↓ ↑↓ ↑↓	↑ ↑ ↑ ↑ ↑	↑

represented by

$$1s^2 2s^2 2p^6 3s^2 3p^6 3d^5 4s^1$$

(22 total electrons, 1 valence). At the next element, manganese, the 4s fills up again,

$$1s^2 2s^2 2p^6 3s^2 3p^6 3d^5 4s^2,$$

(2 valence electrons, out of a total of 25),

1s	2s	—— 2p ——	3s	—— 3p ——	———— 3d ————	4s
↑↓	↑↓	↑↓ ↑↓ ↑↓	↑↓	↑↓ ↑↓ ↑↓	↑ ↑ ↑ ↑ ↑	↑↓

At iron, the d orbitals begin pairing up,

$$1s^2 2s^2 2p^6 3s^2 3p^6 3d^6 4s^2,$$

1s	2s	—— 2p ——	3s	—— 3p ——	———— 3d ————	4s
↑↓	↑↓	↑↓ ↑↓ ↑↓	↑↓	↑↓ ↑↓ ↑↓	↑↓ ↑ ↑ ↑ ↑	↑↓

This continues up to copper. The force of 9 electrons in the d level is strong enough to pull in an electron from the 4s, giving

$$1s^2 2s^2 2p^6 3s^2 3s^2 3p^6 3d^{10} 4s^1$$

1s	2s	—— 2p ——	3s	—— 3p ——	———— 3d ————	4s
↑↓	↑↓	↑↓ ↑↓ ↑↓	↑↓	↑↓ ↑↓ ↑↓	↑↓ ↑↓ ↑↓ ↑↓ ↑↓	↑

At zinc, the 4s fills up again,

$$1s^2 2s^2 2p^6 3s^2 3p^6 3d^{10} 4s^2$$

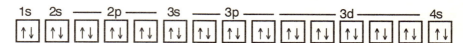

With gallium, we begin filling the 4p's, following the rules given for them. For example, selenium would be

$1s^2 2s^2 2p^6 3s^2 3p^6 3d^{10} 4s^2 4p^4$, shown as

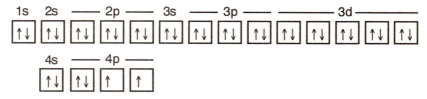

Again, one can apply these rules when moving down vertically on the periodic table. Remember when dealing with d subshells, they are one energy level lower than the outer energy level of the atom. For example, niobium (#41), starting with a neon core, would be

$3s^2 3p^6 3d^{10} 4s^2 4p^6 4d^3 5s^2$,

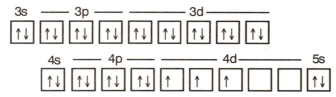

Silver, starting with a neon core would be

$3s^2 3p^6 3d^{10} 4s^2 4p^6 4d^{10} 5s^1$, or

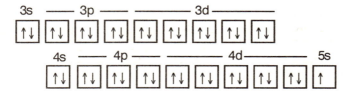

Iodine would be

$3s^2 3p^6 3d^{10} 4s^2 4p^6 4d^{10} 5s^2 5p^5$, or

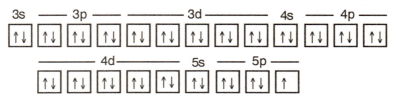

The last set of orbitals that involves another set of rules are those of the *Lanthanoid* and *Actinoid Series*. Again, looking at the quantum numbers, when n = 4, $\ell = 3$, which corresponds to an "f" subshell. The m number of an "f" subshell can

have a value of -3, -3, -1, 0, 1, 2, 3, which gives us at total of seven orbitals in the "f" subshell, at two electrons each; that is, 14 electrons. Lanthanum, predictably, would be (starting with a xenon core) $5d^16s^2$. With the next element, cerium, the "f" orbitals begin to fill, observing Hund's Rule. Note that it is a 4f that is filling, two energy levels below the outer level. This rule holds true for all of these series. Cerium, the first of the lanthanoid series, begins to fill the 4f orbitals. However, the force of one electron in the 4f is enough to pull the electron out of the 5d. The 5d electron joins the 4f. Hence cerium (starting with a xenon core) would be

$4f^25d^06s^2$, or

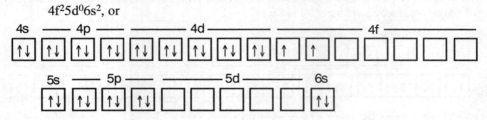

The 4f orbitals continue to fill, obeying Hund's Rule, and the 5d remains empty. Neodymium would be

$4f^45d^06s^2$

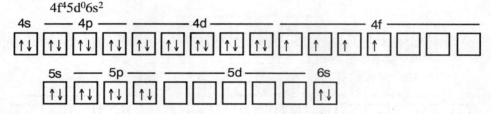

At gadolinium, an electron again goes to the 5d, giving

$4f^75d^16s^2$

4s ——— 4p ——— ————— 4d ——————— ——————— 4f ———————

5s ——— 5p ——— ————— 5d ——————— 6s

With terbium, the lone 5d electron is again pulled down into the 4f, giving

$4f^95d^06s^2$

4s ——— 4p ——— ————— 4d ——————— ——————— 4f ———————

5s ——— 5p ——— ————— 5d ——————— 6s

At lutetium, an electron again goes to the 5d, giving

$4f^{14}5d^16s^2$,

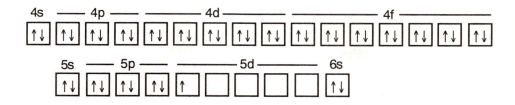

From there we proceed to hafnium, and continue to fill the 5d subshell. The notation for tungsten, starting with a xenon core would be

$4f^{14}5d^56s^1$.

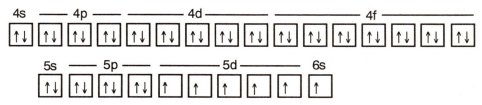

Polonium would be $4f^{14}5d^{10}6s^26p^4$.

The same rules can be applied directly below to the actinoid series. Uranium, starting with a xenon core would be

$4f^{14}5d^{10}5f^46d^07s^2$,

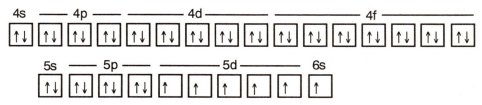

PROBLEM

Write the complete electronic notation and representations showing Hund's Rule for:

a) osmium
b) cadmium
c) calcium
d) strontium
e) curium

Solution

a) Os — $1s^22s^22p^63s^23p^63d^{10}4s^24p^64d^{10}4f^{14}5s^25p^65d^66s^2$

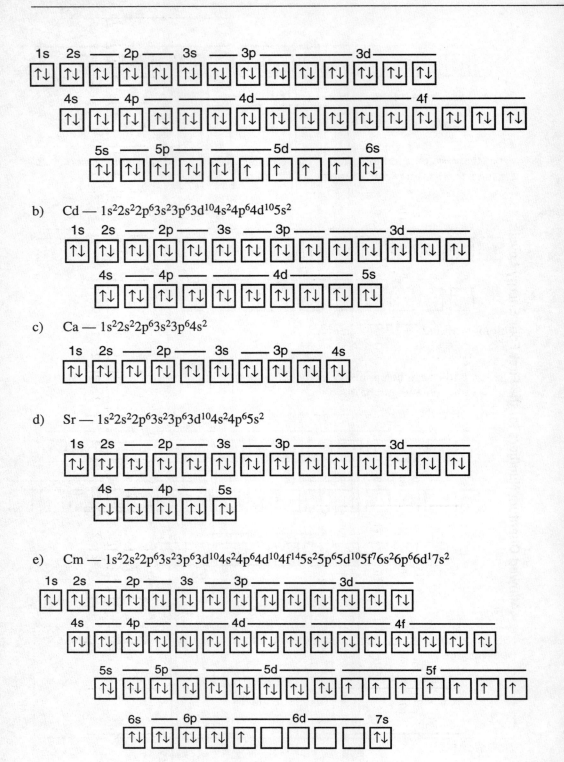

b) Cd — $1s^22s^22p^63s^23p^63d^{10}4s^24p^64d^{10}5s^2$

c) Ca — $1s^22s^22p^63s^23p^64s^2$

d) Sr — $1s^22s^22p^63s^23p^63d^{10}4s^24p^65s^2$

e) Cm — $1s^22s^22p^63s^23p^63d^{10}4s^24p^64d^{10}4f^{14}5s^25p^65d^{10}5f^76s^26p^66d^17s^2$

Allowed Quantum Numbers for the First Four Energy Levels

Energy Level—n: 1

Subshell—l	Orbital—m	Spin—$S\left(\frac{h}{2\pi}\right)$
0 (s)	0	$+\frac{1}{2}$, $-\frac{1}{2}$

Energy Level—n: 2

Subshell—l	Orbital—m	Spin—$S\left(\frac{h}{2\pi}\right)$
0 (s)	0	$+\frac{1}{2}$, $-\frac{1}{2}$
1 (p)	-1	$+\frac{1}{2}$, $-\frac{1}{2}$
	0	$+\frac{1}{2}$, $-\frac{1}{2}$
	+1	$+\frac{1}{2}$, $-\frac{1}{2}$

Energy Level—n: 3

Subshell—l	Orbital—m	Spin—$S\left(\frac{h}{2\pi}\right)$
0 (s)	0	$+\frac{1}{2}$, $-\frac{1}{2}$
1 (p)	-1	$+\frac{1}{2}$, $-\frac{1}{2}$
	0	$+\frac{1}{2}$, $-\frac{1}{2}$
	+1	$+\frac{1}{2}$, $-\frac{1}{2}$
2 (d)	-2	$+\frac{1}{2}$, $-\frac{1}{2}$
	-1	$+\frac{1}{2}$, $-\frac{1}{2}$
	0	$+\frac{1}{2}$, $-\frac{1}{2}$
	+1	$+\frac{1}{2}$, $-\frac{1}{2}$
	+2	$+\frac{1}{2}$, $-\frac{1}{2}$

Energy Level—n: 4

Subshell—l	Orbital—m	Spin—$S\left(\frac{h}{2\pi}\right)$
0 (s)	0	$+\frac{1}{2}$, $-\frac{1}{2}$
1 (p)	-1	$+\frac{1}{2}$, $-\frac{1}{2}$
	0	$+\frac{1}{2}$, $-\frac{1}{2}$
	+1	$+\frac{1}{2}$, $-\frac{1}{2}$
2 (d)	-2	$+\frac{1}{2}$, $-\frac{1}{2}$
	-1	$+\frac{1}{2}$, $-\frac{1}{2}$
	0	$+\frac{1}{2}$, $-\frac{1}{2}$
	+1	$+\frac{1}{2}$, $-\frac{1}{2}$
	+2	$+\frac{1}{2}$, $-\frac{1}{2}$
3 (f)	-3	$+\frac{1}{2}$, $-\frac{1}{2}$
	-2	$+\frac{1}{2}$, $-\frac{1}{2}$
	-1	$+\frac{1}{2}$, $-\frac{1}{2}$
	0	$+\frac{1}{2}$, $-\frac{1}{2}$
	+1	$+\frac{1}{2}$, $-\frac{1}{2}$
	+2	$+\frac{1}{2}$, $-\frac{1}{2}$
	+3	$+\frac{1}{2}$, $-\frac{1}{2}$

2. Classification of Elements and Chemical Properties of Groups and Rows

Elements in the same vertical row of the periodic table have the same number of valence electrons. Group 1A (starting with hydrogen) has one valence electron, 2A (starting with beryllium) has two, 3A (starting with boron) has three, etc. for all of the "A" groups. The transition metals (1B thru 3B) as well as the Lanthanoid and Actinoid Series usually have two valence electrons. The few exceptions to this can easily be predicted using the electron orbital notation mentioned in the last section.

A.   FIRST AND SECOND IONIZATION ENERGIES

All atoms strive to have a full outer shell. For hydrogen and helium, this means two outer electrons. For all other atoms, it is eight. The energy required to remove one electron from an atom is known as its "First Ionization Potential." The energy required to remove a second electron is known as "Second Ionization Potential," etc. Since the group 1A elements need only to lose one electron to have a full outer shell, their first ionization energy is fairly low, ranging from 3.9 electron volts (eV) with cesium to 5.4 eV with lithium. However, giving up a second electron is much more difficult for these atoms, since that will keep their outer shell from being full. The secondary ionization potentials for this group ranges from 25.1 eV for cesium to 75.6 eV for lithium, significantly higher than the first ionization potential. The group 2A elements will want to lose two electrons, hence their secondary ionization potential will be lower than that of the 1A group.

The primary and secondary ionization energies for beryllium are 9.3 and 18.2 eV, respectively. Note that it does take more energy to form a +2 ion from a 2A element than it does a +1 ion from a 1A element. Using this rule it can logically and correctly be deduced that it would take even more energy to form a +3 ion from a 3A element. These ionization potentials will increase as one moves across the periodic table. At the far right-hand side, the noble gases are the most difficult to ionize since they already have a full outer shell. The first and second ionization potentials for neon are 21.6 and 41.1 eV, respectively. It should also be noted that ionization energy decreases slightly as one moves vertically down the table. For all practical purposes, the ionization potentials of the transition metals can be treated as if they belonged to group 2A.

B.   ELECTRON AFFINITIES

The opposite of losing electrons is gaining. The measure of energy released when an electron is added to an atom to form a negative ion is called "electron affinity." As can be expected, the noble gases have zero electron affinity, since their outer shell is full, and they neither want to gain nor lose electrons. The metals, since they tend to lose electrons, would have very low electron affinities. For example, lithium needs only to lose one electron to have a full outer shell, whereas it would have to gain seven. Hence its electron affinity is only 0.54 eV. Contrast this with fluorine, which will have a full outer shell by either gaining just one electron, or losing seven. Its electron affinity is 3.45 eV (remember, this is energy given up, not required). Electron affinity increases as one moves to the upper right-hand corner of the periodic table (The noble gases are not included in this.).

C. ELECTRONEGATIVITY

Electronegativity is the attraction of an atom for the electrons in its outer shell. It is related to ionization potential and electron affinity. Electronegativity will be used later on to predict bonding and polarity of molecules. If the noble gases are removed from the table, electronegativity increases as one moves to the upper right-hand corner of the periodic table, and decreases as one moves to the lower left-hand corner. Hence, among the non-radioactive elements, fluorine is the most electronegative and cesium is the least.

III. BONDING

1. Types of bonds

A. IONIC BONDS

If there is a great difference in electronegativities between atoms, an ionic bond will occur. An ionic bond involves an actual transfer of electrons from one atom to another, creating ions which are held together by electrostatic attraction. For example, cesium has one valence electron, and fluorine, seven. Due to the difference in electronegativities, fluorine can pull the outer electron off cesium, and incorporate it into its own outer shell. The result will be a Cs+ cation and a F- anion. Since opposite charges attract, the two ions come together to form CsF.

Sometimes more than two ions are needed. In the case of potassium and sulfur, K^+ and S^{-2} are formed. To balance out the charges, two sulfurs are needed for every potassium, hence the formula is K_2S. Ionic bonds are the strongest chemical bonds known. It takes a great deal of energy to dissociate them.

B. POLAR COVALENT BONDS

If there is a difference in electronegativities between bonding atoms, an unequal sharing of electrons will occur, and the resultant bond will be neither ionic nor truly covalent. This type of bond is known as a polar covalent bond, as it will have a slightly positive end and a slightly negative end due to the unequal sharing of electrons. For example, in a molecule of iodine fluoride, the atom of fluorine is more electronegative than the atom of iodine. The electrons will therefore spend more time with the fluorine, giving it a slightly negative charge. The iodine atom will consequently have a slightly positive charge.

C. COVALENT BONDS

If the difference in electronegativities between atoms is slight or non-existent, a covalent bond will form. A covalent bond involves a sharing of electrons from one atom to another. Covalent bonds are weaker than ionic bonds. An example of a covalent bond would be the formation of a chlorine molecule, Cl_2, from individual chlorine atoms. The details of covalent bonding will be discussed in section 2-A, Lewis Electron Dot Structures.

D. HYDROGEN BONDING

When hydrogen is involved with the above dipole forces, interacting with such atoms as fluorine, nitrogen, or oxygen, a much stronger bond is established than in ordinary dipole interactions. The attractive force exerted between these atoms is so great that it has been given the special name of "Hydrogen Bonding." There are two reasons why the hydrogen bond is greater than the ordinary dipole.

1) The difference in electronegativity between hydrogen and the elements ni-

trogen, oxygen, and fluorine is quite large. As a result, the electrons are markedly displaced from the hydrogen.

2) The small size of the hydrogen atom allows it to approach the other atoms very closely.

E. DIPOLE INTERACTIONS

Recall that in polar bonding, a dipole moment is established. If there is not another dipole in the same molecule to cancel it, the resulting molecule is polar, (having a positive and a negative end). In polar molecules, the negative end of one molecule is attracted to the positive end of another. An example of this would be iodine chloride. Due to the differences in electronegativity, the chlorine atom will have the shared electrons for a greater period of time than the iodine, placing a negative charge on the chlorine atom and a positive one on the iodine. In solid ICl the molecules are tightly aligned in a matter similar to the sodium chloride crystal.

Iodine is attracted by electrostatic forces on all sides of the neighboring chloride atoms, and the chlorine is equally attracted on all sides by neighboring iodine. Unlike the very strong ionic bonds in NaCl, the dipole forces holding the crystal structure of ICl together are much weaker. As a result, when ICl is heated only to 27°C, the relatively weak dipole forces are no longer able to hold the crystal together, and the solid melts.

F. VAN DER WAALS FORCES

The positively charged nucleus of an atom can attract and alter the electron cloud of a neighboring atom. The momentary shift in the electron creates a momentary dipole moment that can induce a similar, momentary dipole in an adjacent molecule. These very weak forces work not only among polar molecules but non-polar as well. They are termed *van der Waals Forces* or *London Forces,* and increase with the mass of the molecule. The behavior of helium is a good example of how very weak these forces are.

In helium, the only attractive force is a very weak van der Waals. The attraction of one helium atom for another is so slight that even at absolute zero (0 K), helium remains a liquid (at normal pressure)! The attraction of one helium atom for another is so slight that helium atoms will never get close enough at ordinary pressure to form a solid.

Below is a chart that compares the relative strengths of the different types of bonds:

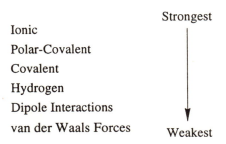

Ionic

Polar-Covalent

Covalent

Hydrogen

Dipole Interactions

van der Waals Forces

Strongest

Weakest

2. Lewis Electron Dot Structures

A. LEWIS ELECTRON DOT STRUCTURES

The Lewis structure simply shows the valence electrons of an atom or ion. A few examples would be

$$\text{Na}^{\cdot} \quad \text{Sr:} \quad :\overset{..}{\text{S}}: \quad :\overset{..}{\text{I}}: \quad \text{Xe}$$

for sodium, strontium, sulfur, iodine, and xenon, respectively. Returning to the above problem of the covalent bonding of chlorine, note from the Lewis structure,

$$:\overset{..}{\text{Cl}}:$$

that each Cl atom has one unpaired electron. Were two Cl atoms to come together and share their unpaired electron with the other, a covalent bond will be formed, and each Cl atom will have a full outer shell. This can be shown as

$$:\overset{..}{\text{Cl}} . \, {}^{\cdot}\overset{..}{\text{Cl}}:$$

shared e–'s

Another example would be oxygen gas, O_2. Note the Lewis structure for O is

$$:\overset{..}{\text{O}}$$

To form a covalent bond two pairs of electrons will have to be shared, creating what is appropriately called a "double bond", giving the resulting structure

$$\overset{..}{\text{O}}::\overset{..}{\text{O}}$$

Sometimes lines are used rather than dots, in this case, each line represents a pair of electrons. Such a structure for Cl_2 and O_2 would be

$$|\,\overline{\text{Cl}} - \overline{\text{Cl}}\,|, \quad \overline{\text{O}} = \overline{\text{O}},$$

respectively. Often unshared electron pairs are not shown, giving the representations as follows

$$\text{Cl} - \text{Cl}, \quad \text{O} = \text{O}.$$

B. RESONANCE STRUCTURES

Sometimes a single structure cannot accurately represent a molecule or ion. An example would be sulfur-dioxide, SO_2, which can have either oxygen double bonded to the sulfur, which could be represented as

The "real" structure is neither of these, but a hybrid structure in between the two. The concept is called "resonance", and the structure is called a "resonance hybrid," and is best represented by

It must be stressed that SO_2 does not spend part of the time in one state and the remainder in the other; it is in a state that is a hybrid between the two.

C.   FORMAL CHARGE

Often a group of atoms can covalently bond, and as a group need to gain or lose electron to fill all outer shells. As a result of these excess or deficient electrons, the group of atoms will have an overall charge, and is called a polyatomic ion. An example of such is sulfate, $SO_4^=$, which needs two additional electrons to fill the outer shells, giving an overall charge of -2, it can be represented as

$$\left[\begin{array}{c} :\ddot{O}: \\ :\ddot{O}: \ddot{S} :\ddot{O}: \\ :\ddot{O}: \end{array} \right]^=$$

Another example is ammonia, NH_4^+, which has to give up an electron to have all outer shells full, resulting in a +1 charge. It can be represented as

$$\left[\begin{array}{c} H \\ H:\ddot{N}:H \\ \ddot{H} \end{array} \right]^+$$

D.   LEWIS ACIDS AND BASES

A Lewis acid is anything that can accept a pair of electrons, such as Cu^{++}. A Lewis base is anything that can donate a pair of electrons, such as $O^=$.

E.   VALENCE SHELL ELECTRONS AND THE PREDICTION OF SHAPES OF MOLECULES

Often in covalent bonding, electrons from an s orbital will join those from a p. As can be expected, the shape of the resultant hybrid orbital will help determine the shape of the molecule that is formed. Recall that the s is spherical and the p dumbbell in shape. Obviously the more p orbitals present, the more the resultant hybrid orbital will resemble a p than an s. Such is a case in methane, CH_4, where one s electron is blended with three electrons from p orbitals. This is called sp^3 hybridization. The resultant orbital is in the shape of a tetrahedon, and so is the shape of a methane molecule. In boron tri-fluoride, BF_3, one s electron is blended with two electrons from p orbitals. This is known as sp^2 hybridization, and the resultant orbital has less p character than the above sp^3. The sp^2 hybrid is a flat, triangular (trigonal planar) shaped orbital, and so is the resultant molecule, with a fluorine atom at each corner of the triangle.

IV. PHASES AND PHASE EQUILIBRIA

1. Standard Temperature, Pressure, and Standard Molar Volume

Since gases will assume not only the shape of their container, but its volume too, standard conditions that can be easily replicated in any laboratory have been agreed upon. Standard temperature is the temperature of melting ice, which is 0°C, or 273 K. Standard pressure is the pressure of the earth's atmosphere at sea level, which is one atmosphere, or 760 Torr. Collectively, standard pressure and temperature are known as STP. One mole of ideal gas at STP will occupy a volume of 22.4 liters. The ideal gas can be used to calculate pressure, temperature, volume, or number of moles of a gas, provided three of these four parameters are known.

The equation for the ideal gas law is

$$PV = nRT,$$

where P is the pressure in atmospheres, V is the volume in liters, n is the number of moles, T is the temperature in Kelvin, and R is the universal gas law constant. R, like π or e, will always have the same value. In the case of this equation, it is 0.0821 L·Atm/mole·K. For example, the ideal gas law can verify the molar volume of an ideal gas. Putting into the equation, $PV = nRT$, standard conditions, we get

$$(1 \text{ Atm}) \, (V) = (1 \text{ mole}) \, (0.0821 \text{ L·Atm/mole·K}) \, (273 \text{ K}).$$

Solving for V yields 22.4 liters. When using this law, it is important to keep the pressure in atmospheres, volume in liters, and temperature in Kelvin. With the above ideal gas law, almost all gas problems can be solved. However, there are simpler laws of more limited applicability, that can be easier to use, and are not so stringent with the units used. The first to be covered is Boyle's Law. Boyle's Law is: The volume of a given gas held at constant temperature is inversely proportional to the pressure under which it is measured. Stated mathematically,

$$P_1V_1 = P_2V_2$$

where P_1 and V_1 are the initial pressure and volume, respectively (in any units), and P_2 and V_2 are the final pressure and volume, respectively (in the same units as P_1 and V_1). For example, if a gas has a volume of 200 ml at 760 Torr pressure, and keeping the temperature constant, what will its volume be if the pressure were lowered to 190 Torr? By simple logic, it can be deduced that the new volume should be greater than the original. Plugging the values into the formula for Boyle's Law, we get

$$(760 \text{ Torr}) \, (200 \text{ ml}) = (190 \text{ Torr}) \, (V_2).$$

Solving for V_2 gives a new volume of 800 ml, which is in agreement with the deduction made earlier. Another useful law is Charles' Law, which is: The volume of a given mass of gas is directly proportional to its temperature on the Kelvin scale when the pressure is constant. Mathematically stated this is

$$V_1/T_1 = V_2/T_2,$$

where V_1 and T_1 are the initial volume and temperature (volume can be in any units, temperature *must* be in Kelvin), and V_2 and T_2 are the final volume and temperature (in whatever units are used for V_1 and Kelvin). For example, if a gas has a volume of 300 ml at 283 K, and the pressure is kept constant, what is the new volume if the temperature is raised to 303 K? As was done before, using logic, one can conclude that at a higher temperature, if the pressure were kept constant, the volume should increase. Hence the new volume should be greater than 300 ml. Plugging into the above equation, we get

$$(300 \text{ ml}) / (283 \text{ K}) = (V_2) / (303 \text{ K}).$$

Solving for V_2 we get

$$V_2 = 321 \text{ ml},$$

which agrees with our initial speculation.

The kinetic molecular theory of gases can be summarized in the three following statements developed from the five postulates for kinetic theory:

1. Gases are composed of separate particles called molecules. The volume occupied by these individual molecules is quite insignificant when compared to the total volume of the gas. These gas molecules are relatively far apart and have little attraction for one another.

2. Gas molecules are in constant motion. The molecules can vary in speed. They travel in straight lines in all directions, and have perfectly elastic collisions with the walls of their containers and each other. The average number of collisions with the walls of their container determines the pressure of the gas.

3. The average kinetic energy of the molecules of different gas molecules is the same at the same temperature. This kinetic energy increases and decreases with the temperature. Since

    $$\text{kinetic energy} = \frac{1}{2}mv^2,$$

    where m = the mass of the molecule and v = the velocity of the molecule, molecules of small mass (e.g. hydrogen) must move at higher speeds than more massive molecules (e.g. chlorine) to have the same kinetic energy.

The laws mentioned above apply to ideal gases, which do not exist. Real gases differ from ideal gases in several ways.

1. Their molecules are not geometric points, i.e., they do occupy space.

2. Real gas molecules do experience a slight attraction for one another.

3. The collisions of real gas molecules are not perfectly elastic. Real gases can behave very much like ideal gases under conditions of low pressure and high temperature.

When a mixture of gases is present, the molar fraction of each gas present exerts its own pressure. These individual gas pressures can be summed to find the total pressure of the system. For example, in a closed system, He, Ar, CO_2 and H_2 are present at pressures of 450, 230, 86, and 3 Torr, respectively. The total pressure of the system is

$$(450 + 230 + 86 + 3) = 769 \text{ Torr.}$$

PROBLEM

a) A gas has a volume of 30.0 ml and a pressure of 420 Torr. What is its new pressure if the temperature is held constant and the volume is changed to 500 ml?

b) A gas occupies 6.0 liters at 200 K. What is its new temperature if the pressure is kept constant and the volume changed to 10 liters?

c) Helium is present in a container at a pressure of 5 atm. Xenon is introduced until the total pressure is 25 atmospheres. What is the pressure of the xenon?

d) How many moles of carbon monoxide are present in a volume of 20.0 liters at 300 K and 2.00 atm. of pressure?

Solution

a) $P_2 = 25.2$ Torr

b) $T_2 = 333K$

c) $P_{Xe} = 20$ atm.

d) 1.62 moles of CO

PROBLEM

a) Hydrochloric acid can react with sodium carbonate to form carbon dioxide by the following unbalanced reaction:

$$HCl + Na_2CO_3 \longrightarrow NaCl + CO_2 + H_2O.$$

290.0 grams of 80.0% pure HCl are reacted with 82.0 grams of pure Na_2CO_3. The impurities will not react at all. What volume of CO_2 will be produced by this reaction at 80° C and 700 Torr pressure?

b) How many grams of steam at 100° C. and 1 atm. pressure will fill a 55.0 gallon drum? (1 gallon = 3.88 liters). How many grams will it hold if the temperature of the steam is raised to 200° C.?

c) Oxygen gas can be produced by the decomposition of potassium chlorate by the following unbalanced reaction

$$KClO_3 \longrightarrow KCl + O_2.$$

2.00 liters of oxygen gas are collected over water at 15° C. The vapor pressure of water at this temperature is 22.0 Torr. The pressure of the wet gas is 1.00 atm. How many grams of pure potassium perchlorate are needed to decompose to produce the above 2.00 liters of O_2?

d) Calculate the density of radon gas at 25° C. and 1.00 atm.

Solution

a)   Calculate the molecular weights;

$HCl = (1 + 35) = 36$ Daltons,

$Na_2CO_3 = [(2 \times 23) + 12 + (3 \times 16)] = 106$ Daltons.

Calculate total grams of HCl;

$290.0 \times 80.0\% = 232$ grams of HCl.

Calculate moles of HCl;

$232/36 = 6.44$ moles HCl.

Calculate moles

$Na_2CO_3;\ 82.0\ /\ 106 = 0.774$ moles of Na_2CO_3.

Balance the equation;

$$2HCl + Na_2CO_3 \longrightarrow 2NaCl + CO_2 + H_2O.$$

Determine the limiting reagent; in this case it is Na_2CO_3, since it will be used up, and HCl will be left over.

Calculate the moles of CO_2 produced; by the balanced equation it can be seen that for every mole of Na_2CO_3 consumed, one mole of CO_2 is produced, hence 0.774 moles of CO_2 are produced.

Convert C to K;

$(80 + 273) = 353$ K.

Convert Torr to atm.;

$(700/760) = 0.921$ atm.

Calculate volume of

$CO_2;\ PV = nRT,\ (0.921)\ (V) = (0.774)\ (0.0821)\ (353) = 24.4$ liters.

OR

Calculate CO_2 volume at STP;

$0.744 \times 22.4 = 17.3$ liters.

Change pressure to 700 Torr;

$P_1V_1 = P_2V_2,\ (760)\ (17.3) = (700)\ (V_2),\ V_2 = 18.8$ liters.

Change temperature to 353 K;

$V_1\ /\ T_1 = V_2\ /\ T_2,\ (18.8\ /\ 273) = (V_2\ /\ 353)\ V_2 = 24.4$ liters.

b)   Calculate number of liters in 55.0 gallons;

$(55.0 \times 3.88) = 213$ liters.

Convert C to K;

$(100 + 273) = 373$ K.

Calculate moles of steam; (assuming steam is an ideal gas)

$$PV = nRT, (1) (213) = \text{n} (0.0821) (373), n = 6.96 \text{ moles of steam.}$$

OR

Change conditions to STP,

$$V_1 / T_1 = V_2 / T_2, (213 / 373) = (V_2 / 273), V_2 = 156 \text{ liters.}$$

Calculate number of moles;

$$22.4 / 156 = 156 = 6.96 \text{ liters.}$$

Calculate M.W. of steam;

$$H_2O, (2 \times 1) + (1 \times 16) = 18 \text{ Daltons.}$$

Calculate mass of steam;

$$6.96 \times 18 = 125 \text{ grams of steam.}$$

Repeating the above at 200°C (473 K) a mass of 98.7 grams is obtained.

c) Convert vapor pressure of water to atm. 22 / 760 = 0.029 atm.

Subtract water pressure from total pressure to get pressure of O_2;

$$1.00 - 0.029 = 0.971 \text{ atm. of } O_2$$

The balanced equation is

$$2KClO_3 \rightarrow 2 \text{ KCl} + 3O_2$$

Find moles O_2 using $PV = nRT$

$$(0.971) (2) = (\text{n}) (0.0821) (288) \text{ n} = 0.0821 \text{ moles } O_2$$

$$\text{Moles KClO}_3 = \frac{\text{moles } O_2}{3} \cdot (2) = 0.05475 \text{ mole KClO}_3 \text{ or 6.7 grams}$$

$$\text{MW KClO}_3 = (1 \times 39.1) + (1 \times 35.4) + (3 \times 16) = 122.5 \text{ Daltons}$$

d) Any amount of radon can be used; one mole is the easiest to work with.

One mole of radon will have a mass of 222 grams under any conditions (look at the atomic weight!).

Convert Celsius to Kelvin;

$$(25 + 273) = 298 \text{ K.}$$

Using $PV = nRT$, we get the volume

$$(1) (V) = (1) (0.0821) (298), \text{ or } V = 24.4 \text{ liters.}$$

Calculate density;

$$(222 / 24.4) = 9.10 \text{ gm / liters.}$$

2. Phase Equilibria

In solids, the molecules are packed tightly together with no room for movement other than slight vibration. Upon heating, the vibrations increase until the molecules can break away from one another. At this point, they are moving fairly rapidly with a fair amount of distance between them. Under such conditions, it is said that the solid has melted. Upon further heating, the molecules move farther apart and travel at greater speeds until they are at relatively great distances from one another and traveling at fairly high speeds. At this point the liquid has become a gas. The change of state, e.g., liquid to gas, solid to liquid, etc., is termed a phase transition. The diagram below shows the changes of state of water. As energy is added to the system, the temperature of the ice increases until it reaches 0°C. At this point, energy is still absorbed by the system, but there is no further increase in temperature, since the energy is used to melt the ice. Ice and water can both exist at 0°C. After the ice has totally melted, addition of further energy results in an increase in the water's temperature until 100°C is reached. Again, energy is absorbed without any increase in temperature. This time the energy is used to convert the liquid to a gas. Water and steam can both exist at 100°C. After all of the water has been converted to steam, addition of further energy increases the temperature of the steam.

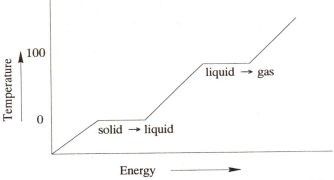

At standard pressure, water boils at 100°C and ice melts at 0°C. However, the boiling point can change drastically at other pressures, whereas the melting point remains fairly constant, decreasing only slightly with a great increase in pressure. The vapor pressure of a liquid increases with its temperature. When the vapor pressure equals atmospheric pressure, boiling occurs. Obviously, if the atmospheric pressure is lowered, the liquid does not have to be heated to as high of a temperature to boil. Conversely, at a higher atmospheric pressure, the liquid will boil at a higher temperature. If a plot is made of temperature vs. pressure for a substance, it is called a "Phase Diagram."

A phase diagram for water is shown below. At the pressures and temperatures in the upper left-hand corner, water can only exist as ice, hence it is labeled "solid." Moving to the right, crossing the vertical line at 0°, but not crossing the line that curves up to the right, are the temperatures and pressures where water will only exist as a liquid, hence it is labeled as such. Beyond the line that curves up, water will exist as a gas. Where the two lines intersect, 0.01° and 4.6 Torr for water, is called the "Triple Point". At this pressure and temperature, the material can exist in equilibrium in all three states of matter.

As was mentioned earlier, the melting and boiling points of pure substances are constant, and can be used to aid in their identification. However, if other materials are present, these and other properties can be altered. The material present in the greatest quantity is called the "solvent," that in the least is called the "solute." Together they make what is called the "solution." In a solution, several colligative

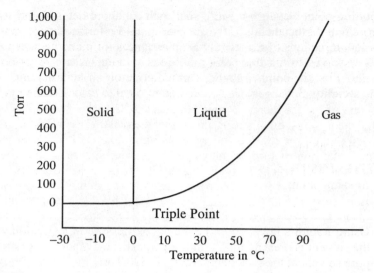

properties of the solvent are altered. Among these are a lowering of vapor pressure, freezing point depression, and boiling point and osmotic pressure elevation. Vapor pressure lowering follows Raoult's Law, which states:

$$P = XP°,$$

where P is the vapor pressure of the solvent over the solution, X is the mole fraction of solvent in the solution, and $P°$ is the vapor pressure of the pure solvent at the same temperature. The osmotic pressure is the minimum pressure that must be applied to a solution bound by a semipermeable membrane to keep osmosis from occurring. This osmotic pressure is denoted by the symbol π, and is calculated as

$$\pi = MRT,$$

where M is the number of moles of solute found per liter of solution, R is the universal gas law constant (0.0821 atm.·liter / mole K), and T is the temperature in Kelvin. At this point, it is useful to introduce a unit of concentration, molality (abbreviated "m"). Molality is defined as the number of moles of solute per kilogram of solvent. For example if 2.00 moles of sodium chloride are dissolved in water, and the total mass of the solvent is one kg, the resulting concentration is 2.00 m. If 0.01 moles of camphor is dissolved in benzene with a mass of 0.150 kg, the concentration is (0.01 / 0.150) = 0.0667 m.

For every mole of solute dissolved per kilogram of solution, the boiling point of the solution is raised a constant amount above that of the pure solvent, and the freezing point is lowered by a constant amount below that of the pure solvent. For water the boiling point elevation, k_b, is 0.52°, and the freezing point depression, k_f, is 1.86°. Hence, a 1.00 m solution of sugar in water would boil at 100.52°, and freeze at -1.86°. A 2.00 m solution of sugar in water would boil at

$$[100 + (2 \times 0.52)] = 101.04°,$$
and would freeze at

$$[0 - (2 \times (1.86))] = -3.72°.$$

If the solute dissociates to form ions in solution, the number of moles of ions formed per mole of solute is multiplied by the molality to calculate the freezing point depression and boiling point elevation. [More shall be said about determining whether or not a material will dissociate into ions at a later time.] For example, if a material that dissociates into three ions (three moles of ions per mole of material) when dissolved in water, is dissolved to make a 1.00 m aqueous solution, what are its boiling and freezing point? First the number of ions formed per mole of material must be multiplied by the molality; $3 \times 1 = 3$. This value is now used to calculate the new b.p. and f.p.;

$$[100 + (3 \times 0.52)] = 101.56°C$$

is the new boiling point,

$$[0 - (3 \times 1.86)] = -5.58°C$$

is the new freezing point.

PROBLEM

a) Using Raoult's law, determine the vapor pressure of a solution where the solvent is present at 95.6 molar percent. The vapor pressure of the pure solvent at the same temperature is 830 Torr.

b) What is the osmotic pressure, π, of a solution at 400 K if the concentration is 0.0016 moles per liter?

c) What is the concentration in molality of 4.68 moles of $CuCl_2$ dissolved in water, so the final mass of the solution is 15.0 kg?

d) If $CuCl_2$ dissociates to form three ions when dissolved in water, what is the boiling point of the solution in question c? What is the freezing point?

Solution

a) 793 Torr

b) 0.052 atm.

c) 0.326 m (Remember total solution mass = solvent mass + solute mass)

d) b.p. = 100.51°C, f.p. = -1.82°C

PROBLEM

a) What is the freezing point of 2.81 liters of water after 5.26 grams of ethanol (CH3OH) are added to it?

b) What is the boiling point of a solution made by adding 9.32 grams of water to 2.68 kg of acetic acid (CH_3COOH)? The normal boiling point of acetic acid is 118°, and the k_b is 2.93.

c) 10.0 grams of an unknown hydrocarbon are dissolved in 1.00 kg of cyclohexane. The freezing point of the solution is 5.09°. What is the molecular weight of the hydrocarbon? The normal freezing point of cyclohexane is 6.50°, and the k_f is 20.2.

Solution

a) Find the total weight of the solvent;

2.81 liters of water has a mass of 2.81 kg.

Calculate M.W. of ethanol;

$(1 \times 12) + (4 \times 1) + (16 \times 1) = 32$ Daltons.

Find number of moles of ethanol;

$5.26 / 32 = 0.0164$ moles.

Calculate molality;

$0.0164 / 2.810 = 0.0584$ m.

Multiply by k_f of water;

$(0.0584 \times 1.86) = 0.109°$.

Subtract this value from the normal f.p. of water;

$0 - 0.109 = -0.109°C$.

b)   The solvent is acetic acid;

Mass of solvent = 2.68 kg.

Calculate M.W. of water (H_2O);

$(1 \times 2) + (16 \times 1) = 16$ amu.

Calculate number of moles of water;

$(9.32/18) = 0.518$ moles of H_2O.

Calculate molality of the solution;

$0.518 / 2.68 = 0.193$ m.

Multiply by k_b for acetic acid;

$(0.193 \times 2.93) = 0.565°C$.

Add this to the normal b.p.;

$(0.565 + 118.000) = 118.565°C$.

c)   Determine the change in f.p.;

$(5.09 - 6.50) = - 1.41°$.

Divide f.p. change by k_f to get molality of solution;

$(1.41 / 20.2) = 0.0698$ m.

Determine total moles of hydrocarbon present; using 1 kg of solvent

$(0.0698 \times 1.00) = 0.0698$ moles of hydrocarbon.

Determine the M.W. of the hydrocarbon;

$(10.0 / 0.0698) = 143$ Daltons.

V. SOLUTION CHEMISTRY

1. Ions in Solution

Any salt that is soluble in water will dissociate into ions. Positively charged ions are called "cations" and negatively charged ions are called "anions." Any salt that is soluble in water will dissociate into anions and cations when dissolved in water. For example, NaCl, when dissolved in water, becomes sodium cations and chloride anions. This is represented as

$$NaCl \longrightarrow Na^+ + Cl^-.$$

Note that two moles of ions are produced per mole of salt dissolved. This is important to keep in mind when doing freezing point depression and boiling point elevation calculations, as well as molecular weight determinations using molality. Na_3PO_4 will give four ions,

$$Na_3PO_4 \longrightarrow 3Na^+ + PO_4^=.$$

Below are rules for naming common ions.

1. Single cations are simply called by the element's name. For example Na^+ would be called a sodium ion, Al^{+++} would be called an aluminum ion.

2. The only common polyatomic cation is NH_4^+, which is called "ammonium."

3. Single anions are named by dropping the ending of the element's name and adding "-ide." Cl^- is chloride, $S^=$ is sulfide, $N^≡$ is nitride. Most of the names of polyatomic anions have to do with the number of oxygen atoms associated with them.

4. For the halogen family (F, Cl, Br, I), nitrogen, and carbon, if three oxygens are combined with the atom, the ending is changed to "-ate." Hence ClO_3^- is chlorate, NO_3^- is nitrate, $CO_3^=$ is carbonate, etc. Note that with the exception of $CO_3^=$, all of these ions have a -1 charge.

5. If four oxygens are combined with the atoms mentioned in rule #4, the prefix "per-" is placed before the name of the atom, followed by the suffix "-ate." ClO_4^- is perchlorate, BrO_4^- is perbromate, etc.

6. If only two oxygen atoms are associated with the atoms mentioned in rule #4, the suffix "-ite" is used. NO_2^- is nitrite, ClO_2^- is chlorite, etc.

7. If the atoms mentioned in rule #4 are associated with only one oxygen atom, the prefix "hypo-" and suffix "-ite" are used. ClO^- is hypochlorite, IO^- is hypoiodite, etc.

8. $SO_4^=$ is sulfate, one less oxygen makes it $SO_3^=$ and is called sulfite.

9. $PO_4^≡$ is phosphate, one less oxygen makes it $PO_3^≡$, and is called phosphite.

10. CN^- is called cyanide.

11. CH_3COO^- is acetate.

2. Solubility

The concentration of solutions can be expressed in many ways. The easiest is percent composition, which can be either by volume or mass. If 5.0 ml of acetone is added to 95.0 ml of water, it is a 5.0% (V) solution. Dissolving 8.0 grams of sugar into 92.0 grams of water yields an 8.0% (W) solution. Molality has been discussed earlier. It is the number of moles of solute per kilogram of solvent. Dissolving 78.0 moles of decane into 3.45 kg of benzene, the concentration is

$$(78.0 / 3.45) = 22.6 \text{ m}.$$

Molarity (abbreviation "M") is the most commonly used units of concentration in chemistry. Molarity is defined as the number of moles of solute per liter of solution. If 10.0 moles of carbon disulfide are dissolved to produce 2.00 liters of solution, the concentration is

$$(10.0 / 2.00) = 5.00 \text{ M}.$$

The solubility of most common salts in water can usually be determined by the following generalization. [Keep in mind, however, these are generalizations!]

1. Most nitrates and acetates are soluble. Silver, chromium (II), and mercury (I) acetate are only slightly soluble.

2. All chlorates are soluble except potassium chlorate, which is slightly soluble.

3. All chlorides are soluble except those of mercury (I), silver, lead, and copper (I).

4. All sulfates are soluble except those of strontium, barium, and lead. Calcium and silver sulfate are slightly soluble.

5. Carbonates, and phosphates are insoluble, except for those of ammonium and the group 1A metals.

6. All sulfides other than ammonium are insoluble.

7. The hydroxides of the group 1A metals, ammonium, barium, and strontium are soluble. Calcium hydroxide is slightly soluble. All other hydroxides are insoluble. For salts considered slightly soluble, a very small amount actually does go into solution. From this can be calculated the solubility product constant, k_{sp}.

It should be noted that the k_{sp} changes with temperature, most are given at 25°C. For an insoluble salt that dissociates as follows:

$$A_xB_y \longrightarrow xA^+ + yB^-$$

the k_{sp} can be calculated as follows:

$$k_{sp} = \frac{[A^+]^x [B^-]^y}{[A_xB_y]^l}.$$

The brackets, [ ], denote "concentration (in molarity) of the entity enclosed therein." Also note that the coefficients, l, x, and y, become exponents. Remember this gives the k_{sp} only for the temperature at which the concentration measurements were made.

For example, MnS has a k_{sp} of 5.6×10^{-16} at 25°C. If 25.0 grams of MnS are mixed into one liter of water, and allowed to settle out, what is the concentration of Mn^{++} ions in the water? We can begin by writing the equation for the dissociation of MnS in water, even though it occurs at a very low rate:

$$MnS \longrightarrow Mn^{++} + S^{=}.$$

Fortunately, the coefficients are all one; this makes the exponents very easy to handle. The

$$k_{sp} = \frac{[Mn^{++}]^1 [S^{=}]^1}{[MnS]^1}.$$

We can also conclude that $[Mn^{++}] = [S^{=}]$. As can be seen by the very low k_{sp}, the vast majority of the MnS will not be in the solution at all. When working with such highly insoluble material, its concentration is taken to be "1". Assigning an algebraic variable, x, to represent the $[Mn^{++}]$, which will also equal $[S^{=}]$, we can solve the equation:

$$5.6 \times 10^{-16} = (X \cdot X) / 1, \text{ or } 5.6 \times 10^{-16} = x^2, x = 2.37 \times 10^{-8}M.$$

Since $x = [Mn^{++}]$, the Mn^{++} concentration is 2.37×10^{-8} moles per liter. Note that with such an insoluble compound, the mass added to the solvent was not even used in the calculation. It can be calculated from the above information that only 2.05 micrograms of MnS went into solution, which is 0.00000822% of the total salt added, a very small amount indeed! How many grams of lead are in 2.50 liters of a saturated solution of PbI_2? The k_{sp} of PbI_2 is

$$8.8 \times 10^{-9} \text{ at this temperature.}$$

A saturated solution has as much of the solute in it as possible. Any additional PbI_2 added will not go into solution. The dissociation is

$$PbI_2 \longrightarrow Pb^{++} + 2I^-, \text{ hence we can write}$$

$$k_{sp} = \frac{[Pb^{++}]^1 [I^-]^2}{[PbI_2]^1}.$$

If $x = [Pb^{++}]$, then it can be seen that $2x = [I^-]$. Substituting values into the equation, we get

$$8.8 \times 10^{-9} = (x) \cdot (2x)^2 / 1, \text{ or } 8.8 \times 10^{-9} = 4x^3, \text{ or } x = 1.30 \times 10^{-3}M = [Pb^{++}].$$

Multiplying by the volume of the solution,

$$(1.30 \times 10^{-3} \cdot 2.50) = 3.25 \times 10^{-3}$$

moles of Pb^{++} present, converting to grams by multiplying by the atomic weight of lead, we get,

$$(3.25 \times 10^{-3} \cdot 207) = 0.670$$

grams of lead cations in the solution. Return to the first example, using MnS. Suppose $S^{=}$ ions were added to the solution from another source. They would help to push the $S^{=}$ (and hence Mn^{++}) out of the solution. This is known as the "Common Ion Effect." Repeating the example, but dissolving the MnS into 0.100 M $(NH_4)_2S$, we can see how much less Mn^{++} is in solution. From our solubility rules, we can see that ammonium sulfide dissociates readily $(NH_4)_2S$ $2NH_4^+ + S^{=}$. Hence, the $[S^{=}]$ from the

$(NH_4)_2S$ is 0.100 M. Plugging this into the equation used above, there are now two sources of $S^=$, that from the MnS (x), and the $(NH_4)_2S$ (0.100).

$$k_{sp} = \frac{[Mn^{++}]^1 [S^=]^1}{[MnS]^1}.$$

now becomes

$$5.6 \times 10^{-16} = (x)(x + 0.100) / 1.$$

Since we know that x for the $S^=$ from the MnS is so very low, it can be neglected. (Whenever a term is very, very small, it can be neglected in an addition or subtraction operation, but NEVER in a multiplication or division operation.) This now gives us

$$5.6 \times 10^{-16} = (x)(0.100) / 1.$$

Solving for x gives a value of

$$[Mn^{++}] = 5.6 \times 10^{-15} M,$$

which is 7 orders of magnitude smaller than the original answer, due to the common ion effect.

PROBLEM

a)   What is the percent concentration of a solution made by dissolving 28.9 grams of napthalene into 437 grams of Benzene?

b)   If 20.9 moles of $CuSO_4$ are dissolved into 4.89 liters of water, what is the molarity of the solution?

c)   If 0.0490 moles of NaCl are dissolved in 25.5 liters of water, what is the molarity and approximate molality of the solution?

d)   If 2.8 moles of $NaNO_3$ are dissolved into 4.90 liters of water, what is the $[NO_3^-]$?

e)   What is the maximum concentration of $BaSO_4$ in water? The $k_{sp} = 1.08 \times 10^{-10}$.

f)   What is the maximum concentration of $BaSO_4$ in a 0.200 M solution of Na_2SO_4?

g)   In a saturated solution of $Tl(OH)_3$, the $[Tl^{+++}]$ was found to be 6.38×10^{-12}, and the $[OH^-]$ was 1.92×10^{-11}. Find the k_{sp} for $Tl(OH)_3$ at this temperature.

Solution

a)   6.20%(W)

b)   4.27 M

c)   0.00194 M and 0.00194 m

d)   0.571 M

e) 1.04×10^{-5} M

f) 5.40×10^{-10} M

g) 4.52×10^{-44}

VI. ACIDS AND BASES

1. Acid/Base Equilibria

By the Brønsted/Lowrey definition an acid is a proton donor, a base is a proton acceptor. Consider the acid, HA, and base, B^-. The acid can donate its proton, and the base accept it by the following reaction:

$$HA + B^- \longrightarrow A^- + HB,$$

where HB is the conjugate acid, and A^- is the conjugate base. For example, the amino acid, glycine, can act as an acid or a base. In the reaction

$$H_2NCH_2COOH + H_3O^+ \longrightarrow {}^+H_3NCH_2COOH + H_2O,$$

it is behaving as a base, accepting a proton from a hyronium ion, and becoming a conjugate acid in the process. In the reaction

$$H_2NCH_2COOH + H_2O \longrightarrow H_2NCH_2COO^- + H_3O^+,$$

it is behaving as an acid, donating a proton to the water molecule, and becoming a conjugate base. Water can behave as both an acid and a base, by the reaction

$$2H_2O \longrightarrow H_3O^+ + OH^-.$$

In pure water, there is always as much H_3O^+ as OH^-. The equilibrium constant for the dissociation of water, k_w, can be calculated as

$$k_w = \frac{[H_3O^+][OH^-]}{[H_2O]^2} = 10^{-14}.$$

From this it can be seen that in pure water the

$$[H_3O^+] = [OH^-] = 10^{-7} \text{ (The } [H_2O] \text{ goes to ``1'')}.$$

A convenient scale for measuring the $[H_3O^+]$ in water is the pH. Any value below 7 is acidic, any value about 7 is basic, and a value of 7 is neutral.

$$pH = -\log[H_3O^+].$$

A solution with a

$$[H_3O^+] = 10^{-3}$$

will have a pH of 3,

$$[H_3O^+] = 10^{-11},$$

the pH is 11. As can be seen from the k_w, $[H_3O^+]$ for pure water is 10^{-7}, hence the pH of water is 7. Another important term, pOH, is defined the same way; $pOH = -\log[OH^-]$. In a solution where the

$$[OH^-] = 10^{-8},$$

the pOH = 8. The pOH of pure water is 7. pOH and pH are related by the formula

$$14-pOH = pH.$$

This is due to the relationship

$$k_w / [OH^-] = [H_3O^+].$$

Strong acids and bases dissociate readily in water. Strong acids include

HCl, H_2SO_4, HNO_3, and $HClO_4$.

Strong bases include any hydroxide of the group 1A metals. Since strong acids completely dissociate, their pH is easy to calculate. HCl dissociates by the reaction

$$HCl + H_2O \longrightarrow H_3O^+ + Cl^-.$$

If a solution of

HCl is 10^{-2}M, then the $[H_3O^+] = 10^{-2}$M, and the pH is 2.0.

Sulfuric acid gives up two protons by the reaction

$$H_2SO_4 + 2H_2O \longrightarrow SO_4^= + 2H_3O^+.$$

If a solution is

2.5×10^{-5}M in H_2SO_4,

then the $[H_3O^+]$ will be twice that, or 5.0×10^{-5}, and the pH will be 4.30. (It is necessary to have a table of common logarithms or calculator for most pH calculations.) There are two ways to calculate the pH of a solution of a strong base. One is to calculate the pOH, and convert it to pH; the other is to convert the $[OH^-]$ to $[H_3O^+]$ and calculate the pH. In a 3.8×10^{-3} M solution of NaOH, the base is entirely dissociated,

$$NaOH \longrightarrow Na^+ + OH^-. \quad [OH^-] = 3.8 \times 10^{-3}.$$

Calculating the pOH gives a value of 2.42. Substituting into the equation

$14 - pOH = pH$,

we get a value of

$(14 - 2.42) = 11.58 = pH$.

Solving by the other method, we convert

$[OH^-]$ to $[H_3O^+]$, $(10^{-14} / 3.8 \times 10^{-3}) = 2.63 \times 10^{-12} = [H_3O^+]$,

the pH is 11.58, the same as with the other method. What is the pH of a solution of HNO_3 that is 10^{-9} M? One might assume that the

$[H_3O^+] = 10^{-9}$,

and therefore the pH = 9. Can an acidic solution have a pH above 7.0? Obviously not. In this case, the $[H_3O^+]$ from the water (normally insignificant) must be included. The total

$[H_3O^+] = 10^{-9}$ (from the HNO_3) $+10^{-7}$ (from the H_2O) $= 1.01 \times 10^{-7}$,

which gives a pH of 6.9957, or for all practical purposes, 7.0.

Weak acids do not dissociate entirely, nor do weak bases. Formic acid will dissociate somewhat,

$$HCOOH + H_2O \longrightarrow HCOO^- + H_3O^+,$$

but the vast majority will stay in molecular form. A dissociation constant k_a can be calculated for a particular weak acid at a particular temperature just as one might do a solubility constant, k_{sp}. For formic acid the equation is

$$k_a = \frac{[HCOO^-]^1 \, [H_3O^+]^1}{[HCOOH]^1}.$$

For formic acid the

$$k_a = 1.8 \times 10^{-4} \text{ at } 25°C.$$

What is the pH of a 7.28×10^{-2} M solution of formic acid at $25°C$.? From the dissociation equation, it can be seen that

$$[HCOO^-] = [H_3O^+].$$

As was done with the k_{sp} values, let the above ion concentrations equal x. The amount of undissociated formic acid will be

$$7.28 \times 10^{-2} - x.$$

Plugging these numbers into the equation yields:

$$1.8 \times 10^{-4} = x^2 / (7.28 \times 10^{-2} - x),$$

which can be solved as a quadratic;

$$x^2 + (1.80 \times 10^{-4})\, x - (1.31 \times 10^{-5}) = 0.$$

Solving for x yields values of

$$+3.53 \times 10^{-3} \text{ M and } -3.71 \times 10^{-3} \text{ m for } x, \text{ hence, the } [H_3O^+].$$

Since any ion concentration cannot be negative, the positive value is chosen. Calculating the pH from this gives a value of 2.45. Solving quadratic equations is easier than it used to be, thanks to calculators, and often one can run into cubics and even quartics in such calculations. Remember that the MCAT does not allow the luxury of a calculator, however. Fortunately, the amount of formic acid lost to the formation of formate and hydronium ions is small, so small that it can be neglected, changing the equation to

$$1.8 \times 10^{-4} = x^2 / 7.28 \times 10^{-2}.$$

This is easy to solve, giving

$$x = 3.62 \times 10^{-3} \text{ M} = [H_3O^+], \text{ pH} = 2.44.$$

As k_a gets even smaller, the accuracy of this method increases even more. If more H_3O^+ is added to the weak acid (e.g. in the form of a strong acid), the molecular species becomes more predominate. The pk_a is defined as $-\log(k_a)$, and is the pH at which the concentration of the molecular form is equal to the concentration of the dissociated form. For formic acid, the pk_a is

$$-\log(1.8 \times 10^{-4}) = 3.74.$$

The pH of solutions of weak bases is determined by the same method. What is the pH of a 0.200 M solution of phenylamine? The dissociation of phenylamine in water can be written as

$$C_6H_5NH_2 + H_2O \rightleftarrows C_6H_5NH_3^+ + OH^-.$$

From this, the equation for dissociation constant (for bases, k_b) can be written as:

$$k_b = \frac{[C_6H_5NH_3^+]^1 \, [OH^-]^1}{[C_6H_5NH_2]^1}.$$

(Note that as with the acids the term $[H_2O]$ does not enter into this equation, as it has an effective concentration of "1".) For phenylamine the k_b is

4.6×10^{-10}. Since $[C_6H_5NH_3^+] = [OH^-]$,

the algebraic variable, x, can be used for the concentration of either of these. The amount lost from the original 0.200 M phenylamine, x, is so small as to be negligible. The resultant equation is

$4.6 \times 10^{-10} = x^2 / 0.200$, or $x = 9.59 \times 10^{-6} = [OH^-]$.

This gives a pOH of 5.02, and a pH of 8.98. The pH could also have been calculated by dividing the k_w by the $[OH^-]$ to obtain the $[H_3O^+]$. The pk_b of a weak base is pH value at which half of it is dissociated, and half of it is in molecular form. It is calculated as

$pk_b = 14- (-\log(k_b))$.

For phenylamine the $pk_b = 4.66$.

PROBLEM

What is the pH of Aqueous Solutions of the following?

a) 0.04 M HCl

b) 0.04 M H_2SO_4

c) 0.04 M benzoic acid

$(C_6H_5COOH + H_2O \longrightarrow C_6H_5COO^- + H_3O^+, k_a = 6.3 \times 10^{-5})$

d) 4.00 M HCl

e) 0.04 M NaOH

f) 4.00 M NaOH

g) 4×10^{-14} M NaOH

h) 0.04 M ethylamine

$(CH_3CH_2NH_2 + H_2O \longrightarrow CH_3CH_2NH_3^+ + OH^-, k_b = 4.3 \times 10^{-4})$

Solution

a)	1.40	b)	1.097
c)	2.80	d)	-0.60
e)	12.60	f)	13.4
g)	7.00	h)	11.62

2. Salts of Acids and Bases

A salt of a strong acid and strong base will yield a neutral solution when dissolved in water, no matter what its concentration is. For example, the pH of a 0.125 M NaCl solution is 7.00.

The salt of a weak acid and strong base will yield a basic solution when dissolved in water. What is the pH of a 0.125M sodium acetate solution? The k_a for acetic acid is 1.75×10^{-5}. Sodium acetate will dissociate to form ions:

$$CH_3COONa \longrightarrow CH_3COO^- + Na^+.$$

The acetate ion will want to take a proton from the water:

$$CH_3COO^- + H_2O \longrightarrow CH_3COOH + OH^-,$$

the equilibrium constant for this can be calculated as

$$\frac{[CH_3COOH]^1 [OH^-]^1}{[CH_3COO^-]^1} = k_{eq}.$$

This is very similar to the expression for the k_a. By multiplying the numerator and denominator by $[H_3O^+]$ we get

$$k_{eq} = \frac{[CH_3COOH][OH^-][H_3O^+]}{[CH_3COO^-][H_3O^+]}$$

Recall that the term in the numerator $[OH^-][H_3O^+] = k_w$, hence the equation can be rewritten as

$$k_{eq} = \frac{[CH_3COOH] k_w}{[CH_3COO^-][H_3O^+]}.$$

Notice the term involving concentrations is now the reciprocal of the k_a times k_w. This could be rewritten as

$$k_{eq} = k_w \quad (1 / k_a) = k_w / k_a.$$

The value for this can now be calculated;

$$10^{-14} / 1.75 \times 10^{-5} = 5.71 \times 10^{-10} = [CH_3COOH] [OH^-].$$

Assigning the algebraic variable, x, to represent the $[OH^-]$, we can also see that

$$x = [CH_3COOH].$$

That is, for every acetate converted to acetic acid, a water molecule is converted to a hydroxide ion.

The $[CH_3COO^-]$ is equal to 0.125 M minus what was lost to form acetic acid, e.g., $0.125-x$. The amount lost to this is so slight that it can be neglected. The final equation is

$$5.71 \times 10^{-10} = x^2 / 0.125,$$

solving for x gives a $[OH^-] = 8.45 \times 10^{-6}$, a pOH = 5.07, and a pH = 8.93.

Calculations involving the salt of a weak base and strong acid are much the same, except the solution will be acidic. What is the pH of a 0.125 M solution of ammonium chloride? The k_b for ammonium hydroxide is 1.80×10^{-5}. Ammonium chloride will dissociate by

$$NH_4Cl \longrightarrow NH_4^+ + Cl^-.$$

The ammonium ions formed will react with the water thus,

$$NH_4^+ + H_2O \longrightarrow NH_3 + H_3O^+,$$

resulting in an acidic solution. As with the previous example, the

$$k_{eq} = \frac{[NH_3][H_3O^+]}{[NH_4^+]}.$$

This time multiplying the numerator and denominator by $[OH^-]$, yields $k_{eg} = k_w / k_b$. (See the previous paragraph for the mathematics.) We know that $[NH_3] = [H_3O^+]$, and can be assigned the value x. The

$$[NH_4^+] = 0.125 - x$$

(x being the amount lost by dissociation), and x is small enough to be neglected. The final formula is

$$\frac{10^{-14}}{1.80 \times 10^{-5}} = x^2 / 0.125.$$

Solving for x gives a $[H_3O^+] = 8.33 \times 10^{-6}$, and a pH of 5.08

For solutions of salts of weak acids and weak bases, the pH can be either acidic or basic, depending upon the salt. What is the pH of a 0.125 M solution of ammonium formate? The k_b for ammonium hydroxide is

$$1.80 \times 10^{-5},$$

and the k_a for formic acid is

$$1.76 \times 10^{-4}.$$

To spare a lot of mathematics,

$$[H_3O^+] = ((k_w \cdot k_a) / k_b)^{1/2}.$$

Notice that this formula does not even concern the concentration of the salt. This is true so long as the concentration of the salt is greater than the $[OH^-]$ and $[H_3O^+]$ in pure water. If it is below these values, the pH is 7.00. Solving for the above problem yields

$$[H_3O^+] = ((10^{-14} \cdot 1.76 \times 10^{-4}) / 1.80 \times 10^{-5})^{1/2}$$

$$= 3.13 \times 10^{-7}, \text{ and a pH of 6.50.}$$

PROBLEM

What is the pH of the following solutions?

a) 0.489 M potassium nitrate (KNO_3)

b) 0.0239 M sodium flouride (NaF). The K_a for HF is 6.7×10^{-4}.

c) 0.159M hydrazine chloride

(H_2NNH_3Cl). The K_b for H_2NNH_2 is 1.3×10^{-10}.

d) 2.65 M aniline acetate ($C_6H_5NH_4OOCH_3$).

The k_a of CH_3COOH is 1.75×10^{-5}, the k_b of $C_6H_5NH_3$ is 4.0×10^{-10}.

Solution

a) 7.00

b) 4.79

c) 5.34

d) 4.68

3. Buffers

A buffer is solution of a weak acid with one of its salts, or a weak base with one of its salts. The purpose of a buffer is to resist changes in pH. (Note the key word is "resist," not *prevent.*) Consider a solution of hydrofluoric acid that is 0.25 M, mixed with a sodium fluoride solution of 0.5 M. What is the pH of the resultant buffer? We know that NaF will dissociate as

$$NaF \longrightarrow Na^+ + F^-.$$

The dissociation of HF,

$$HF + H_2O \longrightarrow H_3O^+ + F^-$$

is not very great. The k_a for the reaction is 6.7×10^{-4}. Recall that

$$k_a = \frac{[F^-][H_3O^+]}{[HF]}.$$

The [HF] will equal 0.25 M minus x, the amount that dissociates. Since x is quite small, it can be neglected. $[H_3O^+] = x$, and [F⁻] is the sum of the F⁻ from the NaF and the HF, 0.50 + X. Again, since X is so small, it can be neglected. The final equation is

$$6.7 \times 10^{-4} = (0.50)\,(x)\,/\,0.25.$$

Solving for x gives $[H_3O^+] = 3.35 \times 10^{-4}$, and pH = 3.47.

Compare the reactions of this with an unbuffered solution of the same initial pH,

$$3.35 \times 10^{-4} \text{ HCl}.$$

Compare the effect on pH of the addition of 10.0 ml of 2.50 M NaOH to 200 ml of each solution. In 200 ml of the unbuffered solution there are 6.7×10^{-5} moles of H_3O^+. This will react with the NaOH in a neutralization reaction. Of the 0.025 moles of NaOH present (0.010 liters $\times$ 2.5 M = 0.025 moles), 6.7×10^{-5} will react with the acid to form NaCl, leaving 0.0249 moles left over. The new concentration is

$$0.0249\,/\,(0.200 + 0.010) = 0.119 \text{ M} = [OH^-].$$

The pOH is 0.925, the pH is 13.07. Compare that to the initial value of 3.47. Now looking at the same amount of the NaOH solution added to 200 ml of the buffered solution. In that volume of buffer there will be 0.05 moles of HF and 0.100 moles of F⁻. The 0.025 moles of NaOH will react as follows,

$$OH^- + HF \longrightarrow H_2O + F^-.$$

After all of the OH⁻ has reacted there will be 0.025 moles of HF left, and 0.125 moles of F⁻ total (0.100 + 0.025). With the new volume of 0.210 liters, the concentrations are 0.119 M for HF, and 0.595 M for F⁻. Putting this into the equation

$$k_a = \frac{[F^-][H_3O^+]}{[HF]}.$$

yields $[H_3O^+] = 1.34 \times 10^{-4}$, and a pH = 3.87.

Note how little this has changed from the original value. Moving in the opposite direction, compare the addition of 10.0 ml of 1.00 M HNO_3 to 200 ml first of the un-buffered HCl solution, then of the above buffer of the same pH. In 200 ml of the unbuffered solution, there are 6.7×10^{-5} moles of $[H_3O^+]$. In 10.0 ml of 1.00 M HNO_3 there are 0.01 moles of $[H_3O^+]$. Adding these values together, this gives a new concentration of

$$(0.01 + 6.7 \times 10^{-5}) / 0.210 = 0.0479 \text{ M} = [H_3O^+], \text{ and a pH} = 1.32.$$

Adding the same amount of the HNO_3 solution to 200 ml of the buffered solution alters the pH less. The reaction will be

$$H_3O^+ + F^- \longrightarrow HF + H_2O.$$

The F^- and HF are initially present at 0.100 and 0.050 moles, respectively. After the above reaction with 0.01 moles of H_3O^+, they will be 0.090 and 0.060 moles, and their concentration in the new volume of 0.210 liters will be 0.428 M and 0.286 M. Plugging these values into the k_a equation yields a

$$[H_3O^+] = 4.48 \times 10^{-4}, \text{ and a pH} = 3.35.$$

The last example will show the effect of simple dilution on buffered and unbuffered solutions. Adding 20.0 liters of pure water to 200 ml of the unbuffered HCl solution (pH = 3.47), dilutes it. The initial 6.7×10^{-5} moles of H_3O^+ are in a new volume of 20.2 liters. The

$$[H_3O^+] = 3.32 \times 10^{-6} \text{ M, and the new pH} = 5.48.$$

Adding the same amount of pure water to 200 ml of the buffered solution changes the concentration of the F^- to 4.95×10^{-3} and HF concentration to 2.48×10^{-3}, and plugging these values into the k_a equation gives

$$[H_3O^+] = 3.36 \times 10^{-4} \text{ M, and a pH} = 3.47.$$

Note that the pH is unchanged from the initial value!

PROBLEM

a)   0.298 moles of methylamine

     $(CH_3NH_2, k_b = 4.8 \times 10^{-4})$

     are mixed with 0.602 moles of methylamine bromide

     (CH_3NH_4Br)

     in a volume of 1.00 liter of water. What is the pH? (Clue: find the $[OH^-]$.)

b)   What is the pH of the solution when 100 ml of the above buffer is mixed with 50.0 ml of 0.100 M HCl? (Clue: remember to correct for the change in volume.)

Solution

a)   10.99

b)   10.88

4. Titrations

Slowly adding small aliquots of a base of known concentration to an acid of unknown concentration, and carefully measuring the pH after each addition, will yield data to determine the concentration of the unknown acid. The opposite can be done with a known acid and unknown base. In either event, such a procedure is known as a "titration." In titrating a strong acid with a strong base, and plotting the volume of the known material added on the x axis, and the resultant pH on the y, the curve will be almost horizontal, until it nears the equivalence point, at which it will shoot up, and then level off almost horizontal again.

Titration of Strong Acid with a Strong Base

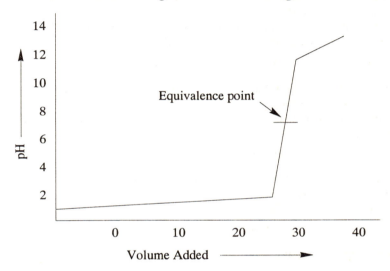

**Titration of a Weak Acid with a Strong Base.
Different Values of k_a are shown**

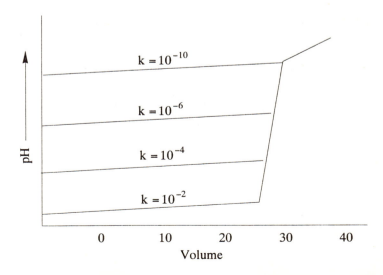

The equivalence point will be at the middle of the almost vertical portion of the plot. At this point the amount of base equals the amount of acid. One can read down to the x axis, find the volume of known material used, and from that calculate the concentration of the unknown. Above is a graph of the titration of a strong acid with a strong base. Titrating a weak acid with a strong base will cause the left-end portion of the curve to flatten out. The smaller the k_a of the acid, the flatter that portion of the curve will be. Titrating a weak base with a strong acid will flatten out the right-hand portion of the curve, again, depending upon k_b of the base. Titrating a weak acid with a weak base broadens the curve on both sides, and titrating a buffered solution broadens it even more.

5. Indicators

Indicators are seldom used in titration anymore, having been replaced by pH meters. However, for the benefit of the MCAT test, below is a list of indicators, and their color changes at various pH ranges:

Name	pH Interval	Acid Color	Base Color
Methyl violet	0.0-1.6	yellow	violet
Methyl yellow	2.9-4.0	red	yellow
Methyl orange	3.2-4.4	red	yellow
Methyl red	4.8-6.2	red	yellow
Bromthymol blue	6.0-8.0	yellow	blue
Thymol blue	8.0-9.6	yellow	blue
Phenolphthalein	8.2-19.9	colorless	pink
Alizarine yellow	10.1-12.0	yellow	red

PROBLEM

a) How many grams of BaF_2 will dissolve in 5.00 liters of water? The k_{sp} for $BaF_2 = 1.7 \times 10^{-6}$.

b) How many grams of BaF_2 will dissolve in 5.00 liters of a 0.879 M NaF solution?

c) 4.70 ml of a 4.80 M HNO_3 solution are added to 1.28 liters of water. What is the pH of the solution?

d) 4.89 grams of KOH are mixed into 28.6 liters of water. What is the pH of the solution?

e) What is the pH of a 0.249 M solution of HIO_3? The k_a for HIO_3 is 0.20.

f) What is the pH of a 0.0987 M solution of KClO? The k_a for HClO is 1.1×10^{-8}.

g) What is the pH of a 0.0987 M solution of NH_4ClO? The k_b for NH_4OH is 1.80×10^{-5}.

h) A solution of HClO has a pH of 4.65. 2.50 liters of this are mixed with 1.62 liters of the KClO solution in problem #6. What is the resultant solution's pH?

i) If 1.00 gram of pure NaOH were dissolved in the above solution (#8), what would the new pH be, assuming no change in volume?

Solution

a) Set up the equation for the dissociation;

$$BaF_2 \longrightarrow Ba^{++} + 2F^-.$$

From this the formula for the k_{sp} can be determined;

$$k_{sp} = \frac{[Ba^{++}]^1 [F^-]^2}{[BaF_2]^1}.$$

Using the variable x to represent

$$[Ba^{++}], \text{ then } 2X = [F-].$$

The $[BaF_2]$ goes to 1. Plugging into the equation;

$$1.7 \times 10^{-6} = (x) (2x)^2 / 1,$$

simplifying yields

$$1.7 \times 10^{-6} = 4x^3,$$

solving for x gives $[Ba^{++}] = 0.00752$ M.

For every mole of BaF_2 in solution there is one mole of Ba^{++}, hence the $[BaF_2]$ in solution is 0.00752 M.

In 5.00 liters there would be

$$(5.00 \times 0.00752) = 0.0376 \text{ moles of } BaF_2.$$

Calculating M.W.;

$$(2 \times 19) + (1 \times 137.3) = 175.3 \text{ Daltons.}$$

Calculating the mass of BaF_2 dissolved;

$$(0.0376 \times 175.3) = 6.59 \text{ grams of } BaF_2 \text{ in the solution.}$$

b) The same set-up is used as on the previous problem;

$$k_{sp} = \frac{[Ba^{++}]^1 [F^-]^2}{[BaF_2]^1},$$

this time the [F-] from the BaF_2 is insignificant when compared to the amount of F- from the NaF, which is 0.879 M.

Plugging into the equation gives,

$$1.7 \times 10^{-6} = (x) (0.879)^2 / 1,$$

solving for x yields $[Ba^{++}] = 2.20 \times 10^{-6}$ M.

For every mole of Ba^{++} in solution, one mole of BaF_2 goes into solution, hence the

$[BaF_2] = 2.20 \times 10^{-6}$ M.

In 5.00 liters of solution there are

$(5.00 \times 2.20 \times 10^{-6}) = 1.10 \times 10^{-5}$ moles of BaF_2 dissolved.

Multiplying by the M.W. yields

$(175.3 \times 1.10 \times 10^{-5}) = 1.92 \times 10^{-3}$ grams,

or 1.93 milligrams dissolve in 5.00 liters.

c)   (4.70 ml = 0.0047 liters 0.0047 ×4.80 = 0.0226 moles of HNO_3 present.

New volume is 1.28 + 0.0047 = 1.2847 liters.

New concentration of HNO_3 is 0.0226 / 1.2847 = 0.0176 M.

$[HNO_3] = [H_3O^+] = 0.0176$ M. V] pH = -log (0.0176) = 1.76.

d)   M.W. of KOH = (39 + 16 + 1) = 56 Daltons.

Numbers of moles of KOH = 4.89 / 56 = 0.0873 moles.

$[KOH] = 0.0873 / 28.6 = 0.00305$ M.

$[KOH] = [OH^-] = 0.00305$ M. v} pOH = -log (0.00305) = 2.52.

pH = 14 - 2.52 = 11.48.

(This could also be calculated by dividing the k_w by the $[OH^-]$ to get the $[H_3O^+]$.)

e)   The dissociation is $HIO_3 + H_2O \longrightarrow H_3O^+ + IO_3^-$.

The k_a is calculated as

$$k_a = \frac{[H_3O^+]^1 \, [IO_3^-]^1}{[HIO_3]^1},$$

Plugging numbers into the equation:

$[H_3O^+] = [IO_3^-] = x$, $[HIO_3] = 0.249 - x$,

this time the k_a is large enough that the amount lost by the HIO_3 cannot be neglected, hence we have to solve a quadratic;

0.20 = (x) (x) / (0.249 -x).

This simplifies to $x^2 = 0.02x - 0.0498 = 0$. Solving for x yields

0.144 M or -0.344 M;

obviously the $[H_3O^+]$ is the positive value.

pH = -log (0.144) = 0.840.

f)   KClO will dissociate almost entirely:

$KClO \longrightarrow K^+ + ClO^-$.

The hypochlorate ions formed will react with water:

$ClO^- + H_2O \longrightarrow HClO + OH^-$.

From the equations it can be seen that

$[OH^-] = [HClO]$.

Assigning values,

$[OH^-] = x$, $[HClO^-] = 0.0987-x$,

x is small enough to be ignored.

$$\frac{k_w}{k_a} = \frac{[HCLO][OH^-]}{[ClO^-]},$$

substituting values,

$(10^{-14} / 1.1 \times 10^{-8}) = x^2 / 0.0987$,

solving for x yields

$[OH^-] = 3.00 \times 10^{-4}$ M.

pOH $= -\log (3.00 \times 10^{-4}) = 3.52$. pH $= 14 - 3.52 = 10.48$.

g)   Concentration has nothing to do with the pH in this case.

$[H_3O^+] = ((k_w k_a) / k_b)^{1/2}$.

Plugging into these numbers gives

$[H_3O^+] = (10^{-14} \cdot 1.1 \times 10^{-8}) / 1.80 \times 10^{-5})^{1/2} = 2.47 \times 10^{-9}$ M.

pH $= -\log (2.47 \times 10^{-9}) = 8.61$.

h)   We are making a buffer solution. First we need to find the concentration of the weak acid solution.

$[H_3O^+]$ = antilog $(-4.65) = 2.25 \times 10^{-5}$ M.

$$k_a = \frac{[H_3O^+][ClO^-]}{[HClO]},$$

$[H_3O^+] = [ClO^-]$,

$[HClO]$ is the unknown, which will be assigned x. This gives

$1.1 \times 10^{-8} = (2.24 \times 10^{-5})^2 / x$,

solving for x yields

$[HClO] = 0.0456$ M.

In 2.50 liters there are

$(2.50 \times 0.0456) = 0.114$ moles of HClO.

In 1.62 liters of the KClO solution there are

$(1.62 \times 0.0987) = 0.160$ moles of ClO$^-$.

The new volume is

$1.62 + 2.50 = 4.21$ liters.

The new concentrations are: for

$[HClO] = 0.114 / 4.21 = 0.0271$ M, for $[ClO^-] = 0.160 / 4.21 = 0.0380$ M.

Putting these into the equation yields

$$1.1 \times 10^{-8} = (x) (0.0380) / 0.0271,$$

solving for x yields

$$[H_3O^+] = 7.84 \times 10^{-9} \text{ M}.$$

$$pH = -\log (7.84 \times 10^{-9}) = 8.10.$$

i)   M.W. of NaOH = 23 + 16 + 1 = 40 Daltons.

In one gram of NaOH there is

$$1/40 = 0.025 \text{ moles of NaOH,}$$

hence 0.025 moles of OH⁻.

The OH⁻ reacts with the buffer by

$$OH^- + HClO \ H_2O + ClO^-.$$

The initial amounts (*NOT concentrations*) of HClO and ClO⁻ are 0.114 and 0.160 moles, respectively. After the OH⁻ is consumed, they are

$$0.114 - 0.025 = 0.089, \text{ and } 0.160 + 0.025 = 0.185 \text{ moles.}$$

The concentrations of HClO and ClO⁻ are

$$0.089 / 4.21 = 0.0211 \text{ M and } 0.185 / 4.21 = 0.0439 \text{ M, respectively.}$$

Plugging into the equation gives

$$1.1 \times 10^{-8} = (x) (0.0439) / (0.0211),$$

solving for x gives $[H_3O^+] = 5.29 \times 10^{-9}$.

$$pH = -\log (5.29 \times 10^{-9}) = 8.28.$$

VII. THERMODYNAMICS AND THERMOCHEMISTRY

1. Thermodynamics

The first law of thermodynamics states that there is a constant amount of energy in the universe. If heat is added to a system, and work is done, then the change in energy of that particular system is equal to the heat added to the system, q, minus the work done by the system, w. Mathematically this is

$$\Delta E = q\text{-}w.$$

The international unit of energy (and hence heat and work) is the Joule, defined as the force of one Newton acting through the distance of one meter. Energy, potential or kinetic can be measured in Joules. This can be energy stored by position, chemical bonds, or locked in the nucleus of an atom. It can also be energy due to motion heat, or electromagnetic radiation. Other units of energy sometimes seen are listed in the table below:

UNIT	1 JOULE = _____ of these units
erg	10^7
foot·pound	0.73756
foot·poundal	23.730
calorie (*very* outdated)	0.2388
electron volt	6.2419×10^{18}

Temperature scales have been mentioned in an earlier section. As a quick review, the two main scales in use are Celsius (formerly centigrade) and Kelvin. On the Celsius scale, water freezes at 0° and boils at 100°. The Kelvin scale starts at absolute zero; hence, it has no negative temperatures. Water freezes at 273 on this scale and boils at 373. When a temperature is given followed by the degree symbol but the scale is not shown, it is presumed to be Celsius (e.g., 25°). Temperature in Celsius can be converted to Kelvin by adding 273.

Thermal energy (heat) can be transferred from one body to another in three ways:

1) **Conduction** — This occurs when one body is placed in direct contact with another, and heat flows from one to the other. An example of conduction might be a block of metal at 85° placed on top of another block of metal at 0°. The heat will flow by conduction from the warmer block to the colder one.

2) **Convection** — This occurs when a warm body heats the air surrounding it, and the air currents carry the heat to other bodies. A hot stove warms a room

chiefly by convection.

3) **Radiation** — A warm body can emit photons of infrared wavelengths. These can travel through space and warm the bodies they strike. Heat travels from the sun through space to the earth by radiation.

When a substance is heated, its molecules move further apart, causing the material to expand. This is quite obvious with gases, as has been covered in an earlier section, and occurs to a much smaller extent in liquids and solids. The increase in volume can be calculated using the coefficient of volume expansion, ex_V, which is unique for each substance. For example the ex_V for ethyl alcohol is 11×10^{-4} / °C. If 40.0 liters of ethyl alcohol are at 0°, and heated to 55°, what will its new volume be? First the change in temperature must be determined; 55 - 0 = 55°. This is multiplied by the ex_V and the original volume;

$$55 \times (11 \times 10^{-4}) \times 40.0 = 2.42 \text{ liters.}$$

This is added to the original volume to give the new volume of 42.4 liters. This is a change of only 6%, compared to a change of 20% had this been 40 liters of gas going from 0 to 55°. For solids, the change in volume is even less with temperature. The ex_V for ice is

$$0.5 \times 10^{-4} / \text{°C.}$$

If 4,000 cm^3 of ice are at -12° and cooled to -190°, what is its new volume? First the temperature change is determined;

$$(-12) - (-190) = 178°.$$

The change in temperature is again multiplied by the ex_V and original volume;

$$(178) \times (0.5 \times 10^4) \times (4,000) = 35.6 \text{ cm}^3.$$

This is subtracted from the original volume to give a new volume of 3,964.4 cm^3. If the solids are greatly larger by one axis than any of the others (e.g., a wire), then a coefficient of linear expansion, ex_l, is used in the same manner as the ex_V to determine the change in length, rather than volume. The ex_l for silver is 2.0×10^{-5}. If a silver needle is 15.0 cm long at 25°, how long will it be at 125°? The change in temperature is 125 - 25 = 100°. We multiply the change in temperature by the ex_l and the original length;

$$(100) \times (2.0 \times 10^{-5}) \times (15) = 0.03 \text{ cm.}$$

Adding this to the original length gives a new length of 15.03 cm.

Recall in a previous section, it was shown that energy must be absorbed by a substance to convert it from a solid to a liquid, and a liquid to a solid. There was an absorption of energy, but no change in temperature, only a change of state. The heat of fusion is the energy required to convert a certain amount of substance from the solid to the liquid state. For example, the heat of fusion for water is 6.03 kJ / mole. How much energy is required to melt 25.0 moles of ice at 0° to water at 0°? A simple multiplication tells us $6.03 \times 25.0 = 151$kJ, or 151,000 Joules are needed to do this.

Note that the units were in kJoules / mole. Sometimes they can be given in kJ / gram, kJ /kg, etc. Be on the watch for this. The energy required to convert a certain amount of a substance from the liquid to the gaseous state is the heat of vaporization.

For example the heat of vaporization of water is 40.6 kJ / mole. How much energy is required to change 29.9 grams of water at 100° to steam at 100°? First we must convert grams to moles; 29.9 / 18 = 1.66 moles.

$$1.66 \times 40.6 = 67.4 \text{ kJ,}$$

or 67,400 Joules are required.

PROBLEM

> a)   If 28.7 liters of mercury are heated from -15° to 25°, what is its new volume? The ex_V for mercury is 1.8×10^{-4} / °C.
>
> b)   An iron nail is 15.0000 cm long at 35°. How long will it be at -200°? The ex_1 for iron is 1.2×10^{-5}.
>
> c)   How much energy is required to melt 29.8 *grams* of mercury? The heat of fusion is 2.34 kJ / mole, and the atomic weight is 200 Daltons.
>
> d)   How much energy must be lost by 56.0 *moles* of mercury vapor to condense to liquid mercury? The heat of vaporization is 56.5 kJ / mole.

Solution

a)   28.9 liters

b)   14.9577 cm

c)   348 Joules

d)   3,160 kJoules

2. Thermochemistry

A property of a system that is not dependent upon how the system got to that state, but is only dependent upon the state itself is called a "state function." For example, if we are heating water from 0° to 15°, it makes no difference whether it is heated directly from 0° to 15°, or if it is heated to 80° first, then allowed to cool to 15°; the end state (15°) is the same.

As was stated in the previous section, there is only a finite amount of energy in the universe. We can take this to mean that energy can be neither destroyed nor created—it can only change its form. Endothermic reactions require energy to go, and they pull in heat from their surroundings. Exothermic reactions will not only run by themselves, but will give heat to their surroundings. To determine whether a reaction is endothermic or exothermic, the change in enthalpy, ΔH, is calculated. Hess's Law states: "For any process which can be looked upon as being the sum of several step-wise processes, the enthalpy change for the total process must be equal to the sum of the enthalpy changes for the various steps." The ΔH for various compounds can be looked up in a table. Most ΔH's are listed in kJ / mole at 298 K. For the reaction

$$CH_4 + 2O_2 \longrightarrow CO_2 + 2H_2O.$$

The energy created in forming the above substances from the necessary elements is given as follows (in kJ / mole):

$$CH_4 = -74.9, O_2 = 0, CO_2 = -394, H_2O \text{ (as vapor)} = -242.$$

The negative sign shows that energy is given up when these bonds are formed. Since this is on a per mole basis, the value for water vapor must be multiplied by two in this instance, since two moles are in the equation. The energy produced by forming one mole of CO_2 and two moles of H_2O vapor is

$$[(1 \times (-394)) + (2 \times (-242))] = -878 \text{ kJ}.$$

The negative signs indicate that energy is given off. However, bonds had to be broken with the O_2 and CH_4 before the products could be made. To find the energy required to do this, the signs of the ΔH values must be reversed. This gives us

$$[(1 \times (+79.4)) + (2 \times 0)] = +79.4 \text{ kJ}.$$

The positive sign shows that energy is required. Hence, for every mole of methane reacted, 79.4 kJ are required, but 878 kJ are given off, so this is a net gain of 799 kJ. Another way of showing this is by adding the sum of the ΔH's for products and reactants; (-878 + 110 kJ. The negative sign shows that energy is being released). Repeating the above steps for the reaction

$$2Ag_2S + 2H_2O \longrightarrow 4Ag + 2H_2S + O_2$$

will give the following results. The heats of formation are:

$$AgS_2 = -32.6, H_2O \text{ (liquid)} = -286, Ag = 0, H_2S = -20.1, O_2 = 0.$$

Summing up the ΔH's for the products gives:

$$[(3 \times 0) + (2 \times (-20.1) + (1 \times 0)] = -40.2 \text{kJ}.$$

Changing the signs for the reactants and summing gives

$$[(2 \times (+32.6)) + (2 \times (+286))] = +637.2 \text{ kJ}.$$

Summing the ΔH's of the products and reactants gives

$$-40.1 + 637.2 = 597 \text{ kJ}.$$

The positive signs tell us that this much energy must be applied before this reaction will run. Sometimes the ΔH value cannot be found for a particular compound. In this case it can be approximated by the ΔH for the bond energies. For example, a single carbon-hydrogen bond has a value of -23.6 kJ / mole. Since methane has four C-H bonds, its ΔH of formation can be calculated as

$$(4 \times (-23.6)) = -94.4 \text{ kJ / mole}.$$

This agrees very closely with the observed value of -79.4. The error comes from the fact that not all C-H bonds are of equal energy, due to surrounding atoms. The value given is an average. The values of ΔH's are determined experimentally using a calorimeter. The particular reaction is carried out in such a device, and the energy liberated heats a known mass of water. Measuring the increase in the temperature of the water yields data that allows the ΔH of the reaction to be calculated.

The "heat capacity" of a substance is the amount of energy required to raise the temperature of a body by 1°C. The "specific heat" is the amount of energy required to raise the temperature of one gram of substance 1°C. One can see that specific heat can actually be used to identify a material. For example, calculate the energy required to raise 125 grams of mercury from -10° to 120°. The specific heat of mercury is 0.138 Joules / gram·°C. This is easily calculated, first by noting the change in temperature;

$$120 - (-10) = 130°. \ (130) \cdot (0.138) \ (125) = 2242.5 \text{ Joules.}$$

Much of the energy involved in chemical reactions can be made to do useful work, but some of it, normally, is not available. A reaction will occur spontaneously at constant pressure and temperature only if it is capable of doing useful work. This amount of useful work that can be done by a reaction at constant temperature and pressure is referred to as the "Gibbs free energy change," ΔG. If the value of ΔG for a particular reaction at a given temperature and pressure is negative, then the reaction is spontaneous, and if it is positive, the reaction will spontaneously run in the opposite direction. If it is zero, the system is in equilibrium. Like enthalpy, ΔH, the Gibbs free energy is a state function, and hence can be calculated much like ΔH. Returning to a previous example of

$$2Ag_2S + 2H_2O \longrightarrow 4Ag + 2H_2S + O_2.$$

Looking up values of ΔG at 298 K and 1 atm., we get:

$$Ag_2S = -40.6 \text{ kJ / mole}, H_2O \text{ (liquid)} = -237 \text{ kJ / mole,}$$

$$Ag = 0, H_2S = -33.5 \text{ kJ / mole}, O_2 = 0.$$

ΔG of the products is

$$(4 \times 0) + (2 \times (-33.5)) + (1 \times 0) = -67.0 \text{ kJ / mole.}$$

Reversing the signs, the ΔG for the reactants is

$$(2 \times (+40.6)) + (2 \times (+237)) = +555.2 \text{ kJ / mole.}$$

Adding together the two values gives

$$-67.0 + 555.2 = 488.2 \text{ kJ / mole.}$$

The positive sign indicates that the reaction will not run spontaneously at 298K and one atmosphere of pressure. However, the reverse reaction will, and will liberate 488.2 kJ of energy. Compare this with the previous value of 597 kJ for ΔH for the same reaction. ΔH gives the total energy change, and ΔG tells how much is available at the given temperature and pressure. While ΔH is relatively constant with temperature and pressure changes, ΔG definitely is not. Neither ΔH nor ΔG are affected by the path which the reaction takes. One might correctly guess that ΔG and ΔH are related. If one subtracts the free energy change from the enthalpy change of the above reaction, a value of 423 kJ is obtained. Where has this energy gone if it did not do useful work? This energy increased the randomness, or disorder of the system, is referred to as the "entropy." As the entropy of a system increases, so does the disorder. The symbol for change in entropy is ΔS, and, like ΔG and ΔH, it is a state function, and values for ΔS can be looked up in tables. $\Delta G = \Delta H - T\Delta S$, where T is the temperature in Kelvin. Note that a positive ΔS value denotes a spontaneous reaction, which is the opposite of ΔH and ΔG.

PROBLEM

23.2 grams of ice are at -15°, and are mixed with 125 grams of water at 85° in an insulated container. Assuming that no heat is lost, what is the final temperature of the contents of the container when equilibrium has been achieved? The specific heats of ice and water are 0.116 J / mole·°C and 0.232 J / mole·°C, respectively, and the heat of fusion for water is 6.03 Joules / mole.

Solution

Since the above values are in per mole units, we first need to convert to moles from grams; 23.2 / 18 = 1.29 moles of ice, 125 / 18 = 6.94 moles of water.

The number of Joules lost by the water will equal the number gained by the ice;

$$J_i = J_w. \tag{1}$$

The Joules gained by the ice will be the number required to raise the ice from

$$-15° \ (\Delta T = 15) \tag{2}$$

to zero, plus the amount required to melt the ice at 0° to water at 0°, plus the amount required to raise the water at 0° to its final temperature,

$$T \ (\Delta T = T - 0). \tag{3}$$

The Joules lost by the water will be the amount needed to lower its temperature from 85° to the final temperature,

$$T \ (\Delta T = 85 - R). \tag{4}$$

Placing these values into the equation from step (2) we get:

$$(15 \times 0.116 \times 1.29) + (1.29 \times 6.03) + (1.29 \times 0.232 \times T)$$

$$= (6.94 \times 0.232 \times [85 - T]).$$

This simplifies to $10.2 + 0.299T = 136.8 - 1.61T$, or $1.909T = 126.8$ or $T = 66.4°$.

VIII. KINETICS AND EQUILIBRIUM

1. Reaction Rate

The rate of a chemical reaction is the amount of product produced per period of time. Most reactions do not run at a constant rate. For two reactants coming together to form a single product such as

$$mA + nB \longrightarrow C,$$

where m and n are the stoichiometric coefficients, we can write the rate law as

$$R = k[A]^m[B]^n.$$

Where R is the rate, k is the rate constant (which is different for each reaction), $[A]$ is the concentration of reactant A, taken to the mth power, $[B]$ is the concentration of reactant B taken to the nth power. The reaction order depends upon the exponents and with the respect to which reactant the exponent is associated. For example, the reaction,

$$3Mg° + N_2 \longrightarrow Mg_3N_2,$$

will have the rate,

$$R = k[Mg]^3[N_2]^1.$$

This reaction is first order with respect to N_2, and third order with respect to Mg. The overall order of the reaction is equal to $n + m$. In the case of the example, it is $(1 + 3)$ = 4, or overall, it is a fourth order reaction. Most chemical reactions involve a number of individual steps between the reactants and the products. We cannot ordinarily write a correct rate equation or establish the order for an overall reaction involving several steps simply by looking at the overall balanced equation. The reaction

$$NO_2 + CO \longrightarrow CO_2 + NO$$

actually occurs in two steps at temperatures below 225°;

$$NO_2 + NO_2 \longrightarrow NO_3 + NO$$

is is the first step, and is very slow.

$$NO_3 + CO \longrightarrow NO_2 + CO_2$$

is the second step, and is very fast. The first step, is the slowest, and hence the "Rate limiting reaction."

Note that the rate of the first reaction

$$(R = k_1 [NO_2]^2),$$

a second order reaction with respect to NO_2. Almost as soon as the NO_3 is formed, it reacts with the CO; hence, the $[CO]$ has little to do with the rate of the second reaction. The rate for this would simply be $R = k_2$ (where k_2 is the rate constant for the second reaction), and we say this is a zero order reaction with respect to CO. One couid not tell this by simply looking at the overall equation; this would have to be determined experimentally. Generally speaking, endothermic reactions increase their rate with temperature, while exothermic reactions reduce their rate as the temperature rises. Often, an activation energy must be applied to get a reaction started. If the reaction is endothermic, the activation energy is greater than that required to keep the reaction going once it is started. If the reaction is exothermic, the energy need no longer be applied once the reaction has started, as it will then be giving off energy. An example of the latter is

$$2Mg + \Delta G_2 \longrightarrow 2Mg + \Delta G.$$

Although this is very exothermic, magnesium can be in contact with oxygen for years at room temperature without any reaction occurring. However, raising the temperature to that of an ordinary match will give sufficient activation energy. Once the energy has been supplied, the match can be removed and the magnesium will burn brightly until either it or the oxygen have all been consumed. This activation energy arranges the molecules involved in a state that is intermediate to that of the reactants and the products, and of higher energy than either. This is known as the transition state. From the transition state, the lower energy products are formed, and the energy given off can be used to activate more reactants to the transition state, and the cycle is repeated.

The presence of a catalyst will lower this activation energy, or eliminate it entirely. Enzymes are a special class of catalysts made of proteins. They also lower the activation energy of a reaction, but usually operate within a narrow pH and temperature range.

2. Equilibrium

For a chemical reaction

$$aA + bB \longrightarrow cC + dD,$$

there will tend to be a certain amount of a back reaction,

$$cC + dD \longrightarrow aA + bB.$$

When the rate of the back reaction equals that of the forward reaction, the system is said to be in equilibrium. Remember, since this is a dynamic equilibrium, the forward and backward reactions are both running, and they are simply running at the same rate, hence the concentrations of the materials do not change. An equilibrium constant k_{eq}, for any given reaction at any given temperature can be calculated. For the above forward reaction, it will be

$$k_{eq} = \frac{[A]^a \, [B]^b}{[C]^c \, [D]^d},$$

This should look familiar, as it is just another form of k_{sp}, k_a, k_b, etc. The Le Chatelier principle states: "If a stress (e.g., change in pressure, concentration, temperature, etc.) is applied to a system in equilibrium, the equilibrium is shifted in a way that tends to undo the effects of the stress." In the above reaction, the addition of A or B, or the removal of C or D will shift the equilibrium to the right. Removal of C or D, or the addition of A or B will shift it to the left.

Think of the equation as a balance, if something is added or removed from one side, material will have to be moved from one side to the other to keep it in balance. An increase in temperature will shift the equilibrium of an endothermic reaction to the right, an exothermic to the left. A decrease in temperature will do just the opposite. For a purely gaseous system increasing the pressure will favor the side of the reaction with the fewest molecules. For example, the reaction

$$N_2 + 3H_2 \longrightarrow 2NH_3$$

has four molecules on the left-hand side, and two on the right. An increase in pressure will shift the equilibria to the right, and a decrease will shift it to the left. This rule applies only to pure gaseous system. The presence of a catalyst will not shift the equilibrium; it will simply allow the system to attain it sooner.

As was mentioned in an earlier section, when a system is at equilibrium, the ΔG = 0. Knowing this, the k_{sp}, k_{eq}, etc. can be calculated using the ΔG. The k calculated will be valid for whatever temperature the G was reported for. The relationship is

$$\Delta G = -RT \ln (k).$$

Where T is the temperature in Kelvin, and R is the ideal gas law constant, but with different units, and hence a different value; 8.314 Joules / mole·Kelvin. For example

AgCl has a ΔG of 55.6 kJ / Mole at 298 K.

Solving for the k_{sp} yields

$$55.6 = -(8.314)(298) \ln (k_{sp}), -22.46 = \ln (k_{sp}), k_{sp} = 175 \times 10^{-10}.$$

PROBLEM

What is the energy of the silver-sulfur bond in silver sulfide? The k_{sp} = 1.0 $\times 10^{-51}$ at 298 k.

Solution

The dissociation is

$$Ag_2S \longrightarrow 2Ag^+ + 2S^=,$$

and from the k_{sp} value, it can be seen that it occurs to a very slight extent, hence the bond must be fairly strong.

$$\Delta G = -RT \ln (k_{sp}), \text{ or } G = -(8.314)(298) \ln (1.0 \times 10^{-51}),$$

solving for ΔG gives 291 kJoules / moles at 298K.

In one formula unit the energy would be

$$291,000 / 6.02 \times 10^{-23} = 4.83 \times 10^{-19} \text{ Joules / formula unit.}$$

In each formula unit there are two AgS bonds;

$$4.83 \times 10^{-19} / 2 = 2.42 \times 10^{-19} \text{ Joules per bond.}$$

IX. ELECTROCHEMISTRY

1. Electrolytic Cells

Electrolytic cells are chemical cells that allow electrical energy to cause chemical reactions. Such an example would be the electrolysis of water. Electrons from a source combine with hydrogen ions to form H_2 gas.

$$(2H^+ + 2e^- \longrightarrow H_2)$$

As a result, hydrogen gas collects at the negative electrode. OH^- will give up its extra electron in the reaction

$$4OH^- \longrightarrow O_2 + 2H_2O + 4e^-,$$

hence oxygen gas will collect at the positive electrode. In reviewing previous chemistry, it can be seen that the H^+ is reduced and the OH^- is oxidized. Rather than using the terms + and - for electrodes, as was done above, in electrochemistry the terms anode and cathode are preferred. The oxidation reaction always occurs at the anode, and the reduction reaction always occurs at the cathode. This is easy to remember since cathode and reduction both begin with a consonant, and anode and oxidation both begin with a vowel. An electrolyte is a material in the cell containing ions.

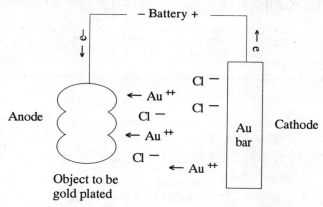

The above illustration shows an electrolytic cell used to gold plate objects. The electrolyte is a solution of gold chloride ($AuCl_2$), which in solution consists of gold and chloride ions. The negative pole of a battery is connected to the anode, which is the object to be electroplated. The positive pole is connected to the cathode, in this case a gold bar. The anode and cathode are then immersed into the electrolyte. Electrons flow from the negative pole of the battery to the anode where they reduce the gold ions in the solution to gold atoms by the reaction

$$Au^{++} + 2e^- \longrightarrow Au°.$$

The gold metal plates out on the target. At the cathode, gold atoms on the surface of the bar lose their valence electrons by the opposite reaction, and become gold ions in the solution. The electrons move to the positive pole of the battery. The flow of electrons and ions are shown in the diagram.

Note that the electron flow is in the opposite direction of the positive ion flow. Note that in the case of gold, two electrons are required to plate out one atom of gold. One mole of electrons will plate out half a mole of gold, or 98.5 grams of gold. Electric charge is measured in coulombs, and one mole of electrons will have a charge of 96,487 coulombs (this value is known as Faraday's constant, or a Faraday of charge). A current of one ampere (abbreviated Amp.) has a charge of one coulomb passing a point every second. How much gold metal can the cell above plate out running for 8.00 hours at 0.120 Amps? Assume that there is no limit to the amount of gold ions available.

8.00 hours = 480 minutes = 28,800 seconds.

At 0.250 amps, this gives a total charge of

28,800 × 0.250 = 7,200 Coulombs

of charge delivered in that amount of time.

7,200 / 96,487 = 0.0746 moles of electrons, or 0.0746 / 2 = 0.0373 moles

of gold plated out.

This corresponds with (0.0373 × 197) = 7.35 grams of gold in that period of time. Note that we could use this procedure to calculate the amount of any material produced by such a cell, whether it is a gas or a metal.

2. Galvanic Cells

A galvanic cell does just the opposite of an electrolytic cell; it uses a chemical reaction to produce an electric current. A more common name is a battery. Again, oxidation occurs at the anode, and reduction at the cathode. In the cell shown below, zinc atoms give up two electrons to become zinc ions, by the reaction

$$Zn° \longrightarrow Zn^{++} + 2e^-.$$

The electrons travel up the anode (the (-) pole of this battery), to the electrical device (e.g., light, meter, motor, etc.) then to the cathode (the (+) terminal). At the cathode they reduce the copper ions to copper atoms by the reaction

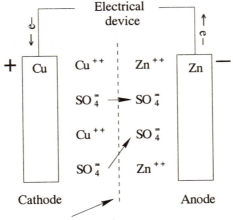

$$Cu^{++} + 2e^- \longrightarrow Cu^\circ.$$

Two electrolytes are used in this cell, separated by a semipermeable membrane. The copper cathode is surrounded by a copper sulfate solution, and the zinc anode is surrounded by a zinc sulfate solution. As the reaction proceeds, the zinc anode will decrease in size while the $ZnSO_4$ solution will increase in concentration. The copper cathode will increase in size, while the $CuSO_4$ solution will become more dilute. As the concentration of the electrolytes change, sulfate ions are free to pass from one solution to the other via the semipermeable membrane. Note that the direction of movement of the sulfate ions is opposite that of the electrons.

Also note that the (+) and (-) designations for the anode and cathode are just the opposite in a galvanic cell than they are in an electrolytic cell. When the reaction has reached equilibrium, the electron flow halts, and the battery is said to be "dead." It can be "recharged" by connecting it to another source of electrons, and now becomes an electrolytic cell, the anode and cathode having exchanged positions.

The potential of a cell is measured in volts. Under standard conditions (298 K, 1 atm, 1 molar concentrations) the standard potential, E°, is easily calculated. Tables exist of Standard Reduction Potentials that list the E° for standard reduction reactions. To convert the value to an oxidation potential, reverse the sign. For the cell above, the following two reactions are found:

$$Zn^{++} + 2e^- \longrightarrow Zn^\circ, E^\circ = -0.763 \text{ volts},$$

$$Cu^{++} + 2e^- \longrightarrow Cu^\circ, E^\circ = +0.337 \text{ volts}.$$

Since in the above cell, zinc is being oxidized, the sign is reversed, giving a potential of $+0.763$ volts. The total potential of the cell, E°, is determined by summing the two values,

$$0.763 + 0.337 = +1.10 \text{ volts}.$$

In other words, the cell described above, under standard conditions, will produce 1.10 volts of electric potential, no matter what physical size it is. The positive value shows that the cell will produce electricity, but were this value zero or less, no electrical current would be produced. In fact, were the E° negative, that would mean the cell was electrolytic, not galvanic, and a current would have to be applied to get the reaction to run.

What if concentrations are not at one molar for the electrolytes of a cell? How can the E be calculated? This is easy to do using the Nernst equation,

$$E = E^\circ - 0.059 / n \cdot \log \frac{[\text{product}]}{[\text{reactant}]}.$$

Where E is the potential under non-standard conditions, E° is the potential under standard conditions, n is the number of electrons exchanged between atoms, and

$$\frac{[\text{products}]}{[\text{reactants}]}$$

is just another equilibrium term. If in the above cell

$$[CuSO_4] = 0.145 \text{ M, and } [ZnSO_4] = 1.80 \text{ M},$$

what would the potential, E, be? Plugging into the equation, we get

$$E = 1.10 - (0.059 / 2) \cdot \log (1.80 / 0.145).$$

($ZnSO_4$ is produced in this reaction, it is the product; $CuSO_4$ is consumed, it is the reactant.) Continuing,

$$E = 1.10 - 0.0295 \cdot \log (12.41), \text{ or } E = 1.10 - (0.0295 \times 1.09),$$

or $E = 1.07$ volts.

PROBLEM

a)   How many grams of Thallium metal can be *plated* out of a solution of Tl^{+++} ions using a current of 4.68 amps for 2.60 hours?

b)   What is the standard potential of a galvanic cell that operates by the reaction

$Cr^{+++} + Al° \longrightarrow Cr° + Al^{+++}$? $Cr^{+++} + 3e^- \longrightarrow Cr°$,

$E° = -0.74$ volts. $Al^{+++} + 3e^- \longrightarrow Al°$, $E° = -1.66$ volts?

c)   What is the potential if the $[Cr^{+++}] = 2.50$ M, and the $[Al^{+++}] = 0.178$ M?

Solution

a)   30.9 grams of thallium

b) $E° = 0.92$ volts

c) $E = 0.95$ volts

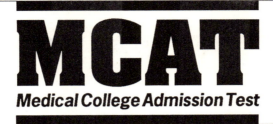

Chapter 4

Physics Review

Chapter 4

I. TRANSLATIONAL MOTION

1. Units and Dimensions

Conversion Factors

1 mile	=	5280 ft
1 ft	=	.305 m
1 in	=	2.54 cm

g = 9.8 m/s ≈ 10 m/s

   = 32.2 ft/s

(See Appendix for a more complete table)

2. Vectors and Scalars

BASIC DEFINITIONS OF VECTORS AND SCALARS

A vector is a quantity that has both magnitude and direction. Some typical vector quantities are: displacement, velocity, force, acceleration, momentum, electric field strength and magnetic field strength.

A scalar is a quantity that has magnitude but no direction. Some typical scalar quantities are: mass, length, time, density, energy and temperature.

ADDITION OF VECTORS ($\bar{a} + \bar{b}$) — GEOMETRIC METHODS

Triangle Method (Head-to-Tail Method)

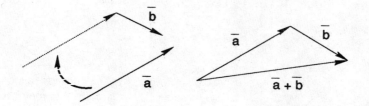

(i) Attach the head of $\bar{a}$ to the tail of $\bar{b}$.

(ii) By connecting the head of $\bar{a}$ to the tail of $\bar{b}$, the vector $\bar{a} + \bar{b}$ is defined.

Figure 1.1 — Triangle Method of Adding Vectors

Parallelogram Method (Tail-to-Tail Method)·

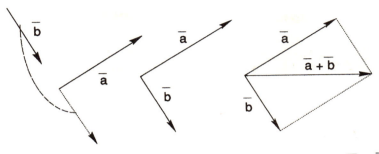

(i) Join the tails of the two vectors.

(ii) Construct a parallelogram having $\overline{a}$ and $\overline{b}$ as two of its sides. The long diagonal of the parallelogram represents the vector $\overline{a} + \overline{b}$.

Figure 1.2 — The Parallelogram Method of Adding Vectors

SUBTRACTION OF VECTORS

The subtraction of a vector is defined as the addition of the corresponding negative vector. Therefore, the vector $\mathbf{P} - \mathbf{F}$ is obtained by adding the vector $(-\mathbf{F})$ to the vector $\mathbf{P}$, i.e., $\mathbf{P} + (-\mathbf{F})$. See the following figure.

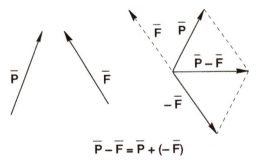

$$\overline{P} - \overline{F} = \overline{P} + (-\overline{F})$$

Figure 1.3 — The Subtraction of a Vector

THE COMPONENTS OF A VECTOR

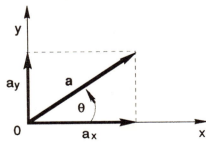

a_x and a_y are the components of a vector **a**. The angle θ is measured counterclockwise from the positive x-axis. The components are formed when we draw perpendicular lines to the chosen axes.

Figure 1.4 – The Formation of Vector Components on the Positive $X - Y$ Axis

The components of a vector are given by

$$A_x = A \cos \theta$$

$$A_y = A \sin \theta$$

A component is equal to the product of the magnitude of vector A and cosine of the angle between the positive axis and the vector.

The magnitude can be expressed in terms of the components.

$$A = \sqrt{A_x{}^2 + A_y{}^2}$$

For the angle θ,

$$\text{Tan } \theta = \frac{A_y}{A_x}$$

PROBLEM

Two hikers set off in an eastward direction. Hiker 1 travels 3 km while hiker 2 travels 6 times the distance covered by hiker 1. What is the displacement of hiker 2?

Solution

From the information given the displacement vector is directed east. The magnitude of the displacement vector for hiker 2 is 6 times the magnitude of the displacement vector for hiker 1. Therefore, its magnitude is

$$6 \times (3 \text{ km}) = 18 \text{ km}$$

PROBLEM

Two wires are attached to a corner fence post with the wires making an angle of 90° with each other. If each wire pulls on the post with a force of 50 pounds, what is the resultant force acting on the post? See Figure 1.5.

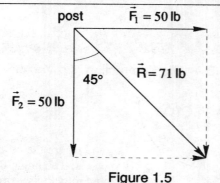

Figure 1.5

Solution

As shown in the figure, we complete the parallelogram. If we measure R and scale it, we find it is equal to about 71 pounds. The angle of the resultant is 45° from either of the component vectors.

If we use the fact that the component vectors are at right angles to each other, we can write

$$R^2 = 50^2 + 50^2$$

whence

$R = 71$ pounds approximately at 45° to each wire.

3. Uniformly Accelerated Motion

Consider the special case of constant or uniform acceleration **a** = rate of change in velocity/time = constant. In one dimension, the statement would be that a = constant and the acceleration-time curve is given by Figure 1.6. The average acceleration would be

$$<a> = \Delta v / \Delta t = (v - v_0) / (t - 0).$$

The meaning of this physics problem-solving technique is that the area under the acceleration-time curve is the change in velocity (hatched area in Figure 1.6).

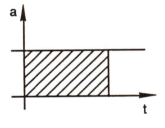

Figure 1.6

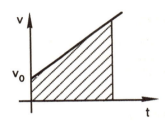

Figure 1.7

In one dimension the first equation for motion would be

$$v = v_0 + at.$$

Hence, if one knows the change and velocity and the time, the acceleration can be found. This means that the slope of the velocity-time curve (Figure 1.7) is the acceleration.

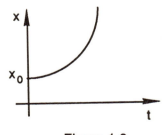

Figure 1.8

Now, the definition of velocity is **v** = rate of change in direction/time. The average velocity is

$$\langle v \rangle = \Delta \mathbf{r} / \Delta t = (\mathbf{r} - \mathbf{r}_0) / (t - 0).$$

Hence, if one knows the distance covered and the time taken, one can find the average velocity. For the special case of uniform acceleration only,

$$\langle v \rangle = (v + v_0) / 2,$$

as one would expect for an average value.

In one dimension, the second important equation is that

$$x = x_0 + v_0 t + \tfrac{1}{2} at^2.$$

(See Figure 1.8 for the position-time curve.) Note that the slope of the position-time curve at any time is the instantaneous velocity.

A third important formula is obtained by solving for the time

$$t = (v - v_0) / a$$

and substituting into

$$x - x_0 = \langle v \rangle t$$

to get

$$v^2 = v_0^2 + 2a (x - x_0).$$

This formula is useful if the time is not part of the given information in the problem.

PROBLEM

An airplane lands on a carrier deck at 150 mi/hr and is brought to a stop uniformly, by an arresting device, in 500 ft. Find the acceleration and the time required to stop.

Solution

Converting units to ft-sec,

$$v_0 = (150 \text{ mi} / \text{hr}) \times \left(\frac{5280 \text{ ft} / \text{mi}}{3600 \text{ sec} / \text{hr}} \right) = 220 \text{ ft} / \text{sec}.$$

Since there is a constant deceleration,

$$2as = v_1^2 - v_0^2$$

$$2a(500 \text{ ft}) = 0 - (220 \text{ ft} / \text{sec})^2$$

$$a = \frac{-(220 \text{ ft} / \text{sec})^2}{2(500 \text{ ft})} = -48.4 \text{ ft} / \text{sec}^2.$$

Solving for t in the following formula,

$$v_1 = v_0 + at$$

$$t = \frac{v_1 - v_0}{a} = \frac{0 - 220 \text{ ft} / \text{sec}}{-48.4 \text{ ft} / \text{sec}^2} = 4.55 \text{ sec}.$$

4. Freely Falling Bodies

Free fall in one dimension is a special case of constant acceleration translational kinematics. If the direction downward is taken as negative, then

$$a = -g = -9.8 \text{ m/s}^2,$$

and the first two formulae become

$$v = v_0 - gt \quad \text{and} \quad y = y_0 + v_0 t - \frac{1}{2} g t^2.$$

The displacement-time curve is thus a parabola. If an object is projected upwards with a positive initial velocity, the time to reach the apex where $v = 0$ is just $t = v_0 / g$.

PROBLEM

A boy leaning over a railway bridge 49 ft high sees a train approaching with uniform speed and attempts to drop a stone down the funnel. He releases the stone when the engine is 80 ft away from the bridge and sees the stone hit the ground 3 ft in front of the engine. What is the speed of the train?

Solution

Applying the equation applicable to uniform acceleration,

$$x - x_0 = v_0 t + \frac{1}{2} a t^2,$$

to the dropping of the stone 49 ft from rest under the action of gravity, we can find the time t the stone is in motion. The initial velocity of the stone v_0 is zero. The distance the stone travels,

$$x - x_0 = 49 \text{ ft.}$$

Therefore,

$$49 \text{ ft} = 0 + \left(\frac{1}{2}\right)(32 \text{ ft/sec}^2)(t^2)$$

$$\therefore t = \sqrt{\frac{2 \times 49 \text{ ft}}{32 \text{ ft / s}^2}} = \frac{7}{4} s.$$

In the time of 7/4 s it takes the stone to drop, the engine has moved with uniform speed u a distance of (80 - 3) ft.

$$\therefore u = \frac{d}{t} = \frac{77 \text{ ft}}{7/4 \text{ sec}} = 44 \text{ ft / sec} = 30 \text{ mph.}$$

5. Projectiles

Projectile motion in two dimensions follows from keeping track of the components in the first two kinematic formulae

$$v_y = v_{0y} - gt \quad \text{and} \quad y = y_0 + v_{0y} t - \frac{1}{2} g t^2$$

$$v_x = v_{0x} = \text{constant} \quad \text{and} \quad x = x_0 + v_{0x} t.$$

The y versus x curve may be shown to be parabolic. Note that because velocity is a vector,

$$v_{0x} = v_0 \cos \theta \quad \text{and} \quad v_{0y} = v_0 \sin \theta,$$

where θ is the initial angle of projection (see Figure 1.9). The time to reach the apex of the path is again $t = v_{0y} / g$, and the height may be found by substituting into the $y = y(t)$ equation. Also, the range is found by substituting $t_R = 2t$ into the equation $x = x_0 + v_x t$.

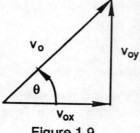

Figure 1.9

PROBLEM

A ball is thrown with an initial velocity, v_0, of 160 ft/sec, directed at an angle, θ_0, of 53° with the ground.

a) Find the x- and y-components of v_0.

b) Find the position of the ball and the magnitude and direction of its velocity when $t = 2$ sec.

c) At the highest point of the ball's path, what is the ball's altitude (h) and how much time has elapsed?

d) What is the ball's range d? (See Figure 1.10.)

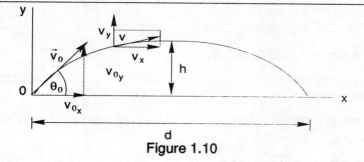

Figure 1.10

Solution

a) Using the figure

$$v_{0_x} = v_0 \cos\theta_0; \quad v_{0_y} = v_0 \sin\theta_0$$

Hence,

$$v_{0_x} = 160 \text{ ft / sec} \cdot \cos 53° = 160 \text{ ft / sec } (3/5) = 96 \text{ ft / sec}$$

$$v_{0_y} = 160 \text{ ft / sec} \cdot \sin 53° = 160 \text{ ft / sec } (4/5)$$

$$= 128 \text{ ft / sec}$$

b) The acceleration due to gravity is constant. Furthermore, there is no force acting on the projectile in the x-direction, and its acceleration in the x-direction is therefore zero. Hence

$$a_x(t) = 0 \qquad\qquad a_y(t) = -g$$

$$v_x(t) = v_{0_x} \qquad\qquad v_y(t) = v_{0_y} - gt$$

$$x(t) = x_0 + v_{0_x}t \qquad\qquad y(t) = y_0 + v_{0_y}t - \tfrac{1}{2}gt^2$$

Here, x_0, y_0 are the initial coordinates of the projectile, and v_{0_x}, v_{0_y} are the initial x and y components of the ball's velocity. Taking the origin (0) as shown in the figure, we have, at $t = 2$ sec

$$v_x = 96 \text{ ft/sec}$$

$$x = (96 \text{ ft/sec}) (2 \text{ sec}) = 192 \text{ ft}$$

$$v_y = 128 \text{ ft/sec} - (32 \text{ ft/sec}^2) (2 \text{ sec}) = 64 \text{ ft/sec}$$

$$y = (128 \text{ ft/sec}) (2 \text{ sec}) - (1/2) (32 \text{ ft/sec}^2) (4 \text{ sec}^2)$$

$$y = 256 \text{ ft} - 64 \text{ ft} = 192 \text{ ft}.$$

The magnitude of the ball's velocity is

$$v = (v_x^2 + v_y^2)^{1/2}$$

$$v = ((64 \text{ ft/sec})^2 + (96 \text{ ft/sec})^2)^{1/2}$$

$$v = 115.4 \text{ ft/sec}.$$

The direction of the velocity relative to the x-axis is

$$\tan\theta = \frac{v_y}{v_x} = \frac{64}{96} = \frac{2}{3}$$

$$\theta = 34°$$

c)   At the highest point of the path, the ball has no vertical velocity. Then, by our kinematics equations,

$$v_y = 0 = v_0 - gt$$

$$t = \frac{v_{0_y}^{-0}}{g} = \frac{128 \text{ ft / sec}}{32 \text{ ft / sec}^2} = 4 \text{ sec}.$$

It takes 4 sec for the ball to reach its maximum height. It has traveled a vertical distance,

$$y_{max} = v_{0_y}t - \tfrac{1}{2}gt^2$$

$$= (128 \text{ ft/sec}) (4 \text{ sec}) - 1/2(32 \text{ ft/sec}^2) (4 \text{ sec})^2$$

$$= 512 \text{ ft} - 256 \text{ ft} = 256 \text{ ft}.$$

d)   It takes the ball as much time to fall as it does to rise. Hence, the entire trajectory requires 8 sec. By the kinematics equations, we find its horizontal position at the end of its trajectory,

$$x(t) = v_{0_x}t = 96 \text{ ft / sec} \cdot 8 \text{ sec} = 768 \text{ ft}.$$

II. FORCE AND MOTION, GRAVITATION

1. Mass and Weight

Mass → units: (Kilograms (kg))

For a given body, the ratio of the magnitude of the force to that of the acceleration is a constant and is called its mass:

$$m = \frac{F}{a} = \text{constant (for a given body).}$$

Weight → units: (Newtons)

The weight of a body is the gravitational force exerted on the body by the earth and is given by the product of the mass and the gravitational acceleration.

$$W = mg$$

2. Newton's Second Law

$$\mathbf{F} = m\mathbf{a}$$

If the forces, **F**, acting on a particle of mass, *m*, are different from zero, the particle will have an acceleration, **a**. The direction of the acceleration will be in the same direction as the force as shown in the above equation.

3. Newton's Third Law

$$F_A = -F_B$$

For every action, there is a corresponding *equal* and opposing reaction.

PROBLEM

A car on a country road in Maryland passes over an old-fashioned hump-backed bridge. The center of gravity of the car follows the arc of a circle of radius 88 ft. Assuming that the car has a weight of 2 tons, find the force exerted by the car on the road at the highest point of the bridge if the car is traveling at 30 mph. At what speed will the car lose contact with the road? (See Figure 2.1)

Solution

The forces acting on the car at the highest point of the bridge are its weight W = *m*g downward and the normal force N exerted by the bridge upward. These cannot be equal, since there must be a net downward force to provide the acceleration necessary to keep the car traveling in a circle. Thus

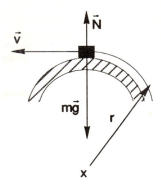

Figure 2.1

$mg - N = m(v^2/r)$,

by Newton's Second Law.

$$N = m\left(g - \frac{v^2}{r}\right) = \frac{W}{g}\left(g - \frac{v^2}{r}\right) = W\left(1 - \frac{v^2}{rg}\right).$$

where W is the height of the car.

Here $v = 30$ mph $= 44$ ft/s.

$$\therefore N = 2 \text{ tons} \left(1 - \frac{44^2 \text{ ft}^2/\text{s}^2}{88 \times 32 \text{ ft}/\text{s}^2}\right)$$

$$= 2\left(1 - \frac{11}{16}\right) \text{ ton} = \frac{5}{8} \text{ ton}.$$

But action and reaction are equal and opposite. Thus, if the road exerts a force of 5/8 ton on the car, the car exerts the same force on the road.

The car loses contact with the road when $N = 0$, that is, when $v^2 = rg$. Thus the speed required is

$$v = \sqrt{rg} = \sqrt{88 \text{ ft} \times 32 \text{ ft}/\text{s}^2} = 16\sqrt{11} \text{ ft}/\text{s}$$

$$= 53.1 \text{ ft}/\text{s} = 36 \text{ mph}.$$

4. Newton's Law of Gravitation

$$F = \frac{Gm_1 m_2}{r^2}$$

$$G = 6.7 \times 10^{-11} \frac{\text{Nm}^2}{\text{kg}^2}$$

Between every two objects in the universe, there exists an attractive force of gravitation, which is proportional to the masses of the objects and inversely proportional to the distance squared between them.

At what distance from the center of the earth does the acceleration due to gravity have one half of the value that it has on the surface of the earth?

Solution

Newton's Second Law implies that $W = mg$. W is the weight of an object of mass m (that is, the gravitational force of attraction between the earth and the object), and g is the acceleration due to gravity. Then, by Newton's Law of Universal Gravitation,

$$W = \frac{GM_e m}{R^2} = mg$$

where R is the distance of the object of mass m from the center of the earth, and M_e is the mass of the earth. Therefore

$$g(R) = \frac{GM_e}{R^2}$$

At the surface of the earth,

$$g(R_e) = \frac{GM_2}{R_e^2}$$

But we want $g(R) = {}^1/_2\, g(R_e)$. Therefore,

$$\frac{GM_e}{R^2} = \frac{1}{2}\frac{GM_e}{R_e^2}$$

$$R^2 = 2R_e^2$$

$$R = \sqrt{2}R_e$$

$$= 1.414 \times 6.38 \times 10^6\,\text{m} = 9.02 \times 10^6\ m$$

The acceleration due to gravity is reduced to one half of its usual value at a distance of 9.02×10^6 meters from the center of the earth. This is equivalent to a height of 2.64×10^6 meters or 1640 miles above the surface of the earth.

5. Uniform Circular Motion, Centripetal Force

The force acting on a body of mass m undergoing uniform circular motion is the centripetal force, given by

$$F = ma = m\frac{v^2}{r}$$

A body of mass m is traveling in uniform circular motion. The body is pulled toward the center of the circle of radius r with a force $F = \frac{mv^2}{r}$

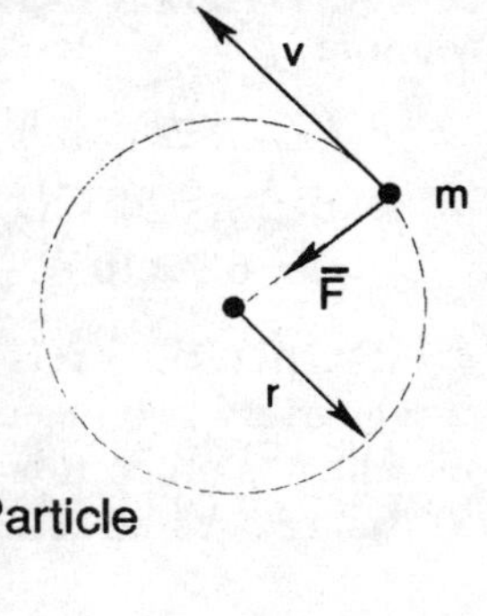

Figure 2.2 — Centripetal Force of a Particle

Here, v is the magnitude of velocity, which is constant, and r is the radius of the circle.

6. Friction

For impending motion,

Frictional Force $= F_s = \mu_s N$

where μ_s = Coefficient of Static Friction

     N = Normal Force

For a body already in motion,

$F_k = \mu_k N$

where μ_k = Coefficient of Kinetic Friction

PROBLEM

If the coefficient of sliding friction for steel on ice is 0.05, what force is required to keep a man weighing 150 pounds moving at constant speed along the ice?

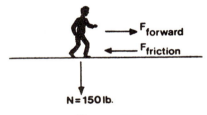

Figure 2.3

Solution

To keep the man moving at constant velocity, we must oppose the force of friction tending to retard his motion with an equal but opposite force (see Figure 2.3).

The force of friction is given by:

$F = \mu_{kinetic} N$

By Newton's Third Law

$F_{forward} = F_{friction}$

Therefore

$F_{forward} = \mu_{kinetic} N$

$F_{forward} = (.05)(150 \text{ lb}) = 7.5 \text{ lb}.$

7. Inclined Planes

The key to solving incline problems is to resolve all the forces acting on the object to their components along and perpendicular to the plane.

PROBLEM

What is the acceleration of a block on a frictionless plane inclined at an angle θ with the horizontal?

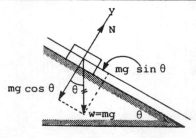

Figure 2.4

Solution

In order to find the acceleration, a, of the block, we must calculate the net force, F, on the block, and relate this to its acceleration via Newton's Second Law, $F = ma$. (Here m is the mass of the block).

The only forces acting on the block are its weight mg and the normal force N exerted by the plane (See Figure 2.4). Take axes parallel and perpendicular to the surface of the plane and resolve the weight into x- and y- components. Then

$$\Sigma F_y = N - mg \cos \theta,$$

$$\Sigma F_x = mg \sin \theta.$$

But we know that the acceleration is in the y direction, $a_y = 0$, since the block doesn't accelerate off the surface of the inclined plane. From the equation $\Sigma F_y = ma_y$ we find that $N = mg \cos \theta$. From the equation $\Sigma F_x = ma_x$, where a_x is the acceleration of the block in the x direction, we have

$$mg \sin \theta = ma_x,$$

$$a_x = g \sin \theta.$$

The mass does not appear in the final result, which means that any block, regardless of its mass, will slide on a frictionless inclined plane with an acceleration down the plane of $g \sin \theta$. (Note that the velocity is not necessarily down the plane).

8. Pulley Systems

Remember that tension at all points along a rope in a pulley system is the same.

PROBLEM

For the block and tackle shown in Figure 2.5:

a) Find the displacement ratio.

b) What force, F, must be exerted on the free end of the rope to lift a 200 lb load?

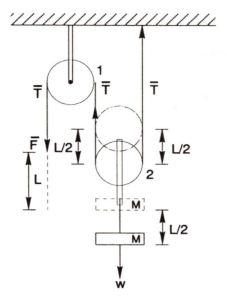

Figure 2.5

Solution

a)   When **F** pulls down the rope by an amount L, pulley 2 moves up by $\frac{1}{2}L$ (as shown in Figure 2.5) since the shortening of the rope is shared by the two segments of rope that hold the pulley. Therefore, the ratio of the displacement of load to the displacement of rope is

$$\frac{\frac{1}{2}L}{L} = \frac{1}{2}.$$

b)   From the figure, we see that the load is held up by a force $2T$ where **T** is the tension in the rope. Hence, in order to lift the load, the minimum tension should satisfy

$$W = 2T$$

or $T = \frac{1}{2}W$

where W is the weight of the load.

F is equal to **T** as long as the rope does not break since the stress in the rope is caused by the action of **F**. We have

$$F = T = \frac{W}{2}$$

$$= \frac{200 \text{ lb}}{2} = 100 \text{ lb}$$

III. EQUILIBRIUM AND MOMENTUM

1. Equilibrium

A. TRANSLATIONAL EQUILIBRIUM

Fundamental to physics is the concept of a force. Intuitively, a force is a push or a pull acting on some object. More precisely, Newton's laws help us to define a force. Newton's First Law states that an object at rest remains at rest and an object in motion remains in motion with constant velocity in the absence of external forces. Newton's Second Law is the basis of dynamics, but one consequence of it is that the weight force of any mass is $W = mg$, where g is the gravitational acceleration = 9.8 m/s^2 near the surface of the Earth.

Other than weight, several important forces are tension (the force in a string or cable), the normal force N acting perpendicular to a surface, the force of static friction

$$F_s \leq \mu_s N,$$

the force of kinetic friction

$$F_k = \mu_k N$$

and a pivot or reaction force R acting at an angle θ with respect to the surface. For example, in standing on the floor, you exert a force of magnitude W on the floor; the floor responds by exerting a force $N = R$ on you. The reaction force of the floor prevents you from falling through the floor.

In order to solve a statics (or any) physics problem, first write down the information in terms of numbers and symbols. Then draw a figure showing the relevant objects and angles. Next, choose points in the system and draw free body diagrams for those points. For example, in Figure 3.1, two important free body diagrams are shown for the case of a mass suspended by a cord from a ceiling.

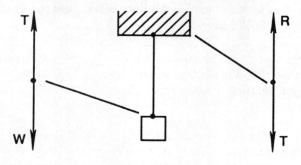

Figure 3.1

In statics, we now apply the two conditions of equilibrium. The first condition is that the sum of the forces in each direction is zero:

$$\Sigma F = 0.$$

The equilibrium is said to be static if also the velocity

$$v = 0.$$

For example, in Figure 3.1, choosing the positive direction as down, we get

$$\Sigma F_y = W - T = 0 \quad \text{and} \quad T - R = 0.$$

Hence, $T = W$ and $R = T$; the weight determines both the tension in the string and the reaction force of the ceiling. In Figure 3.2, a force F pushes an object of mass m on a flat but rough surface with coefficient of static friction μ_s and coefficient of kinetic friction μ_k. Resolving F into its x and y components, we find

$$F_x = F \cos \theta \quad \text{and} \quad F_y = F \sin \theta.$$

Static equilibrium in the y-direction gives

$$\Sigma F_y = F_y + N - W = 0 \quad \text{or} \quad N = mg - F \sin \theta$$

to find the normal force. Note that the normal force is not always equal to mg! If the object starts out at rest, then it will begin to move when

$$\Sigma F_x = F_x - F_s = 0 \quad \text{or} \quad F \cos \theta = \mu_s N.$$

If the object is moving at constant velocity, then

$$\Sigma F_x = F_x - F_k = 0 \quad \text{or} \quad \mu_k N = F \cos \theta.$$

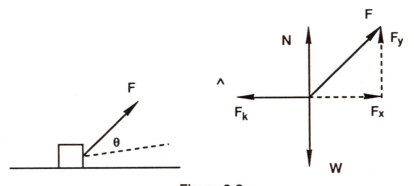

Figure 3.2

PROBLEM

A 200 lb man hangs from the middle of a tightly stretched rope so that the angle between the rope and the horizontal direction is 5°, as shown in Figure 3.3(A). Calculate the tension in the rope. (Figure 3.3(B).)

Solution

Since the two sections of the rope are symmetrical with respect to the man, the tensions in them must have the same magnitude, (Figure 3.3(B)). This can be arrived at by summing the forces in the horizontal direction and setting them equal to zero since the system is in equilibrium. Then

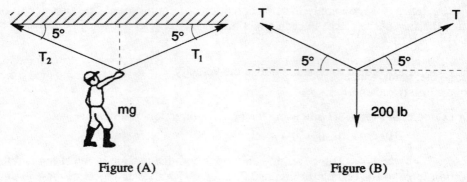

Figure (A)   Figure (B)

Figure 3.3

$$\Sigma F_x = T_1 \cos 5° - T_2 \cos 5° = 0$$

and $T_1 = T_2 = T$

Considering the forces in the vertical direction,

$$\Sigma F_y = T \sin 5° + T \sin 5° - 200 \text{ lb} = 0$$

$$200 \text{ lb} = 2T \sin 5° = 2T(0.0871)$$

$$T = \frac{(200)}{(2)(0.0871)} = 1150 \text{ lbs.}$$

Note the significant force that can be exerted on objects at either end of the rope by this arrangement. The tension in the rope is over five times the weight of the man. Had the angle been as small as 1°, the tension would have been

$$T = \frac{200}{2 \sin 1°} = \frac{200}{(2)(0.0174)} = 5730 \text{ lbs.}$$

This technique for exerting a large force would only be useful to move something a very small distance, since any motion of one end of the rope would change the small angle considerably and the tension would decrease accordingly.

B.   ROTATIONAL EQUILIBRIUM

The second condition, that of rotational equilibrium, is that the sum of all torques is zero:

$$\Sigma \tau = 0$$

where the torque

$$\tau = \mathbf{r} \times \mathbf{F}$$

is a cross product. Note that position vector **r** where the force acts and the force **F** must be drawn with a common origin to find the angle θ between them; then the right hand rule is used to find the direction of the torque. Figure 3.4 shows a standard boom problem, where the boom has a weight $B = m_b g$ and the person has weight $W = mg$. The first equilibrium gives

$$\Sigma F_x = R_x - T_x = 0 \quad \text{hence} \cdot \quad R_x = T \cos \theta.$$

Also,

$$\Sigma F_y = R_y + T_y - W - B = 0 \quad \text{or} \quad R_y = W + B - T \sin \theta.$$

If R and T are unknown, one cannot find them just from these two equations. Hence, choose the point where the boom contacts the wall as the origin for calculating torques. Rotational equilibrium then implies

$$\Sigma \tau = \Sigma r F \sin \theta$$
$$= (0)\,(R) - xW \sin 90 - d/2\,B \sin 90 + dT \sin (180 - \theta)$$
$$= 0$$

or solving for the tension

$$T = (xW + bD/2) / (d \sin \theta).$$

The positive and negative directions come from the right hand rule. The angles come from moving the position vector such that it and the force have a common origin (Figure 3.5).

The concept of rotational equilibrium can also be used to locate the center of gravity or gravitational center of a system of objects. This is just the pivot point where the system balances as in the childhood seesaw. More importantly, the center of gravity often coincides with the center of mass of an object where

$$r_{cm} = \Sigma mr / \Sigma m.$$

In the boom problem, Figure 3.4, we assumed the weight of the boom acted at the center of the mass of the boom $d/2$.

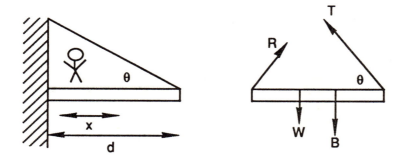

Figure 3.4

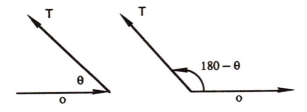

Figure 3.5

PROBLEM

What scale readings would you predict when a uniform 120 lb plank 6.0 ft long is placed on two balances as shown in Figure 3.6, with 1.0 ft extending beyond the left support and 2.0 ft extending beyond the right support?

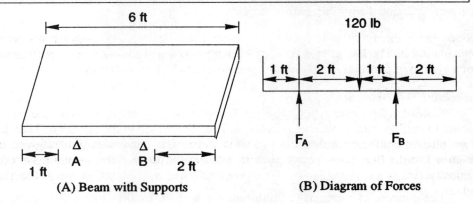

(A) Beam with Supports   (B) Diagram of Forces

Figure 3.6

Solution

From the first condition for equilibrium, the forces upward must equal the forces downward.

$$F_A + F_B - 120 \text{ lb} = 0$$

The plank is uniform, meaning that the center of mass is at the center of the beam, three feet from each end. This is the point at which the 120 lb gravitational force can be considered to act.

Torque about a point is defined as the tendency of a force to cause rotation about the point. The magnitude of the torque is given by the product of the magnitude of the force and the perpendicular distance of the line of action of the force (the line along which the force acts) from the point of rotation. The direction of the torque can be found using the right hand rule. Place the fingers of the right hand in the direction of the distance vector. Rotate the distance vector into the direction of the force vector. If this rotation is in the clockwise direction, the torque is negative. For counterclockwise rotation, the torque is positive. For equilibrium, the sum of all the torques about any point in the body must equal zero.

To apply this second condition for equilibrium, we may choose to write torques about an axis through A, noting that the center of mass of the plank is 2.0 ft from A.

$$- 120 \text{ lb} \times 2.0 \text{ ft} + F_B (3.0) \text{ ft} = 0 \quad \text{or} \quad F_B = 80 \text{ lb}$$

Substitution of 80 lb for F_B in the first equation gives $F_A = 40$ lb. Alternatively, we may write a second torque equation, this time about an axis through B.

$$+ 120 \text{ lb} \times 1.0 \text{ ft} - F_A (3.0 \text{ ft}) = 0 \quad \text{or} \quad F_A = 40 \text{ lb}$$

2. Momentum

A.   CONSERVATION OF LINEAR MOMENTUM

Recall that the momentum of an object is given by

$$\mathbf{p} = m\mathbf{v}.$$

Since the momentum is a vector, one must keep track of the components when calculating it. The law of conservation of momentum states that the total momentum of a system of particles is conserved in the absence of external forces:

$$\Sigma \mathbf{p}_0 = \Sigma \mathbf{p}.$$

Consider the problem of Figure 3.7. One object of mass m_1 and speed v_1 is about to collide with another of mass m_2 at rest. This is the initial situation. Then the two objects collide or interact via internal forces. The final situation is given by Figure 3.8: the first mass moves off with velocity (v'_1, θ) and the second mass with velocity $(v'_2, -\phi)$. From Figure 3.7, conservation of momentum in the x-direction gives

$$m_1 v_1 = m_1 v'_1 \cos \theta + m_2 v'_2 \cos \theta.$$

Similarly, in the y-direction we have

$$0 = m_1 v'_1 \sin \theta - m_2 v'_2 \sin \phi.$$

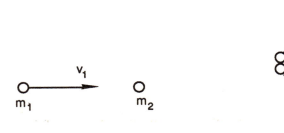

Figure 3.7   Figure 3.8

B.   ELASTIC AND INELASTIC COLLISIONS

If the collision is elastic, then the kinetic energy also is conserved:

$$\Sigma K_0 E = \Sigma KE.$$

This means that

$$\tfrac{1}{2} m_1 v_1^2 = \tfrac{1}{2} m_1 v_1'^2 + \tfrac{1}{2} m_2 v_2'^2$$

and so given v_1 one can solve for v'_2 (for example) in terms of v'_1. The momentum conservation equations then become two equations in two unknowns.

If the collision is inelastic, then the loss of kinetic energy is given by

$$\Delta KE = KE - K_0 E$$

$$= \tfrac{1}{2} m_1 v_1'^2 + \tfrac{1}{2} m_2 v_2'^2 - \tfrac{1}{2} m_1 v_1^2 - \tfrac{1}{2} m_2 v_2^2.$$

PROBLEM

A cue ball traveling at a speed of 3 m/s collides with a stationary billiard ball and imparts a speed of 1.8 m/s to the billiard ball. If the billiard ball moves in the same direction as the oncoming cue ball, what is the velocity of the cue ball after the collision? Assume that both balls have the same mass.

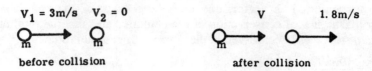

$V_1 = 3m/s$ $V_2 = 0$ v   1.8m/s

m   m   m

before collision   after collision

Figure 3.9

Solution

Linear momentum must be conserved in this isolated, two particle system. Thus, the initial momentum of the system must equal the system's final momentum. Since the collision is 1-dimensional, we may drop the vector nature of momentum and write

$$P_f = P_i$$

$$mv + m\,(1.8\ \text{m/sec}) = m\,(3\ \text{m/sec}) + m(0\ \text{m/sec})$$

$$m(v + 1.8\ \text{m/sec}) = m\,(3\ \text{m/sec})$$

$$v + 1.8\ \text{m/sec} = 3\ \text{m/sec}$$

$$v = 1.2\ \text{m/sec}$$

C.   IMPULSE

The impulse momentum theorem follows from Newton's Second Law

$$F = \Delta p / \Delta t$$

Therefore, the impulse is

$$I = \Delta p = Ft$$

PROBLEM

A 100 kg man jumps into a swimming pool from a height of 5 m. It takes 0.4 sec for the water to reduce his velocity to zero. What average force did the water exert on the man?

Solution

The man's initial velocity (before jumping) is zero. Therefore, as he strikes the water, his velocity v is

$$v^2 = v_0^2 + 2gh,$$

which reduces to $v^2 = 2gh$

$$v = \sqrt{2gh} = \sqrt{2 \times (9.8\ \text{m} / \text{sec}^2) \times (5\ \text{m})}$$

$$= 10\ \text{m} / \text{sec}$$

Therefore, the man's momentum on striking the water was

$$p_1 = mv$$
$$= (100 \text{ kg}) \times (10 \text{ m/sec})$$
$$= 1000 \text{ kg} - \text{m/sec}$$

The final momentum was $p_2 = 0$, so that the average force was

$$\mathbf{F} = \frac{\Delta p}{\Delta t} = \frac{p_2 - p_1}{\Delta t}$$
$$= \frac{0 - 1000 \text{ kg} - \text{m} / \sec^2}{0.4 \text{ sec}}$$
$$= -2500 \text{ N}$$

The negative sign means that the retarding force was directed opposite to the downward velocity of the man.

IV. WORK AND ENERGY

1. Work

Work is given by the dot product of the force and displacement; if the force and displacement are in the same direction, then the work is simply the force times the distance. In general, one must calculate

$Fd \cos \theta$

as in Figure 4.1. The work can also be negative, for example, frictional work is energy dissipative and in the simplest case given by $-\mu_k Nx$.

$W = (F \cos \theta)d$

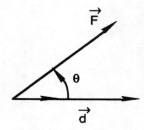

Figure 4.1

2. Kinetic and Potential Energy

Kinetic energy is energy of motion and for a single particle given by

$KE = \frac{1}{2} mv^2 = p^2 / 2m.$

Hence, given the speed, momentum, and mass, one can calculate numerically the kinetic energy. Consider the kinematics of a single particle subject to acceleration:

$v^2 = v_0^2 + 2a(x - x_0).$

By multiplying this equation by $\frac{1}{2}m$, we get the result

$W = \Delta T = T - T_0$

which is the work energy theorem. Work done on an object changes the kinetic energy of that object.

The concept of work leads immediately to the idea of potential or stored energy

$PE = Fs.$

For the gravitational force, in moving an object up, the force and the displacement point in opposite directions; hence the potential energy is just *mgh* near the surface of the Earth.

For every conservative force, we can define a potential energy. If a spring is compressed or stretched a distance x from equilibrium, the Hooke's Law potential energy is $\frac{1}{2} kx^2$. One may simply plug numbers into formulae to calculate the potential energy in solving a problem. Or one may have to use the fact that potential energy can be transformed. For example, a mass can fall and compress a spring transforming the gravitational potential energy mgh into compressional potential energy $\frac{1}{2} kx^2$.

PROBLEM

Air consists of a mixture of gas molecules which are constantly moving. Compute the kinetic energy K_E of a molecule that is moving with a speed of 500 m/s. Assume that the mass of this particle is 4.6×10^{-26} kg.

Solution

The mass of the gas molecule, $m = 4.6 \times 10^{-26}$ kg, and its speed $v = 5 \times 10^2$ m/s, are the known observables. Using the equation:

$$K_E = \frac{1}{2} mv^2$$
$$K_E = (\frac{1}{2}) (4.6 \times 10^{-26} \text{ kg}) (5.0 \times 10^2 \text{ m/s})^2$$
$$= 5.75 \times 10^{-21} \text{ J}.$$

PROBLEM

How much work is required to raise a 100 g block to a height of 200 cm and simultaneously give it a velocity of 300 cm/sec?

Solution

The work done is the sum of the potential energy,

$$PE = mgh,$$

and the kinetic energy,

$$KE = \frac{1}{2} mv^2$$
$$PE = mgh$$
$$= (100 \text{ g}) \times (980 \text{ cm/sec}^2) \times (200 \text{ cm})$$
$$= 1.96 \times 10^7 \text{ g-cm}^2/\text{sec}^2$$
$$= 1.96 \times 10^7 \text{ ergs}$$
$$KE = \frac{1}{2} mv^2$$
$$= \frac{1}{2} \times (100 \text{ g}) \times (300 \text{ cm/sec})^2$$
$$= 4.5 \times 10^6 \text{ g-cm}^2/\text{sec}^2$$
$$W = PE + KE$$
$$= 1.96 \times 10^7 \text{ ergs} + 0.45 \times 10^7 \text{ ergs}$$
$$= 2.41 \times 10^7 \text{ ergs}$$
$$= 2.41 \text{ J}$$

3. Conservation of Energy

The law of conservation of mechanical energy states that the total mechanical energy

$$E = KE + PE$$

is conserved:

$$\Sigma E_0 = \Sigma E.$$

For a single particle, this means that

$$\Delta KE = - PE.$$

For the mass on a spring system of Figure 4.2, this means that

$$^1/_2\, kA^2 = {}^1/_2\, mv^2 + {}^1/_2\, kx^2$$

for any value of the displacement x. For example, as a mass on a spring moves from $x = A$ to $x = 0$ to $x = -A$, the potential energy $^1/_2\, kx^2$ is transformed into kinetic energy

$$KE = {}^1/_2\, mv^2$$

and then back again into stored energy. A good method of attack in solving energy problems is to draw two pictures, one showing the initial situation (e.g., mass on spring stretched to $x = A$) and the other showing the final situation (e.g., mass on spring at $x = 0$).

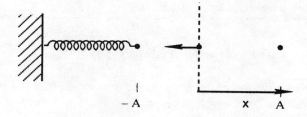

Figure 4.2

For an object projected upward (Figure 4.3), one can use this principle to find the height since

$$^1/_2\, mv_0^2 = mgh + {}^1/_2\, mv_{0x}^2, \quad \text{or } {}^1/_2\, mv_{0y}^2 = mgh;$$

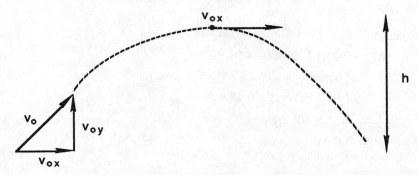

Figure 4.3

note that the energy problem-solving method gives the same answer as we get from kinematics:

$$h = v_{0y}^2 / 2g.$$

For distances in between $y = 0$ and $y = h$, for an object projected straight upward ($\theta = 90°$), we have

$$\tfrac{1}{2} \, mv^2 + mgy = mgh.$$

If friction is involved in a problem, then one must take into account that some energy is lost or goes into frictional heat. For example, in sliding down the incline of Figure 4.4, the law of conservation of energy must be written as

$$mgh = mgy + \tfrac{1}{2} \, mv^2 + \mu_k N_x$$

and the usual dynamics approach used to find N.

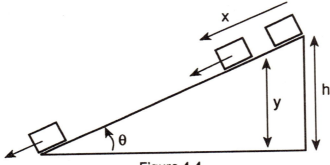

Figure 4.4

PROBLEM

A 1 kg block slides down a rough inclined plane whose height is 1 m. At the bottom, the block has a velocity of 4 m/sec. Is energy conserved?

Solution

Energy will be conserved if the kinetic energy gained by the block is equal to the potential energy lost. At top:

$$PE = mgh$$
$$= (1 \text{ kg}) \times (9.8 \text{ m/sec}^2) \times (1 \text{ m})$$
$$= 9.8 \text{ J}.$$

At bottom:

$$KE = \tfrac{1}{2} mv^2$$
$$= \tfrac{1}{2} \times (1 \text{ kg}) \times (4 \text{ m/sec})^2$$
$$= 8 \text{ J}.$$

Apparently, energy is not conserved. But we know that friction is present between the block and the rough plane. A certain amount of energy (1.8 J) has evidently been expended in overcoming this friction. This amount of energy appears as thermal energy and could be detected by measuring the temperature rise in the block and the plane after the slide is completed.

4. Power

Power is the work done per unit time

$\Delta W / \Delta t$

In the simplest case, one can find the work done by simply multiplying the power times the time. For translational motion, power is

$P = \mathbf{F} \cdot \mathbf{v}.$

In our electric bills we pay for kilowatt-hours of energy used, or 10^3 W·3600 s = 3.6 × 10^6 J or 3.6 Megajoules.

PROBLEM

A constant horizontal force of 10 *N* is required to drag an object across a rough surface at a constant speed of 5 m/sec. What power is being expended? How much work would be done in 30 min?

Solution

Power is the rate of doing work,

$$P = \frac{\Delta W}{\Delta t} = \frac{F \Delta s}{\Delta t}.$$

(Note that in this problem the work reduces to the force multiplied by the distance the object is moved.) But $\Delta s/_{\Delta t}$ is just the velocity. Therefore,

$P = Fv$

$\quad = (10 \text{ N}) \times (5 \text{ m/sec})$

$\quad = 50 \text{ J/sec}$

$\quad = 50 \text{ W}$

$W = Pt$

$\quad = (50 \text{ W}) \times (^1/_2 \text{ hr})$

$\quad = 25 \text{ W-hr.}$

The work, of course, is done against the force of sliding friction.

V. WAVE CHARACTERISTICS AND PERIODIC MOTION

1. Wave Characteristics

A wave is considered to be a disturbance that propagates through some material medium or space. There are two classifications of waves. Waves which travel through a material medium are called mechanical waves. Waves which carry the various forms of light are electromagnetic waves, and travel at the speed of light through a vacuum.

A. TRANSVERSE AND LONGITUDINAL MOTION

Both mechanical and electromagnetic waves can travel by means of a transverse type wave. Transverse waves cause matter to move in a direction perpendicular to the direction of wave propagation. Figure 5.1 shows 4 points along a wave medium. As the wave travels to the right, the matter within the medium moves up, then down as the wave passes. Thus, the wave is transverse.

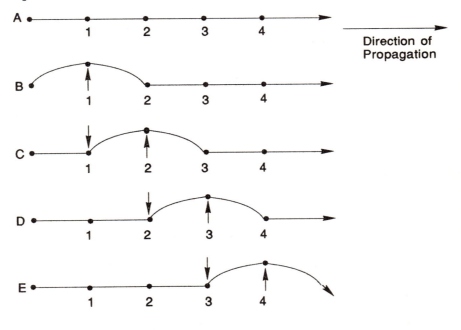

Figure 5.1

A second type of mechanical wave is the longitudinal or compression wave. Longitudinal waves cause material in the medium to move parallel to wave propagation. Figure 5.2 shows a compression wave pulse through a coil spring. When released, the compressed area attempts to spread out which will compress the coils to their right. This process continues throughout the length of the spring.

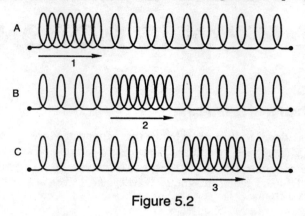

Figure 5.2

Sound waves are the best example of compression waves. The shock from a sound compresses the air near the source which sends a compression wave through the air in all directions. You hear the sound when the compression shock hits your eardrum.

2. WAVELENGTH, FREQUENCY, VELOCITY

If a source which creates a wave does so repeatedly at equal time intervals, then a periodic wave will result. Figure 5.3 shows a periodic transverse wave with equal disturbances over equal time periods.

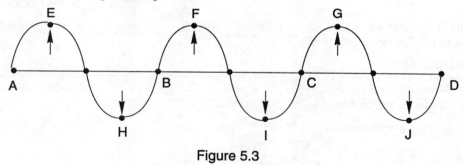

Figure 5.3

Shown are three complete waves, each having an upper displacement crest, and a lower displacement trough. The distance from a point on a wave to the same point on the next is called one wavelength. For our wave, the wavelength, λ, (lambda), could be measured from A to B, one crest and one trough; from E to F, crest to crest; or from H to I, trough to trough.

A wave which travels through one crest and one trough has completed one cycle. If we measure the number of waves which pass a given point in a specified time interval, then this is known as wave frequency. Frequency, f, is measured in cycles per second which is a hertz. The period, T, for a wave is the time for one complete wave to pass a reference point. Finally, a wave that moves in a given direction must have velocity in that direction. Wavelength, frequency, period, and velocity all relate to each other. Figure 5.4 shows two waves traveling one meter

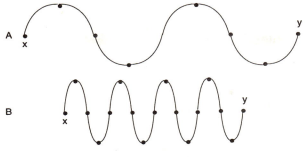

Figure 5.4

from *X* to *Y*. Each wave can travel from *X* to *Y* in one second.

Looking at wave *A*, we find that in one second, two complete waves will pass point *Y* which gives a frequency equal to 2 hz. For wave *B*, four waves pass *Y* in one second which gives a frequency of 4 hz. Since the waves are traveling 2 per second in *A*, the period for wave *A* is $^1/_2$ second. In *B*, waves pass 4 per second and the period is $^1/_4$ second. Note that the frequency and period are reciprocals. Thus,

$$f = 1/T \quad \text{and} \quad T = 1/f$$

Since each wave travels a distance, λ, in time *T*,

$$v = \lambda/T.$$

Substituting for $1/T$ gives

$$v = \lambda/T = (1/T)\,(\lambda) = f\lambda$$

$$v = f\,\lambda$$

This final equation is true for all periodic waves, transverse or longitudinal, regardless of medium material.

PROBLEM

A wave is represented by the equation $y = 0.20 \sin .40\pi\,(x - 60t)$, where all distances are measured in centimeters and time in seconds. Find:

a) the amplitude,

b) the wavelength,

c) the speed, and

d) the frequency of the wave.

e) What is the displacement at $x = 5.5$ cm and $t = 0.020$ sec?

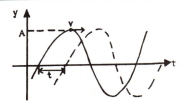

Figure 5.5

Solution

The displacement y of the medium due to wave motion at a position x at a time t is (see Figure 5.6)

$$y = A \sin \frac{2\pi}{\lambda}(x - vt)$$

where A is the amplitude, λ is the wavelength, and v is the velocity with which the wave is traveling along the x-axis. If we compare this equation with the expression given in the question, we see that

a) $A = 0.20$ cm

b) $\dfrac{2\pi}{\lambda} = 0.40\pi$ $\qquad\qquad \lambda = \dfrac{2}{0.40}$ cm $= 5.0$ cm

c) $v = 60$ cm/sec

d) $f = \dfrac{v}{\lambda} = \dfrac{60 \text{ cm / sec}}{5.0 \text{ cm}} = 12 \text{ / sec}$

e)
$$y = (0.20 \text{ cm}) \sin [0.40\pi (5.5 - 60 \times 0.020)]$$
$$= (0.20 \text{ cm}) \sin [0.40\,\pi\,(5.5 - 1.2)]$$
$$= (0.20 \text{ cm}) \sin (0.40 \times 4.3\,\pi)$$
$$= (0.20 \text{ cm}) \sin 1.72\pi$$
$$= (0.20 \text{ cm}) (-0.77) = -0.15 \text{ cm}$$

C. SUPERPOSITION OF WAVES, INTERFERENCE, AND PHASE

Superposition is the algebraic summing of the amplitudes of two travelling waves when they pass through each other. The waves then travel on past each other unchanged. If the sum of the two waves is greater than the amplitudes of each individual wave, then the waves are said to *constructively interfere*. *Destructive interference* occurs if the algebraic sum of the waves is less than the amplitude of each individual wave.

For two waves travelling in the same direction at the same speed, superposition will also occur. The waves in this case will not pass each other, but the effects of

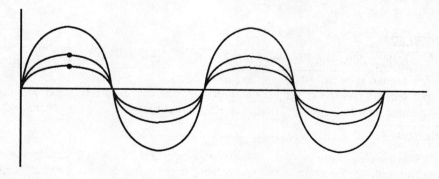

Figure 5.6

constructive or destructive interference will be seen for as long as the two waves are travelling at the same speed. The amount of interference will depend on the *phase* difference between the two waves. For example, in Figure 5.6 the two waves with equal wavelength travelling at the same speed are in phase because the maximum point at the crests of both waves line up.

Two waves in phase have a phase difference ϕ, between them, of zero and constructively interfere to produce a resultant wave shown in Figure 5.6 by the heavier line.

When a phase difference of $\phi = 180°$ occurs the waves will destructively interfere. In fact, waves with equal amplitudes will completely cancel each other out as shown in Figure 5.7.

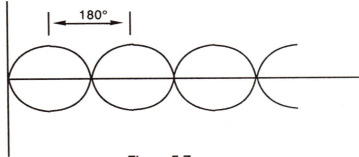

Figure 5.7

Phase differences between $\phi = 0°$ and $\phi = 180°$ will form a resultant wave that is the algebraic sum of the two original waves, because at some points the waves move constructively interefere and at other points the waves may destructively interfere.

D. BEATS

If two waves do not have the same wavelength (frequency), but their frequencies are very close, the waves will continuously constructively and destructively interfere. As a result a wave with a beat frequency

$$f_{beat} \quad |f_1 - f_2|$$

will be formed.

PROBLEM

When two tuning forks are sounded simultaneously, a beat note of 5 cycles per second is heard. If one of the forks has a known frequency of 256 cycles per second, and if a small piece of adhesive tape fastened to this fork reduces the beat note to 3 cycles per second, what is the frequency of the other fork?

Solution

This problem involves the phenomenon of beats. When two similar waves are superimposed, the beat frequency represents the numerical difference in their frequencies. Hence, for the case in question,

$$n = (256 \pm 5) \text{ cycles/sec}$$

where n represents the unknown frequency.

It appears that n has two possible values, either 251 or 261. Now, when the standard fork is loaded with the tape, its frequency will decrease. Since the best frequency is then reduced to 3 cycles per second, the unknown frequency must be less rather than more than 256. Hence,

$$n = 251.$$

2. Periodic Motion

A. HOOKE'S LAW

$$F_s = - kx$$

where F_s is the force produced by the spring along its length, x is the displacement of the spring, and k is the spring's constant. The force of the spring is always opposite to the direction of displacement, therefore a negative sign is included in the formula.

B. SIMPLE HARMONIC MOTION

Equations of Motion — The Variables for S.H.M.

The Period of Motion

$$T = \frac{2\pi}{\omega} = 2\pi\sqrt{\frac{m}{k}} \rightarrow \text{units: Seconds}$$

The Frequency of Motion

$$f = \frac{1}{T} = \frac{\omega}{2\pi} = \frac{1}{2\pi}\sqrt{\frac{k}{m}} \rightarrow \text{units: } \frac{1}{\text{seconds}}$$

The Angular Frequency of Motion

$$\omega = 2\pi f = \frac{2\pi}{T} = \sqrt{\frac{k}{m}} \rightarrow \text{units: } \frac{\text{Rads}}{\text{sec}}$$

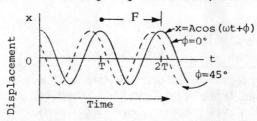

Figure 5.8 — Simple Harmonic Oscillation

Differential Equations of Motion

Displacement

$$\mathbf{x} = A \cos (\omega t + \phi)$$

Velocity

$$\frac{dx}{dt} = v = -\omega A \sin(\omega t + \phi)$$

PROBLEM

One end of a fingernail file is clamped in a vise and the other end is given a to-and-fro vibration. The motion of the free end is approximately S.H.M. If the frequency is 10 vibrations per second and the amplitude is 4 millimeters, what is the velocity when the displacement of the free end is 2 millimeters?

Solution

The problem states that the motion is S.H.M. Therefore, we know that the displacement of the file is

$$x = A \sin(\omega t + \alpha) \tag{1}$$

where A is the amplitude and α is a constant. ω is the angular frequency of the vibration. If f is the frequency of the motion

$$\omega = 2\pi f.$$

The velocity of the end of the file is, differentiating (1),

$$v = A\omega \cos(\omega t + \alpha) \tag{2}$$

We need the velocity when $x = 2$ mm. At this position, using (1)

$$2\text{ mm} = 4\text{ mm} \sin(\omega t + \alpha)$$

$$\sin(\omega t + \alpha) = \tfrac{1}{2}$$

whence $(\omega t + \alpha) = 30°$

Hence, using (2),

$$v = A\omega \cos(30°)$$

or $\qquad v = A(2\pi f) \cos(30°)$

$$v = (4\text{ mm})(6.28)(10\text{ per sec})(\sqrt{3}/2)$$

$$v = \left(\frac{40\text{ mm}}{\text{sec}}\right)(6.28)(.866) = 218\text{ mm}/\text{sec}.$$

C. PENDULUM MOTION

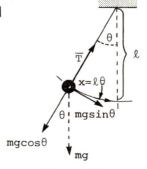

Figure 5.9

Force, F

$$\mathbf{F} = -mg\theta = \frac{-mg}{L}\,x$$

Period T

$$T = 2\pi\sqrt{\frac{L}{g}}$$

VI. SOUND

1. Production of Sound

Sound waves are treated exactly like other waves with the frequency and wavelength related by

$$v = f\lambda.$$

Sound waves, however, are mechanical waves. They are longitudinal waves corresponding to the compression and rarefaction (expansion) of the medium in which the waves are travelling.

PROBLEM

What is the wavelength of the sound wave emitted by a standard 440 cycles per second turning form?

Solution

Noting that the velocity (v), frequency (f), and wavelength (λ) of sound are related by $v = f\lambda$, and assuming the velocity of sound to be 34,000 cm/sec, or approximately 1100 ft/sec, we find

$$\lambda = v\,/\,f = \frac{1100\ \text{ft}}{440} = 2.5\ \text{ft}\quad(\text{approx.})$$

PROBLEM

What is the frequency of a 2-cm sound wave in sea water? The velocity of sound in sea water is $v = 1.53 \times 10^5$ cm/sec.

Solution

The 2 cm is the wavelength l of the sound wave. The frequency is given by

$$f = \frac{v}{\lambda}$$

$$= \frac{1.53 \times 10^5\ \text{cm}\,/\,\text{sec}}{2\ \text{cm}}$$

$$= 7.6 \times 10^4\ \text{Hz} = 76\ \text{kHz}$$

which is an ultrasonic wave (that is, above the human audible range). A 2 cm sound wave in air would be audible.

2. Relative Speed of Sound in Solids, Liquids, and Gases

Wave Speed in a Fluid

$$v = \sqrt{\frac{B}{\rho}}$$

v = Speed of sound in a fluid

B = Modulus of elasticity

ρ = Density of medium

Wave Speed in a Solid

To determine the speed a wave travelling in a solid the value of B is replaced by a parameter appropriate to the particular situation. For a wave travelling along a taut rope B is replaced by the tension T.

Wave Speed in a Gas

$$v_g = \sqrt{\frac{\gamma p}{\rho}}$$

v_g = Speed of sound in a gas

γ = Ratio of specific heats for a gas

p = Undisturbed pressure

ρ = Density of medium

3. Intensity of Sound

Average Intensity — I

$$I = \frac{1}{2} \frac{P_m^2}{\sqrt{B\rho}}$$

P_m = Pressure amplitude

B = Bulk modulus of elasticity

ρ = Density of medium

Loudness of sound is measured in decibels and defined as

$$\text{loudness} = 10 \log \frac{I}{I_0}$$

where $I_0 = 10^{-12}$ Wb/m^2 which is the lowest sound a human ear can hear.

As a comparison, a very loud stereo system can crank out 100 dB which corresponds to an intensity $I = 10^{-2}$ Wb/m^2. An intensity of 1 Wb/m^2 or 120 dB is at the threshold of pain for a human ear.

4. Doppler Effect

One interesting idea regarding wave velocity is the Doppler Effect. This effect refers to a wave which originates from a source which is traveling with some velocity. In essence, the source velocity appears to be added to or subtracted from the wave velocity. The Doppler Effect is best explained by examining sound waves.

The frequency of a sound wave determines a characteristic known as pitch. Interpreting pitch is how the human ear distinguishes among frequencies. The higher the frequency, the higher the pitch. If the source of sound is in motion relative to the listener, then the Doppler Effect occurs, and the pitch heard is not the true pitch of the wave. Figure 6.1 shows the Doppler Effect. Remember that sound travels by compression waves, but for this diagram they are shown as transverse.

The listeners at positions X and Y hear the wave perpendicular to the motion of the train. These waves are unaffected by the motion of the source, and the true pitch is heard. Listener F hears a wave which is traveling the same direction as the course. As the source approaches, the frequency heard increases and the pitch is higher. Listener B hears the opposite effect. Since the sound is moving opposite the source, the frequency heard decreases and the pitch is lower.

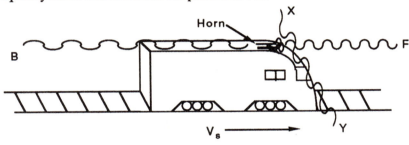

Figure 6.1

To describe the Doppler effect more analytically, let v_s be the velocity of the source and v_0 that of the observer. Then, the frequency observed by the observer is

$$f' = f(v \pm v_0) / (v \pm v_s).$$

For example, in the situation of Figure 6.2, since $v_s = 0$ and the observer is moving away from the source, we expect that $\lambda' > \lambda$ or $f' < f$. More precisely,

$$f' = f(v - v_0)/v.$$

In the situation of Figure 6.3, where $v_0 = 0$ and the source is moving towards the observer, we expect that $\lambda' < \lambda$ and hence $f' > f$. More precisely,

$$f' = f\ v/(v - v_s).$$

Figure 6.2   Figure 6.3

PROBLEM

A researcher notices that the frequency of a note emitted by an automobile horn appears to drop from 284 cycles·s⁻¹ to 266 cycles·s⁻¹ as the automobile passes him. From this observation he is able to calculate the speed of the car, knowing that the speed of sound in air is 1100 ft·s⁻¹. What value does he obtain for the speed?

Solution

This is an example illustrating the Doppler effect. When there is no movement of the surrounding medium the relation between the frequency as heard by a moving observer and that emitted by a moving source is

$$\frac{f_L}{u \pm v_L} = \frac{f_s}{u \mp v_s}$$

where f_L is the frequency heard by the listener, f_s the frequency emitted by the moving source, v_L the velocity of the listener, v_s the velocity of the source, and u the velocity of sound (= 1100 ft·s⁻¹). The upper signs (+ left side of equation, – right side) corresponds to the source and observer moving along the line joining the two and approaching each other and the lower signs (- left, + right) correspond to source and observer receding from one another.

In this case the frequencies heard by the stationary listener ($v_L = 0$) will be

$$f_L = u f_s / (u \mp v_s).$$

As the automobile approaches the observer he records a frequency of 284 cycles·s⁻¹, and as the automobile moves away from him, he records 266 cycles ·s⁻¹. Thus

$$284 \, s^{-1} = \frac{u f_s}{u - v_s} \tag{1}$$

and

$$266 \, s^{-1} = \frac{u f_s}{u + v_s} \tag{2}$$

Dividing (1) by (2)

$$\frac{u + v_s}{u - v_s} = \frac{284}{266}$$

$$266 (u + v_s) = 284(u - v_s)$$

$$(266 + 284)v_s = (284 - 266)u$$

or

$$\frac{v_s}{u} = \frac{18}{550}.$$

$$\therefore v_s = \frac{18}{550} \times 1100 \text{ ft} \cdot \text{s}^{-1} = 36 \text{ ft} \cdot \text{s}^{-1}$$

$$= 36 \text{ ft} \cdot \text{s}^{-1} \times \frac{1 \text{ mile}}{5280 \text{ ft}} \times \frac{60 \text{ s}}{1 \text{ min}} \times \frac{60 \text{ min}}{1 \text{ hr}} = 24.5 \text{ mph}$$

5. Resonance in Pipes and Strings, and Harmonics

As mentioned in the last chapter, a travelling wave moving to the right and one moving to the left may interfere to produce standing waves of amplitude A. For a string of length L the usual condition is $L = n\lambda/2$, where the $n = 1, 2$, and 3 waveforms are shown in Figure 6.4. The points where $y = \pm A$ are called antinodes and the points where $y = 0$ termed nodes. Hence, the number n gives the number of antinodes.

The situation in a pipe closed at both ends is exactly the same $L = n\lambda/2$ as Figure 6.4. Only now we are speaking about pressure or sound waves interfering. For a pipe open at both ends, we also have $L = n\lambda/2$ as in Figure 6.5. Finally, for a pipe open at one end and closed at the other, the reader may draw the waveforms and see that $L = n\lambda/4$ where $n = 1, 3, 5$, etc.

Since $f = v/\lambda$, we get for the frequencies

$$f_n = n\, v/2L = n f_1$$

where f_1 is called the fundamental frequency or the first harmonic. The term harmonic is used here since we have a harmonic series or quantized equation. Similarly, f_2 and f_3 are the second and third harmonics.

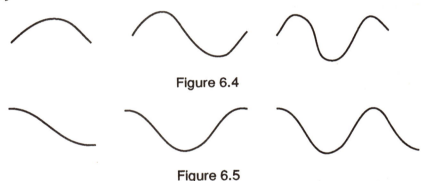

Figure 6.4

Figure 6.5

VII. FLUIDS AND SOLIDS

This review section assumes a basic understanding of the physical properties of fluids and solids, as well as an understanding of fluids in motion and solids acted on by forces.

1. Fluids

A. DENSITY, SPECIFIC GRAVITY

Density is the ratio of mass over volume. Specific gravity is the ratio of the density of a substance to that of a reference substance, usually water.

$$\rho = M/V$$

$$s = \rho/\rho_{ref}$$

The most commonly used reference density is that of water, 1 gram per cubic centimeter.

$$\rho(\text{water, } 4.0°C) = 1g/cm3.$$

PROBLEM

The specific weight of water at ordinary pressure and temperature is 62.4 lb/ft³ (9.81 kN/m³). The specific gravity of mercury is 13.55. Compute the density of water and the specific weight and density of mercury.

Solution

Knowing that density and specific weight of a fluid are related as follows:

$$\rho = \frac{\gamma}{g} \quad \text{or} \quad \gamma = \rho g$$

and that specific gravity s of a liquid is the ratio of its density to that of pure water at a standard temperature, we can calculate:

$$\rho_{water} = \frac{\gamma_{water}}{g} = \frac{62.4 \, lb/ft^3}{32.2 \, ft/s^2} = 1.94 \, slugs/ft^3$$

$$= \frac{9.81 \, kN/m^3}{9.81 \, m/s^2} = 1.00 \, Mg/m^3 = 1.00 \, g/cm^3$$

$\gamma_{mercury} = s_{mercury} \, \gamma_{water} = 13.55 \, (62.4) = 846 \, lb/ft^3$
13.55 (9.81) = 133 kN/m³

$\rho_{mercury} = s_{mercury} \, \rho_{water} = 13.55 \, (1.94) = 26.3 \, slugs/ft^3$
13.55 (1.00) = 13.55 Mg/m³

B.   ARCHIMEDES' PRINCIPLE

Archimedes' principle describes the effects of buoyancy. The mass of a floating object equals the mass of the fluid displaced. Also, the upward force of an immersed object equals the volume displaced times the difference between the weight of fluid displaced and that of the object.

PROBLEM

In order to determine their density, drops of blood are placed in a mixture of xylene of density 0.867 g·cm^{-3}, and bromobenzene of density 1.497 g·cm^{-3}, the mixture being altered until the drops do not rise or sink. The mixture then contains 72% of xylene and 28% of bromobenzene by volume. What is the density of the blood?

Solution

Using the definition of density

$$\text{density} = \frac{\text{mass}}{\text{volume}}$$

every 72 cm^3 of xylene has a mass of

$$72 \text{ cm}^3 \times 0.867 \text{ g·cm}^{-3} = 62.424 \text{ g,}$$

and every 28 cm^3 of bromobenzene has a mass of

$$28 \text{ cm}^3 \times 1.497 \text{ gm·cm}^{-3} = 41.916 \text{ g.}$$

Thus, 100 cm^3 of the mixture has a mass of

$$(62.424 + 41.916)\text{g} = 104.340 \text{ g.}$$

Thus the density of the mixture is 1.0434 g·cm^{-3}.

But blood neither rises nor sinks in this mixture, showing that the blood has no net force acting on it. Thus the weight of any drop of blood is exactly equal to the upthrust acting on it. But, by Archimedes' principle, the upthrust is the weight of an equal volume of mixture. Hence the blood and the mixture have the same densities; thus the density of blood is 1.0434 g·cm^{-3}.

C.   HYDROSTATIC PRESSURE

Hydrostatic pressure is the pressure exerted at the bottom of a column of fluid divided by the area of the base. It is equal to the pressure at the top of the column plus the force exerted by the fluid.

$$P = P_0 + w/A = P_0 + \rho g h \quad (V = A * h)$$

D.   BERNOULLI'S EQUATION

Bernoulli's equation is a simplified form of the mechanical energy equation used when changes in the kinetic and potential energies of a fluid are to be determined. It relates changes in pressure, height and velocity.

$$p_1 + \frac{1}{2}\rho v_1^2 + \rho g y_1 = p_2 + \frac{1}{2}\rho v_2^2 + \rho g y_2 = \text{constant}$$

PROBLEM

An open tank containing water has an orifice which is located near the bottom of the tank as shown in the figure. Show that for ideal flow, the discharge velocity at the orifice is $\sqrt{2gh}$. Assume steady flow.

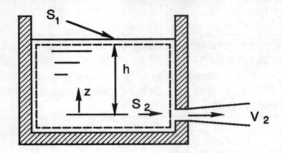

Figure 7.1

Solution

Consider the control volume shown in Figure 7.1 Apply the Bernoulli equation to sections s_1 and s_2.

$$\frac{p_1}{\rho} + \frac{v_1^2}{2g_c} + \frac{gz_1}{g_c} = \frac{p_2}{\rho} + \frac{v_2^2}{2g_c} + \frac{gz_2}{g_c} \tag{1}$$

Experiments indicate that the pressure at any section open to the atmosphere can be taken to be at atmospheric pressure. Therefore,

$$p_1 = p_2 = p_{atm}$$

Also, using continuity equation,

$$v_1 A_1 = v_2 A_2 \tag{2}$$

and by the fact that $A_1 \gg A_2$, we can take $v_1 \ll v_2$. Thus v_1 can be neglected. Under these circumstances, Equation (1) reduces to

$$\frac{v_2^2}{2g} = z_1 - z_2 = h$$

or

$$v_2 = \sqrt{2gh}$$

E. VISCOSITY

Viscosity (η) of a fluid relates the force required to produce motion in a fluid. The units are force * time/area.

$$F = \eta \frac{Av}{L}$$

A = Area of liquid over which forces applied

L = Transverse Dimension

v = Velocity

PROBLEM

The space between two parallel plates 1.5 cm apart is filled with an oil of viscosity η = 0.050 kg/ms. A thin 30 × 60 cm rectangular plate is pulled through the oil 0.50 cm from one plate and 1.00 cm from the other. What force is needed to pull the plate at 0.40 m/s?

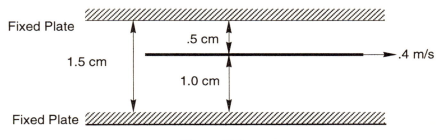

Fixed Plate

.5 cm

1.5 cm   .4 m/s

1.0 cm

Fixed Plate

Figure 7.2

Solution

The total force overcomes the viscous shear over both the upper and the lower surface of the moving plate as indicated in Figure 7.2. Thus,

$$F_{total} = F_{upper} + F_{lower}$$

$$= \text{(upper shear stress) (area)} + \text{(lower shear stress) (area)}$$

$$= \eta(V/h_{upper})\,(A) + \eta(V/h_{lower})\,(A)$$

$$= (0.050)\,(0.40/0.005)\,(0.180) + (0.050)\,(0.40/0.010)\,(0.180)$$

$$= 0.72 + 0.36$$

$$= 1.08\ N$$

F. CONTINUITY EQUATION

The equation of continuity states that the rate of accumulation of mass equals the rate of mass in minus the rate of mass out. Taken over a fixed volume and assuming steady state conditions this simplifies to

$$(pAv)_{in} = (pAv)_{out}$$

v = velocity of the fluid.

G. TURBULENCE

There are two flow regimes in the typical newtonian fluid. Laminar flow describes fluids as flowing in layers over one another. In a typical pipe flow the flow at the boundary (the pipe wall) fluid velocity is taken to be zero. At the center of the pipe, flow is at the highest velocity. Flow becomes turbulent at higher flow rates because of mixing between the layers and eddy currents. Turbulent flow tends to occur when the Reynolds number exceeds 2100. The dimensionless Reynolds number is the diameter times the bulk flow times the density divided by the viscosity.

$$N_R = \frac{\rho v D}{\eta}$$

ρ = Density of fluid

v = Average velocity

D = Diameter of pipe

η = Coefficient of viscosity

H. SURFACE TENSION

The attractive forces between molecules pull them closer to each other to form more stable, lower energy forms — similar to the way atoms combine to form molecules to decrease their energy. These molecular attractions will cause the molecules to form shapes with the lowest possible energy. For a liquid, this shape is a sphere, which is why water droplets always have a spherical shape. At the surface of a glass of water the molecules are not bound on all sides, like the water molecules below them, so they try to reduce the surface area as much as possible. Surface tension decreases with increasing temperature and will change depending on the gas in contact with the surface.

Surface tension is a cause of capilarity, the creeping up of water on the inside of a filled test tube. In the case of water, the attraction of the water to the glass is greater than the surface tension and a concave *meniscus* forms in the tube. For mercury, the attraction between Hg molecules is greater than the attraction of Hg to the glass so the mercury forms a convex meniscus. The convex shape keeps all the mercury molecules as close to each other as possible.

2. Solids

A. ELASTIC PROPERTIES

When the *stress* on a solid object is linearly proportional to the *strain* of the object, this stress-strain relationship is governed by Hooke's law

$\sigma = E\varepsilon$

$\sigma \equiv$ axial stress

$\varepsilon \equiv$ axial strain

$E =$ modulus of elasticity.

A little beyond the point where stress is linearly proportional to strain the *elastic deformation limit* occurs. Further stress applied beyond this limit will result in a permanent or *plastic* deformation of the solid object.

VIII. ELECTROSTATICS AND ELECTROMAGNETISM

1. Electrostatics

A. COULOMB'S LAW

Electrostatics is the study of discrete or continuous systems of electric charge at rest. Electric charge comes in two varieties, positive and negative, the MKS unit being the Coulomb $\equiv C$. Like charges repel one another and unlike charges attract each other. Fundamental to electricity is Coulomb's law, which states that between every two charges, there exists an electric force given by (see Figure 8.1)

$$\mathbf{F} = k_e\, q_1 q_2 / r^2\, \mathbf{r}$$

where $k_e = 9.0 \times 10^9$ N - m²/C² is the MKS Coulomb force constant. If using the CGS system of units, $k_e = 1$ exactly, and the charge is measured in esu or electrostatic units. If there is more than one charge in the vicinity, then one must sum up the vector force from each nearby charge to get the resultant force (see Vectors); this is called the principle of superposition.

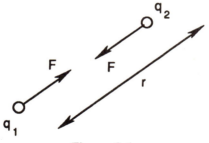

Figure 8.1

PROBLEM

Calculate the resultant force on the charge q_3 in the figure.

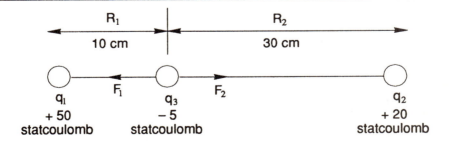

Figure 8.2

Solution

The force exerted by q_1 on q_3 is

$$F_1 = \frac{q_1 q_3}{R_1^2}$$

$$= \frac{(50)(-5)}{(10)^2} = -2.5 \text{ dyne}$$

The negative sign denotes an attractive force. The force exerted on q_3 by q_2 is

$$F_2 = \frac{q_2 q_3}{R_2^2}$$

$$= \frac{(20)(-5)}{(30)^2} = \frac{-100}{900}$$

$$= -0.111 \text{ dyne}$$

Since q_2 is positive and q_3 is negative this force is attractive and is directed to the right toward q_2.

The resultant force on q_3 is

$$F_R = F_1 - F_2 = -2.5 - (-0.111)]$$

$$= -2.389 \text{ dyne}$$

and is directed to the left.

B. CHARGE ON CONDUCTORS AND INSULATORS

To better understand electrostatics, one should examine how an object first obtained a charge. Most everything in nature is electrically neutral, meaning that they contain an equal amount of positive and negative charges. However, if an additional charge is added to a normally neutral object by touching the object with a charged rod, the neutral object will then have an extra positive or negative charge. This is known as charging by contact. All extra charges, now on the previously neutral object, are of the same type all positive or negative. Each charge of the same type will repel one another so they will spread out, as much as they can, throughout the object. This is why charge can be removed from an object by grounding it to the earth. The earth is very large allowing the charges to spread out far away from each other so they will leave the small charged object, making it neutral again.

PROBLEM

Show how two metallic balls that are mounted on insulating glass stands may be electrostatically charged with equal amounts but opposite sign charges.

Solution

The two metal balls are assumed to be initially uncharged and touching each other. (Any charge on them may first be removed by touching them to the earth. This will provide a path for the charge on the spheres to move to the ground). A charged

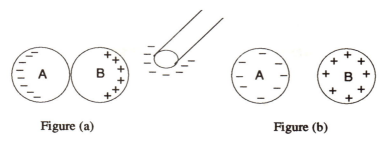

Figure (a)   Figure (b)

Figure 8.3

piece of amber is brought near one of the balls (B) as shown in the figure. The negative charge of the amber will repel the electrons in the metal and cause them to move to the far side of A, leaving B charged positively. If the balls are now separated, A retains a negative charge and B has an equal amount of positive charge. This method of charging is called charging by induction, because it was not necessary to touch the objects being electrified with a charged object (the amber). The charge distribution is induced by the electrical forces associated with the excess electrons present on the surface of the amber.

C.   ELECTRIC FIELD

The electric field acting on a charge is defined as the electric force acting on that charge divided by the magnitude of the charge. Hence, for a single point charge the electric field is given by

$$\vec{E} = k_e q / r^2 \hat{r}.$$

The electric field at a point in space due to a system of point charges can also be found using superposition, summing up the electric fields of the individual point charge. Positive charges are sources of electric field and negative charges are sinks (See Figure 8.4), which means that electric field vectors point away from positive charges ($\hat{r}$ direction) and towards negative charges ($-\hat{r}$ direction). Electric field lines are found by connecting electric field vectors, as shown in Figure 8.5

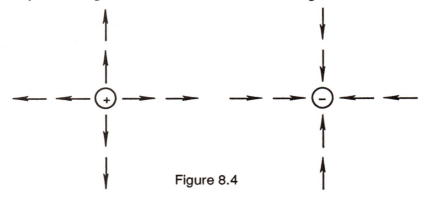

Figure 8.4

D.   POTENTIAL DIFFERENCE

In order to better study the effect of an electric charge, we can use the concept of an electrical potential. This is known to most people as voltage. Electric potential

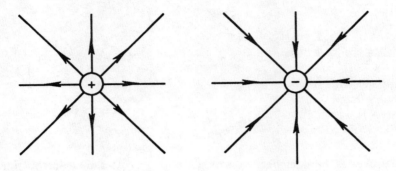

Figure 8.5

is the amount of work done when you move a single charge, let's call it a test charge, near an area with other charges. The surrounding charges will attract or repel the test charge. Therefore, work must be done to move the charge while all the other charges are acting on it. If you move the test charge from position A to position B, the amount of work done is the electrical potential or

$V = W/Q.$

Using the electric field, the potential difference

$V = Va - Vb = -Ed,$

where E is a constant electric field and d is the distance from B to A.

2. Magnetics

A. MAGNETIC FIELDS

Magnetics is familiar to all of us from the childhood magnet, which has a north and south pole. The magnetic field lines extend from the north pole to the south pole as shown in Figure 8.6. Like poles repel and unlike poles attract one another. A magnetic field is produced by the motion of electric charges. So in addition to the electric field surrounding an electron, if that electron is moving, a magnetic field will also be created around the electron.

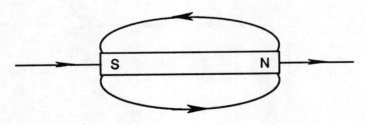

Figure 8.6

If another electron is brought close to the electron in motion and crosses its magnetic field, the magnetic field will apply a force on the second electron. The strength and direction of this force is given by

$$\mathbf{F} = q\mathbf{v} \times \mathbf{B}.$$

F is the force on the electron, **v** is the velocity of the electron's motion and B is the magnetic field produced. The cross product of **v** and **B** is given by the right-hand rule (see Figure 8.7). If the vector **v** is moved counterclockwise toward **B** and if you place your right hand with your fingers curled counterclockwise, the force will be in the direction your thumb is pointing. Remember the force is related by a cross product so if an electron is travelling parallel to the magnetic field then no magnetic force will act on it. For a direction other than parallel to the field, the perpendicular component of the velocity will determine the strength of the force. However, regardless of the electron's motion an electric force will always occur between two electrons.

When dealing with problems involving both electric and magnetic forces the two forces can be solved for separately. Then their influence on another object can be summed together. A wire carrying current will also produce a magnetic field because it has a flow of electrons passing through it. To find the magnetic field around the wire, use the formula

$$B = \mu I / 2\pi r.$$

The direction of the magnetic field is again given by the right-hand rule. By holding the wire with your right hand and making sure your thumb is pointing in the direction of the current, your fingers will be curled around the wire in the direction of the magnetic field.

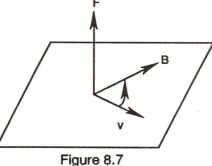

Figure 8.7

PROBLEM

The current from a dc supply is carried to an instrument by two long parallel wires, 10 cm apart. What is the magnetic flux density midway between the wires when the current carried is 100 A?

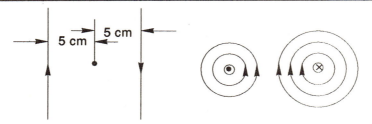

Figure (A): Side View   Figure (B): Top View

Figure 8.8

Solution

The magnetic field due to each wire in the diagram at the point midway between them will be into the paper. This may be seen by use of the right hand rule. If the thumb of the right hand points in the direction of current through the wire, then the fingers will curl in the direction of the magnetic field (or magnetic flux density) created by the current. Application of this rule to both current carrying wires indicates that the field of each is into the page (see Figure 8.8). The effects due to the wires are therefore additive at that point and the total effect is twice the effect of either alone. Hence, midway between the wires the magnetic field due to one wire is

$$B = \frac{\mu_0}{2\pi}\frac{I}{r}$$

where the permeability

$$\mu_0 = 4\pi \times 10^{-7}\ N \text{-} A^{-2},$$

I is the current through the wire, and r is the distance from the point being considered to the wire. Thus

$$B = 2 \times 10^{-7} N - A^{-2} \times \frac{100\ A}{0.05\ m} = 4 \times 10^{-4}\ Wb - m^{-2}$$

The magnetic field due to both wires is then

$$B_T = 2\,B = 8 \times 10^{-4}\ \text{Wb - m}^{-2}.$$

B. ELECTROMAGNETIC SPECTRUM

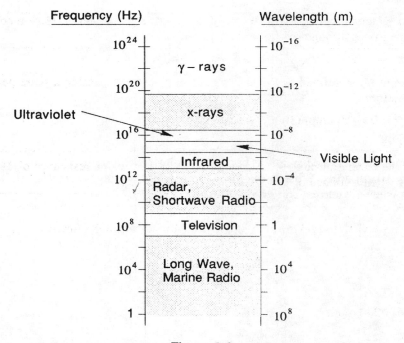

Figure 8.9

IX. ELECTRIC CIRCUITS

1. Current, Voltage, Resistance

RESISTANCE

The basic element of all electric circuits is resistance, because all elements in a circuit will have some resistance. However, current technology has found some devices which have zero resistance; these are called superconductors. The use of superconductors still needs some development so we still must deal with resistance. Resistance is the slowing down of the flow of energy throughout a circuit.

OHM'S LAW

Current, I, is the motion of charge through a conductor. A conductor has a current of 1 Ampere when a charge of 1 Coulomb per second flows through it. Voltage, V, is the force or potential that pushes charge through the circuit. For most material, the ratio of V/I is a constant. This is Ohm's Law

$$R = V/I \quad \text{or} \quad V = IR.$$

For example, a 10 Ohm resistor requires 10 volts across it in order for a current of 1 Ampere to flow.

PROBLEM

A car battery supplies a current I of 50 amp to the starter motor. How much charge passes through the starter in $1/_2$ min?

Solution

Current (I) is defined as the net amount of charge, Q, passing a point per unit time. Therefore,

$$Q = It = (50 \text{ amp}) (30 \text{ sec}) = 1500 \text{ c.}$$

PROBLEM

Find the current through the filament of a light bulb with a resistance of 240 ohms when a voltage of 120 volts is applied to the lamp.

Solution

Since we wish to find the current, we use Ohm's Law in the form

$$I = \frac{V}{R}.$$

$V = 120$ volts,

$R = 240$ ohms

Therefore

$$I = \frac{120 \text{ volts}}{240 \text{ ohms}} = 0.5 \text{ ampere.}$$

PROBLEM

The voltage across the terminals of a resistor is 6.0 volts and an ammeter connected as in the diagram reads 1.5 amp.

a) What is the resistance of the resistor?

b) What would the current be if the potential difference were raised to 8.0 volts?

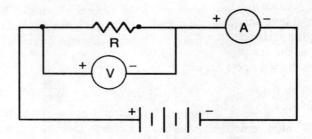

Figure 9.1

Solution

a) $$R = \frac{V}{I} = \frac{6.0 \text{ volts}}{1.5 \text{ amp}} = 4.0 \text{ ohms}$$

b) $$I = \frac{V}{R} = \frac{8.0 \text{ volts}}{4.0 \text{ ohms}} = 2.0 \text{ amp.}$$

In part a) of this solution we have used merely the definition of resistance. But in part b) we have used Ohm's Law, that is, the fact that R is constant.

2. Resistors

The value of a resistor is determined by its physical dimensions and a characteristic of the material called resistivity. For a conducting wire the resistance is given by

$$R = \rho L/A,$$

where L is the wire length and A is its cross-sectional area. The resistance is temperature dependent

$$\Delta R = \alpha R \Delta T$$

because the resistivity varies with temperature. This variation is known for different materials and is given by the factor α, the temperature coefficient of resistance.

PROBLEM

What is the resistance of a piece of nichrome wire 225 centimeters long with a cross-sectional area of 0.015 square centimeter?

Solution

To solve this problem we use the relation

$$R = \rho \frac{L}{A}$$

where R = Resistance

ρ = Resistivity

L = Wire length

A = Cross-sectional area

This basic relationship tells us that resistance is directly proportional to resistivity and length and inversely proportional to cross-sectional area. In the case of a wire this means that the resistance depends on the nature of the substance (which appears in the equation as the resistivity), that the resistance increases as the wire gets longer and decreases as the wire gets thicker.

The resistivity (ρ) for nichrome is 100×10^{-6} ohm-centimeter. The length is 225 centimeters, and the area is 0.015 square centimeter. Then

$$R = \frac{10^{-4} \text{ ohm - cm} \times 225 \text{ cm}}{0.015 \text{ cm}^2} = 1.5 \text{ ohms}.$$

3. Parallel-Plate Capacitors

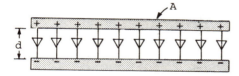

Parallel-plate capacitor

Figure 9.2

$$C = \frac{Q}{V} = \frac{\varepsilon_0 A}{d} \rightarrow \text{units:} \frac{\text{coulomb}}{\text{volt}} = \text{farad}$$

C = Capacitance

Q = Electric Charge

V = Electric Potential

ε_0 = Permittivity Constant

A = Cross-sectional Area of Plates

d = Distance Between Plate Surfaces

4. Kirchoff's Voltage and Current Laws for a Circuit

The voltage and currents in a circuit can be explained by Kirchoff's laws. Kirchoff's voltage law states that the sum of all the voltage drops around a closed loop must equal zero. Thus, for the voltages in Figure 9.3

$$V_1 + V_2 + V_3 + V_4 = 0.$$

Kirchoff's current law states that the sum of all the currents into a node, a point where three or more circuit elements are connected, must equal zero. Therefore, for the circuit of Figure 9.4, Kirchoff's law tells us that

$$I_1 + I_2 + I_3 = 0.$$

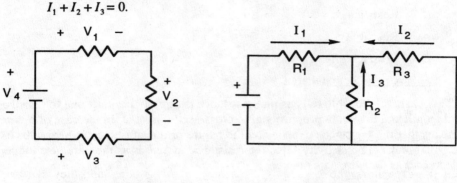

| Figure 9.3 | Figure 9.4 |

5. Series and Parallel Connections

Electric circuits or parts of electric circuits involving series resistances can be simplified by using the fact that series resistances add up

$$R_T = \Sigma R_i .$$

For example, the resistance of three resistors in Figure 9.3 can be replaced by one resistor

$$R_T = R_1 + R_2 + R_3.$$

Parallel resistors in a circuit, such as R_2 and R_3 in Figure 9.4 add with the reciprocal rule:

$$1/R_P = 1/R_2 + 1/R_3.$$

Thus the total resistance across the battery in Figure 9.4 is

$$R_T = R_1 + R_P = R_1 + \frac{R_2 + R_3}{R_2 R_3}.$$

PROBLEM

Find the equivalent resistor R and equivalent capacitor C as shown in Figure 9.5, where μF denotes a microfarad, equivalent to 10^{-6} farad.

Solution

First, examine the resistors. Note that the 2Ω and 6Ω resistors are in series and can be replaced by a single resistance of $6 + 2 = 8\Omega$. Now the 8Ω and 4Ω resistors are in parallel. Combine them to get a single resistance R given by

$$\frac{1}{R} = \frac{1}{8} + \frac{1}{4}$$

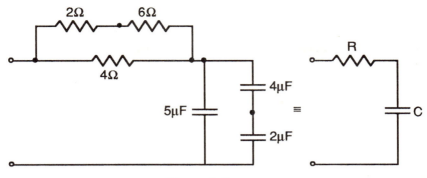

Figure 9.5

$$R = \frac{8 \cdot 4}{8+4} = \frac{32}{12} = \frac{8}{3}\,\Omega.$$

For the capacitors, the 2μF and 4μF capacitors are in series and they can be combined to give a capacitor

$$\frac{2 \cdot 4}{2+4}\,\mu F \quad \text{or} \quad \frac{4}{3}\,\mu F.$$

This will be in parallel with a 5μF capacitor. Hence

$$C = 5 + \frac{4}{3} = \frac{19}{3}\,\mu F.$$

Note: The rule for capacitors is different. Capacitors in series add like resistors in parallel by the reciprocal rule, and capacitors in parallel add like resistors in series.

6. Power

In order to find the power used by a circuit element, the voltage across that element is multiplied by the current through it or $P = VI$, where P is the power in watts.

7. Root-Mean Square Current and Voltage

To compare the energy an AC signal can deliver to a circuit with the energy a DC signal delivers an effective or RMS value of current and voltage is used

$$I_{rms} = \frac{I_m}{\sqrt{2}}$$

$$V_{rms} = \frac{V_m}{\sqrt{2}}$$

I_m = peak current value (max amplitude)

V_m = peak voltage value

X. LIGHT AND GEOMETRIC OPTICS

1. Refraction, Refractive Index, Snell's Law

Recall that light propagates at speed

$$c = f\lambda$$

in a vacuum, or speed

$$v = c/n$$

in a medium of index of refraction n. Usually, the propagation of light is also represented as a ray moving in a straight line. For many problems in optics, one may use the fact that for a ray of light the angle of incidence is equal to the angle of reflection from a mirrored surface. Hence, the first part of solving an optics problem is always to draw an accurate ray diagram.

To solve problems involving the propagation of light from one medium (or index of refraction n_i) to another (or index of refraction n_r). Snell's Law is used. Refer to Figure 10.1. Snell's Law states that

$$n_i \sin \theta_i = n_r \sin \theta_r.$$

Hence, given any three of the four variables, one can solve for the other. Note that for a vacuum or near vacuum (sometimes a good approximation for air), the index of refraction is one.

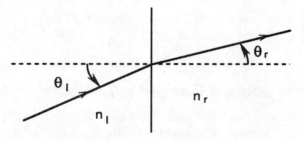

Figure 10.1

PROBLEM

How fast does light travel in glass of refractive index 1.5?

Solution

By definition, refractive index n is the ratio of the velocity of light in vacuum (3.00×10^{10} cm/sec) to the velocity of light in the medium in question. Therefore

$$n = \frac{3 \times 10^{10} \text{ cm/s}}{v} = 1.5$$

Therefore

$$v = \frac{3 \times 10^{10} \text{ cm/s}}{1.5}$$

$$= 2.00 \times 10^{10} \text{ cm/sec.}$$

2. Total Internal Reflection

Notice from Figure 10.1 that it is conceivable to have $\theta_r = 90°$. When this happens, θ_i is called the critical angle θ_c given by $\sin \theta_c = n_r / n_i$. If the angle of incidence is greater than the critical angle, then we have total internal reflection: the light will not escape from the first medium. This principle is used to transmit pulses of light in fiber optic communication.

Critical angle θ_c.

$$\sin \theta_c = \frac{n_2}{n_1} \ , \quad \frac{n_2}{n_1} < 1$$

PROBLEM

What is the critical angle between carbon disulfide and air?

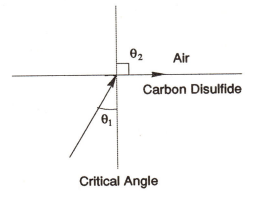

Critical Angle

Figure 10.2

Solution

Carbon disulfide is a more optically dense material than air. Therefore, as a beam of light passes from carbon disulfide to air, the angle of refraction is larger than the angle of incidence. There is an angle of incidence smaller than 90° for which the angle of refraction is equal to 90°, meaning that the beam of light emerges parallel to the boundary between the two mediums. This angle of incidence is called the critical angle. If the angle of incidence is greater than this value, the light will not escape from the carbon disulfide. It will be reflected back into the carbon disulfide following the regular law of reflection. Solving for the critical angle θ_1, let θ_2 be 90°. The index of refraction for carbon disulfide is 1.643 and for air it is 1.00. Using Snell's Law

$$n_1 \sin \theta_1 = n_2 \sin \theta_2$$

$$1.643 \sin \theta_1 = 1.00 \sin 90°$$

$$\sin \theta_1 = \frac{1.00}{1.643} = 0.608$$

$$\theta_1 = 37.4°.$$

3. Lenses and Optical Instruments

The optics of thin lenses may be understood using Snell's Law. Again, one must always draw a careful ray diagram in attacking the problem. From Snell's Law we can derive a relation called the thin lens equation

$$1/s + 1/s' = 1/f$$

where

$1/f \equiv (n - 1)\ (1/R_1 - 1/R_2)$ is the reciprocal of the focal length.

This thin lens equation applies to both concave (diverging) and convex (converging) lenses. Convex lenses have positive focal length (see Figure 10.3 for a typical ray diagram), whereas concave lenses have $f < 0$. The object seen by the lens is said to be real if the object distance is positive. The image is said to be real if the image distance is positive. Otherwise, the object/image is called virtual. The image is erect if the magnification is positive; inverted if $m_1 < 0$.

The simple microscope consists of one lens placed near the eye with the object just inside the focal point of the lens and the image at the near point of the eye. Using the thin lens equation, we have $1/s = 1/f + 1/25$ or for the magnification

$$m_1 = h'/h = -s'/s = 1 + 25/f.$$

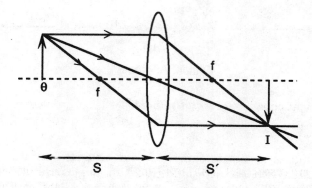

Figure 10.3

When the eye is relaxed, the object at the focal point of the lens and the image is at infinity. In that case, we obtain a smaller magnification $m_1 = 25/f$.

The compound microscope consists of two lenses, an objective and an eyepiece. The two lenses are separated by a distance l very much greater than f_e or

$$f_0 : 1 >> f_0, f_e.$$

The object is placed just outside the focal length of the objective forming an image close to the focal length of the eyepiece. The eyepiece serves as a simple magnifier for this first image. The net magnification is thus

$$m_1 = m_0 m_e = - l/f_0 \cdot 25/f_e.$$

The telescope also makes use of an objective and an eyepiece separated by a distance l. But here, we have

$$l = f_0 + f_e.$$

The first image is formed at the focal point of the objective because the object is at ∞. The magnification is then

$$m_1 = - f_0 / f_e.$$

Hence, it is essential for the telescope that the objective focal length be greater than the eyepiece focal length.

PROBLEM

A converging lens with a focal length of 3 m forms an image of an object placed 9 m from it. Find the position of the image and the magnification.

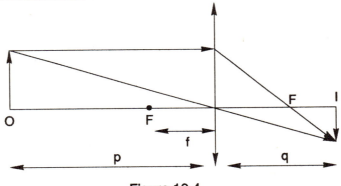

Figure 10.4

Solution

The simple lens equation for the covering lens of this problem is

$$\frac{1}{f} = \frac{1}{p} + \frac{1}{q}$$

where f, p and q are respectively the focal length of the lens and the distances of the object and the image from the lens. The image is real and inverted (see the figure). Substituting the given values in the above equation, we get

$$\frac{1}{q} = \frac{1}{f} - \frac{1}{p} = \frac{1}{3m} - \frac{1}{9m} = \frac{2}{9} \, m^{-1}$$

and

$$q = \frac{9}{2}m = 4.5m.$$

Since the value of q is positive, the image occurs on the right side of the lens. The magnification M is

$$M = \frac{q}{p} = \frac{4.5 \text{ m}}{9 \text{ m}} = 0.5$$

so the image is one-half as high as the object.

PROBLEM

When an object is placed 10 in from a certain lens, its virtual image is formed 10 in from the lens. Determine the focal length and character of the lens.

Solution

Since the image is virtual, on the same side of the lens as the object, its distance from the lens, q, is negative. Substitution in the general equation for lenses yields

$$\frac{1}{p} + \frac{1}{q} = \frac{1}{f}$$

$$\frac{1}{20 \text{ in}} + \frac{1}{-10 \text{ in}} = \frac{1}{f}$$

$$\frac{1}{f} = \frac{-10 \text{ in} + 20 \text{ in}}{(20 \text{ in}) \times (-10 \text{ in})} = -\frac{10}{200 \text{ in}}$$

$$f = -20 \text{ in}.$$

The negative sign for the focal length indicates that the lens is diverging. Diverging lenses are concave.

4. Polarization

Polarized light is light which has waves in only one plane. This light can be obtained by passing unpolarized light through a material that only allows light to pass through in one plane.

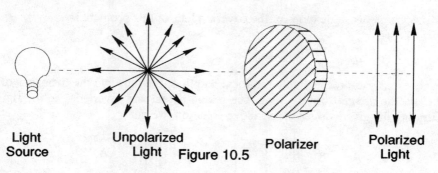

| Light Source | Unpolarized Light | Figure 10.5 | Polarizer | Polarized Light |

5. Dispersion

Because for some transparent materials the index of refraction depends on frequency, the speeds of the different wavelengths of light will not be the same when passing through this transparent material. This fact that the speeds of different wavelengths of light are different in a refracting medium is called dispersion.

6. Visual Spectrum, Color

Color	Wavelength Å
Ultraviolet	< 4000
Violet	4000 - 4250
Blue	4250 - 4900
Green	4900 - 5750
Yellow	5750 - 5850
Orange	5850 - 6500
Red	6500 - 7000
Infrared	> 7000

XI. ATOMIC AND NUCLEAR STRUCTURE

1. Quantized Energy Levels and Atomic Spectra

The simplest atom, hydrogen, has a spectrum with wavelengths at 6562, 4860, 4339, and 4101 Å. This is the well-known Balmer series. These spectral lines are produced by photons given off when electrons in the hydrogen atom change from an excited state to a lower energy state. The reason there are only specific wavelengths given off and not a continuous range of values between 6500Å and 4000Å is that the electron can only have certain discrete energy values. To understand this discretization of energy levels, consider the more general problem of Figure 11.1. An electron of charge $-e$ and mass m orbits around a central nucleus of charge Ze at radius r. This is called an *H*-like atom.

By Newton's Second Law for Centripetal Motion

$$F = ma = mv^2 / r.$$

Furthermore, the source of the centripetal force is the Coulomb force

$$F = k_e Z_e^2 / r^2.$$

With only these two equations, one could find the force given the distance and nucleus (e.g., $Z = 1$ for hydrogen). Then the force could be used to find the speed

$$v = \sqrt{Fr / m}.$$

However, with the quantization of angular momentum postulate of Bohr theory, we can go beyond this. The concept of the de Broglie wavelength $\pi\lambda = h$ (h is Planck's constant) can be used with the non-interference condition $n\lambda = 2\pi r$ to derive this postulate. The postulate says that

$$L = mvr = n\hbar \quad n = 1, 2, 3, \ldots$$

where $\hbar = h/2\pi$. n is called the principal quantum number. Using this, we can eliminate the speed ($v = n\hbar / mr$) from our equation

$$mv^2 / r = k_e Ze^2 / r^2$$

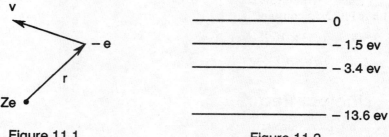

Figure 11.1   Figure 11.2

to get

$$r_n = n^2 a_0 / Z$$

where $a_0 = \hbar^2 / k_e me^2 = .5292$ Å is the $n = 1$ hydrogen Bohr radius.

One can also determine the total energy of the H-like atom using this problem-solving method. The total mechanical energy is

$$E = KE + U = \frac{1}{2} mv^2 - k_e Ze^2/r$$
$$= - k_e Ze^2 / r.$$

Using our result for the radius $r = r_n$, we get

$$E_n = - Z^2/n^2\, 13.6 \text{ eV}.$$

Consider as an example the hydrogen atom with $Z = 1$. One may then obtain an energy level diagram (Figure 11.2) by substituting $n = 1, 2, 3$, etc.

Atomic and molecular spectra arise from transitions between energy levels on similar diagrams. In Bohr theory, we can use the Einstein relation

$$\Delta E = h\nu = hc/\lambda,$$

where ν is the frequency to find the wavelength of a transition from level n_i to n_f (Figure 11.3).

$$hc / \lambda = E_{n_i} - E_{n_f}$$
$$= Z^2 13.6 \text{ eV } (1/ n_f^2 - 1/ n_i^2).$$

For example, taking $Z = 1$ (hydrogen), $n_f = 2$ (Balmer series), $n_i = 3$, and $hc = 12{,}400$ eV - Å, we get $1 = 6561$ Å the first line in the Balmer series!

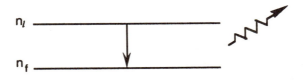

Figure 11.3

PROBLEM

What is the energy of a photon of green light (frequency = 6×10^{14} vps)?

Solution

Planck's hypothesis states that $E = h\nu$, where ν is the frequency of the radiation, and h is Planck's constant. Therefore

$$E = (6.63 \times 10^{-34} \text{ joule/sec}) (6 \times 10^{14} \text{ vps})$$

$$E = 3.98 \times 10^{-19} \text{ joules}.$$

2. Nuclear Reactions

In a typical nuclear reaction $I + T \rightarrow R + E$ where an incident particle interacts with a target particle to produce an emitted particle and a residual particle, one can define a Q-value

$$Q = (m_I + m_t - m_i - m_R) C^2.$$

If $Q > 0$, then the reaction is exoergic; for $Q < 0$, it is endoergic or requires energy. This approach is useful in the radioactive decay of one particle by taking $m_I = 0$.

When dealing with nuclear reactions, the key is to keep track of which particles are emitted and how much of the mass of the elements involved changes. Each particle in a reaction is assigned a symbol with a superscript giving the mass number and a subscript for the atomic number. Also some reactions will involve the loss of energy in the form of gamma rays. In this case, the particles involved do not change mass, but instead change in energy.

PROBLEM

B^{10} is bombarded with neutrons, and a particles are observed to be emitted. What is the residual nucleus?

Solution

Only α particles (helium nuclei) are observed to be emitted in the reaction. The reaction can be described as follows:

$$^{10}_{5}B + {}^{1}_{0}n \rightarrow {}^{A}_{Z}(X) + {}^{4}_{2}He$$

where the superscript gives the mass number A. It is the total number of protons and neutrons in that nucleus. In a nuclear reaction the total nucleon number and the total charge is conserved, therefore the mass number A of the unknown nucleus must be such that

$$10 + 1 = A + 4.$$

Hence $A = 7$.

The subscripts refer to the atomic numbers, total number of protons in each nucleus. Since the above reaction involves protons and neutrons only, the protons carry the total charge. The conservation of total electric charge in that case reduces to the conservation of the total number of protons. Therefore,

$$5 + 0 = Z + 2$$

or $Z = 3$.

The nucleus with $A = 7$, $Z = 3$ is ${}^{7}_{3}Li$.

3. Einstein's Relation

$$E = mc^2$$

An object's mass can also be described as an amount of energy.

PROBLEM

What is the energy content of 1 gm of water?

Solution

If the mass of the gram of water was completely converted to energy, the amount of energy released would be

$$E = mc^2$$
$$= 1 \times 10^{-3} \times (3 \times 10^8)^2$$
$$= 9 \times 10^{13} \text{ joules}$$

4. Radioactive Decay, Half-Life

Radiation is pervasive in the world around us in various forms: light (4000 - 8000 Å photons), radio waves, black-body protons, cosmic ray particles, etc. Many forms of radiation, especially particles, follow an exponential law

$$N = N_0 e^{-\lambda t}$$

where λ is the decay constant.

This exponential decay can be related to the half-life $t_{1/2}$ since

$$N_0 / 2 = N_0 e^{-\lambda t_{1/2}}.$$

Using the natural logarithm gives

$$t_{1/2} = \ln 2 / 1$$

PROBLEM

The half-life of radon is 3.80 days. After how many days will only one-sixteenth of a radon sample remain?

Solution

A half-life of 3.80 days means that every 3.80 days, half the amount of radon present decays. Since one-sixteenth is a power of one-half, this problem can be solved by counting. After 3.80 days, one-half the original sample remains. In the next 3.80 days, one-half of this decays so that after 7.60 days one-fourth the original amount remains. After 11.4 days, one-eighth the original amount remains, and after four half-lives (15.2 days), one-sixteenth the original amount remains.

As an alternative solution, the formula for decaying matter can be used.

$$\frac{N}{N_0} = e^{-\lambda t_{(1/2)}}$$

λ is an experimental constant which can be determined from the half-life. Therefore, for

$$\frac{N}{N_0} = \frac{1}{2},$$

$$\ln \frac{N}{N_0} = -\lambda t_{(1/2)}$$

$$\lambda = \frac{\ln \frac{N_0}{N}}{t_{(1/2)}} = \frac{\ln 2}{t_{(1/2)}} = \frac{0.693}{3.80 \text{ days}} = 0.182 / \text{day}.$$

We want $N/N_0 = 1/16 = e^{-\lambda t} = e^{-0.182t}$.

$$\frac{N}{N_0} = \frac{1}{16},$$

$$\ln \frac{N}{N_0} = --0.182t$$

$$\frac{\ln \frac{N_0}{N}}{0.182} = t$$

$$\frac{\ln 16}{0.182} = \frac{2.77}{0.182} = 15.2 \text{ days.}$$

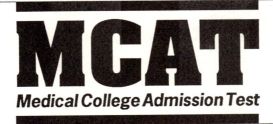

Chapter 5
Mathematics Review

Chapter 5

I.   ARITHMETIC

1. Integers and Real Numbers

Most of the numbers used in algebra belong to a set called the **real numbers** or **reals**. This set can be represented graphically by the real number line.

Given the number line below, we arbitrarily fix a point and label it with the number 0. In a similar manner, we can label any point on the line with one of the real numbers, depending on its position relative to 0. Numbers to the right of zero are positive, while those to the left are negative. Value increases from left to right, so that if a is to the right of b, it is said to be greater than b.

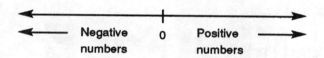

If we now divide the number line into equal segments, we can label the points on this line with real numbers. For example, the point 2 lengths to the left of zero is - 2, while the point 3 lengths to the right of zero is + 3 (the + sign is usually assumed, so + 3 is written simply as 3). The number line now looks like this:

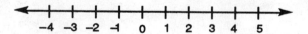

These boundary points represent the subset of the reals known as the **integers**. The set of integers is made up of both the positive and negative whole numbers: $\{... - 4, - 3, - 2, - 1, 0, 1, 2, 3, 4, ...\}$. Some subsets of integers are:

Natural Numbers or Positive Numbers - the set of integers starting with 1 and increasing: $\mathcal{N} = \{1, 2, 3, 4, ...\}$.

Whole Numbers - the set of integers starting with 0 and increasing: $\mathcal{W} = \{0, 1, 2, 3, ...\}$.

Negative Numbers - the set of integers starting with - 1 and decreasing: $\mathcal{Z} = \{- 1, - 2, - 3 ...\}$.

Prime Numbers - the set of positive integers greater than 1 that are divisible only by 1 and themselves: $\{2, 3, 5, 7, 11, ...\}$.

Even Integers - the set of integers divisible by 2: $\{..., - 4, - 2, 0, 2, 4, 6, ...\}$.

Odd Integers - the set of integers not divisible by 2: { ..., - 3, - 1, 1, 3, 5, 7, ...}.

PROBLEM

Classify each of the following numbers into as many different sets as possible. Example: real, integer ...

a)   0   b)   9   c) $\sqrt{6}$

d) $\frac{1}{2}$ e) $\frac{2}{3}$ f)   1.5

Solution

a)   Zero is a real number and an integer.

b)   9 is a real, natural number, and an integer.

c) $\sqrt{6}$ is a real number.

d) $\frac{1}{2}$ is a real number.

e) $\frac{2}{3}$ is a real number.

f)   1.5 is a real number, and a decimal.

2. Ratios and Proportions

The ratio of two numbers x and *y written* x:y is the fraction x/y where $y \neq 0$. A proportion is an equality of two ratios.

Given a proportion $a:b = c:d$, then a and d are called the extremes, b and c are called the means and d is called the fourth proportional to a, b and c. If the two means are equal, as in the proportion $a:b = b:c$, then c is called the third proportional to a and b.

FUNDAMENTAL PROPERTIES OF PROPORTIONS

If $a:b = c:d$, then:

1. $ad = bc$, the product of the means is equal to the product of the extremes. For example, if

$$4 : 8 = 9 : x, \text{ then}$$

$$4x = 72 \text{ and } x = 18$$

2. $a:b = c:d$. Following from Property 1 $ad = bc$, either pair can be made the means and the other pair the extremes.

In this case $a:b = c:d$, bc are the means and ad are the extremes.

3. $b:a = d:c$, inversion.

4. $(a + b):b = (c + d):d$, addition.

5. $(a - b):b = (c - d):d$, subtraction.

PROBLEM

Write the following ratios reduced to simplest form.

a) 12 inches to 2 feet   b) 15 minutes to 2 hours

c) 1100 yards to 1 mile

d) $(x^3 + x^2 - 6x) : (x^3 - 4x^2 + 4x)$

Solution

a) Convert the quantities being compared to the same units. Convert 2 feet to inches

12 inches to 24 inches = 12:24 = 1:2

b) Convert 2 hours to minutes

15 minutes to 120 minutes = 15:120 = 1:8

c) Convert 1 mile to yards

1,100 yards to 1,760 yards = 1,100:1,760 = 5:8

d) Factor each polynomial separately

$$\frac{x^3 + x^2 - 6x}{x^3 - 4x^2 + 4x} = \frac{x(x^2 + x - 6)}{x(x^2 - 4x + 4)} = \frac{x(x-2)(x+3)}{x(x-2)(x-2)}$$

Cancel equivalent terms

$$= \frac{x+3}{x-2} \text{ or } (x+3) : (x-2)$$

PROBLEM

Find the fourth proportional to 2, 5, and 6.

Solution

Set up the proportion

2:5 = 6:x,

then by definition x is the fourth proportional

2x = 30,

x = 15.

PROBLEM

Find the third proportional to 9 and 5.

Solution

Set up the proportion

9:5 = 5:x

then by definition x is the third proportional.

9x = 25,

$x = 2^7/_9$.

PROBLEM

> Find the mean proportional between 4 and 16.

Solution

Set up the proportion

$$4{:}x = x{:}16$$

x is the mean proportional, solve for x

$$x^2 = 64$$

$$x = \pm 8$$

PROBLEM

> Find the value of x in the proportion
>
> $$(x + 2){:}(2x - 8) = 5{:}(x - 5)$$

Solution

Using Property 1, $ad = bc$.

$$(x + 2)(x - 5) = 5(2x - 8)$$

multiply out both sides

$$x^2 - 3x - 10 = 10x - 40$$

$$x^2 - 13x + 30 = 0$$

$$(x - 3)(x - 10) = 0$$

$$x = +3, x = +10$$

PROBLEM

> If $9x = 4y$ find the ratio of $x{:}y$.

Solution

Using Property 2, $a{:}b = c{:}d$, either pair can be made the means and the other pair the extremes.

Choosing $9x$ as the extremes will have $x{:}y = 4{:}9$.

PROBLEM

> Solve the proportion $\dfrac{x+1}{4} = \dfrac{15}{12}$.

Solution

Cross multiply to determine x; that is, multiply the numerator of the first fraction by the denominator of the second, and equate this to the product of the numerator of the second and the denominator of the first.

$$(x + 1)\,12 = 4 \cdot 15$$

$$12x + 12 = 60$$

$$x = 4.$$

3. Percentages

A percent is a number out of 100. A percent can be defined by fractions with a denominator of 100. Decimals can also represent a percent. For instance,

$$56\% = 0.56 \text{ or } {}^{56}/_{100}.$$

PROBLEM

Compute the value of

a)   90% of 400

b)   180% of 400

c)   50% of 500

d)   200% of 4

Solution

The symbol % means per hundred, therefore $5\% = {}^{5}/_{100}$.

a) $90\% \text{ of } 400 = {}^{90}/_{100} \times {}^{400}/_{1} = 90 \times 4 = 360$

b) $180\% \text{ of } 400 = {}^{180}/_{100} \times {}^{400}/_{1} = 180 \times 4 = 720$

c) $50\% \text{ of } 500 = {}^{50}/_{100} \times {}^{500}/_{1} = 50 \times 5 = 250$

d) $200\% \text{ of } 4 = {}^{200}/_{100} \times {}^{4}/_{1} = 2 \times 4 = 8$

PROBLEM

What percent of

a)   100 is 99.5?

b)   200 is 4?

Solution

a)
$$99.5 = x \times 100$$
$$99.5 = 100x$$
$$99.5 = x,$$

but this is the value of x per hundred. Therefore

$$x = 99.5\%.$$

b)
$$4 = x \times 200$$
$$4 = 200x$$
$$.02 = x.$$

Again this must be changed to percent, so

$$x = 2\%.$$

4. Reciprocals

The reciprocal of a number x is the fraction $^1/_x$. x can be any real number.

PROBLEM

Find the reciprocal of each of the following numbers and express them as decimals.

a)   5

b) $^4/_9$

c) $2^4/_5$

d)   4.25

Solution

a)   The reciprocal of 5 is $^1/_5$. In decimal notation $^1/_5 = 0.2$.

b)   The reciprocal of $^4/_9$ is

$$\frac{1}{^4/_9} = 1 \div \frac{4}{9} = 1 \times \frac{9}{4} = \frac{9}{4} = 2.25.$$

c)   First express $2^4/_5$ as a fraction, which is $2^4/_5 = {}^{14}/_5$. The reciprocal of $^{14}/_5$ is

$$\frac{1}{^{14}/_5} = 1 \div \frac{14}{5} = 1 \times \frac{5}{14} = \frac{5}{14} = 0.357.$$

d)   First express 4.25 as a fraction, which is $4^1/_4 = {}^{17}/_4$. The reciprocal of $^{17}/_4$ is

$$\frac{1}{^{17}/_4} = 1 \div \frac{17}{4} = 1 \times \frac{4}{17} = \frac{4}{17} = 0.235.$$

II. SCIENTIFIC CALCULATIONS

1. Exponents

Given the expression $a_n = b$, where a, n, and $b \in R$, a is called the base, n is called the exponent or power.

In 3^2, 3 is the base, 2 is the exponent. If n is a positive integer and if x and y are real numbers such that $x^n = y$, then x is said to be an nth root of y, written

$$x = \sqrt[n]{y} = y^{\frac{1}{n}}.$$

POSITIVE INTEGRAL EXPONENT

If n is a positive integer, then a^n represents the product of n factors each of which is a.

NEGATIVE INTEGRAL EXPONENT

If n is a positive integer,

$$a^{-n} = \frac{1}{a^n} \quad a \neq 0$$

so,

$$2^{-4} = \frac{1}{2^4} = \frac{1}{16}$$

POSITIVE FRACTIONAL EXPONENT

$$a^{\frac{m}{n}} = \sqrt[n]{a^m}$$

where m and n are positive integers. For example

$$4^{\frac{3}{2}} = \sqrt[2]{4^3} = \sqrt{64} = 8$$

NEGATIVE FRACTIONAL EXPONENT

$$a^{-\frac{m}{n}} = \frac{1}{a^{\frac{m}{n}}}$$

For example

$$27^{-\frac{2}{3}} = \frac{1}{27^{\frac{2}{3}}} = \frac{1}{\sqrt[3]{27^2}} = \frac{1}{\sqrt[3]{729}} = \frac{1}{9}$$

ZERO EXPONENT

$$a^0 = 1, \quad a \neq 0$$

General Laws of Exponents:

A) $a^p a^q = a^{p+q}$

B) $(a^p)^q = a^{pq}$

C) $\dfrac{a^p}{a^q} = a^{p-q}, \quad a \neq 0$

D) $(ab)^p = a^p b^p$

E) $\left(\dfrac{a}{b}\right)^p = \dfrac{a^p}{b^p}, \quad b \neq 0$

PROBLEM

Simplify the following expressions:

a) -3^{-2}

b) $(-3)^{-2}$

c) $\dfrac{-3}{4^{-1}}$

Solution

a)   Here the exponent applies only to 3. Since

$$x^{-y} = \frac{1}{x^y}, \quad -3^{-2} = -(3^{-2}) = -\frac{1}{3^2} = -\frac{1}{9}.$$

b)   In this case the exponent applies to the negative base. Thus,

$$(-3)^{-2} = -\frac{1}{(-3)^2} = \frac{1}{(-3)(-3)} = \frac{1}{9}.$$

c) $\dfrac{-3}{4^{-1}} = \dfrac{-3}{\left(\frac{1}{4}\right)^1} = \dfrac{-3}{\frac{1}{4^1}} = \dfrac{-3}{\frac{1}{4}}.$

Division by a fraction is equivalent to multiplication by that fraction's reciprocal, thus

$$\frac{-3}{\frac{1}{4}} = -3 \cdot \frac{4}{1} = -12,$$

and

$$\frac{-3}{4^{-1}} = -12.$$

PROBLEM

Find the indicated roots.

a) $\sqrt[5]{32}$

b) $\sqrt[3]{-125}$

c) $\pm \sqrt[4]{625}$

d) $\sqrt[4]{-16}$

Solution

The following two laws of exponents can be used to solve these problems:

$$(1) \ \left(\sqrt[n]{a}\right)^n = \left(a^{1/n}\right) = a^1 = a, \quad \text{and} \quad (2) \ \left(\sqrt[n]{a}\right)^n = \sqrt[n]{a^n}.$$

a) $\sqrt[5]{32} = \sqrt[5]{2^5} = \left(\sqrt[5]{2}\right)^5 = 2.$

This result is true because $(2)^5 = 32$, that is, $2 \cdot 2 \cdot 2 \cdot 2 \cdot 2 = 32$.

b) $\sqrt[4]{625} = \sqrt[4]{5^4} = \left(\sqrt[4]{5}\right)^4 = 5.$

This result is true because $(5)^4 = 625$, that is, $5 \cdot 5 \cdot 5 \cdot 5 = 625$.

$$\sqrt[4]{625} = -\left(\sqrt[4]{5^4}\right) = \left[\left(\sqrt[4]{5}\right)\right]^4 = -[5] = -5.$$

This result is true because $(-5)^4 = 625$, that is, $(-5) \cdot (-5) \cdot (-5) \cdot (-5) = 625$.

c) $\sqrt[3]{-125} = \sqrt[3]{(-5)^3} = \left(\sqrt[3]{-5}\right)^3 = -5.$

This result is true because $(-5)^3 = -125$, that is, $(-5) \cdot (-5) \cdot (-5) = -125$.

d)   There is no solution to $\sqrt[4]{-16}$ because any number raised to the fourth power is a positive number, that is, $N^4 = (N) \cdot (N) \cdot (N) \cdot (N) =$ a positive number $\neq$ a negative number, -16.

2. Logarithms

The logarithm of a number N is the power a which the base b must be raised to get the number N. The exponent a must be positive.

Exponential Form

$b_a = N$

Logarithmic Form

$\log_b N = a$

PROBLEM

Express $2^6 = 64$ in logarithmic form.

Solution

Find the base b, exponent a, and number N. Place in the form

$\log_b N = a$

base $b = 2$

number $N = 64$

exponent $a = 6$

Therefore the logarithmic form is $\log_2 64 = 6$.

PROBLEM

Express $3^{-4} = \frac{1}{81}$ in logarithmic form.

Solution

base $\qquad b = 3$

number $\qquad N = \frac{1}{81}$

exponent $\quad a = -4$

Place in form $\log_b N = a$

$\qquad \log_3 \frac{1}{81} = -4$

PROBLEM

Express $\log_5 625 = 4$ in exponential form.

Solution

base $\qquad b = 5$

number $\qquad N = 625$

exponent $\quad a = 4$

Place in form $b^a = N$

$\qquad\qquad 5^4 = 625.$

PROBLEM

Express $\log_{16} \frac{1}{32} = \frac{5}{4}$ in exponential form.

Solution

base $\qquad b = 16$

number $\qquad N = \frac{1}{32}$

exponent $\quad a = -\frac{5}{4}$

Place in form $b^a = N$

$\qquad 16^{-5/4} = \frac{1}{32}.$

PROBLEM

Find the value of x

$\qquad \log_{128} 16 = x$

Solution

First find the base, exponent, and number

base $\qquad b = 128$

exponent $\quad a = x$

number $\qquad N = 16$

Place in exponential form $b^a = N$

$$128^x = 16$$

Find a common base between the numbers. In this case, the base is 2

$$(2^7)^x = 2^4$$

Equate the exponents

$$7x = 4$$

$$x = {}^4/_7$$

PROPERTIES OF LOGARITHMS

A) $\log_a MN = \log_a M + \log_a N$

B) $\log_a {}^M/_N = \log_a M - \log_a N$

C) $\log_a M^k = k \log_a M$

PROBLEM

Express $\log_a \dfrac{\sqrt[3]{17}}{\sqrt{10}}$ in terms of logarithms of prime numbers.

Solution

Use Property B)

$$\log_a \frac{\sqrt[3]{17}}{\sqrt{10}} = \log_a \sqrt[3]{17} - \log_a \sqrt{10}$$

Express radicals as exponents

$$\log_a (17)^{1/3} - \log_a (10)^{1/2}$$

Express the number 10 as prime numbers

$$\log_a (17)^{1/3} - \log_a (5 \cdot 2)^{1/2}$$

Use Property A)

$$\log_a (17)^{1/3} - (\log_a 5^{1/2} + \log_a 2^{1/2})$$

Use Property C)

$$\tfrac{1}{3} \log_a 17 - \tfrac{1}{2} \log_a 5 - \tfrac{1}{2} \log_a 2$$

LOGARITHMS WITH BASE 10

Any positive number except 1 can be used as the base, but for computational purposes, it is convenient to use 10 as the base. When the base is omitted, base 10 is understood.

The logarithms of numbers which are integral powers of 10 are very easy to find. For example,

$\log 1 = 0, \log 10 = 1, \log 100 = 2, \log 1000 = 3, \log 0.1 = -1, \log 0.01 = -2.$

For some general number, which is not a power of 10, the logarithm has a whole number (integer) part called the **characteristic**, and a decimal part called the **man-**

tissa. For example,

$$2580 = 10^{3.4116} \quad \text{or} \quad \log 2580 = 3.4116$$

so the characteristic is 3 and the mantissa is .4116

NATURAL LOGARITHMS

For scientific and mathematical purposes, sometimes another base is used instead of base 10. This base is denoted by "e," where $e = 2.71828$. The logarithm with base e is called the natural logarithm.

To find out the natural logarithm, it is convenient to use the following formula:

$$\log_e x = \log_e 10 \cdot \log_{10} x = 2.303 \log_{10} x.$$

3. Scientific Notation

To simplify the expressing of very large or very small numbers scientific notation is used.

A real number expressed in scientific notation is written as a product of a real number n and an integral power of 10; the value of n is $1 \le n < 10$.

PROBLEM

Express the distance of the earth to the moon, 236,121 miles in scientific notation.

Solution

First find the n between 1 and 10.

n is 2.3

Then move the decimal point 5 places to the right to get 236,121. Each movement to the right represents a multiplication by 10. Therefore, 5 places equals a multiplication by 10^5.

Expressed in scientific notation

$$236,121 = 2.3 \times 10^5 \text{ miles}$$

PROBLEM

Express the wavelength of the new Ka band police radar .011 m in scientific notation.

Solution

The number n between 1 and 10 is 1.1 The decimal must now be moved 2 places to the left. Two places to the left equals a multiplication of 10^{-2}.

Expressed in scientific notation

$$.011 = 1.1 \times 10^{-2} \text{ m}$$

PROBLEM

Convert the number 6.38×10^6 to ordinary decimal notation.

Solution

The multiplication by 10^6 is equivalent to moving the decimal point 6 places to the right. Therefore $6.38 \times 10^6 = 6,380,000$.

4. Metric Units

The international system of units (abbreviated SI) commonly known as the metric system, is divided into three classes: base units, supplementary units, and derived units. While the list of all the units is very long, the following table gives the most basic units used.

TABLE 1— Basic Metric Units

Quantity	Unit	Symbol
length	meter	m
mass	kilogram	kg
time	second	s
angle	radian	rad
temperature	celsius	C
volume	liter	L

PREFIX

Prefixes are used to form the multiple and submultiple of the SI units. The following table gives the most commonly used prefixes.

TABLE 2 — Metric Prefixes

Multiplication Factor	Prefix	Abbreviation
10^9	giga	G
10^6	mega	M
10^3	kilo	k
10^2	hecto	h
10^1	deka	da
10^{-1}	deci	d
10^{-2}	centi	c
10^{-3}	milli	m
10^{-6}	micro	μ
10^{-9}	nano	n

CONVERSION FACTORS

The following table lists the multiplying factors necessary to convert from one unit of measure to another for the basic metric units in Table 1.

TABLE 3 — Conversion Factors

To Convert	Into	Multiply by	Conversely, Multiply by
meters	feet	3.28	30.48×10^{-2}
meters	inches	39.37	2.54×10^{-2}
meters	miles	6.212×10^{-4}	1609.35
meters	yards	1.094	0.9144
kilograms	pounds	2.205	0.4536
radians	degrees	57.27	1.746×10^{-2}
kelvin	Fahrenheit	1.8 K - 459.67	(°F + 459.67)/1.8
kelvin	Celsius	K - 273.1 = °C	°C + 273.1 = K
liters	gallons (U.S.)	0.2642	3.785
liters	pints (U.S. Fluid)	2.113	0.4732

III. ALGEBRA AND TRIGONOMETRY

1. Simplifying Algebraic Expressions

The following concepts are important while factoring or simplifying algebraic expressions.

The factors of an algebraic expression consist of two or more algebraic expressions which when multiplied together produce the given algebraic expression.

Some important formulae, useful for the factoring of algebraic expressions, are listed below.

$$a(c + d) = ac + ad$$

$$(a + b)(a - b) = a^2 - b^2$$

$$(a + b)(a + b) = (a + b)^2 = a^2 + 2ab + b^2$$

$$(a - b)(a - b) = (a - b)^2 = a^2 - 2ab + b^2$$

$$(x + a)(x + b) = x^2 + (a + b)x + ab$$

$$(ax + b)(cx + d) = acx^2 + (ad + bc)x + bd$$

$$(a + b)(c + d) = ac + bc + ad + bd$$

$$(a + b)(a + b)(a + b) = (a + b)^3 = a^3 + 3a^2b + 3ab^2 + b^3$$

$$(a - b)(a - b)(a - b) = (a - b)^3 = a^3 - 3a^2b + 3ab^2 - b^3$$

$$(a - b)(a^2 + ab + b^2) = a^3 - b^3$$

$$(a + b)(a^2 - ab + b^2) = a^3 + b^3$$

$$(a + b + c)^2 = a^2 + b^2 + c^2 + 2ab + 2ac + 2bc$$

$$(a - b)(a^2 + ab + b^2) = a^3 - b^3$$

$$(a - b)(a^3 + a^2b + ab^2 + b^3) = a^4 - b^4$$

$$(a - b)(a^4 + a^3b + a^2b^2 + ab^3 + b^4) = a^5 - b^5$$

$$(a - b)(a^5 + a^4b + a^3b^2 + a^2b^3 + ab^4 + b^5) = a^6 - b^6$$

$$(a - b)(a^{n-1} + a^{n-2}b + a^{n-3}b^2 + \ldots + ab^{n-2} + b^{n-1}) = a^n - b^n$$

where n is any positive integer $(1, 2, 3, 4, \ldots)$.

$$(a + b)(a^{n-1} - a^{n-2}b + a^{n-3}b^2 - \ldots - ab^{n-2} + b^{n-1}) = a^n + b^n$$

where n is any positive odd integer $(1, 3, 5, 7, \ldots)$.

The procedure for factoring an algebraic expression completely is as follows:

Step 1: First find the greatest common factor if there is any. Then examine each factor remaining for greatest common factors.

Step 2: Continue factoring the factors obtained in Step 1 until all factors other than monomial factors are prime.

EXAMPLE

Factoring $4 - 16x^2$,

$$4 - 16x^2 = 4(1 - 4x^2) = 4(1 + 2x)(1 - 2x)$$

PROBLEM

Express each of the following as a single term.

a) $3x^2 + 2x^2 - 4x^2$ b) $5axy^2 - 7axy^2 - 3xy^2$

Solution

a) Factor x^2 in the expression.

$$3x^2 + 2x^2 - 4x^2 = (3 + 2 - 4)x^2 = 1x^2 = x^2.$$

b) Factor xy^2 in the expression and then factor a.

$$5axy^2 - 7axy^2 - 3xy^2 = (5a - 7a - 3)xy^2$$
$$= [(5 - 7)a - 3]xy^2$$
$$= (-2a - 3)xy^2.$$

PROBLEM

Simplify $\dfrac{\frac{1}{x-1} - \frac{1}{x-2}}{\frac{1}{x-2} - \frac{1}{x-3}}$.

Solution

Simplify the expression in the numerator by using the addition rule:

$$\frac{a}{b} + \frac{c}{d} = \frac{ad + bc}{bd}$$

Notice bd is the Least Common Denominator, LCD. We obtain

$$\frac{x - 2 - (x - 1)}{(x - 1)(x - 2)} = \frac{-1}{(x - 1)(x - 2)}$$

in the numerator.

Repeat this procedure for the expression in the denominator:

$$\frac{x - 3 - (x - 2)}{(x - 2)(x - 3)} = \frac{-1}{(x - 2)(x - 3)}$$

We now have

$$\frac{\frac{-1}{(x-1)(x-2)}}{\frac{-1}{(x-2)(x-3)}},$$

which is simplified by inverting the fraction in the denominator and multiplying it by the numerator and cancelling like terms

$$\frac{-1}{(x - 1)(x - 2)} \cdot \frac{(x - 2)(x - 3)}{-1} = \frac{x - 3}{x - 1}.$$

2. Equations

An equation is defined as a statement of equality of two separate expressions.

Equations with the same solutions are said to be equivalent equations.

A)   Replacing an expression of an equation by an equivalent expression results in an equation equivalent to the original one. Given the equation below

$$3x + y + x + 2y = 15$$

We know that for the left side of this equation we can apply the commutative and distributive laws to get:

$$3x + y + x + 2y = 4x + 3y.$$

Since these are equivalent, we can replace the expression in the original equation with the simpler form to get:

$$4x + 3y = 15.$$

B)   The addition or subtraction of the same expression on both sides of an equation results in an equivalent equation to the original one: E.g., given the equation

$$y + 6 = 10,$$

we can add (- 6) to both sides

$$y + 6 + (- 6) = 10 + (- 6)$$

to get $y + 0 = 10 - 6 \Rightarrow y = 4$. So $y + 6 = 10$ is equivalent to $y = 4$.

C)   The multiplication or division on both sides of an equation by the same expression results in an equivalent equation to the original. E.g.,

$$3x = 6 \Rightarrow 3x/3 = 6/3 \Rightarrow x = 2.$$

$3x = 6$ is equivalent to $x = 2$.

D)   If both members of an equation are raised to the same power, then the resultant equation is equivalent to the original equation. Example:

$$a = x^2y, \quad (a)^2 = (x^2y)^2, \text{ and } a^2 = x^4y^2.$$

This applies for negative and fractional powers as well. E.g.,

$$x^2 = 3y^4.$$

If we raise both members to the -2 power we get

$$(x^2)^{-2} = (3y^4)^{-2}$$

$$\frac{1}{(x^2)^2} = \frac{1}{(3y^4)^2}$$

$$\frac{1}{x^4} = \frac{1}{9y^8}$$

If we raise both members to the $^1/_2$ power which is the same as taking the square root, we get:

$$(x^2)^{\frac{1}{2}} = (3y^4)^{\frac{1}{2}}$$
$$x = \sqrt{3}y^2$$

E)   The reciprocal of both members of an equation are equivalent to the original equation. Note: The reciprocal of zero is undefined.

$$\frac{2x+y}{z} = \frac{5}{2} \qquad \frac{z}{2x+y} = \frac{2}{5}$$

PROBLEM

Solve, justifying each step. $3x - 8 = 7x + 8$.

Solution

$$3x - 8 = 7x + 8$$

Adding 8 to both members, $3x - 8 + 8 = 7x + 8 + 8$

Additive inverse property, $3x + 0 = 7x + 16$

Additive identity property, $3x = 7x + 16$

Adding $(-7x)$ to both members, $3x - 7x = 7x + 16 - 7x$

Commuting, $-4x = 7x - 7x + 16$

Additive inverse property, $-4x = 0 + 16$

Additive identity property, $-4x = 16$

Dividing both sides by -4, $x = {}^{16}/_{-4}$

$$x = -4$$

Check: Replacing x by -4 in the original equation:

$$3x - 8 = 7x + 8$$
$$3(-4) - 8 = 7(-4) + 8$$
$$-12 - 8 = -28 + 8$$
$$-20 = -20$$

LINEAR EQUATIONS

A linear equation with one unknown is one that can be put into the form $ax + b = 0$, where a and b are constants, $a \neq 0$.

To solve a linear equation means to transform it in the form $x = {}^{-b}/_a$.

A)   If the equation has unknowns on both sides of the equality, it is convenient to put similar terms on the same sides. E.g.,

$$4x + 3 = 2x + 9$$
$$4x + 3 - 2x = 2x + 9 - 2x$$
$$(4x - 2x) + 3 = (2x - 2x) + 9$$

$$2x + 3 = 0 + 9$$
$$2x + 3 - 3 = 0 + 9 - 3$$
$$2x = 6$$
$$^{2x}/_2 = ^6/_2$$
$$x = 3.$$

B)   If the equation appears in fractional form, it is necessary to transform it, using cross-multiplication, and then repeating the same procedure as in A), we obtain:

$$\frac{3x+4}{3} \quad\diagdown\!\!\!\!\diagup\quad \frac{7x+2}{5}$$

By using cross-multiplication we would obtain:

$$3(7x + 2) = 5(3x + 4).$$

This is equivalent to:

$$21x + 6 = 15x + 20,$$

which can be solved as in A):

$$21x + 6 = 15x + 20$$
$$21x - 15x + 6 = 15x - 15x + 20$$
$$6x + 6 - 6 = 20 - 6$$
$$6x = 14$$
$$x = ^{14}/_6$$
$$x = ^7/_3$$

C)   If there are radicals in the equation, it is necessary to square both sides and then apply A)

$$\sqrt{3x+1} = 5$$
$$(\sqrt{3x+1})^2 = 5^2$$
$$3x + 1 = 25$$
$$3x + 1 - 1 = 25 - 1$$
$$3x = 24$$
$$x = ^{24}/_3$$
$$x = 8$$

PROBLEM

Solve the equation $2(x + 3) = (3x + 5) - (x - 5)$.

Solution

We transform the given equation to an equivalent equation where we can easily recognize the solution set.

$$2(x + 3) = 3x + 5 - (x - 5)$$

Distribute, $\qquad\qquad 2x + 6 = 3x + 5 - x + 5$

Combine terms, $\qquad\quad 2x + 6 = 2x + 10$

Subtract $2x$ from both sides, $\quad 6 = 10$

Since $6 = 10$ is not a true statement, there is no real number which will make the original equation true. The equation is inconsistent and the solution set is ϕ, the empty set.

PROBLEM

Solve the equation $2(^2/_3\, y + 5) + 2(y + 5) = 130$.

Solution

The procedure for solving this equation is as follows:

$^4/_3\, y + 10 + 2y + 10 = 130$, Distributive property

$^4/_3\, y + 2y + 20 = 130$, Combining like terms

$^4/_3\, y + 2y = 110$, Subtracting 20 from both sides

$^4/_3\, y + ^6/_3\, y = 110$, Converting $2y$ into a fraction with denominator 3

$^{10}/_3\, y = 110$, Combining like terms

$y = 110 \cdot ^3/_{10} = 33$, Dividing by $^{10}/_3$

Check: Replace y by 33 in the original equation,

$2(^2/_3(33) + 5) + 2(33 + 5) = 130$

$2(22 + 5) + 2(38) = 130$

$2(27) + 76 = 130$

$54 + 76 = 130$

$130 = 130$

Therefore the solution to the given equation is $y = 33$.

TWO LINEAR EQUATIONS

Equations of the form $ax + by = c$, where a, b, c are constants and $a, b \neq 0$ are called linear equations with two unknown variables.

There are several ways to solve systems of linear equations in two variables:

Method 1: Addition or subtraction — if necessary multiply the equations by numbers that will make the coefficients of one unknown in the resulting equations numerically equal. If the signs of equal coefficients are the same, subtract the equation, otherwise add.

The result is one equation with one unknown; we solve it and substitute the value into the other equations to find the unknown that we first eliminated.

Method 2: Substitution — find the value of one unknown in terms of the other, substitute this value in the other equation and solve.

Method 3: Graph — graph both equations. The point of intersection of the drawn lines is a simultaneous solution for the equations and its coordinates correspond to the answer that would be found analytically.

If the lines are parallel they have no simultaneous solution.

Dependent equations are equations that represent the same line, therefore every point on the line of a dependent equation represents a solution. Since there is an infinite number of points there is an infinite number of simultaneous solutions, for example

$$2x + y = 8$$

$$4x + 2y = 16$$

The equations above are dependent, they represent the same line, all points that satisfy either of the equations are solutions of the system.

A system of linear equations is consistent if there is only one solution for the system.

A system of linear equations is inconsistent if it does not have any solutions.

Example of a consistent system. Find the point of intersection of the graphs of the equations:

$$x + y = 3,$$

$$3x - 2y = 14$$

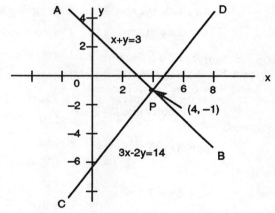

To solve these linear equations, solve for y in terms of x. The equations will be in the form $y = mx + b$, where m is the slope and b is the intercept on the y-axis.

$$
\begin{aligned}
x + y &= 3 \\
y &= 3 - x \qquad \text{subtract } x \text{ from both sides} \\
3x - 2y &= 14 \qquad \text{subtract } 3x \text{ from both sides} \\
-2y &= 14 - 3x \qquad \text{divide by } -2. \\
y &= -7 + {}^3/_2 x
\end{aligned}
$$

The graphs of the linear functions, $y = 3 - x$ and $y - 7 + {}^3/_2 x$ can be determined by plotting only two points. For example, for $y = 3 - x$, let $x = 0$, then $y = 3$. Let $x = 1$, then $y = 2$. The two points on this first line are $(0, 3)$ and $(1, 2)$. For $y = -7 + {}^3/_2 x$, let $x = 0$, then $y = -7$. Let $x = 1$, then $y = -5^1/_2$. The two points on this second line are $(0, -7)$ and $(1, -5^1/_2)$.

To find the point of intersection P of

$$x + y = 3 \quad \text{and} \quad 3x - 2y = 14,$$

solve them algebraically. Multiply the first equation by 2. Add these two equations to eliminate the variable y.

$$2x + 2y = 6$$
$$3x - 2y = 14$$
$$5x \quad\ = 20$$

Solve for x to obtain $x = 4$. Substitute this into $y = 3 - x$ to get $y = 3 - 4 = -1$. P is $(4, -1)$. AB is the graph of the first equation, and CD is the graph of the second equation. The point of intersection P of the two graphs is the only point on both lines. The coordinates of P satisfy both equations and represent the desired solution of the problem. From the graph, P seems to be the point $(4, -1)$. These coordinates satisfy both equations, and hence are the exact coordinates of the point of intersection of the two lines.

To show that $(4, -1)$ satisfies both equations, substitute this point into both equations.

$x + y = 3$	$3x - 2y = 14$
$4 + (-1) = 3$	$3(4) - 2(-1) = 14$
$4 - 1 = 3$	$12 + 2 = 14$
$3 = 3$	$14 = 14$

Example of an inconsistent system. Solve the equations $2x + 3y = 6$ and $4x + 6y = 7$ simultaneously.

We have 2 equations in 2 unknowns,

$$2x + 3y = 6 \qquad (1)$$

and

$$4x + 6y = 7 \qquad (2)$$

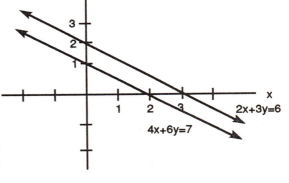

There are several methods to solve this problem. We have chosen to multiply each equation by a different number so that when the two equations are added, one of the variables drops out. Thus

multiplying equation (1) by 2:	$4x + 6y = 12$	(3)
multiplying equation (2) by -1:	$-4x - 6y = -7$	(4)
adding equations (3) and (4):	$0 = 5$	

We obtain a peculiar result!

Actually, what we have shown in this case is that if there were a simultaneous solution to the given equations, then 0 would equal 5. But the conclusion is impossible; therefore there can be no simultaneous solution to these two equations, hence no point satisfying both.

The straight lines which are the graphs of these equations must be parallel if they never intersect, but not identical, which can be seen from the graph of these equations (see the accompanying diagram).

Example of a dependent system. Solve the equations $2x + 3y = 6$ and $y = -\left(^{2x}/_3\right) + 2$ simultaneously.

We have 2 equations in 2 unknowns.

$$2x + 3y = 6 \tag{1}$$

and

$$y = -\left(^{2x}/_3\right) + 2 \tag{2}$$

There are several methods of solution for this problem. Since equation (2) already gives us an expression for y, we use the method of substitution. Substituting $-\left(^{2x}/_3\right) + 2$ for y in the first equation:

$$2x + 3(-^{2x}/_2 + 2) = 6$$

Distributing, $\qquad 2x - 2x + 6 = 6$

$$6 = 6$$

Apparently we have gotten nowhere! The result $6 = 6$ is true, but indicates no solution. Actually, our work shows that no matter what real number x is, if y is determined by the second equation, then the first equation will always be satisfied.

The reason for this peculiarity may be seen if we take a closer look at the equation $y = -\left(^{2x}/_3\right) + 2$. It is equivalent to $3y = -2x + 6$, or $2x + 3y = 6$.

In other words, the two equations are equivalent. Any pair of values of x and y which satisfies one satisfies the other.

It is hardly necessary to verify that in this case the graphs of the given equations are identical lines, and that there are an infinite number of simultaneous solutions of these equations.

A system of three linear equations in three unknowns is solved by eliminating one unknown from any two of the three equations and solving them. After finding two unknowns substitute them in any of the equations to find the third unknown.

PROBLEM

Solve the system

$$2x + 3y - 4z = -8 \tag{1}$$
$$x + y - 2z = -5 \tag{2}$$
$$7x - 2y + 5z = 4 \tag{3}$$

Solution

We cannot eliminate any variable from two pairs of equations by a single multiplication. However, both x and z may be eliminated from equations 1 and 2 by multiplying equation 2 by -2. Then

$$2x + 3y - 4z = -8 \tag{1}$$
$$-2x - 2y + 4z = 10 \tag{4}$$

By addition, we have $y = 2$. Although we may now eliminate either x or z from another pair of equations, we can more conveniently substitute $y = 2$ in equations 2 and 3 to get two equations in two variables. Thus, making the substitution $y = 2$ in equations 2 and 3, we have

$$x - 2z = -7 \tag{5}$$

$$7x + 5z = 8 \tag{6}$$

Multiply (5) by 5 and multiply (6) by 2. Then add the two new equations. Then $x = -1$. Substitute x in either (5) or (6) to find z.

The solution of the system is $x = -1$, $y = 2$, and $z = 3$. Check by substitution.

A system of equations, as shown below, that has all constant terms b_1, b_2, ..., b_n equal to zero is said to be a homogeneous system:

$$\begin{cases} a_{11}x_1 + a_{12}x_2 + \ldots + a_{1n}x_m = b_1 \\ a_{21}x_1 + a_{22}x_2 + \ldots + a_{2n}x_m = b_2 \\ \vdots \quad\quad \vdots \quad\quad\quad \vdots \quad\quad \vdots \\ a_{n1}x_1 + a_{n2}x_2 + \ldots + a_{nn}x_m = b_n. \end{cases}$$

A homogeneous system always has at least one solution which is called the trivial solution that is $x_1 = 0$, $x_2 = 0$, ..., $x_m = 0$.

For any given homogeneous system of equations, in which the number of variables is greater than or equal to the number of equations, there are non-trivial solutions.

Two systems of linear equations are said to be equivalent if and only if they have the same solution set.

PROBLEM

Solve for x and y.

$$x + 2y = 8 \tag{1}$$

$$3x + 4y = 20 \tag{2}$$

Solution

Solve equation (1) for x in terms of y:

$$x = 8 - 2y \tag{3}$$

Substitute $(8 - 2y)$ for x in (2):

$$3(8 - 2y) + 4y = 20 \tag{4}$$

Solve (4) for y as follows:

Distribute: $\quad 24 - 6y + 4y = 20$

Combine like terms and then subtract 24 from both sides:

$$24 - 2y = 20$$

$$24 - 24 - 2y = 20 - 24$$

$$-2y = -4$$

Divide both sides by - 2:

$$y = 2$$

Substitute 2 for y in equation (1):

$$x + 2(2) = 8$$
$$x = 4$$

Thus, our solution is $x = 4$, $y = 2$.

Check: Substitute $x = 4$, $y = 2$ in equations (1) and (2):

$$4 + 2(2) = 8$$
$$8 = 8$$
$$3(4) + 4(2) = 20$$
$$20 = 20$$

PROBLEM

Solve algebraically:

$$4x + 2y = -1 \tag{1}$$
$$5x - 3y = 7 \tag{2}$$

Solution

We arbitrarily choose to eliminate x first.

Multiply (1) by 5: $20x + 10y = -5$ $\qquad$ (3)

Multiply (2) by 4: $20x - 12y = 28$ $\qquad$ (4)

Subtract (3) - (4): $\qquad 22y = -33$ $\qquad$ (5)

Divide (5) by 22: $y = -\,^{33}/_{22} = -\,^{3}/_{2}$,

To find x, substitute $y = -\,^{3}/_{2}$ in either of the original equations. If we use Eq. (1), we obtain $4x + 2(-\,^{3}/_{2}) = -1$, $4x - 3 = -1$, $4x = 2$, $x = {}^{1}/_{2}$.

The solution $({}^{1}/_{2}, -\,^{3}/_{2})$ should be checked in both equations of the given system.

Replacing $({}^{1}/_{2}, -\,^{3}/_{2})$ in Eq. (1):

$$4x + 2y = -1$$
$$4({}^{1}/_{2}) + 2(-\,^{3}/_{2}) = -1$$
$${}^{4}/_{2} - 3 = -1$$
$$2 - 3 = -1$$
$$-1 = -1$$

Replacing $({}^{1}/_{2}, -\,^{3}/_{2})$ in Eq. (2):

$$5x - 3y = 7$$
$$5({}^{1}/_{2}) - 3(-\,^{3}/_{2}) = 7$$
$${}^{5}/_{2} + {}^{9}/_{2} = 7$$

$$^{14}/_2 = 7$$

$$7 = 7$$

(Instead of eliminating x from the two given equations, we could have eliminated y by multiplying Eq. (1) by 3, multiplying Eq. (2) by 2, and then adding the two derived equations.)

QUADRATIC EQUATIONS

A second degree equation in x of the type $ax^2 + bx + c = 0$, $a \neq 0$, a, b and c are real numbers, is called a quadratic equation.

To solve a quadratic equation is to find values of x which satisfiy $ax^2 + bx + c = 0$. These values of x are called solutions, or roots, of the equation.

A quadratic equation has a maximum of 2 roots. Methods of solving quadratic equations:

A)   Direct solution:

Given $x^2 - 9 = 0$.

We can solve directly by isolating the variable x:

$$x^2 = 9$$

$$x = \pm 3.$$

B)   Factoring:

Given a quadratic equation $ax^2 + bx + c = 0$, a, b, $c \neq 0$, to factor means to express it as the product $a(x - r_1)(x - r_2) = 0$, where r_1 and r_2 are the two roots.

Some helpful hints to remember are:

a) $r_1 + r_2 = {}^{-b}/_a$.

b) $r_1 r_2 = {}^c/_a$.

Given $x^2 - 5x + 4 = 0$.

Since $r_1 + r_2 = {}^{-b}/_a = {}^{-(-5)}/_1 = 5$, so the possible solutions are (3, 2), (4, 1) and (5, 0). Also $r_1 r_2 = {}^c/_a = {}^4/_1 = 4$; this equation is satisfied only by the second pair, so $r_1 = 4$, $r_2 = 1$ and the factored form is $(x - 4)(x - 1) = 0$.

If the coefficient of x^2 is not 1, it is necessary to divide the equation by this coefficient and then factor.

Given $2x^2 - 12x + 16 = 0$

Dividing by 2, we obtain:

$$x^2 - 6x + 8 = 0$$

Since $r_1 + r_2 = {}^{-b}/_a = 6$, the possible solutions are (6, 0), (5, 1), (4, 2), (3, 3). Also $r_1 r_2 = 8$, so the only possible answer is (4, 2) and the expression $x^2 - 6x + 8 = 0$ can be factored as $(x - 4)(x - 2)$.

C)   Completing the Squares:

If it is difficult to factor the quadratic equation using the previous method, we can complete the squares.

Given $x^2 - 12x + 8 = 0$.

We know that the two roots added up should be 12 because $r_1 + r_2 = -b/a = -(-12)/1 = 12$. The possible roots are $(12, 0)$, $(11, 1)$, $(10, 2)$, $(9, 3)$, $(8,4)$, $(7,5)$, $(6, 6)$.

But none of these satisfy $r_1 r_2 = 8$, so we cannot use (B).

To complete the square, it is necessary to isolate the constant term,

$$x^2 - 12x = -8.$$

Then take $1/2$ coefficient of x, square it and add to both sides

$$x^2 - 12x + \left(\frac{-12}{2}\right)^2 = -8 + \left(\frac{-12}{2}\right)^2$$

$$x^2 - 12x + 36 = -8 + 36 = 28.$$

Now we can use the previous method to factor the left side: $r_1 + r_2 = 12$, $r_1 r_2 = 36$ is satisfied by the pair $(6, 6)$, so we have:

$$(x - 6)^2 = 28.$$

Now extract the root of both sides and solve for x.

$$(x - 6) = \pm \sqrt{28} = \pm 2\sqrt{7}$$
$$x = \pm 2\sqrt{7} + 6$$

So the roots are:

$$x = 2\sqrt{7} + 6, \quad x = -2\sqrt{7} + 6.$$

PROBLEM

Solve the equation $x^2 + 8x + 15 = 0$.

Solution

Since $(x + a)(x + b) = x^2 + bx + ax + ab = x^2 + (a + b)x + ab$, we may factor the given equation, $0 = x^2 + 8x + 15$, replacing $a + b$ by 8 and ab by 15. Thus,

$$a + b = 8, \quad \text{and} \quad ab = 15.$$

We want the two numbers a and b whose sum is 8 and whose product is 15. We check all pairs of numbers whose product is 15:

(a) $1 \cdot 15 = 15$; thus $a = 1$, $b = 15$ and $ab = 15$.

   $1 + 15 = 16$, therefore we reject these values because $a + b \neq 8$.

(b) $3 \cdot 5 = 15$, thus $a = 3$, $b = 5$, and $ab = 15$.

   $3 + 5 = 8$. Therefore $a + b = 8$, and we accept these values.

Hence $x^2 + 8x + 15 = 0$ is equivalent to

$$0 = x^2 + (3 + 5)x + 3 \cdot 5 = (x + 3)(x + 5)$$

Hence, $x + 5 = 0$ or $x + 3 = 0$

since the product of these two numbers is zero, one of the numbers must be zero. Hence, $x = -5$, or $x = -3$, and the solution set is $x = \{-5, -3\}$.

The student should note that $x = -5$ or $x = -3$. We are certainly not making the statement, that $x = -5$, and $x = -3$. Also, the student should check that both these numbers do actually satisfy the given equations and hence are solutions.

Check: Replacing x by (-5) in the original equation:

$$x^2 + 8x + 15 = 0$$
$$(-5)^2 + 8(-5) + 15 = 0$$
$$25 - 40 + 15 = 0$$
$$-15 + 15 = 0$$
$$0 = 0$$

Replacing x by (-3) in the original equation:

$$x^2 + 8x + 15 = 0$$
$$(-3)^2 + 8(-3) + 15 = 0$$
$$9 - 24 + 15 = 0$$
$$-15 + 15 = 0$$
$$0 = 0.$$

PROBLEM

Solve the following equations by factoring.

a) $2x^2 + 3x = 0$ b) $y^2 - 2y - 3 = y - 3$

c) $z^2 - 2z - 3 = 0$ d) $2m^2 - 11m - 6 = 0$

Solution

a) $2x^2 + 3x = 0$. Factoring out the common factor of x from the left side of the given equation,

$$x(2x + 3) = 0.$$

Whenever a product $ab = 0$, where a and b are any two numbers, either $a = 0$ or $b = 0$. Then, either

$$x = 0 \quad \text{or} \quad 2x + 3 = 0$$
$$2x = -3$$
$$x = -3/2$$

Hence, the solution set to the original equation $2x^2 + 3x = 0$ is: $\{-3/2, 0\}$.

b) $y^2 - 2y - 3 = y - 3$. Subtract $(y - 3)$ from both sides of the given equation:

$$y^2 - 2y - 3 - (y - 3) = y - 3 - (y - 3)$$
$$y^2 - 2y - 3 - y + 3 = y - 3 - y + 3$$
$$y^2 - 3y = 0.$$

Factor out a common factor of y from the left side of this equation:

$$y(y - 3) = 0.$$

Thus, $y = 0$ or $y - 3 = 0, y = 3$.

Therefore, the solution set to the original equation $y^2 - 2y - 3 = y - 3$ is: $\{0,3\}$.

c) $z^2 - 2z - 3 = 0$.

Factor the original equation into a product of two polynomials:

$$z^2 - 2z - 3 = (z - 3)(z + 1) = 0$$

Hence, $(z - 3)(z + 1) = 0$; and $z - 3 = 0$ or $z + 1 = 0$

$$z = 3 \qquad z = -1$$

Therefore, the solution set to the original equation $z^2 - 2z - 3 = 0$ is: $\{-1, 3\}$.

d) $2m^2 - 11m - 6 = 0$.

Factor the original equation into a product of two polynomials:

$$2m^2 - 11m - 6 = (2m + 1)(m - 6) = 0$$

Thus, $2m + 1 = 0$ or $m - 6 = 0$

$$2m = -1 \qquad\qquad m = 6$$

$$m = {}^{-1}/_2$$

Therefore, the solution set to the original equation $2m^2 - 11m - 6 = 0$ is: $\{-^1/_2, 6\}$.

3. Functions

Constant: A constant is a symbol which represents one particular number during a discussion. For example, numbers 5, -3, π and $2^6/_7$ are constants.

Variable: A variable is a symbol to which may be assigned any of several numbers during the course of a discussion.

Function: If two variables, x and y, are so related that to each permissible value of x, there corresponds one or more values of a second variable, then y is called a function of x.

In the formulation, x is called the **independent** variable, while y is called the **dependent** variable. In order to express the fact that y is a function of x, the symbol used is $y = f(x)$.

PROBLEM

If $f(x) = x^2 + 3x - 7$, find $f(2)$.

Solution

$f(2)$ indicates that 2 is to be substituted for x.

$$f(2) = 2^2 + 3.2 - 7 = 4 + 6 - 7 = 3$$

PROBLEM

If $f(x) = x^3 + 2x - 6$

a) $f(-1)$ b) $f(0)$ c) $f(^1/_a)$

Solution

$$f(x) = x^3 + 2x - 6$$

a) $f(-1)$ means that $x = -1$ is substituted into $f(x)$.

$$\begin{aligned} f(-1) &= (-1)^3 + 2(-1) - 6 \\ &= -1 - 2 - 6 \\ &= -9 \end{aligned}$$

b) $f(0)$ substitute in $x = 0$

$$\begin{aligned} f(0) &= (0)^3 + 2(0) - 6 \\ &= 0 + 0 - 6 \\ &= -6 \end{aligned}$$

c) $$f\left(\frac{1}{a}\right) = \left(\frac{1}{a}\right)^3 + 2\left(\frac{1}{a}\right) - 6$$

$$= \frac{1}{a^3} + \frac{2}{a} - 6$$

$$= \frac{1}{a^3} + \frac{2a^2}{a^3} - \frac{6a^3}{a^3}$$

$$= \frac{1 + 2a^2 - 6a^3}{a^3} \qquad \text{get common denominator}$$

PROBLEM

If $f(x) = x^2 - 3x + 9$

a) $f(y + 1)$ \qquad\qquad\qquad b) $f(a + b)$

Solution

$$f(x) = x^2 - 3x + 9$$

a) $f(y + 1)$ means that $x = y + 1$ is substituted into $f(x)$

$$\begin{aligned} f(y + 1) &= (y + 1)^2 - 3(y + 1) + 9 \\ &= y^2 + 2y + 1 - 3y - 3 + 9 \qquad \text{expand terms} \\ &= y^2 - y + 7 \qquad\qquad\qquad \text{add like terms} \end{aligned}$$

b) $f(a + b)$ substitute in $x = a + b$

$$\begin{aligned} f(a + b) &= (a + b)^2 - 3(a + b) + 9 \\ &= a^2 ab + b^2 - 3a - 3b + 9 \qquad \text{expand terms} \end{aligned}$$

4. Graphs

The graph shown is called the Cartesian coordinate plane. The graph consists of a pair of perpendicular lines called coordinate axes. The vertical axis is the y-axis and the horizontal axis is the x-axis. The point of intersection of these two axes is called the origin; it is the zero point of both axes. Furthermore, points to the right of the

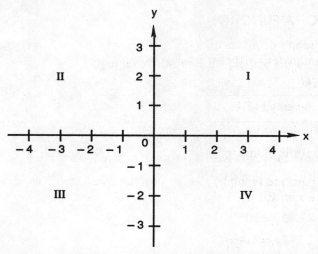

origin on the x-axis and above the origin on the y-axis represent positive real numbers. Points to the left of the origin on the x-axis or below the origin on the y-axis represent negative real numbers.

The four regions cut off by the coordinate axes are, in counterclockwise direction from the top right, called the first, second, third and fourth quadrant. The first quadrant contains all points with two positive coordinates.

In the graph shown, two points are identified by the ordered pair, (x, y) of numbers. The x-coordinate is the first number and the y-coordinate is the second number. In this case, point A has the coordinates (4, 2) and the coordinates of point B are (-3, -5).

The number indicating how many units a point is to the right or to the left of y-axis is called the abscissa. In the case of point A, the abscissa is 4, while for point B the abscissa is -3.

The number indicating how many units a point is above or below the x-axis is called the ordinate. The ordinate for point A is 2, while for point B, the ordinate is -5.

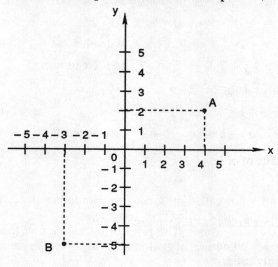

GRAPH OF A FUNCTION

The graph of a function $y = f(x)$ consists of all points and only those points whose coordinates satisfy the relationship $y = f(x)$.

PROBLEM

Plot the graph of $4x - 2y = 10$

Solution

To make the graph we need a set of ordered pairs (x, y).

The pairs are found by first solving the equation for y and substituting in appropriate values for x.

$$4x - 2y = 10$$
$$2y = 4x - 10$$
$$y = 2x - 5$$

Then form a table by substituting values for x

x	-2	-1	0	1	2	3
y	-9	-7	-5	-3	-1	1

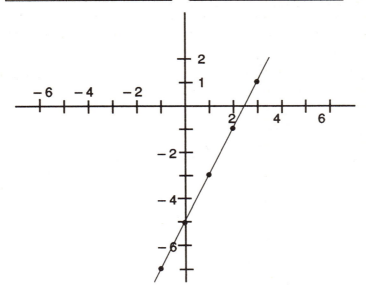

Plot the points of ordered pairs

5. Scales

There are three kinds of scales usually used for plotting functions. They are

1. **Arithmetic:** When the abscissa is x and the ordinate is y. This kind of scale is the most commonly used.

2. **Semilog:** When either the abscissa is log x and the ordinate is y, or when the abscissa is x and the ordinate is log y. This type of scale is used when either x is larger than y, or vice versa.

3. **Log-Log:** When the abscissa is log x and the ordinate is log y. This type of scale is used when both x and y are large numbers.

6. Distance

For any two points A and B with coordinates (X_A, Y_A) and (X_B, Y_B), respectively, the distance between A and B is represented by:

$$AB = \sqrt{(X_A - X_B)^2 + (Y_A - Y_B)^2}$$

This is commonly known as the distance formula or the Pythagorean Theorem.

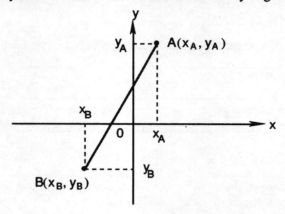

PROBLEM

Find the distance between the point $A(1, 3)$ and $B(5, 3)$.

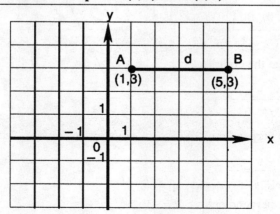

Solution

In this case, where the ordinate of both points is the same, the distance between the two points is given by the absolute value of the difference between the two abscissas. In fact, this case reduces to merely counting boxes as the figure shows.

Let, x_1 = abscissa of A y_1 = ordinate of A

         x_2 = abscissa of B y_1 = ordinate of B

         d = the distance.

Therefore, $d = |\, x_1 - x_2\, |$. By substitution, $d = |\, 1 - 5\, | = |\, -4\, | = 4$. This answer can also be obtained by applying the general formula for distance between any two points

$$d = \sqrt{(x_1 - x_2)^2 + (y_1 - y_2)^2}$$

By substitution,

$$d = \sqrt{(1-5)^2 + (3-3)^2} = \sqrt{(-4)^2 + (0)^2} = \sqrt{16} = 4.$$

The distance is 4.

7. Slope of a Straight Line

The slope of a straight line containing two points (x_1, y_1) and (x_2, y_2) is given by

$$\text{slope} = m = \frac{y_2 - y_1}{x_2 - x_1}.$$

Horizontal lines have a slope of zero and the slope of vertical lines is undefined. Parallel lines have equal slopes and perpendicular lines have slopes which are negative reciprocals.

PROBLEM

> Find the slope of the straight line which contains points A and B. Also determine the slope of the perpendicular line.
>
> a) $A\,(-1, 2),\, B\,(-2, -1)$
>
> b) $A\,(1, 0),\, B\,(0, 1)$
>
> c) $A\,(-1, 0),\, B\,(1, 0)$

Solution

a)   We can treat the coordinates of A as $A\,(x_1, y_1)$ and of B as $B\,(x_2, y_2)$. Then

$$m = \frac{y_2 - y_1}{x_2 - x_1} = \frac{-1-2}{-2-(-1)} = \frac{-3}{-2+1} = \frac{-3}{-1} = 3.$$

The slope of the perpendicular line is the negative reciprocal of m which is $-1/_3$.

b) $m = \dfrac{1-0}{0-1} = \dfrac{1}{-1} = -1$

The slope of the perpendicular line $= -1/_m = 1$

c) $m = \dfrac{0-0}{1-(-1)} = \dfrac{0}{1+1} = \dfrac{0}{2} = 0$

Because m is 0, this line is a horizontal line, and therefore its perpendicular line is a vertical line whose slope is undefined.

8. Trigonometric Ratios

Given a right triangle $\triangle ABC$ as shown in the following figure

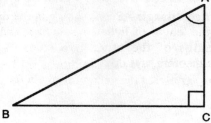

Definition 1:

$$\sin A = \frac{BC}{AB} = \frac{\text{measure of side opposite } \angle A}{\text{measure of hypotenuse}}$$

Definition 2:

$$\cos A = \frac{AC}{AB} = \frac{\text{measure of side adjacent } \angle A}{\text{measure of hypotenuse}}$$

Definition 3:

$$\tan A = \frac{BC}{AC} = \frac{\text{measure of side opposite } \angle A}{\text{measure of side adjacent to } \angle A}$$

Definition 4:

$$\cot A = \frac{AC}{BC} = \frac{\text{measure of side adjacent to } \angle A}{\text{measure of side opposite } \angle A}$$

$$\sec A = \frac{AB}{AC} = \frac{\text{measure of hypotenuse}}{\text{measure of side adjacent to } \angle A}$$

$$\csc A = \frac{AB}{BC} = \frac{\text{measure of hypotenuse}}{\text{measure of side opposite } \angle A}$$

The following table gives the values of sine, cosine, tangent and cotangent for some special angles.

TABLE (Value of Common Trigonometric Functions)

α	Sin α	Cos α	Tan α	Cot α
$0°$	0	1	0	∞
$\frac{\pi^R}{6} = 30°$	$\frac{1}{2}$	$\frac{\sqrt{3}}{2}$	$\frac{1}{\sqrt{3}}$	$\sqrt{3}$
$\frac{\pi^R}{4} = 45°$	$\frac{1}{\sqrt{2}}$	$\frac{1}{\sqrt{2}}$	1	1
$\frac{\pi^R}{3} = 60°$	$\frac{\sqrt{3}}{2}$	$\frac{1}{2}$	$\sqrt{3}$	$\frac{1}{\sqrt{3}}$
$\frac{\pi^R}{2} = 90°$	1	0	∞	0

PYTHAGOREAN THEOREM

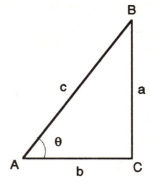

In the right triangle ABC as shown in the diagram, C is the length of hypotenuse and a and b are the lengths of the other two sides. The Pythagorean theorem says that

$$c^2 = a^2 + b^2$$

PROBLEM

For the right triangle shown above $\sin \theta = {}^4/_5$. Find

a) $\cos \theta$ b) $\tan \theta$.

Solution

By definition,

$$\sin \theta = {}^a/_c = {}^4/_5.$$

Therefore we can take $a = 4$ and $c = 5$. Applying the Pythagorean theorem,

$$b^2 = c^2 - a^2 = 5^2 - 4^2 = 25 - 16 = 9$$

or $b = \sqrt{9} = 3$.

a)   Therefore, $\cos \theta = {}^b/_c = {}^3/_5$.

b) $\tan \theta = {}^a/_b = {}^4/_3$.

We can find the relationships between the sides of a right triangle by using the table for the common trigonometric functions. For example

if $\theta = 30$, then

$$\sin \theta = {}^a/_c = {}^1/_2$$

which implies that $2a = c$. So for a right triangle with $\theta = 30$, the length of the hypotenuse is twice the length of a. Similarly if $\theta = 45°$, then

$$\tan 45 = {}^a/_b = 1$$

which implies $a = b$. If $\theta = 60°$, then

$$\cos \theta = {}^b/_c = {}^1/_2,$$

which implies that $2b = c$.

9. Inverse Trigonometric Functions

If we know the value of some trigonometric functions as defined above, then we can find the corresponding angles by taking the inverse trigonometric function. A unique value is assigned to each inverse trigonometric function in each quadrant. Usually, when the trigonometric function of some angle A is given, and nothing more is specified, it is assumed that angle A is in the first quadrant. In other words it is assumed that angle A is between $0°$ and $90°$. However, in general there are an infinite number of angles corresponding to the same trigonometric values.

Here are the trigonometric functions and their inverses:

If $y = \sin x$,   then $x = \sin^{-1} y = \text{Arcsin } y$

       $y = \cos x$, $x = \cos^{-1} y = \text{Arccos } y$

       $y = \tan x$, $x = \tan^{-1} y = \text{Arctan } y$.

The others are written the same way.

PROBLEM

> For the triangle ABC as shown in the diagram find all the remaining sides and the angles.

Solution

We know $b = 2\sqrt{3}$ and $c = 4$. Applying the Pythagorean theorem,

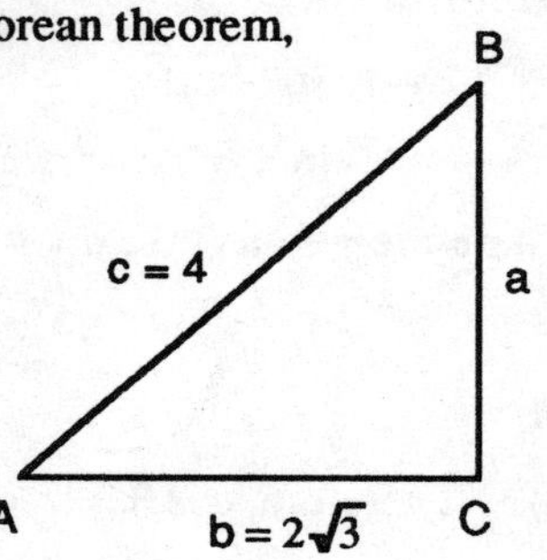

$$a^2 = c^2 - b^2$$

$$= 4^2 - (2\sqrt{3})^2 = 16 - 12 = 4$$

or $a = \sqrt{4} = 2$

To find angle A

$$\sin A = {}^a/_c = {}^2/_4 = {}^1/_2$$

or $A = \sin^{-1}({}^1/_2)$

Looking in the table for the angle whose sin is ${}^1/_2$, we find $A = 30°$.

Since the sum of all the angles in a triangle are 180, and we know $A = 30°$, and $C = 90°$, so $B = 60°$.

IV. VECTORS AND SCALARS

A vector is a quantity that has both magnitude and direction, for example, displacement, velocity, force, acceleration, momentum, electric field strength, magnetic field strength, etc.

A scalar is a quantity that has magnitude but no direction, for example, mass, length, time, density, energy, temperature, etc.

1. Addition and Subtraction of Vectors-Geometric Methods

Triangle Method (Head-To-Tail Method)

The following two steps describe the triangle method of vector addition.

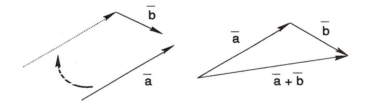

(i) Attach the head of $\bar{a}$ to the tail of $\bar{b}$.

(ii) By connecting the head of $\bar{a}$ to the tail of $\bar{b}$, the vector $\bar{a} + \bar{b}$ is defined.

Triangle Method of Adding Vectors

Parallelogram Method (Tail-To-Tail Method)

The following two steps describe the parallelogram method of vector addition.

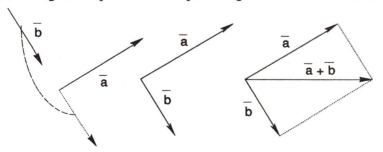

(i) Join the tails of the two vectors.

(ii) Construct a parallelogram having $\bar{a}$ and $\bar{b}$ as two of its sides. The long diagonal of the parallelogram represents the vector $\bar{a} + \bar{b}$.

The Parallelogram Method of Adding Vectors

SUBTRACTION OF VECTORS

The subtraction of a vector is defined as the addition of the corresponding negative vector. Therefore, the vector **P** - **F** is obtained by adding the vector (-**F**) to the vector **P**, i.e., **P** + (-**F**).

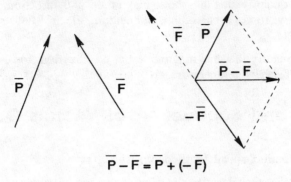

$$\overline{P} - \overline{F} = \overline{P} + (-\overline{F})$$

The Subtraction of a Vector

MULTIPLICATION OF A VECTOR BY A SCALAR

The product of a vector **a** and a scalar k, written as k**a**, is a new vector whose magnitude is k times the magnitude of **a**; if k is positive, the new vector has the same direction as **a**; if k is negative, the new vector has a direction opposite that of **a**.

The following rules also hold

$$k\,(\mathbf{a} + \mathbf{b}) = k\mathbf{a} + k\mathbf{b}$$

$$k\,(a - \mathbf{b}) = k\mathbf{a} - k\mathbf{b}$$

PROBLEM

A bicyclist is moving northward at 30 mi/hr and a wind of 40 mi/hr is blowing directly from the east. What is the apparent magnitude and direction of the wind experienced by the bicyclist?

Solution

Construct the two vectors representing the motion of the bicyclist and the wind as follows:

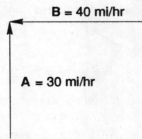

The effective magnitude and direction of the wind is the vector **B** - **A**. Applying the triangle rule for vector subtraction, we have to add **B** and - **A**. The following diagram shows the resultant vector.

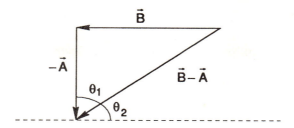

Applying the Pythagorean theorem, we can find the magnitude of **B - A**, which is

$$|B - A|^2 = |B|^2 + |-A|^2$$
$$= 40^2 + 30^2 = 2500$$

or $\qquad |B - A| = 50$

To find the direction, apply the trigonometric ratios:

$$\sin \theta_1 = \frac{\text{magnitude of } B}{\text{magnitude of } B \text{ - } A} = \frac{40}{50} = \frac{4}{5}$$

$$\theta_1 = \sin^{-1} {}^4\!/_5 = 53°$$
$$\theta_2 = 90° - 53° = 37°$$

2. The Components of a Vector

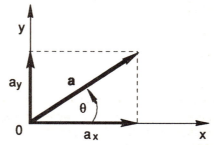

a_x and a_y are the components of a vector **a**. The angle θ is measured counterclockwise from the positive x-axis. The components are formed when we draw perpendicular lines to the chosen axes.

The Formation of Vector Components on the Positive *X-Y* Axis

A) The components of a vector are given by

$$A_x = A \cos \theta$$
$$A_y = A \sin \theta$$

A component is equal to the product of the magnitude of vector A and cosine of the angle between the positive axis and the vector.

B) The magnitude can be expressed in terms of the components.

$$A = \sqrt{A_x^2 + A_y^2}$$

For the angle θ,

$$\text{Tan } \theta = \frac{A_y}{A_x}$$

C) A vector **F** can be written in terms of its components F_x and F_y

$$\mathbf{F} = \mathbf{i}F_x + \mathbf{j}F_y$$

where **i** and **j** represent perpendicular unit vectors (magnitude = 1) along the x- and y-axis.

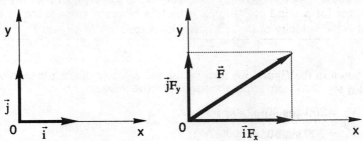

(a) The unit vectors **i** and **j** of the two-dimensional rectangular coordinate system.

(b) The components F_x and F_y.

Vector Components and the Unit Vector

A Unit Vector in the direction of a vector **a** is given by

$$\mathbf{u} = \frac{\mathbf{a}}{|\mathbf{a}|} = \frac{\mathbf{a}}{a} = \left(\frac{a_x}{a} \mathbf{i} + \frac{a_y}{a} \mathbf{j} \right)$$

3. Adding Vectors Analytically

Analytical addition involves adding the components of the individual vectors to produce the sum, expressed in terms of its components.

To find $\mathbf{a} + \mathbf{b} = \mathbf{c}$ analytically:

i) Resolve **a** in terms of its components:

$$\mathbf{a} = \mathbf{i}a_x + \mathbf{j}a_y$$

ii) Resolve **b** in terms of its components:

$$\mathbf{b} = \mathbf{i}b_x + \mathbf{j}b_y$$

iii) The components of **c** equal the sum of the corresponding components of **a** and **b**:

$$\mathbf{c} = \mathbf{i}(a_x + b_x) + \mathbf{j}(a_y + b_y)$$

and

$$\mathbf{c} = \mathbf{i}c_x + \mathbf{j}c_y$$

and the magnitude

$$|c| = \sqrt{c_x^2 + c_y^2}$$

with θ given by

$$\text{Tan } \theta = \frac{c_y}{c_x}.$$

PROBLEM

> An airplane would be flying in a direction 30° northeast at 200 mi/hr if it were not for a wind of 50 mi/hr which is blowing from south to north. What is the velocity of the airplane with respect to the ground?

Solution

As shown in the figure, we resolve the air velocity of the plane into its components V_x and V_y.

$$V_x = 200 \cos 30° = 173 \text{ mi/hr}$$
$$V_y = 200 \sin 30° = 100 \text{ mi/hr}$$

We then combine the y components to obtain the total velocity in the y-direction which is

$$100 \text{ mi/hr} + 50 \text{ mi/hr} = 150 \text{ mi/hr}.$$

The only velocity component in the x-direction, V_x is 173 mi/hr. Hence the magnitude of the resultant velocity is

$$V = \sqrt{(150)^2 + (173)^2} = 230 \text{ mi / hr.}$$

The resultant velocity is in a direction which makes an angle θ with the positive x-direction, where

$$\tan \theta = \frac{150}{173} \quad \text{or} \quad \theta = \tan^{-1} \frac{150}{173} = 41°$$

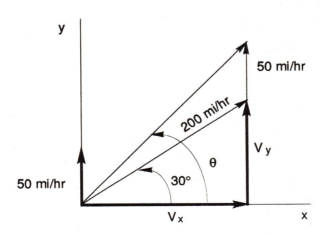

V. PROBABILITY AND STATISTICS

1. Probability

Let e denote an event which can happen in k ways out of a total of n ways. All n ways are equally likely. The probability of occurrence of the event e is defined as

$$p = pr\{e\} = \frac{k}{n}$$

The probability of occurrence of e is called its success. The probability of failure (non-occurrence) of the event is denoted by q.

$$q = pr\{\text{not } e\} = \frac{n-k}{n} = 1 - \frac{k}{n} = 1 - p$$

Hence, $p + q = 1$. The event "not e" is denoted by $\tilde{e}$ or $\sim e$.

EXAMPLE

A toss of a coin will produce one of two possible outcomes (heads, tails). Let e be the event that tails will turn up in a single toss of a coin. Then

$$p = \frac{1}{1+1} = \frac{1}{2}.$$

EXAMPLE

We define the event e to be number 5 or 6 turning up a single toss of a die. There are six equally likely outcomes of a single toss of a die

$$\{1, 2, 3, 4, 5, 6\}$$

Thus, $n = 6$. The event e can occur in two ways

$$p = pr\{e\} = \frac{2}{6} = \frac{1}{3}$$

Probability of failure of e is

$$q = pr\{\sim e\} = 1 - \frac{1}{3} = \frac{2}{3}.$$

For any event e

$$0 \le pr\{e\} \le 1$$

If the event cannot occur, its probability is 0. If the event must occur, its probability is 1.

Next we define the odds. Let p be the probability that an event will occur. The odds in favor of its occurrence are $p : q$ and the odds against it are $q : p$.

EXAMPLE

We determine the probability that at least one tail appears in two tosses of a coin. Let h denote heads and t tails. The possible outcomes of two tosses are

$$(h, h), (h, t) (t, h), (t , t)$$

Three cases are favorable. Thus

$$p = \frac{3}{4}$$

EXAMPLE

The event e is that the sum 8 appears in a single toss of a pair of dice. There are $6 \cdot 6 = 36$ outcomes

$$(1, 1), (2, 1), (3, 1), \ldots, (6, 6).$$

The sum 8 appears in five cases

$$(2, 6), (6, 2), (3, 5), (5, 3), (4, 4)$$

Then

$$p\{e\} = \frac{5}{36}$$

The concept of probability is based on the concept of random experiment. A random experiment is an experiment with more than one possible outcome, conducted such that it is not known in advance which outcome will occur. The set of possible outcomes is denoted by a capital letter, say, X. Usually, each outcome is either a number (a toss of a die) or something to which a number can be assigned (head = 1, tail = 0 for a toss of a coin).

2. Mean, Median, Mode

MEAN

The mean is the arithmetic average. The sum of the variables divided by the number of variables is the mean. For example:

$$\frac{4+3+8}{3} = 5$$

PROBLEM

Find the mean salary for four company employees who make $5/hr., $8/hr., $12/hr., and $15/hr.

Solution

The mean salary is the average.

$$\frac{\$5 + \$8 + \$12 + \$15}{4} = \frac{\$40}{4} = \$10 / \text{hr.}$$

PROBLEM

> Find the mean length of five fish with lengths of 7.5 in., 7.75 in., 8.5 in., 8.5 in., 8.25 in.

Solution

The mean length is the average length.

$$\frac{7.5+7.75+8.5+8.5+8.25}{5} = \frac{40.5}{5} = 8.1 \text{ in.}$$

MEDIAN

The median is the middle value of a set of an odd number of values. There are an equal amount of values larger and smaller than the median. When the set is an even number of values, the average of the two middle values is the median. For example:

The median of (2, 3, 5, 8, 9) is 5.

The median of (2, 3, 5, 9, 10, 11) is $\frac{5+9}{2} = 7$.

MODE

The mode is the most frequently occurring value in the set of values. For example the mode of 4, 5, 8, 3, 8, 2 would be 8.

PROBLEM

> For this series of observations find the mean, median, and mode.
>
> 500, 600, 800, 800, 900, 900, 900, 900, 900, 1000, 1100

Solution

The mean is the value obtained by adding all the measurements and dividing by the number of measurements.

$$\frac{500+600+800+800+900+900+900+900+900+1000+1100}{11}$$

$$= \frac{9300}{11} = 845.45.$$

The median is the observation in the middle We have 11, so here it is the sixth, 900.

The mode is the observation that appears most frequently. That is also 900, which has 5 appearances.

All three of these numbers are measures of central tendency. They describe the "middle" or "center" of the data.

PROBLEM

Nine rats run through a maze. The time each rat took to traverse the maze is recorded and these times are listed below.

1 min., 2.5 min., 3 min., 1.5 min., 2 min., 1.25 min., 1 min., 9 min., 30 min.

Which of the three measures of central tendency would be the most appropriate in this case?

Solution

We will calculate the three measures of central tendency and then compare them to determine which would be the most appropriate in describing these data.

The mean is the sum of observations divided by the number of observations. In this case,

$$\frac{1+2.5+3+1.5+2+1.25+1+.9+30}{9} = \frac{43.15}{9} = 4.79.$$

The median is the "middle number" in any array of the observations from the lowest to highest.

0.9, 1.0, 1.0, 1.25, 1.5, 2.0, 2.5, 3.0, 30.0

The median is the fifth observation in this array of 1.5. There are four observations larger than 1.5 and four observations smaller than 1.5.

The mode is the most frequently occurring observation in the sample. In this data set the mode is 1.0.

mean = 4.79

median = 1.5

mode = 1.0

The mean is not appropriate here. Only one rat took more than 4.79 minutes to run the maze and this rat took 30 minutes. We see that the mean has been distorted by this one large observation.

The median or mode seem to best describe this data set better and would be more appropriate to use.

3. Standard Deviation

The standard deviation is a measure of the dispersion of data with respect to its mean or average value. By definition the standard deviation of a set $x_1, x_2, \ldots, x_n$ of n numbers is defined by

$$s = \sqrt{\frac{\sum_{i=1}^{n}(x_i - \bar{x})^2}{n}}$$

where $\bar{x}$ is the mean of $x_1, x_2, \ldots, x_n$.

If some number x_i in the data set occurs f_i times, then f_i is called the frequency of the number x_i. The above formula for the standard deviation holds when the frequency of each number is 1. When the frequency of some or all of the numbers is greater than 1, then the data is called grouped data. For grouped data we use the modified formula for the standard deviation. Let the frequencies of the numbers x_1, x_2, ..., x_n be $f_1, f_2, ..., f_n$ respectively, then

$$s = \sqrt{\frac{\sum_{i=1}^{n} f_i (x_i - \bar{x})^2}{\sum_{i=1}^{n} f_i}}$$

The variance of a set of numbers is the square of the standard deviation.

Simplified formulas exist for finding the standard deviation. These are

$$s = \sqrt{\frac{\sum_{i=1}^{n} x_i^2}{n} - \left(\frac{\sum_{i=1}^{n} x_i}{n}\right)^2}$$

and, for grouped data,

$$s = \sqrt{\frac{\sum_{i=1}^{n} f_i x_i^2}{\sum_{i=1}^{n} f_i} - \left(\frac{\sum_{i=1}^{n} f_i x_i}{\sum_{i=1}^{n} f_i}\right)^2}$$

PROBLEM

Find the standard deviation of the numbers 3, 5, 6, 8, 13, 21.

Solution

$$\sum_{i=1}^{n} x_i^2 = 3^2 + 5^2 + 6^2 + 8^2 + 13^2 + 21^2 = 744$$

$$\sum_{i=1}^{n} x_i = 56$$

$$S = \sqrt{\frac{744}{6} - \left(\frac{56}{6}\right)^2} = 6.07$$

PROBLEM

We find the standard deviation for the data shown below. The height of 100 students was measured and recorded.

Height (inches)	Class Mark x	x²	Frequency f	fx²	fx
60 - 62	61	3,721	7	26,047	427
63 - 65	64	4,096	21	86,016	1,344
66 - 68	67	4,489	37	166,093	2,479
69 - 71	70	4,900	26	127,400	1,820
72 - 74	73	5,329	9	47,961	657

Solution

We apply the formula

$$s = \sqrt{\frac{\sum fx^2}{\sum f} - \left(\frac{\sum fx}{\sum f}\right)^2}$$

Sum the data in the appropriate columns

$$\sum f = 100 \quad \sum fx^2 = 453,517 \quad \sum fx = 6,727$$

and substitute into the equation

$$s = \sqrt{4,535 - 4,525} = 3.16$$

4. Correlation Coefficient

The correlation coefficient is a measure of the relationship between two sets of data. The most commonly used relationship is the linear relationship. The corresponding correlation coefficient r for two sets of data $\{x_1, x_2, ..., x_n\}$ and $\{y_1, y_2, ..., y_n\}$ is given by

$$r = \frac{\sum_{i=1}^{n}(x_i - \bar{x})(y_i - \bar{y})}{\sqrt{\sum_{i=1}^{n}(x_i - \bar{x})^2 \sum_{i=1}^{n}(y_i - \bar{y})^2}}$$

where $\bar{x}$ is the mean of $\{x_1, x_2, ..., x_n\}$ and $\bar{y}$ is the mean of $\{y_1, y_2, ..., y_n\}$.

The value of the correlation coefficient is always between - 1 and 1. Negative values show that the two data sets are "opposite" to each other. This is one type of correlation. Hence, if $r = - 1$, it means that the two sets of data are strongly negatively correlated. If $r = 0$, it means that there is no correlation. In some cases, it means that the data sets are independent of each other. Positive values show that two data sets are "similar" to each other. If $r = 1$, it means that the two data sets are almost similar.

PROBLEM

Compute the correlation coefficient for the following sets of data.

x	y	$x_i - \bar{x}$	$y_i - \bar{y}$	$(x_i - \bar{x})(y_i - \bar{y})$	$(x_i - \bar{x})^2$	$(y_i - \bar{y})^2$
9.2	9.6	2.41	1.16	2.80	5.81	1.35
9.7	8.6	2.91	0.16	0.47	8.47	0.03
8.1	11.2	1.31	2.76	3.62	1.72	7.62
5.5	8.7	- 1.29	0.26	- 0.34	1.66	0.07
7.7	10.2	0.91	1.76	1.60	0.83	3.10
5.6	8.4	- 1.19	- .04	0.05	1.42	0.0016
5.7	4.4	- 1.09	- 4.04	4.40	1.19	16.32
5.4	7.6	- 1.39	- 0.84	1.17	1.93	0.71
2.3	10.1	- 4.49	1.66	- 7.45	20.16	2.76
8.7	5.6	1.91	- 2.84	- 5.42	3.65	8.07

Solution

Apply the formula

$$r = \frac{\sum_{i=1}^{n}(x_i - \bar{x})(y_i - \bar{y})}{\sqrt{\sum_{i=1}^{n}(x_i - \bar{x})^2 \sum_{i=1}^{n}(y_i - \bar{y})^2}}$$

Take the averages of x and y

$$\bar{x} = 6.79, \quad \bar{y} = 8.44$$

Perform the necessary summations

$$\sum_{i=1}^{n}(x_i - \bar{x})(y_i - \bar{y}) = 0.90$$

$$\sum_{i=1}^{n}(x_i - \bar{x})^2 = 46.84$$

$$\sum_{i=1}^{n}(y_i - \bar{y})^2 = 40.03$$

Substitute totals into formula

$$r = \frac{0.90}{\sqrt{(46.84)(40.03)}} = \frac{0.90}{43.30} = 0.02$$

Since r is close to 0, this leads us to conclude that the data sets x and y are very weakly related to each other.

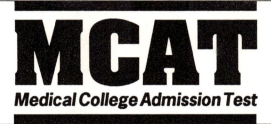

Chapter 6
Writing Sample Review

Chapter 6

WRITING SAMPLE REVIEW

Composing a Well-Written Essay

Physicians must be able to communicate with their patients, clientele, staff, and colleagues. Not only must they be able to convey facts, findings, their thoughts and feelings, but they must be able to respond to the important questions asked by those with whom they come into contact. Doctors must be able to receive information efficiently in both oral and written form. They must be able to organize this information, give directives, and provide clear, relevant answers to questions, particularly those asked by their patients. Even factual information can confuse and frighten patients — who may already be anxious, uninformed, or misinformed — if this information is carelessly presented.

Patients expect satisfactory verbal skills from their physicians. Tabulations from surveys done by the National Research Corporation (NRC) show that a physician's ability to communicate effectively is of prime concern to the general public. Those surveyed deem this "bedside manner" to be of greater importance than any other factor, including cost and location. *Social Science and Medicine* reports a finding that the physician's behavior (including communication) had more of an impact on patient outcome than did the patient's own behavior. The best physicians encourage the understanding and participation of their patients. Clearly, effective communication is vital.

Most medical schools consider the writing ability and analytical synthesizing skills of their applicants as part of their required admission criteria. One important part of the MCAT focuses on demonstrating these skills.

The MCAT Writing Sample

Each MCAT Writing Sample consists of a statement — often a direct quotation from a well-known figure or from a work of literature. The selected reading is not, however, directly related to the biological or physical sciences, religious issues, topics that tend to generate strong emotions in the readers, the application process for medical schools, or to the rationale/motives for the examinee's decision to pursue medical school admission.

Following the quotation or statement are three specific tasks for the reader to complete in a 30-minute period. There are usually two Writing Samples (each with a quotation/statement and three writing tasks) on the MCAT. During an hour testing session the examinee normally is expected to complete both MCAT Writing Samples.

Purpose of the MCAT Writing Samples

The MCAT Writing Samples require the examinee to demonstrate expository writing, a type of writing that focuses the reader's attention on objects, people, events, or ideas, rather than on one's feelings or attitudes about them. Expository writing must contain information or cover important points. This is the usual type of writing demanded on standardized exams requiring essay writing. Expository writing differs from expressive writing (which places its emphasis on the writer's feelings and reactions to the world, people, objects, events, and ideas) and from writing which is done strictly for the pleasure of the reader/writer. The expository writing called for on the MCAT differs from persuasive writing, which is often called for on the Law School Admission Test (LSAT). The purpose of persuasive writing is to influence the reader's attitudes and actions by arguing for or against a position. Consider how this differs from expository writing.

The Writing Samples included on the MCAT test many levels of knowledge. The reader is required to read at the literal level; for instance, in order to answer the question(s) asked, the writer must be able to demonstrate an understanding of what is asked. The writer is also required to comprehend; for example, the writer must be able to explain unusual terms. The writer must analyze (break into parts) what is expected of him/her and synthesize (put together) concepts and ideas. The examinee must develop a central idea and present ideas logically, using correct grammar, sentence and paragraph structure, punctuation, capitalization, and spelling.

Certain steps are necessary in preparing a good answer to the MCAT Writing Sample and in meeting these goals.

Preparing to Write

Before successful examinees begin to write an answer to an essay question, they complete certain preparatory steps.

1.   READ THE STATEMENT/QUESTION CAREFULLY

The examinee may re-read the question/statement several times before and during the writing of the essay. Examinees may wish to underline key words or phrases of the statement/question in the test booklet. If the source of the statement/question is given, the examinee should pay attention to the author, the date/period when the statement was made, and/or the reference from which it was taken.

2.   CONSIDER THE AUDIENCE

Successful writers determine which of the three types of audiences they will be addressing and address their writing to that audience. An audience might be

1) a general audience,

2) a mixed audience, or

3) a specialized audience.

A general audience consists of people who may not be experts on a subject but who are willing to read the material. This is usually not the group that will mark the MCAT essays. A mixed audience may consist of both specialists and general readers; again, this is not likely to be the group that will score the MCAT essays. It is the third group — a specialized audience — that will likely score the essays; they have considerable knowledge of the subject and will be looking for certain things. A savvy test-taker will be aware of the concerns of the specialized audience. These concerns include

- correct grammar,

- correct spelling,

- logical organization,

- generalizations supported by specific details, and

- an objective tone that is not too personal or too informal.

3.   STUDY THE WRITING TASKS THAT FOLLOW THE STATEMENT

Each statement/quotation is followed by three writing tasks. In order to receive full credit for the essay, the examinee must address each writing task. It is helpful, in writing the essay, to use wording similar to that of the question so that the scorer can see immediately which task is being addressed.

4.   PREPARE A ROUGH OUTLINE FOR THE ESSAY WHICH ADDRESSES FULLY EACH OF THE THREE TASKS

With a time limit of only 30 minutes, the examinee will not be able to prepare a detailed outline such as might be used for an untimed essay. However, jotting down main points (with specifics that are to be included) may help the writing go more quickly and easily. Such an outline helps the writer develop a logical sequence for assembling the data. With the rough outline the writer is not likely to forget to include one of the writing tasks, to omit a specific supporting statement, or to have to pause to try to remember a point she/he intended to make.

Only after the preliminary steps are completed is the examinee ready to begin actually writing the paper by writing the introductory paragraph.

Writing the Introductory Paragraph

The first paragraph (the introductory paragraph) keeps the question(s) in focus for the writer and restates the question(s) for the reader. The introductory paragraph contains a thesis statement that should do two things:

1)   Give the main idea(s) of the essay

2)   Provide the organization for the reader

In the introductory paragraph the three writing tasks should be obvious to the writer and the reader.

Developing the Paragraphs in the Body of the Essay

The body of the essay will usually include three paragraphs — one for each of the three writing tasks given in the MCAT Writing Sample. Ideally, each paragraph should contain a topic sentence to which all the sentences in the paragraph will relate. Each of these paragraphs will relate to the thesis sentence as stated in the introductory paragraph.

Preparing the Concluding Paragraph of the Essay

The successful examinee includes a concluding paragraph in the essay. This paragraph should review the main points of the answer(s), sum up the answer(s), and restate the thesis sentence. This concluding paragraph is an important part of a well-written essay.

Proofreading and Revising the Essay

The examinee should allow a few minutes at the end of the 30-minute period as a time to proofread and (if necessary) revise the essay. The specialized audience scoring the essay reads the essay as a first draft; a perfect copy is not expected. Nevertheless, the successful examinee should make sure of the following:

- All writing is clear and legible
- All sentences have a subject and a verb and express a clear thought
- Run-on sentences have been avoided
- The antecedent of each pronoun is clear
- Each pronoun agrees with its antecedent in number
- Each subject and verb agree in number
- The same tense is used throughout the essay
- Words are spelled correctly
- Items in a series have been separated by commas
- All proper nouns and the first word of each sentence have been capitalized
- Each sentence ends with its proper mark of punctuation
- Apostrophes have been used correctly for possession. (Contractions are avoided in formal writing.)
    — Singular nouns are made to show possession by adding *'s*
    — Plural nouns ending in *s* are made to show possession by adding *'*; plural nouns not ending in *s* are made to show possession by adding *'s*
- *It's* is a contraction meaning "it is" and should be avoided since contractions should be avoided in formal writing
- *Its* is a possessive pronoun and requires no apostrophe (*'*)
- To add a word, use the caret (^); to add a whole section, make a note in the paper where the insertion is to be made and write the section at the end
- To delete a word or a section, a line through the word or a large *X* through a paragraph is quicker and neater than scratching out each word.

CAUTION: An English grammar book should be consulted by the prospective examinee who needs a more intensive review of writing and mechanics.

Scoring the Essays

Readers of the Writing Samples use a holistic method of scoring the essays. Each essay is regarded as a unit and is assigned a single score based on what is considered to be its total quality. Some mistakes are expected on the timed essays, so an occasional mistake will not affect the evaluation of the essay. Readers of the papers are trained. Retraining is given at intervals to assure that accurate scoring is continued.

Each paper is scored by two readers using a six-point scale. If the paper receives two scores that are more than one point apart, a third reader will determine the total score for the paper. Clarity, depth, and unity are used to determine the score. If an essay fails to address one of the writing tasks, a score no higher than 3 can be assigned. Papers may be reported as "Not scorable" if they are blank, not written in English, illegible, or totally disregard the writing tasks.

Score reports, percentile data, score distributions, and an explanation of the general writing characteristics of each score level are provided to the medical schools. Listed below are the typical characteristics of each of the six-point classifications.

1) Problems with organization and mechanics in these essays make them difficult for the reader to follow. The essays may fail to address the topic altogether.

2) These essays seriously fail to address adequately one or more than one of the writing tasks. They may contain recurring mechanical errors. Problems with organization and analysis are typical.

3) These essays may neglect or distort one or even more of the writing tasks or may present only a minimal treatment of the topic. These essays may show some clarity of thought but may be classified as simplistic. Organizational problems may be obvious. The essays demonstrate a basic control of both sentence structure and vocabulary, but the language may not serve to communicate the writer's ideas effectively.

4) All three tasks are addressed; the topic is given only moderate (not thorough) exploration. Clarity (but not complexity) of thought is present. Some digressions may be present, but coherent organization is evident. Vocabulary and sentence structure is acceptable.

5) All three tasks are addressed by these essays. The treatment of the topic is substantial (but not thorough). Some depth of thought, control of vocabulary, control of sentence structure, and coherent organization are present but not to the same degree as an essay meriting six points.

6) Thorough exploration of the topic and fully addressed tasks are features of the essay scoring six points. These essays show depth of thought, superior vocabulary and sentence control, complexity of thought, and coherent, focused organization.

Read, plan, write, proofread, and revise! The result will be a good essay for the MCAT Writing Sample!

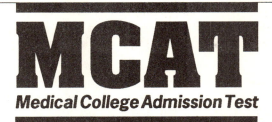

Test I

TEST 1
ANSWER SHEET

Section 1:
Verbal Reasoning

1. Ⓐ Ⓑ Ⓒ Ⓓ
2. Ⓐ Ⓑ Ⓒ Ⓓ
3. Ⓐ Ⓑ Ⓒ Ⓓ
4. Ⓐ Ⓑ Ⓒ Ⓓ
5. Ⓐ Ⓑ Ⓒ Ⓓ
6. Ⓐ Ⓑ Ⓒ Ⓓ
7. Ⓐ Ⓑ Ⓒ Ⓓ
8. Ⓐ Ⓑ Ⓒ Ⓓ
9. Ⓐ Ⓑ Ⓒ Ⓓ
10. Ⓐ Ⓑ Ⓒ Ⓓ
11. Ⓐ Ⓑ Ⓒ Ⓓ
12. Ⓐ Ⓑ Ⓒ Ⓓ
13. Ⓐ Ⓑ Ⓒ Ⓓ
14. Ⓐ Ⓑ Ⓒ Ⓓ
15. Ⓐ Ⓑ Ⓒ Ⓓ
16. Ⓐ Ⓑ Ⓒ Ⓓ
17. Ⓐ Ⓑ Ⓒ Ⓓ
18. Ⓐ Ⓑ Ⓒ Ⓓ
19. Ⓐ Ⓑ Ⓒ Ⓓ
20. Ⓐ Ⓑ Ⓒ Ⓓ
21. Ⓐ Ⓑ Ⓒ Ⓓ
22. Ⓐ Ⓑ Ⓒ Ⓓ
23. Ⓐ Ⓑ Ⓒ Ⓓ
24. Ⓐ Ⓑ Ⓒ Ⓓ
25. Ⓐ Ⓑ Ⓒ Ⓓ
26. Ⓐ Ⓑ Ⓒ Ⓓ
27. Ⓐ Ⓑ Ⓒ Ⓓ
28. Ⓐ Ⓑ Ⓒ Ⓓ
29. Ⓐ Ⓑ Ⓒ Ⓓ
30. Ⓐ Ⓑ Ⓒ Ⓓ
31. Ⓐ Ⓑ Ⓒ Ⓓ

32. Ⓐ Ⓑ Ⓒ Ⓓ
33. Ⓐ Ⓑ Ⓒ Ⓓ
34. Ⓐ Ⓑ Ⓒ Ⓓ
35. Ⓐ Ⓑ Ⓒ Ⓓ
36. Ⓐ Ⓑ Ⓒ Ⓓ
37. Ⓐ Ⓑ Ⓒ Ⓓ
38. Ⓐ Ⓑ Ⓒ Ⓓ
39. Ⓐ Ⓑ Ⓒ Ⓓ
40. Ⓐ Ⓑ Ⓒ Ⓓ
41. Ⓐ Ⓑ Ⓒ Ⓓ
42. Ⓐ Ⓑ Ⓒ Ⓓ
43. Ⓐ Ⓑ Ⓒ Ⓓ
44. Ⓐ Ⓑ Ⓒ Ⓓ
45. Ⓐ Ⓑ Ⓒ Ⓓ
46. Ⓐ Ⓑ Ⓒ Ⓓ
47. Ⓐ Ⓑ Ⓒ Ⓓ
48. Ⓐ Ⓑ Ⓒ Ⓓ
49. Ⓐ Ⓑ Ⓒ Ⓓ
50. Ⓐ Ⓑ Ⓒ Ⓓ
51. Ⓐ Ⓑ Ⓒ Ⓓ
52. Ⓐ Ⓑ Ⓒ Ⓓ
53. Ⓐ Ⓑ Ⓒ Ⓓ
54. Ⓐ Ⓑ Ⓒ Ⓓ
55. Ⓐ Ⓑ Ⓒ Ⓓ
56. Ⓐ Ⓑ Ⓒ Ⓓ
57. Ⓐ Ⓑ Ⓒ Ⓓ
58. Ⓐ Ⓑ Ⓒ Ⓓ
59. Ⓐ Ⓑ Ⓒ Ⓓ
60. Ⓐ Ⓑ Ⓒ Ⓓ
61. Ⓐ Ⓑ Ⓒ Ⓓ
62. Ⓐ Ⓑ Ⓒ Ⓓ
63. Ⓐ Ⓑ Ⓒ Ⓓ
64. Ⓐ Ⓑ Ⓒ Ⓓ
65. Ⓐ Ⓑ Ⓒ Ⓓ

Section 2:
Physical Sciences

66. Ⓐ Ⓑ Ⓒ Ⓓ
67. Ⓐ Ⓑ Ⓒ Ⓓ
68. Ⓐ Ⓑ Ⓒ Ⓓ
69. Ⓐ Ⓑ Ⓒ Ⓓ
70. Ⓐ Ⓑ Ⓒ Ⓓ
71. Ⓐ Ⓑ Ⓒ Ⓓ
72. Ⓐ Ⓑ Ⓒ Ⓓ
73. Ⓐ Ⓑ Ⓒ Ⓓ
74. Ⓐ Ⓑ Ⓒ Ⓓ
75. Ⓐ Ⓑ Ⓒ Ⓓ
76. Ⓐ Ⓑ Ⓒ Ⓓ
77. Ⓐ Ⓑ Ⓒ Ⓓ
78. Ⓐ Ⓑ Ⓒ Ⓓ
79. Ⓐ Ⓑ Ⓒ Ⓓ
80. Ⓐ Ⓑ Ⓒ Ⓓ
81. Ⓐ Ⓑ Ⓒ Ⓓ
82. Ⓐ Ⓑ Ⓒ Ⓓ
83. Ⓐ Ⓑ Ⓒ Ⓓ
84. Ⓐ Ⓑ Ⓒ Ⓓ
85. Ⓐ Ⓑ Ⓒ Ⓓ
86. Ⓐ Ⓑ Ⓒ Ⓓ
87. Ⓐ Ⓑ Ⓒ Ⓓ
88. Ⓐ Ⓑ Ⓒ Ⓓ
89. Ⓐ Ⓑ Ⓒ Ⓓ
90. Ⓐ Ⓑ Ⓒ Ⓓ
91. Ⓐ Ⓑ Ⓒ Ⓓ
92. Ⓐ Ⓑ Ⓒ Ⓓ
93. Ⓐ Ⓑ Ⓒ Ⓓ
94. Ⓐ Ⓑ Ⓒ Ⓓ
95. Ⓐ Ⓑ Ⓒ Ⓓ
96. Ⓐ Ⓑ Ⓒ Ⓓ

97. Ⓐ Ⓑ Ⓒ Ⓓ
98. Ⓐ Ⓑ Ⓒ Ⓓ
99. Ⓐ Ⓑ Ⓒ Ⓓ
100. Ⓐ Ⓑ Ⓒ Ⓓ
101. Ⓐ Ⓑ Ⓒ Ⓓ
102. Ⓐ Ⓑ Ⓒ Ⓓ
103. Ⓐ Ⓑ Ⓒ Ⓓ
104. Ⓐ Ⓑ Ⓒ Ⓓ
105. Ⓐ Ⓑ Ⓒ Ⓓ
106. Ⓐ Ⓑ Ⓒ Ⓓ
107. Ⓐ Ⓑ Ⓒ Ⓓ
108. Ⓐ Ⓑ Ⓒ Ⓓ
109. Ⓐ Ⓑ Ⓒ Ⓓ
110. Ⓐ Ⓑ Ⓒ Ⓓ
111. Ⓐ Ⓑ Ⓒ Ⓓ
112. Ⓐ Ⓑ Ⓒ Ⓓ
113. Ⓐ Ⓑ Ⓒ Ⓓ
114. Ⓐ Ⓑ Ⓒ Ⓓ
115. Ⓐ Ⓑ Ⓒ Ⓓ
116. Ⓐ Ⓑ Ⓒ Ⓓ
117. Ⓐ Ⓑ Ⓒ Ⓓ
118. Ⓐ Ⓑ Ⓒ Ⓓ
119. Ⓐ Ⓑ Ⓒ Ⓓ
120. Ⓐ Ⓑ Ⓒ Ⓓ
121. Ⓐ Ⓑ Ⓒ Ⓓ
122. Ⓐ Ⓑ Ⓒ Ⓓ
123. Ⓐ Ⓑ Ⓒ Ⓓ
124. Ⓐ Ⓑ Ⓒ Ⓓ
125. Ⓐ Ⓑ Ⓒ Ⓓ
126. Ⓐ Ⓑ Ⓒ Ⓓ
127. Ⓐ Ⓑ Ⓒ Ⓓ
128. Ⓐ Ⓑ Ⓒ Ⓓ
129. Ⓐ Ⓑ Ⓒ Ⓓ
130. Ⓐ Ⓑ Ⓒ Ⓓ
131. Ⓐ Ⓑ Ⓒ Ⓓ
132. Ⓐ Ⓑ Ⓒ Ⓓ
133. Ⓐ Ⓑ Ⓒ Ⓓ
134. Ⓐ Ⓑ Ⓒ Ⓓ
135. Ⓐ Ⓑ Ⓒ Ⓓ
136. Ⓐ Ⓑ Ⓒ Ⓓ
137. Ⓐ Ⓑ Ⓒ Ⓓ
138. Ⓐ Ⓑ Ⓒ Ⓓ
139. Ⓐ Ⓑ Ⓒ Ⓓ

140. Ⓐ Ⓑ Ⓒ Ⓓ
141. Ⓐ Ⓑ Ⓒ Ⓓ
142. Ⓐ Ⓑ Ⓒ Ⓓ

Section 4:
Biological Sciences

143. Ⓐ Ⓑ Ⓒ Ⓓ
144. Ⓐ Ⓑ Ⓒ Ⓓ
145. Ⓐ Ⓑ Ⓒ Ⓓ
146. Ⓐ Ⓑ Ⓒ Ⓓ
147. Ⓐ Ⓑ Ⓒ Ⓓ
148. Ⓐ Ⓑ Ⓒ Ⓓ
149. Ⓐ Ⓑ Ⓒ Ⓓ
150. Ⓐ Ⓑ Ⓒ Ⓓ
151. Ⓐ Ⓑ Ⓒ Ⓓ
152. Ⓐ Ⓑ Ⓒ Ⓓ
153. Ⓐ Ⓑ Ⓒ Ⓓ
154. Ⓐ Ⓑ Ⓒ Ⓓ
155. Ⓐ Ⓑ Ⓒ Ⓓ
156. Ⓐ Ⓑ Ⓒ Ⓓ
157. Ⓐ Ⓑ Ⓒ Ⓓ
158. Ⓐ Ⓑ Ⓒ Ⓓ
159. Ⓐ Ⓑ Ⓒ Ⓓ
160. Ⓐ Ⓑ Ⓒ Ⓓ
161. Ⓐ Ⓑ Ⓒ Ⓓ
162. Ⓐ Ⓑ Ⓒ Ⓓ
163. Ⓐ Ⓑ Ⓒ Ⓓ
164. Ⓐ Ⓑ Ⓒ Ⓓ
165. Ⓐ Ⓑ Ⓒ Ⓓ
166. Ⓐ Ⓑ Ⓒ Ⓓ
167. Ⓐ Ⓑ Ⓒ Ⓓ
168. Ⓐ Ⓑ Ⓒ Ⓓ
169. Ⓐ Ⓑ Ⓒ Ⓓ
170. Ⓐ Ⓑ Ⓒ Ⓓ
171. Ⓐ Ⓑ Ⓒ Ⓓ
172. Ⓐ Ⓑ Ⓒ Ⓓ
173. Ⓐ Ⓑ Ⓒ Ⓓ
174. Ⓐ Ⓑ Ⓒ Ⓓ
175. Ⓐ Ⓑ Ⓒ Ⓓ
176. Ⓐ Ⓑ Ⓒ Ⓓ

177. Ⓐ Ⓑ Ⓒ Ⓓ
178. Ⓐ Ⓑ Ⓒ Ⓓ
179. Ⓐ Ⓑ Ⓒ Ⓓ
180. Ⓐ Ⓑ Ⓒ Ⓓ
181. Ⓐ Ⓑ Ⓒ Ⓓ
182. Ⓐ Ⓑ Ⓒ Ⓓ
183. Ⓐ Ⓑ Ⓒ Ⓓ
184. Ⓐ Ⓑ Ⓒ Ⓓ
185. Ⓐ Ⓑ Ⓒ Ⓓ
186. Ⓐ Ⓑ Ⓒ Ⓓ
187. Ⓐ Ⓑ Ⓒ Ⓓ
188. Ⓐ Ⓑ Ⓒ Ⓓ
189. Ⓐ Ⓑ Ⓒ Ⓓ
190. Ⓐ Ⓑ Ⓒ Ⓓ
191. Ⓐ Ⓑ Ⓒ Ⓓ
192. Ⓐ Ⓑ Ⓒ Ⓓ
193. Ⓐ Ⓑ Ⓒ Ⓓ
194. Ⓐ Ⓑ Ⓒ Ⓓ
195. Ⓐ Ⓑ Ⓒ Ⓓ
196. Ⓐ Ⓑ Ⓒ Ⓓ
197. Ⓐ Ⓑ Ⓒ Ⓓ
198. Ⓐ Ⓑ Ⓒ Ⓓ
199. Ⓐ Ⓑ Ⓒ Ⓓ
200. Ⓐ Ⓑ Ⓒ Ⓓ
201. Ⓐ Ⓑ Ⓒ Ⓓ
202. Ⓐ Ⓑ Ⓒ Ⓓ
203. Ⓐ Ⓑ Ⓒ Ⓓ
204. Ⓐ Ⓑ Ⓒ Ⓓ
205. Ⓐ Ⓑ Ⓒ Ⓓ
206. Ⓐ Ⓑ Ⓒ Ⓓ
207. Ⓐ Ⓑ Ⓒ Ⓓ
208. Ⓐ Ⓑ Ⓒ Ⓓ
209. Ⓐ Ⓑ Ⓒ Ⓓ
210. Ⓐ Ⓑ Ⓒ Ⓓ
211. Ⓐ Ⓑ Ⓒ Ⓓ
212. Ⓐ Ⓑ Ⓒ Ⓓ
213. Ⓐ Ⓑ Ⓒ Ⓓ
214. Ⓐ Ⓑ Ⓒ Ⓓ
215. Ⓐ Ⓑ Ⓒ Ⓓ
216. Ⓐ Ⓑ Ⓒ Ⓓ
217. Ⓐ Ⓑ Ⓒ Ⓓ
218. Ⓐ Ⓑ Ⓒ Ⓓ
219. Ⓐ Ⓑ Ⓒ Ⓓ

TEST 1

Section 1 — Verbal Reasoning

TIME: 85 Minutes
QUESTIONS: 1-65

> **DIRECTIONS:** The verbal reasoning section contains seven passages, each followed by a series of questions. Based on the information given in a passage, choose the one best answer to each question. If you are not sure of an answer, eliminate those choices that you know are incorrect and choose an answer from among those remaining. Fill in the corresponding circle on the answer sheet to indicate your answer.

PASSAGE I (Questions 1-10)

A good scientific law or theory is falsifiable simply because it makes definite claims about the world. For the falsificationist, it follows readily that the more falsifiable a theory is, the better. The more claims a theory makes, the more potential there is for showing that the world does not, in fact, behave in the way laid down by that theory. A very good theory is one that makes very wide-ranging claims about the world, and which is, consequently, highly falsifiable. This is a theory that resists falsification whenever it is put to the test.

This point can be illustrated by means of a trivial example. Consider the two laws:

(a) Mars moves in an ellipse around the sun.

(b) All planets move in ellipses around their sun.

It is clear that (b) has a higher status than (a) as a piece of scientific knowledge. Law (b) tells us what law (a) tells us and more. Law (b), the preferable law, is more falsifiable than (a). If observations of Mars should turn out to falsify (a), then they would falsify (b) also. Any falsification of (a) will be a falsification of (b), but the reverse is not the case. Observation statements referring to the orbits of Venus, Jupiter, etc. that might conceivable falsify (b) are irrelevant to (a). If we follow Popper and refer to those sets of observation statements that would serve to falsify a law or theory as potential falsifiers of that law or theory, then we can say that the potential falsifiers of (a) form a class that is a subclass of the potential falsifiers of (b). Law (b) is more falsifiable than law (a), which is tantamount to saying that it claims more, that it is the better law.

A less-contrived example involves the relation between Kepler's theory of the solar system and Newton's theory of the solar system. Kepler's theory consists of three laws of planetary motion. Potential falsifiers of this theory consist of sets of statements referring to planetary positions, relative to the sun, at specified times. Newton's theory, a better theory that supersedes Kepler's, is more comprehensive. It consists of Newton's law of motion, plus his law of gravitation, with the latter asserting that all pairs of bodies in the universe attract each other with a force that varies inversely as the square of their separation. Some of the potential falsifiers of Newton's theory are sets of statements of planetary positions at specified times, but there are many others. These include those referring to the behavior of falling bodies and pendulums, the correlation between the tides and the locations of the sun and moon, and so on. There are many more opportunities to falsify Newton's theory than there are to falsify Kepler's theory. As the falsificationist's theory goes, Newton's theory is able to resist falsification attempts, thereby establishing its superiority over Kepler's theory.

Highly falsifiable theories should be preferred over less falsifiable ones, provided they have not, in fact, been falsified. This qualification is important to the falsificationist. Theories that have been falsified must be ruthlessly rejected. The enterprise of science consists in the proposal of highly falsifiable hypotheses, followed by deliberate and tenacious attempts to falsify them.

"We learn from our mistakes. Science progresses by trial and error." Falsifications become important landmarks, striking achievements, and major growing-points in science because of this logical process. This renders impossible the derivation of universal laws and theories from observation, but makes possible the deduction of their falsity.

Adapted from A.F. Chalmers. *What Is This Thing Called Science?*, 2nd edition. New York: University of Queensland Press, 1982. pp. 42-43.

1.   According to the author, the most important advances in science occur by

    (A)   proposing highly falsifiable theories.

    (B)   falsifying existing theories.

    (C)   finding general theories of motion.

    (D)   identifying theories of planetary motion.

2.   The author's example in paragraph two is intended to

    (A)   inform the reader of the shape of Mars' orbit.

    (B)   describe how all planets move about the sun.

    (C)   show how a theory can be falsified.

    (D)   illustrate how a theory can be more falsifiable.

3.   Based on the passage, which of the following is a *potential falsifier?*

    (A)   An observation statement that falsifies an existing theory

    (B)   A description of a general theory

    (C)   A statement describing a narrowly defined theory

    (D)   A statement describing the shape of Mars' orbit

4.   Based on the passage, it can be reasonably inferred that a bad scientific theory does which of the following?

    (A)   Limits the advance of scientific knowledge

    (B)   Fails to make definite claims about the world

(C)   Has been falsified

(D)   Inaccurately describes planetary motion

5.   According to the author, Newton's theory is superior to Kepler's because of which of the following?

(A)   Kepler's theory was proven false.

(B)   Kepler's theory inaccurately describes the motion of Mars.

(C)   Newton's theory makes broader claims than Kepler's.

(D)   Newton's theory makes specific claims.

6.   According to the author, one scientific theory is considered better than another if it does which of the following?

(A)   Makes more claims about the world

(B)   Has been falsified

(C)   Is limited to descriptions of planetary motion

(D)   Contains a subset of Newton's theory

7.   Based on the passage, which of the following would a falsificationist consider necessary for a very good scientific theory?

I.   A theory making wide-ranging claims about the world

II.   A theory that resists falsification

III.   A theory containing false claims

(A)   I only.   (B)   I and II.

(C)   I and III.   (D)   II and III.

8.   The author's suggestion that we learn from our mistakes refers to

(A)   the way habits are formed.

(B)   learning to propose broader theories.

(C)   the preference for highly falsifiable theories.

(D)   the trial and error nature of scientific progress.

9.   Based on the passage, which of the following is the most falsifiable theory?

(A)   Judges make decisions based on a small number of environmental cues.

(B)   Supreme Court justices make decisions based on a small number of environmental cues.

(C)   Appellate judges make decisions based on a small number of environmental cues.

(D)   People make decisions based on a small number of environmental cues.

10. According to the passage, which of the following would not be considered a potential falsifier of Kepler's theory?

   (A) An observation that Mars was not in the correct place at a given time

   (B) An observation that neither Mars nor Venus were in the predicted places at a specified time

   (C) An observation that there was no correlation between the tides and the positions of the sun and moon

   (D) An observation that none of the planets in the solar system conformed to their predicted positions at any point in time

PASSAGE II (Questions 11–19)

It is a fundamental claim of feminism that women are oppressed. The word 'oppression' is a strong word that repels and attracts. It is dangerous, dangerously fashionable, and in danger of losing its meaning. It is also misused intentionally in many instances.

The statement that women are oppressed is frequently met with the claim that men are also oppressed. We hear that the act of oppressing is oppressive to those who oppress, as well as to those who are oppressed. Some men cite as evidence of their oppression their much-advertised inability to cry. It is difficult, women are told, to be masculine. When the stress and frustration of being a man are cited as evidence that they, as oppressors, are oppressed by their oppressive actions, the word 'oppression' is being stretched to meaninglessness. It is treated as though its scope includes any and all human experience of limitation or suffering, no matter the cause, degree or consequence. Once such usage has been put on us, then, if we ever deny that any person or group is oppressed. We seem to imply that we think they never suffer or have feelings. We are accused of insensitivity; even of bigotry. For women, such accusation is particularly intimidating, since sensitivity is one of the few virtues that has been assigned to us. If we are found insensitive, we may fear we have no redeeming traits at all, and perhaps are not real women. Thus, we are silenced before we begin: the name of our situation, drained of meaning, and our guilt mechanisms tripped.

But this is nonsense. Human beings can be miserable without being oppressed. It is perfectly consistent to deny that a person or group is oppressed without denying that they have feelings or that they suffer.

One is marked for application of oppressive pressures by one's membership in some group or category. Much of one's suffering and frustration befalls one partly, or largely, because one is a member of that category. In the case at hand, it is the category, "woman." "Being a woman is a major factor in my not having a better job than I do; being a woman selects me as a likely victim of sexual assault or harassment; it is my being a woman that reduces the power of my anger to a proof of my insanity." If a woman has little, or no, economic or political power, and/or achieves little of what she wants to achieve, a major causal factor is that she is a woman. For any women of any race or economic class, being a woman is significantly attached to whatever disadvantages and deprivations she suffers, be they great or small.

This is not the case with respect to a person being a man. Simply being a man is not what stands between him and a better job. Whatever assaults and harassments a man is subject to, being male is not what selects him for victimization. Being male is not a factor which would make his anger impotent; in fact quite the opposite. If a man has little, or no, material or political power, and/or achieves little of what he wants to achieve, his being male is not part of the explanation. Being male is something he has working for him, even if race, class, age, or disability is working against him.

Women are oppressed for being women. Members of certain racial and/or economic groups and classes, both the males and the females, are oppressed for being members of those races and/or classes. But men are not oppressed for being men.

Adapted from Marilyn Frye. *The Politics of Reality: Essays in Feminist Theory.* Trumansburg, New York: The Crossing Press, 1983. pp. 1-2, 15-16.

11. Based on the passage, which of the following is an accurate statement of the author's feeling about the word 'oppression'?

   (A) It should not be used to describe what has happened to women.

   (B) It can never be applied to men.

   (C) It loses meaning when applied to describing mere misery.

   (D) It has no application to feminist theory.

12. The author argues that to claim oppressing is oppressive to the oppressors is

   (A) nonsense.

   (B) an unrealistic description of the state of affairs produced in an oppressive environment.

   (C) unfair to those being oppressed.

   (D) contrary to feminist theory.

13. Based on the passage, which of the following does the author argue?

   (A) Men are never oppressed.

   (B) Men do not oppress women.

   (C) Women never oppress men.

   (D) Men are not oppressed simply due to their gender.

14. Which of the following problems does the author claim is caused in large part by her being a woman?

   I. Not having a better job

   II. Being subject to sexual harassment

   III. Suffering any deprivations

   (A) I only.   (B) II only.

   (C) I and II.   (D) I, II, and III.

15. The author argues one is marked for oppression due to which of the following?

   (A) Because one is a man

    (B)   Due to membership in some group

    (C)   Because one is a woman

    (D)   Due to individual characteristics

16.   The author argues which of the following with respect to being a man?

    I.   Men are not oppressed.

    II.   One is not oppressed for being a man.

    III.   Men can be miserable without being oppressed.

    (A)   I only.   (B)   II and III.

    (C)   I and III.   (D)   I, II, and III.

17.   Which of the following does the author argue occurs when women deny that some group is oppressed?

    (A)   Women are oppressed.

    (B)   Men are oppressed.

    (C)   Women are accused of being insensitive.

    (D)   Women are seen as being oppressors.

18.   Women may sometimes be accused of bigotry when they deny some group has been oppressed. Based on the passage, what is an underlying cause of such an accusation?

    (A)   Distortion of the word 'oppression'

    (B)   The dangerousness of the word 'oppression'

    (C)   The truth of the accusation

    (D)   The lack of economic power of women

19.   The author notes women may fear they have no redeeming traits if they are considered insensitive. To be true, this argument must be based on the assumption that

    (A)   women see themselves as being sensitive.

    (B)   men see women as being sensitive.

    (C)   women only have one redeeming trait.

    (D)   women are insensitive.

PASSAGE III (Questions 20–29)

    In the first quarter of this century two momentous theories were proposed: the theory of relativity and the quantum theory. From them sprang most of twentieth-century physics. But the new physics soon revealed much more than simply a better model of the physical world. Physicists began to realize that their discoveries demanded a radical reformulation of the most fundamental aspects of reality. They learned to approach their subject in totally unexpected and novel ways that seemed to turn common sense on its head and find accord with mysticism rather than materialism.

The fruits of this revolution are only now starting to be plucked by philosophers and theologians. Many ordinary people too, searching for a deeper meaning behind their lives, find their beliefs about the world very much in tune with the new physics. The physicist's outlook is even finding sympathy with psychologists and sociologists, especially those who advocate a holistic approach to their subjects.

In giving lectures and talks on modern physics I have discerned a growing feeling that fundamental physics is pointing the way to a new appreciation of man and his place in the universe. Deep questions of existence — "How did the universe begin and how will it end? What is matter? What is life? What is mind?" — are not new. What is new is that we may at last be on the verge of answering them. This astonishing prospect stems from some spectacular recent advances in physical science — not only the new physics, but its close relative, the new cosmology.

For the first time, a unified description of all creation could be within our grasp. No scientific problem is more fundamental or more daunting than the puzzle of how the universe came into being. Could this have happened without any supernatural input? Quantum physics seems to provide a loophole to the age-old assumption that "you can't get something for nothing." Physicists are now talking about "the self-creating universe": a cosmos that erupts into existence spontaneously, much as a subnuclear particle sometimes pops out of nowhere in certain high energy processes. The question of whether the details of this theory are right or wrong is not so very important. What matters is that it is now possible to conceive of a scientific explanation for all creation. Has modern physics abolished God altogether?

Yet, this is not a book about religion. Nor is this a science book. Rather, it is about the impact of the new physics on what were formerly religious issues. In particular, I make no attempt to discuss religious experiences or questions of morality. This is a book about science and its wider implications. Inevitably, it is necessary to explain some technicalities in careful detail, but I do not claim that the scientific discussions are either systematic or complete. The reader should not be deterred by the thought that he or she is in for some punishing mathematics or strings of specialist terminology. I have tried to avoid technical jargon as much as possible.

The central theme of the book concerns what I call the Big Four Questions of Existence. Toward the end of the book, tentative answers to these questions begin to emerge — answers based on the physicist's conception of nature. The answers may be totally wrong, but I believe that physics is uniquely placed to provide them. It may seem bizarre, but in my opinion science offers a surer path to God than religion. Right or wrong, the fact that science has actually advanced to the point that, what were formerly religious questions, can be seriously tackled, in itself indicates the far-reaching consequences of the new physics.

Adapted from Paul Davies. *God and the New Physics*. New York: Simon & Schuster, 1983. pp. vii-ix.

20.   According to the passage, the author's book considers which of the following?

   (A)   Science

   (B)   Religion

    (C)   The implications of science

    (D)   Two momentous theories of physics

21.   Which of the following does the author suggest about quantum theory and the theory of relativity?

    (A)   Relativity proved useless after quantum theory was discovered.

    (B)   They caused a reexamination of fundamental theories of reality.

    (C)   Their implications were confined to the physical world.

    (D)   They had little impact on the scientific community.

22.   According to the author, which of the following groups have benefited by the new physics?

    I.   Theologians

    II.   Psychologists

    III.   Ordinary people

    (A)   I and II.   (B)   I and III.

    (C)   II and III.   (D)   I, II, and III.

23.   In the passage, which of the following does the author argue is the most fundamental puzzle in science?

    (A)   The creation of the universe

    (B)   The basis of quantum theory

    (C)   The nature of matter

    (D)   The nature of God

24.   As evidence for the proposition of a self-creating universe, the author notes the existence of which of the following?

    (A)   The existence of black holes

    (B)   Darwin's theory of evolution

    (C)   The pattern of planetary motion

    (D)   The behavior of subnuclear particles

25.   Which of the following does the author assert with respect to answers to the Big Four Questions of Existence?

    (A)   He has the correct answers to these questions.

    (B)   These questions are unanswerable.

    (C)   Physics is in a good position to attempt to answer them.

    (D)   These questions are irrelevant to the new physics.

26. By suggesting the physicist's outlook is finding sympathy with sociologists, the author means which of the following?

    (A) Sociologists feel sorry for physicists.

    (B) Some sociologists agree with the physicist's outlook.

    (C) Physicists agree with the sociological viewpoint.

    (D) Sociologists now study the new physics.

27. The author asks whether the new physics has abolished God. Based on the passage what does the author most likely believe about the question?

    (A) The author believes it is true.

    (B) The author believes it is false.

    (C) The author believes this will be the eventual conclusion reached by the new physics.

    (D) The author believes the question has no relevance to the new physics.

28. According to the author, new discoveries in physics forced physicists to do which of the following?

    (A) Concentrate their energies on particle physics

    (B) Begin to examine religion

    (C) Reject psychological notions of mind and matter

    (D) Examine physics in ways contrary to common-sense

29. In the passage, which of the following does the author claim his book will do?

    (A) Provide a complete scientific discussion of the topic

    (B) Discuss the nature of religious experiences

    (C) Explain some technicalities of the topic in detail

    (D) Examine the moral implications of the new physics

PASSAGE IV (Questions 30–38)

Each year millions of people die of malnutrition and related health problems. For those of us in the affluent countries, this poses an acute moral problem. We spend money on ourselves, not only for the necessities of life but for innumerable luxuries. The problem is that we could forgo our luxuries and give the money for famine relief instead. The fact that we don't suggests that we regard our luxuries as more important than feeding the hungry.

Instead of asking the question, "Why do we behave as we do?" we should ask, "What is our duty? What should we do?" We might think of this as the "common-sense" view of the matter: morality requires that we balance our own interests against the interests of others. It is understandable, of course, that we look out for our own interests, and no one can be faulted for attending to his own basic needs. But at the same time the needs of others are also important, and when we can help others, especially at little cost to ourselves, we should do so.

But, one person's common sense is another person's naive platitude. Some thinkers have maintained that, in fact, we have no "natural" duties to other people. Ethical Egoism is the idea that each person ought to pursue his or her own self-interest exclusively. It is different from Psychological Egoism, which is a theory of human nature concerned with how people do behave — Psychological Egoism says that people do in fact always pursue their own interests. Ethical Egoism, by contrast, is a normative theory — that is, a theory about how we ought to behave. Regardless of how we do behave, Ethical Egoism says we have no moral duty except to do what is best for ourselves.

Ethical Egoism does not say that one should promote one's own interests as well as the interests of others. That would be an ordinary, unexceptional view. Ethical Egoism is the radical view that one's only duty is to promote one's own interests. According to Ethical Egoism, there is only one ultimate principle of conduct: the principle of self-interest. This principle sums up *all* of one's natural duties and obligations.

However, Ethical Egoism does not say that you should avoid actions that help others, either. It may very well be that in many instances your interests coincide with the interests of others, so that in helping yourself you will be aiding others. Or it may happen that aiding others is an effective means for creating some benefit for yourself. Ethical Egoism does not forbid such actions; in fact, it may demand them. The theory insists only that in such cases the benefit to others is not what makes the act right. What makes the act right is, rather, the fact that it is to one's own advantage.

Finally, Ethical Egoism does not imply that in pursuing one's interests one ought always to do what one wants to do, or what gives one the most pleasure in the short run. Someone may want to do something that is not good for himself or that will eventually cause himself more grief than pleasure — he may want to drink a lot or smoke cigarettes or take drugs or waste his best years at the race track. Ethical Egoism would frown on all this, regardless of the momentary pleasure it affords. It says that a person ought to do what really is to his or her own best interest over the long run. It endorses selfishness, but it doesn't endorse foolishness.

Adapted from James Rachels. *The Elements of Moral Philosophy.* New York: Random House, 1986. pp. 65–67.

30.   The author's purpose in this passage is to do which of the following?

(A)   Discuss the problem of world hunger

(B)   Consider the moral implications of not contributing to stop world hunger

(C)   Argue that Ethical Egoism is the correct moral position

(D)   Introduce Ethical Egoism as an alternative to common-sense morality

31.   According to the author, the common-sense view of morality holds which of the following?

(A)   Act to provide the greatest good to the most people

(B)   Act to help others, especially when it costs us little

(C)   Consider only the interests of others in deciding how to act

(D)   Act according to our own common sense

32. Based on the passage, the author would most probably say which of the following is our duty with respect to world hunger?

    (A) Give up our luxuries and give the money to the world hunger relief effort

    (B) Continue to enjoy our luxuries

    (C) Ignore the problem

    (D) The passage gives no indication as to how the author thinks we should act.

33. According to the author, Ethical Egoism is best described by which of the following?

    (A) The idea that one should pursue one's own interests

    (B) A theory of human nature describing how people behave

    (C) A belief that one should put others' interests first

    (D) The notion that one should avoid helping others

34. With respect to helping others, the author tells us that Ethical Egoism holds which of the following?

    (A) Such actions should always be avoided.

    (B) Actions which help others may sometimes be necessary.

    (C) Actions which help others should only be undertaken if they involve no cost to ourselves.

    (D) It is our natural duty to avoid helping others.

35. From the passage, we can gather that a normative theory is one which does which of the following?

    (A) Describes how things are

    (B) Tells how things should be

    (C) Explains why things are the way they are

    (D) Describes the norms of Americans

36. Based on the passage, which of the following is most likely to be consistent with Ethical Egoism?

    I. Playing video games

    II. Opening a savings account

    III. Smoking cigarettes

    (A) I only.   (B) II only.

    (C) III only.   (D) I, II, and III.

37. As described by the author which of the following is true with respect to Ethical Egoism's view of natural duties?

    (A) No natural duties are recognized by Ethical Egoism.

    (B) Immediate gratification is the primary natural duty.

    (C) Self-interest is the only natural duty recognized by Ethical Egoism.

    (D) Ethical Egoism recognizes the need for utilitarianism.

38. Which of the following problems is most likely to occur when applying Ethical Egoism in real world situations?

    (A) Identifying long-term and short-term interests

    (B) Avoiding helping others

    (C) Eliminating common-sense actions

    (D) Logistical interpretation of natural duty

PASSAGE V (Questions 39–48)

A nurse I know believes that more babies are born during the full moon than at any other time. She recently told me, "The moon was full last week, and we had double the normal number of births. It happens all the time." Someone else I know canceled a trip to Europe this past summer for fear of a terrorist hijacking but thinks nothing of commuting to work every day. An acquaintance who has played the stock market for two decades swears by a certain fund: "Any money manager who can consistently outperform the market eight years in a row gets my money!"

The foregoing examples illustrate various forms of "math abuse": the inability or unwillingness to apply a simple logical analysis to certain situations that arise in everyday life. Someone who cannot deal with simple numerical ideas is innumerate, just as someone who cannot read or write is illiterate. I prefer the term "math abuse" because it has a wider scope. It includes errors that are not strictly numerical, and it also has a moral dimension. We abuse mathematics by failing to apply even the little we know of it to the false or questionable ideas that we encounter. We do not want to be duped, but most of us are fooled on a regular basis by politicians, the media and even friends.

What is wrong, for example, with the notion that more babies are born during the full moon? The idea certainly has charm, and I for one would not be upset in the slightest if it turned out to be true. Suppose for the moment, though, that it is not true. Why might the nurse still claim that the peak baby-delivery period comes during the full moon?

Suppose that after watching the delivery of 15 babies in one day, the nurse looks out the window and sees a full moon. A month later the maternity ward is relatively quiet, but the nurse does not bother to check the phase of the moon. If one watches only for the events that reinforce a belief, one is screening out all the events that falsify it. This phenomenon of belief is what Paulos calls a filter.

Filters can be found everywhere. Casinos that contain dozens of slot machines ring with the sound of winning. Every time the three little cherries line up, a machine disgorges a bunch of quarters that clatter into a tray. Losing makes no sound. Someone entering a casino may well be overwhelmed by the impression that everyone is winning. Yet even a few quarters won every 10 tries on average would produce a more or less continuous clatter from just 10 active machines.

The filtering phenomenon accounts for a good deal more than the "charitable casino" illusion. It can misguide us in our investment strategies. Was my friend right to place such confidence in a fund that beat the odds eight years in a row? Here is a simple way to judge the issue. First assume that the success of a fund depends on just plain luck—say, the flip of a coin. If the coin comes up heads one year, the fund will outperform the market index. If the coin comes up tails, on the other hand, the fund will drop below the index. Now if 1,024 funds were operating in 1982, consider their fate over eight years. By 1983, say, out of one-half of the funds, 512, had outper-formed the index. By 1984 half of these, 256, had again beaten the index. Each year the number of funds that continued to show superior returns was halved: 128, 64, 32, 16, 8, 4. The last number represents the "hot funds," those that produced unusually good profits every year from 1982 through 1989.

It was amusing to watch a television interview of the manager of a hot fund. To what did he attribute his unusual success? The manager carried on at some length about waves, cycles, bulls and bears. But the fact is that his success might have been just luck. A simple probabilistic model accounts for the hot-fund phenomenon quite well. In the face of this model, investors are well advised to view any and all claims with a certain degree of skepticism.

Adapted from A.K. Dewdney. "Mathematical Recreations." *Scientific American*, March 1990. pp. 118-119.

39. Based on the passage, which of the following terms refers to the problem concerning the author?

(A) Birth conditions   (B) Innumeracy

(C) Illiteracy   (D) Math abuse

40. Based on the passage, which of the following can we reasonably conclude about the author's beliefs concerning birth rates?

(A) The nurse is in a position to know the details of birth rate cycles.

(B) It is more likely that fewer, rather than more, babies are born during a full moon.

(C) It is unlikely there is any statistical basis for the nurse's belief.

(D) Birth rates have nothing to do with math abuse.

41. Which of the following best describes the problem concerning the author?

(A) Not applying simple logical analysis to commonplace situations

(B) Incorrect estimation of birth rates

(C) Poor investment strategies

(D) Inappropriate travel plans

42. According to the author, how prevalent is the problem he describes in the passage?

    (A)   It only occurs in pediatrics.

    (B)   It occurs occasionally to some people.

    (C)   It occurs to most of us on a regular basis.

    (D)   It only occurs in the media.

43.   Which of the following does the author suggest is a reason for the nurse's belief about birth rates?

    (A)   Actual differences based on the moon's cycles

    (B)   A misunderstanding of the law of probability

    (C)   Undue emphasis on events which reinforce her belief

    (D)   The probabilities involved in casino games

44.   According to the passage, which of the following best describes the role filters play in math abuse?

    (A)   They cause people to avoid mathematics.

    (B)   They cause people to ignore events which are contrary to what they want to believe.

    (C)   They cause people to lose money.

    (D)   Filters have nothing to do with math abuse.

45.   According to the author, what is the filtering process occurring in casinos?

    (A)   Gamblers tend to win more often playing slot machines.

    (B)   There is a low probability of winning at slot machines.

    (C)   It is only obvious when people win playing slot machines.

    (D)   Casinos make the least amount of money on slot machines.

46.   Based on the passage, which of the following would the author most likely say does not suffer from math abuse?

    (A)   The probability of a coin toss

    (B)   Playing the lottery

    (C)   Media advertising

    (D)   Political statements

47.   What is the author suggesting by explaining the probabilities of coin tosses with respect to hot funds?

    (A)   That investing is based on chance

    (B)   That the laws of probability do not apply to investing

    (C)   That investing in hot funds is a wise strategy

    (D)   That some hot funds will occur simply by chance

48. If the suggestion about hot funds is correct, which of the following is most likely to be the author's advice about investing in a fund which has beat the market for eight years in a row?

   (A) Invest in it immediately.

   (B) Do not invest in it for the sole reason that it is hot.

   (C) Invest only a small amount in the hot fund.

   (D) Wait a year before investing.

PASSAGE VI (Questions 49–57)

Opponents of abortion often profess deep concern for the health of women. In literature and speeches, they suggest that abortion poses greater physical and psychological risks than childbirth. John C. Willke, president of the National Right to Life Committee, recently reiterated these claims to *Scientific American*. He said his belief in them rests on his experience as an obstetrician and on anecdotal reports, primarily from others in the anti-abortion movement. "There are no good, hard statistics on this," he said, "but there are none on the other side either."

In fact, government statistics clearly show legal abortion to be safer than giving birth. Data compiled by the National Center for Health Statistics from 1981 to 1985 indicate that abortion was 11 times less likely than childbirth to lead to a woman's death. Researchers at the Centers for Disease Control reported in 1982 that women undergoing abortions are 100 times less likely to have complications requiring major abdominal surgery than women bearing children.

The question of psychological harm has been more difficult to assess. Indeed, C. Everett Koop, the former Surgeon General, judged past studies to be inconclusive. Now, however, a group at the Johns Hopkins School of Hygiene and Public Health has provided "hard statistics" on this issue.

The researchers studied 334 black urban teenagers who entered clinics in Baltimore to be tested for pregnancy. The homogeneity of the group reduced the chances that the study's results would be skewed by other variables, according to Laurie Schwab Zabin, who performed the study with Marilyn B. Hirsch. The teenagers were initially interviewed before they or the researchers knew the results of the pregnancy tests. They were then divided into three groups—those who bore a child, those who had an abortion and those who were not pregnant—and tracked for two years.

The investigators' report in *Family Planning Perspectives* concluded that those who chose abortion were less likely to undergo adverse psychological episodes (as measured by three separate psychological tests) than either those who bore children or those who had not been pregnant. They were also more likely to remain in school and less likely to become pregnant again.

"The right-to-lifers have been saying that it is terrible to let young women go through abortions," Zabin says. "Our study shows we should lay that ghost to rest. Not only is abortion a medically safe procedure; we now know it is psychologically safe."

Poor urban teenagers represent an important minority of all those who elect to have abortions, Zabin notes. They are the most likely to be affected by laws proposed in a number of states that would limit the use of public funds for abortion, require minors to gain consent from parents or otherwise restrict the practice of abortion.

Moreover, such laws could help give more substance to Willke's claims if they hinder women from obtaining timely abortions. Numerous studies show that the risks of medical complications rise significantly when abortions are performed after 16 weeks of pregnancy.

Adapted from John Horgan. "Right to Lie?" *Scientific American*, April 1990, pp. 14, 18.

49. Based on the passage, from which of the following are "hard statistics" most likely derived?

(A) Personal experience

(B) Research studies

(C) Anecdotal reports

(D) Patient histories

50. Based on the information in the second and last paragraph, it can be inferred that a legal abortion

(A) must be court-ordered.

(B) is risk-free.

(C) would be performed before the 16th week of pregnancy.

(D) would be 11 times more likely than childbirth to lead to a woman's death.

51. Based on the passage, which of the following types of abortion statistics were gathered without difficulty?

I. Death due to abortions versus childbirth

II. Medical complications following abortions versus childbirth

III. Psychological effects following abortions versus childbirth

(A) I and II.

(B) I and III.

(C) II and III.

(D) I, II, and III.

52. According to the author, which of the following is true with respect to studies, prior to the Johns Hopkins study, attempting to determine the psychological effects of having an abortion?

(A) The Johns Hopkins study was the first on the topic.

(B) A former Surgeon General found previous studies did not reach any reliable conclusions.

(C) The author determined that all previous studies were unscientific and did not use statistics.

(D) Previous studies only dealt with anecdotal data.

53. Based on the passage, which of the following statements best describes the findings of the National Center for Health Statistics and the Centers for Disease Control?

(A) Death and complications following an abortion are much less likely than after childbirth.

(B) Death and complications following an abortion are much more lilely than after childbirth.

(C) Death and complications following an abortion are slightly less likely than after childbirth.

(D) Death is less likely following an abortion, but the probability of complications increases.

54. According to the author, which of the following is true with respect to the findings of Zabin and Hirsch?

(A) Subjects having abortions were more likely to suffer psychological episodes than those who were not pregnant, but no more likely than those who gave birth.

(B) Subjects having abortions were less likely to suffer psychological episodes than those in either of the other groups.

(C) Subjects having abortions were more likely to suffer psychological episodes than those in either of the other groups.

(D) Their findings were inconclusive.

55. The author quotes Zabin as saying, "Our study shows we should lay that ghost to rest." What "ghost" is Zabin referring to?

(A) Right-to-lifers

(B) The person who actually wrote up the report

(C) The fear of death due to abortion

(D) The fear of psychological harm to young women

56. The Zabin and Hirsch study focused exclusively on black urban teenagers. Which of the following was not specifically mentioned as an advantage of such a limited focus?

I. Avoid the influence of other variables

II. Extension of the findings to other groups

III. This group is most likely to be affected by certain anti-abortion laws

(A) I only.   (B) II only.

(C) III only.   (D) I and II.

57. Based on the passage, why does the author suggest anti-abortion laws might actually cause the problems claimed by Willke?

(A) They will force those wanting an abortion to commit crimes.

(B) They will allow the performance of illegal abortions.

(C) They will keep women from obtaining abortions before it becomes dangerous.

(D) They will force women to lose their privacy when they request public funding to have an abortion.

PASSAGE VII (Questions 58–65)

Although democratic nations are founded on the principle of individual liberties and rights, there clearly must be a balance between the scope of individual freedom and the needs of government. Theoretically, individual rights must be curtailed where their exercise constitutes a threat to the very preservation of the nation or of the states and local communities within it. Whether a nation, a state, or a locality, the community at large does have a public interest that it can and should pursue with diligence. In the broadest sense, the decisions made by legislative majorities reflect community interests, although such interests are also represented by the executive and the judiciary. Only at the federal level is the judiciary independent of direct political control, under the system of separation of powers and checks and balances. At the state and local levels, judges are still mostly elected, making them directly accountable to the people. An elected judiciary is less likely to stand apart from the political process in making its decisions on the scope of individual liberties and rights. Such rights therefore are more likely to be limited if there is a public clamor for their restriction (as, for example, where the elected officials of localities respond to local public opinion by demanding controls over "obscene" magazines, movies, and books).

While there may be political excesses that threaten to limit civil liberties and rights, there are also legitimate governmental needs that may call for a modification of individual freedoms. This occurs when these civil freedoms are used, or misused, to attack the very foundations of the system itself. This problem becomes most acute during times of war or civil unrest. During such times the Supreme Court has given the government wide powers to curb individual freedom.

Perhaps the most extraordinary abridgment of the rights of citizens occurred in 1941, when a Japanese attack was considered by large numbers of people within and outside the government, including military leaders, to be an imminent possibility on the West Coast. An even more likely probability considered was sabotage and subversion by Japanese infiltrators. These fears eventually led to the establishment of concentration camps for Japanese-Americans, largely based upon an executive order by President Roosevelt, a decision that was upheld by the Supreme Court, against constitutional challenges in *Korematsu v. United States* in 1944. Writing for the majority of the Court, Justice Hugo Black said that during wartime, military necessity justified the order, which excluded Japanese-Americans from the West Coast. Did the exclusionary order constitute racial discrimination? No. The Court said that although only the Japanese-Americans were excluded, the reason was not of race but of military necessity. *Korematsu* was an extreme case, but it illustrates the degree to which civil rights have been denied on the basis of the public interest.

In drawing the line between public interest and individual freedom, the Supreme Court has relied upon the "balancing test," which attempts to weigh the needs of government against the rights of individuals to determine the proper balance between permissible government restraints and individual freedom. One of the most important spheres of civil liberties, where the balancing test has been applied, regards the civil liberties and rights enumerated in the First Amendment, particularly the liberties of speech, press, and the right of assembly. In addition to the balancing test, the "clear and present danger" test is used in determining the permissible scope of political speech, press, and assembly. In this political sphere the clear and present danger test is used to judge the extent to which Congress or the state legislatures may regulate and control the expression of political ideas.

Adapted from Peter Woll and Robert H. Binstock. *America's Political System*, 4th edition. New York: Random House, 1984. pp. 95-96.

58. Based on the passage, with which of the following statements would the authors be most likely to agree?

    (A) Individual rights are superior to governmental needs

    (B) Governmental needs are superior to individual rights

    (C) A balance must be struck between individual rights and governmental needs

    (D) Political excesses can never limit civil liberties

59. Based on the passage, we can reasonably infer which of the following?

    (A) Local judges are mostly elected.

    (B) Federal judges are mostly elected.

    (C) State judges are not accountable to the people.

    (D) Federal judges are not elected.

60. According to the authors, which of the following are in a better position to protect individual liberties?

    (A) Members of Congress   (B) Federal judges

    (C) State judges   (D) The president

61. Based on the passage, what type of governmental needs can justify limitations on individual liberties?

    (A) Any type of governmental need

    (B) Those needs which restrict civil rights

    (C) Those which threaten the nation

    (D) No governmental need justifies limitations on individual liberties.

62. According to the authors, what was the justification for the abridgment of rights in *Korematsu*?

    (A) Fear of Japanese invasion   (B) Racial discrimination

    (C) Public opinion   (D) Electoral pressures

63. Based on the passage, the establishment of concentration camps for Japanese-Americans was found to be which of the following?

    (A) Justified   (B) Illegal

    (C) Unconstitutional   (D) Unnecessary

64. Which of the following liberties is not specifically mentioned in the passage as a First Amendment liberty?

(A)   Speech   (B)   Press

(C)   Religion   (E)   Assembly

65.   Based on the passage, which of the following tests may allow restrictions on civil rights and liberties?

I.   Balancing test

II.   Rational basis test

III.   Clear and present danger test

(A)   I and II.   (B)   I and III.

(C)   II and III.   (D)   I, II, and III.

STOP

If time still remains, you may review work only in this section.

When the time allotted is up, you may go on to the next section.

Section 2 — Physical Sciences

TIME: 100 Minutes
QUESTIONS: 66-142

> **DIRECTIONS:** Most of the questions in this section are arranged in groups, each corresponding to a descriptive passage. Based on the information given in a passage, choose the one best answer to each question in the group. Some questions are independent of a descriptive passage and of each other. Choose the one best answer to each of these questions. If you are not sure of an answer, eliminate those choices that you know are incorrect and choose an answer from among those remaining. Fill in the corresponding circle on the answer sheet to indicate your answer. You may refer to the periodic table at any time.

PASSAGE I (Questions 66-72)

Starch is a polymer consisting of many glucose monomer units. The enzyme amylase, found in human saliva, catalyzes the hydrolysis (reaction with water) of starch to form simple glucose molecules (molecular formula $C_6H_{12}O_6$. molar mass 180 g/mol). Within the human body, a series of complex reactions oxidizes glucose to carbon dioxide and water with the liberation of energy. The overall chemical equation for the oxidation of glucose is:

$$C_6H_{12}O_6 \text{ (s)} + 6O_2 \text{ (g)} \longrightarrow 6CO_2 \text{ (g)} + 6H_2O \text{ (l)}$$

$\Delta H° = -2803$ kJ   (Reaction 1)

Glucose is a very important source of energy in humans and other animals. Another source of metabolic energy is fat. A typical fat, glyceryl trimyristate (from oil of nutmeg) has the molecular formula $C_{45}H_{86}O_6$ (molar mass 723 g/mol.). The equation for the combustion of this fat is:

$$C_{45}H_{86}O_6 \text{ (s)} + 63\frac{1}{2}O_2 \text{ (g)} \longrightarrow 45CO_2 \text{ (g)} + 43H_2O \text{ (l)}$$

$\Delta H° = -27820$ kJ   (Reaction 2)

In general, fats have much higher molar enthalpies of combustion than glucose and hence a small amount of fat may "contain a large number of calories." Food "calories" are usually measured as the heat of combustion of the food and expressed in kilocalories:

1 kcal = 4.18 kJ.

66. What percentage, by mass, of glyceryl trimyristate is carbon?

(A)   33%   (B)   45%

(C)   75%   (D)   92%

67. According to the equation for Reaction 1, how many moles of oxygen gas are required for the combustion of 60 g of glucose?

    (A) 1 mol   (B) 2 mol

    (C) 3 mol   (D) 6 mol

68. According to the equation for Reaction 2, what volume, measured at standard conditions (STP), of oxygen gas (assumed to behave as an ideal gas) is required for the combustion of 1.00 mol of glyceryl trymyristate? The molar volume of an ideal gas at STP is 22.4 L/mol.

    (A) 1.4 m^3 (B) 6.7 m^3

    (C) 22.4 m^3 (D) 63.5 m^3

69. All the energy liberated in the combustion of 0.100 mol of glucose (Reaction 1) is transferred to 1.00 kg of water in a well-insulated container. The initial temperature of water was 21.0°C. Assuming no heat loss or gain, what will be the final water temperature? The specific heat of water is 4.18 J/g °C.

    (A) 25.3°C   (B) 37.0°C

    (C) 50.5°C   (D) 88.1°C

70. The combustion of a certain amount of glucose liberated 125 mL of carbon dioxide gas measured at 37°C and 0.90 atm pressure. At what temperature will this sample of carbon dioxide gas occupy a volume of 175 mL at a pressure of 851 mm Hg?

    (A) 58°C   (B) 149°C

    (C) 267°C   (D) 540°C

71. In Reaction 1 glucose is oxidized. The oxidation number (oxidation state) of carbon increases in this reaction. By how much does the oxidation number of carbon change in Reaction 1?

    (A) 2   (B) 4

    (C) 6   (D) 8

72. How many "food calories" correspond to 5.0 g (about a teaspoonful) of glyceryl trimyristate?

    (A) 45 kcal   (B) 192 kcal

    (C) 247 kcal   (D) 522 kcal

PASSAGE II (Questions 73-78)

A chemist found an old bottle, containing a white powder, on the reagent shelf of her laboratory. The label on the bottle was partly worn away, leaving only the last three letters of the name of the contents of the bottle. These letters, "ose," suggested that the bottle might contain a sugar. In order to identify the white powder in the bottle, the chemist did several experiments.

Experiment 1. A solution was prepared by dissolving 1.500 g of the white powder in 10.00 g of water. It was noted that the temperature of the system decreased as the solution formed. The freezing point of the solution was measured to be − 1.90°C. It was noted that the solution did not conduct an electric current.

Experiment 2. Qualitative elemental analysis indicated that the white powder contained only carbon, hydrogen and oxygen. The white powder melted with a sharp, well-defined melting point, indicating that it is a pure compound.

Experiment 3. A 30.0 mg sample of the white powder was burned with excess oxygen in a combustion analysis apparatus. The carbon dioxide and water formed were collected and weighed. The mass of carbon dioxide obtained was 44.0 mg and that of water was 18.0 mg.

73. The solubility of the white powder in water

    (A) increases with increasing temperature.

    (B) decreases with increasing temperature.

    (C) remains the same with changing temperature.

    (D) changes with changing temperature, but the nature of the change cannot be deduced on the basis of the information given in Passage 2.

74. The density of the solution prepared in experiment 1 was 1.05 g/mL. What was its volume?

    (A) 9.5 mL   (B) 10.0 mL

    (C) 10.5 mL   (D) 11.0 mL

75. What is the approximate molecular weight of the white powder? The molal freezing point lowering constant for water is 1.86C°/m.

    (A) 98   (B) 147

    (C) 181   (D) 342

76. What is the simplest or empirical formula of the white powder?

    (A) CHO   (B) CH_2O

    (C) C_2H_2O (D) $C_{12}H_{22}O_{11}$

77. Knowledge of the approximate molecular weight, such as might be obtained from the data of experiment 1, and the simplest formula, such as might be obtained from experiment 3, may be combined to determine the molecular formula of a substance. If the approximate molecular weight of a substance which has the simplest formula CH is determined to be about 67, what is the molecular formula of the substance?

    (A) C_4H_4 (B) C_5H_5

    (C) C_6H_6 (D) C_7H_7

78. Which of the following best describes the interunit bonding within the crystals of the white powder?

(A)   Ionic

(B)   Metallic

(C)   Dispersive (London) forces only

(D)   Dipole-dipole forces

PASSAGE III (Questions 79-84)

An isotope of the fictitious, transuranium element mysterium has the following properties: Atomic number: 119; Mass number: 300; First ionization energy: 300 kJ/ mol; Alpha particle decay half life: 600 s.

Note that its atomic number places mysterium directly below francium, atomic number 87, in the periodic table. Mysterium was produced by bombardment of a uranium target with high energy uranium nuclei. The target, containing unreacted uranium, mysterium, and many other reaction products was dissolved and the mysterium separated by a series of precipitation and ion exchange reactions. The first time mysterium was produced, the chemical separation required 30.0 minutes and the quantity of mysterium recovered was 1.0 mg.

79.   Which of the following properties is *least likely* to be true of mysterium chloride?

(A)   It is a white, crystalline solid at 25°C.

(B)   It is soluble in cold water.

(C)   It forms ionically bonded crystals.

(D)   It forms elemental mysterium when strongly heated.

80.   If the production of mysterium involved the reaction of $^{238}_{92}U$ with $^{238}_{92}U$ and only one product in addition to the $^{300}_{119}My$ was produced, what is the symbol for the other product?

(A) ^{300}Zn (B) ^{176}Tb

(B) ^{191}At (E) ^{258}Md

81.   Using the symbol My for mysterium, what is the formula of mysterium sulfate?

(A) My_2SO_4 (B) $MySO_4$

(C) $My_2(SO_4)_3$ (D) $My(SO_4)_2$

82.   What is the second ionization energy of mysterium?

(A)   150 kJ/mol   (B)   300 kJ/mol

(C)   320 kJ/mol   (D)   1250 kJ/mol

83.   What is the atomic number of the alpha particle decay product of mysterium?

(A)   115   (B)   117

(C)   121   (D)   123

84. The first time mysterium was produced, what mass of mysterium was present in the target at the end of the bombardment just before the start of the chemical separation? Assume no loss in the separation process.

(A) 0.1 mg   (B) 1.0 mg

(C) 3.0 mg   (D) 8.0 mg

QUESTIONS 85-90 are NOT based on a descriptive passage.

---

85. A car travels at a rate of 30 kilometers/hour for 15 kilometers. It then increases its average speed to 60 kilometers/hour for the next 30 kilometers. The overall average speed for the 45 km is

(A) 30 km/hr.   (B) 35 km/hr.

(C) 40 km/hr.   (D) 45 km/hr.

86. A brick falls from the top of a tall building (1200 ft). How many seconds will it take for the brick to hit the ground?

(A) 8.66 sec   (B) 75 sec

(C) 7.5 sec   (D) 32 sec

87. A gas placed under 1 atmosphere absolute pressure occupies a volume of 2 cubic meters at 250°K. What will be the new volume if the temperature is increased to 294°K?

(A) $5.8 \, m^3$ (B) $2.35 \, m^3$

(C) $2 \, m^3$ (D) $588 \, m^3$

88. Cellulose is a natural polymer composed of monomer

(A) glucagon.   (B) amino acids.

(C) glucose.   (D) amides.

89. What is the product of the following reaction?

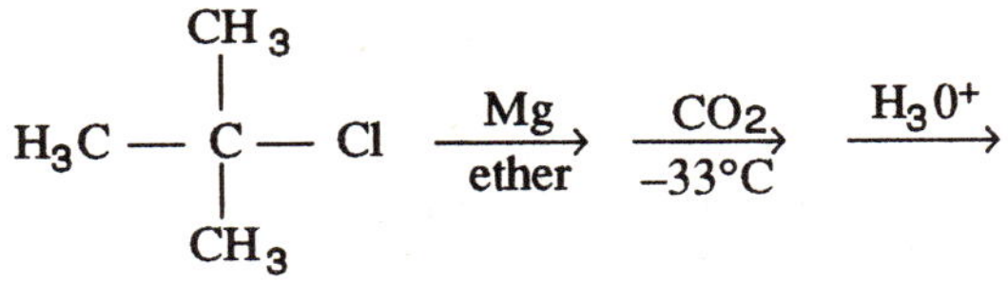

$$H_3C - \underset{\underset{CH_3}{|}}{\overset{\overset{CH_3}{|}}{C}} - Cl \xrightarrow[\text{ether}]{Mg} \xrightarrow[-33°C]{CO_2} \xrightarrow{H_3O^+}$$

(A) 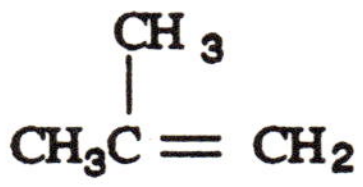 $CH_3\underset{\overset{|}{CH_3}}{C} = CH_2$

(B) 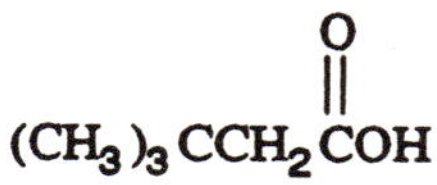 $(CH_3)_3 CCH_2 \overset{\overset{O}{||}}{C}OH$

(C) $(CH_3)_3 C\overset{\overset{O}{||}}{C}CH_3$

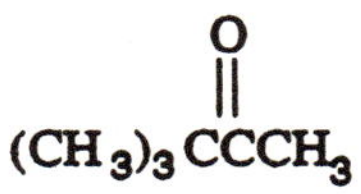

(D) 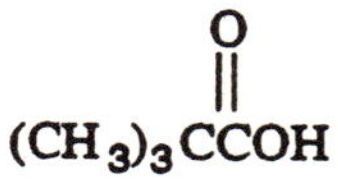 $(CH_3)_3 C\overset{\overset{O}{||}}{C}OH$

90. Glycine and glucose are similar in that

    (A) they are sugars.

    (B) they are ketones.

    (C) they react with Grignard reagent.

    (D) they have similar heats of combustion.

PASSAGE IV (Questions 91-97)

An independent testing laboratory tested the effectiveness of four antacids. The procedure used was to first dissolve the antacid in standard hydrochloric acid solution and then titrate the excess, unreacted hydrochloric acid with standard sodium hydroxide solution. Phenolphthalein indicator was used. Phenolphthalein has an acid-base pH range such that the titration was stopped, i.e., the end point of the titration was reached, at pH = 9.0. The table below lists the average volume of 0.100 M sodium hydroxide solution needed to titrate the excess hydrochloric acid. In each case, 0.750 g of the antacid was reacted with 25.00 mL of 0.5000 HCl solution.

Antacid	Volume of NaOH/mL
Brand A	39.84
Brand B	40.12
Brand C	37.50
Baking soda	35.70

The baking soda was pure sodium hydrogen carbonate (sodium bicarbonate, $NaHCO_3$) and brand C was milk of magnesia, a suspension of magnesium hydroxide $[Mg(OH)_2]$ in water. The baking soda acts as a weak base through the hydrolysis of the bicarbonate ion:

$$HCO_3^- + H_2O \longrightarrow H_2CO_3 + OH^- \quad Kb = 2.4 \times 10^{-8}.$$

Magnesium hydroxide is a strong base but has low solubility in water. Its solubility product constant is $Ksp = 1.8 \times 10^{-11}$.

91. What volume of 0.1000 M sulfuric acid solution could be neutralized to the phenolphthalein end point by 0.750 g of brand B antacid?

    (A) 9.88 mL

    (B) 25.0 mL

    (C) 35.7 mL

    (D) 42.5 mL

92. According to the Bronsted-Lowry theory of acids and bases, what is the conjugate acid of hydroxide ion in the hydrolysis of bicarbonate ion?

    (A) HCO_3^-

    (B) H_2O

    (C) H_2CO_3

    (D) There is none.

93. What is the hydroxide ion concentration at the end point of the titration of HCl solution with NaOH solution using phenolphthalein as the indicator?

    (A) 1×10^{-5}

    (B) 1×10^{-7}

    (C) 1×10^{-9}

    (D) 1×10^{-11}

94. Which of the titration curves below best represents the titration of HCl solution with NaOH solution (the NaOH solution is added from a buret to the HCl solution)?

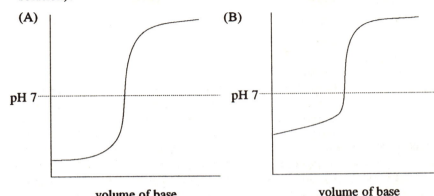

(A) pH 7 ... volume of base

(B) pH 7 ... volume of base

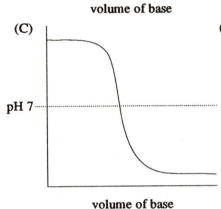
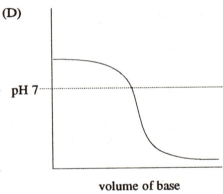

(C) pH 7 ... volume of base

(D) pH 7 ... volume of base

95. If the chemical equation for the naturalization of magnesium hydroxide by hydrochloric acid is balanced using the smallest possible set of integer coefficients, what is the coefficient of HCl?

(A) 1   (B) 2

(C) 3   (D) 4

96. Assuming that the only reaction which takes place is the hydrolysis of bicarbonate ion, what is the pH of a 0.42 M sodium bicarbonate solution?

(A) 4.0   (B) 6.0

(C) 8.0   (D) 10.0

97. What is the pH of a solution that is saturated in magnesium hydroxide and also 0.18 M in magnesium chloride?

(A) 7.0   (B) 9.0

(C) 11.0   (D) 13.0

PASSAGE V (Questions 98-102)
The rates of many biochemical reactions may be analyzed using the Michaelis-

Menton mechanism for enzyme kinetics. This model uses a two-step mechanism. In the first step the enzyme (E) reacts with the substrate (S) to form an enzyme-substrate complex (ES). In the second step the enzyme-substrate complex decomposes to regenerate the enzyme and form the product (P).

$$\text{Step 1} \quad E + S \overset{k}{\underset{k'}{\rightleftharpoons}} ES$$

$$\text{Step 2} \quad ES \overset{k''}{\rightleftharpoons} E + P$$

Note that the total concentration of enzyme (TE = E + ES) is constant. An expression for the rate of formation of product may be obtained using the steady state approximation. It is assumed that the rate of formation of ES is equal to its rate of disappearance.

$$k[E] [S] = k'[ES] + k''[ES] \qquad \text{(Reaction 3)}$$

Substituting [TE] - [ES] for [E], rearranging, and letting Km = (k' + k'')/k leads to:

$$[ES] = [TE] [S] / (Km + [S]) \qquad \text{(Reaction 4)}$$

The rate of product formation, from step 2, is equal to k''[ES]. Substituting for [ES] using equation (4) gives

$$\text{Rate of product formation} = k''[TE][S] / (Km + [S]) \qquad \text{(Reaction 5)}$$

This somewhat awkward expression for the rate of product formation may be simplified for two limiting cases. If the concentration of substrate is very small, i.e., [S] << Km, then

$$\text{Rate of product formation} = k''[TE] [S] / Km \qquad \text{(Reaction 6)}$$

On the other hand, if the substrate concentration is very large, i.e., [S] >> Km, then

$$\text{Rate of product formation} = k''[TE] \qquad \text{(Reaction 7)}$$

98. The first step of the Michaelis-Menton mechanism is a bimolecular, second-order reaction. If the initial concentrations of both the enzyme (E) and substrate (S) are doubled, by what factor will the initial rate of formation of enzyme-substrate complex (ES) change?

   (A)   2   (B)   4

   (C)   8   (D)   16

99. What are the overall reaction orders for the rate expressions given in equations (6) and (7)?

   (A)   (6) is second order and (7) is first order.

   (B)   (6) is third order and (7) is first order.

   (C)   (6) is first order and (7) is zeroth order.

   (D)   Both are first order.

100. Equation (3) may be rearranged into the form of an equilibrium constant:

$K_{eq} = [ES]/[E] [S].$

What is K_{eq} expressed in terms of rate constants?

(A) $k/(k'k'')$ (B) $k'k''/k$

(C) $1/Km$ (D) Km

101. Which graph below best represents the dependence of the rate of product formation (R) on the substrate concentration ([S]) according to the Michaelis-Menton mechanism, equation (5)?

(A)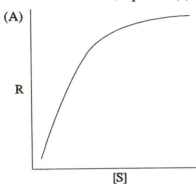

(B)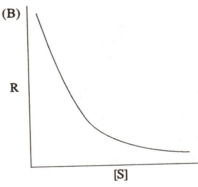

(C)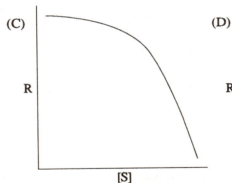

(D)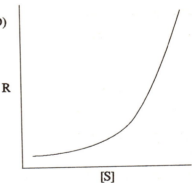

102. Equation (6) leads to the following expression for the concentration of substrate with time:

$\ln[S] = \ln[So] - Ct$

where [So] is the initial substrate concentration and C is a constant which depends on the rate constants and total enzyme concentration. What is the half time for the disappearance of substrate under these conditions?

(A) $\ln C/2$ (B) $2/\ln C$

(C) $C/\ln 2$ (D) $\ln 2/C$

PASSAGE VI Questions 103-107)
    In the old dollar bill game, one person (the dropper) suspends a dollar bill by one end, so that its midpoint is between the separated thumb and forefinger of a second

person (the catcher). The rules of the game are as follows: The catcher must keep his/her hand stationary, but as soon as the bill has been released by the dropper, he/she may catch it between the thumb and forefinger. If the bill is caught, the catcher may keep it.

The dimensions of a dollar bill are such (about 6 cm by 16 cm) that the distance from the top where it is held by the dropper, to the position of the thumb and forefinger of the catcher is 8 cm. The mass of a dollar bill is about 2.5 g.

Air resistance may be ignored for the first 16 cm of fall because the speed of the bill is very small. At higher speeds, after the bill has fallen further, air resistance is important. However, to analyze the game, free fall, with constant acceleration of 9.80 m/s², due to gravity, may be assumed.

The average person's reaction time is 0.2 s. Usually the game is played in a stationary room, but it could be played in an elevator that is either ascending or descending.

103. Starting from rest, how long does it take the bill to fall freely a distance of 8 cm?

(A)   0.03 s   (B)   0.09 s

(C)   0.13 s   (D)   0.20 s

104. What is the kinetic energy of the bill after it has fallen freely, starting from rest, through a distance of 8 cm?

(A)   2 mJ   (B)   7 mJ

(C)   15 mJ   (D)   25 mJ

105. If the dollar bill game were played in an elevator ascending at a uniform speed of 4.9 m/s

(A)   the catcher would have a 50% better chance of success.

(B)   the catcher would have a 25% better chance of success.

(C)   the catcher would have a 25% poorer chance of success.

(D)   the catcher would have the same chance of success as when the game was played in the elevator while at rest.

106. If the catcher were allowed to place his/her thumb and forefinger near the bottom of the bill, 16 cm from the top edge, the catcher would have more time to react. By what factor does the free fall time increase if the distance increases from 8 cm to 16 cm?

(A) $\frac{1}{2}$ (B) $\sqrt{2}$

(C)   2   (D)   4

107. The resisting force, due to air resistance, as the bill falls through distances greater than its own length is proportional to the bill's speed. If after falling more than 100 cm the bill attains a constant terminal speed of 7.0 m/s, what is the value of the proportionality constant between the resisting force and the bill's speed?

(A) 0.5 g/s   (B) 1.5 g/s

(C) 2.5 g/s   (D) 3.5 g/s

QUESTIONS 108-112 are NOT based on a descriptive passage.

108. What is the product of the following reaction?

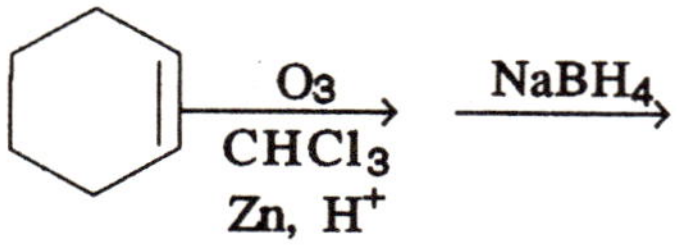

(A)

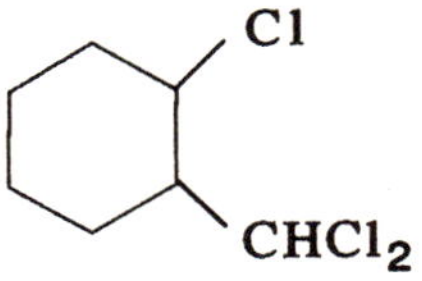

(B)

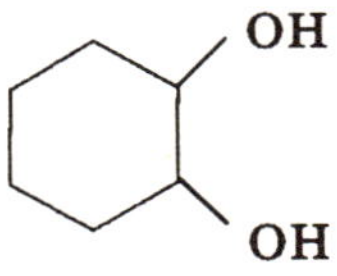

(C) 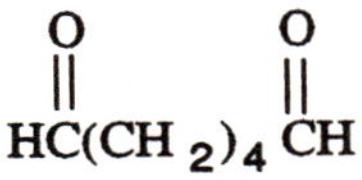 $HC(CH_2)_4CH$ (with two O double bonds)

(D) $HO(CH_2)_6OH$

109. Which of the following has the greatest vapor pressure?

(A) CH_3CL (B) CH_3CH_2Cl

(C) $CH_3CH_2CH_2CL$ (D) $(CH_3)_3CCl$

110. All of the following share the same crystal structure except:

(A) LiCl   (B) NaCl

(C) KCl   (D) CsCl

111. Which of the following is not characteristic of an exothermic reaction?

(A) The potential energy of the reactants is lower than the potential energy of the products.

(B) There is a positive ΔH.

(C) There is no energy of activation.

(D) (A), (B), and (C).

112. The density of a steel alloy is 7.8 gm/cm^3. What would be the mass of a 2 meter × 3 meter × 5 meter block constructed out of this alloy?

(A) 2.34 gm   (B) 2.34×10^8 gm

(C) 234 gm   (D) 3900 gm

PASSAGE VII (Questions 113–118)

A person holds a 10 pound (4.54 kg) steel ball in his hand, with the forearm horizontally extended and the upper arm vertically extended. The elbow joint exerts a force, *F*, downward on the forearm. The biceps muscle exerts an upward tension, T, on the forearm, at a distance of 2″ (5.08 cm) from the elbow joint. The center of mass of the forearm is located 6″ (15.24 cm) from the elbow joint. The weight of the forearm is 3 pounds (mass 1.36 kg). The center of mass of the steel ball resting in the person's hand is 15″ (38.1 cm) from the elbow joint. The whole system is motionless, thus the two conditions of static equilibrium apply: the net force must be zero and the net torque must be zero. The situation is diagrammed in the figure below.

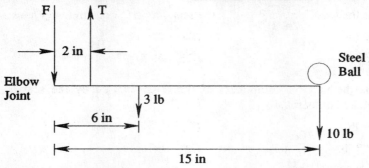

If the person drops the steel ball he may then hold his arm in an outstretched, horizontal position through the action of the deltoid muscle. The deltoid muscle is connected from the scapula (shoulder blade) to the humerus at a point 6″ (15.24 cm) from the shoulder joint. The angle between the tension (*T′*) in the deltoid muscle and the humerus is 17° (sin 17° = 0.29, cos 17° = 0.96). The scapula exerts a force (*F′*) on the humerus at the shoulder joint. This force makes an angle of 9.3° (sin 9.3° = 0.16, cos 9.3° = 0.99) with the horizontal. The center of mass of the outstretched arm is located 13″ (23.02 cm) from the shoulder joint and the weight of the arm is 8 pounds (mass 3.63 kg). This situation is diagrammed below. The acceleration due to gravity is 9.8 m/s²

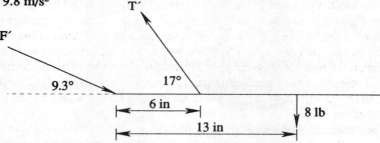

113. What is the weight of the steel ball in newtons?

    (A)   0.46 N   (B)   1.02 N

    (C)   44 N   (D)   98 N

114. What is the tension in the biceps muscle as the person holds the steel ball?

    (A)   13 lb   (B)   29 lb

    (C)   47 lb   (D)   84 lb

115. What is the force exerted on the forearm at the elbow joint as the person holds the steel ball?

    (A) 71 lb   (B) 97 lb

    (C) 115 lb   (D) 227 lb

116. What is the tension exerted by the deltoid muscle on the outstretched humerus?

    (A) 20 lb   (B) 60 lb

    (C) 75 lb   (D) 115 lb

117. What is the total force exerted by the scapula on the outstretched humerus?

    (A) 9 lb   (B) 27 lb

    (C) 58 lb   (D) 66 lb

118. What is the vertical component of the force exerted by the scapula on the outstretched humerus?

    (A) 9 lb   (B) 27 lb

    (C) 58 lb   (D) 66 lb

PASSAGE VIII (Questions 119-126)

In the human eye, light is focused on the retina by the combined action of the cornea and lens. A simplified model of the eye, the reduced eye, ignores the lens by assuming that the cornea is filled with a fluid of index of refraction 1.47 rather than the actual value of 1.33. For angles small enough such that the sine of the angle may be approximated by the value of the angle in radians, the object (p) and image (q) distances are related to the radius of curvature of the cornea by:

$$n'/p + n/q = (n - n')/R \qquad \text{(Equation 1)}$$

For (p) very large, this leads to the focal length (f) of the reduced eye: $f = nR/(n-n')$ where R is the radius of curvature of the cornea, n is the index of refraction of the fluid within the eyeball ($n = 1.47$), and n' is the index of refraction of the medium outside the eye ($n'' = 1.00$ for an object viewed in air.) The distance from the cornea to the retina is 24 mm for a typical eye. The radius of curvature of the cornea, when viewing an object at a very great distance, is 7.7 mm. You may wish to verify that the image of an object infinitely far away will be focused on the retina, by the cornea, in this model of the eye.

The retina consists of a large number of closely spaced, light-sensitive, receptor cells. These cells vary slightly in size and spacing. In the most acute part of the eye (the fovea centralis), where the color sensitive cells are packed tightly, they are about one micrometer between centers. Outside this region they are 3 μm to 5 μm apart. Also, away from the fovea are the rod cells used in night vision. Two points of light from an object will not be seen as two distinct points, unless the images fall on non-adjacent receptors. In a typical eye, the distance between non-adjacent cells is 2 μm. Since the distance from the center of curvature of the cornea to the retina is about 16 mm, the angular separation, in radians, of two object points which can just be resolved is $r = x/16$ mm, where x is the linear separation of non-adjacent receptor cells. Visual acuity is the reciprocal of the angular resolution expressed in minutes of arc.

119. The speed of light is 3.0×10^8 m/s in vacuum. What is the speed of light in a medium with index of refraction 1.47?

    (A) 1.0×10^8 m/s   (B) 2.0×10^8 m/s

    (C) 3.0×10^8 m/s   (D) 4.0×10^8 m/s

120. Light traveling in air strikes the surface of a medium with index of refraction 1.47 at an angle of incidence of 5°. What is the angle of refraction, in radians?

    (A) 0.059   (B) 0.087

    (C) 0.128   (D) 0.243

121. For the reduced eye model, to what value must the radius of curvature of the cornea change if the image of an object at 250 mm in air is to fall on the retina 24 mm behind the cornea?

    (A) 5.6 mm   (B) 7.2 mm

    (C) 7.7 mm   (D) 8.2 mm

122. The focal length of the "normal" reduced eye is 24 mm corresponding to the cornea to retina distance. If the focal length of an "abnormal" reduced eye were 30 mm, but the cornea to retina distance still 24 mm, what must be the focal length of a corrective lens (eye glasses)?

    (A) 30 mm   (B) 60 mm

    (C) 120 mm   (D) 240 mm

123. If an object of length 20 cm is viewed from a distance of 120 cm by a normal reduced eye (cornea to retina distance of 24 mm), what is the size of the image on the retina?

    (A) 2 mm   (B) 3 mm

    (C) 4 mm   (D) 5 mm

124. For receptor spacing of 1 μm, the visual acuity is 2.3. That is, the angular resolution is about 26 seconds of arc. How closely spaced may two dots be, if when viewed from a distance of 250 mm, they can just be resolved with visual acuity 2.3?

    (A) 2 μm   (B) 31 μm

    (C) 1.02 mm   (D) 109 mm

125. The human eye responds to visible light in the approximate wavelength range 400 nm to 700 nm. To what region of the electromagnetic spectrum does radiation of wavelength 1 μm, approximately the spacing of receptor cells in the fovea centralis, correspond?

    (A) X-ray   (B) Ultraviolet

    (C) Infrared   (D) Microwave

126. The human eye is very sensitive to light which has an energy per quantum of 3.6×10^{-19} J. What is the wavelength of this light? The speed of light is 3.0×10^8 m/s and Planck's constant is 6.6×10^{-34} j s.

    (A) 500 nm

    (B) 550 nm

    (C) 700 nm

    (D) 850 nm

PASSAGE IX (Questions 127-132)

   The electrical circuit in an X-ray room is 120 V and has a 20 A circuit breaker. The small X-ray unit plugged into this circuit draws a current of 8 A. In addition to the X-ray unit, a 1200 W coffee maker is plugged into this circuit. The X-ray unit contains both a step-up and a step-down transformer. The step-down transformer converts the 120 V to 6 V to heat the cathode of the X-ray tube to produce electrons. The step-up transformer converts the 120 V to 48000 V, which is then rectified, and used to accelerate the electrons within the X-ray tube where they collide with the anode to produce the X-rays. The X-ray unit contains many electrical circuits. A small part of one of these circuits is diagrammed below. In this portion of the circuit, a 10 ohm resistor is connected in series with a 5 ohm resistor and this combination is in parallel with a 15 ohm resistor.

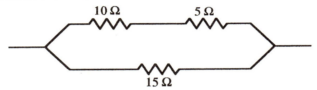

127. What power is used by the X-ray unit when it operates at 8 A and 120 V?

    (A) 15 S

    (B) 240 W

    (C) 960 W

    (D) 7680 W

128. What is the resistance of the coffee maker?

    (A) 2 ohm

    (B) 6 ohm

    (C) 10 ohm

    (D) 12 ohm

129. What is the ratio of the number of turns of wire on the primary to the number of turns on the secondary of the step-down transformer (120 V to 6 V) in the X-ray unit?

    (A) 1/720

    (B) 1/20

    (C) 20/1

    (D) 720/1

130. What single resistor is equivalent to the combination of resistors described and diagrammed above?

    (A) 7.5 ohm

    (B) 15 ohm

    (C) 22.5 ohm

    (D) 30 ohm

131. What is the kinetic energy of an electron which has been accelerated from rest through a potential difference of 48000 V? The mass and charge of an electron

are 1.60×10^{-19} C and 9.11×10^{-31} kg, respectively.

(A)   6 keV

(B)   12 keV

(C)   24 keV

(D)   48 keV

132.   If 75% of the power used by the 1200 W coffee maker heats the water (25% is lost to the surroundings), how much time will be required to heat 968 g of water from 20°C to 100°C? The specific heat of water is 4.18 J/°C g.

(A)   2 min

(B)   4 min

(C)   6 min

(D)   8 min

PASSAGE X (Questions 133-138)

Sound is a longitudinal pressure wave in the medium through which it is transmitted. The speed of sound depends on the density of the medium and temperature. For gases, the speed of sound is proportional to the square root of the absolute temperature. Approximate values of the speed of sound, near room temperature, in three materials, is given in the table below.

Material	Speed of Sound (m/s)
air	340
helium	1020
tissue	1600

The human ear can detect sound over a wide range of frequencies, extending from as low as 50 Hz to as high as 20 kHz. Ultrasound, with frequencies of a few megahertz, and wavelength of the order of 0.1 mm in tissue, is used as a diagnostic tool. For example, the reflection of a focused beam of ultrasound from a tumor may be used to locate the depth and size of the tumor.

The intensity level of sound is usually measured in decibels. The intensity level in decibels (db) is related to the intensity (I) or sound pressure (P) by db = 10 log

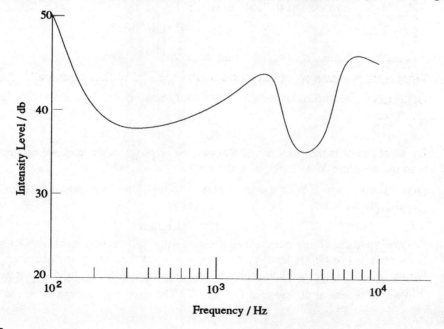

$(I/I_0) = 20 \log(P/P_0)$. The most commonly used reference is to take $P_0 = 200$ picobar $= 2 \times 10^{-5}$ N/m². The loudness of a sound, as detected by the human ear, varies with the intensity level and with the frequency or pitch of the sound. The loudness level, measured in a unit called a phon, is defined such that at a frequency of 1000 Hz, the intensity level in decibels is numerically equal to the loudness level in phons. At other frequencies the loudness level may be greater or smaller than the intensity level. The figure below shows the variation of the intensity level with frequency for a constant loudness level of 40 phons.

133. For a given wavelength and temperature, what is the ratio of the frequency of sound in helium to that in air?

    (A)   1/3

    (B)   3/1

    (C) $1/\sqrt{3}$

    (D) $\sqrt{3/1}$

134. The time interval between the ultrasound echos from the front and rear surfaces of a tumor was measured to be 10 μs. What is the thickness of the tumor?

    (A)   2 mm

    (B)   4 mm

    (C)   8 mm

    (D)   16 mm

135. The speed of sound in air is 340 m/s at 14°C. At what temperature is the speed of sound in air 310 m/s?

    (A)   - 34°C

    (B)   - 14°C

    (C)   0°C

    (D)   10°C

136. A violin string of length *L* is plucked and vibrates as shown below:

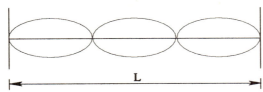

L

What is the wavelength of the sound wave produced by this vibration?

    (A)   *L*/3

    (B)   2*L*/3

    (C)   *L*/2

    (D)   3*L*/2

137. By what factor is the pressure of a sound wave of intensity level 40 db greater than the pressure of a 20 db intensity level sound wave?

    (A)   2

    (B)   5

    (C)   10

    (D)   20

138. According to the figure showing the relationship of intensity level to frequency for a constant loudness level of 40 phons, at what frequency in the range 100 Hz to 10 kHz is the human ear most sensitive to sound at a loudness level of 40 phons?

(A) 100 Hz	(B) 1000 Hz
(C) 4000 Hz	(D) 9000 Hz

QUESTIONS 139-142 are NOT based on a descriptive passage.

---

139. What is the kinetic energy of a 100 gram projectile traveling with a velocity of 60 m/sec?

(A) 60 joules	(B) 80 joules
(C) 100 joules	(D) 180 joules

140. The Newton is an expression of which relationship?

(A) $kg \cdot m/s$	(B) $grams \cdot cm/s^2$
(C) $slugs \cdot ft/s^2$	(D) $kg \cdot m/s^2$

141. Substances acting to reduce the actions of catalysts are known as

(A) anti-catalysis agents.	(B) inhibitors.
(C) regressors.	(D) homologs.

142. A thermally insulated ideal gas is compressed quasi-statically from an initial macrostate of volume V_0 and pressure p_0 to a final macrostate of volume V_f and pressure p_f. Calculate the work done on the gas in this process.

(A) $c_V / R \, (p_f V_f - p_0 V_0)$	(B) 0
(C) $(c_p - c_V) / R \, (p_f V_f - p_0 V_0)$	(D) $c_p / R \, (p_f V_f - p_0 V_0)$

STOP

If time still remains, you may review work only in this section.

When the time allotted is up, you may go on to the next section.

Section 3 — Writing Sample

TIME: 60 minutes
2 essays, separately timed
30 minutes each

DIRECTIONS: This section tests your writing skills by asking you to write two essays. You will have 30 minutes to write each one.

During the first 30 minutes, work only on the first essay. If you finish it in less than 30 minutes, you may review what you have written, but do not begin the second essay. During the second 30 minutes, work only on the second essay. If you finish it in less than 30 minutes, you may review what you have written for that essay only. Do not go back to the first essay.

Read each assigned topic carefully. Make sure your essays respond to the topics as they are assigned.

Make sure your essays are written in complete sentences and paragraphs, and are as clear as you can make them. Make any corrections or additions between the lines of your essays. Do not write in the margins.

On the day of the test, you are given three pages to write each essay. You are not required to use all of the space provided, but do not skip lines so you will not waste space. Illegible essays cannot be scored.

Part 1

Consider this statement:

"That government is best which governs least."

From *On The Duty of Civil Disobedience*, by Henry David Thoreau.

Write a comprehensive essay in which you accomplish the following objectives. Explain what you think the above statement means. Describe one or two specific situations in which the powers of government should be increased. Discuss what you think should be the basis for increasing or decreasing a government's powers.

STOP

If time still remains, you may review work only in this section.

When the time allotted is up, you may go on to the next section.

Part 2

Consider this statement:

"[Humans} cannot subsist on the scanty satisfaction which they can extort from reality."

From *Introductory Lectures on Psychoanalysis*, by Sigmund Freud.

Write a comprehensive essay in which you accomplish the following objectives. Explain what you think the above statement means. Describe one or two specific situations in which individuals have remained human while experiencing extreme frustration. Discuss what you think is the possibility of living a meaningful life while confronting the reality of suffering.

STOP

If time still remains, you may review work only in this section.

When the time allotted is up, you may go on to the next section.

Section 4 — Biological Sciences

TIME: 100 Minutes
QUESTIONS: 143-219

> **DIRECTIONS:** Most of the questions in this section are arranged in groups, each corresponding to a descriptive passage. Based on the information given in a passage, choose the one best answer to each question in the group. Some questions are independent of a descriptive passage and of each other. Choose the one best answer to each of these questions also. If you are not sure of an answer, eliminate those choices that you know are incorrect and choose an answer from among those remaining. Fill in the corresponding circle on the answer sheet to indicate your answer. You may refer to the periodic table at any time.

PASSAGE I (Questions 143-148)

Fluids within the body account for approximately 60% of body weight and are contained within several different compartments. Two-thirds of the body fluids are located intracellularly and the remaining one-third is extracellular. The extracellular fluid is divided into two components: the circulating blood plasma and the interstitial fluid. The body fluid compartments do not exist in isolation. Exchange of fluids can occur internally between compartments and between the external environment and the body fluid compartments as shown in Figure 1.

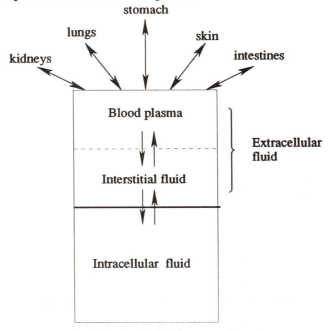

Figure 1 — The body fluid compartments.
The arrows indicate possible sites of fluid exchange.

It is possible to measure the size of the various body fluid compartments by injecting a substance into the compartment of interest, allowing adequate time for mixing to occur and then obtaining a sample of fluid from the compartment. The concentration of the injected substance in the sample is then determined. Using this information, the volume of fluid in which the substance was distributed can be calculated. The substance used should ideally remain only in the compartment of interest, distribute quickly and uniformly within the compartment, be removed slowly from the body, be non-toxic and easy to measure.

Extracellular fluid volume is difficult to measure because the boundaries of this space are difficult to define and few substances mix rapidly in all parts of the extracellular fluid (i.e., bone, cartilage). Interstitial fluid volume cannot be measured directly because substances that equilibrate in the interstitial fluid will also equilibrate in the plasma. It can, however, be calculated by subtracting plasma volume from extracellular fluid volume. In the same manner, intracellular fluid volume cannot be measured directly, but can be calculated by subtracting the extracellular fluid volume from total body water.

143. The primary force producing movement of water among the various body fluid compartments is

(A) Brownian motion.

(B) active transport.

(C) osmosis.

(D) facilitated diffusion.

144. Evans blue is an aniline dye that binds to proteins circulating in the blood. Which body fluid compartment could it be used to measure?

(A) Extracellular fluid

(B) Plasma volume

(C) Intracellular fluid

(D) Interstitital fluid

145. With the exception of blood cells, exchange of water and solutes between the intracellular compartment and the plasma

(A) can occur directly.

(B) does not take place at all.

(C) occurs only in highly perfused organs, such as the lungs and kidneys.

(D) can occur only indirectly, via movement through the interstitial fluid.

146. Normally the various body fluid compartments are in osmotic equilibrium. Therefore, a net loss of solute from the extracelluar fluid

(A) leads to hypotonicity of the extracellular fluid relative to the intracellular fluid.

(B) leads to hypotonicity of the intracellular fluid relative to the extracellular fluid.

(C) leads to hypertonicity of the extracellular fluid relative to the intracellular fluid.

(D) does not change the tonicity of the extracellular fluid or intracellular fluid.

147. Which of the following body fluid compartments is most susceptible to change?

   (A) Intracellular fluid

   (B) Interstitial fluid

   (C) Plasma volume

   (D) All compartments are equally susceptible.

148. The extracellular fluid volume of a 70 kg man was determined to be 14 liters. In this same individual, plasma volume was 3.5 liters. Therefore, interstitial fluid volume

   (A) is 17.5 liters.

   (B) is 10.5 liters.

   (C) cannot be determined because total body water was not measured.

   (D) is 7.0 liters.

PASSAGE II (Questions 149-154)

   Protein synthesis begins in the nucleus of a cell with the transfer of the genetic code from DNA to RNA via the process of transcription. Before leaving the nucleus, messenger RNA (mRNA) often undergoes post-transcriptional modification. Once the mRNA moves out of the nucleus, it associates with ribosomes and dictates the formation of a polypeptide chain via the process of translation. After the polypeptide chain is formed, it can be post-translationally modified by a variety of reactions to produce the final protein product.

   Insulin is a pancreatic hormone which undergoes the processes outlined above during its synthesis. The proinsulin gene located on chromosome 11 in humans serves as the template for mRNA synthesis in the nucleus. The mRNA is processed by removing 2 introns and adding a poly-A tail. In the cytoplasm, this mRNA chain serves as a template for the formation of a preproinsulin polypeptide chain. As this molecule enters the endoplasmic reticulum, its 23-amino acid leader sequence is removed. The molecule is then folded and 2 disulfide bonds form between the A and B chains to make proinsulin. Cleavage of a connecting segment between the A and B chains yields the insulin molecule which is secreted by the pancreas.

149. During which state of protein synthesis is the poly-A tail added?

   (A) Translation

   (B) Transcription

   (C) Post-translational modification

   (D) Post-transcriptional modification

150. Actinomycin D binds to DNA, preventing the polymerization of RNA on DNA. If actinoymcin D was added to a pancreatic tissue culture, which of the following molecules would be present inside the pancreatic cells 1 hour later?

   (A) Preproinsulin   (B) Proinsulin gene

   (C) Connecting peptide   (D) Insulin

151. Which of the following cellular structures is essential for transcription to occur?

   (A)   Nucleus   (B)   Ribosomes

   (C)   Endoplasmic reticulum   (D)   Golgi apparatus

152. The entire process of protein synthesis

   (A)   occurs only within the cell nucleus.

   (B)   is accomplished in a single step.

   (C)   requires many steps, some of which modify the protein.

   (D)   occurs only in the cell cytoplasm.

153. Post-translational modification of insulin involves

   (A)   adding a poly-A tail to the proinsulin gene.

   (B)   nothing; there is no post-translational modification of insulin.

   (C)   removal of 2 introns.

   (D)   removal of a leader sequence and folding.

154. In eukaryotes, the portions of the genes used for protein synthesis are usually located in several segments called exons which are separated by segments that are not translated called introns. The final mRNA which enters the cytoplasm

   (A)   is an unmodified transcription of the genetic code.

   (B)   is composed solely of introns because the exons have been removed during processing.

   (C)   contains alternating segments of introns and exons.

   (D)   is composed only of exons because the introns have been removed during processing.

PASSAGE III (Questions 155-160)

The long-term regulation of blood pressure is controlled by the kidneys because of an exquisite relationship which exists between blood pressure and urinary sodium output (Figure 2). If there is a rise in blood pressure above the normal, resting level, sodium and water excretion (output) will increase. This occurs in order to reduce blood volume, and hence, to return blood pressure to its normal level. If there is a fall in blood pressure, the kidneys will retain sodium and water and sodium excretion will decrease. The retention of sodium and water will cause blood volume to increase and blood pressure will rise back to its normal level. This regulatory mechanism operates around a constant level of blood pressure at which urinary sodium excretion is approximately equal to dietary sodium intake. Should blood pressure deviate from this set point, the kidneys will alter sodium excretion accordingly in an effort to restore blood pressure to normal. Conversely, if dietary sodium intake is changed, blood pressure must adjust to restore the balance between sodium intake and output. The shape, slope and set point of the curve shown in Figure 2 will vary from individual to individual.

A disease such as hypertension (high blood pressure) alters the relationship between sodium excretion and blood pressure such that a higher blood pressure is needed to excrete the same amount of sodium (i.e., sodium intake has not changed). Thus, the set point has been shifted upward and to the right on the curve. Diuretics, drugs that cause the kidneys to increase sodium and water excretion and thus tend to lower blood pressure, are commonly used to treat hypertension.

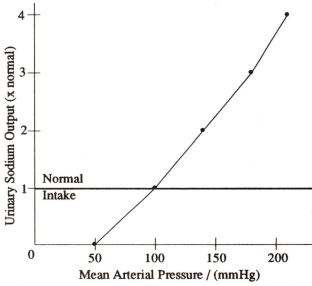

Figure 2 - Relationship between sodium output and blood pressure.

155. If a person with high blood pressure switches to a low sodium diet, which of the following should occur theoretically?

   (A) The kidneys will oppose the decrease in dietary sodium by retaining more sodium and blood pressure will rise even further.

   (B) Blood pressure will remain the same.

   (C) In order to maintain sodium balance, blood pressure should decrease.

   (D) Blood pressure will initially increase, but then will decrease back to the original hypertensive level.

156. Angiotensin, a powerful vasoconstrictor, shifts the entire curve shown in Figure 2 to the right on the x-axis. At the same level of sodium intake, the presence of angiotensin would

   (A) shift blood pressure to a higher level without changing sodium output.

   (B) have no effect upon the level of blood pressure.

   (C) increase urinary sodium output.

   (D) shift blood pressure to a lower level and decrease sodium output.

157. Patient A is more sensitive to change in dietary sodium than Patient B. When both are placed on a high salt diet, Patient A will

(A) exhibit a fall in blood pressure while Patient B's blood pressure will rise.

(B) have a rise in blood pressure similar to Patient B.

(C) show no change in blood pressure, while Patient B's blood pressure will fall.

(D) exhibit a greater rise in blood pressure than Patient B.

158. The relationship between sodium excretion and blood pressure is an example of a

(A) hormonally mediated event.

(B) negative feedback system.

(C) counter-current system.

(D) positive feedback system.

159. Would it be possible to remain hypertensive if there was no change in the set point between blood pressure and sodium excretion?

(A) No, because the kidneys would increase sodium and water excretion until blood pressure returned to normal, non-hypertensive level.

(B) Yes, because the set point is never altered.

(C) Yes, since blood pressure and kidney function are unrelated.

(D) Yes, because an increase in blood pressure does not have any long-term effect on kidney function.

160. If a person who is using diuretics to control blood pressure stops taking them for a period of several days, which of the following would most likely occur?

(A) Blood pressure would return to a hypertensive level because the kidneys would excrete less salt and water.

(B) Sodium and water excretion by the kidneys would increase leading to a further reduction in blood pressure.

(C) Renal function would remain unchanged because diuretics do not affect the kidneys.

(D) Blood pressure would remain at a normotensive level because the underlying defect in kidney function would have been corrected by the prior diuretic therapy.

QUESTIONS 161-166 are NOT based on a descriptive passage.

---

161. The connective tissue sac enclosing the heart is called the

(A) endothelium   (B) myocardium.

(C) pericardium   (D) vena cava.

162. The pumping chambers of the heart are called the

    (A)   atria.   (B)   ventricles.

    (C)   pacemakers.   (D)   cardiac muscles.

163. The process by which gases are exchanged in the alveoli of our lungs is called

    (A)   external respiration.   (B)   indirect respiration.

    (C)   internal respiration.   (D)   direct respiration.

164. Vitamin A is associated with

    (A)   blood coagulation.   (B)   liver function in some animals.

    (C)   bone growth.   (D)   skin epithelial maintenance.

165. Why do α-amino acids differ from β-amino acids?

    (A)   They constitute an enantiomeric pair.

    (B)   They constitute a diastereomeric pair.

    (C) α-Amino acids exist as Zwitterions.

    (D)   None of the above.

166. Which of the following Newman projections illustrates the most thermo-dynamically stable conformation of iso-pentane?

    (A)

    (B)

    (C)

    (D)

PASSAGE IV (Questions 167-172)

   Skeletal muscle tissue is composed of actin and myosin filaments arranged in an orderly, overlapping fashion within each muscle fiber. When actin and myosin interact, muscle contraction occurs and tension develops. Due to the arrangement of the actin and myosin filaments, there is an optimum muscle length at which maximal tension can be developed. At muscle lengths longer or shorter than this, the tension developed is less than maximal.

   To study the length-tension relationship, an isolated muscle experiment can be performed. The gastrocnemius muscle of a frog is removed from the leg and placed in an isometric transducer. The transducer measures the tension which the muscle develops when stimulated to contract. The muscle is originally placed in the transducer at approximately the same length as it would have at rest in the body. It is then shortened and lengthened in 1 millimeter increments. At each muscle length, the same stimulus is applied and the tension which develops when the muscle contracts is measured. The total tension developed can be separated into 2 components: active tension and passive tension. Active tension is generated when the muscle itself contracts. Passive tension develops as the muscle is stretched beyond its resting length. It is due to stretch of supporting structures in the muscle, such as connective tissue and elastic fibers. Total tension is equal to the sum of the active and passive tensions.

Change in Muscle Length (mm)	Active tension (kg)	Passive tension (kg)	Total tension (kg)
- 3	0.5	0	0.5
-2	2.0	0	2.0
-1	11.0	0	11.0
0	15.0	0	15.0
+1	13.5	2.0	15.5
+2	7.0	10.0	17.0
+3	3.0	16.0	19.0

Table 1

Active, passive and total tension developed when an isolated muscle is stimulated to contract at its resting length (0) and at lengths shorter (- 1, - 2, - 3) and longer (+1, +2, +3) than resting length.

167. If the isolated muscle used in the experiment was stretched by 5 miilimeters from the resting length, which of the following would be true?

(A) Active tension = 10; passive tension = 0; total tension = 10

(B) Active tension = 0; passive tension = 20; total tension = 20

(C) Active tension = 0; passive tension = 0; total tension = 0

(D) Active tension = 10; passive tension = 20; total tension = 30

168. What is the advantage to using an isolated muscle in the experiment instead of leaving the muscle intact in the body?

(A) The properties of just the muscle itself can be studied since it is devoid of neural and hormonal influences.

(B) Muscle length can be easily changed, whereas in the body muscles do not change length.

(C) The muscle is better able to contract and develop tension when removed from the body.

(D) There is no advantage; the results would be the same.

169. Why is there no passive tension developed when the muscle is shortened to less than its resting length?

(A)   Passive tension is developed, but it is obscured by the greater active tension

(B)   Muscle contraction cannot occur when the muscle is shorter than its resting length

(C)   Tension cannot develop at all if the muscle is at less than its resting length

(D)   There is no stretch of connective tissue and elastic fibers

170.   If the active tension data were plotted on the ordinate versus the change in muscle length on the abscissa, the graph would resemble

(A)   a straight line.   (B)   an S-shaped curve.

(C)   a bell shaped curve.   (D)   a U-shaped curve.

171.   When a muscle contracts, tension develops because of

(A)   interaction between the actin and myosin filaments.

(B)   the overlapping arrangement of the actin and myosin filaments.

(C)   a slackening within the connective tissue elements.

(D)   the length-tension relationship.

172.   Why does total tension continue to increase while at the same time active tension is decreasing when a muscle is stretched beyond its resting length?

(A)   Total tension and active tension are not related and may change independently of one another.

(B)   Total tension is equal to passive tension minus active tension, so as the muscle is stretched, passive tension will increase, active tension will decrease and total tension will therefore increase.

(C)   Although active tension decreases, this is offset by the increase in passive tension generated by stretch of the muscle.

(D)   Total tension increases because the muscle itself generates a greater force when stimulated to contract at longer lengths.

PASSAGE V (Questions 173-178)

About 1.5% of body weight in an adult human is due to the mineral calcium. Calcium is necessary for important physiological processes, such as muscle contraction, nerve function and blood clotting. Approximately 99% of calcium in the body is located in the skeleton. Some of this calcium is available as a readily exchangeable reservoir, while the rest forms a large pool of stable calcium that is only slowly exchangeable. To maintain adequate plasma levels, calcium moves in and out of the readily exchangeable pool, in the bone, every day. Low blood calcium levels result in a condition known as hypocalcemic tetany which is characterized by skeletal muscle spasms that can become severe enough to block the airway and lead to asphyxia.

In humans, there are usually 4 parathyroid glands located on the dorsal surface of the thyroid gland. Each gland has an abundant supply of blood vessels and is about 3 × 6 × 2 millimeters in size. The parathyroid glands produce and secrete parathyroid hormone (PTH). PTH is essential for life because it is involved in the regulation of calcium metabolism. Specifically, PTH acts directly on bone to mobilize calcium leading to an increase in blood calcium levels. Secretion of PTH from the parathyroid glands is regulated by the level of plasma calcium. When plasma calcium levels fall, PTH secretion will increase. When plasma calcium levels are high, PTH secretion is inhibited.

173. An excess of PTH would

(A) lead to calcium deposition in the bone.

(B) cause plasma calcium to decrease.

(C) be manifested as tetany.

(D) eventually lead to bone demineralization.

174. PTH is a classical hormone because

(A) it is essential for life.

(B) its site of action is distant from its site of secretion.

(C) of its ability to regulate calcium metabolism.

(D) it is produced and secreted by an exocrine gland.

175. Calcium is extremely important, since it is necessary for

(A) tetany, which is normal muscle contraction.

(B) the regulation of PTH secretion.

(C) the normal function of nerve and muscle tissue.

(D) the process of bone resorption to occur.

176. The fact that the parathyroid glands are so small

(A) has no significance because hormones are effective in minute quantities.

(B) means that they are relatively unimportant glands.

(C) is so that all 4 can fit on the dorsal surface of the thyroid gland.

(D) is because they tend to shrink in size as a person ages.

177. After eating a meal high in calcium, which of the following will occur?

(A) PTH secretion will increase and calcium will be deposited in bone.

(B) PTH secretion will decrease and calcium will be deposited in bone.

(C) PTH secretion will increase to mobilize calcium from bone.

(D) None of the above will occur because the plasma calcium level does not affect PTH secretion.

178. When the plasma calcium level is high, secretion of the hormone calcitonin increases. Calcitonin inhibits the mobilization of calcium from bone. As plasma calcitonin increases

(A) plasma calcium will increase due to bone resorption.

(B) plasma PTH will decrease because these hormones have antagonistic actions.

(C) the parathyroids will increase secretion of PTH so that plasma PTH also increases.

(D) plasma calcium will decrease as a result of increased PTH activity.

PASSAGE VI (Questions 179-185)

In many species, the differences between the sexes depend primarily on a single chromosome (Y) and a single pair of endocrine structures (testes and ovaries). Of the 23 chromosomes found in germ cells, one is known as the sex chromosome. This chromosome may be one of two types, either an X or Y. Gender is determined by the sex chromosome of the sperm which fertilizes the egg. Each ovum contains a single X chromosome. Fifty percent of normal sperm contain X chromosomes and the other half contain Y chromosomes. The combination of two X chromosomes results in a genetic female. A genetic male is the product when an ovum combines with a Y-containing sperm.

The differentiation of the primitive gonads into testes in the case of a male, or into ovaries in the female, is determined genetically. Until the sixth week of development, the primitive gonads are identical in both sexes. They are bipotential, meaning they are capable of developing into either testes or ovaries at this point. In genetic males, the presence of a specific cell-surface protein, the H-Y antigen, stimulates the primitive gonads to develop into testes. The absence of the H-Y antigen in genetic females causes the ovaries to develop instead. The embryonic ovary does not secrete any hormones. The fetal testes, however, begins to produce and secrete the hormone testosterone in response to placental chorionic gonadotropin. The complete formation of the male internal and external genitalia depends upon the presence of testosterone. In the absence of testosterone, female internal and external genitalia will develop.

After birth, both male and female gonads are quiescent until adolescence when they are stimulated by the anterior pituitary to begin producing and secreting hormones. These hormones are responsible for the appearance of the features typical of adult males and females known as secondary sexual characteristics. The masculinizing androgens and feminizing estrogens are produced by both sexes, however, androgens predominate in males, while estrogens predominate in females.

179. A pseudohermaphrodite is an individual with the genetic constitution and glands of one sex and the genitalia of the other sex. Which of the following could result in a female pseudohermaphrodite?

(A) Exposure of a genetic female to testosterone at birth

(B) Exposure of a genetic male to estrogens during the 5th-6th week of gestation

(C) Exposure of a genetic male to placental chorionic gonadotropin

(D) Exposure of a genetic female to androgens during the 8th-13th week of gestation.

180. The number of males born annually is generally slightly higher than the number of females. Which of the following statements provides a plausible expla-

nation for this phenomenon?

(A)   There are more X-containing sperm than Y-containing sperm, so an XX combination will occur more frequently than an XY combination.

(B)   There are more Y-containing sperm produced than X-containing ones, so the odds of an XY combination occurring are greater than an XX combination.

(C)   There are approximately equal numbers of X- and Y-containing sperm, therefore the reason must lie elsewhere, perhaps in differences of motility between X and Y sperm.

(D)   Since all eggs contain a Y chromosome, the odds of producing a male are better than a female.

181.   The two primary functions of the mature gonads are

(A)   production of germ cells and secretion of hormones.

(B)   secretion of androgens and estrogens.

(C)   production of ova and maintenance of secondary sex characteristics.

(D)   secretion of testosterone and production of sperm.

182.   Up until the sixth week of gestation the primitive gonads in both sexes are identical. What causes the internal and external genitalia to develop differently in males and females?

(A)   Estrogen secreted by the immature ovaries

(B)   The presence of the H-Y antigen on the surface of cells in males

(C)   Testosterone and estrogen secreted by the testes

(D)   Chemical signals sent from the developing brain

183.   Why do germ cells contain half the number of chromosomes found in all of the other cells of the body?

(A)   Because germ cells are diploid cells

(B)   So that the combination of an egg and sperm results in the full complement of 46 chromosomes

(C)   Their small size permits them to contain only half the number of chromosomes of other cells

(D)   Because during mitosis, which is the process of germ cell formation, the chromosome number is cut in half.

184.   If an X-containing sperm fertilizes an egg, the resultant offspring will be

(A)   an XY combination, which is a male.

(B)   a genetic male.

(C)   an XYY combination, which is a female.

(D)   a genetic female.

185. In order for secondary sexual characteristics to appear at the time of adolescence

 (A) the testes must secrete estrogen in males and the ovaries must secrete testosterone in females.

 (B) the testes must stop producing androgens.

 (C) the gonads must be producing and secreting hormones.

 (D) the ovaries must stop producing estrogens.

PASSAGE VII (Questions 186-192)

The fundamental unit of all living things is the cell. Each individual cell is capable of reproducing, metabolizing and adapting to changes in its environment. Cells are separated from one another by their cell membranes, however, they are not isolated because materials may pass through the cell membranes to move in and out of the cells. Cells in the human body are organized into tissues and organs where they act collectively to accomplish activities basic to life such as energy production, movement, communication and reproduction.

The two major components of a cell are the nucleus and cytoplasm. The nucleus is separated from the rest of the cell by the nuclear membrane. It is the control center of the cell because it contains the genetic material DNA. Also found within the nucleus is an RNA producing structure called the nucleolus, which is not bound by a membrane. Filling the space between the nucleus and the cell membrane is the cytoplasm. Membrane bound structures called organelles and a complex network of protein filaments and microtubules called the cytoskeleton are suspended in the cytoplasmic fluid. The cytoskeleton gives the cell its shape and also provides the basis for movement of the entire cell and its individual organelles.

The organelles are highly organized physical structures, each of which is specialized to perform a function in a more efficient manner than could be achieved simply by chemicals dispersed in the cytoplasm. The mitochondria provide energy for the cell in the form of ATP. These structures are self-replicating and can increase in number when the demand for energy increases. The endoplasmic reticulum and the Golgi apparatus are both composed of a network of flattened sacs. Rough endoplasmic reticulum (RER) has attached ribosomes and serves as a site for protein synthesis. Smooth endoplasmic reticulum (SER) does not have attached ribosomes. It is involved in lipid metabolism, steroid synthesis and drug detoxification. Proteins and other substances formed in the endoplasmic reticulum are often transported to the Golgi where they are modified, sorted and packaged for delivery elsewhere in the cell or for secretion out of the cell. Lysosomes provide an intracellular digestive system. They are membrane bound vesicles filled with hydrolytic enzymes that are

Component	Percentage of cellular mass
Water	80%
Protein	15%
Lipid	3%
Carbohydrate	1%
Electrolytes and minerals	1%

Table 2 — The composition of a generalized eukaryotic cell.

capable of digesting proteins, nucleic acids, lipids and glycogen. Lysosomes remove unwanted substances from the cell, such as damaged organelles or foreign bacteria.

186. Most of the cellular organelles are surrounded by membranes. The purpose of this is to

    (A) completely separate the organelles from one another since there is no need for interaction among these structures.

    (B) provide a series of compartments in which chemical reactions can take place.

    (C) decrease the surface area available for chemical reactions to occur.

    (D) subdivide the cell into a series of smaller parts, each of which can exist on its own.

187. According to Table 2, most of a cell is made up of

    (A) protein, lipid and carbohydrate.

    (B) electrolytes, minerals and water.

    (C) carbohydrate.

    (D) water and protein.

188. Why would cells be unable to survive for any substantial length of time without a functional lysosomal system?

    (A) An accumulation of cellular debris or invasion by infectious agents would likely kill the cells.

    (B) The cells would be unable to properly package and secrete proteins.

    (C) Reproduction could not occur because DNA is contained within the lysosomes.

    (D) Energy production would be too slow to sustain life.

189. Rough and smooth endoplasmic reticula are distinguished from each other by the

    (A) attachment of the cytoskeleton to the RER, which anchors it in place.

    (B) fact that SER is membrane bound while RER is not.

    (C) proximity to the Golgi apparatus — RER is closer than SER.

    (D) presence of ribosomes on RER and their absence on SER.

190. Of all the organelles in the cell, the mitochondria are usually the most abundant. Which of the following statements best explains why?

    (A) Mitochondria are the control centers of the cell.

    (B) Digestive enzymes are contained within the mitochondria.

    (C) Practically all cellular processes require ATP as an energy source.

    (D) These structures shuttle proteins and other substances between the endoplasmic reticulum and Golgi apparatus.

191. One of the few structures in the cell which is not surrounded by a membrane is the

(A) Golgi apparatus.

(B) nucleus.

(C) nucleolus.

(D) lysosome.

192. Numerous membrane bound vesicles are frequently found around the Golgi apparatus. Their function probably is to

(A) digest the substances released from the Golgi.

(B) carry material between the Golgi and other organelles or to the cell membrane.

(C) shuttle ATP between the ribosomes and the Golgi.

(D) direct the flow of materials form the Golgi to the endoplasmic reticulum.

QUESTIONS 193-196 are NOT based on a descriptive passage.

---

193. Translocation is a type of chromosomal mutation where

(A) a segment of the chromosome is missing.

(B) a portion of the chromosome is represented twice.

(C) a segment of one chromosome is transferred to another non-homologous chromosome.

(D) a segment is removed and reinserted.

194. The thin barrier at Bowman's capsule allows for filtration of

(A) whole blood.

(B) ammonia.

(C) plasma.

(D) oxygen.

195. The phenomenon of rigor mortis is a direct result of

(A) the breaking of myosin bonds by ATP.

(B) the breaking of actin bonds by ATP.

(C) the inability of the myosin cross bridges to combine with single amino acids.

(D) the loss of ATP in dead muscle cells.

196. Which of the following is a meta-directing, deactivating substituted benzene?

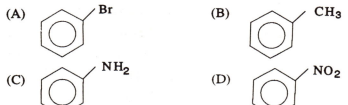

PASSAGE VII (Questions 197-202)

Proteins are made up of various combinations of the 20 amino acids. All of the amino acids are constructed with a central carbon atom called the *a* carbon. Bonded to the *a* carbon are an amino group, carboxyl group, hydrogen atom and one variable group called a side chain or R group. Because only the side chains vary from one amino acid to another, it is these groups which impart individuality to each amino acid.

The amino acids can be classified conveniently using the physical properties of the side chain. At physiological pH (≈ 7), amino acids are grouped according to their electric charge when ionized, and according to their affinity for water. Five of the amino acids have charged side chains at pH 7. Two of these are negatively charged and are the acidic amino acids. The other three are the basic amino acids which are positively charged. The non-ionic (uncharged) polar amino acids have side chains which are hydrophilic and thus tend to be located on the surface of the protein molecule which is exposed to the aqueous medium. Nonpolar amino acids are only slightly soluble in water and are usually confined to the interior of the protein molecule.

The α carbon is the center of asymmetry for all of the amino acids except glycine. Therefore, each amino acid can exist in two nonsuperimposable mirror image forms, or enantiomers. All of the amino acids found in proteins possess the same absolute configuration as L-alanine, which corresponds to the arrangement of analagous groups in the structure of L-glyceraldehyde. D-amino acids have an absolute configuration corresponding to D-glyceraldehyde. These are found in the cell walls of bacteria and in a number of antibiotics of bacterial origin.

197. Which of the following amino acids has a negatively charged side chain?

(A)   Glycine

(B)   Alanine

$$\begin{array}{c} NH_2 \\ | \\ H-CH-COOH \end{array}$$

$$\begin{array}{c} NH_2 \\ | \\ CH_3-CH-COOH \end{array}$$

(C)   Aspartic acid

(D)   Phenylalanine

$$\begin{array}{c} NH_2 \\ | \\ HOOC-CH_2-CH-COOH \end{array}$$

$$\begin{array}{c} NH_2 \\ | \\ \text{(benzene ring)}-CH_2-CH-COOH \end{array}$$

198. Amino acids are classified as either D- or L-forms based upon

(A)   the sign of rotation of plane polarized light.

(B)   the percentage of ionized versus non-ionized molecules in solution.

(C)   their hydrophobicity or hydrophilicity.

(D)   the structural relationship to D- or L-glyceraldehyde.

199. Amino acids with side chains that consist only of hydrocarbons are

(A)   hydrophobic.

(B)   enantiomers.

(C)   zwitterions.

(D)   hydrophilic.

200. The unchanged polar side chains of several of the amino acids are most likely involved in

    (A)   peptide bonds.   (B)   hydrogen bonds.

    (C)   covalent bonds.   (D)   hydrophobic interactions.

201. At the pH typically found in most cells, the amino group of an amino acid is in which of the following forms?

    (A) $-NH_2$ (B) $=NH_2$

    (C) $-HN_4+$ (D) $-NH_3+$

202. A particular position in a protein chain derives its physical and chemical properties from (the)

    (A)   R group.   (B) α-amino group.

    (C)   Factor XIV.   (D)   carboxyl group.

PASSAGE IX (Questions 203-208)

In order to study a compound in isolation, it must be separated from the thousands of components with which it normally occurs. The desired substance may be quite labile and cannot be exposed to extremes of pH, temperature or pressure. Isolation is made more difficult when only micro amounts of the substance are available and by the presence of other molecules that differ slightly from the desired compound. This has led to the development of highly selective methods for isolating and purifying biological compounds.

Many of the separation methods involve the distribution of a mixture of solutes between two immiscible solvents. The molecules in the mixture are propelled through a channel of solvent by a force which acts equally on each molecule. Other forces retard movement of the molecules through the channel. If the retarding forces are different for different molecules in the solute mixture, separation of the molecules will occur as the mixture passes through the length of the channel.

Chromatography includes a number of separation methods based upon the technique described above that involve the percolation of a solute mixture through a porous solid support. In thin-layer chromatography (TLC), a variation of liquid-liquid chromatography, a thin film of solid support of uniform thickness, usually alumina or silica gel, is prepared on a glass or plastic surface. One of the immiscible solvents, the stationary phase, is immobilized on the inert solid support. A small amount of the solute mixture to be separated is spotted near one end of the plate. The other solvent, the mobile phase, is applied to the end of the plate closest to the spot. As the mobil phase moves along the support by capillary action, the individual components of the solute mixture will separate based upon their partition coefficients in the two phases. The order of migration of compounds can be changed by using different solvents, but in general less polar compounds move the fastest. To increase the rate at which more polar compounds move, a more polar solvent must be used.

203. Four different samples consisting of mixtures of unknown compounds were prepared for TLC. On the right side of each plate the unknown was spotted. On the left side, a sample of a known compound (A) was spotted. Which of the following plates contains compound A in the unknown mixture?

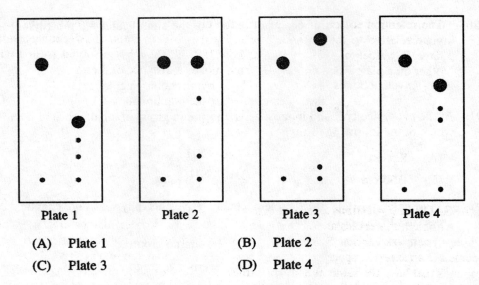

Plate 1   Plate 2   Plate 3   Plate 4

(A)   Plate 1   (B)   Plate 2
(C)   Plate 3   (D)   Plate 4

204. Which of the plates in question 203 contains the mixture with the most polar compounds?

(A)   Plate 1   (B)   Plate 2
(C)   Plate 3   (D)   Plate 4

205. To increase the rate at which more polar compounds move up the plate, which of the following solvents would be used?

(A)   Benzene   (B)   Ethanol
(C)   Acetic acid   (D)   Hexane

206. Which of the following class of compounds will move the furthest on a TLC plate?

(A)   Aldehydes RCH= O

(B)   Carboxylic acids

(C)   Halogenated hydrocarbons RX

(D)   Alkenes $R_2C=CR_2$

207. Spots from colorless organic compounds will not be visible on a TLC plate. Why does exposure of the plate to iodine vapor allow the spots to be visualized?

(A)   Iodine forms colored complexes with most organic compounds.

(B)   Iodine causes the spots to fluoresce.

(C)   Iodine forms colored complexes with most of the plate coatings commonly used.

(D)   Iodine forms colored complexes with the mobile phase.

208. The retention factor, or R_f value, is the distance that a spot moves up a TLC plate relative to the distance moved by the solvent front. If two compounds have R_f values of 0.50 and 0.61, how far will they be separated from each other on a plate when the solvent front moves a distance of 5 cm?

$$R_f = \frac{\text{distance travelled by the compound}}{\text{distance travelled by the solvent}}$$

(A) 2.5 cm

(B) 0.11 cm

(C) 0.55 cm

(D) 3.05 cm

PASSAGE X (Questions 209-214)

Although molecules are often drawn in only one or two dimensions, they exist in three-dimensional forms. Stereochemistry is the study of how the atoms in a molecule are arranged in space relative to one another. Isomers are two or more compounds that have the same molecular formulas. If the atoms are attached in different orders, the compounds have different structures and are called structural isomers of each other.

A second type of isomerism is geometric isomerism, which occurs in only two classes of compounds: alkenes and cyclic compounds. These compounds contain double bonds, or pi bonds, which generally cannot be broken at room temperature. The groups attached to pi-bonded carbons are therefore fixed in space relative to one another. Consider for example, the two possible structures of 1, 2-dichloroethene:

These two compounds are not structural isomers because the order of attachment of the atoms and the location of the double bond is the same in both cases. Instead, they are called stereoisomers. These isomers are different compounds that have the same structure, but differ in the arrangement of the atoms in space. The structure on the left represents a *cis*-isomer in which the two Cl atoms are on the same side of the pi bond and the two H atoms are on the other side. The structure on the right is a *trans*-isomer. Here, the Cl groups are on opposite sides of the pi bond. Due to the rigidity of the double bond, the *cis*- and *trans*-isomers are not easily interconvertible.

209. Why are there no structural isomers of unsubstituted alkanes with three or fewer carbon atoms?

(A) The ring structure does not permit structural isomerization.

(B) Compounds containing double bonds cannot have structural isomers.

(C) The functional groups are always attached in the same position.

(D) There is only one possible way in which the atoms can be arranged.

210. Which of the following is a structural isomer of 1-propanol ($CH_3CH_2CH_2OH$)?

(A) $CH_2 {=} CHCH_2 OH$

(B) $CH_3 CH_2 \overset{\overset{\displaystyle OH}{\displaystyle |}}{C} HCH_3$

(C) $CH_3 \overset{\overset{\displaystyle OH}{\displaystyle |}}{C} HCH_3$

(D) $CH_3 CH_2 \overset{\overset{\displaystyle O}{\displaystyle \|}}{C} H$

211. Which of the following pairs of formulas represent the same compound and therefore do not represent isomers?

(A) $CH_3 \overset{\overset{\displaystyle Cl}{\displaystyle |}}{C} HCHCl_2$ and $Cl_2 \overset{\overset{\displaystyle Cl}{\displaystyle |}}{C} HCHCH_3$

(B) $Cl{-}\langle\text{ring}\rangle{-}Cl$ and   [ring with Cl and Cl substituents]

(C) $CH_3 \overset{\overset{\displaystyle CH_3}{\displaystyle |}}{C} HCH_2 CH_3$ and $CH_3 \underset{\underset{\displaystyle CH_3}{\displaystyle |}}{\overset{\overset{\displaystyle CH_3}{\displaystyle |}}{C}} CH_3$

(D) $CH_3 OCH_3$ and $CH_3 CH_2 OH$

212. Which of the following pairs of structures are stereoisomers of each other?

(A)
$$\underset{H}{\overset{Cl}{\diagdown}}C{=}C\underset{CH_3}{\overset{CH_3}{\diagup}}$$
and
$$\underset{Cl}{\overset{H}{\diagdown}}C{=}C\underset{CH_3}{\overset{CH_3}{\diagup}}$$

(B)
$$\underset{H}{\overset{CH_3}{\diagdown}}C{=}C\underset{H}{\overset{CH_2CH_3}{\diagup}}$$
and
$$\underset{H}{\overset{CH_3}{\diagdown}}C{=}C\underset{CH_2CH_3}{\overset{H}{\diagup}}$$

(C)
$$\underset{Cl}{\overset{Cl}{\diagdown}}C{=}C\underset{H}{\overset{Cl}{\diagup}}$$
and
$$\underset{H}{\overset{Cl}{\diagdown}}C{=}C\underset{Cl}{\overset{Cl}{\diagup}}$$

(D)
$$\underset{H}{\overset{Cl}{\diagdown}}C{=}C\underset{CH_2Cl}{\overset{H}{\diagup}}$$
and
$$\underset{Cl}{\overset{H}{\diagdown}}C{=}C\underset{H}{\overset{CH_2Cl}{\diagup}}$$

213. A requirement of stereoisomers in alkenes is that each of the carbon atoms involved in the pi bond must

  (A) have identical groups attached to it.

  (B) lie on the same side of the double bond.

  (C) rotate freely around the pi bond.

  (D) have two different groups attached to it.

214. Why are *trans*-isomers generally more stable at room temperature than *cis*-isomers?

  (A) All of the groups attached to the pi-bonded carbons are the same in *trans*-isomers.

  (B) There is more steric hindrance in the *cis*-isomers.

  (C) Smaller groups, such as H atoms, are attached to the pi-bonded carbons in *cis*-isomers.

  (D) There is more electrostatic interaction among groups in the *trans* form.

QUESTIONS 215-219 are NOT based on a descriptive passage.

---

215. When bone formation takes place in pre-existing cartilage, it is called

  (A) intramembranous bone formation.

  (B) primary ossification.

  (C) endochondral ossification.

  (D) subchondral ossification.

216. Which of the following is part of the appendicular skeleton?

  (A) Humerus   (B) Vertebrae

  (C) Ribs   (D) Sternum

217. Which of the following birth control methods is closest to being 100% effective?

  (A) Rhythm   (B) IUD

  (C) Diaphragm   (D) The pill

218. Which of the following undergoes saponification?

  (A) Glucose   (B) Starches

  (C) Glycogen   (D) Fats

219. Which of the following may exist as optical isomers?

I. $CH_3CH_2CHOHCH_3$

II. $CH_3CHClCH_3$

III. $CH_3CH_2CHOHCOH$

IV.

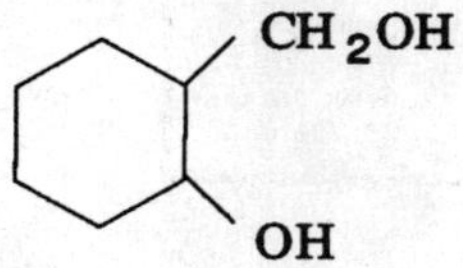

(A)   I.

(B)   II.

(C)   II and IV.

(D)   I, III.and IV.

STOP

If time still remains, you may review work only in this section.

TEST 1

ANSWER KEY

1.	(B)	26.	(B)	51.	(A)	76.	(B)
2.	(D)	27.	(B)	52.	(B)	77.	(B)
3.	(A)	28.	(D)	53.	(A)	78.	(D)
4.	(B)	29.	(C)	54.	(B)	79.	(D)
5.	(C)	30.	(D)	55.	(D)	80.	(B)
6.	(A)	31.	(B)	56.	(B)	81.	(A)
7.	(B)	32.	(D)	57.	(C)	82.	(D)
8.	(D)	33.	(A)	58.	(C)	83.	(B)
9.	(D)	34.	(B)	59.	(D)	84.	(D)
10.	(C)	35.	(B)	60.	(B)	85.	(D)
11.	(C)	36.	(B)	61.	(C)	86.	(A)
12.	(A)	37.	(C)	62.	(A)	87.	(B)
13.	(D)	38.	(A)	63.	(A)	88.	(C)
14.	(D)	39.	(D)	64.	(C)	89.	(D)
15.	(B)	40.	(C)	65.	(B)	90.	(C)
16.	(B)	41.	(A)	66.	(C)	91.	(D)
17.	(C)	42.	(C)	67.	(B)	92.	(B)
18.	(A)	43.	(C)	68.	(A)	93.	(A)
19.	(C)	44.	(B)	69.	(D)	94.	(A)
20.	(C)	45.	(C)	70.	(C)	95.	(B)
21.	(B)	46.	(A)	71.	(B)	96.	(D)
22.	(D)	47.	(D)	72.	(A)	97.	(B)
23.	(A)	48.	(B)	73.	(A)	98.	(B)
24.	(D)	49.	(B)	74.	(D)	99.	(C)
25.	(C)	50.	(C)	75.	(B)	100.	(C)

101.	(A)	131.	(D)	161.	(C)	191.	(C)
102.	(D)	132.	(C)	162.	(B)	192.	(B)
103.	(C)	133.	(B)	163.	(B)	193.	(C)
104.	(A)	134.	(D)	164.	(D)	194.	(C)
105.	(D)	135.	(A)	165.	(D)	195.	(D)
106.	(B)	136.	(B)	166.	(B)	196.	(D)
107.	(D)	137.	(C)	167.	(B)	197.	(C)
108.	(D)	138.	(C)	168.	(A)	198.	(D)
109.	(A)	139.	(D)	169.	(D)	199.	(A)
110.	(D)	140.	(D)	170.	(C)	200.	(B)
111.	(D)	141.	(B)	171.	(A)	201.	(D)
112.	(B)	142.	(A)	172.	(C)	202.	(A)
113.	(C)	143.	(C)	173.	(D)	203.	(B)
114.	(D)	144.	(B)	174.	(B)	204.	(A)
115.	(A)	145.	(D)	175.	(C)	205.	(C)
116.	(B)	146.	(A)	176.	(A)	206.	(D)
117.	(C)	147.	(C)	177.	(B)	207.	(A)
118.	(B)	148.	(B)	178.	(B)	208.	(C)
119.	(B)	149.	(D)	179.	(D)	209.	(D)
120.	(A)	150.	(B)	180.	(C)	210.	(C)
121.	(B)	151.	(A)	181.	(A)	211.	(A)
122.	(C)	152.	(C)	182.	(B)	212.	(B)
123.	(C)	153.	(D)	183.	(B)	213.	(D)
124.	(B)	154.	(D)	184.	(D)	214.	(B)
125.	(C)	155.	(C)	185.	(C)	215.	(C)
126.	(B)	156.	(A)	186.	(B)	216.	(A)
127.	(C)	157.	(D)	187.	(D)	217.	(D)
128.	(D)	158.	(B)	188.	(A)	218.	(D)
129.	(C)	159.	(A)	189.	(D)	219.	(D)
130.	(A)	160.	(A)	190.	(C)		

DETAILED EXPLANATIONS
OF ANSWERS

Section 1 — Verbal Reasoning

PASSAGE I (Questions 1-10)

The author of this passage describes what makes one scientific theory superior to another in terms of its falsifiability. We are given two examples to illustrate the difference. The author concludes by arguing that science proceeds by trial and error.

1.   **(B)**   The author makes this clear in the sixth paragraph by emphasizing the words *mistakes, error*, and *falsifications*. Proposing highly falsifiable theories is preferable to proposing nonfalsifiable ones, but, according to the author's claims in paragraph six, we do not learn from either type of theory until it is falsified. Thus, (A) is incorrect. For the same reason, (D) and (C) are incorrect and, in addition, are too narrowly phrased. Science includes more than just theories of planetary motion.

2.   **(D)**   The author begins paragraph two by telling us he will illustrate the point he made in paragraph one. This point is: "A very good theory will be one that makes very wide-ranging claims about the world, and which is consequently highly falsifiable...." He then presents in the second paragraph two theories of planetary motion, and explains in paragraph three why the second theory is more falsifiable than the first. (A) and (B) are incorrect because the two theories are used only for purposes of illustration. The author does not particularly care about planetary orbits, except as an example of the falsifiability of two theories. (C) is incorrect because the author does not proceed to falsify either theory.

3.   **(A)**   The author defines this term in the sixth sentence of the third paragraph by telling us, "If we follow Popper and refer to those sets of observation statements that would serve to falsify a law or theory as *potential falsifiers* of that law or theory ..." (B), (C), and (D) are all incorrect because potential falsifiers are not theories themselves, but statements that, if observed, would serve to falsify an existing theory.

4.   **(B)**   The author begins the passage by telling us what a good scientific theory does: it makes definite claims about the world. By inference, a bad scientific theory does not make definite claims about the world. (A) may in fact be true, but we are given no information about theories which limit the advance of scientific knowledge. One might reason, that theories which do not make definite claims about the world are nonfalsifiable. Since it is the falsification of theories which leads to the striking achievements in science (sixth paragraph), we might conclude that theories which do not make definite claims about the world do limit the advance of scientific knowledge. Selecting (B), however, yields the same result more directly, and is, thus, the better answer. Although we are told in the fifth paragraph that falsified theories must be ruthlessly rejected, this does not make them *bad* scientific theories. Falsified theories have made enough definite claims about the world to be falsified, and

thereby advance science. Thus, (C) is incorrect. (D) describes a theory which has not yet, but soon will be, falsified. It thus falls into the same category as (C), making (D) incorrect.

5.   **(C)**   The author's description of the theories of Kepler and Newton are intended to provide a second example of how one scientific theory can be superior to another. As we are told in the first paragraph and shown in the example in the second paragraph, theories which make broader claims are superior. The author explains in the fourth paragraph why Newton's theory is considered broader, and therefore superior, to Kepler's. (A), (B), and (D) are all incorrect because the passage makes no mention of whether either of the theories have been falsified.

6.   **(A)**   This is the conclusion which should be reached after the author has presented his two examples to illustrate the point. (C) and (D) are incorrect because they merely refer to the two examples. (B) is incorrect because we are told in the fifth paragraph that falsified theories "must be ruthlessly rejected." From the author's statements in paragraph six, the value is in what we learn by falsifying a theory, not the falsified theory itself.

7.   **(B)**   The author tells us this directly in the first paragraph, and again less directly in the fifth. We are also told in the fifth paragraph why (III) is not part of a good scientific theory.

8.   **(D)**   The author makes this point directly in the sixth paragraph. (A) is incorrect because there is no mention in the passage of how one learns to propose broader theories. Although there is a preference for highly falsifiable theories, (C) is nevertheless incorrect because we do not learn from a theory until it has been falsified.

9.   **(D)**   In this question the reader is asked to determine which of the four options makes the broader claims about the world. From this problem it can be deduced which of the four options contains the largest set of decision makers. Although the reader may not know the size of the subsets, Supreme Court justices, appellate judges, and judges, it should be clear that all the members of the first three categories are people, but not all people are one type of judge or another. Thus, (D) has the largest set of decision makers and makes the broadest claims about the world. Based on the passage, this makes (D) the most falsifiable theory.

10.   **(C)**   As described in the passage, Kepler's theory dealt exclusively with planetary motion. Since (C) is not an observation relating to planetary motion, it is not a potential falsifier of Kepler's theory (though it is of Newton's). (A), (B), and (D) are all statements suggesting the locations of various planets were not as predicted. These all relate to planetary motion and are, thus, potential falsifiers of Kepler's theory.

PASSAGE II (Questions 11-19)
     The author of this passage describes the word 'oppression' and how it should be properly applied to various groups. We are given examples of how the word is misapplied and how this misapplication can lead to accusations of insensitivity and bigotry on the part of women.

11.　**(C)**　The author first makes this point in the fifth sentence of paragraph two. She makes the point more directly in the second sentence of the third paragraph when she says, "Humans beings can be miserable without being oppressed. ..." The first sentence of the sixth paragraph shows (A) to be clearly incorrect. Although in the sixth paragraph the author tells us men are not oppressed as men, she does allow in the fourth and fifth paragraphs that men might be oppressed (just not because they are men). Thus, (B) is incorrect. The first sentence of the passage makes it clear that "oppression' has direct application to feminist theory, making (D) incorrect.

12.　**(A)**　The author tells us of this claim in the second paragraph, and in the first sentence of the third paragraph tells us directly that the claim is nonsense. (B) fails to make the distinction between mere misery and oppression. The author admits (or at least does not deny) that men might be miserable even though they are oppressors. The author's concern is the label attached to that misery, not the description of the misery itself (C) and (D) may very well be true, but they are not mentioned in the passage.

13.　**(D)**　This point is made directly in the last sentence of the passage. In the sixth paragraph the author allows for the possibility that men can be oppressed for reasons other than that they are men, making (A) incorrect. (B) and (C) are incorrect because the author does not specifically tell us who she thinks is oppressing women. We can reasonably infer that the author believes men to be oppressing women, but, aside from making (B) false, it appears she is assuming men oppress women rather than arguing the point.

14.　**(D)**　The author makes this point directly in the fourth and sixth sentences of the fourth paragraph.

15.　**(B)**　The author makes this point in the first sentence of the fourth paragraph. (A) is clearly incorrect due to the author's statement in the last sentence of the passage. The author does assert that she is marked for oppression because she is a woman, but this is because she is a member of a group which she feels has been marked for oppression (women). Thus, although (C) is true, (B) is the better answer. (D) is incorrect because the author makes no mention of individual characteristics, as opposed to group characteristics, as marking one for oppression.

16.　**(B)**　We know (II) is true from the last sentence of the passage. In the third paragraph the author tells us humans can be miserable without being oppressed. This statement is intended to counter the claim presented in the second paragraph that men are oppressed because they are oppressors. The conclusion is that men can be miserable without being oppressed (III). (I) is false because in the sixth paragraph the author allows that men might be oppressed if they belong to certain groups, but not because they are men.

17.　**(C)**　This point is made in the sixth and seventh sentences of the second paragraph. (A) is incorrect. The author certainly believes women are oppressed. Although there is no mention of this in the passage, it is inferred women are oppressed *because* they may deny that some group is oppressed. (B) is incorrect because there is no mention of men being oppressed only the possibility that they will if they belong to certain groups (sixth paragraph). For (B) to be correct, women would have to be the oppressors, which is option (D). (D) is incorrect, however, because there is no mention in the passage of women ever being oppressors.

18.   **(A)**   The author's point in the second paragraph is that the word 'oppression' has been "stretched to meaninglessness." According to the author one effect of this distortion is that if women attempt to use the word correctly, they run the risk of being called insensitive, or even bigots. Although the author clearly states in the first paragraph that the word 'oppression' is dangerous, there is no connection between this belief and accusing women of bigotry. Thus, (B) is incorrect. The implication of the author's argument in the second paragraph is that women are *not* bigots, making (C) incorrect. (D) refers to one of the problems the author associates with how women are oppressed (fourth and fifth paragraphs). There is no connection in the passage between this argument and accusing women of bigotry.

19.   **(C)**   The initial assumptions are that women see themselves as sensitive (A) and being sensitive is a redeeming trait. If women are considered insensitive, to reach the conclusion that they have no redeeming traits, one must also assume that they have no redeeming traits other than sensitivity. Although (A) is an assumption of the above argument, it is neither a necessary nor a sufficient condition for the conclusion to hold. Even if women did not see themselves as being sensitive, they may not think they have any redeeming traits, thus making the conclusion true (the necessary condition). Even assuming (A) to be correct it does not necessarily follow that women will believe they have no redeeming traits *unless* they also believe it is their only redeeming trait. For similar reasons, (B) and (D) are also incorrect.

PASSAGE III (Questions 20-29)
    The author of this passage introduces the reader to some of the broader implications and areas affected by momentous discoveries in the area of physics. In particular, he suggests discoveries in the physical world may bring us closer to an understanding of several questions which were previously thought of as solely religious in nature.

20.   **(C)**   The author states this directly in the fifth sentence of the fifth paragraph when he states: "It is a book *about* science and its wider implications." (A) is incorrect because of the fourth sentence of the fifth paragraph. (B) is incorrect because of the first sentence of the fifth paragraph. The author tells us in the sixth sentence of the fifth paragraph that the scientific discussion will not be complete, making (D) incorrect.

21.   **(B)**   The author makes this point in the fourth sentence of the first paragraph. (A) is incorrect because there is no mention in the passage of the value of the theory of relativity after quantum theory was proposed. (C) is incorrect because of the author's statement in the third sentence of the first paragraph. In addition, in the second paragraph the author tells us the effects of these discoveries have been felt by philosophers, theologians, psychologists, and sociologists—none of whom deal exclusively with the physical world—as well. (D) is clearly incorrect from the first paragraph.

22.   **(D)**   In the second paragraph the author notes theologians have benefitted from the new physics by saying they have plucked the fruits of the scientific revolution. Later in the paragraph, he tells us psychologists find sympathy with the new

view of science. The author also indicates in the second paragraph that the beliefs of ordinary people are often in tune with the view of the world presented by the new physics. Thus, (D) is correct.

23. **(A)** The author tells us this in the second sentence of the fourth paragraph. (B) is incorrect because we are given no information as to the basis for quantum theory. In the third paragraph the author notes that asking, "What is matter?" is a deep question. Several other questions are also identified as deep, but the author indicates none are as fundamental as how the universe came to be. Thus, (C) is incorrect. In the first sentence of the fifth paragraph the author tells us his book is not about religion. In the third sentence of the same paragraph he tells us he will make no attempt to discuss religious experiences. By implication this includes discussing the nature of God, making (D) incorrect.

24. **(D)** In the fifth sentence of the fourth paragraph the author compares the idea of a self-creating universe to "a subnuclear particle [that] sometimes pops out of nowhere in certain high energy processes." (A), (B), and (C) are all incorrect because the passage does not mention black holes, Darwin's theory of evolution, or the pattern of planetary motion.

25. **(C)** The author makes this point in the third sentence of the sixth paragraph. (A) is incorrect because in the same sentence the author admits that the answers physicists find may be wrong. Despite the possibility that the answers provided by the new physics to the Big Four Questions may be wrong, there is no indication in the passage that the author believes them to be unanswerable. Thus (B) is incorrect. (D) is clearly incorrect from the author's statement in the third sentence of the sixth paragraph.

26. **(B)** In the context of the passage (in particular the third sentence of the second paragraph), the author is using the word *sympathy* to indicate agreement. (A) is incorrect because there is no indication sociologists have any reason to feel sorry for physicists. (C) is incorrect because it has the relationship backwards. (D) is incorrect because it is the physicists' view of the world which is gaining popularity, not necessarily the study of physics. It is unlikely sociologists will give up their discipline and turn to physics. It is more likely they will begin to study how the implications of the new physics affects sociology.

27. **(B)** This answer is reached by eliminating the other answers. (A) and (C) are very unlikely given the author's willingness to still consider some questions of a religious nature (fifth and sixth paragraphs) even though they may be answered by the new physics. This conclusion is supported by the author's unwillingness to discuss religious phenomena. If he believed the new physics to have abolished God, he would be more likely to try to explain such phenomena in scientific terms. From the sixth paragraph it should be clear the author believes the question *is* relevant to the new physics, making (D) incorrect.

28. **(D)** The author makes this point in the fifth sentence of the first paragraph. Certainly many physicists do concentrate their energies on particle physics, but the only mention of this subarea of physics is in the form of a brief reference to subnuclear particles in the forth paragraph. Thus, (A) is incorrect. In the sixth paragraph

the author argues physicists may begin to answer some questions formerly thought to be solely religious, but this does not mean physicists are examining religion. Rather, it means they are viewing physics in a new way which may have an impact on religious questions. Thus, (B) is incorrect. (C) is incorrect because we are given no information about psychological notions of mind and matter or whether they have been rejected by physicists.

29. **(C)** This question is answered by the fifth paragraph. In the sixth sentence he tells us we may have to delve into some areas in detail. In that same sentence we are told that the scientific discussions will be neither systematic nor complete, making (A) incorrect. In the third sentence the author tells us he will make no attempt to "discuss religious experiences or questions of morality." Thus, both (B) and (D) are incorrect.

PASSAGE IV (Questions 30-38)
The author of this passage is introducing the idea of Ethical Egoism. He gives an example and describes how most people would react when confronted with the problem, then suggests how an Ethical Egoist would react. He goes into some detail as to exactly what Ethical Egoism holds.

30. **(D)** This becomes clear in the third paragraph. In the first two paragraphs the author presents a moral problem and suggests how most would react. In the third paragraph he introduces Ethical Egoism as an alternative to what he calls common-sense morality. In the following paragraphs the author explains at length exactly what is required by Ethical Egoism. (A) is incorrect because the example of world hunger is used only as an example of a moral problem to which most people are sympathetic, and yet do not do much about. (B) is incorrect for similar reasons. The point of mentioning world hunger is to present a moral dilemma so the author can contrast common-sense morality with Ethical Egoism. Other than as a good example, there is nothing of particular importance about mentioning world hunger in this passage. (C) is incorrect because the author never uses language to suggest he believes one way or the other about Ethical Egoism. Even in introducing the concept he uses very neutral language: "Some thinkers have maintained ..." (second sentence, third paragraph).

31. **(B)** In the fifth sentence of the second paragraph the author tells us that common-sense morality holds, "when we can help others—especially at little cost to ourselves—we should do so." (A) is a utilitarian position and is not mentioned in the passage. (C) might be considered an extreme form of altruism, and is also not mentioned in the passage. Although the implication of *common-sense* morality is that it is based on common sense, (D) is incorrect because common-sense morality assumes a specific view of what constitutes common sense (i.e., helping others when it costs us little). No individual variation is allowed.

32. **(D)** In this passage the author introduces the concept of Ethical Egosim. He does not use any language to suggest he personally believes in Ethical Egoism or that it is the correct moral view. He also gives no indication that he prefers the common-sense view of morality. Thus, since (A) represents the common-sense view of morality and (B) represents Ethical Egoism, both are incorrect. The problem of world

hunger is used only as an example in the passage and there is no indication as to how the author feels about the problem, making (C) incorrect as well.

33. **(A)** The author makes this point by initially defining Ethical Egoism in the third sentence of the third paragraph. (B) is incorrect because it describes Psychological Egoism, as the author describes it in the fourth sentence of the third paragraph. From the third sentence of the third paragraph it is clear (C) does not describe Ethical Egoism. (C) also does not describe common-sense morality (fifth sentence of the second paragraph). In the first sentence of the fifth paragraph the author specifically rejects the idea that Ethical Egosim says we should avoid helping others. Thus, (D) is incorrect.

34. **(B)** This is the point of the fifth paragraph. According to the author, it may sometimes be necessary to advance the interests of others to pursue one's own interests. If one cannot separate the interests of others from one's own interests, it will be necessary to help others while helping oneself. The first sentence of the fifth paragraph makes it clear that (A) is incorrect. (C) is incorrect because Ethical Egoism does not take into consideration the interests of others. As explained in the third and fourth paragraphs, the Ethical Egoist pursues his or her self-interest exclusively. The interests of others are irrelevant. Paragraph four, and in particular the last sentence, make it clear that under Ethical Egosim one's only natural duty is to advance one's own interests. (D) is not mentioned. Also, this has nothing to do with (C). (D) does not say anything about the interests of others.

35. **(B)** This is explained in the fifth sentence of the third paragraph. A normative theory is one that tells us how we should or ought to behave. Psychological Egosim is a theory that describes the way people *do* behave. The author specifically points out the difference between these two theories. (A) is a description of Psychological Egosim, and is, thus, incorrect. For similar reasons, (D) is also incorrect. Describing the norms of Americans merely tells us how they behave. It would not tell us how they ought to behave. (C) goes beyond mere description to explanation, but is still incorrect. In the first sentences of the second paragraph the author makes it clear he is not concerned with *why* people do not contribute to world hunger. Rather, he wants to discuss whether it is their duty to do so.

36. **(B)** In the final sentences of the passage the author tells us that Ethical Egoism tells us to advance our *long-term* interests. Momentary pleasure, unless of course it also has long-term gains, is frowned upon. The author specifically indicates in this paragraph that smoking cigarettes is not an activity condoned by Ethical Egoism (III). (I) is also an activity with only short-term pleasures. Only (II) holds any long-term advantage for the actor.

37. **(C)** This point is made in the sixth sentence of the third paragraph where the author says, "Regardless of how we do behave, Ethical Egosim says we have no moral duty except to do what is best for ourselves." This statement clearly makes (A) incorrect. The author's discussion in the sixth paragraph of the preference for long-term interests makes (B) incorrect. (D) is incorrect because the passage makes no mention of utiltarianism. Even if one knows utilitarianism generally holds one should act to achieve the greatest good for the most people, this is clearly contrary to Ethical Egoism's view of natural duties.

38.   (A)   In the final paragraph the author tells us Ethical Egosim only advocates that individuals pursue their *long-term* interests. The problem is in determining their long-term interests. The smoker might argue the years of pleasurable smoking is a long-term interest despite the inevitable result. For lottery winners, it was certainly in their long-term interests to have played, even though for everyone else it was not. The author speaks as if there is some objective standard which people can use to gauge whether a particular course of action *really is* in their interests. Unfortunately, people can only go by their own subjective view of what their interests are. (B) is incorrect because, as pointed out in the fifth paragraph, Ethical Egosim does not suggest one should avoid helping others. Similarly, (C) is incorrect because there may be instances where common-sense morality and Ethical Egoism coincide. Just as Ethical Egoism does not say we should avoid helping others, common-sense morality does not say we cannot act in our own interests as well as help others. (D) is nonsense and has nothing to do with the passage.

PASSAGE V (Questions 39-48)
    In this passage the author gives us some examples of what he terms math abuse. He then tells us why these examples are abusing mathematics. Later in the passage he begins to explain how filtering leads to math abuse. He ends the passage by giving an example of how pure luck can lead to results similar to those explained by methods that abuse math.

39.   (D)   In the third sentence of the second paragraph the author introduces the term math abuse. In the following sentence the author explains that this term includes those who do not know mathematical concepts as well as those who are unwilling to apply even the ones they know. (A) is incorrect because the author uses the example of the nurse's belief as an example of math abuse. It is not the central theme of the passage. The author tells us innumeracy is the inability to deal with simple numerical ideas (second sentence of the second paragraph). In the next sentence the author tells us that the term math abuse includes the problem of innumeracy and *also* a moral component. Thus, (B) is incorrect. The author refers to illiteracy in the second paragraph only to compare it to innumeracy. It is not the problem concerning the author, making (C) incorrect.

40.   (C)   In the second sentence of the third paragraph the author admits that it really does not matter whether more babies are born during a full moon. Nevertheless, by using births as an example of math abuse, and later explaining the filtering process using the same example, we can reasonably conclude the author is skeptical of any statistical relationship between birth rate and a full moon. (A) is incorrect because of the above, and because there is no mention in the passage of deferring to the nurse because of her expertise. In fact, the author uses the nurse's expertise and that of the acquaintance who has invested for twenty years to emphasize that these people should know better. Given the explanation for (C), (B) is also incorrect. In addition, there is no mention in the passage of the possibility of *fewer* babies being born during a full moon. (D) is clearly incorrect. If it were true, the author would not have selected it to illustrate the problem.

41.   (A)   The author defines math abuse in the fourth and fifth sentences of the second paragraph. In the first paragraph the author notes (B), (C), and (D) as specific

examples of math abuse. (A) is more general and includes the examples of (B), (C), and (D), making it the better answer.

42. **(C)** The author makes this point in the last sentence of the second paragraph by telling us, "We do not want to be duped, but most of us are fooled on a regular basis by politicians, the media, and even friends." This statement clearly makes (B) incorrect. The statement also makes (D) incorrect since it includes politicians and friends in addition to the media. (A) is incorrect because the author has provided several examples of math abuse (first paragraph) out of which only one involves pediatrics.

43. **(C)** The author explains how the filtering process can cause the nurse's belief in the fourth paragraph. A second example of the process is given in the fifth paragraph, and the discussion is continued in the sixth paragraph. (A) is incorrect because the whole tenor of the passage suggests the author does not believe there to be actual differences in birth rates corresponding to the phases of the moon. (B) is incorrect because there is no indication in the passage that the nurse applied probability to the situation to reach her conclusion. In fact, if she had, the author would not likely have used her belief as an example. Applying the law of probability to the situation, even incorrectly, would not constitute math abuse according to the author's definition in the second paragraph. (D) is incorrect because the author does not indicate any connection between the nurse's belief and the later example of the casino.

44. **(B)** This is summed up in the third sentence of the fourth paragraph where the author says, "If one watches only for the events that reinforce a belief, one is screening out all the events that falsify it." (A) is incorrect because there is no indication that filtering necessarily avoids mathematics, but only abuses it. Consider the casino example. One may very well know probabilities are involved in slot machines, but the filtering process acts to distort our perception of the actual probability of winning. Although it may be true that filtering *can* work to lose people's money, it does not necessarily *cause* such losses. For example, the nurse does not lose money directly as a result of her belief (unless she makes bets or investments based on her belief). (D) is clearly incorrect. The point of the author's fourth, fifth, and sixth paragraphs is that filtering is a major cause of math abuse.

45. **(C)** We can reach this conclusion based on the fifth paragraph. In particular, by telling us, "Losing makes no sound," the implication is that winning does. It is the sound of winning, quarters hitting the tray, that people hear and use as a filter to distort their expectations of winning. (A) is incorrect because there is no information in the passage that gamblers win more often at slot machines than other people, nor is there any suggestion that gamblers win more often at slot machines than other games. (B) is incorrect because the *actual* probability of winning at a slot machine does not matter. The point is that filtering causes the *perceived* probability to be higher than the actual. (D) is incorrect because we are given no information on how much money casinos make on slot machines or any other games.

46. **(A)** Since the author favorably uses this probability to illustrate an example of math abuse, it is likely the author feels it does not suffer from math abuse. In

addition, math abuse occurs in how mathematics is applied (or not). The probability of a coin toss itself cannot suffer from math abuse. It may, however, be *applied* in such a way that abuses mathematics. The author specifically mentions politicians and the media as frequent math abusers (last sentence of the second paragraph). Thus (C) and (D) are incorrect. Given the examples the author has presented, it should be clear that claims of winning big and successful strategies for picking lottery numbers also suffer from math abuse. In playing the lottery, most people do not stop to calculate their actual chances of winning. If they did, the author would probably argue that they wouldn't play.

47.   **(D)**   The discussion in the sixth paragraph makes this point. If the determination of whether a fund succeeds or fails is based on pure luck and has an even chance of doing either, each year about half the funds will succeed and the other half fail. If one begins with a large enough number of funds, even after several years some of them, simply by chance, will have succeeded every year. (A) is incorrect because the author is not suggesting that investing *is* based on chance, only that chance *might* be the explanation for a hot fund rather than the expertise of the fund manager. (B) is simply a restatement of (A) and is also incorrect. (C) is incorrect for two reasons. First, the author makes no judgment about investing in hot funds. The author's concern lies in the reasons why one chooses one fund over another. The author wants the investor to avoid math abuse in making an investment decision. Second, as will be explained in greater detail in question 48, if hot funds can be explained by chance, the investor is better off not investing in them after they become hot.

48.   **(B)**   Continuing the author's example in paragraph six, in the next year we expect only two of the remaining funds to have succeeded. In the following year, only one of the two that are left. In the next year perhaps, none. Thus, if chance guides which funds are successful, in any given year there is a 50 percent chance that any fund will gain, *and* a 50 percent chance that the same fund will lose. Our expectations cannot guarantee that exactly half of all successful funds will fail the next year, but over many trials this is the expectation. Thus, we can reasonably expect hot funds to eventually lose money. Thus, one should not invest in hot funds for the sole reason that they are hot. (One should also not avoid them just because they are hot. This would be a form of math abuse known as the Gambler's Fallacy.) (A), (C), and (D) are all incorrect to the extent that such a strategy is based upon whether or not the fund is hot. To the extent they are not based on whether the fund is hot, they are specific examples of (B), making (B) the better answer.

PASSAGE VI (Questions 49-57)
        The author of this passage is concerned about what he thinks are misinterpretations being spread by John C. Willke, president of the National Right to Life Committee. Specifically, the author argues that there are hard statistics to support the claim that legal abortions are medically safer than childbirth. In addition, the author describes a study which found that in a select group of teenagers there were fewer adverse psychological episodes among those who had abortions as opposed to those who gave birth.

49.   **(B)**   In the first paragraph the author tells us of John C. Willke who says his evidence comes from his own experience and anecdotal reports, and then is quoted as

saying neither side has hard statistics to support its claims. This distinguishes personal experience and anecdotal reports from hard statistics. In the third paragraph the author tells us there are hard statistics on psychological harm, and in the fourth paragraph describes a research study by Zabin and Hirsch. This explanation makes (A) and (C) incorrect. (D) is incorrect because there is nothing in the passage which suggests patient histories have anything to do with hard statistics.

50.   **(C)**   In the final paragraph of the passage, the author informs us that the medical risks due to abortion rise significantly after the sixteenth week of pregnancy. In the second paragraph the author tells us deaths and medical complications are much less likely with *legal* abortions than childbirth. Together these two bits of information suggests that a legal abortion would be performed before the 16th week of pregnancy. (A) is incorrect because there is no mention that an abortion must be court ordered to be legal. (B) is incorrect because it is not indicated that an abortion is risk-free. (D) is also incorrect because the exact opposite is stated: abortions are "11 times less likely than childbirth to lead to a woman's death."

51.   **(A)**   In the second paragraph the author tells us of statistics relating to deaths and medical complications due to abortions versus childbirth. In the first sentence of the third paragraph the author tells us that psychological harm "has been more difficult to assess." Nowhere in the passage is there any indication that the other statistics were difficult to obtain. Thus, (I) and (II) are true and (III) is not.

52.   **(B)**   In the third paragraph we are told that C. Everett Koop, the former Surgeon General, found past studies dealing with psychological harm to be inconclusive. This means they did not reach any reliable conclusions. The fact that there were previous studies to be considered inconclusive makes (A) incorrect. (C) is incorrect because we are not told *why* Koop found the previous studies to be inconclusive, only that he did. For the same reason, (D) is incorrect. We do not know how the previous studies were conducted, so we cannot make any conclusions based on their methods.

53.   **(A)**   In the second paragraph we are told that data compiled by the National Center for Health Statistics indicate "abortion was 11 times *less* likely than childbirth to lead to a woman's death" (emphasis added). In the same paragraph the author notes that the Centers for Disease Control reported "women undergoing abortions are 100 times *less* likely to have complications requiring major abdominal surgery than women bearing children" (emphasis added). The factors 11 and 100 justify the use of the word *much* rather than *slightly*, as the latter is used in (C). Thus, (C) is incorrect. That both institutions found abortions less likely to lead to the indicated problem, (B) which says *more*, is incorrect. (D) suggests the results were mixed, which is also incorrect.

54.   **(B)**   In the fifth paragraph the author tells us of Zabin and Hirsch's findings. According to the author, they report "those who chose abortion were *less* likely to undergo adverse psychological episodes ... than *either* those who bore children or those who had not been pregnant" (emphasis added). From paragraph four we know there were only three groups in the study: those who had abortions, those who bore a child, and those who were not pregnant. The results were not mixed for those who

had abortions compared to the other two groups, making (A) incorrect. The author clearly states adverse psychological episodes were *less* likely for those who had abortions compared to the other two groups, making (C) incorrect. (D) is incorrect because the Zabin and Hirsch study was not one of the ones declared inconclusive by Koop. In addition, there is no indication in the passage that the author believes the results to be inconclusive. On the contrary, in introducing the Zabin and Hirsch study the author indicates the study provides hard statistics on psychological harm (last sentence of the third paragraph).

55. **(D)** The reference to *ghost* appears in the second sentence of the sixth paragraph. The following sentence goes on to clarify the ghost reference and clarifies that it means the fear of psychological harm. According to Zabin, her study shows abortions are psychologically safe. (A) is incorrect because, according to Zabin, the right-to-lifers were the ones arguing abortions were psychologically harmful to young women (first sentence of the sixth paragraph). Neither Zabin nor the author claims the right-to-lifers are ghosts. (B) is incorrect because there is no indication in the passage that Zabin and Hirsch used a ghost writer to draft their report. (D) is incorrect because the Zabin and Hirsch study did not examine the connection between deaths and abortion, rather they studied the psychological effects of abortion.

56. **(B)** In the fourth paragraph we are told the homogeneity of the group studied (black urban teenagers) reduced the chances that the results would be skewed by the influence of other variables. Thus, avoiding the influence of other variables is considered an advantage (I). In the seventh paragraph we are told this group consists of those "most likely to be affected by laws ... that would limit ... abortion. ..." If the findings of Zabin and Hirsch are correct, it is important to know what the psychological effects will be on this group if access to abortions is restricted. Thus, (III) is an advantage. (II) is not mentioned as an advantage. In fact, it is a disadvantage. The homogeneity of the group studied will make extension of the findings to other groups difficult.

57. **(C)** In the last paragraph the author suggests that restrictions on the access of abortions will hinder women from obtaining them quickly. The author notes that despite the findings presented earlier in the passage, the risks associated with having an abortion increase significantly when the abortion is performed past the sixteenth week of pregnancy. Willke's argument is that abortions are more harmful than bearing a child. Thus, by advocating restrictions which slow down the process, Willke is causing his arguments to come true. (A) and (B) are incorrect because there is no consideration in the passage of the possibility of women having illegal abortions, and thus committing a crime, as a result of restrictions. The implication is that even legal abortions performed later in the pregnancy are riskier than those performed early. (D) is incorrect because there is no indication in the passage that privacy rights will be hampered by restrictions on abortion. In addition, this is not an argument attributed to Willke in the passage.

PASSAGE VII (Questions 58-65)
The authors of this passage explain the balance between governmental needs and individual rights and liberties. We are told that neither can dominate, but there are times when one must give way to the other. We are given an example where several abridge-

ments of individual rights was justified on the basis of military necessity. The authors end the passage by identifying two tests used by the Supreme Court to strike the necessary balance.

58.   **(C)**   The authors tell us this in the first sentence of the passage when they say, "there clearly must be a balance between the scope of individual freedom and the needs of government." The authors note there may be instances when either individual rights or governmental needs dominate, but these are extreme cases (e.g., *Korematsu*) and the usual case is to strike a balance between the two. Thus, both (A) and (B) are incorrect. (D) is incorrect because the authors admit in the first sentence of the second paragraph that "there may be political excesses that threaten to limit civil liberties and rights...." Although it is true that a threatened limitation is not necessarily a limitation, if it did not sometimes occur the author would have been remiss in mentioning the possibility without indicating it hasn't happened. (In addition, anyone with a general understanding of the political process knows that political excesses quite often limit individual rights yet this should be taken into account.)

59.   **(D)**   In the fourth sentence of the first paragraph the authors tell us that federal judges are independent of direct political control. In the next sentence the authors contrast this by telling us most state and local judges are elected "making them directly accountable to the people." We can thus infer that federal judges are not elected (which is true). Thus, (B) is incorrect. This same statement also makes (C) incorrect. Although (A) is true, we do not have to *infer* that local judges are mostly elected. We are directly told this is the case in the fifth sentence of the first paragraph.

60.   **(B)**   In the first sentence of the second paragraph the authors mention the concern of political excesses. In the sixth sentence of the first paragraph, the authors suggest elected judges might be influenced by the political process in making its decisions. In the fourth sentence of the first paragraph we are told federal judges are not subject to direct political control. Thus, federal judges are better able to make decisions protecting individual liberties even though such decisions may run counter to public preferences. (A), (C), and (D) are all incorrect because each of these groups is elected and therefore subject to political influences.

61.   **(C)**   The authors address this question in the second paragraph when they tell us, "there are also legitimate governmental needs that may call for a modification of individual freedoms. This occurs when these civil freedoms are used or misused to attack the very foundations of the system itself." In the third paragraph the authors discuss how World War II concentration camps for Japanese Americans were justified on the basis of the fear the Japanese would attack the West Coast. Thus, when the nation is threatened, individual liberties may be limited. It is clear, then, that (D) is incorrect. It should be equally clear that (A) is incorrect. The third paragraph illustrates that the governmental need must be great to justify the magnitude of the restrictions placed on Japanese Americans. In addition, in the first sentence of the second paragraph the authors note the limitation that the governmental need must be *legitimate*. (B) is incorrect because it suggests that the government may restrict civil rights when it needs to restrict civil rights. This merely restates the question and does not answer it.

62.   **(A)**   This point is made in the first sentence of the third paragraph. The fear of the Japanese invading the West Coast, along with the fear of subversive activities, justified the extraordinary limitation of the rights of the Japanese Americans relocated to concentration camps. (B) is incorrect because we are told the Supreme Court specifically rejected the possibility that the exclusion of Japanese Americans was racially motivated. Rather, it was based on military necessity (sixth sentence of the third paragraph). (C) and (D) are incorrect because there is no mention of electoral pressures or public opinion in the discussion of the exclusion and *Korematsu*.

63.   **(A)**   In the third sentence of the third paragraph we are told the order excluding Japanese Americans from the West Coast was upheld by the Supreme Court against constitutional challenges (making (C) incorrect). In the following sentences we are told the exclusion was justified by military necessity. If the exclusion was upheld and justified, it cannot be considered either unnecessary or illegal, making both (B) and (D) incorrect.

64.   **(C)**   The second sentence of the fourth paragraph indicates, "One of the most important spheres of civil liberties where the balancing testing has been applied is with regard to the civil liberties and rights enumerated in the First Amendment, particularly the liberties of *speech, press,* and *the right of assembly*" (emphasis added). Although the free exercise of religion *is* a First Amendment liberty, it is *not* specifically mentioned in the passage. Since (A), (B), and (D) are all mentioned, they are all incorrect.

65.   **(B)**   The fourth paragraph of the passage introduces the balancing and clear and present danger tests. Since the authors hare previously indicated in both discussion and by example that restrictions on civil rights and liberties may sometimes be allowed, the purpose of these tests is to aid in the determination of when restrictions are justified. Thus, application of both the balancing test (I) and the clear and present danger test (III) may allow restrictions on civil rights and liberties. The rational basis test (II) is not mentioned in the passage, so we cannot make any judgments as to what it allows.

Section 2 — Physical Sciences

66.   **(C)**   One mole of the compound $C_{45}H_{86}O_6$ contains 45 moles of carbon atoms and therefore (45 mol) (12 g/mol) = 540 g C. Since one mole of the compound has a total mass of 723 g (the given molar mass), the percentage of carbon by mass is

(540 g/723 g) × 100 = 75%.

67.   **(B)**   According to the equation for reaction 1, six moles of oxygen gas are required for each mole of glucose consumed. First, use the molar mass of glucose (180 g/mol) to find the number of moles corresponding to 60 g of glucose, and then use the mole ratio from the equation to find the moles of oxygen gas required.

$$60 \text{ g } C_6H_{12}O_6 \times \frac{1 \text{ mol } C_6H_{12}O_6}{180 \text{ g } C_6H_2O_6} \times \frac{6 \text{ mol } O_2}{1 \text{ mol } C_6H_{12}O_6} = 2 \text{ mol } O_2$$

68.   **(A)**   According to the equation for reaction 2, $63\frac{1}{2}$ moles of oxygen gas are required to react with one mole of glyceryl trimyristate. At STP, each mole of oxygen gas occupies a volume 22.4 L or 22.4×10^{-3} m³ (there are 1000 L in a m³.) The total volume of oxygen gas required is $(63.5 \text{ mol})(22.4 \times 10^{-3} \text{ m}^3) = 1.4$ m³

69.   **(D)**   The H° value represents the amount of heat liberated (the negative sign indicates that the reaction is exothermic) when one mole of glucose burns. For 0.100 mol glucose, the heat liberated is $(0.100 \text{ mol})(2803 \text{ kJ/mol}) = 280.3$ kJ $= 2.803 \times 10^5$ J. The specific heat, C, is the quantity of heat energy needed to raise the temperature of a unit mass of material by unit temperature. Thus the total heat, Q, for total mass m and temperature change

$$\Delta T = T_f - T_i \text{ is } Q = Cm \ \Delta T = Cm(T_f - T_i).$$

T_f is the final temperature and T_i is the material's initial temperature. Substituting the values $Q = 2.803 \times 10^5$ J, $m = 1000$ g, $C = 4.18$ J/g c°, and $T_i = 21.0°$C yields:

$$2.803 \times 10^5 = (4.18)(1000)(T_f - 21.0)$$

$$T_f = (2.803 \times 10^5)/(4.18)(1000) + 21.0$$

$$T_f = 67.1 + 21.0 = 88.1°C$$

70.   **(C)**   The absolute temperature of a gas sample varies directly with both its volume and pressure. Convert the given temperature to Kelvin, $37°C + 273 = 310$ K, and convert one of the given pressures to the units of the other:

(0.90 atm) (760 mm Hg / atm) = 684 mm Hg or

(851 mm Hg) (1 atm / 760 mm Hg) 1.12 atm,

then apply the combined gas laws:

$$T_{final} = (310 \text{ K})(851 \text{ mm Hg} / 684 \text{ mm Hg})(175 \text{ mL} / 125 \text{ mL}) = 540 \text{ K}$$

or

$$T_{final} = (310 \text{ K})(1.12 \text{ atm} / 0.90 \text{ atm})(175 \text{ mL} / 125 \text{ mL}) = 540 \text{ K}$$

and convert to Celsius: 540 K - 273 = 267°C

71.   **(B)**   The oxidation numbers of oxygen and hydrogen, both in glucose and in carbon dioxide, are -2 and +1, respectively. Since the sum of the oxidation numbers in a neutral molecule must equal zero, the oxidation number of carbon in glucose (x) is given by: $6(x) + (12(+1) + 6(-2)) = 0$ or $x = 0$. The oxidation number of carbon, in carbon dioxide (y), is given by: $y + 2(-2) = 0$ or $y = +4$. Therefore, the oxidation number of carbon has increased by four.

72.   **(A)**   Convert the given mass to moles, use the enthalpy for reaction 2, which corresponds to the energy liberated in the combustion of one mole of the fat, and finally convert the energy to kilocalories.

(5.0 g) (1 mol/723 g) (27280 kJ / mol) (1 kcal / 4.18 kJ) = 45 kcal

73.   **(A)**   The decrease in temperature, as the white powder dissolves, shows that

the solution process is endothermic. Since heat is required to form the solution, adding heat to raise the temperature will promote solution, thus increasing the solubility at the higher temperature.

74. **(D)** The total mass of the solution was 1.5 g + 10.0 g = 11.5 g. The volume is this mass divided by the density.

$$(11.5 \text{ g}) (1 \text{ mL} / 1.05 \text{ g}) = 11.0 \text{ mL}$$

75. **(B)** The freezing point, lowering of a dilute solution of a non-volatile solute, is proportional to the molal concentration of the solute:

$$T_f = (K_f) (Cm).$$

Using this relationship, the moles of solute per kilogram of solvent (molality, Cm) may be found: $Cm = (T_f) / (K_f) = [0°C - (- 1.90°C)] / (1.86°C/m) = 1.02$ m. = 1.02 mole white powder per kg of water. The solution was made by dissolving 1.500 g of white powder in 10.00 g = 0.01000 kg of water. The solution contains 1.500g white powder / 0.01000 kg water = 150 g solute per kilogram of solvent. Therefore 150 g of white powder corresponds to 1.02 mol of white powder. The molar mass, numerically equal to the molecular weight, is 150 g/1.02 mol = 147 g/mol.

76. **(B)** In experiment 3 it was found that 44.0 mg or 44.0 mg (1 mmol/44.0 mg) = 1.00 mmol of CO_2 and 18.0 mg or 18.0 mg (1 mmol/18.0 mg) = 1.00 mmol of H_2O were formed in the combustion of 30.0 mg of the white powder. Since one millimole of CO_2 contains one millimole of carbon, and one millimole of H_2O contains two millimoles of hydrogen atoms, the 30.0 mg of white powder contains 1.00 mmol C (12.0 mg C/ mmol C) = 12.0 mg C and 2.00 mmol H (1.0 mg H/mmol H) 2.0 mg H. Experiment 2 indicated that the white powder contained only C, H, and O. The mass of oxygen can be found by difference: 30.0 mg - 12.0 mg - 2.0 = 16.0 mg O. Converting this mass to millimoles of oxygen yields 16.0 mg O (1mmol O/16.0 mg O) = 1.00 mmol. The mole ratio of the elements in the white power is 1.00 mmol C/2.00 mmol H/1.00 mmol O which leads to the simplest formula CH_2O.

77. **(B)** The molecular weight, corresponding to the molecular formula, must be a whole number multiple of the molecular weight of the simplest formula (e.g. 13 for CH.)

$$67 / 13 = 5.2 \sim 5$$

Therefore the molecular formula must contain five simplest formula units: $(CH)_5$ or C_5H_5.

78. **(D)** Solids which have metallic bonding, or dispersive forces only (i.e., nonpolar molecules), generally have very low solubility in polar solvents such as water. Solutions of ionically bonded solids in water conduct an electric current. Since experiment 1 showed that the white power is readily soluble in water but that the solution is nonconducting, the only reasonable choice is that the interunit bonding is through dipole-dipole interactions. This is consistent with the bottle label (which said that the white powder might be a sugar) and with the molecular formula found in question 77.

79. **(D)** From its position in the periodic table, mysterium is an alkali metal and hence its chloride is expected to be similar to NaCl and KCl. That is, MyCl is expected to be a very stable, ionically bonded, water soluble, white crystaline solid near room temperature. The alkali metals (and other active metals) form chlorides (and other salts) which are very stable and which do not decompose even when heated to very high temperatures (>2000 K).

80. **(B)** In a balanced equation for a nuclear reaction, both the sum of the mass numbers (A) and the atomic numbers (Z) for the products and reactants must be equal.

$$A \text{ (reactants)} = 238 + 238 = 476 = A \text{ (products)} = 300 + x \quad x = 476 - 300 = 176$$

$$Z \text{ (reactants)} = 92 + 92 = 184 + Z \text{ (products)} = 119 + y \quad y = 184 - 119 = 65$$

Atomic number 65 corresponds to the element terbium, Tb.

$$2 \, {}^{239}_{92}\text{U} \rightarrow {}^{300}_{110}\text{My} + {}^{176}_{75}\text{Tb}$$

81. **(A)** Since mysterium is in the first column of the periodic table, it would be expected to form compounds similar to those of potassium and sodium. That is, mysterium would be expected to form ionic compounds, in which it exists as a singly positive ion. Sulfate is a doubly negative ion, hence two My^+ ions are required for one $SO_4^=$ ion: My_2SO_4.

82. **(D)** The elements of the first group of the periodic table easily lose one electron to form singly positive ions; they have low first ionization energies. The resulting singly positive ion has a stable, noble gas-like electron configuration and a very large second ionization energy. Choices (A), (B), and (C), since they are less than, equal to, and only very slightly greater than the first ionization energy, are all unreasonable. Choice (D), more than a factor of four, greater than the first ionization energy, must be the second ionization energy of mysterium.

83. **(B)** The emission of an alpha particle, the nucleus of a helium-4, removes two protons and decreases the atomic number of the parent nuclide by two: 119 - 2 = 117.

84. **(D)** Assuming no chemical or mechanical loss, only radioactive decay during the separation process must be considered. The 30.0 minute separation time represents 3.0 half lives (one half life = 600 s = 10.0 minute). Over a period of three half lives the mass of My decreases by a factor of $(1/2)^3 = 1/8$ or the mass must have been 8 times as great at the beginning of the separation as it its end: 8×1.0 mg = 8.0 mg. An alternate approach is to use the radioactive decay equation

$$A = A_0 \exp (-0.693 \, t/t^{1/}2)$$

solved for A_0:

$$A_0 = A \exp(+0.693 \, t/t^{1/}2).$$

$$A_0 = (1.0 \text{ mg})[\exp(+0.693(30.0 \text{ min}/10.0 \text{ min}))] = 8.0 \text{ mg}.$$

85. **(D)** Average speed is the speed at which the car would travel the given distance in the given time:

$$t_1 = \frac{d_1}{v_1} \qquad\qquad t_2 = \frac{d_2}{v_2}$$

$$t_1 = \frac{15 \text{ km}}{30 \text{ km} / \text{hr}} = \frac{1}{2} \text{ hr} \qquad t_2 = \frac{30 \text{ km}}{60 \text{ km} / \text{hr}} = \frac{1}{2} \text{ hr}$$

$$t_{\text{total}} = \frac{1}{2} + \frac{1}{2} = 1 \text{ hr to cover 45 km}$$

therefore:

$$v_{\text{avg}} = \frac{d_{\text{total}}}{t_{\text{total}}} = \frac{45 \text{ km}}{1 \text{ hr}} = 45 \text{ km} / \text{hr} \, .$$

86. **(A)** Given the following equation for a free-falling body,

$$d = v_i t + \frac{1}{2} g t^2$$

$$d = 1200 \text{ ft.}$$

$$v_i = 0$$

$$g = 32 \text{ ft/sec}^2$$

then,

$$1200 \text{ ft} = 0 + \frac{1}{2}(32 \text{ ft/sec}^2)(t^2)$$

$$1200 \text{ ft/16 ft/sec}^2 = t^2$$

$$75 \text{ sec}^2 = t^2$$

$$8.66 \text{ sec} = t.$$

87. **(B)** The relationship between temperature and volume of a gas is stated in Charles' Law:

$$\frac{V_1}{T_1} = \frac{V_2}{T_2}$$

Note: All temperatures must be in ° Kelvin.

$$\frac{2 \text{ m}^3}{250° \text{K}} = \frac{V}{294° \text{K}}$$

$$588 \text{ m}^3 \cdot °\text{K} = 250°\text{K} \, V_2$$

$$V_2 = 2.35 \text{ m}^3$$

88. **(C)** Glucose is the monomer of cellulose as well as starch.

89. **(D)** The reaction given describes the reaction of an alkyl halide with magnesium in dry ether to produce the Grignard reagent. The Grignard reagent subse-

quently reacts with solid CO_2, or dry ice, to produce a carboxylic acid. The reaction process is illustrated below:

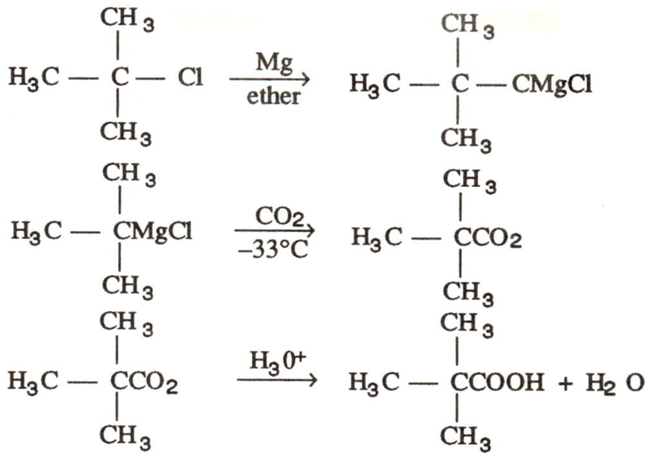

90. **(C)** Both glycine and glucose react with the Grignard reagent. The aldehyde group of glucose reacts with the Grignard reagent to produce an alcohol while the carbonyl group of glycine reacts with the Grignard reagent to produce a ketone.

91. **(D)** Calculate the amount of hydrogen ion neutralized by 0.750 g of brand B based on the data in the table, and then use this amount of hydrogen ion to calculate the volume of sulfuric acid solution required.

Amount of H^+ in 25.00 mL of 0.5000 M HCl solution.

(25.00 mL) (0.5000 mmol / mL) = 12.5 mmol H^+

Amount of OH^- used in back titration for brand B.

(40.12 mL) (0.1000 mmol/mL) = 4.0 mmol OH^- = 4.0 mmol H^+ not reacted.

Amount of H^+ reacted with 0.750 g brand B.

12.5 mmol - 4.0 mmol = 8.5 mmol H^+ that did react with brand B.

Volume of sulfuric acid solution containing this amount of H^+.

(8.5 mmol H^+) (1 mmol H_2SO_4/2 mmol H^+) (1 mL/0.1000 mmol) = 42.5 mL

92. **(B)** According to the Bronsted-Lowry acid-base theory, an acid becomes its conjugate base when it donates a proton to a base, and a base becomes its conjugate acid when it accepts a proton.

Hydroxide ion is the conjugate base of water, or water is the conjugate acid of hydroxide ion for this reaction.

93. **(A)** Note that the indicator signals the end point of the titration at pH = 9.0. First calculate the hydrogen ion concentration from the pH and use the ion product of water to find the hydroxide ion concentration.

$$pH = 9.0 = -log[H^+]$$

$$[H^+] = 10^{-9p} = 1.0 \times 10^{-9} \text{ M}$$

$$Kw = 1.0 \times 10^{-14} = [H^+][OH^-]$$

$$[OH^-] = Kw / [H^+] = (1.0 \times 10^{-14}) / (1.0 \times 10^{-9}) = 1.0 \times 10^{-5} \text{ M}$$

94. **(A)** Hydrochloric acid is a strong acid and sodium hydroxide is a strong base. The inflection point of their titration curve will occur at pH = 7.0. Since the base was added to the acid, the pH will start low (near pH = 1), rise through the inflection point at pH = 7, and gradually approach the pH of the base (near pH = 13).

95. **(B)** Two moles of HCl are needed per mole of magnesium hydroxide.

$$Mg(OH)_2 + 2HCl \longrightarrow MgCl_2 + 2H_2O.$$

96. **(D)** For the given hydrolysis reaction:

$$Kb = 2.4 \times 10^{-8} = [H_2CO_3] [OH^-] / [HCO_3^-]$$

Assuming that $[HCO_3^-] = 0.42$ M and that $[H_2CO_3] = [OH^-]$

$$\frac{[OH^-]^2}{(0.42)} = 2.4 \times 10^{-8}$$

$$[OH^-] = [(0.42)(2.4 \times 10^{-8})]^{1/2} = 1.0 \times 10^{-4} \text{ M}$$

$$pOH = -\log (1.0 \times 10^{-4}) = 4.0; \quad pH = 14.0 - pOH = 10.0$$

97. **(B)** The solubility reaction is $Mg(OH)_2 \longleftrightarrow Mg^{++} + 2OH^-$ and the solubility product is $Ksp = 1.8 \times 10^{-11} = [Mg^{++}] [OH^-]^2$, with $[Mg^{++}] = 0.18$ M.

$$(0.18 [OH^-]^2) = 1.8 \times 10^{-11}$$

$$[OH^-] = [1.8 \times 10^{-11} / 0.18]^{1/2} = 1.0 \times 10^{-5} \text{ M}$$

$$pOH = 5.0; \quad pH = 9.0$$

98. **(B)** From step 1, or equation 3, the rate of formation of ES is proportional to the product [E] [S]. If both [E] and [S] are doubled, the rate of formation of ES will increase by a factor of (2) (2) = 4.

99. **(C)** Note that k'', Km, and [TE] are all constant. Equation (6) reduces to RATE = (constant)[S] (first order in S) and equation (7) reduces to RATE = constant (zeroth order.)

100. (C) $K[E][S] = K'[ES] + k''[ES] = (K' + k'')[ES]$

$$K_{eq} = \frac{[ES]}{[E][S]} = \frac{K}{K' + K^m} = \frac{1}{Km}$$

101. (A) Use equations 6 and 7 to analyze the dependence of R on [S]. Equation 6 shows that R increases in proportion to [S] for small values of [S], and equation 7 shows that R approaches a constant value for large values of [S].

102. (D) For a first order reaction the rate law is $\ln[S] = \ln[So] - Ct$. If $t = h$, the half time, then $[S] = \frac{1}{2}[So]$.

$\ln[\frac{1}{2}So] = \ln[So] - Ch$

$\ln[\frac{1}{2}So] = \ln[So] = - Ch$

$\ln(\frac{1}{2}) = \ln - Ch = - \ln(2)$

$h = \ln(2) / C$

103. (C) With the initial displacement and initial velocity both zero, the displacement, x, of an object subjected to constant acceleration, a, as a function of time, t, is $x = \frac{1}{2}at^2$. Solving for time.

$$t = \sqrt{2x/a}.$$

Substituting $x = 0.08$ m and $a = g = 9.8$ m/s^2

$$t = \sqrt{(2)(0.08)/(9.8)} = 0.13 \text{ s}.$$

104. (A) By conservation of mechanical energy, the kinetic energy after falling must equal the gravitational potential energy at the start of the fall.

kinetic energy after = potential energy before = mgh,

where h is the height or distance fallen.

kinetic energy $= (2.5 \times 10^{-3}$ kg$)(9.8$ m/s$^2)(0.08$ m$) = 2 \times 10^{-3}$ J $= 2$ mJ.

An alternate method is to calculate the speed of the bill after falling 8 cm and then use the definition of kinetic energy.

$$v = at = \sqrt{2ax} = \sqrt{(2)(9.8)(0.8)} = 1.25 \text{ m/s}$$

$$T = \frac{1}{2}mv^2 = \frac{1}{2}(2.5 \times 10^{-3})(1.25)^2 = 2 \times 10^{-3} \text{ J} = 2 \text{ mJ}$$

105. (D) Since the dropper, catcher, and dollar bill are all moving with the same uniform (non-accelerated) speed, the game is the same as when the elevator is at rest.

106. (B) See question 103:

$$\text{time} = \sqrt{2x/a} \, \alpha \sqrt{x}.$$

If x increases by a factor of two, from 8 cm to 16 cm, then the time increases by a factor of $\sqrt{2}$.

107. **(D)**   When a falling object reaches its terminal speed, s, the resisting force, R, must equal the downward force, that is, the object's weight, mg. With k as the sought-for proportionality constant:

$$R = ks = mg = k(7.0 \text{ m/s}) = 2.5 \text{ g}) (9.8 \text{ m/s}^2)$$

$$k = (2.5) (9.8) / (7.0) = 3.5 \text{ g/s}$$

108. **(D)**   Ozonolysis is a characteristic reaction of alkenes. It degrades alkenes to aldehydes:

$$\underset{\text{}}{R-\overset{\displaystyle O}{\overset{\|}{C}}-H}$$

and ketones:

$$\underset{\text{}}{R-\overset{\displaystyle O}{\overset{\|}{C}}-R'}$$

by cleaving the double bond with ozone (O_3) in the presence of zinc dust (Zn) and acid (H^+).

The mechanism of the reaction is as follows: ozone is passed through the alkene which causes the formation of an ozonide; the ozonides, which are explosive, are converted into aldehydes and ketones in the presence of zinc dust and acid:

$$R_2C = CR_2 + O_3 \longrightarrow R_2C \overset{O-O}{\underset{O}{\diagup \quad \diagdown}} CR_2$$

alkene   ozone   ozonide

$$R_2C \overset{O-O}{\underset{O}{\diagup \quad \diagdown}} CR_2 \xrightarrow[\text{H+}]{\text{Zn}} R_2C \; O + HRC = O + H_2O$$

The position of the double bond in the original alkene will be indicated by the carbonyl group $(C = O)$ formed in the products after ozonolysis. Sodium borohydride $(NaBH_4)$ is a reagent used to reduce the carbonyl group of aldehydes, ketones and carboxylic acids to the hydroxyl group of the corresponding alcohol. With the metal hydrides, the key step is the transfer of a hydride ion to the carbonyl carbon of the substance being reduced. The acidic hydrogen first reacts to liberate hydrogen gas. The carbonyl group is then attacked by the BH_4 q ion, and the group is reduced to the primary alkoxide. Overall, the reaction may be written as:

$$4 \text{ RCHO} + 3NaBH_4 \longrightarrow 4H_2 + (RCH_2O)_4BNa \longrightarrow 4 \text{ RCH}_2OH$$

In this problem, the following occurs:

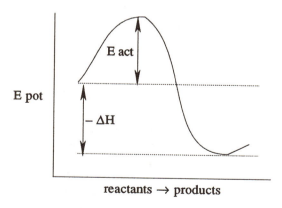

109. (A) Examining the given compounds, one observes that they are all alkyl chlorides. Recalling the fact that vapor pressure is related to boiling point and in turn, the relationship between boiling point and molecular weight, this problem may now be solved. The boiling point of a substance is defined by the temperature at which the vapor pressure of the substance is equal to the atmospheric pressure. Hence, the compound with the greatest vapor pressure has the lowest boiling point. The boiling point is also related to the molecular weight as boiling points increase along a homologous series in direct relation to molecular weights. Therefore, the compound with the greatest vapor pressure would be that compound which has the smallest molecular weight. Of the compounds given, the one of smallest molecular weight is CH_3Cl.

110. (D) LiCl, NaCl, and KCl all have the 6PO(NaCl) structure. Because of the large ionic radius of Cs, CsCl takes on the 3.2PTOT(CsCl) structure.

111. (D) All reactions, exothermic or endothermic, that involve any type of bond breaking will have an energy of activation, though it may be very low. An exothermic reaction has a negative ΔH (change in enthalpy). Since heat is being liberated it is only logical that the potential energy of the products should be lower than the potential energy of the reactants. This is summarized in the following diagram:

E pot

E act

$-\Delta H$

reactants → products

112. (B) Using the equation

$$Density = \frac{Mass}{Volume}$$

we obtain

Mass = (Density)(Volume).

Since density is in gm/cm^3 let us use the CGS system. Hence, we must convert the measurements of the block into centimeters.

2 meters = 200 centimeters

3 meters = 300 centimeters

5 meters = 500 centimeters

Now, finding the volume of the block $V = l \times w \times h = 200 \times 300 \times 500$

$V = 3.0 \times 10^7 \text{ cm}^3$

Finally, we can find the mass:

Mass = $(7.8 \text{ gm/cm}^3)(3.0 \times 10^7 \text{ cm}^3)$

Mass = 2.34×10^8 gm

113. **(C)** Weight is the force resulting from the acceleration due to gravity:

$F = ma = (4.54 \text{ kg})(9.8 \text{ m/s}^2) = 44 \text{ N} = \text{weight}.$

114. **(D)** Applying the static condition that the sum of the torques about a point must be zero, using the elbow joint as the point about which the torques are calculated gives:

$(T)(2'') = (3 \text{ lb})(6'') + (10 \text{ lb})(15'')$

$T = (18 + 150)/2 = 84 \text{ lb}.$

115. **(A)** Applying the static condition that the net force must be zero and using the result of question 38:

$F = 84 \text{ lb} - 3 \text{ lb} - 10 \text{ lb} = 71 \text{ lb}.$

An alternate method is to use the sum of torques about the point at which the biceps muscle is attached:

$(F)(2'') = (3 \text{ lb})(4'') + (10 \text{ lb})(13'')$

$F = (12 + 130)/2 = 71 \text{ lb}.$

116. **(B)** Equate the counterclockwise torques to the clockwise torques about the shoulder joint. Only the vertical component of the tension in the deltoid muscle is used.

$(8 \text{ lb})(13'') = (T' \sin 17°)(6'')$

$T' = (8)(13)/(0.29)(6) = 60 \text{ lb}.$

117. **(C)**   Since they are the only horizontal forces, the horizontal component of the force exerted by the shoulder blade must be equal to the horizontal component of the tension in the deltoid muscle:

$$F'\cos 9.3° = T'\cos 17°$$

$$F'(0.99) = (60 \text{ lb}) (0.96)$$

$$F'= (60) (0.96) / (0.99) = 58 \text{ lb}.$$

An alternate method, which avoids using the result of question 116, is to equate the clockwise to counterclockwise torques about the point at which the deltoid muscle is attached to the humerus:

$$(F'\sin 9.3°) (6'') = (8 \text{ lb}) (7'')$$

$$F'= (8) (7) / (0.16) (6) = 58 \text{ lb}.$$

118. **(B)**   For the humerus to remain stationary, the sum of the vertical component of F' and the weight of the humerus must equal the vertical component of the tension in the deltoid muscle. Using $T'= 60$ lb found in question 116.

$$F'\sin 9.3° + 8 \text{ lb} = T'\sin 17° = 60(0.29) = 17.4 \text{ lb}$$

$$F'\sin 9.3° = 17.4 - 8 = 9 \text{ lb}.$$

119. **(B)**   The index of refraction of a medium is the ratio of the speed of light in vacuum to the speed of light in the medium. Therefore, the speed of light in the medium is the speed of light in vacuum, divided by the index of refraction.

$$(3.0 \times 10^8 \text{ m/s}) / (1.47) = 2.9 \times 10^8 \text{ m/s}.$$

120. **(A)**   Snell's law states that when light travels from one medium into a second medium, the index of refraction of the first medium, times the sine of the angle of incidence, is equal to the index of refraction of the second medium, times the sine of the angle of refraction. For small angles, the sine of the angle may be replaced by the value of the angle in radians. When light moving through air ($n = 1.00$) is incident at an angle of $5° = 5\pi/180 = 0.0873$ radians passes into a medium with index of refraction 1.47, the angle of refraction, r, is given by

$$n \sin\theta_2 = n'\sin\theta_r$$

$$(1.00) (0.0873) = (1.47) (r)$$

$$r = 0.0875 / 1.47 = 0.059 \text{ radians}$$

121. **(B)**   Use equation 1 with the index of refraction of air $n'= 1.00$, the object distance $p = 250$ mm, the index of refraction of the fluid within the eyeball $n = 1.47$, and the image distance q = 24 mm. $1.00 / 250 \text{ mm} + 1.47 / 24 \text{ mm} = (1.47 - 1.00) / R$

$$\{(1.00)(24) + (1.47) (250)\} / (24) (250) = 0.47 / R$$

$$R = (0.47) (24) (250) / (24 + 367) = 7.2 \text{ mm}$$

122. **(C)**   The focal length, f'', of a combination of lenses which have individual focal lengths f and f' is given by

$$1/f'' = 1/f + 1/f'$$

The focal length of the eye plus corrective lens must be $f'' = 24$ mm and the focal length of the "abnormal" eye is given as $f = 30$ mm.

$$1/24 \text{ mm} = 1/30 \text{ mm} + 1/f$$

$$1/f = 1/24 - 1/30 = (30 - 24)/(24)(30) = 1/120 \text{ mm}$$

$$f = 120 \text{ mm}$$

123. **(C)**   As a ray diagram will show, the ratio of the image size, I, to the object size, O, is the same as the ratio of the image distance, q, to the object distance, p: $I/O = q/p$. For this case $O = 20$ cm $= 200$ mm, $q = 24$ mm, and $p = 120$ cm $= 1200$ mm.

$$I/200 \text{ mm} = 24 \text{ mm}/1200 \text{ mm}$$

$$I = (200 \text{ mm})(24 \text{ mm})/(1200 \text{ mm}) = 4 \text{ mm}$$

124. **(B)**   The angular resolution of 26 seconds of arc corresponds to $26/(60)(60) = 0.00722$ degrees of arc or $0.00722\pi/180 = 1.26 \times 10^{-4}$ radians.

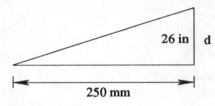

For this small angle, $1.26 \times 10^{-4} = d/250$

$$d = (250)(1.26 \times 10^{-4}) = 0.031 \text{ mm} = 31 \text{ μm}.$$

125. **(C)**   Since 1 μm $= 1000$ nm, radiation of wavelength 1 μm is slightly longer in wavelength than visible light. It is beyond the red end of the visible spectrum or in the infrared region. Both x-rays and ultraviolet radiation are of shorter wavelength than visible light. Microwaves are of substantially longer wavelength than visible light, of the order of mm to cm.

126. **(B)**   Planck's quantum equation combined with the relationship that the product of the frequency times wavelength is equal to the speed of light is $E = hc/\lambda$.

$$\lambda = hc/E = (6.6 \times 10^{-34} \text{ J s})(3.0 \times 10^8 \text{ m/s})/(3.6 \times 10^{-19} \text{ J})$$

$$\lambda = 5.5 \times 10^{-7} \text{ m} = 550 \text{ nm}.$$

Even without doing the above calculation the only reasonable choice is 550 nm because, as stated in question 125, the limits of visible light are 400 nm to 700 nm.

127. **(C)**   Electric potential (voltage) is energy per charge, electric current is

charge per time, and their product is electric power:

$$P = IV = (8 \text{ C/s}) (120 \text{ J/s}) = 960 \text{ J/s} = 960 \text{ W}.$$

128. **(D)**   Combining Ohm's law, $V = IR$, with the power equation, $P = IV$, leads to $R = V/I = V/(P/V) = V^2/P$. Substituting $V = 120$ V and $P = 1200$ W; $R = (120)^2/(1200) = 12$ ohms.

129. **(C)**   The voltage ratio of the primary to secondary cores of a transformer is the same as the ratio of the number of turns of wire on the cores:

$$Vp/Vs = Np/Ns = 120/6 = 20$$

130. **(A)**   The two resistors, in series, can be replaced by a single resistor equal to their sum: $R_1 = 5$ ohm + 10 ohm = 15 ohm. The given circuit reduces to an equivalent circuit of two 15 ohm resistors, in parallel. The reciprocals of the two resistors in parallel add to give the reciprocal of the resistance of a single resistor, which is equivalent to them.

$$1/R_2 = 1/15 + 1/15 = 2/15, R_2 = 15/2 = 7.5 \text{ ohm}.$$

131. **(D)**   The energy unit "electron volt" is defined such that an electron accelerated through a potential difference of one volt acquires a kinetic energy of one electron volt (eV). An electron accelerated through a potential difference of 48000 V reaches a kinetic energy of 48000 eV = 48 KeV.

132. **(C)**   Taking 75% of 1200 W gives 900 W or 900J/s which heats the water. The total energy needed to raise the temperature of the 968 g of water 80°C (from 20°C to 100°C) is (968 g) (4.18 J/°C g) (80°C) = 3.24×10^5 J. Combining this result with the rate at which energy is added to the water gives time = (3.24×10^5 J) / (900 J/s) = 360 s = 6 minutes.

133. **(B)**   The product of the frequency and wavelength of sound is equal to the speed of sound. The speed of sound, in a particular medium, is, therefore, proportional to its frequency for a fixed wavelength.

(frequency in He) / (frequency in air)

= (speed in He)/(speed in air) (1020 m/s)/(340 m/s) = 3

134. **(D)**   From the table, the speed of sound in tissue is 1600 m/s. In 10 μs, sounds travels a distance of (1600 m/s) $(10 \times 10^{-6}\text{s})$ = 0.016 m = 16 mm.

135. **(A)**   The speed of sound in a gas is proportional to the square root of the absolute temperature of the gas. At 14°C + 273 = 287 K, the speed of sound in air is 340 m/s. For the speed of sound in air to be 310 m/s, the temperature must satisfy the following:

$$\sqrt{T/287 \text{ K}} = (310 \text{ m/s}) / (340 \text{ m/s})$$

$$T = (287 \text{ K}) (310/340)^2 = 239 \text{ K}$$

$t = 239 - 273 = -34°C$

136. (B) Since the distance between nodes (points of zero wave amplitude) is one half the wavelength, the conventional illustration shows three half-waves in the distance L. Thus, the wavelength must be two thirds of L or $2L/3$.

137. (C) The intensity level is db = 20 log(P/P_o). Solving for the pressure, P, by taking antilogarithms, gives $P = P_o \, 10^{-db/20}$. The ratio of the pressures for two intensity levels is

$$P_1/P_2 = 10^{(db1 - db2)/20} = 10^{(40-20)/20} = 10$$

138. (C) The lower the intensity level of a sound that is perceived at a given loudness level, the more sensitive the ear is to that type of sound. Examination of the figure shows that for 40 phons loudness level, there is a minimum intensity level at 4000 Hz. Hence the ear is most sensitive to sound of frequency 4000 Hz at a loudness level of 40 phons.

139. (D)

$$KE = {}^1\!/_2 \, mv^2$$

Using the MKS system we obtain

$$m = 0.1 \text{ kg} \qquad v = 60 \text{ m/sec}$$

then, $KE = {}^1\!/_2(0.1 \text{ kg}) (60 \text{ m/sec})^2$

$$KE = +1/_2 \, (0.1 \text{ kg}) (3600(\text{m/sec})^2)$$

$$KE = 180 \, \frac{\text{kg} \cdot \text{m}^2}{\text{sec}^2} = 180 \text{ N} \cdot \text{m}$$

$KE = 180$ joules.

140. (D) The newton is that unbalanced force which acts upon one kilogram mass, and produces an acceleration of one meter per second squared.

141. (B) The substances used to reduce the action of catalysts are known as inhibitors. Inhibitors are useful because they allow a reaction to be stopped after an intermediate product has been produced. This is useful when the intermediate product can further react to form another product. This type of reaction inhibition or "poisoning" may be seen in the example of the catalytic hydrogenation of acetylene:

$$HC \equiv CH \xrightarrow[\text{Pd}]{H_2} H_2C = CH_2 \xrightarrow[\text{Pd}]{H_2} H_3C - CH_3$$

As can be seen from the previous reaction, acetylene is completely hydrogenated to ethane with no ethene left in the reaction mixture. However, ethene may be obtained as the final product by either limiting the amount of H_2 to one mole per one mole of acetylene, or by adding an inhibitor to the catalyst (Pd). A suitable inhibitor for this reaction is quinoline. This "poisoning" of the catalyst reduces its effectiveness so that the intermediate product of the previous reaction becomes the final product.

142. **(A)** The gas is thermally insulated

$$\Rightarrow dQ = 0$$

and hence the expansion is adiabatic.

$$W = -\int_{V_0}^{V_f} p\, dV = -\int_{V_0}^{V_f} kV^{-\gamma}\, dV \text{ since } pV^\gamma = k$$

$$= \frac{k}{-\gamma+1} V^{-\gamma+1} \Big|_{V_f}^{V_0} = \frac{k}{\gamma-1} \left(\frac{V_f}{V_f^\gamma} - \frac{V_0}{V_0^\gamma} \right)$$

$$= \frac{1}{\gamma-1} (p_f V_f - p_0 V_0)$$

Now $\gamma - 1 = \dfrac{C_p}{C_V} - 1 = \dfrac{C_p - C_V}{C_V} = \dfrac{R}{C_V}$

$$W = \frac{C_V}{R} (p_f V_f - p_0 V_0)$$

Section 3 — Writing Sample

SAMPLE ESSAY 1

This statement reflects the suspicion of government, which has been so common throughout the history of the United States. The statement suggests that government is essentially in opposition to the interests of the free individual, and that, at best, a government's use of power is a necessary evil. Ideally, each individual would take care of his or her own affairs, without interference from anyone. In reality, however, individuals need to be protected from others who attempt to violate their rights. Government, then, has the right to protect individuals from interference but no right to extend its powers and activities beyond this function. In other words, government should not interfere in the lives of individuals, except to prevent them from infringing upon the rights of one another. Any other exercise of power, the statement implies, would be excessive.

Since the beginnings of this nation, citizens of the United States have been on the lookout for government interference in their lives. The Revolutionary War was fought to gain independence from excessive governmental power. With this experience behind them, the framers of the Constitution of the United States sought to limit the power of government. The Bill of Rights lists ways in which individual freedom is guaranteed against such interference. The legislative, judicial, and executive branches of government were separated so that each might prevent the others from becoming too powerful. More recently, the tenure in office of a president was limited to two consecutive terms, to prevent any individual from gaining too much personal power over the government of its citizens. Since government can overpower individual interests, it has been treated with the same caution and constraint which one might use when handling a dangerous animal.

This attitude toward government is not always healthy, for there are circumstances in which the powers of government should be enhanced, rather than limited. In periods of national emergency, such as in time of war, or after a natural disaster, the federal government must assume extraordinary powers for the good of citizens who otherwise would not be able to help themselves. During a war, for the good of everyone in the nation, the government must be able to conscript troops for battle, and to impose severe penalties on individuals who, without very good reason, refuse to obey. After a community has been devastated by a flood, the federal government should provide aid to those who would not be able to recover without it. In such instances, it seems clear that government should do more than just protect individuals from one another. It must, in addition, use its power to provide aid, and to compel individuals to engage in activities required for the good of everyone.

The quote above, then, expresses a view of government that is too extreme. While we can sympathize with a desire to restrain government from becoming too powerful, we can still agree that there are circumstances in which individuals can only be helped by an increase in governmental power. No simple formula can decide what the correct amount of governmental power should be. The statement could be revised in the following manner, to express a more reasonable understanding of government: "That government is best which governs for the well-being of the governed." This statement subordinates government to "the governed," without suggesting that government would ideally not exist. Whether the power of government in any specific circumstance should be great, or small, would depend upon the circumstances in which its power is to be exercised.

Explanation of Essay 1

This essay directly addresses the issue of the statement, and accomplishes the required tasks. Paragraphs 1 and 2 explain clearly the fundamental meaning of the statement, indicated as the first task ("Explain what you think the above statement means"). The second task ("Describe one or two specific situations in which the powers of government should be increased") is accomplished in the third paragraph. Finally, the third task ("Discuss what you think should be the basis for increasing or decreasing a government's powers") is accomplished in the fourth paragraph.

The essay develops the theme of the statement with insight, explaining not only the fundamental meaning of the statement, but exploring other important implications as well. The first three sentences indicate the attitude of rugged individualism which is the basis for distrusting governmental power. The fourth sentence indicates a basis for properly coercing individuals, and thus provides a basis, made explicit in the fifth sentence, for the coercive power of government. The final two sentences of the first paragraph return to the topic of distrust of governmental power, basing this, again, on the right of individuals to independence. The second paragraph provides historical examples of the attitude toward individuality and government, expressed in the first paragraph. The third paragraph looks at governmental power in a more positive light, thus, apparently contradicting the almost purely negative attitude toward it, expressed in the first two paragraphs. This sets the stage for a criticism, in the fourth paragraph of the statement, and allows for a reasonable correction of the statement.

The ideas in this essay are clearly and logically developed. Each paragraph leads naturally into the next, such that the ideas developed in each seem spontaneously to call forth the ideas that follow. The idea of government interference, for example, expressed in sentence 1 of paragraph 2, is anticipated by sentence 6 of the first paragraph. The basic attitude toward government, expressed in the statement, is expressed again in the last sentence of paragraph 2, setting the stage for the criticism of the statement expressed in paragraph 3. The essay thus acquires structural unity.

The essay uses correct grammar and, while using sentences which are clearly organized, it varies their length and cadence to provide an interesting flow. For example, the final sentence of paragraph 1 is short and to the point, driving home the ideas developed through the longer and more complex sentences that precede it. The vocabulary employed is appropriate for expressing the ideas clearly and accurately, neither drawing attention to itself by being pretentious, nor giving the impression of talking down to the reader by being too stinted or simplistic (for example, in sentence 1 of paragraph 3: "the powers of government should be enhanced ..."; and in sentence 4 of paragraph 3: "After a community has been devastated ...").

Sample Essay 2

Humans require more for life than simply sustaining a heartbeat. Someone could, for example, have enough food to keep from starving to death and still be unable to live humanly. Without a variety of gratifying experiences, human life can become monotonous, and even hopeless. An individual unable to do more than stay alive physically would be dead psychologically and emotionally. The brain of such a person might be physically sound, but it would be operating only at a level required to sustain a monotonous, repetitious existence. It would not be surprising if such a person were unable to sustain, for very long, even a biological existence; for we need to experience more satisfaction from life than that which we can receive from barely surviving.

The statement asserts that it is impossible for people to generally find what they need for a satisfying human existence through reality and the world around them. History seems to support this assertion, with its accounts of war and human suffering in all regions and throughout all periods of the world. Great literature such as the *Iliad*, or *Madame Bovary*, has portrayed human destruction through frustration in love. Our own personal experiences, if carefully and honestly reviewed, indicate that few, if any, of our dreams have been fully realized. Being "realistic," or "facing reality," means becoming resigned to the great distance between what we want and what we can realistically get. It may seem only reasonable, then, that great numbers of people must resign themselves to a life barely lived, if lived at all, in a human manner.

Such pessimism hardly seems justified, however, when we recall the masses of people who left their homelands to settle in this country, looking for a new and better life. Not all were successful, but many were able to improve their condition, and most, at least, were enlivened by new hopes and dreams. Recently, masses in eastern Europe have fought for, and won, new opportunities for a fuller life. If such people have had to confront a real world which has not easily yielded to their efforts, they have nevertheless been able to discover, in this world, opportunities for imagining and attempting to realize efforts for improving their lives.

It must be admitted that frustration and suffering are constant features of human life, and that it is only in fantasy that they are absent for long. It is also true that, no matter how much suffering humans experience, they often, in large numbers, find the power to resist being dominated by their pain, and are able to struggle with their reality in the hope of changing it. If the statement is correct in assuming that reality for most people is harsh, it nevertheless incorrectly assumes that most people are crushed by reality. Undoubtedly, the reality of some individuals' lives has been so frustrating as to destroy their humanity. However, reality, is, for most people, a varied interweaving of fulfillment and frustration, providing many, if not most individuals, the ability to plan and struggle beyond periods of frustration toward periods of greater fulfillment.

Explanation of Essay 2

This essay directly addresses the central issue of the statement, and addresses each of the three writing tasks. The first task is addressed in the first two paragraphs, the second in the third paragraph, and the final task is addressed in the fourth paragraph. The first paragraph clearly establishes the meaning of "subsist," as it is used in the statement, and indicates the relationship between "satisfaction" and human subsistence. The second paragraph explains the statement's reference to "reality," and the lack of satisfaction to be gained from it. The third paragraph provides clearly identifiable examples of situations in which reality is frustrating, without causing loss of human subsistence. The fourth paragraph generalizes from the points made in the first three paragraphs, to provide a unified view of reality as a negative, as well as a positive, influence on peoples' attempts to live humanly.

This essay proceeds logically through sentences and paragraphs which center consistently on the theme of the statement. Each paragraph leads to the one that follows, preparing for the ideas expressed in it, as well as referring to previously developed ideas. This unity is indicated in the transitions employed ("Such pessimism hardly seems justified ...," at the beginning of paragraph 3, and "It must be admitted that frustration and suffering ...," at the beginning of paragraph 4, refer back to the central issue of paragraphs 1, 2, and 3, and the fundamental issue of the statement).

The essay is written clearly and thoughtfully. Sentences directly state the ideas which they are intended to convey (for example sentences 1, 6, 10, and 18). The language of the essay states precisely what is intended (for example, sentence 3: "Without a variety of gratifying experiences, human life can become monotonous, and even hopeless"). The complexity of the issue is treated with clearly organized sentence and paragraph development.

Section 4 — Biological Sciences

PASSAGE I (Questions 143-148)

143. **(C)**   This question requires an understanding of the forces that dictate the movement of water within the body. Osmosis is the movement of water from an area of greater concentration across a semipermeable barrier, to an area of less concentration. Most of the membranes in the body are semipermeable, i.e., permeable to water, but not to most ions. Answer (A) is incorrect because it refers to the random movement of particles within a solution caused by collisions with fluid molecules. Answers (B) and (D) are incorrect because these types of movement require energy to move molecules against a concentration gradient. They also often require carrier proteins to transport the substance being moved.

144. **(B)**   An understanding of the various body fluid compartments is needed to answer this question. The only compartment in which there is a true circulating fluid that contains proteins is the blood plasma. Although the plasma volume is a part of the extracellular fluid, answer (A) is incorrect because the extracellular fluid also includes answer (D), interstitial fluid. Answer (C) is wrong because intracellular fluid does not circulate, although it does contain proteins.

145. **(D)**   This question requires interpretation of Figure 1, which shows exchange between intracellular fluid, and the plasma must be indirect since it can only occur if the fluids have first passed through the interstitial space. Answer (A) is incorrect because fluids may be exchanged directly only between the intracellular compartment and the interstitial fluid, not the plasma. Answer (B) is incorrect because exchange of fluids between compartments is constantly occurring in an effort to maintain homeostasis. Exchange of fluids can occur throughout the body, not just in isolated organs, which is why answer (C) is wrong.

146. **(A)**   To answer this question, the nature of equilibrium must be understood. Since the two compartments are initially in osmotic balance, removing solute from one of the compartments will upset this balance. The extracellular fluid will contain less solute, relative to the intracellular fluid, yet the absolute amount of water in both compartments is equal. The extracellular fluid has thus become hypotonic, meaning it has less osmotically active particles, when compared to the intracellular fluid. Answer (C) is the exact opposite of the correct answer. Answer (B) is incorrect because the intracellular fluid would become hypertonic relative to the extracellular fluid. Answer (D) is incorrect because removing solute from one of the compartments will upset the osmotic equilibrium and, therefore, the tonicity of the compartments, relative to each other, must change.

147. **(C)**   To answer this question, Figure 1 should be used. It can be seen that the blood plasma is the only compartment which can directly exchange fluids with the interstitial fluid and with the external environment via a number of organs. Plasma volume will be affected if there is a change in either the internal or the external environment. It is therefore most susceptible to change. Answer (A) is least susceptible to change, while answer (B) is intermediate between intracellular fluid and plasma.

148. **(B)**   This question requires an understanding of the relationship among the body fluid compartments. Interstitial fluid volume is equal to extracellular fluid volume, minus plasma volume (14 liters - 3.5 liters = 10.5 liters). Answer (C) is incorrect because total body water does not have to be measured to determine interstitial fluid volume, in this case.

PASSAGE II (Questions 149-154)

149. **(D)**   The poly-A tail is added to the mRNA before it leaves the nucleus and, thus, it must occur during the process of post-transcriptional modification. Answer (A) is the stage during which mRNA serves as the template for polypeptide chain formation. Answer (B) occurs when DNA transfers the genetic code to mRNA, and answer (C) is modification of the protein after it has been translated.

150. **(B)**   Since actinomycin D prevents the first stage of protein synthesis from occurring, only the proinsulin gene, which is part of the DNA molecule, would be present within the cell. Although mRNA molecules transcribed prior to actinomycin D addition would continue unimpeded through protein synthesis, the final product, insulin, is secreted (i.e., no longer in the cell). Answers (A), (C) and (D) are all produced during later stages of protein synthesis and would not be present if transcription never took place.

151. **(A)**   Transcription of DNA to mRNA occurs in the nucleus of the cell, the only place where DNA is normally found. Answers (B) and (C) are involved with translation, while answer (D) is where post-translational modification occurs.

152. **(C)**   Protein synthesis occurs in many stages and during some of these stages the protein is modified by addition or elimination of amino acids, by folding or by the formation of bridges between amino acid side chains. These modifications are important because they tend to stabilize the protein and to confer a specific configuration or conformation which is necessary for the protein to function properly. Answers (A) and (D) are incorrect because the entire process of protein synthesis takes place in both the nucleus and cytoplasm.

153. **(D)**   Post-translational modification occurs after the polypeptide chain has been formed by translation of the genetic code carried by the mRNA. In the case of insulin, it is during this stage that the leader sequence is removed and the protein is folded. Answers (A) and (C) occur during post-transcriptional modification of the mRNA before it leaves the nucleus.

154. **(D)**   During post-transcriptional modification of the mRNA, the introns are removed. Thus, the mRNA which enters the cytoplasm consists only of exons. An-

swer (A) is wrong because the mRNA is modified prior to leaving the nucleus. Answers (B) and (C) are wrong because the introns are removed from the mRNA.

PASSAGE III (Questions 155-160)

155. **(C)** Answering this question requires an understanding of the relationship between sodium excretion (output) and blood pressure, as depicted in Figure 2. If the amount of sodium in the diet (intake) is reduced, urinary sodium excretion must also be reduced to maintain sodium balance. When sodium excretion decreases, blood pressure will also decrease. If blood pressure remained high, sodium excretion would proceed at a greater rate than sodium intake and depletion of total body sodium would occur. Answer (B) is wrong because a change in sodium intake/excretion should, theoretically, produce a change in blood pressure. Answer (A) is incorrect because the kidneys will not avidly retain sodium unless there is a sodium deficiency. A low salt diet can be maintained, as long as the diet contains adequate sodium. Answer (D) is wrong because blood pressure should not increase, but rather it should decrease.

156. **(A)** If the whole curve in Figure 2 was shifted to the right, blood pressure would rise at the same level of sodium intake. Answer (B) is incorrect because blood pressure must change when the entire curve is shifted either to the right, or left, of normal. Answer (C) is incorrect because urinary sodium output should not change, since sodium intake did not change. Answer (D) is wrong because the curve was shifted to the right, not the left, and sodium output should not change.

157. **(D)** An increase in dietary sodium would cause blood pressure to rise, in an effort to restore sodium balance. In a person more sensitive to the effect of sodium on blood pressure, blood pressure will increase to an even greater extent. Answer (A) is wrong because an increase in dietary salt will lead to an increase in blood pressure, not a decrease. Answer (B) is incorrect because Patient A is more sensitive to changes in sodium than Patient B, thus, they should not have the same blood pressure response. Answer (C) is wrong because both Patients A and B should exhibit a rise in blood pressure.

158. **(B)** To answer this question, the concept of a feedback system must be understood. Negative feedback occurs when a change in a variable sets in motion a series of events which are designed to restore the variable to its original condition. In this case, when blood pressure increases, sodium excretion will increase until blood pressure decreases back to its original level. Answer (A) is incorrect because hormones are not directly involved in the relationship between sodium excretion and blood pressure. Answer (C) is incorrect because counter-current systems generally refer to fluid exchange systems, in which fluid and solutes exchange rapidly between parallel streams of flow. Answer (D) is the opposite of negative feedback, and in effect it promotes disequilibrium.

159. **(A)** The set point must change in order for blood pressure to remain elevated. Otherwise, sodium and water excretion would increase until blood pressure was returned to a normal level. Answer (B) is wrong because the set point can change for many reasons. Answers (C) and (D) are incorrect because blood pressure and kidney function are related as shown by Figure 2.

160. **(A)**   Diuretics act upon the kidneys to increase sodium and water excretion. If diuretic therapy were discontinued, more salt and water would be retained by the kidneys, blood volume would increase and blood pressure would rise. Answer (B) is incorrect because sodium and water excretion would decrease. Answer (C) is wrong because diuretics specifically act upon the kidneys to alter their function. Answer (D) is incorrect because even though diuretics can alter renal function, they do not correct any underlying defects in the kidneys.

161. **(C)**   The pericardium is the membranous sac that encloses the heart. Endothelium is a term that refers to endothelial cells. Endocardium and myocardium refer to the heart muscle. The vena cava is the largest vein in the body.

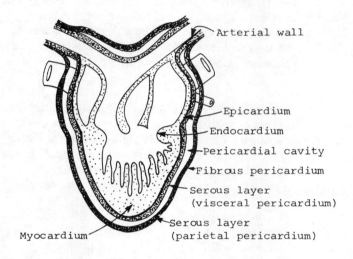

The Surrounding Heart Layers

162. **(B)**   The ventricles are the two lower chambers of the heart and are responsible for the pumping of the blood; the right ventricle pumps blood through the pulmonary artery into the lungs, and the left ventricle pumps blood to the aorta into systemic circulation. The atria are the two upper chambers of the heart responsible for the receipt of blood from the body. Pacemakers initiate the beating of the heart. Cardiac muscles make up the walls of all four chambers of the heart. Intercalated discs are histological components of the heart. (See figure on following page.)

163. **(B)**   In the alveoli, indirect respiration occurs. There are two phases of indirect respiration: the internal phase and the external phase. Direct respiration involves the direct exchange of gases by an organism with the external environment. This is done by lower organisms such as paramecia or hydra. (See figure on following page.)

164. **(D)**   Vitamin A is necessary for the growth and maintenance of the epithelial cells of the skin. Vitamin K assists in blood coagulation. Vitamin E is associated with liver function in some animals. Vitamin E is also responsible for male sterility in rats and possibly other animals.

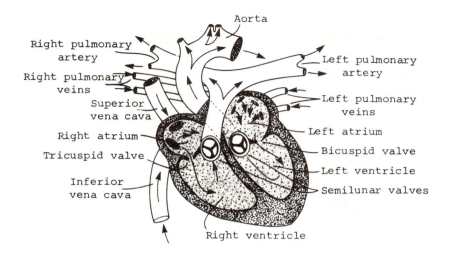

The Structure of the Human Heart

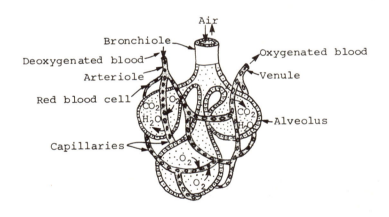

A Magnified Alveoli of Humans

165. **(D)** α-amino acids have the amino group bonded to the carbon adjacent to the carboxyl group while β-amino acids have the amino group bonded to the second carbon from the carboxyl group.

166. **(B)** Steric interactions between atoms in a molecule are the direct cause of certain conformations of that molecule to be unstable. These various conformations and their steric interactions may be visualized through the use of Newman projections. Using a molecular model kit in conjunction with Newman projections is an immense help in discerning which structures will be stable and which will not.

PASSAGE IV (Questions 167-172)

167. **(B)** This question requires interpretation of Table 1, in which the active, passive and total tensions developed at various muscle lengths is listed. If the muscle were stretched 5 millimeters (+5) beyond its resting length, there would be no active tension. Passive tension would still develop and total tension would equal passive tension plus 0. Answers (A) and (D) are incorrect because active tension would not develop. Answer (C) is wrong because passive and total tensions would not be 0.

168. **(A)** This question requires an understanding of the fact that relatively few processes in the body occur independently or isolated from the influences of other processes. It would be very difficult to study just the properties of skeletal muscle in the intact body because there are so many other variables that need to be controlled. There is no basis for answers (B) and (C), since the function of muscles is to contract and develop tension, and this can occur at a variety of different muscle lengths.

169. **(D)** The differences between active and passive tension must be understood to answer this question. Passive tension develops when connective tissue and elastic elements within the muscle are stretched, as opposed to active tension which is produced by the actual muscle contraction. Thus, there is no passive tension when a muscle is shortened to less than its resting length because the muscle is not being stretched. Answer (A) is wrong because passive tension does not develop. Answers (B) and (C) are incorrect because muscle contraction and thus, tension development, can occur at shorter muscle lengths.

170. **(C)** This question requires an understanding of basic graphing techniques. Plotting active tension versus the change in muscle length would result in a bell shaped curve, with the greatest active tension developed at the resting length (0) and lesser tensions when the muscle is shortened (-1, -2, -3,or lengthened (+1, +2, +3).

171. **(A)** A basic understanding of muscle structure and function is needed to answer this question. Tension development in a muscle is a function of the interaction which occurs between actin and myosin filaments. Answer (B) is incorrect because a physical interaction must occur not merely in overlapping of the filaments, in order for contraction to occur. Answer (C) is wrong because a slackening would not contribute to tension development at all. Answer (D) explains the differences in tension development at different muscle lengths, but, not why tension develops.

172. **(C)** Total tension is equal to the sum of active and passive tensions. As a muscle is stretched, the increase in passive tension is greater than the decrease in active tension and total tension will, therefore, increase. Answer (A) is wrong because total and active tension are not independent of one another. Answer (B) is incorrect because total tension is equal to active plus passive tension. Answer (D) is incorrect because active tension decreases when a muscle is stretched.

PASSAGE V (Questions 173-178)

173. **(D)** This question requires an understanding of the role played by PTH in the regulation of calcium metabolism. An overabundance of PTH would mobilize

large amounts of calcium from the skeleton, hence leading to bone demineralization. Answer (A) is incorrect because it is the opposite effect that PTH would have on bone. Answer (B) is wrong because PTH removes calcium from bone, which then enters the plasma, thus raising plasma calcium levels. Answer (C) is wrong because tetany occurs when plasma calcium levels are low, not high.

174. **(B)** Answering this question requires an understanding of the definition of a hormone. Hormones generally are regulatory proteins that are produced by endocrine glands. They are secreted into the bloodstream, act upon targets distant from the site of secretion and are effective in minute quantities. Answer (A) is incorrect because not all hormones are essential for life. Answer (C) is wrong because hormones regulate a large number of processes, not just calcium metabolism. Answer (D) is wrong because PTH is produced by an endocrine gland.

175. **(C)** This question requires knowledge of the role of calcium in various physiological processes. Calcium is extremely important for proper functioning of nerve and muscle tissue. Answer (A) is incorrect because tetany results from a lack of calcium. Although the level of plasma calcium regulates PTH secretion, this is not the most important function of calcium, therefore, answer (B) is wrong. Answer (D) is incorrect because calcium does not regulate bone resorption.

176. **(A)** To answer this question, it must be understood that the anatomic size of an organ does not necessarily reflect its importance. Answer (B) is incorrect because the parathyroid glands are extremely important in the regulation of calcium metabolism. Answers (C) and (D) are wrong because they are not factual.

177. **(B)** Following the ingestion of a meal which is high in calcium, PTH secretion will decrease because the level of plasma calcium regulates PTH secretion in a negative feedback fashion. Deposition of calcium in the skeleton will increase at PTH levels fall. Answers (A) and (C) are incorrect because PTH secretion will decrease. Answer (D) is wrong because plasma calcium levels do regulate PTH secretion.

178. **(B)** This question requires an understanding of the concept of antagonistic hormones. When plasma calcium is high, calcitonin will increase and PTH will decrease since they have opposite effects upon the blood calcium level. Answer (A) is wrong because plasma calcium will decrease, due to calcitonin stimulated uptake by the bones. Answers (C) and (D) are incorrect because plasma PTH will decrease.

PASSAGE VI (Questions 179-185)

179. **(D)** In order for a genetic female to develop male genitalia, the fetus must have been exposed to androgens during the period of gestation when the genitalia form (after the 7th week). Answer (A) is wrong because exposure to testosterone at birth would not affect development of the genitalia. Answer (B) is incorrect because estrogens are not secreted by either sex during gestation. Answer (C) is incorrect since exposure of a male to chorionic gonadotropin stimulates normal development of the testes.

180. **(C)** Approximately half of sperm contain the X chromosome and half contain a Y. It is thought that Y-containing sperm have greater motility and therefore a better chance of fertilizing an egg. This could explain why more males are born than females. Answers (A) and (B) are incorrect because there are approximately equal numbers of X and Y sperm. Answer (D) is wrong because eggs contain X chromosomes, not Y.

181. **(A)** Mature gonads produce ova and secrete estrogens in the female and in the male they produce sperm and secrete androgens. Answer (B) is incorrect because the gonads also produce germ cells. Answers (C) and (D) are wrong because they describe the functions of the gonads in one sex, but not in both.

182. **(B)** Testes develop in genetic males due to the presence of the H-Y antigen. Since females lack this antigen, ovaries develop instead of testes. Answer (A) is incorrect because the immature ovaries do not secrete any hormones. Answer (C) is incorrect because the testes do not secrete estrogen. Answer (D) is wrong because the brain does not control development of the genitalia in the fetus.

183. **(B)** Germ cells contain half of the number of chromosomes found in somatic cells so that when an egg and sperm unite, the zygote will contain all 46 chromosomes (23 + 23 = 46). Answer (A) is wrong because germ cells are haploid. Answer (C) is wrong because size does not determine chromosome number. Answer (D) is incorrect because meiosis is the process of germ cell formation, not mitosis.

184. **(D)** Since all eggs contain an X chromosome, the union of an X-containing sperm and an egg results in a genetic female (XX). Answers (A) and (B) are incorrect because the offspring is female. Answer (C) is wrong because an XYY combination results in a male.

185. **(C)** The reproductive hormones, androgens (primarily testosterone) in males and estrogen in females stimulate the development of the secondary sex characteristics during puberty. Answer (A) is wrong because the testes secrete testosterone and the ovaries secrete estrogen. Answers (B) and (D) are incorrect because the gonads must begin, not stop, producing hormones.

PASSAGE VII (Questions 186-192)

186. **(B)** The function of cellular membranes is to compartmentalize the enzymes and substrates necessary for specific chemical reactions. This increases the efficiency with which the reactions can occur. Answer (A) is wrong because most of the membranes are semi-permeable, allowing for a great deal of interaction among organelles. Answer (C) is wrong because membranes increase the available surface area. Answer (D) is wrong because the organelles cannot exist independently of one another.

187. **(D)** This question requires interpretation of Table 2. Water and protein account for 95% of the total cellular mass (80 + 15). Answer (A) accounts for only 19% (15 + 3 + 1), answer (B) 81% (1 + 80) and answer (C) 1%.

188. **(A)**   Lysosomes function as digestive organelles by removing unwanted and harmful substances from the interior of the cell. Without them, toxic materials would quickly build up and eventually kill the cell. Cells would also be unable to fight bacterial infection in the absence of lysosomes. Answers (B), (C), and (D) are wrong because lysosomes are not involved in protein packaging, reproduction, or energy production.

189. **(D)**   Rough ER is characterized by the attachment of ribosomes which gives it a rough appearance. The portion of endoplasmic reticulum which is not associated with ribosomes is smooth in appearance. Answer (A) is incorrect because the cytoskeleton attaches to both rough and smooth ER. Answer (B) is wrong because both smooth and rough ER are bound by membranes. Answer (C) is wrong because smooth ER is usually closer to the Golgi than rough ER.

190. **(C)**   Mitochrondria are the "power houses" of the cell. They provide the cell with energy in the form of ATP, so that the cell can perform basic life functions. To insure a continual supply of ATP, there must be numerous mitochrondia. Answers (A), (B), and (D) are incorrect because mitochrondia are not directly involved in these processes.

191. **(C)**   The nucleolus, located in the nucleus, is unique in that it is not surrounded by its own membrane. Answers (A), (B), and (D) are wrong because all of these organelles are membrane bound.

192. **(B)**   The Golgi packages materials, which are then transported, via vesicles, to other organelles or to the cell membrane for secretion. Answer (A) is incorrect because these vesicles do not digest the material that they carry. Answers (C) and (D) are wrong because the vesicles transport material away from the Golgi, not toward it.

193. **(C)**   When a segment of one chromosome is transferred to another non-homologous chromosome, the mutation is known as a translocation. A deletion is a mutation in which a segment of the chromosome is missing. In duplication, a portion of the chromosome is represented twice. An inversion results when a segment is removed and reinserted in the same location, but in the opposite direction. (See figure below.)

A B C D E F	Normal
A B C E F	Deletion of segment D
A B C C D E F	Duplication of segment C
A E D C B F	Inversion of segment B-E
G H I J K L A B C	Translocation from A-C to chromosome GHIJKL

Mutations Involving Chromosome Structure

194. **(C)** The thin barrier around Bowman's capsule is composed of two extremely thin layers: (A) the single-celled capillary wall and (2) the one-celled lining of Bowman's capsule. The filtration of plasma can occur through this thin barrier because plasma contains no large blood cells.

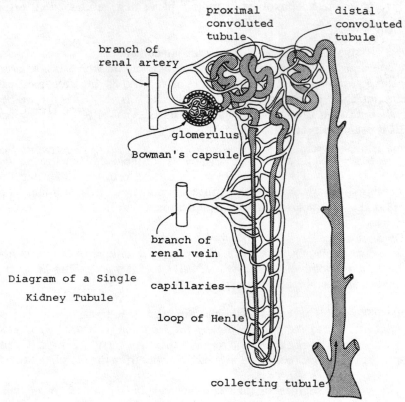

Diagram of a Single
Kidney Tubule

195. **(D)** Rigor mortis is a phenomenon in which the muscles become very stiff after death. It results directly from the loss of ATP in the dead muscle cells; the myosin crossbridges are unable to combine with actin and those bonds already formed are unable to be broken. Thus, the rigid condition results.

196. **(D)** Aromatic compounds with activating groups are ortho, para directors. They are also electron releasing groups and will direct electrophiles to add ortho and para to the substituent. Deactivating groups are meta directors with the exception of the halogens. They are electron withdrawing groups and they will direct the electrophile to add meta to the substituent.

The halogens are an exception; they are deactivating groups, but they are ortho, para directors. A methyl group on a benzene ring is activating and orth, para directing. The amino group of aniline is also activating and ortho, para directing, The nitro group of nitrobenzene is deactivating and meta directing.

PASSAGE VIII (Questions 197-202)

197. **(C)**   At pH 7, the amino acids exist in the following ionized forms:

glycine

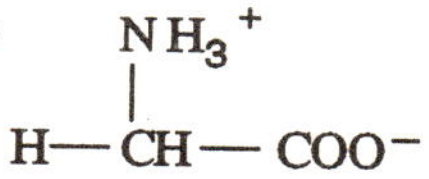

$$\overset{\overset{\displaystyle NH_3^+}{|}}{H-CH-COO^-}$$

alanine

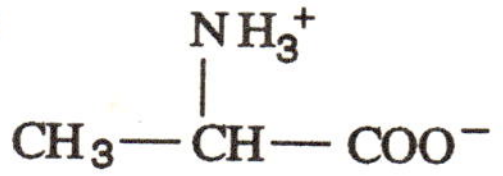

$$\overset{\overset{\displaystyle NH_3^+}{|}}{CH_3-CH-COO^-}$$

aspartic acid

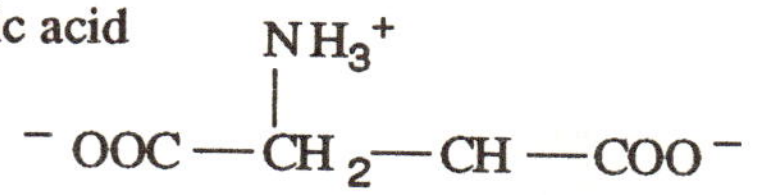

$$^-OOC-\overset{\overset{\displaystyle NH_3^+}{|}}{CH_2-CH-COO^-}$$

phenylalanine

$$\langle\!\bigcirc\!\rangle-CH_2-\overset{\overset{\displaystyle NH_3^+}{|}}{CH}-COO^-$$

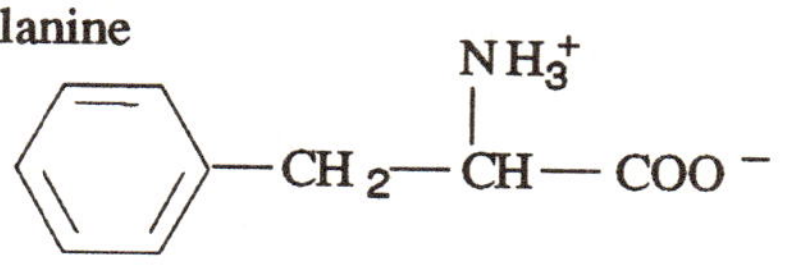

Aspartic acid is the only amino acid of the 4 shown which has a negatively charged side chain.

198. **(D)**   The stereochemistry of amino acids is based upon their structural relationship of D- or L-glyceraldehyde as shown below:

D-Glyceraldehyde

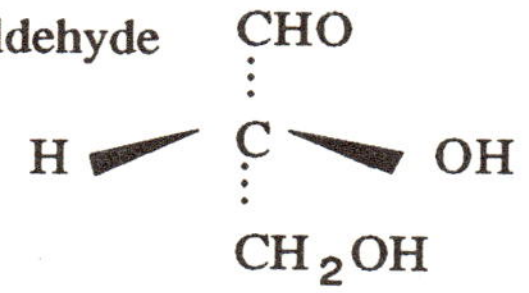

$$\overset{\displaystyle CHO}{\underset{\displaystyle CH_2OH}{H-C-OH}}$$

L-Glyceraldehyde

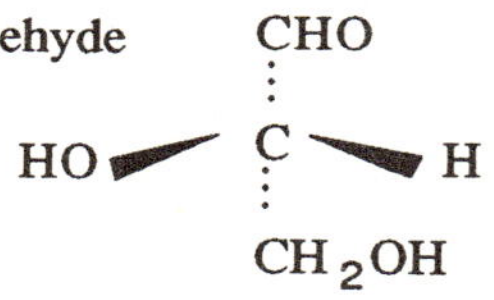

$$\overset{\displaystyle CHO}{\underset{\displaystyle CH_2OH}{HO-C-H}}$$

D-Alanine

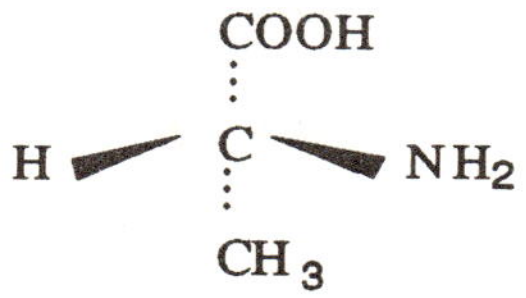

$$\overset{\displaystyle COOH}{\underset{\displaystyle CH_3}{H-C-NH_2}}$$

L-Alanine

$$\overset{\displaystyle COOH}{\underset{\displaystyle CH_3}{H_2N-C-H}}$$

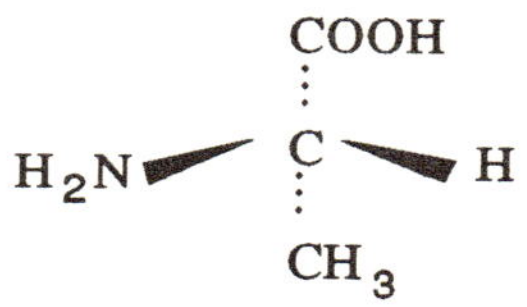

Answers (A), (B), and (C) are wrong because classification as a D- or L-form has nothing to do with the sign of rotation of polarized light, percentage of ionized molecules, or attraction to water.

199. **(A)**   Hydrocarbons do not readily interact with water. Amino acids with hydrocarbon side chains will thus be hydrophobic. Answers (B) and (C) are incorrect because they are terms which may be used to describe all of the amino acids, not just those with hydrocarbon side chains. Answer (D) is wrong because these amino acids will not be attracted to water.

200. **(B)**   Neutral or uncharged polar side chains are most likely to hydrogen bond with water. Answer (A) is wrong because the side chains do not participate in peptide bond formation. Answer (C) is incorrect because neutral molecules will not be involved in covalent bonding. Answer (D) is wrong because these amino acids will by hydrophilic, not hydrophobic.

201. **(D)**   At pH 7, the amino group of all of the amino acids is in the form of an ammonium ion ($-NH_3^+$). This occurs because the basic amino group and acidic carboxyl group of each amino acid undergoes an acid-base reaction in which the amino

group accepts an H atom donated by the carboxyl group. This results in protonation of the amino group.

202. **(A)** Proteins are basically chains of amino acids linked end to end. Since the only part of each of the 20 amino acids which differs is the side chain or R group, it is this portion of the amino acid which imparts the different physical and chemical properties to each position in the protein chain.

PASSAGE IX (Questions 203-208)

203. **(B)** Plate 2 contains compound A, in the unknown mixture, because it is the only plate in which a spot from the unknown, on the right side of the plate, corresponds exactly to the known spot, on the left side, following separation.

204. **(A)** More polar compounds tend to move up a TLC plate at a slower rate, than less polar compounds. Therefore, the mixture which contains the most polar compounds will have spots which have moved the least from the original spot on the plate. Plate 1 contains the most polar compounds because there are more spots (3), closer to the original spot, than on any of the other plates.

205. **(C)** Polar compounds move at a relatively slow rate because they are more attracted to the stationary phase then to the mobile phase. In order to increase the rate at which a polar compound moves on a plate, a more polar mobile phase must be used. Of the compounds listed, acetic acid is the most polar. Answers (A) and (D) would be poor choices because they are nonpolar solvents.

206. **(D)** Nonpolar compounds move the fastest on a TLC plate because they are more attracted to the mobile phase, then to the stationary phase. Of the compounds listed, the alkenes are the only nonpolar group and thus will travel the fastest and furthest on a plate.

207. **(A)** Iodine will react with most organic compounds to form a colored complex, which is why it is commonly used to visualize spots on a TLC plate. Answer (B) is incorrect because iodine forms colored complexes, not fluorescent ones. Iodine will react with most of the late coatings to form colored complexes, however, this reaction takes longer than the reaction with the organic compounds and will only occur if the plate is exposed to iodine for too long. Answer (D) is incorrect because the plate is removed from the mobile phase following separation and so, there is no mobile phase present when visualization takes place.

208. **(C)** Rearranging the equation for R_f yields the following:

distance travelled by the compound = (R_f) (distance travelled by the solvent)

If the solvent travels a distance of 5 cm, the distance travelled by any given compound is equal to its R_f multiplied by 5 cm. The distance travelled by the first compound is (0.50) (5 cm), which equals 2.50 cm. The distance travelled by the second compound is (0.61) (5 cm), which equals 3.05 cm. The determine how far apart these two compounds are on the plate, simply subtract the distances that they have travelled: 305 cm - 2.50 cm = 0.55 cm.

PASSAGE X (Questions 209-214)

209. **(D)**   Alkanes with three or fewer carbons (methane: CH_4, ethane: CH_3CH_3 and propane: $CH_3CH_2CH_3$) can only be arranged in one way and, therefore, do not have structural isomers. Answers (A) and (B) are wrong because these alkanes do not have a ring structure and do not contain double bonds. Answer (C) is incorrect because there are no functional groups associated with alkanes.

210. **(C)**   This is the only possible structural isomer because it contains the same atoms found in 1-propanol (3 C, 6 H and 1 O), however, they are arranged in different order. Answers (A), (B) and (D) all contain different atoms than 1-propanol and therefore cannot be structural isomers of it.

211. **(A)**   These two formulas represent the same structure because the atoms are attached in the same order, only the orientation has been changed. Answers (B), (C) and (D) are pairs of structural isomers because the order of attachment of the atoms is different for both formulas of each pair.

212. **(B)**   These structures differ in the arrangement of their atoms in space and are stereoisomers. The structure on the left is the *cis*-isomer in which the CH_3 and CH_2CH_3 groups are on the same side of the pi bond. The structure on the right is the *trans*-isomer where the CH_3 and CH_2CH_3 groups are located on opposite sides of the double bond. Answers (A) and (C) are incorrect because in order for stereoisomers to exist, there must be two different groups attached to each carbon of the double bond. Answer (D) is wrong because both of the structures are *trans*-isomers.

213. **(D)**   In order for stereoisomers to exist, there must be two different groups attached to each of the pi-bonded carbons. Answer (A) is incorrect because the groups cannot be the same. Answers (B) and (C) are wrong because the carbon atoms involved in the pi bond do not lie on either side of it or rotate around it.

214. **(B)**   *Trans*-isomers are more stable because they are less sterically hindered than *cis*-isomers. This is because the groups attached to the carbons of the double bond are located on opposite sides of the pi bond in *trans*-isomers but, on the same side in *cis*-isomers. Answer (A) is incorrect because different groups must be attached to the pi-bonded carbons in order for stereoisomers to exist. Answer (C) is incorrect because the same atoms, whether H, or another, are attached to the pi-bonded carbons in both *cis*- and *trans*-forms. Answer (D) is wrong because there is less interaction among groups in the *trans*-isomer because the groups are located on opposite sides of the double bond.

215. **(C)**   Bone formation that takes place in pre-existing cartilage is called endochondral ossification. The cartilage, which is present in infants, is replaced by bone in later years. Bones at the base of the skull in the vertebral column, the pelvis, and the limbs are all called cartilage bones because they form in this manner.

216. **(A)**   The appendicular skeleton is comprised of the shoulder girdle, upper extremities, pelvic girdle, and lower extremities. The humerus is the bone in the upper arm and is, therefore, part of the appendicular skeleton. The vertebra, ribs, sternum (breast bone), and skull are all part of the axial skeleton.

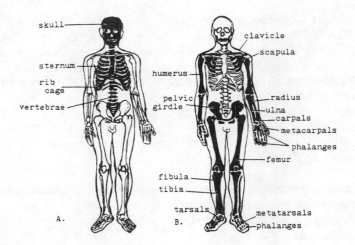

skull

clavicle

scapula

sternum

humerus

rib
cage

vertebrae

pelvic
girdle

radius

ulna

carpals

metacarpals

phalanges

femur

fibula

tibia

tarsals

metatarsals

phalanges

A.

B.

Diagrams of the human body showing, A, the bonds of the axial skeleton and B, the bones of the appendicular skeleton.

217. (D) The pill, an oral contraceptive, acts to prevent ovulation in women. The pill is taken from the fifth to the twenty-fifth day of a woman's menstrual cycle. The efficiency of the pill is nearly 100%. Condoms and diaphragms have an approximately 12% - 14% pregnancy rate (12 - 14 pregnancies out of 100). An IUD interferes with the endometrial preparation for accepting the embryo. The IUD has an approximately 2% pregnancy rate. The rhythm method involves the restriction of intercourse to a "safe" period. This is the least effective method and has a pregnancy rate of approximately 24%.

218. (D) Saponification is the alkaline hydrolysis of esters to produce the salt of the ester (a soap) and an alcohol. Fats are esters of glycerol so they do undergo saponification.

The general reaction for this process is:

$$\underset{\text{ester}}{R-\underset{\underset{O}{\parallel}}{C}-O-R'} + NaOH \xrightarrow{\text{aq}} \underset{\text{ester salt}}{R-\underset{\underset{O}{\parallel}}{C}-\overset{\ominus\oplus}{O}Na} + \underset{\text{alcohol}}{R'OH}$$

219. (D) A carbon atom to which are attached four different atoms or groups is called a chiral carbon. A molecule containing a chiral carbon cannot be superimposed on its mirror image. Therefore, the two isomers are not identical. Isomers whose molecules differ only in the positioning of groups around a chiral carbon are called optical isomers.

In (I), 2-butanol, there exists an optical isomer, since there are four different groups attached to a central carbon atom:

$$CH_3\,CH_2 \overset{\displaystyle OH}{\underset{\displaystyle H}{-\,C\,-}} CH_3$$

In (II), 2-chloropropane, the compound has no optical isomer since two of the four groups are the same.

$$CH_3 \overset{\displaystyle H}{\underset{\displaystyle Cl}{-\,C\,-}} CH_3$$

In (III), α-hydroxybutanol, the compound has an optical isomer, since it has four different groups attached to a central carbon atom.

$$\overset{\displaystyle O}{\overset{\displaystyle \|}{\overset{\displaystyle CH}{\underset{\displaystyle CH_2\,CH_3}{H-\,C\,-OH}}}}$$

In (IV), 2-hydroxymethylcyclohexanol, the compound has an optical isomer since it has four different groups attached to its central carbon atom.

$$\overset{\displaystyle CH_2\,OH}{\underset{\displaystyle CH_2\,CH_2\,CHOH}{CH_2CH_2-\,C\,-H}}$$

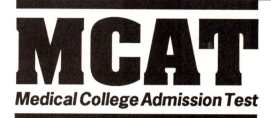

Test 2

MEDICAL COLLEGE ADMISSION TEST
TEST 2
ANSWER SHEET

Section 1:
Verbal Reasoning

1. Ⓐ Ⓑ Ⓒ Ⓓ
2. Ⓐ Ⓑ Ⓒ Ⓓ
3. Ⓐ Ⓑ Ⓒ Ⓓ
4. Ⓐ Ⓑ Ⓒ Ⓓ
5. Ⓐ Ⓑ Ⓒ Ⓓ
6. Ⓐ Ⓑ Ⓒ Ⓓ
7. Ⓐ Ⓑ Ⓒ Ⓓ
8. Ⓐ Ⓑ Ⓒ Ⓓ
9. Ⓐ Ⓑ Ⓒ Ⓓ
10. Ⓐ Ⓑ Ⓒ Ⓓ
11. Ⓐ Ⓑ Ⓒ Ⓓ
12. Ⓐ Ⓑ Ⓒ Ⓓ
13. Ⓐ Ⓑ Ⓒ Ⓓ
14. Ⓐ Ⓑ Ⓒ Ⓓ
15. Ⓐ Ⓑ Ⓒ Ⓓ
16. Ⓐ Ⓑ Ⓒ Ⓓ
17. Ⓐ Ⓑ Ⓒ Ⓓ
18. Ⓐ Ⓑ Ⓒ Ⓓ
19. Ⓐ Ⓑ Ⓒ Ⓓ
20. Ⓐ Ⓑ Ⓒ Ⓓ
21. Ⓐ Ⓑ Ⓒ Ⓓ
22. Ⓐ Ⓑ Ⓒ Ⓓ
23. Ⓐ Ⓑ Ⓒ Ⓓ
24. Ⓐ Ⓑ Ⓒ Ⓓ
25. Ⓐ Ⓑ Ⓒ Ⓓ
26. Ⓐ Ⓑ Ⓒ Ⓓ
27. Ⓐ Ⓑ Ⓒ Ⓓ
28. Ⓐ Ⓑ Ⓒ Ⓓ
29. Ⓐ Ⓑ Ⓒ Ⓓ
30. Ⓐ Ⓑ Ⓒ Ⓓ
31. Ⓐ Ⓑ Ⓒ Ⓓ

32. Ⓐ Ⓑ Ⓒ Ⓓ
33. Ⓐ Ⓑ Ⓒ Ⓓ
34. Ⓐ Ⓑ Ⓒ Ⓓ
35. Ⓐ Ⓑ Ⓒ Ⓓ
36. Ⓐ Ⓑ Ⓒ Ⓓ
37. Ⓐ Ⓑ Ⓒ Ⓓ
38. Ⓐ Ⓑ Ⓒ Ⓓ
39. Ⓐ Ⓑ Ⓒ Ⓓ
40. Ⓐ Ⓑ Ⓒ Ⓓ
41. Ⓐ Ⓑ Ⓒ Ⓓ
42. Ⓐ Ⓑ Ⓒ Ⓓ
43. Ⓐ Ⓑ Ⓒ Ⓓ
44. Ⓐ Ⓑ Ⓒ Ⓓ
45. Ⓐ Ⓑ Ⓒ Ⓓ
46. Ⓐ Ⓑ Ⓒ Ⓓ
47. Ⓐ Ⓑ Ⓒ Ⓓ
48. Ⓐ Ⓑ Ⓒ Ⓓ
49. Ⓐ Ⓑ Ⓒ Ⓓ
50. Ⓐ Ⓑ Ⓒ Ⓓ
51. Ⓐ Ⓑ Ⓒ Ⓓ
52. Ⓐ Ⓑ Ⓒ Ⓓ
53. Ⓐ Ⓑ Ⓒ Ⓓ
54. Ⓐ Ⓑ Ⓒ Ⓓ
55. Ⓐ Ⓑ Ⓒ Ⓓ
56. Ⓐ Ⓑ Ⓒ Ⓓ
57. Ⓐ Ⓑ Ⓒ Ⓓ
58. Ⓐ Ⓑ Ⓒ Ⓓ
59. Ⓐ Ⓑ Ⓒ Ⓓ
60. Ⓐ Ⓑ Ⓒ Ⓓ
61. Ⓐ Ⓑ Ⓒ Ⓓ
62. Ⓐ Ⓑ Ⓒ Ⓓ
63. Ⓐ Ⓑ Ⓒ Ⓓ
64. Ⓐ Ⓑ Ⓒ Ⓓ
65. Ⓐ Ⓑ Ⓒ Ⓓ

Section 2:
Physical Sciences

66. Ⓐ Ⓑ Ⓒ Ⓓ
67. Ⓐ Ⓑ Ⓒ Ⓓ
68. Ⓐ Ⓑ Ⓒ Ⓓ
69. Ⓐ Ⓑ Ⓒ Ⓓ
70. Ⓐ Ⓑ Ⓒ Ⓓ
71. Ⓐ Ⓑ Ⓒ Ⓓ
72. Ⓐ Ⓑ Ⓒ Ⓓ
73. Ⓐ Ⓑ Ⓒ Ⓓ
74. Ⓐ Ⓑ Ⓒ Ⓓ
75. Ⓐ Ⓑ Ⓒ Ⓓ
76. Ⓐ Ⓑ Ⓒ Ⓓ
77. Ⓐ Ⓑ Ⓒ Ⓓ
78. Ⓐ Ⓑ Ⓒ Ⓓ
79. Ⓐ Ⓑ Ⓒ Ⓓ
80. Ⓐ Ⓑ Ⓒ Ⓓ
81. Ⓐ Ⓑ Ⓒ Ⓓ
82. Ⓐ Ⓑ Ⓒ Ⓓ
83. Ⓐ Ⓑ Ⓒ Ⓓ
84. Ⓐ Ⓑ Ⓒ Ⓓ
85. Ⓐ Ⓑ Ⓒ Ⓓ
86. Ⓐ Ⓑ Ⓒ Ⓓ
87. Ⓐ Ⓑ Ⓒ Ⓓ
88. Ⓐ Ⓑ Ⓒ Ⓓ
89. Ⓐ Ⓑ Ⓒ Ⓓ
90. Ⓐ Ⓑ Ⓒ Ⓓ
91. Ⓐ Ⓑ Ⓒ Ⓓ
92. Ⓐ Ⓑ Ⓒ Ⓓ
93. Ⓐ Ⓑ Ⓒ Ⓓ
94. Ⓐ Ⓑ Ⓒ Ⓓ
95. Ⓐ Ⓑ Ⓒ Ⓓ
96. Ⓐ Ⓑ Ⓒ Ⓓ

97. Ⓐ Ⓑ Ⓒ Ⓓ
98. Ⓐ Ⓑ Ⓒ Ⓓ
99. Ⓐ Ⓑ Ⓒ Ⓓ
100. Ⓐ Ⓑ Ⓒ Ⓓ
101. Ⓐ Ⓑ Ⓒ Ⓓ
102. Ⓐ Ⓑ Ⓒ Ⓓ
103. Ⓐ Ⓑ Ⓒ Ⓓ
104. Ⓐ Ⓑ Ⓒ Ⓓ
105. Ⓐ Ⓑ Ⓒ Ⓓ
106. Ⓐ Ⓑ Ⓒ Ⓓ
107. Ⓐ Ⓑ Ⓒ Ⓓ
108. Ⓐ Ⓑ Ⓒ Ⓓ
109. Ⓐ Ⓑ Ⓒ Ⓓ
110. Ⓐ Ⓑ Ⓒ Ⓓ
111. Ⓐ Ⓑ Ⓒ Ⓓ
112. Ⓐ Ⓑ Ⓒ Ⓓ
113. Ⓐ Ⓑ Ⓒ Ⓓ
114. Ⓐ Ⓑ Ⓒ Ⓓ
115. Ⓐ Ⓑ Ⓒ Ⓓ
116. Ⓐ Ⓑ Ⓒ Ⓓ
117. Ⓐ Ⓑ Ⓒ Ⓓ
118. Ⓐ Ⓑ Ⓒ Ⓓ
119. Ⓐ Ⓑ Ⓒ Ⓓ
120. Ⓐ Ⓑ Ⓒ Ⓓ
121. Ⓐ Ⓑ Ⓒ Ⓓ
122. Ⓐ Ⓑ Ⓒ Ⓓ
123. Ⓐ Ⓑ Ⓒ Ⓓ
124. Ⓐ Ⓑ Ⓒ Ⓓ
125. Ⓐ Ⓑ Ⓒ Ⓓ
126. Ⓐ Ⓑ Ⓒ Ⓓ
127. Ⓐ Ⓑ Ⓒ Ⓓ
128. Ⓐ Ⓑ Ⓒ Ⓓ
129. Ⓐ Ⓑ Ⓒ Ⓓ
130. Ⓐ Ⓑ Ⓒ Ⓓ
131. Ⓐ Ⓑ Ⓒ Ⓓ
132. Ⓐ Ⓑ Ⓒ Ⓓ
133. Ⓐ Ⓑ Ⓒ Ⓓ
134. Ⓐ Ⓑ Ⓒ Ⓓ
135. Ⓐ Ⓑ Ⓒ Ⓓ
136. Ⓐ Ⓑ Ⓒ Ⓓ
137. Ⓐ Ⓑ Ⓒ Ⓓ
138. Ⓐ Ⓑ Ⓒ Ⓓ
139. Ⓐ Ⓑ Ⓒ Ⓓ

140. Ⓐ Ⓑ Ⓒ Ⓓ
141. Ⓐ Ⓑ Ⓒ Ⓓ
142. Ⓐ Ⓑ Ⓒ Ⓓ

Section 4:
Biological Sciences

143. Ⓐ Ⓑ Ⓒ Ⓓ
144. Ⓐ Ⓑ Ⓒ Ⓓ
145. Ⓐ Ⓑ Ⓒ Ⓓ
146. Ⓐ Ⓑ Ⓒ Ⓓ
147. Ⓐ Ⓑ Ⓒ Ⓓ
148. Ⓐ Ⓑ Ⓒ Ⓓ
149. Ⓐ Ⓑ Ⓒ Ⓓ
150. Ⓐ Ⓑ Ⓒ Ⓓ
151. Ⓐ Ⓑ Ⓒ Ⓓ
152. Ⓐ Ⓑ Ⓒ Ⓓ
153. Ⓐ Ⓑ Ⓒ Ⓓ
154. Ⓐ Ⓑ Ⓒ Ⓓ
155. Ⓐ Ⓑ Ⓒ Ⓓ
156. Ⓐ Ⓑ Ⓒ Ⓓ
157. Ⓐ Ⓑ Ⓒ Ⓓ
158. Ⓐ Ⓑ Ⓒ Ⓓ
159. Ⓐ Ⓑ Ⓒ Ⓓ
160. Ⓐ Ⓑ Ⓒ Ⓓ
161. Ⓐ Ⓑ Ⓒ Ⓓ
162. Ⓐ Ⓑ Ⓒ Ⓓ
163. Ⓐ Ⓑ Ⓒ Ⓓ
164. Ⓐ Ⓑ Ⓒ Ⓓ
165. Ⓐ Ⓑ Ⓒ Ⓓ
166. Ⓐ Ⓑ Ⓒ Ⓓ
167. Ⓐ Ⓑ Ⓒ Ⓓ
168. Ⓐ Ⓑ Ⓒ Ⓓ
169. Ⓐ Ⓑ Ⓒ Ⓓ
170. Ⓐ Ⓑ Ⓒ Ⓓ
171. Ⓐ Ⓑ Ⓒ Ⓓ
172. Ⓐ Ⓑ Ⓒ Ⓓ
173. Ⓐ Ⓑ Ⓒ Ⓓ
174. Ⓐ Ⓑ Ⓒ Ⓓ
175. Ⓐ Ⓑ Ⓒ Ⓓ
176. Ⓐ Ⓑ Ⓒ Ⓓ

177. Ⓐ Ⓑ Ⓒ Ⓓ
178. Ⓐ Ⓑ Ⓒ Ⓓ
179. Ⓐ Ⓑ Ⓒ Ⓓ
180. Ⓐ Ⓑ Ⓒ Ⓓ
181. Ⓐ Ⓑ Ⓒ Ⓓ
182. Ⓐ Ⓑ Ⓒ Ⓓ
183. Ⓐ Ⓑ Ⓒ Ⓓ
184. Ⓐ Ⓑ Ⓒ Ⓓ
185. Ⓐ Ⓑ Ⓒ Ⓓ
186. Ⓐ Ⓑ Ⓒ Ⓓ
187. Ⓐ Ⓑ Ⓒ Ⓓ
188. Ⓐ Ⓑ Ⓒ Ⓓ
189. Ⓐ Ⓑ Ⓒ Ⓓ
190. Ⓐ Ⓑ Ⓒ Ⓓ
191. Ⓐ Ⓑ Ⓒ Ⓓ
192. Ⓐ Ⓑ Ⓒ Ⓓ
193. Ⓐ Ⓑ Ⓒ Ⓓ
194. Ⓐ Ⓑ Ⓒ Ⓓ
195. Ⓐ Ⓑ Ⓒ Ⓓ
196. Ⓐ Ⓑ Ⓒ Ⓓ
197. Ⓐ Ⓑ Ⓒ Ⓓ
198. Ⓐ Ⓑ Ⓒ Ⓓ
199. Ⓐ Ⓑ Ⓒ Ⓓ
200. Ⓐ Ⓑ Ⓒ Ⓓ
201. Ⓐ Ⓑ Ⓒ Ⓓ
202. Ⓐ Ⓑ Ⓒ Ⓓ
203. Ⓐ Ⓑ Ⓒ Ⓓ
204. Ⓐ Ⓑ Ⓒ Ⓓ
205. Ⓐ Ⓑ Ⓒ Ⓓ
206. Ⓐ Ⓑ Ⓒ Ⓓ
207. Ⓐ Ⓑ Ⓒ Ⓓ
208. Ⓐ Ⓑ Ⓒ Ⓓ
209. Ⓐ Ⓑ Ⓒ Ⓓ
210. Ⓐ Ⓑ Ⓒ Ⓓ
211. Ⓐ Ⓑ Ⓒ Ⓓ
212. Ⓐ Ⓑ Ⓒ Ⓓ
213. Ⓐ Ⓑ Ⓒ Ⓓ
214. Ⓐ Ⓑ Ⓒ Ⓓ
215. Ⓐ Ⓑ Ⓒ Ⓓ
216. Ⓐ Ⓑ Ⓒ Ⓓ
217. Ⓐ Ⓑ Ⓒ Ⓓ
218. Ⓐ Ⓑ Ⓒ Ⓓ
219. Ⓐ Ⓑ Ⓒ Ⓓ

TEST 2

Section 1 — Verbal Reasoning

TIME: 85 Minutes
QUESTIONS: 1-65

DIRECTIONS: The verbal reasoning section contains seven passages, each followed by a series of questions. Based on the information given in a passage, choose the one best answer to each question. If you are not sure of an answer, eliminate those choices that you know are incorrect and choose an answer from among those remaining. Fill in the corresponding circle on the answer sheet to indicate your answer.

PASSAGE I (Questions 1-10)

The philosopher Socrates is put on trial in Athens in 400 B.C. on two charges: corrupting the youth and impiety. Socrates begins his defense, as recorded in Plato's dialogue The Apology, by saying how he is going to "speak plainly and honestly," unlike the eloquent sophists the Athenian jury is accustomed to hearing. This appeal to unadorned language offends the jurors, who are expecting to be entertained.

Next, Socrates identifies two sets of accusers that he must face: past and present. The former, who filled the jurors' heads with lies about him when they were young, Socrates finds most dangerous because they cannot be cross-examined and because they influenced the jurors when they were young and impressionable. This offends the jury because it calls into question their ability to be objective and render a fair judgment.

Now Socrates addresses the charges themselves and dismisses them as mere covers for the deeper attack on his philosophical activity. That activity, which involves questioning others until they reveal contradictions in their beliefs, gave rise to Socrates' motto, "The unexamined life is not worth living" and the "Socratic Method," which is still employed in many law schools. This critical questioning of leading Athenians has made Socrates very unpopular with the powers that be and, he insists, led to his trial. This challenge to the legitimacy of the legal system itself further alienates his judges.

Socrates tries to explain that his philosophical life came about quite by accident. He was content to be a humble stone mason until the day that a friend informed him that the Oracle of Delphi said that "Socrates is the wisest man in Greece." Socrates was so surprised by the statement, and so sure of its inaccuracy, that he set about disproving it by talking to the reputed wise men of Athens and showing how much more knowledge they possessed. Unfortunately, as he tells the jury, those citizens reputed to be wise (politicians, businessmen, artists) turned out to be ignorant, either by knowing absolutely nothing, or by having limited knowledge (in their fields of expertise) and assuming knowledge of everything else. Of these, Socrates had to admit, "I am wiser, because although all of us have little knowledge, I am aware of my ignorance, while they are not." But this practice of revealing prominent citizens' ignorance and arrogance did not earn Socrates their affection, especially when the bright young men of Athens began following him around and delighting in the disgracing of their elders. Hence, in his view, the formal charges of "corrupting the youth" and "impiety" were a pretext to retaliate for the deeper offense of challenging the pretensions of the establishment.

Although Socrates views the whole trial as a sham, he cleverly refutes the charges by using the same method of questioning that landed him in the docket. Against the charges of corrupting the youth, Socrates asks his chief accuser, Meletus, if anyone wants to harm himself, to which Meletus answers "no." Then, Socrates asks if one's associates have an effect on one: good people for good, and evil people for evil, to which Meletus answers "yes." Then, Socrates asks if corrupting one's companions makes them better or worse, to which Meletus answers "worse." Finally, Socrates springs the trap by asking Meletus if he corrupted the youth intentionally or unintentionally, to which Meletus, wanting to make the charge as bad as possible, answers "intentionally." Now Socrates shows the contradictory nature of the charge, since by intentionally corrupting his companions he makes them worse, thereby bringing harm on himself. He refutes the second charge of impiety the same way, by showing that its two components (teaching about strange gods and atheism) are inconsistent.

Although Socrates has logically refuted the charges against him, the Athenian jury finds him guilty, and Meletus proposes the death penalty. The defendant Socrates is allowed to propose an alternative penalty and Socrates proposes a state pension, so he can continue his philosophical activity to the benefit of Athens. He states that this is what he "deserves." The Athenian jury, furious over his presumption, vote the death penalty and one of the great philosophers of the Western heritage is executed.

1. Socrates was an

    (A) ancient Roman philosopher.   (B) ancient Roman lawyer.

    (C) ancient Greek philosopher.   (D) ancient Greek researcher.

2. Socrates' appeal to simple, honest speech implies that the sophists' style of speaking is

    (A) persuasive.   (B) dishonest.

    (C) appealing.   (D) vulgar.

3. By identifying his past accusers as more dangerous than his present ones, Socrates suggests that his current jurors

    (A) are old men.

    (B) were impressionable when young.

    (C) like to gossip.

    (D) are nostalgic.

4. The Socratic method is still used in

    (A)   many medical schools.   (B)   police academies.

    (C)   military training.   (D)   many law schools.

5. Before beginning his defense, Socrates offends the Athenian jury

    (A)   once.   (B)   twice.

    (C)   three times.   (D)   four times.

6. Socrates' situation occurs anytime

    (A)   a stone mason attempts to become a philosopher.

    (B)   an individual challenges authority by revealing its ignorance.

    (C)   an old man asks a lot of questions.

    (D)   society allows trial by jury.

7. For the Socratic Method, consistency is

    (A)   the hobgoblin of small minds.

    (B)   the sign of a trumped-up charge.

    (C)   the sign of a genuine charge.

    (D)   impossible in a court of law.

8. The fact that Socrates is found guilty shows that

    (A)   he did corrupt the youth.

    (B)   rationality always wins.

    (C)   rationality may not always win.

    (D)   Athens did not have a Supreme Court.

9. Socrates' suggestion of an alternative penalty of a state pension is viewed by the jury as

    (A)   the ramblings of a disturbed man.

    (B)   an appropriate award.

    (C)   an insult to Meletus and reward to Socrates.

    (D)   an insult to Socrates and reward to Meletus.

10. Socrates' trial is relevant throughout the Western heritage whenever

    (A)   courts are corrupt.

    (B)   defendants are intellectual.

    (C)   youthful juries decide on the elderly.

    (D)   established authority executes its critic.

PASSAGE II (Questions 11-16)

The system of American federalism, because it established two distinct levels of government, each with its own jurisdiction, will inevitably create tension and conflict. The division between national and state authorities was designed, partly because of James Madison's fear of absolute political power, to distribute sovereignty among several bodies and, thereby, to prevent concentration of power and tyranny. However, this has caused historical controversies over the precise distribution of power between the central and decentralized governments. Such a controversy eventually led to the Civil War.

One interpretation of American federalism, originally held by the Anti-Federalists and later by the Confederacy, was the "compact theory." According to this view, the states had entered into a compact after the Revolution and had established the national government to perform specific and limited functions (primarily foreign affairs and interstate commerce). Most of the lawmaking authority over domestic policy, then, resided in the states. If a conflict over the division of federal and state authority arose, the compact theory held that the states, through a convention, could interpret the exact meaning of the Constitution. It also implied that any state could secede from the Union.

Another view of American federalism, held by the Federalists and later the Northern advocates of Union, argued that the Constitution was created by "The People," apart from their membership in the various states, and therefore it was not beholden to the states for its authority. This perspective, which eventually prevailed, held that the national government was separate from, and superior to, the state governments. It also believed that the United States Supreme Court should decide any disputes over the meaning of federalism in the Constitution through its power of "judicial review." This view justified many incursions into state sovereignty including most of the Civil Rights laws and much of police procedure, under the doctrine that the federal Bill of Rights took precedence over state law.

A third conception of American federalism, often called "cooperative federalism," holds that each level of government has its own jurisdiction but that they inevitably overlap (in policies associated with health, welfare, education, etc.) and therefore the two tiers of government must work together. This view helped form many of the 1960s "social welfare" policies, in which the national government would design and fund programs for the poor, elderly, and so on, and the states would implement them according to local needs. The federal categorical grant programs, and later, block grants and revenue sharing programs grew out of this "partnership" between Washington and the states. President Reagan's "New Federalism" cut many of these programs, shifting authority and funding to the states alone.

The dynamism and adaptability of the American system is partly due to the ambiguous nature of American federalism; but this also necessitates continual tension and accommodation.

11. According to Madison, American federalism would divide political power in order to

   (A) give categorical grants.

   (B) prevent concentration of power.

   (C) allow Southern states to secede.

   (D) allow the South to retain slavery.

12. According to the "compact theory" the conclusion of the Civil War was

   (A) unjust.   (B) just.
   (C) a mistake.   (D) inevitable.

13. When a conservative Supreme Court grants greater jurisdiction to states and localities, it is supporting the idea of

   (A) compact federalism.   (B) judicial federalism.
   (C) cooperative federalism.   (D) dual federalism.

14. "Judicial review" allows the Supreme Court to assume which function of the states from the "compact theory" perspective?

   (A) Constitutional convention (B) *Habeas Corpus*
   (C) Block grants   (D) Desegregation

15. President Reagan's "New Federalism" subscribed to which notion of federalism?

   (A) Compact theory   (B) Judicial federalism
   (C) Dual federalism   (D) Cooperative federalism

16. The nature of American federalism makes the relationship between the United States government and the states

   (A) confused, but authoritarian.   (B) tense, but permanent.
   (C) stable, but undefined.   (D) adaptable, but conflictual.

PASSAGE III (Questions 17-25)

Although Plato's book *The Republic* is one of the most famous works in political theory, its vision of humanity and society are radically different from contemporary ideas. Indeed, in a twentieth century world that values democracy, equality and freedom, Plato's ideal state seems shocking.

Plato conceives of human nature as made up of three elements or dispositions: (1) the philosophic, (2) the spirited and (3) the appetitive. The philosophic part of a person is his or her desire and capacity for acquiring knowledge, the passionate search for truth fueled by curiosity. The spirited element is the love of combat and fighting—it loves the struggle of battle and the thrill of triumphing over an opponent. The appetitive side of human nature is concerned with material things: possessions, comforts and the economy in general. For Plato, all three elements are present in everyone but one predominates in each individual, forming his or her character. This distribution of dominant traits renders humanity essentially *unequal,* although this inequality is not, for Plato, based on gender, as both men and women can be philosophic, spirited, or appetitive.

The natural division of humanity into three dominant characteristics creates, for Plato, a natural class system in society. The philosophic people, whose virtue is wisdom, should govern society; the spirited people, whose virtue is courage, should form the military; and the appetitive people, whose virtue is moderation, should work in the economic sector: production, distribution, and so on. Justice, for Plato, consists of the "right ordering" of psychic and social, elements and classes. The individual is subordinate to the needs of the whole society and should occupy a proper "place" in the social order. This explains Plato's rationale for a "philosopher-king" ruling over society because his or her wisdom is of this order and the virtues that accompany it.

Plato devises a "myth of the metals" which explains and justifies this class society, based on internal dispositions and functional excellence. According to this myth, or "noble lie," each person born is mixed with some metal from the earth: gold with the philosophic nature, silver with the spirited nature and bronze with the appetitive nature. This myth makes it easier for common people to understand their "place" in society.

However, because dominant natures are not passed on through heredity (i.e., gold parents can have a silver or bronze child, bronze parents can have a silver or gold child), Plato devises an elaborate educational system (often called "communism in children") that discerns and cultivates each child's natural propensities and abilities. In this scheme, it is best for the individual to be told what their nature is by the State and to be developed in a certain way, rather than to be able to choose freely on limited knowledge. For Plato, this social system will guarantee the most harmonious country and the happiest citizens. A democracy, by contrast, in which everyone is left free to decide their own occupation, will be chaotic, leading to disorder and eventually to tyranny. Only an all-wise philosopher-king can determine each person's true capacity and order society accordingly.

Plato's inegalitarian theory, with its emphasis on individuals' fixed natures and inevitable class status, seems odd and even offensive to twentieth century minds which value free choice, equality, democracy, and protection from authoritarian government. However, as Western democracies suffer from uncertainty, and individuals feel alienated from any secure "place" in society, Plato's ideas forever haunt humanity.

17. A human quality that Plato does not include in his catalogue of human dispositions is

    (A)   the spirited.   (B)   the philosophic.

    (C)   the humorous.   (D)   the appetitive.

18. A business entrepreneur would most likely fall into the Platonic category of

    (A)   the philosophic.   (B)   the appetitive.

    (C)   the spirited.   (D)   the innovative.

19. Which remark by Thomas Jefferson most contrasts with Plato's philosophy about class differences?

    (A)   "The blood of patriots waters the tree of liberty ..."

    (B)   "All men are created equal."

    (C)   "We are all federalists, all republicans."

    (D)   "There is a natural aristocracy ..."

20. The wisdom that characterizes the philosopher and qualifies him or her for rule is

(A) knowledge of moderation.

(B) knowledge of combat.

(C) knowledge of the stock market.

(D) knowledge of virtue.

21. The feature of American society that most embodies Plato's social principles is

(A) free enterprise.

(B) presidential elections.

(C) public education.

(D) the Congress.

22. One virtue that Plato's *Republic* does not always endorse is

(A) courage.

(B) moderation.

(C) honor.

(D) truthfulness.

23. A country that recruits young people into the army by appealing to their desires for money, benefits, and training that will help them "land a job" is applying which class standards to the military, in Plato's view?

(A) The philosophic

(B) The appetitive

(C) The spirited

(D) The virtuous

24. If a man aged nineteen said; "I don't know what to do with my life, and I haven't got any skills," Plato would say

(A) he is lazy.

(B) he is stupid.

(C) he is corrupt.

(D) his society has failed him.

25. One public belief that would cause Americans to reject Plato's system is

(A) support of the military.

(B) love and property.

(C) skepticism of an all-wise leader.

(D) respect for education.

PASSAGE IV (Questions 26-34)

America in the 1990s is entering a social period that might be called Neo-Victorian. Like the original Victorian period of the latter nineteenth century in England and the United States, this period just ahead will be characterized by an emphasis on traditional values and morality, stable families, conventional religion and economic conservatism. The reasons for this new period of Neo-Victorianism are complex, but some of the most obvious causes are: the middle age status of the baby-boom generation and their having children of their own; the continuing spread of the AIDS epidemic—even into small towns, rural areas and among people with "traditional" lifestyles; and the loss of rapid economic growth, as the decade experiences recession or slow growth. All three of these factors will contribute to the emerging Neo-Victorian *zeitgeist,* or spirit of the times.

The baby-boom generation — that enormous group of Americans born during the 1950s — entered middle age during the late 1980s. Television programs like "Thirtysomething," and others characterized the mood of this graying generation, as its ages rose to late thirties and even early forties. This was the generation that experienced its adolescent rebellion *en masse* during the 1960s, causing the enormous social turmoil of the rock era, the free love movement, the drug culture, anti-war protests, radical political groups, etc. This generation then had "seen it all," had lost its innocence, and found itself with a bad hangover by the 1970s. Those that survived the drug deaths, political bombings, and fractured personal relationships entered middle age as "born again" conservatives, like the notorious reformed prostitute who is holier-than-thou and ready to stamp out sin and immorality everywhere. Compounding this reaction against their own past, the baby-boom generation started settling down and having babies of its own. In 1989 there were as many births in this country as during the biggest year of the baby-boom era. With children comes a sense of responsibility and the need for stability, reliability, and order. Graying baby boomers had experienced the destructiveness of mass rebellion, of tearing down established morality and authority. Now they will repent with a vengeance. *Catcher in the Rye* may have been their Bible, but their children will be raised on *Peter Rabbit*. Disney is the thing today. The middle-aged baby boomers are the new advocates of traditional family values, social decency, religious ethics, and especially public safety.

The AIDS epidemic threatens public safety more than any other single problem. Its association with illicit sex will bring a return to traditional monogamous relationships, sex after marriage, and suspicion of nontraditional lifestyles. Again, the Neo-Victorian ethos of sobriety and propriety will prevail. The children growing up in the 1990s (like those of the 1890s and 1950s) will be taught the sanctity of the family, and fidelity.

Finally, the impending economic recession and, after that, continued slow growth in the American economy, will encourage frugality and conservatism. No extravagant public spending plans or private indulgences will be tolerated. The Puritan ethic of hard work and saving will descend on America.

Social trends work in cycles, however, and this Neo-Victorian period too shall pass. In fact, if history is a guide, the children growing up in the 1990s should have quite a wild time (à la the 1920s and 1960s) around 2008.

26. A possible cause of the Neo-Victorian era that was not mentioned by the author is

   (A) economic recession. (B) AIDS.

   (C) drugs. (D) aging baby boomers.

27. A flaw in the author's historical analysis of the Victorian era (and therefore the Neo-Victorian era) may be

   (A) its absence in England. (B) its hypocritical morality.

   (C) its boring nature. (D) its *zeitgeist*.

28. According to the author's logic, those who advocate a return to traditional values tend to be people who

   (A) are good Christians.

(B) were raised by clergy.

(C) are well educated.

(D) have experienced excess and changed their lifestyles.

29. The act of raising children, as presented in this essay, leads people to become

(A) neurotic.   (B) responsible.

(C) bossy.   (D) irreverent.

30. In this essay, the book *Catcher in the Rye* is portrayed as

(A) a fairy tale.   (B) a Walt Disney movie.

(C) a book of critical rebellion.   (D) the Bible.

31. An issue raised in the first paragraph as a dimension of a cause of the Neo-Victorian period, but not fully developed later in the essay, is

(A) AIDS in small towns and rural areas.

(B) slowed economic growth.

(C) baby-boomer parenthood.

(D) the AIDS epidemic.

32. If the author's views of social and psychological change are correct, the proper course to produce a *radical* adult would be to

(A) give them a conservative upbringing.

(B) give them a radical upbringing.

(C) let them rebel as adolescents.

(D) keep them from political involvement.

33. Winston Churchill's remark, "If you are not a radical at age 20 you have no heart, and if you are not a conservative at age 40 you have no head" would seem to

(A) support the logic of the essay.

(B) oppose the logic of the essay.

(C) be irrelevant to the essay.

(D) prove that the essay was written by Churchill.

34. If the author's historical prediction is correct and the baby boomers' children rebel in 2008 they should become conservative themselves around the year

(A) 2028.   (B) 2058.

(C) 1968.   (D) 2098.

PASSAGE V (Questions 35-45)

The nineteenth century British philosopher John Stuart Mill provides arguments for intellectual liberty, and against social conformity that have greatly affected American notions of free speech, free press, and academic freedom.

In his essay, *On Liberty,* John Stuart Mill argues that it is not enough to lift formal legal and ecclesiastical restrictions on freedom of thought and expression; the individual must be protected against informal *social* prohibitions on unconventional ideas. The "tyranny of society" can exert more severe penalties such as ostracism, on the nonconformist, than can any number of laws against unconventional or unpopular ideas. To avoid such tyranny of opinion, Mill advocates a free, tolerant atmosphere in a progressive civilized and humane society. The advantages of such a liberal society are manifold for Mill, especially in the advancement of knowledge.

In *On Liberty,* John Stuart Mill gives two primary reasons for allowing complete expression of all ideas, no matter how radical. First, he claims, the new ideas or viewpoints might be *correct,* and so, their suppression by law or popular prejudice could rob the world of original, innovative ideas. A new and more useful conception of nature, the universe (as Galileo's), medicine, or politics could be denied mankind and the innovator's society could fall behind the development of others. Secondly, Mill asserts, even if the new radical idea is wrong, the right view will be strengthened by refuting. The established truth, if it is truth, should not fear or resent challenges, but rather welcome them as another opportunity to reassert its own validity. Thus, Mill sees the ongoing debate between established beliefs and their radical challengers as clarifying and sharpening the truth. The open-minded intellectual will actually relish such contests and affirm with Mill the view that "he who knows only his own side of the case, knows little of that."

Of course, Mill does not extend this idea of complete intellectual liberty to the total freedom to *act* on all of our beliefs. It is one thing to advocate the overthrowing of the United States government through violent revolution as Marxists do, but to engage in the actual killing that such a revolution entails is rightfully prohibited, both legally and socially, for Mill. Even the verbal expression of such a belief may be suppressed if the society (such as during a Depression) is in a situation where the ideas will lead people to act upon them. This forms the Supreme Court's standard of a "clear and present danger" to the society that permits punishment of inflammatory speech, as enunciated by Oliver Wendell Holmes.

John Stuart Mill's conception of liberty underlies American free speech and free press in which all viewpoints are permitted to be aired. The recent suppression of rock music groups on obscenity charges (based on "community standards") might concern Mill as an example of the "tyranny of the majority" squelching individual liberty of expression.

American academic freedom, in which university and college professors are protected in teaching controversial ideas and theories, also rests on Mill's conception of intellectual liberty. Moves to disallow discussion of certain ideas in college classrooms because they "offend" some individual or group, may seem to Mill a dangerous step away from intellectual liberty.

John Stuart Mill's ideas on liberty will always be in conflict with conformist opinions, and the struggle between conventional and radical speech will continue to occur in a free society.

35. An area of American society that might be influenced by Mill's *On Liberty* **not** mentioned in the essay is

    (A)   journalism.   (B)   academia.

    (C)   law.   (D)   None of the above.

36. Social prohibitions on unconventional ideas and expressions may be more severe than legal restrictions for Mill because

    (A)   their range of punishment is broader.

    (B)   they include the death penalty.

    (C)   they include ostracism.

    (D)   (A) and (C).

37. Mill asserts that a free, open, and tolerant society

    (A)   will advance knowledge.   (B)   will be more humane.

    (C)   will be more civilized.   (D)   All of the above.

38. The value, for Mill, in the expression of radical ideas that are wrong is

    (A)   their eventual acceptance.

    (B)   their obnoxious character.

    (C) their sharpening of the truth.

    (D)   their inability to persuade.

39. If a Mormon man outside of Utah advocated polygamy and then took three wives, American society according to Mill could

    (A)   legally prosecute him.

    (B)   leave him free.

    (C)   invoke the doctrine of clear and present danger.

    (D)   ask if he is a communist.

40. If a single man gave a speech before an angry mob, in Washington, D.C., in front of the federal courthouse, shouting, "Burn the Courthouse," American society could, according to Mill,

    (A)   legally prosecute him.

    (B)   leave him free.

    (C)   invoke ecclesiastical restrictions.

    (D)   ask if he is a communist.

41. The "clear and present danger" test of legally protected speech was developed on the Supreme Court by

    (A)   Justice Marshall.   (B)   Justice Brandeis.

    (C)   Justice Holmes.   (D)   Justice Burger.

42. An example of the Millian tradition might be

    (A) a newspaper.   (B) an assembly line.

    (C) a news program.   (D) a city council debate.

43. Another example of the Millian approach to truth in American society is

    (A) elementary education.   (B) the adversary judicial system.

    (C) medical schools.   (D) boot camp.

44. John Stuart Mill might be concerned about the prosecution of rock groups on obscenity charges because "community standards" could represent

    (A) bigotry.   (B) decent people.

    (C) the tyranny of the majority. (D) immoral smut.

45. A law requiring university professors to only teach the popular side of an issue would deny Mill's contention that

    (A) truth arises from the Bible.

    (B) truth arises out of scholarly research.

    (C) truth arises from intelligent philosophers.

    (D) truth arises out of the clash of right and wrong views.

PASSAGE VI (Questions 46-55)

Organizational theory in American public administration relies on two very different approaches to understanding, structuring, and managing governmental agencies. The traditional institutional approach focuses on the organization itself: offices, positions, structures, and functions. The newer "humanist" approach emphasizes the people in the organization: their psychological needs, aspirations, performance, etc. Reconciling these two very distinctive approaches to public administration is not easy, but a closer examination of each theory's orientation may be helpful.

The classic structural approach to governmental organizations comes from the writings of the German sociologist Max Weber. Weber's theory of bureaucracy presents an ideal administrative structure that would produce efficient, equitable public services. Weber's bureaucracy involves a clear hierarchy of official positions, each with clearly specified duties and authority. This for Weber would make for a smooth-running organization in which everyone knows their place, their superiors, and their subordinates. These official positions would be defined and limited by specific rules and regulations so the authority of the official would not be personal (as that of a prince) and less subject to abuse. All positions in the bureaucracy would be filled according to objective criteria: training, experience, etc. Salary would be tied to position; the result being that educational level, expertise, authority, and income would all correspond with each other. The organization's relations with the public, in Weber's view, would be characterized by rational, impartial and equitable treatment of all citizens as defined by specific procedures and policies, rules, and regulations. Together, the internal and external workings of this kind of government agency would create a just and efficient regime — for Weber.

The humanist approach to public management rejects the institutional approach to administration with its emphasis on structures and functions and offers a vision of organizations growing out of the psychology of the individuals involved. Abraham Maslow, an American psychologist, exemplifies this humanist approach with his famous "ladder of human needs." According to Maslow, human beings have a succession of needs, from lower, economic needs, to higher, emotional needs, that must be satisfied if one is to work effectively in any organization. Maslow identifies the first human need as basic economic sustenance: food, clothing, shelter, etc. But after this need has been met, a need for assurances of future security must be satisfied. Then, the individual needs to be loved by others. After that need is satisfied, a human need for self-esteem or a feeling of self-worth, must be addressed. Finally, the person needs to be "self-actualized," which entails developing and using all of one's talents and ability. The public administration that subscribes to this humanist theory of management cares less about organizational structures and positions, and more about the individual psychological development of the people in the organization. He or she sees administrative work as nurturing the people's needs and believes that this will make for a more productive and effective organization.

The traditional and humanist approaches are so radically dissimilar that it is inconceivable that they can ever be reconciled in the future.

46. A feature not common to the traditional, structural approach to organizational theory is

   (A)   official positions.   (B)   rules and regulations

   (C)   self-esteem.   (D)   impartial treatment clientele.

47. For Max Weber, his bureaucracy would create

   (A)   abuses of power.   (B)   excessive rules and regulations.

   (C)   inefficient government.   (D)   smoothly operating agencies.

48. Historically, one reason that Weber may have found his ideal bureaucracy attractive was its contrast with

   (A)   Nazi Germany.   (B)   decentralized feudal principalities.

   (C)   modern America.   (D)   ancient Rome.

49. Historically, one reason that the world is fearful of Weber's efficient bureaucracy is

   (A)   Nazi Germany.   (B)   decentralized feudal principalities.

   (C)   modern America.   (D)   ancient Rome.

50. Humanist organizational theory focuses on

   (A)   animal rights.   (B)   education and experience.

   (C)   procedural due process.   (D)   individual psychology.

51. A manager who periodically tells his or her subordinates that he/she "cares" about them is probably trying to satisfy their need for

(A) love.   (B) self-esteem.

(C) self-actualization.   (D) boredom.

52. For a Maslowian manager, an organization full of self-actualized people would be

(A) intolerable.   (B) productive.

(C) chaotic.   (D) boring.

53. A common criticism of Maslowian theory is that it requires administrators to be

(A) efficient.   (B) psychologists.

(C) tyrannical.   (D) boring.

54. The writer's analysis of these two dominant schools of administrative theory fails to

(A) describe the theories.   (B) show their differences.

(C) name their proponents.   (D) show how they might be reconciled.

55. This passage shows organization theory in American public administration to be

(A) consistent.   (B) confused.

(C) complex.   (D) boring.

PASSAGE VII (Questions 56-65)

   Public administration studies leadership styles and traits in order to determine which produce more effective administrative leadership and, therefore, more effective organizational relations and employee morale. This field of management leadership asks such basic questions as: Are good leaders born or made? What traits are characteristic of all good leaders? How are subordinates' abilities able to affect leadership?

   A common typology of administrative leadership grew out of a study of different management styles. This involved a study, conducted in the 1930s with three groups of boys, each assigned to complete a certain project. One group's leader was characterized as "authoritarian," which meant that he made all the decisions by himself, assigned tasks and work partners, was limited in power by neither rules nor other people, and employed a highly personal or *ad hominem* form of correction. The second group was led by a "democratic" style leader who encouraged input from the group members, established objective rules and schedules, served as a guide or facilitator rather than a dictator, and corrected people in terms of actions rather than persons. The third group had a leader characterized as "laissez-faire" which meant that he left the group members free to do whatever they wanted individually, without orders or guidance, and basically projected a "do your own thing" attitude. The boys in this third group were free to come and go as they pleased, work with whom they pleased, and perform tasks as they pleased. At the end of the projects (which were identical), the members of each group were measured according to two variables: efficiency in completing the project and satisfaction in doing so. The first group, under the authoritarian leader, ranked high in efficiency, but low in satisfaction; the second group under the democratic leader ranked high in efficiency *and* high in satisfaction; and the third group under the laissez-faire leader was low in both efficiency and satisfaction. This seemed to suggest that "democratic" administrators produced the best results and the highest morale, which gave rise to the "participatory management" school.

Another approach to leadership styles measures concern for two variables: people and production. In this model, a leader with high concern for the people in the organization, but low concern for production, will be termed a "Country Club" manager. An administrator with high concern for production, but low concern for people, will be called an "Authoritarian" manager. A high concern for both production and people is "Team Leadership" and a low concern for production and the organization's employees is "Impoverished" leadership.

The study of leadership styles in public administration should contribute to a better understanding of what makes up effective leadership and render America more competitive.

56. The first study of leadership styles in the passage lists which number of leaders?

    (A)   Two   (B)   Three

    (C)   Four   (D)   Five

57. The type of leader in the first study most likely to correct the workers using personal insults is

    (A)   "Impoverished."   (B)   "Laissez-faire."

    (C)   "Authoritarian."   (D)   "Democratic."

58. The results of the first study of leadership styles suggest that having complete freedom to do what you want in a group project

    (A)   is fun.   (B)   is anarchy.

    (C)   is unfulfilling.   (D)   is unusual.

59. A type of leader found in both leadership studies is

    (A)   "Laissez-faire."   (B)   "Impoverished."

    (C)   "Democratic."   (D)   "Authoritarian."

60. An organizational manager who worked for high pay and benefits for his or her employees, and did not make serious demands on their work, would most closely resemble which type of leader?

    (A)   "Country club"   (B)   "Authoritarian"

    (C)   "Totalitarian"   (D)   "Laid-back"

61. If the Secretary of Health and Human Services made the statement, "I think that most of these programs are a waste of time and money, and most of the people who work here are lazy, bureaucratic bums," this would most likely

qualify that leader as

(A)   "Country Club."   (B)   "Authoritarian."

(C)   "Impoverished."   (D)   "Totalitarian."

62.   The "Team Leadership" model in the second typology most resembles which style in the first typology?

(A)   "Democratic"   (B)   "Authoritarian"

(C)   "Laissez-faire"   (C)   "The New York Mets"

63.   A topic mentioned in the introductory paragraph not developed in the essay is

(A)   administrative effectiveness.

(B)   administrative traits.

(C)   whether good leaders are born or made.

(D)   how leadership affects morale.

64.   The passage implies that a better understanding of effective leadership would help

(A)   Eastern Europe.   (B)   the American economy.

(C)   Gorbachev.   (D)   President Bush.

65.   A deceitful "Machiavellian" leader that appears good and kind when he is, in fact, wicked and cruel would fall into which category discussed in this passage?

(A)   "Country Club"   (B)   "Laissez-faire"

(C)   "Authoritarian"   (D)   None of the above.

STOP

If time still remains, you may review work only in this section.

When the time allotted is up, you may go on to the next section.

Section 2 — Physical Sciences

TIME: 100 Minutes
QUESTIONS: 66-142

DIRECTIONS: Most of the questions in this section are arranged in groups, each corresponding to a descriptive passage. Based on the information given in a passage, choose the one best answer to each question in the group. Some questions are independent of a descriptive passage and of each other. Choose the one best answer to each of these questions. If you are not sure of an answer, eliminate those choices that you know are incorrect and choose an answer from among those remaining. Fill in the corresponding circle on the answer sheet to indicate your answer. You may refer to the periodic table at any time.

PASSAGE I (Questions 66-70)

A company is testing a new polymer material to be used as a covering on golf balls. An experiment is set up so that a machine strikes the golf ball at known angles to the ground, with varying initial speeds. Making the assumption that the golf ball moves only in a vertical plane, and knowing $V_y = V_0 \sin \theta_0 - at$ where a is acceleration, t is time and V is velocity, it is possible to obtain values capable of quantifying the performance of the products. Also, assume g (the acceleration due to gravity) = 9.75 m/s^2.

66.   At what time will the golf ball reach the highest point in its trajectory, assuming an angle of 37° and an initial speed of 50 m/s.? (sin 37° = 0.602/cos 37° = 0.799)

(A)   Not enough information.   (B)   290 sec

(C)   3.1 sec   (D)   4.1 sec

67.   Given that maximum height is reached after a time of 7.25 seconds and $y = y_0 + (V_0 \sin \theta_0)t + \frac{1}{2} at^2$, what is the maximum height reached if the ball is struck at 45° with an initial velocity of 100 m/sec?

(A)   Not enough information.   (B)   769 m

(C)   512 m   (D)   256 m

68.   If the golf ball is hit at an angle of 45° and an initial speed of 100 m/sec, how long will the ball be in the air?

(A)   14.5 sec   (B)   7.25 sec

(C)   10.25 sec   (D)   20.5 sec

69.   If the distance travelled in the air is defined as the range and equals $(V_0 \cos \theta_0)t$, how far does a golf ball travel if struck at 100 m/sec at an angle of 37°?

    (A)   Not enough information.   (B)   493 m

    (C)   79.9 m   (D)   982 m

70.   If the ball is in the air for 12.44 seconds and travels a distance of 311 meters, what was the angle at which the ball was hit if the initial velocity was 50 m/sec?

    (A)   30°   (B)   60°

    (C)   90°   (D)   80°

PASSAGE II (Questions 71-75)

    A new circuit company is investigating new multiple component circuits for use in leading edge equipment. They are examining a multiple capacitance circuit and a multiple resistor circuit shown below (Figures 1 and 2 respectively).

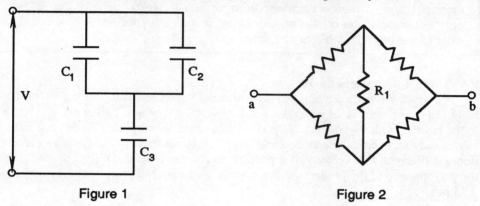

Figure 1   Figure 2

It is possible to vary a number of these components and observe interesting results. A systematic study of some of the more interesting ideas are yours to complete.

71.   Find the equivalent capacitance of the combination shown in Figure 1 knowing that $C_1 = 20$ μF, $C_2 = 10$ μF and $C_3 = 5.0$ μF.

    (A)   35 μF   (B)   4.3 μF

    (C)   2.9 μF   (D)   11.7 μF

72.   During testing, suppose that capacitor C_2 in Figure 1 is removed. What is the charge for capacitor C_3 assuming $V = 100V$, $C_1 = 20$ μF, and $C_3 = 5.0$ μF?

    (A)   Not enough information.   (B) 2.5×10^{-3} C

    (C) 4.0×10^{-4} C   (D) 5.0×10^{-4} C

73.   What is the potential difference on capacitor C_3 (Figure 1) assuming that $C_1 = 10$ μF, $C_2 = 5.0$ μF, $C_3 = 4.0$ μF, and the voltage is 100 V?

    (A)   80 V   (B)   73 V

    (C)   45 V   (D)   480 V

74. What is the measured current on resistor R_1 in the circuit in Figure 2 assuming every resistor is 10 Ω and there is an applied voltage of 50 V?

(A) 5.0 A   (B) 1.7 A

(C) 2.5 A   (D) 0 A

75. What is the equivalent resistance between points a and b of the circuit in Figure 2 if the resistor R_1 is removed? Assume each of the other resistors is 100 Ω.

(A) 400 Ω   (B) 1.00×10^{-2} Ω

(C) 100 Ω   (D) 50 Ω

PASSAGE III (Questions 76-80)

As a theoretical physicist in an optics company, your responsibilities include new designs in mirrors, lenses, and filters. You know that the focal point for a thin lens is

$$\frac{1}{s} + \frac{1}{s'} = (n-1)\left(\frac{1}{r_1} - \frac{1}{r_2}\right)$$

where s is the object's distance from the lens, s' is the image's distance from the lens, $r_1 + r_2$ are the curvature of radius of the surface of the lens, and n is the refractive index of the lens material. As a specialist in the area of lenses, you also know that

$$\frac{1}{s} + \frac{1}{s'} = \frac{1}{f}$$

where f is the focal length of the lens. The last thing you want to investigate is the magnification (m) which is given by $m = -(s'/s)$.

76. You have recently observed that spherical mirrors exhibit behavior similar to thin lenses. The equation

$$\frac{1}{s} + \frac{1}{s'} = \frac{2}{r},$$

where r = radius of curvature of the mirror, holds when investigating a number of reflective surfaces. What condition must hold true to lead to the result that $r/2 = s'$?

(A) The radius of curvature is greater than the object's distance.

(B) The mirror must be flat (r approaches 0).

(C) The object's distance is greater than the radius of curvature.

(D) The object's distance is equal to the radius of curvature.

77. What would the radius of curvature of a spherical mirror be if you wanted an object at 50 cm from the mirror to cast an image at half the distance to the mirror?

(A) .060 cm   (B) 33 cm

(C) 17 cm   (D) .12 cm

78. What does the negative sign in the magnification mean?

    (A) The image is smaller than the original object.

    (B) The image is on the same side of the lens as the object.

    (C) The image is on the opposite side of the lens as the object.

    (D) The image is inverted compared to the original object.

79. A double convex thin lens made of glass with a refractive index of 2.0 has both radii of curvature of magnitude 25 cm. Find the focal length of the lens.

    (A) 12.5 cm   (B) 25 cm

    (C) Focal length is undefined.   (D) .020 cm

80. If a thin lens like the one described in problem 78 has a focal length of 10 cm and the original object is located 30 cm from the lens, what is the lateral magnification?

    (A) .50   (B) - .25

    (C) - 4.0   (D) - .50

QUESTIONS 81-86 are NOT based on a descriptive passage.

---

81. According to the law of inertia, an object will travel in a straight line if there is no force which pushes or pulls the object into a curved path. What is this force?

    (A) Centrifugal force   (B) Kinetic friction

    (C) Moment of inertia   (D) Centripetal force

82. If a 25 kg object is raised 10 meters, what is the work being done?

    (A) 1250 J   (B) 2400 J

    (C) 2450 J   (D) 250 J

83. A man stands 3 meters from a small, intense source of light at the same level as his feet. If the man is 2 meters tall, how big will his shadow be on a wall 18 meters from the light source?

    (A) 5 m   (B) 10 m

    (C) 12 m   (D) 15 m

84. Which of the following elements would you expect to have the highest electro-negativity?

    (A) Carbon   (B) Zinc

    (C) Aluminum   (D) Silicon

85. All of the following assumptions would be in agreement with the existence of ideal gases, except one, which is:

    (A) the particles of such a gas are in random motion.

    (B) collisions between the gas particles are elastic.

    (C) there are no mutual interactions between the particles of such a gas.

    (D) the gas particles have zero volume.

86. Three moles of an ideal diatomic gas occupy a volume of 20 m^3 at 300 K. If the gas expands adiabatically to 40 m^3, then find the final pressure.

    (A) $1.62 \times 10^3 d/cm^2$

    (B) $1.82 \times 10^3 d/cm^2$

    (C) $1.42 \times 10^3 \, d/cm^2$

    (D) $3.74 \times 10^3 d/cm^2$

PASSAGE IV (Questions 87-91)

As the experimental physicist for the Circular Notion Pulley and Lever Company you have been asked to investigate some light weight, high impact plastic, solid disk pulleys. The experiment you have set up has a nylon rope, wound around the rim of the uniform disk, pivoted to rotate around a frictionless fixed axis, through the disk's center. The mass of the disk is 515 g, with a radius of 25 cm. Also, a carefully measured 10 N force is applied to the rope.

From previous experimentation and theory, you have established the following relationships: Angular velocity

$$\omega = \omega_0 + \alpha_0 t$$

where α_0 is the constant angular acceleration and the applied torque

$$\tau = Tr$$

where T is the tension and r is the radius of the disk. Furthermore, you've shown that for a solid disk, the moment of inertia

$$I = \frac{1}{2} mr^2.$$

87. For your experiment, calculate the moment of inertia.

    (A) $3.2 \times 10^{-2} \, kg \cdot m^2$

    (B) $1.6 \times 10^{-2} \, kg \cdot m^2$

    (C) $6.4 \times 10^{-2} \, kg \cdot m^2$

    (D) $1.6 \times 10^1 \, kg \cdot m^2$

88. From your experiment, what is the value for the applied torque?

    (A) $2.5 \, N \cdot m$

    (B) $2.5 \times 10^2 \, N \cdot m$

    (C) $4.0 \times 10^1 \, Nm^{-1}$

    (D) $4.0 \times 10^{-1} \, Nm^{-1}$

89. If, in your experiment, you measured the angular acceleration to be 1.56×10^2 rad/sec^2, what would the angular velocity of the disk be after 10.0 sec, assuming that the disk was initially at rest?

    (A) Not enough information.

    (B) 1.56×10^4 rad/sec

    (C) 1.56×10^3 rad/sec

    (D) 1.56×10^1 rad/sec

90. Knowing the angular momentum (L) is equal to the amount of inertia times the angular velocity, what would the angular momentum after 5 sec be if the disk had a radius of 50 cm, with the same mass and a $\omega = 3.91 \times 10^2$ rad/s at 5 sec?

    (A) 6.3 kg $\cdot$ m^2/sec

    (B) 5.0×10^1 kg $\cdot$ m^2/sec

    (C) 1.3×10^2 kg $\cdot$ m^2/sec

    (D) 2.5×10^1 kg $\cdot$ m^2/sec

91. If the power (P) is equal to the applied torque times the angular velocity, what would the power input be at 20 sec, given $\omega = 3.13 \times 10^3$ rad/sec?

    (A) 1.6×10^5 W

    (B) 3.1×10^4 W

    (C) 7.8×10^5 W

    (D) 7.8×10^3 W

PASSAGE V (Questions 92-96)

Mercury vapor lamps, used for street lights, produce light when excited with an electrical discharge corresponding to the atomic spectrum of mercury. We want to investigate other gases that could also exhibit these properties. The gas of interest to us behaves very similarly to hydrogen and obeys all hydrogen energy equations. We know that

$$E_{photon} = h\upsilon,$$

$$c = \upsilon\lambda$$

$$c = \text{speed of light} = 3.00 \times 10^8 \text{ m/sec}$$

and h = Planck's constant = 6.626×10^{-34} J sec.

92. What wavelength region corresponds to the visible region of the electromagnetic spectrum?

    (A)   200 - 400 nm

    (B)   4000 - 200 cm^{-1}

    (C)   4000 - 7000 Å

    (D)   50,000 - 25,000 cm^{-1}

93. If the frequency of the light is 6.17×10^{14} Hz, what is the wavelength of the light (in nm)?

    (A)   486 nm

    (B) 4.86×10^{-7} nm

    (C) 2.06×10^6 nm

    (D) 4.09×10^{-19} nm

94. If the frequency of the light is 6.17×10^{14} Hz, what is the energy of the photon?

    (A) $4.86 \times \quad 10^{-7}$ J

    (B) 4.09×10^{-19} J

    (C) 1.07×10^{-48} J

    (D) 1.85×10^{23} J

95. If we believe Einstein's equation that $E = mc^2$, then what would the mass of that photon be if the frequency is 6.17×10^{14} Hz?

    (A) 4.54×10^{-36} kg

    (B) 6.86×10^{-3} kg

    (C) 1.36×10^{-27} kg

    (D) 4.54×10^{-36} g

96.   Employing the Rydberg equation

$$\left(\frac{1}{\lambda} = 109,678 \text{ cm}^{-1} \left(\frac{1}{n_1^2} - \frac{1}{n_2^2}\right)\right),$$

what would the wavelength of a photon be (in nm) if we observed a change from $n_1 = 2$ to $n_2 = 3$?

(A) 1.52331×10^4 nm   (B)   252.487 nm

(C) 3.96059×10^4 nm   (D)   656.467 nm

PASSAGE VI (Questions 97-103)

We are investigating the pressure vs. temperature behavior of new materials for underwater applications. Below is a phase diagram obtained through measurements of the pressure vs. temperature.

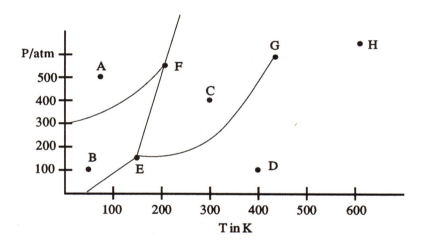

97.   Which point(s) is/are defined as the triple point?

(A)   Point F only.   (B)   Point E only.

(C)   Points E and F.   (D)   Point G only.

98.   From the plot, what is the critical temperature?

(A)   600 K   (B)   200 K

(C)   150 K   (D)   450 K

99.   If you evaluate the temperature from 100 K to 300 K at 200 atm what occurs?

(A)   The solid becomes a gas directly.

(B)   The solid becomes a different solid.

(C)   The solid melts and then turns into a gas.

(D)   The solid melts and becomes a liquid.

100.   If you hold the temperature at 300 K and go from 250 atm to 400 atm what do you observe?

(A)   The liquid becomes a gas.

(B)   The liquid becomes a solid.

(C)   No physical changes are observed.

(D)   The liquid freezes and then turns into a different solid.

101.   What is the name of the process going directly from point B to point D?

(A)   Fusion   (B)   Sublimation

(C)   Melting   (D)   Boiling

102.   How many phases exist at Point H?

(A)   1   (B)   2

(C)   3   (D)   4

103.   How many different phases exist at Point F?

(A)   1   (B)   2

(C) · 3   (D)   4

QUESTIONS 104-108 are NOT based on a descriptive passage.

---

104.   The acid concentration of solution A is roughly measured to be 0.95N ± 10%. When equal amounts of solution A and a standardized 1.00M KOH solution are mixed, the resulting solution will be

(A)   slightly basic.   (B)   slightly acidic.

(C)   strongly basic.   (D)   Cannot be determined

105.   Which of the salts below will produce an alkaline solution when dissolved in water?

(A) NH_4Cl (B) $NaCl$

(C) Na_2CO_3 (D) $NaNO_3$

106.   If 20 ml of 0.5N salt solution is diluted to 1 liter, what is the new concentration?

(A)   0.01N   (B)   0.001N

(C)   1N   (D)   10N

107. The work required to move 2 coulombs of charge through a potential difference of 5 volts is

    (A)   10 joules.   (B)   2 joules.

    (C)   25 joules.   (D)   50 joules.

108. The phenomenon which occurs when a wave spreads into the region behind an obstruction is known as

    (A)   refraction.   (B)   diffraction.

    (C)   dispersion.   (D)   superposition.

PASSAGE VII (Questions 109-114)

An atmospheric science company is interested in investigating the chemistry of nitric oxide (NO) with varying halogens. Several experiments were performed and the results were outlined as follows:

Experiment 1:

The reaction is $2NO_{(g)} + Cl_{2(g)} \longrightarrow 2NOCl_{(g)}$

Observations (at 25° C)	Initial Conc. (M) NO	Cl_2	Initial Rate of Formation of NOCl (Ms^{-1})
1	.10	.10	8.0
2	.10	.20	16
3	.20	.10	32

Experiment 2:

The reaction is $2NO_{(g)} + I_{2(g)} \longrightarrow 2NOI_{(g)}$

Observations (at 25° C)	Initial Conc. (M) NO	I_2	Initial Rate of Formation of NOCl (Ms^{-1})
1	.10	.10	1.5
2	.10	.20	1.5
3	.20	.10	6.0

Experiment 3:

The reaction is $2NO_{(g)} + At_{2(g)} \longrightarrow 2NOAt_{(g)}$ is shown to have a rate law of rate $= k[NO]$ at 25°C. The rate constant for the reaction was found to be 3.5×10^{-2} s^{-1} using an initial concentration of 0.50 M NO.

109. What is the rate law for the reaction carried out in Experiment 1?

    (A)   Rate = $k[NO]_2$ (B)   Rate = $k[NO]^2$

    (C)   Rate = $k[NO][Cl_2]$ (D)   Rate = $k[NO]^2[Cl_2]$

110. Knowing that the rate law for the reaction carried out in Experiment 2 is rate = $k[NO]^2$, calculate the rate constant at 25°C for this reaction.

    (A) $1.5 \, M \, s^{-1}$

    (B) $1.5 \times 10^1 \, M \, s^{-1}$

    (C) $3.8 \times 10^1 \, M \, s^{-1}$

    (D) $1.5 \times 10^2 \, M^{-1} s^{-1}$

111. What is the half-life of NO at 25° C in Experiment 3?

    (A) 20 sec

    (B) 1.2×10^{-3} sec

    (C) 14 sec

    (D) 7.1×10^{-2} sec

112. What if the rate law for Experiment 3 turned out to be rate = $k[NO]^2$? Find the 1st half-life for the reaction assuming the same value for the rate constant mentioned in the problem, except the units will be $M^{-1} s^{-1}$.

    (A) 2.8×10^2 sec

    (B) 1.7×10^{-2} sec

    (C) 4.0 sec

    (D) 57 sec

113. In Experiment 1, what does knowing the rate law tell us about the mechanism of the reaction?

    (A) Nothing about mechanism is determined.

    (B) Every detail about mechanism is capable of being determined knowing the rate law.

    (C) Only the species reacting in the rate determining step are determined.

    (D) Only the final step in a mechanism is determined.

114. If the rate law of the reaction in Experiment 2 is determined to be rate = $k[NO]^2[Cl]^2$, what is the overall order of the reaction?

    (A) 0

    (B) 1

    (C) 2

    (D) 4

PASSAGE VIII (Questions 115-118)

Potential new molecules for refrigeration, to replace chlorofluorocarbons (CFC), include a group of sulfur halide compounds. Furthermore, this group exhibits a wide variety of chemistry, including selective fluorination. A young company feels it can market chemicals like these and wants to learn more about their structure and possible ways to exploit its chemistry.

115. What is the correct Lewis dot structure for SF_4?

    (A)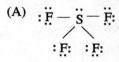

    (B)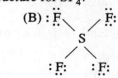

(C)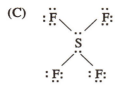

(D)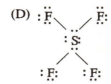

116. What structure would you predict for SCl_4 employing VSEPR theory?

(A) Square Planar

(B) Tetrahedral

(C) Trigonal Bipyramid

(D) See-Saw

117. In SF_6 what is the hybridization of the orbitals?

(A) sp^3

(B) d^2sp^3

(C) sp^3d

(D) sp^3d^2

118. What structure would you predict for SF_2 employing only VSEPR?

(A) Bent

(B) Trigonal Bipyramid

(C) Trigonal Planar

(D) Linear

PASSAGE IX (Questions 119-123)

As a research scientist for a plastics company you have been asked to conduct some experiments with vinyl chloride (C_2H_3Cl) which is used in the manufacture of polyvinyl chloride (PVC) plastics. The reaction you have been asked to study is the formation of the C_2H_3Cl from C_2H_2 (acetylene-molecular mass = 26.04 g/mole) and HCl (hydrochloric acid-molecular mass = 36.46 g/mole) (reaction shown below). Your research budget is limited, however, so you must use what is available. You have found 40.0 L of 6.0 M HCl and a tank with 250 L of acetylene gas.

$$C_2H_2 + HCl \longrightarrow C_2H_3Cl$$

119. How much of the acetylene gas do you have, by weight, assuming that acetylene behaves as an ideal gas, the room temperature is 25° C, and the atmospheric pressure is 0.970 atm?

(A) 3.08×10^3 g

(B) 9.92 g

(C) 2.58×10^2 g

(D) 2.63 g

120. How much HCl by weight do you possess?

(A) 8.75×10^3 g

(B) 2.19×10^2 g

(C) 6.58 g

(D) 1.52×10^{-1} g

121. If 41.0 g of C_2H_2 is reacted with 55.0 g of HCl what is the maximum amount of product that can be obtained?

(A) 96.0 g

(B) 94.4 g

(C) 98.1 g

(D) 55.0 g

122. If, for a certain reaction performed, the maximal amount of product possible was 66.6 g and you received 49.8 g, what is the percentage yield for this reaction?

    (A) .748%   (B) 25.2%

    (C) 74.8%   (D) .252%

123. Later you find a small tank of Cl_2 gas (chlorine-molecular mass = 70.9 g/mole). If 25.6 g of C_2H_2 are reacted with 10.1 g of Cl_2 gas, what is the maximal amount of product formed?

    (A) 61.5 g   (B) 17.75 g

    (C) 10.1 g   (D) 8.88 g

PASSAGE X (Questions 124-130)
    The study of oxygenated hydrocarbons has been of great interest for many years. As an analytical chemist, it is required that several different types of measurements be taken and the results combined to get a factual picture of what is really occurring. A problem of this sort has now fallen to you.

Experiment 1:
    A 5.00 g sample of an unknown compound, containing only carbon, hydrogen, and oxygen, is burned completely in oxygen yielding 9.55 g of CO_2 and 5.86 g of water.

Experiment 2:
    A 5.00 g sample of the same unknown compound is dissolved in 100 g of water. The measured freezing point is depressed by 2.02°C.

Experiment 3:
    Carbon (graphite) is reacted with $H_{2(g)}$ and $O_{2(g)}$ to yield the standard enthalpy of formation (ΔH_f) of the unknown compound. The measured $\Delta H°_f = $ - 278 kJ/mole and the standard entropy of formation ($\Delta S°_f$) = - 346 J/k mole.

Experiment 4:
    All of the reactants (carbon as graphite, hydrogen gas, and oxygen gas) are placed into a bomb calorimeter which has a heat capacity of 6.11×10^4 J/C. The initial temperature of the calorimeter is set at 25.00°C. After the reaction, the temperature is 29.55°C.

124. From Experiment 1, what is the empirical formula of the unknown compound?

    (A) C_2H_3O (B) C_2H_6O

    (C) $C_3H_5O_2$ (D) $C_4H_{12}O$

125. If the molecular weight of the unknown compound is 86.1 g/mole, and the empirical formula is C_2H_3O, what is the molecular formula?

    (A) $C_4H_6O_2$ (B) C_2H_3O

    (C) $C_5H_{10}O$ (D) $C_3H_2O_3$

126. From experiment 2, what is the calculated molecular weight of the unknown substance, knowing k_f for water = 1.86°C/molal?

(A) Not enough information. (B) 460 g/mole

(C) 4.60 g/mole (D) 46.0 g/mole

127. If the molarity of a different oxygenated hydrocarbon is 1.00×10^{-3} M, what is the osmotic pressure at 25°C?

(A) 2.48 atm (B) 2.05×10^{-3} atm

(C) .021 atm (D) .024 atm

128. From Experiment 3, what is the standard Gibb's Free Energy of Formation ($\Delta G°_F$) at 25°C?

(A) - 381 kJ/mole (B) 1.03×10^5 kJ/mole

(C) - 175 kJ/mole (D) 381 kJ/mole

129. For a different oxygenated hydrocarbon, the measured $\Delta H°_f$ is - 255 kJ/mole. What is the sum of the $\Delta H°_f$ for all the reactants?

(A) 255 kJ/mole (B) - 255 kJ/mole

(C) - 85.0 kJ/mole (D) 0 kJ/mole

130. From Experiment 4, what is the amount of heat given off in the reaction?

(A) 1.81×10^3 kJ (B) 1.70×10^4 kJ

(C) 2.78×10^2 kJ (D) 1.34×10^1 kJ

PASSAGE XI (Questions 131-138)
As an electro-analytical chemist, you have conducted the following experiments:

Experiment 1:
In an electrolytic cell, you placed a solution of $CuSO_4$, a cathode, and an anode. A current of 5.0 A was passed through the solution for 6.0 hours.

Experiment 2:
A Ni/Cu galvanic cell is constructed by placing a 1 M $NiSO_4$ in one side of a 2 chambered cell, with a 1 M $CuSO_4$ solution in the other. A copper electrode is placed in the chamber with the Cu^{2+} solution, and a nickel electrode is placed in the side with the Ni^{2+} solution. Cell potentials are measured using a potentiometer.

Experiment 3:
A Sn/Ni galvanic cell is constructed, as outlined in Experiment 2. However, the Ni^{2+} and Sn^{2+} solutions are under varying concentration conditions. Furthermore, at set concentrations, the dependence of the cell potential vs. temperature is investigated. The following relationship is established:

$$\varepsilon = \varepsilon° - \frac{2.303\,RT}{nF} \log Q$$

where F = Faraday's constant (96,500 C/mole of e^-) and Q is the reaction quotient.

131. In an electrolytic cell, which way do electrons flow?

    (A) From the cathode to the anode

    (B) Through the salt bridge

    (C) Through the conducting solution

    (D) From the anode to the cathode

132. How many grams of copper will be deposited from the copper sulfate solution in Experiment 1?

    (A) 79 g

    (B) 9.9×10^{-3} g

    (C) 35 g

    (D) 3.5×10^6 g

133. What are the signs of the electrodes in galvanic cells?

    (A) Cathode is (-), anode is (+)

    (B) Cathode is (+), anode is unchanged

    (C) Anode is (+), cathode is unchanged

    (D) Cathode is (+), anode is (-)

134. What is the measured cell potential in the galvanic cell in Experiment 2, knowing that the standard reduction potential of Cu^{2+} is 0.34 V and Ni^{2+} is - 0.25 V?

    (A) 0.34 V

    (B) 0.59 V

    (C) 0.09 V

    (D) - 0.09 V

135. In Experiment 3, the standard cell potential $\varepsilon°_{cell}$ was found to be + 0.11 V when 1.0 M Sn^{2+} and 1.0M Ni^{2+} solutions were used. What is the standard free energy change ($\Delta G°$) for the reaction?

    (A) - 1.1×10^1 kJ

    (B) - 4.2×10^1 kJ

    (C) - 2.1×10^1 kJ

    (D) 1.1×10^1 kJ

136. For the reaction in the galvanic cell in Experiment 3, what would the reaction quotient expression look like?

    (A) $[Sn^{2+}]/[Ni^{2+}]$

    (B) $[Ni^{2+}][Sn_{(s)}]/[Sn^{2+}][Ni_{(s)}]$

    (C) $[Sn_{(s)}]/[Ni_{(s)}]$

    (D) $[Ni^{2+}]/[Sn^{2+}]$

137. Using the experimentally confirmed Nernst equation in Experiment 3 and the value for ε°_{cell} from question 135, calculate the cell potential if you started with a 0.10M Sn^{2+} solution and a 0.50M Ni^{2+} solution at 25° C.

(A)   0.09 V

(B)   0.07 V

(C)   0.11 V

(D)   0.13 V

138. If Pb^{2+} is substituted for Sn^{2+} in Experiment 3, the standard cell potential for the new Pb/Ni galvanic cell is measured to be +0.12 V with a $\Delta G° = -2.3 \times 10^1$ kJ/mole. What is the equilibrium constant for the spontaneous reaction shown below at 25°C?

$$Ni°_{(s)} + Pb^{2+} \rightleftharpoons Ni^{2+} + Pb°_{(s)}$$

(A)   0.0

(B) 1.1×10^4

(C)   1.0

(D) 9.3×10^{-5}

QUESTIONS 139-142 are NOT based on a descriptive passage.

---

139. Which of the following has an effective dipole moment?

(A)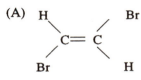

(B) CCl_4

(C)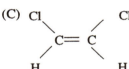

(D) CO_2

QUESTIONS 140-142 refer to the statement below.

A string of 12 freight cars weighs 200 tons and has a coefficient of rolling friction of 0.005. Assume the rail bed is completely level.

140. How fast can an engine of 400 hp pull the string of cars along?

(A)   25 mi/hr

(B)   40 mi/hr

(C)   50 mi/hr

(D)   75 mi/hr

141. How much horsepower is needed to move the train at a rate of 45 mi/hr?

(A)   240 hp

(B)   270 hp

(C)   320 hp

(D)   375 hp

142. Using the information obtained in Question 141, calculate the force exerted by the engine.

    (A)   100 lbs   (B)   50 lbs

    (C)   2,000 lbs   (D)   75 lbs

STOP

If time still remains, you may review work only in this section.

When the time allotted is up, you may go on to the next section.

Section 3 — Writing Sample

TIME: 60 minutes
2 essays, separately timed
30 minutes each

DIRECTIONS: This section tests your writing skills by asking you to write two essays. You will have 30 minutes to write each one.

During the first 30 minutes, work only on the first essay. If you finish it in less than 30 minutes, you may review what you have written, but do not begin the second essay. During the second 30 minutes, work only on the second essay. If you finish it in less than 30 minutes, you may review what you have written for that essay only. Do not go back to the first essay.

Read each assigned topic carefully. Make sure your essays respond to the topics as they are assigned.

Make sure your essays are written in complete sentences and paragraphs, and are as clear as you can make them. Make any corrections or additions between the lines of your essays. Do not write in the margins.

On the day of the test, you are given three pages to write each essay. You are not required to use all of the space provided, but do not skip lines so you will not waste space. Illegible essays cannot be scored.

Part 1

Consider this statement adapted from William James's "The Moral Philosopher and the Moral Life":

> One could not accept a happiness shared with millions if the condition of that happiness were the suffering of one lonely soul.

Write a comprehensive essay in which you accomplish the following objectives. (1) Explain what you think the statement above means. (2) Describe a specific situation in which people *do* accept happiness based on the suffering of others. (3) Discuss the criteria under which one could find happiness without causing the suffering of others.

STOP

If time still remains, you may review work only in this section.

When the time allotted is up, you may go on to the next section.

Part 2

Consider this statement from Jane Howard's *Families* (1978):

Good families are much to all their members, but everything to none.

Write a comprehensive essay in which you accomplish the following objectives: (1) Explain what you think the statement above means. (2) Describe a specific situation in which the good family may be everything to its members. (3) Discuss the criteria implied in the statement in order to have a "good" family, and suggest how groups other than biological or foster families may be considered families.

STOP

If time still remains, you may review work only in this section.

When the time allotted is up, you may go on to the next section.

Section 4 — Biological Sciences

TIME: 100 Minutes
QUESTIONS: 143-219

DIRECTIONS: Most of the questions in this section are arranged in groups, each corresponding to a descriptive passage. Based on the information given in a passage, choose the one best answer to each question in the group. Some questions are independent of a descriptive passage and of each other. Choose the one best answer to each of these questions. If you are not sure of an answer, eliminate those choices that you know are incorrect and choose an answer from among those remaining. Fill in the corresponding circle on the answer sheet to indicate your answer. You may refer to the periodic table at any time.

PASSAGE I (Questions 143-147)

It is sometimes said that the movement of molecules across cell membranes occurring in response to a concentration gradient, and termed "passive transport," requires no metabolic energy. The term "passive transport" is misleading, as no directional movement, across a cell membrane, can occur without the expenditure of energy by the molecules involved. If one assumes the structure of the membrane includes a lipid layer, then passage of molecules from aqueous to lipid phase, and lipid to aqueous phase, presents barriers to the molecules which can be overcome only if the molecules have appropriate energy of activation. If a molecule entering a cell has a high lipid solubility, neither its energy, nor its passage through the membrane presents an obstacle. However, entry of the molecule from the membrane into the aqueous cytoplasm does present an obstacle because of the cohesive bonds it has formed with the lipid molecules of the membrane that must be broken before it can leave the membrane. If, on the other hand, a molecule entering the cell membrane is highly soluble in water, its strong hydrogen bonds with the water, in which it is dissolved outside of the cell, must be broken before the molecule can enter the lipoid membrane. Its movement through the lipoid membrane also presents an obstacle. However, such a molecule readily passes from the membrane into the aqueous cytoplasm inside the cell.

Permeant	ΔH (kcal/mole)	Number of hydrogen bonds
Glycerol	24	6
Ethylene glycol	18.5	4
Diethylene glycol	18.5	4
Triethylene glycol	20.5	4
1,2, - Propandiol	19.5	4
1,3, -Propandiol	19	4

Propanol	4.5	2
Thiourea	13.5	4
Urea	6	5

143. Energy is required to transport molecules across cell membranes

    (A) only in active transport.

    (B) in all instances.

    (C) only for non-polar molecules.

    (D) only when moving them against a concentration gradient.

144. When a molecule of high lipoidal solubility is passing through a cell membrane, what is the most energy demanding portion of this journey?

    (A) Entering the membrane from outside the cell

    (B) Leaving the cell membrane, entering the cytoplasm

    (C) Passing through the cell membrane

    (D) Both (B) and (C).

145. According to the above chart, why might the transport of propanol require less energy than either of the propandiols?

    (A) It lacks an -OH group.

    (B) It is nonpolar.

    (C) It has three carbons.

    (D) It has few hydrogen bonds to break with the water.

146. Which of the following molecules would have the least problem passing through the lipoidal layer?

    (A) Water   (B) Methanol

    (C) Decanol   (D) Propanol

147. One can see from the table that thiourea has only one less hydrogen bond than urea to break, yet it requires 7.5 kcal/mole more energy to transport. A possible explanation might be that

    (A) although urea has more hydrogen bonds to break, differences in polarity between it and thiourea allow it to pass more readily through the membrane.

    (B) thiourea is a larger molecule, hence it requires more energy to transport a larger mass.

    (C) thiourea forms a stronger hydrogen bond with water.

    (D) there is no reasonable explanation for this.

PASSAGE II (Questions 148-153)

The diagram below shows a Fenn-Winterstein Respirometer.

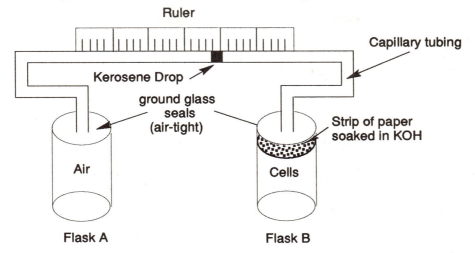

Living cells are sealed in flask B, along with a strip of paper soaked in potassium hydroxide. As the cells consume oxygen, the kerosene drop moves. If the volume of the capillary tube is known, the amount of oxygen consumed can be calculated.

148. What is the purpose of the potassium hydroxide (KOH) in flask B?

    (A) To absorb carbon dioxide produced

    (B) To keep the pH high

    (C) To keep the pH low

    (D) To act as a nutrient for the cells

149. What is the purpose of flask A, filled with air and sealed to the system?

    (A) It is there in case one wishes to measure two cell cultures at once.

    (B) It is there to catch the kerosene drop when it reaches the end of the tubing.

    (C) It is there to cancel the effects of temperature change.

    (D) Its purpose is not readily apparent.

150. Which of the following is not true?

    (A) The above apparatus is not affected by temperature change.

    (B) The above apparatus is not affected by barometric change.

    (C) As oxygen is consumed, the bubble moves away from the cells.

    (D) The rate the bubble moves, with regard to oxygen consumption, varies with the square of the radius of the tubing.

151. Which type of cells would cause the largest shift of the bubble, in the smallest amount of time?

    (A)   Rapidly growing yeast cells

    (B)   Striated muscle tissue from a rabbit

    (C)   Unfertilized amphiox eggs

    (D)   Murine neural tissue

152. The above device can probably be modified for measuring oxygen production during photosynthesis by using cells containing chloroplasts and

    (A)   working in the dark.

    (B)   substituting an oxygen absorbing species for the KOH.

    (C)   using a mercury drop instead of kerosene.

    (D)   it cannot be modified for such a purpose.

153. If the bubble moves 4.6 mm, and the tubing has a uniform diameter of 0.20 mm, how many liters of oxygen are consumed?

    (A) $[(0.02/2)^{2\pi} (0.46)] / 1000$ (B) $[0.2^2/2^{\pi} (4.6)] / 1000$

    (C) $[0.02^{2\pi} \cdot 4.6] / 1000$ (D) $[0.2^{2\pi} \cdot 4.6] \cdot 1000$

PASSAGE III (Questions 154-158)

The spirochetes comprise a small group of non-photosynthetic and non-chemo-synthetic bacteria with a very distinctive structure. The helical cells are extremely long relative to their width. They are capable of movement in a liquid medium by bending back and forth in broad coils, and at all times retaining their fine helical structure. Reproduction is always by transverse binary fission. No resting stages are known. Some of the smaller spirochetes are so thin that they are close to the limits of resolution with the light microscope. Axial fibrils are attached to the cells' poles and wrapped around the coiled, cylindrical cell. Both the axial fibrils and the cells are surrounded by a three-layered membrane called the outer sheath. The outer sheath and axial fibrils are usually not visible by light microscopy. From two to more than one hundred axial fibrils are present per cell, depending upon the type of spirochete. The ultra-structure and chemical composition of the axial fibrils are similar to those of bacterial flagella. Indeed, in preserved specimens, the axial filament can become partially detached from the body of the cell and fray out into a multi-strained structure, with the individual fibrils looking very much like eubacterial flagella. The appearance of such artifacts led early researchers to believe that some spirochetes have flagella. This is now known to be false. The free-living spirochetes are aquatic organisms, commonly found in muddy, polluted waters with low dissolved oxygen content. The largest known spirochetes live in the digestive tracts of clams and other mollusks. There is no indication that they are harmful to the mollusks. Many, but not all, of the smaller spirochetes are pathogenic and are responsible for diseases in humans and other animals.

GENERA OF SPIROCHETES AND THEIR CHARACTERISTICS

Genus	Dimensions (μm)	General Characteristics	Number of Axial Fibrils	Habitat	Diseases
Cristispira	30 - 150 × 0.3 - 0.5	3-10 complete coils	> 100	G.I. tract of mollusks	None
Spirochaeta	5 - 500 × 0.2 - 0.75	Anaerobic or faculative anaerobic	2-40	Aquatic, free living	None
Treponema	5 - 15 × 0.1 - 0.5	Anaerobic	unknown	Parasitic in in animals	Syphillis Yaws
Borrelia	3 - 15 × 0.2 - 0.5	Anaerobic	unknown	Parasitic in mammals and anthropods	Releasing fever
Leptospira	6 - 20 × 0.1	Aerobic	2	Free living or parasitic	Lepto- spirosis

154. What can be inferred from the above passage about the internal structure of spirochetes?

 (A) They resemble eukaryotic flagella.

 (B) Their nucleus and mitochondria are spiral.

 (C) Little was known until the advent of electron microscopy.

 (D) It must be studied under dark-field microscopy.

155. What is true of all spirochetes?

 (A) They are heterotrophs.

 (B) They cause disease in animals.

 (C) They contain axial filaments.

 (D) Both (A) and (C).

156. Which statement is false about spirochetes?

 (A) They have 2 to > 100 axial fibrils.

 (B) They can form spores and other vegetative stages.

 (C) They do not possess flagella.

 (D) Free-living spirochetes prefer brackish waters.

157. Where might one obtain a culture of *Cristispira?*

 (A) In muddy water

 (B) In salt water

 (C) In the blood of a syphilis patient

 (D) In the digestive tract of a healthy clam

158. Which genus of spirochete might one be able to see without the benefit of an oil-immersion lens?

    (A) *Cristispira*   (B) *Spirochaeta*

    (C) *Triponema*   (D) *Leptospira*

QUESTIONS 159-164 are NOT based on a descriptive passage.

---

159. The genetic code is

    (A) commaless.   (B) degenerate.

    (C) non-overlapping.   (D) All of the above.

160. Which of the following is not part of a prophase chromosome?

    (A) Centromere   (B) Centrosome

    (C) Chromatid   (D) DNA

161. Albinism is a recessive trait. In a certain community of 200 people, 18 persons are albinos. How many people are normal homozygotes?

    (A) 182   (B) 164

    (C) 100   (D) 98

162. The most recent theories of the origin of life include all of the following elements in the primitive atmosphere except

    (A) free oxygen.   (B) hydrogen.

    (C) methane.   (D) ammonia.

163. What is the product of the competing reaction of ether production through dehydration by nucleophilic substitution?

    (A) Alkane   (B) Alkene

    (C) Alkyne   (D) Alcohol

164. Which of the following reacts most rapidly with HI by the S_N1 mechanism?

    (A) CH_3CH_2OH (B) $CH_3CHOHCH_3$

    (C) $(CH_3)_3COH$ (D) $CH_3CH_2C(CH_3)_2CH_2OH$

PASSAGE IV (Questions 165-171)

In the pedigree shown below, two autosomal, recessive traits on separate chromosomes are shown. If the top half of a figure is shaded, the individual shows trait a (possibilities: AA, Aa, aa). If the bottom half of a figure is shaded, the individual shows trait b (possibilities: BB, Bb, bb). Figures totally shaded represent individuals that show both traits a and b. As usual, circles represent females, squares represent males, capital letters denote dominant genes, lower case letters denote recessive genes.

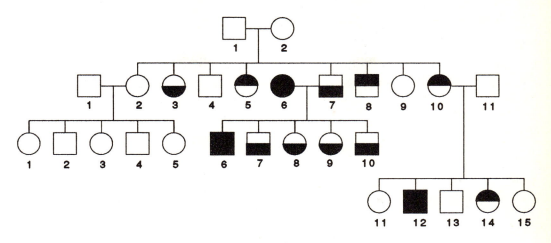

165. What is the genotype of C12?

    (A) aabb

    (B) AaBb

    (C) AABB

    (D) It cannot be determined.

166. What is the genotype of A1?

    (A) aabb

    (B) AaBb

    (C) AABB

    (D) It cannot be determined.

167. What is the genotype of B2?

    (A) aabb

    (B) AaBb

    (C) AABB

    (D) It cannot be determined.

168. What is the genotype of B11?

    (A) aabb

    (B) AaBb

    (C) AABB

    (D) It cannot be determined.

169. What is the genotype of B7?

    (A) Aabb

    (B) AAbb

    (C) AaBb

    (D) AABB

170. What is the genotype of B10?

    (A) AaBb

    (B) aabb

    (C) aaBb

    (D) Aabb

171. What are the chances of C13 being Aabb?

    (A) 50%

    (B) 25%

    (C) 12.5%

    (D) 0%

PASSAGE V (Questions 172-181)

In the pedigree below, trait C/c is autosomal, and trait D is on a sex-chromosome with D dominant over d, the normal condition. A figure with the upper half shaded displays trait C/c and a figure with the lower half shaded displays trait D. A figure with both top and bottom shaded displays both traits. Assume normal mammalian sex determination. As usual, circles are females, squares are males, capital letters denote dominant genes, lower case represent recessive.

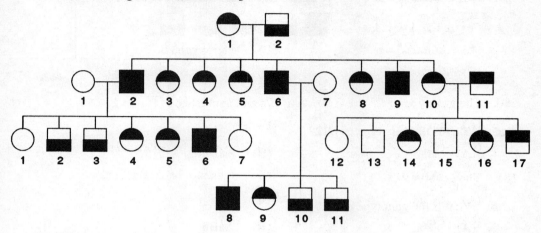

172. Trait C/c appears to be

    (A) recessive.   (B) dominant.

    (C) non-dominant.   (D) It cannot be determined.

173. With regard to trait C/c, individual B2 must be

    (A) Cc.   (B) cc.

    (C) CC.   (D) It cannot be determined.

174. With respect to C/c, individual A2 must be

    (A) Cc.   (B) cc.

    (C) CC.   (D) It cannot be determined.

175. With respect to C/c, individual A1 must be

    (A) Cc.   (B) cc.

    (C) CC.   (D) It cannot be determined.

176. With respect to C/c, individual C11 must be

    (A) Cc.   (B) cc.

    (C) CC.   (D) It cannot be determined.

177. Trait D appears to be located on

    (A) the Y chromosome.

    (B) the X chromosome.

(C)   Both the X and Y chromosome.

(D)   It cannot be determined.

178. For trait D, individual A2 must be

(A)   homozygous.   (B)   heterozygous.

(C)   hemizygous.   (D)   It cannot be determined.

179. For trait D, individual C11 must be

(A)   homozygous.   (B)   heterozygous.

(C)   hemizygous.   (D)   It cannot be determined.

180. The genotype of C3 with respect to C/c and D must be

(A)   ccDd.   (B)   ccdd.

(C)   ccD.   (D)   It cannot be determined.

181. The genotype of B11 must be

(A)   CCdd.   (B)   CcDd.

(C)   Ccd.   (D)   CcD.

PASSAGE VI (Questions 182-187)

Cyclohexene is reacted with ozone, and the product of this reaction is reacted with zinc and water to produce compound X. Cyclohexene is also reacted with $KMnO_4$ to produce compound Y.

For QUESTIONS 182 and 183, use the following choices:

(A) $OHC(CH_2)_4CHO$

(B) $HOOC(CH_2)_4COOH$

(C) $CH_3(CH_2)_4CH_3$

(D)

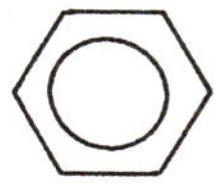

182. What is the formula for compound X?

183. What is the formula for compound Y?

184. 2 ml of a 5% $AgNO_3$ solution is mixed with a drop of a 10% NaOH solution and a few drops of a 2% NH_4OH solution. If this is mixed with compound X, what will most likely happen?

(A) NH_3 gas will be evolved.

(B)   The Ag will precipitate.

(C)   No reaction will occur.

(D)   Both (A) and (B) will occur.

185. Which compound will be soluble in a basic solution?

    (A) Compound X   (B) Compound Y

    (C) Both (A) and (B).   (D) Neither (A) nor (B).

186. If compound X were reacted with $KMnO_4$, what product will be formed?

    (A) Product Y   (B) There will be no further reaction.

    (C) $CH_3(CH_2)_4CH_3$ (D)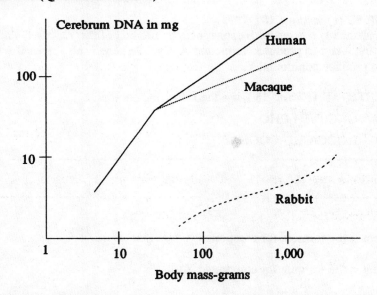

187. Compound Y is further reacted with $SOCl_2$ and then with NH_3. What can be expected of this new product?

    (A) It will be soluble in an organic solvent such as hexane.

    (B) It will be soluble in a basic solution.

    (C) It will be soluble in an acidic solution.

    (D) It will be insoluble in most solvents.

PASSAGE VII (Questions 188-142)

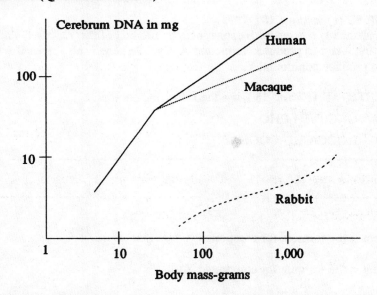

188. In the graph above, body mass is plotted against mg of DNA in cerebrum. What information might mg of DNA contain that grams of cerebrum does not?

    (A) The number of cells present in the cerebrum

    (B) The mitotic rate of neurons in the cerebrum

    (C) The amount of memory in the cerebrum

    (D) The amount of protein synthesized by the cerebrum.

189. Where might the curve for a cat fit on this graph?

    (A) Above the rabbit

    (B) Below the rabbit

    (C) Above the macaque

    (D) There is not enough data to determine this.

190. What is the maximum body weight where humans and macaques have the same ratio of cerebrum DNA to body weight?

    (A) 10 grams   (B) 15 grams

    (C) 35 grams   (D) 50 grams

191. In obtaining this data, what is the most important factor listed below to limit experimental error?

    (A) The amount of time elapsed between the killing of the animals and the extraction and measurement of their DNA

    (B) The diet of the animals before they were killed

    (C) The temperature at which the animals were kept while alive

    (D) The amount of RNA present in the cells

192. Where did the data on this graph come from for humans in the 10 gram region?

    (A) The curve is extrapolated from heavier specimens.

    (B) Although a person cannot weigh 10 grams, a cerebrum can.

    (C) The graph contains fetal data.

    (D) The line for humans does not go down as small as 10 grams.

Questions 193-197 are NOT based on a descriptive passage.

193. Which of the following is an example of a fat?

(A)

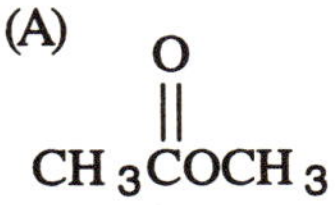

$$CH_3COCH_3$$
(with O double bonded to central C)

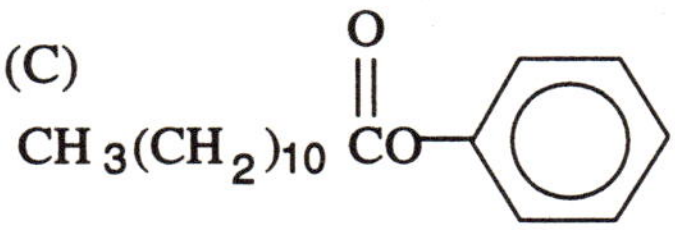

(B)

$$CH_2-O-C-CH_3$$
$$|\quad\quad CH-O-C-CH_3$$
$$|\quad\quad CH_2-O-C-CH_3$$
(each C=O)

(C)

$$CH_3(CH_2)_{10}CO-\bigcirc$$
(with C=O)

(D)

$$\bigcirc-CONH-\bigcirc$$
(with C=O)

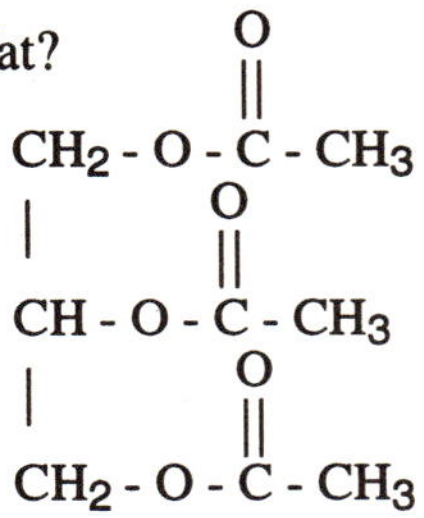

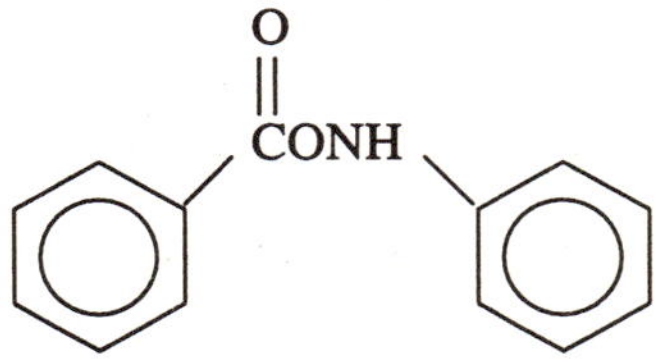

194. Which of the following will form a racemic mixture if combined with an equal amount of its enantiomer?

(A)

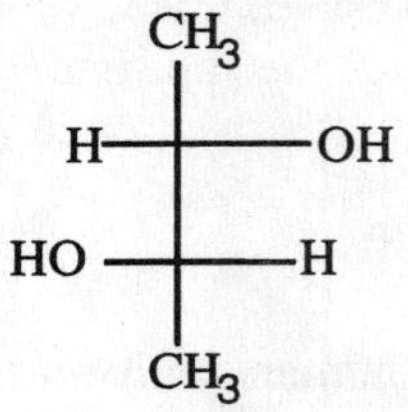

$$CH_3$$
H—————OH
HO —————H
$$CH_3$$

(B)

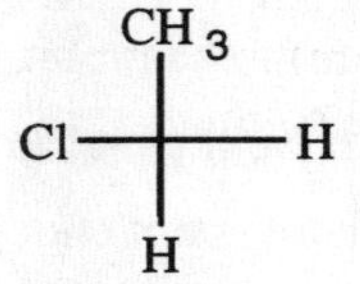

$$CH_3$$
Cl—————H
H

(C)

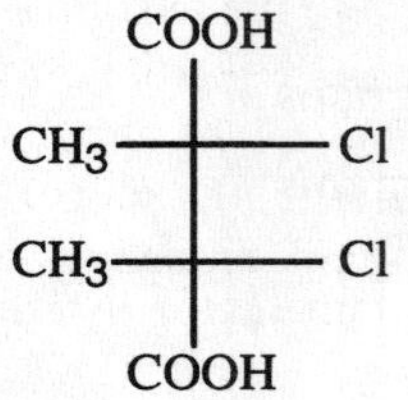

COOH
$$CH_3$$—————Cl
$$CH_3$$—————Cl
COOH

(D)

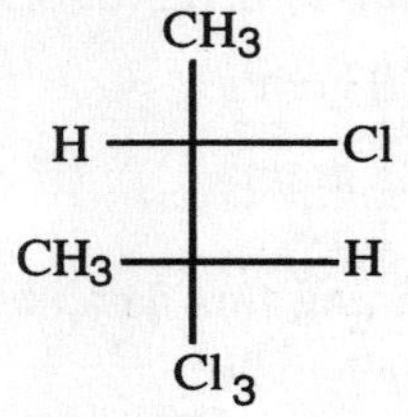

$$CH_3$$
H —————Cl
$$CH_3$$—————H
$$Cl_3$$

195. An organism that makes its own food from carbon dioxide and water is

(A) a green mold.   (B) a green plant.

(C) a mushroom.   (D) yeast.

196. Which of the following items is not part of the human ear?

(A) Tectorial membrane   (B) Cochlea

(C) Hyoid   (D) Oval window

197. The fovea consists of

(A) equal amounts of rods and cones.

(B) more rods than cones.

(C) more cones than rods.

(D) no rods.

PASSAGE VIII (Questions 198-204)
Experiment 1:

75 grams of fresh potatoes and 500 ml of water were homogenized in a blender. Three drops of this "potato juice" were each added to: plain water, a dextrose solution, a sodium chloride solution, and a solution of pyrocathechol. After five minutes, all of the solutions remained colorless except for the pyrocathechol, which had turned yellow.

Experiment 2:

Three solutions of pyrocathechol, of the same concentration, were kept either on ice (0°), room temperature (25°), or in boiling water (100°). Keeping them at these temperatures, and adding three drops of the above "potato juice" to each solution, gave the following results within five minutes: solution on ice – faint yellow; solution at room temperature – yellow; solution in boiling water – still colorless.

Experiment 3:

Solutions of equal concentrations of pyrocathechol were adjusted to have pH values of 4, 7, or 10. When three drops of the above "potato juice" were added (at room temperature) to each solution, within five minutes the solution at pH 4 was dark yellow, the solution at pH 7 was faint yellow, and the solution at pH 10 was still colorless.

Experiment 4:

Four test tubes were set up containing a pyrocathechol solution at the same concentration. Twenty drops of phenylthiourea were added to the first tube, ten drops were added to the second tube, and only one drop was added to the third tube. No phenylthiourea was added to the fourth tube. Three drops of the above "potato juice" were added to each of the above tubes. Within five minutes, the fourth tube had turned yellow, the third tube was slightly yellow, the second tube was very slightly yellow, and the first tube remained colorless.

198. The material in the potato juice that causes the pyrocathechol solutions to turn yellow is most likely a(n)

   (A) enzyme.   (B) protein.

   (C) catalyst.   (D) All of the above.

199. The optimal pH for the substance in potato juice is

   (A) 7.   (B) 4.

   (C) 3.   (D) somewhere in the acidic range.

200. If the potato juice was boiled for ten minutes, cooled to room temperature, and then added to a pyrocathechol solution, within five minutes the solution would

   (A) remain colorless.   (B) turn pale yellow.

   (C) turn yellow.   (D) turn a color other than yellow.

201. When phenylthiourea was added to the pyrocathechol solution, it acted as a(n)

   (A) substrate.   (B) enzyme.

   (C) inhibitor.   (D) All of the above.

202. A pyrocathechol solution containing phenylthiourea and potato juice can be made to turn yellow by

   (A) boiling.   (B) adding more phenylthiourea.

   (C) adding more pyrocathechol. (D) adding more potato juice.

203. Which statement is true?

   (A) The substance in the potato juice causes the pyrocathechol to turn yellow.

   (B) The substance in the potato juice aids the pyrocathechol in turning yellow.

     (C)   The substance in the potato juice reacts with the pyrocathechol to produce a yellow color.

     (D)   More information needs to be given.

204.   If a solution of pyrocathechol was left alone for a very long time, without the addition of potato juice, it would most likely

     (A)   remain colorless.

     (B)   turn yellow.

     (C)   turn a color other than yellow.

     (D)   More information needs to be given.

PASSAGE IX (Questions 205-209)

    Mice, eleven weeks of age, were given 800 rads of X-irradiation. Half of the mice were then inoculated with 2×10^6 fetal liver cells from a $12\frac{1}{2}$ to $13\frac{1}{2}$ day gestation mouse embryo. This was given within a few hours after irradiation. The graph below shows the number of B cells found in the spleen, at various times, after irradiation. The remaining mice received no further treatment after irradiation. The number of B cells found in their spleen is also shown on the graph.

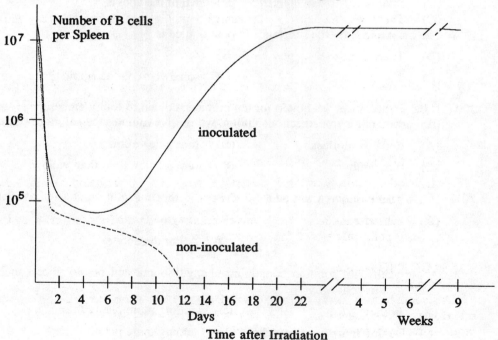

205.   How long do the non-inoculated mice seem to live after irradiation?

     (A)   No more than 12 days

     (B)   12 days

     (C)   At least 12 days

     (D)   It cannot be determined from this graph.

206. In the treated group, how long does it take for the B cells in the spleen to reach half of their pre-irradiated level?

(A)   10 days   (B)   16 days

(C)   18 days   (D)   22 days

207. How long do the inoculated mice seem to live after irradiation?

(A)   At least 9 weeks

(B)   9 weeks

(C)   No more than 9 weeks

(D)   It cannot be determined from this graph.

208. An analysis of the fetal liver cells, injected into the mice, shows that they contain no B cells. What is the most probable explanation for the observed regeneration of B cells?

(A)   The fetal liver cells repair the radiation damage.

(B)   The fetal liver cells contain a stem cell precursor that matures into a B cell.

(C)   There was an error in the analysis of the fetal liver cells; they must contain B cells.

(D)   There is no explanation for this.

209. B cells are seen to grow much more rapidly in normally developing mice than in the same mice after irradiation. The most probable explanation for this is

(A)   the mice are starting a B cell population at a later age than they normally would.

(B)   the radiation slowed cell growth.

(C)   other, more vital, life preserving functions are probably put in order before time is spent with B cell development.

(D)   the radiation has actually increased the growth rate of other cells, so the B cells only appear to be growing slower.

PASSAGE X (Questions 210-215)
Experiment 1:

A student heats 3-methyl-2-butanol in HBr. The reaction generates a single product. However, NMR spectroscopy reveals that the product was not the expected 2-bromo-3-methylbutane, but instead 2-bromo-2-methylbutane.

Experiment 2:

The student notes that if 2-methyl-3-pentanol is treated with concentrated H_2SO_4, at 107°C, the major product is 2-methyl-2-pentene. He also notes that small amounts of 2-methyl-pentene are also formed, as are trace amounts of 4-methyl-2-pentene.

Experiment 3:

The student reacts (2R, 3R) 3-methyl-3-d-2-butanol with hot HRr. The major product is a racemic mixture of 2-bromo-2-methyl-3-deuteriobutane. A small amount of (3R) 2-bromo-3-methyl-3-deuteriobutane is also produced.

210. The production of 2-bromo-2-methylbutane from 3-methyl-2-butanol in hot HBr is an example of what kind of reaction?

    (A) Sn2

    (B) E_2

    (C) Carbocation rearrangement

    (D) Carbanion rearrangement

211. In the above described reaction, why is 2-bromo-2-methylbutane the major product?

    (A) Tertiary carbanions are more stable than secondary carbanions.

    (B) Secondary carbocations are more stable than primary carbocations.

    (C) Secondary carbocations are less stable than tertiary carbocations.

    (D) Via an S_n2 reaction, Br attacks the 3-carbon, displacing a hydrogen. The hydroxyl group is simultaneously protonated with the net effect of a loss of one molecule of H_2O per molecule of reactant.

212. What did the experiment with 3-methyl-3-D-2-Butanol reveal?

    (A) The reaction is an S_n2 reaction.

    (B) There is a carbocation intermediate.

    (C) The hydrogen on the 3-carbon is the migration species.

    (D) Both (B) and (C) are correct.

213. Assuming the reaction in Experiment 2 has a carbocation intermediate, which of the below statements is supported by the experiment's results?

    (A) Tertiary carbocations are more stable than secondary carbocations.

    (B) Tertiary carbocations are more stable than primary carbocations.

    (C) The reaction proceeds via an E_2 mechanism.

    (D) Both (A) and (C) are correct.

214. In Experiment 2, if the student had used 2-methyl-2-pentanol instead of 2-methyl-3-pentanol, what would be the distribution of products?

    (A) The major product would be 2-methyl-1-pentene with a small amount of 2-methyl-2-pentene.

    (B) The major product would be 4-methyl-2-pentene plus a small amount of 2-methyl-2-pentene.

    (C) There would be no reaction. Tertiary alcohols are unreactive under these conditions.

    (D) The distribution of products would be very similar.

215. What products would you expect in the following reaction?

$$CH_3CH_2CH_2CHOHCH_3 \xrightarrow{\text{HBr}} \text{PRODUCTS}$$

I. $CH_3CH_2CH_2CHBrCH_3$
II. $CH_3CH_2CHBrCH_2CH_3$
III. $CH_3CH_2CH_2CH_2CH_2Br$
IV. $CH_3CH_2CHBrCH_3$

(A) I only   (B) I and II
(C) I, II and III   (D) III and IV

Questions 216-219 are NOT based on a descriptive passage.

---

216. The first stage of embryonic development, in which three distinct germ layers are seen, is the

(A) morula.   (B) gastrula.
(C) blastula.   (D) embryo.

217. Migration in birds is guided, in part, by

(A) celestial navigation.

(B) temperature changes.

(C) olfactory cues.

(D) day length changes caused by latitude.

218. The greatest similarity in structure occurs between members belonging to the same

(A) class.   (B) phylum.
(C) family.   (D) species.

219. What is the structural formula of the hydrogenation product of 2-methyl-2-pentene if deuterium was used as a tracer and Pt as a catalyst?

(A)

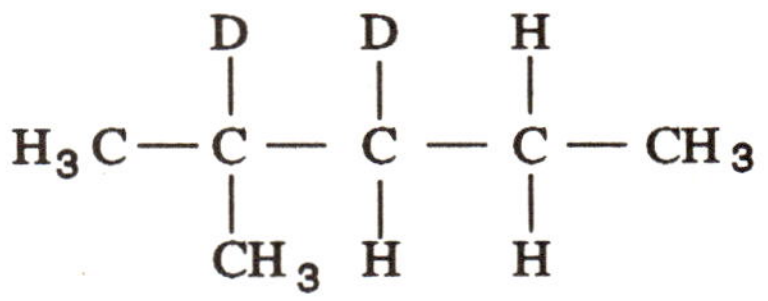

(B)

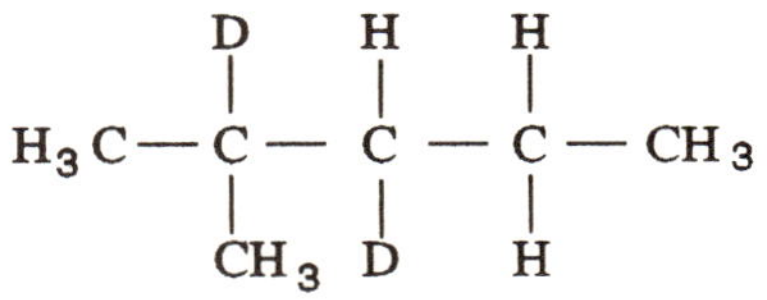

(C)

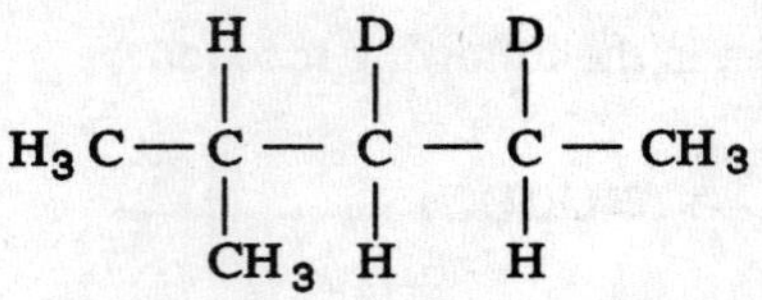

$$H_3C - \underset{\underset{CH_3}{|}}{\overset{\overset{H}{|}}{C}} - \underset{\underset{H}{|}}{\overset{\overset{D}{|}}{C}} - \underset{\underset{H}{|}}{\overset{\overset{D}{|}}{C}} - CH_3$$

(D)

$$H_3C - \underset{\underset{CH_3}{|}}{\overset{\overset{H}{|}}{C}} - \underset{\underset{D}{|}}{\overset{\overset{D}{|}}{C}} - \underset{\underset{H}{|}}{\overset{\overset{H}{|}}{C}} - CH_3$$

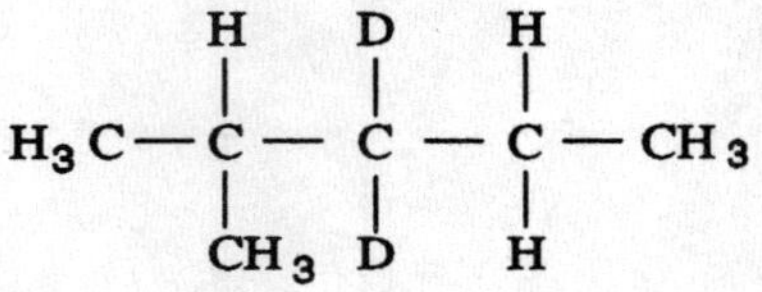

STOP

If time still remains, you may review work only in this section.

TEST 2

ANSWER KEY

1.	(C)	26.	(C)	51.	(A)	76.	(C)
2.	(B)	27.	(B)	52.	(B)	77.	(B)
3.	(B)	28.	(D)	53.	(B)	78.	(D)
4.	(D)	29.	(B)	54.	(D)	79.	(A)
5.	(C)	30.	(C)	55.	(C)	80.	(D)
6.	(B)	31.	(A)	56.	(B)	81.	(D)
7.	(C)	32.	(A)	57.	(C)	82.	(C)
8.	(C)	33.	(A)	58.	(C)	83.	(C)
9.	(C)	34.	(A)	59.	(D)	84.	(A)
10.	(D)	35.	(D)	60.	(A)	85.	(D)
11.	(B)	36.	(D)	61.	(C)	86.	(C)
12.	(A)	37.	(D)	62.	(A)	87.	(B)
13.	(A)	38.	(C)	63.	(C)	88.	(A)
14.	(A)	39.	(A)	64.	(B)	89.	(C)
15.	(A)	40.	(A)	65.	(D)	90.	(D)
16.	(D)	41.	(C)	66.	(C)	91.	(D)
17.	(C)	42.	(D)	67.	(D)	92.	(C)
18.	(B)	43.	(B)	68.	(A)	93.	(A)
19.	(B)	44.	(C)	69.	(D)	94.	(B)
20.	(D)	45.	(D)	70.	(B)	95.	(A)
21.	(C)	46.	(C)	71.	(B)	96.	(D)
22.	(D)	47.	(D)	72.	(C)	97.	(C)
23.	(B)	48.	(B)	73.	(A)	98.	(D)
24.	(D)	49.	(A)	74.	(D)	99.	(D)
25.	(C)	50.	(D)	75.	(C)	100.	(C)

101.	(B)	131.	(A)	161.	(D)	191.	(A)
102.	(A)	132.	(C)	162.	(A)	192.	(C)
103.	(C)	133.	(D)	163.	(B)	193.	(B)
104.	(D)	134.	(B)	164.	(C)	194.	(A)
105.	(C)	135.	(C)	165.	(A)	195.	(B)
106.	(A)	136.	(D)	166.	(B)	196.	(C)
107.	(A)	137.	(A)	167.	(D)	197.	(C)
108.	(B)	138.	(B)	168.	(B)	198.	(D)
109.	(D)	139.	(C)	169.	(A)	199.	(D)
110.	(D)	140.	(D)	170.	(C)	200.	(A)
111.	(A)	141.	(A)	171.	(D)	201.	(C)
112.	(D)	142.	(C)	172.	(B)	202.	(D)
113.	(C)	143	(B)	173.	(A)	203.	(B)
114.	(D)	144.	(B)	174.	(B)	204.	(B)
115.	(A)	145.	(D)	175.	(D)	205.	(A)
116.	(D)	146.	(C)	176.	(B)	206.	(C)
117.	(D)	147.	(A)	177.	(A)	207.	(A)
118.	(D)	148	(A)	178.	(C)	208.	(B)
119.	(C)	149.	(C)	179.	(C)	209.	(C)
120.	(A)	150	(C)	180.	(C)	210.	(C)
121.	(B)	151.	(A)	181.	(C)	211.	(C)
122.	(C)	152.	(B)	182.	(A)	212.	(D)
123.	(B)	153.	(A)	183.	(B)	213.	(A)
124.	(B)	154.	(C)	184.	(B)	214.	(D)
125.	(A)	155.	(D)	185.	(B)	215.	(B)
126.	(D)	156.	(B)	186.	(A)	216.	(B)
127.	(D)	157.	(D)	187.	(C)	217.	(A)
128.	(C)	158.	(B)	188.	(A)	218.	(D)
129.	(D)	159.	(D)	189.	(D)	219.	(A)
130.	(C)	160.	(B)	190.	(C)		

DETAILED EXPLANATIONS
OF ANSWERS

Section 1 — Verbal Reasoning

PASSAGE I (Questions 1-10)

This passage describes the trial of Socrates, as presented in Plato's *Apology*. It provides Socrates' explanation of his philosophical activity and his defense against the charges of heresy and corrupting the youth. The passage suggests why this philosopher, and this description of his life, have become classic archetypes of the conflict between wisdom and authority in the Western heritage.

1.   **(C)**   The first paragraph indicates that Socrates lived in Athens, a city-state of Greece, in 400 B.C. and that he was a philosopher.

2.   **(B)**   By saying that Socrates' simple, honest speech is "unlike the eloquent sophists," the passage contrasts it most clearly with the "dishonest" nature of sophistic rhetoric. The sophists' speech was also persuasive (A) and potentially appealing (C), and possibly vulgar (D), but in this context its elaborate, deceiving qualities are most important.

3.   **(B)**   The reason his past accusers are so dangerous (paragraph two) is that they spread lies about Socrates when the jurors were "young and impressionable." The fact that they now may be old (A), enjoy gossip (C), or be nostalgic (D) is irrelevant to the charges.

4.   **(D)**   The distinguishing feature of the Socratic method is the pursuit of knowledge through questioning, as opposed to straight explanation or exposition. Many law schools employ this method, but it is not common in medical schools (A). The police (B) and military (D) do not use questioning but, rather, orders in routine operations and training.

5.   **(C)**   The passage (paragraphs 1-3) shows how Socrates offends his jury three times even before he refutes the charges. His appeal to simple speech rejects the custom of flowery, emotional appeals in court; his reference to past accusers affecting the jurors in their youth calls into question their fair judgment; and his calling the formal charges a pretext for the real charge of embarrassing the establishment discredits the whole Athenian legal system.

6.   **(B)**   The perennial message of Socrates' life, as can be inferred from the passage, is the threat to any status quo of critical examination and questioning of authority. Socrates' trade (A), age (C), and the jury system (D) are not central to that message.

7.   **(C)**   Socrates' logical refutation of Meletus' charges, by showing their internal inconsistency, shows that consistency is a measure of authenticity and not a characteristic of small minds (A), false charges (B), or necessarily a court of law (D).

8.   **(C)**   The fact that a guilty verdict follows in spite of Socrates' disproving of the charges against him shows that reason does not always win the day (B). Since he refuted the charge of corrupting the youth, (A) is not correct and a Supreme Court (D) is not mentioned.

9.   **(C)**   The key here is that Socrates' alternative penalty of a state pension is either an insult or a proper reward, depending on who is involved. For the Athenians offended by his philosophical activity, it is an insult; to Socrates, who conducts his philosophical activity out of love for Athens and an attempt to improve it, it is a suitable compensation.

10.   **(D)**   The essential lesson of the life of Socrates, which explains its enduring appeal, is that all established authority resents criticism. That courts are corrupt (A), defendants are intellectual (B), or juries youthful (C) does not bear on that essential lesson.

PASSAGE II (Questions 11-16)
This passage describes the basic nature of the American federal system. It provides various interpretations of the relationship between national and state governments within federalism and some of the consequences, both good and bad, of such a political system.

11.   **(B)**   In the first paragraph, it is stated that James Madison saw the advantage of federalism as distributing power among several bodies, thereby preventing tyranny. Categorical grants (A) did not appear until the 1860s; the right to secede and the right to retain slavery, (C) and (D), were not foremost in Madison's plan.

12.   **(A)**   Since the compact theory allows states to secede, the conclusion of the Civil War, which forced the Southern states to remain in the Union, would be considered unjust. It would not be considered just (B), inevitable (D), or merely a mistake (C).

13.   **(A)**   Compact federalism calls for strong state governments and a weaker federal government. (B) Judicial federalism does not exist. Cooperative federalism (C) is diminished by the Court's actions and dual federalism (D) is not mentioned.

14.   **(A)**   Judicial review is the Court's practice of interpreting the Constitution generally and the nature of federal relations specifically. This replaces the Constitutional convention which was intended to serve the same purpose in compact theory. *Habeas corpus* (B) and desegregation (D), are irrelevant, and block grants (C) are a feature of cooperative federalism.

15.   **(A)**   By returning authority and funding to the states, Reagan's policy endorsed the compact theory. Judicial federalism (B) does not exist. Dual federalism (C) calls for sharing responsibility for the social programs discontinued by Reaganism. Cooperative federalism (D) is rejected by this approach.

16.   **(D)**   Every other pair has one incorrect characteristic: authoritarian (A), permanent (B), and undefined (C).

PASSAGE III (Questions 17-25)
   This essay summarizes the political ideas in Plato's *Republic*: his division of the soul into three elements or dispositions with corresponding classes in society. It discusses some of the characteristics of Plato's thought that conflict with twentieth century political ideas.

17.   **(C)**   The second paragraph details Plato's psychological elements which include all but humor.

18.   **(B)**   A business entrepreneur's interest in the production and distribution of goods or money and his primary motive for making a profit would place him or her in the appetitive category. The philosophic (A) loves knowledge for its own sake while the spirited (C) loves military exploit. The innovative is not one of Plato's categories.

19.   **(B)**   Jefferson's assumption of human equality contrasts most sharply with Plato's belief in innate inequality. The revolutionary sentiments of (A) do not address the issue of class differences. Answer (C) about "federalists" also does not discuss class differences. The idea of a natural aristocracy (D) agrees with Plato's views on class differences.

20.   **(D)**   It is the knowledge of the virtue appropriate to each class in society that constitutes the philosopher's wisdom and qualifies him or her for governance. Choices (A) – (C) detail the virtues of other classes (philosophic, spirited, appetitive, respectively).

21.   **(C)**   American public education claims to take children from all backgrounds and discern their natural propensities and occupational abilities, much like Plato's educational system. The chaos and freedom of a market economy (A) does not follow Plato's scheme. Election of leaders (B) is not part of Plato's theory (since the majority of appetitive citizens could not recognize philosophical wisdom). The Congress (D) is wrong because Plato did not believe in electing leaders from the masses.

22.   **(D)**   Plato's "myth of the metals" is premised on a "noble lie" (paragraph 4) which suggests that maintaining the "just order" is more important than always telling the truth. Courage and honor (A), (C) are military virtues; moderation (B) is an appetitive virtue.

23.   **(B)**   By appealing to material incentives for army recruiting that country is applying appetitive or economic rather than military values of honor and courage. The virtuous (D) did not exist.

24.   **(D)**   Because Plato defines a just society (paragraph five) as one that discovers and cultivates each individual's talents, he would see the young man's dilemma as a social rather than an individual (A) – (C) failure.

25.   **(C)**   American public opinion tends to support the military (A), prosperity (B) and education (D) — all of which Plato's *Republic* includes. Americans tend to be skeptical, however, of all-knowing, infallible rulers like Plato's philosopher-king.

PASSAGE IV (Questions 26-34)
        This passage argues that America in the 1990s is entering a Neo-Victorian social period characterized by traditional morality, stable family life and economic conservatism. The essay details several causes of this phenomenon and its probable results in the next century.

26.   **(C)**   Paragraph one details all of the mentioned causes (A), (B), (D) but drugs.

27.   **(B)**   A frequent criticism of the Victorian era which eventually eroded its influence was the hypocritical nature of its morality (for example, "family men" frequently had mistresses). It was obviously present in England, being named after Queen Victoria, making (A) incorrect; it may have been boring (C) but that is not a flaw in the historical analysis. *Zeitgeist* simply means "spirit of the times" (D).

28.   **(D)**   Paragraph two describes the return to traditional values of the baby-boom generation as a result of a reaction to its wild youth and loss of innocence. Being Christian before that reversal (A) is not mentioned, nor is education level (C); being raised by clergy is irrelevant (B).

29.   **(B)**   A primary cause of the Neo-Victorian emphasis on stability and morality is the baby boomers having children of their own and the sense of responsibility that brings. Having children may make one neurotic (A) and bossy (C) but those are not central to the analysis. The theme of the essay suggests that parenthood does not cause people to become irreverent, so (D) is also incorrect.

30.   **(C)**   Near the end of paragraph 2, the book *Catcher in the Rye* is presented as an archetypical 60's book of critical rebellion. It is distinctly contrasted with a fairy tale (A) and Walt Disney (B). It is referred to as the 60's rebels' Bible, but not as "the Bible" (D).

31.   **(A)**   Although the AIDS epidemic and its effect on sexual morality is developed later in the essay (D), its specific spread in small towns and rural areas, traditionally conservative, is not mentioned later. Slowed economic growth (B) and baby boomer parenthood (C) are both developed later in the essay as explanations for Neo-Victorianism.

32.   **(A)**   If the baby boomers become conservative after a radical youth, the logic would suggest that a consistently conservative upbringing (A) would produce a radical, unstable adulthood. A radical upbringing (B) or adolescent rebellion (C) should allow them to choose to be conservative later.

33.   **(A)**   The passage's emphasis on life cycle changes, with a rebellious adolescence and stable adulthood, conforms with Churchill's remark, making (B) incorrect. Its relevance renders (C) incorrect and, by itself, it does not prove Churchill's authorship (D).

34. **(A)**   If the Victorian children of the 1890s rebelled in the 1920s ·and the baby boomers rebelled in the 1960s and conformed in the 1990s it takes 20-30 years to go full cycle, making 2028 the only viable date.

PASSAGE V (Questions 35-45)
This passage describes John Stuart Mill's arguments for free thought and expression and shows their applicability to America.

35. **(D)**   All of the American institutions—journalism, academia, and law (A), (B), (C)—are mentioned in the essay.

36. **(D)**   Mill's argument includes ostracism in the essay (paragraph 2) (C) and implies a broader range of punishment (A); it does not mention the death penalty, making (B) incorrect.

37. **(D)**   In the second paragraph, near the end, the passage shows that Mill identified tolerance and intellectual liberty with a knowledgeable, humane, and civilized society.

38. **(C)**   Mill claims in paragraph 3 that the refutation of wrong ideas will strengthen the correct ideas. He does not see the value of wrong radical ideas as their eventual acceptance (A) (unless they become right) or their obnoxious quality (B) or their inability to persuade (D).

39. **(A)**   Paragraph four says that Mill did not extend liberty of belief and expression to liberty of action, so the Mormon could be prosecuted for practicing polygamy. He should not be left free in his actions (B). The doctrine of clear and present danger (C) does not apply in this instance; his political affiliation (D) is irrelevant.

40. **(A)**   Mill allows for prosecution, even of mere speech, if the social situation could, by the speech, be led to destructive action, which the angry crowd in front of the courthouse represents. The state should not leave the inflammatory speaker free (B) and cannot invoke ecclesiastical restrictions (C); his political affiliation is irrelevant (D).

41. **(C)**   Paragraph four identifies Oliver Wendell Holmes as the progenitor of the "clear and present danger" doctrine.

42. **(D)**   A city council debate encourages expression of conflicting viewpoints to establish the truth, as opposed to mere reporting in newspapers (A) or on television broadcast news programs (C). An assembly line (B) allows no input from individuals.

43. **(B)**   The adversary legal system, like Mill, sees truth coming out of clashing viewpoints. Elementary education tends to rely on teaching basics directly (A); medical schools primarily teach directly, though some debate occurs (C); military boot camp relies on orders and obedience (D).

44.   **(C)**   Mill's concern would not be over the character of the community, bigoted (A), decent (B), or immoral (D), but that the majority of it could constitute a tyranny over individual thought and expression.

45.   **(D)**   Mill's thesis that knowing only one side of an issue (even the correct one) is not to really know it (end of paragraph three) would object to a law requiring university professors to teach only the popular side of an issue and thereby violate academic freedom. Regardless of whether or not the truth is contained in a book or research, (A) or (B), or in other persons (C), Mill would contend that without familiarity with various incorrect views, knowledge of the correct is impossible.

PASSAGE VI (Questions 46-55)
    This passage describes two of the main approaches to organizational theory in American public administration: the traditional institutional approach exemplified in Max Weber's writings and the modern humanist school displayed in Maslow's theories.

46.   **(C)**   Paragraphs one and two show that traditional structural administrative theory includes official positions, rules and regulations and impartial treatment of the public, but not self-esteem, which is characteristic of the humanist approach (paragraph three).

47.   **(D)**   Although the current view of bureaucracy is often negative (A), (B), (C) Weber saw it as rational and efficient, according to paragraph two of the passage.

48.   **(B)**   Weber wrote in the late 19th and early 20th centuries, shortly after the unification of the petty German principalities, and he contrasted, favorably, the bureaucracy's efficiency and rationality to a prince's arbitrary rule. Nazi Germany (A) came after Weber's death; modern America (C) and ancient Rome (D) were not part of his analysis.

49.   **(A)**   The cold efficiency of German bureaucracy was horrible when used by the Nazis in the 1930s and during World War II, causing the world thereafter to be suspicious of bureaucratic "efficiency." Modern American bureaucracy (C) is mild by comparison; ancient Rome (D) and decentralized feudal principalities (B) are not relevant to this modern concern.

50.   **(D)**   The characteristic that distinguishes Humanist administration is (paragraph three, first sentence) the psychology of the individual in the organization. Animal rights are not a concern of Humanist thought (A) and education, experience and procedural due process, (B) and (C), are typical of the formal, institutional model.

51.   **(A)**   In Maslow's ladder of needs the love need is satisfied by "caring." Self-esteem is addressed through respect for accomplishments (B), and self-actualization through use of talents (C). Boredom is not a need in Maslow's theory (D).

52.   **(B)**   At the end of paragraph three of the passage, the writer states that the Maslowian administrator sees the satisfaction of everyone's needs as creating a more efficient, productive organization. Some may find this intolerable (A), chaotic (C), or boring (D), but in Maslow's theory it would be productive (B).

53.   **(B)**   It can be assumed from the passage's description of Maslow's theory that it expects managers to be psychologists in the sense of knowing and promoting employees' psychological needs and potentials. Unlike Weber, his approach does not emphasize efficiency (A) and certainly does not advocate managerial tyranny.

54.   **(D)**   In the first three paragraphs the passage adequately summarizes the two theories (A) and explains their differences (B) while naming two of their proponents (Weber and Maslow) (C), but its conclusion inadequately provides any means of reconciling the two approaches.

55.   **(C)**   The conflicting schools of thought in public administration theory, all of which have some good qualities and advocates, shows the subject to be complex. It is, therefore, not nearly consistent (A). The theories, though different, are not confused (B) and the subject may be boring to some (D), but that is not a distinguishing feature of the subject itself.

PASSAGE VII (Questions 56-65)
    This passage describes management leadership studies in general and two specific administrative leadership models.

56.   **(B)**   Paragraph two describes the first study of leadership styles, which involves three groups and three leaders respectively. No study mentioned involved two (A) or five (D) leaders. The second study, described later in the passage, involved four (C) leaders.

57.   **(C)**   The authoritarian leader is mentioned as employing a "highly personal or *ad hominem* form of correction" which is most likely to involve insulting the worker. The democratic leader (D) is said to correct in terms of "actions rather than persons" and the laissez faire leader (B) offers no correction whatsoever. Impoverished (A) does not apply as it refers to a lack of concern.

58.   **(C)**   The laissez faire leader provided complete freedom for individuals to do what they wanted and was ranked low in efficiency and satisfaction; hence, complete freedom in such a setting is "unfulfilling." It may also produce anarchy (B) and be fun (A) but those are not measured by the study results. Unusual (D) is wrong because the study did not focus on the frequency of use of the leadership styles.

59.   **(D)**   Both leadership studies (paragraphs two and three) contain an "authoritarian" type. Only the first has laissez faire (A) and democratic (C). Only the second study mentions an "impoverished" (B) type.

60.   **(A)**   The "Country Club" manager is described in paragraph three as having a high concern for people (represented here as providing high pay and benefits) and a low concern for production (represented here as not making serious demands on employees' work). The authoritarian type of leader, in both models, has little concern for people and makes many demands (B); neither totalitarian, (C) nor "laid-back" (D), are mentioned in the models described.

61.   **(C)**   The low regard for the agency's work and people expressed in that

statement best qualifies the Secretary as an "impoverished" leader which in paragraph three of the passage is described as having low concern for production and people. "Country Club" leaders (A) have high concern for people and "authoritarian" leaders (B) have high concern for work. Totalitarian leaders (D) are not mentioned.

62. **(A)** Team Leadership concern for both people (implying participation) and production most resembles the high level of worker satisfaction and efficiency in the earlier "democratic" leadership style. Authoritarian leadership's concentration of power (B) denies a concern for people, laissez-faire's low efficiency and satisfaction deny Team leadership's concern for production and people (C); and the New York Mets are not the team mentioned.

63. **(C)** The passage does not discuss the subject of whether good leaders are born or made. It does, in the discussion of leadership models, examine administrative effectiveness or efficiency/productivity (A), administrative traits (concern for people, etc.) (B), and how different forms of leadership affect morale (i.e. satisfaction) (D).

64. **(B)** By saying in the conclusion that the study of leadership styles would contribute to American "competiveness," it is implied that it would help the American economy. Better understanding of leadership might well help Eastern Europe (A), Gorbachev (C), and President Bush (D), but these are not implied in the passage, as is economic competitiveness.

65. **(D)** Machiavelli's Prince deceptively appears to be good and kind while being actually evil and cruel, and none of the leadership styles discussed really fits this description. The "Country Club" manager (A) is genuinely good and kind to his or her employees, the laissez-faire leader (B) simply leaves people alone, and the authoritarian leader (C) is not *deceptively* cruel; he or she is *openly* dictatorial.

Section 2 — Physical Sciences

66. **(C)** is the correct answer because you know $V_y = 0$ at the highest point. All other values are contained within the question.

$$t = \frac{V_0 \sin\theta_0 - V_y}{g} = \frac{(50\text{m}/\sec)(\sin 37) - 0}{9.75\,\text{m}/\sec^2} = 3.1\sec$$

The other three answers are incorrect because: (A) If you make the connection $V_y = 0$ then there is enough information. (B) This assumes you multiplied $(V_0 \sin\theta_0 - V_y)$ by g (note: the units will be wrong!)

$$[(50\text{ m/sec})(\sin 37) - 0] * 9.75\text{ m/sec}^2 = 290\text{ m}^2/\sec^3$$

(D) This assumes you used $\cos\theta_0$ in your calculation.

$$\frac{[(50\text{m}/\sec)(\cos 37) - 0]}{9.75\,\text{m}/\sec^2} = 4.1\sec$$

67. **(D)** is the correct answer setting $y_0 = 0$ and $a = -g$ you can solve this problem with the other information given.

$$Y_{max} = (V_0 \sin \theta_0)t - 1/2\, gt^2$$

$$Y_{max} = [(100 \text{ m/sec}) (\sin 45)] (7.25 \text{ sec}) - 1/2\ (9.75 \text{ m/s}^2)\ (7.25 \text{ s})^2$$

$$Y_{max} = 256 \text{ meters}$$

The other three answers are incorrect because: (A) If you make the connection that $Y_0 = 0$ then you do have enough information to solve the problem. (B) This is wrong due to the fact that you used $a = g$ rather than $a = -g$.

$$Y_{max} = (V_0 \sin \theta_0)t + 1/2\, gt^2$$

$$= [(100 \text{ m/sec}) (\sin 45)] (7.25) + 1/2(9.75 \text{ m/s}^2)\ (7.25 \text{ s})^2$$

$$Y_{max} = 769 \text{ meters}$$

(C) This assumes you made no correction for the initial contact conditions; i.e., $(V_0 \sin \theta_0)t = 0$.

68. **(A)** is the correct answer because you solve for t at $V_y = 0$ as in question one. Then multiply that time t by 2 since the same time is required for the golf ball to go up as it is for the golf ball to come down.

$$t = \frac{(V_0 \sin \theta_0) - V_y}{g}$$

$$= \frac{(100 \text{ m/sec})(\sin 45°) - 0}{9.75 \text{ m/s}^2}$$

Total time $= 2t = 14.5 \text{ sec}$

The other three answers are incorrect because: (B) 7.25 sec does account for the time to come down. This is the time it takes to get to its maximum height. (C) This answer doesn't account for the 45° angle of initial contact, i.e., $\sin \theta_0 = 1$ or for the total time equalling $2t$.

$$\frac{(100 \text{ m/sec})}{9.75 \text{ m/sec}^2} = t = 10.25 \text{ sec}$$

(D) This answer is the same as (C) except you have corrected for $2t$.

$$t = 10.25 \text{ sec} \therefore 2t = 20.5 \text{ sec}.$$

69. **(D)** is the correct answer since the total time of flight can be calculated and used in the equation with the other information given to yield the range.

$$\frac{(100 \text{ m/sec})(\sin 37°) - 0}{9.75 \text{ m/sec}^2} = t = 6.17 \text{ sec}$$

Total time $= 2t = 12.3 \text{ sec}$

$$R = (V_0 \cos \theta_0)\ (2t)$$

$$= (100 \text{ m/sec}) (\cos 37) (12.3) = 982 \text{ m}$$

The other three answers are incorrect because: (A) We are able to calculate the total time using equations as seen in Question 66. Employing this value in the range equation yields a correct valid answer. (B) This answer is possible if you use t from the first equation $1/2$ total time.

$$R = V(\cos \theta_0)t = (100 \text{ m/sec}) (\cos 37°) (6.17 \text{ sec}) = 493 \text{ m}$$

(C) This answer occurs if you forget to multiply by the total time. (Note: Your units would not work out correctly.)

$$R = V_0 \cos \theta_0 = (100 \text{ m/sec}) (\cos 37°) = 79.9 \text{ m/sec}$$

70. **(B)** is the correct answer because from Question 69 the equation $R = (V_0 \cos \theta_0)t$ gives all the parameters together so all we need is to calculate θ_0.

$$R = (V_0 \cos \theta_0)t \quad \text{or} \quad \cos^{-1}\left[\frac{R}{V_0 t}\right] = \theta_0$$

$$\cos^{-1}\left(\frac{311 \text{ m}}{(50 \text{ m/sec})(12.44 \text{ sec})}\right) = \theta_0 = 60°$$

The other three answers are incorrect because: (A) This answer occurs if you take inverse sin (sin $^{-1}$).

$$\sin^{-1}\left(\frac{311 \text{ m}}{(50 \text{ m/sec})(12.44 \text{ sec})}\right) = \theta_0 = 30°$$

(C) This answer is obtained if you don't employ the value R in the equation.

$$\cos^{-1}\left(\frac{1}{V_0 t}\right) = \cos^{-1}\left(\frac{1}{(50 \text{ m/sec})(12.44 \text{ sec})}\right) = \theta_0 = 90°$$

(D) This answer occurs if you leave the time t out of the equation and invert the correct equation.

$$\cos^{-1}\left(\frac{V_0}{R}\right) = \theta_0 = \cos^{-1}\left[\frac{50 \text{ m/sec}}{311 \text{ M}}\right] = 80°$$

71. **(B)** is the correct answer. The capacitance for capacitors in circuits in parallel is $C = C_1 + C_2 + \ldots$ so

$$C' = C_1 + C_2 = 20 \text{ μF} + 10 \text{ μF} = 30 \text{ μF}$$

The capacitance for capacitors in series is $1/C = 1/C_1 + 1/C_2 + \ldots$ so

$$\frac{1}{C} = \frac{1}{C'} + \frac{1}{C^3} = \frac{1}{30} + \frac{1}{5} = 2.33 \times 10^{-1} \text{μF}^{-1}$$

or $C = 4.3 \text{μF}$

The other three answers are incorrect because: (A) is obtained if you simply add all capacitances together.

$$C = C_1 + C_2 + C_3 = 20 \text{ μF} + 10 \text{ μF} + 5 \text{ μF} = 35 \text{ μF}$$

(C) is obtained if you use the formula for all the capacitors in series.

$$\frac{1}{C} = \frac{1}{20} + \frac{1}{10} + \frac{1}{5} = 3.5 \times 10^{-1} \mu F^{-1}$$

$$C = 2.9 \mu F$$

(D) is obtained if you reversed the formula sequence outlined in the correct answer (you used the wrong formula for capacitors in series and parallel).

$$\frac{1}{C'} = \frac{1}{20\mu F} + \frac{1}{10\mu F} = 1.5 \times 10^{-1} \quad \text{or} \quad C' = 6.7\mu F$$

$$C = C' + C_3 = 6.7\mu F + 5.0\mu F = 11.7\mu F$$

72. **(C)** is the correct answer. If C_2 is removed then essentially the circuit is 2 capacitors in series with an equivalent capacitance given by

$$\frac{1}{C} = \frac{1}{C_1} + \frac{1}{C_3} = \frac{C_1 C_3}{C_1 + C_3} = \frac{(20\mu F)(5\mu F)}{(20+5)\mu F} = 4\mu F$$

Knowing that $q = CV$ for C_3 we observe that

$$q = (4 \times 10^{-6} F)(100 V) = 4.0 \times 10^{-4} C$$

The other three answers are incorrect because: (A) is only true if you forgot how to calculate either the overall capacitance or the charge ($q = CV$). (B) is obtained if you used $C = C_1 + C_3 = 25 \mu F$ and calculate q from this value for capacitance.

$$q = (25 \times 10^{-6} F)(100 V) = 2.5 \times 10^{-3} C$$

(D) is obtained if you only used $C = C_3$ for the capacitance.

$$q = (5 \times 10^{-6} F)(100 V) = 5 \times 10^{-4} C$$

73. **(A)** is the correct answer. It is obtained by obtaining the capacitance for $C_1 + C_2$ in parallel. Then using C'

$$C' = C_1 + C_2 = 10 \mu F + 5 \mu F = 15 \mu F$$

plus C_3 as 2 capacitors in series to obtain the overall capacitance.

$$C = \frac{C' C_3}{C' + C_3} = \frac{(15\mu F)(4\mu F)}{(15+4)\mu F} = 3.2\mu F$$

Solving for q yields ($q = CV$)

$$q = (3.2 \times 10^{-6} F)(100 V) = 3.2 \times 10^{-4} C$$

Lastly, finding $V_3 = q/C_3$

$$V_3 = \frac{3.2 \times 10^{-4} C}{4.0 \times 10^{-6} F} = 80V$$

The other three answers are incorrect because: (B) Employs only C_1 in the C' calculation:

$$C' = C_1 = 10\mu F$$

$$C = \frac{C' C_3}{C' + C_3} = \frac{(10\mu F)(4\mu F)}{10\mu F + 4\mu F} = 2.9\mu F$$

$$q = (2.9 \times 10^{-6} F)(100V) = 2.9 \times 10^{-4} C$$

$$\therefore V_3 = \frac{2.9 \times 10^{-4} C}{4.0 \times 10^{-6} F} = 73V$$

(C) is obtained if C' is miscalculated employing

$$C' = \frac{C_1 C_2}{C_1 + C_2}$$

$$C' = \frac{(10\mu F)(5\mu F)}{(10+5)\mu F} = 3.3 \mu F$$

Following the calculation shown in (B) above yields $C = 1.8 \ \mu F$

$$\therefore V_3 = 45 \ V$$

(D) is obtained if you miscalculate C (as if they are in parallel).

$$C' = C_1 + C_2 = 15 \ \mu F$$

$$C = C' + C_3 = 19 \ \mu F$$

$$q = (19 \times 10^{-6} F)(100 \ V) = 1.9 \times 10^{-3} C$$

$$\therefore V_3 = \frac{1.9 \times 10^{-3} C}{4.0 \times 10^{-6} F} = 480V$$

74.   **(D)**   is the correct answer. Since the circuit is balanced (all resistors are equal) no current flow will go through R_1. The other three answers are incorrect because: (A) is obtained if you use $i = E/R$ where $E = 50$ V and $R = 10 \ \Omega$.

$$i = \frac{50V}{10\Omega} = 5.0A$$

(B) is obtained if you use only 3 resistors in series so that $R = 30 \ \Omega$.

$$i = \frac{50V}{30\Omega} = 17A$$

(C) is obtained if you use 2 resistors in series.

$$i = \frac{50V}{20\Omega} = 2.5A$$

75.   **(C)**   is the correct answer. For the resistors in series the formula for equivalence resistance is $R_{eq} = R_1 + R_2 = 100 + 100 = 200 \ \Omega$. After that solve for the two R_{eq} in parallel with the formula

$$\frac{1}{R} = \frac{1}{R_1} + \frac{1}{R_2} = \frac{R_2 + R_1}{R_2 R_1}.$$

$$R = \frac{R_2 R_1}{R_1 + R_2} = \frac{(200)(200)}{200 + 200} = 100\Omega$$

The other three answers are incorrect because: (A) is obtained if you simply add all 4 resistors together.

$$(4)(100 \ \Omega) = 400 \ \Omega$$

(B) is obtained if you calculate $1/R$ instead of R.

$$\frac{1}{R} = \frac{200+200}{(200)(200)} = 1.0 \times 10^{-2} \,\Omega$$

(D) is obtained if you calculate in parallel resistors (R) with the wrong number.

$$R_{eg} = \frac{R_1 R_2}{R_1 + R_2} = \frac{(100)(100)}{100+100} = 50\Omega$$

76.   **(C)**   is the correct answer. When the object's distance is much greater than the radius of curvature, then the $1/s$ term is negligible (≈ 0).

$$\frac{1}{s} + \frac{1}{s'} \approx \frac{1}{s'} = \frac{2}{r}$$

$$\therefore \quad \frac{r}{2} = s'$$

The other three answers are incorrect because: (A) This answer yields a non-negligible s term and the equation can *not* be further reduced. (B) This yields a value of $1/s + 1/s' \approx \infty$. (D) Again this leads to a non-negligible s term and the equation can *not* be further reduced.

77.   **(B)**   is the correct answer. If $s = 50$ cm then $s' = (1/2)s$ or 25 cm. Simply use the equation which holds for spherical mirrors.

$$\frac{1}{s} + \frac{1}{s'} = \frac{2}{r}$$

$$\frac{1}{50} + \frac{1}{25} = \frac{2}{r} = .060 \text{ cm}^{-1}$$

$$\text{or } r = \frac{2}{.060 \text{ cm}^{-1}} = 33 \text{ cm}$$

The other three answers are incorrect because: (A) This is obtained if you just calculate $1/s + 1/s'$ (note wrong units).

$$\frac{1}{50} + \frac{1}{25} = .060 \text{ cm}^{-1}$$

(C) This is obtained if you don't multiply by the factor 2.

$$r = \frac{1}{.060 \text{ cm}^{-1}} = 17 \text{ cm}^{-1}$$

(D) This is obtained if you calculate $2(1/s + 1/s')$.

$$2 \left(\frac{1}{50 \text{ cm}^{-1}} + \frac{1}{25 \text{ cm}^{-1}} \right) = .12 \text{ cm}^{-1}$$

78.   **(D)**   is the correct answer. A negative sign in the magnification term tells you that an image has been inverted. The other three answers are incorrect because: (A) would be true if the magnification term were < 1.0. (B) is a reference to the value of s' not m. (C) See choice (B).

79. **(A)** is the correct answer. Using the equations in the passage with the information in the problem allows for solution by simply plugging in the numbers (note: r_1 and r_2 will have different signs since its a *double* convex lens).

$$\frac{1}{f} = (n-1)\left(\frac{1}{r_1} - \frac{1}{r_2}\right) = (2-1)\left(\frac{1}{25} - \left(-\frac{1}{25 \text{ cm}}\right)\right) = \frac{2}{25 \text{ cm}}$$

$$\therefore \quad f = 12.5 \text{ cm}$$

The other three answers are incorrect because: (B) is obtained if you don't subtract 1 off the index of refraction value.

$$\frac{1}{f} = (2)\left(\frac{1}{25} - \left(-\frac{1}{25 \text{ cm}}\right)\right) = \frac{1}{25} \text{ cm}$$

$$f = 25 \text{ cm}$$

(C) is obtained if you don't realize that $r_1 = -r_2$ thus giving

$$\frac{1}{r_1} - \frac{1}{r_2} = 0$$

Therefore $1/f = 0$ or f would be undefined. (D) is obtained if you only calculate $1/f$ not f which is

$$\frac{1}{50} \text{ cm or } .020 \text{ cm}$$

80. **(D)** is the correct answer. If you first calculate s' using $1/f = 1/s + 1/s'$ then utilizing $m = -(s'/s)$ you can solve for the magnification.

$$\frac{1}{f} = \frac{1}{s} + \frac{1}{s'} \qquad \therefore \frac{1}{s'} = \frac{1}{f} - \frac{1}{s}$$

$$\frac{1}{s'} = .067 \text{ cm}^{-1} \qquad \therefore s' = 15 \text{ cm}$$

$$\text{finally } m = -\frac{15 \text{ cm}}{30 \text{ cm}} = -.50$$

The other three answers are incorrect because: (A) is obtained if you calculate everything correctly but forget the (-) sign in the magnification expression $m = -(s'/s)$. (B) is obtained if you add $1/s$ instead of subtracting in the $1/s'$ expression.

$$\frac{1}{s'} = \frac{1}{10} + \frac{1}{30} = .133 \qquad \therefore s' = 7.5 \text{ and } m = -0.25$$

(C) is obtained if you miscalculate as in (B) but use an inverse for m in the magnification calculation $m = s/s'$.

$$m = \frac{-30}{7.5} = -4.0$$

81. **(D)** According to Newton's law of inertia, a body in motion tends to move in a straight line. To change straight-line motion into circular motion, an outside force must constantly pull the body toward the center of rotation. Such a central force is called a centripetal force.

82.   **(C)**

Work = Force × distance

We know the distance is 10 meters. We must, however, find F. We use the relationship:

$$F = \text{mass} \times \text{acceleration}$$

$$a = 9.8 \text{ m/sec}^2$$

$$m = 25 \text{ kg}$$

$$F = (25 \text{ kg}) (9.8 \text{ m/sec}^2)$$

$$F = 245.0 \text{ kg} \cdot \text{m/sec}^2 = 245.0 \text{ newtons}$$

Now, we can substitute into the first equation:

$$\text{Work} = 245.0 \text{ N} \times 10 \text{ m}$$

$$\text{Work} = 2450 \text{ N} \cdot \text{m}$$

$$= 2450 \text{ joules}$$

83.   **(C)**   Setting up a ratio between the two similar triangles:

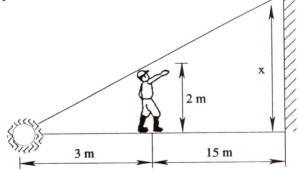

$$\frac{2\,\text{m}}{3\,\text{m}} = \frac{x}{18\,\text{m}}$$
$$3\text{m}\, x = 36\text{m}^2$$

$$x = 12\text{m}$$

The height of the shadow is 12 meters.

84.   **(A)**   In general, electronegativity increases from the left to the right and from the bottom to the top of the periodic table. Of the choices given, carbon is the closest to the top right corner.

85.   **(D)**   The volumes of the particles of an ideal gas are negligible compared to the volume of the space enclosing the gas. However, the particles could not have zero volume. If they did, there could be no collisions (elastic or otherwise) hence, there

would be nothing to impede the flow of the gas particles from one place to another at rates proportional to their speeds.

86. **(C)** The ideal gas law is

$$pV = nRT$$

Initially, $p_0 = nRT_0 / V_0$

$$= 3(8.314 \times 10^7)(300) / (2 \times 10^7)$$

$$= 3.741 \times 10^3 \, d/cm^2$$

In an adiabatic process $\Rightarrow pV^\gamma = $ constant, thus

$$p_0V_0^\gamma = p_fV_f^\gamma, \, p_f = p_0 \left(\frac{v_0}{V_f} \right)^\gamma$$

where the exponent is

$$\gamma = (C_V + R) / C_V = (\frac{5}{2}R + R) / (\frac{5}{2}R) = \frac{7}{5}$$

since a diatomic gas has 2 extra degrees of freedom.

$$p_f = (3.741 \times 10^3) \left(\frac{2 \times 10^7}{4 \times 10^7} \right)^{7/5}$$

$$= 1.42 \times 10^3 \, d/cm^2$$

87. **(B)** is the correct answer. It is calculated directly by using the equation $I = mr^2$ using the values from the passage.

$$I = \frac{1}{2} (.515 \, kg)(.25 \, m)^2 = 1.6 \times 10^{-2} \, kg \cdot m^2$$

The other three answers are incorrect because: (A) is obtained if you do not divide by 2.

$$I = (.515 \, kg)(.25 \, m)^2 = 3.2 \times 10^{-2} \, kg \cdot m^2$$

(C) is obtained if you do not square the radius term (note wrong units).

$$I = \frac{1}{2} (.515 \, kg)(.25 \, m) = 6.4 \times 10^{-2} \, kg \cdot m$$

(D) is obtained if you do not convert to kilograms (note wrong units).

$$I = \frac{1}{2} (515 \, g)(.25 \, m)^2 = 1.6 \times 10^1 \, g \cdot m^2$$

88. **(A)** is the correct answer. Again simply use the equation given and the values in the passage.

$$\tau = TR = (10 \, N)(.25 \, m) = 2.5 \, N \cdot m$$

The other three answers are incorrect because: (B) is obtained if you do not change to meters (wrong units).

$$\tau = (10\ N) * 25\ cm = 250\ N \cdot cm$$

(C) is obtained if you solve for T by dividing by r (units are wrong for τ).

$$\tau = \frac{10\ N}{.25\ m} = 4.0 \times 10^1\ Nm^{-1}$$

(D) is just like (C) except you have also not converted to meters.

$$\tau = \frac{10\ N}{25\ cm} = 4.0 \times 10^{-1}\ Ncm^{-1}$$

89.　**(C)**　is the correct answer. Using the angular velocity equation and substituting zero for ω_0 it is possible to solve this problem.

$$\omega = \omega_0 + \alpha_0 t = 0 + (1.56 \times 10^2\ rad/sec^2)\ (10.0\ sec)$$

$$\omega = 1.56 \times 10^3\ rad/sec$$

The other three answers are incorrect because: (A) in light of choice (C), it is obviously false. (B) is obtained by squaring the time (t) (note wrong units).

$$\omega = 0 + (1.56 \times 10^2\ rad/sec^2)\ (10\ sec)^2 = 1.56 \times 10^4\ rad$$

(D) is obtained by dividing α_0 by t (again units wrong).

$$\omega = 0 + \frac{(1.56 \times 10^2\ rad/sec^2)}{10\ sec} = 1.56 \times 10^1\ rad/sec^3$$

90.　**(D)**　is the correct answer. You first calculate I using the new radius and then use the values in the equation given.

$$I = \tfrac{1}{2}\ mr^2 = \tfrac{1}{2}\ (.515\ kg)\ (.50\ m)^2 = 6.4 \times 10^{-2}\ kg \cdot m^2/sec$$

$$L = IW = (6.4 \times 10^{-2}\ kg \cdot m^2)\ (3.91 \times 10^2\ rad/sec) = 2.5 \times 10^1\ kg \cdot m^2/sec$$

The other three answers are incorrect because: (A) is obtained if you use the radius of 25 cm.

$$L = (1.6 \times 10^{-2}\ kg \cdot m^2)\ (3.91 \times 10^2\ rad/sec) = 6.3\ kg \cdot m^2/sec$$

(B) is obtained if you use $I = mr^2$

$$I = 1.28 \times 10^{-1}\ kg \cdot m^2$$

$$L = (1.28 \times 10^{-1}\ kg \cdot m^2)\ (3.91 \times 10^2\ rad/sec) = 5.0 \times 10^1\ kg \cdot m^2/sec$$

(C) is obtained if you multiply the correct answer outlined in (E) by the time (note wrong units).

$$L = (2.5 \times 10^1\ kg \cdot m^2/sec)\ (5\ sec) = 1.3 \times 10^2\ kg \cdot m^2$$

91.　**(D)**　is the correct answer. Using $\tau = Tr$ to get τ and then putting that value into the equation will yield the solution.

$$\tau = (10\ N)\ (.25\ m) = 2.5\ N \cdot m$$

$$P = \tau \cdot \omega = (2.5\ N \cdot m)\ (3.13 \times 10^3\ rad/s)$$

$P = 7.8 \times 10^3$ W

The other three answers are incorrect because: (A) is obtained if you multiply the answer from (D) by the time (wrong units).

$P = (7.8 \times 10^3 \text{ W}) (20 \text{ sec}) = 1.6 \times 10^5 \text{ N} \cdot \text{m}$

(B) is obtained if you mistakenly use 10 N as the applied torque (wrong units).

$P = (10 \text{ N}) (3.13 \times 10^3 \text{ rad/s}) = 3.11 \times 10^4 \text{ N/s}$

(C) is obtained if you miscalculate τ by not changing to m.

$\tau = (10 \text{ N}) (25 \text{ cm}) = 250 \text{ N} \cdot \text{cm}$

$P = (250 \text{ N} \cdot \text{cm}) (3.13 \times 10^3 \text{ rad/s}) = 7.8 \times 10^5 \text{ N} \cdot \text{cm/s}$

92. **(C)** is the correct answer since the visible region is defined as being from 4000Å - 7000Å or 400-700 nm (where 1 nm = 10Å). The other three answers are incorrect because: (A) defines the ultra-violet region of the spectrum. (B) defines the infra-red region of the spectrum (2500 nm - 50,000 nm). (D) also defines the ultra-violet region of the spectrum (200-400 nm).

93. **(A)** is the correct answer. If you use $c = \upsilon\lambda$ and solve for λ the operational relationship is $\lambda = c/\upsilon$ where υ is the frequency.

$$\lambda = \frac{3.0 \times 10^8 \text{ m/sec}}{6.17 \times 10^{14} \text{ Hz}} = 4.86 \times 10^{-7} \text{ m} \quad \text{or} \quad 486 \text{ nm}$$

The other three answers are incorrect because: (B) solves the problem correctly but does not put into proper units. (C) is obtained if you incorrectly rearrange the relationship $c = \upsilon\lambda$ to $\lambda = \upsilon/c$ (note: units would not work out).

$$\lambda = \frac{6.17 \times 10^{14} \text{ Hz}}{3.0 \times 10^8 \text{ m/sec}} = 2.06 \times 10^6 \text{ 1/m}$$

(D) is obtained if you calculated the energy using $E = h\upsilon$ (again units would be incorrect).

$E = (6.626 \times 10^{-34} \text{ J s}) (6.17 \times 10^{14} \text{ Hz}) = 4.09 \times 10^{-19} \text{ J}$

94. **(B)** is the correct answer. Employing $E_{photon} = h\upsilon$ the energy can be calculated directly.

$E_{photon} = (6.626 \times 10^{-34} \text{ J s}) (6.17 \times 10^{14} \text{ Hz}) = 4.09 \times 10^{-19} \text{ J}$

The other three answers are incorrect because: (A) is obtained by using the wrong equation and solving for λ (note: units are wrong).

$$\lambda = \frac{c}{\upsilon} = \frac{3.0 \times 10^8 \text{ m/sec}}{6.17 \times 10^{14} \text{ Hz}} = 4.86 \times 10^{-7} \text{ m}$$

(C) is obtained if you use a wrong relationship (units will again be wrong).

$$E = \frac{h}{\upsilon} = \frac{6.626 \times 10^{-34} \text{ J/s}}{6.17 \times 10^{14} \text{ Hz}} = 1.07 \times 10^{48} \text{ J s}^2$$

(D) is obtained if you use *c* instead of *h* in the equation (wrong units yet again).

$$E = c\upsilon = (3.0 \times 10^8 \text{ m/sec})(6.17 \times 10^{14} \text{ Hz}) = 1.85 \times 10^{23} \text{ m/sec}^2$$

95. (A) is the correct answer. Knowing $E = h\upsilon$ and $E = mc^2$ we derive the relationship $m = h\upsilon/c^2$ and there is enough information to solve the mass (1 J = 1 kg m²/s²).

$$m = \frac{(6.626 \times 10^{-34} \text{ J/s})(6.17 \times 10^{14} \text{ Hz})}{(3.0 \times 10^8 \text{ m/s})^2} = 4.54 \times 10^{-36} \text{ kg}$$

The other three answers are incorrect because: (B) is obtained using υ in place of E in the $E = mc^2$ equation (note that units will not work out).

$$m = \frac{\upsilon}{c^2} = 6.86 \times 10^{-3} \text{ s/m}^2$$

(C) is obtained if you didn't square *c* in the denominator of the operative equation (units are off again).

$$m = \frac{h\upsilon}{c} = \frac{(6.626 \times 10^{-34} \text{ J/s})(6.17 \times 10^{14} \text{ Hz})}{3.0 \times 10^8 \text{ m/s}}$$

$$m = 1.36 \times 10^{-27} \text{ kg m/s}$$

(D) assumes you incorrectly used the wrong units in Planck's constant substituting g in place of kg.

96. (D) is the correct answer. Simply plug in the variables and convert to nm to get the correct answer.

$$\frac{1}{\lambda} = (109.678 \text{ cm}^{-1})\left(\frac{1}{2^2} - \frac{1}{3^2}\right) = 1.52331 \times 10^4 \text{ cm}^{-1}$$

$$\lambda = 6.56467 \times 10^{-5} \text{ cm or } 656.467 \text{ nm}$$

The other three answers are incorrect because: (A) is in the wrong units. It has not been converted to nm. (B) is obtained if you switch $n_1 + n_2$ and add instead of subtract.

$$\frac{1}{\lambda} = (109.678 \text{ cm}^{-1})\left(\frac{1}{3^2} + \frac{1}{2^2}\right) = 3.96059 \times 10^4 \text{ cm}^{-1}$$

$$\lambda = 2.52487 \times 10^{-5} \text{ cm or } 252.487 \text{ nm}$$

(C) is obtained if you add instead of subtract in the Rydberg Equation (as in choice (B)) but you do not correct to nm.

97. (C) is the correct answer. Three phases exist at both points *F* (solid phase I, solid phase II and liquid) and *E* (solid Phase I, liquid and gas). The other three answers are incorrect because: (A) Point *F* is a triple point but so is point *E*. (B) Point *E* is a triple point but so is Point *F*. (D) Point *G* is *not* a triple point.

98. (D) is the correct answer. At point *G* the distinction between liquid and gas breaks down. This is known as the critical point and occurs at 450 K. The other three answers are incorrect because: (A) is at point *H* and is well above the critical tem-

perature. (B) is well below the critical temperature (several phases exist depending on the pressure). (C) See choice (B).

99. **(D)** is the correct answer. You start in solid phase I and cross the equilibrium line and finish in the liquid phase of our material. The other three answers are incorrect because: (A) occurs only if we cross at a point below 150 atm. (B) can only occur if we elevate the pressure at the temperature given in the problem. (C) The solid does indeed melt but does not cross the equilibrium barrier to become a gas.

100. **(C)** is the correct answer because we've never left the liquid phase according to our phase diagram. The other three answers are incorrect because: (A) We don't cross into the gas phase by increasing the pressure. (B) We don't cross into either the solid phases during these changes. (D) See choice (B).

101. **(B)** is the correct answer. Going directly from a solid to a gaseous phase is by definition called sublimation. The other three answers are incorrect because: (A) Fusion is the process of bringing atoms together where sublimation actually is breaking them apart. (C) Melting would be in going from a solid to a liquid. (D) Boiling would be in going from a liquid to a gas.

102. **(A)** is the correct answer. Since this point is above the critical temperature it is defined as a single phase that is neither a liquid or gas but something between the two. The other three answers are incorrect because: (B) is obtained if you thought the liquid and gas phase existed together at point H. (C) and (D) are impossible since up to point H only 2 phases existed at these higher pressures and temperatures (liquid and gas).

103. **(C)** is the correct answer. At point F we have solid phase I, solid phase II and liquid in equilibrium. The other three answers are incorrect because: (A) At the boundary lines, multiple phases in equilibrium must be present. (B) Since there are two different solids, each constitutes a unique phase of the material (each solid defines a unique phase). (D) There are only three possible phases present at this point, so there could not be greater than three phases present.

104. **(D)** Our very rough measurement of the normality of solution A tells us that the true value could be anywhere between $0.95 - 10\%$ and $0.95 + 10\%$, that is, .86N and 1.05N. If the normality of A is less than 1.00 the final mixture will be basic; if it is greater than 1.00, acidic. Since we are not certain, the correct answer is (D).

105. **(C)** Na_2CO_3 when dissolved in water forms the compound $NaHCO_3$ and sodium hydroxide, both compounds are alkaline. e.g.,

$$Na_2CO_3 + H_2O \longleftrightarrow NaHCO_3 + NaOH$$

(C) is therefore the correct choice here.

106. **(A)**

$$N_A V_A = N_B V_B$$

$$0.5N \times 20ml = N_B \times 1000 \, ml$$

$$N_B = \frac{0.5 \times 20 \, ml}{1000 \, ml} = 0.01N$$

107. **(A)**   The work required to move a charge through a potential difference is equal to the product of the potential difference and the charge,

Work $= Vq$

$\quad = $ (5 volts) (2 coulombs)

$\quad = $ 10 joules.

108. **(B)**   Diffraction is the tendency of a wave to spread into a region behind an obstruction. This also includes a tendency of a wave to spread out when passing through a small aperture.

109. **(D)**   is the correct answer. We see that if the [NO] is held constant and we double the $[Cl_2]$ there is an increase in the rate of a factor of 2. Using general rate law rate $= k[NO]^x[Cl_2]^y$ find $x + y$.

$$\text{rate}^1 = k[NO]^x[Cl_2]^y$$

$$\text{rate}^2 = k[NO]^x[Cl_2]^y$$

$$\therefore \frac{\text{rate}^1}{\text{rate}^2} = \frac{[Cl_2]^y}{2^y[Cl_2]^y} = \frac{1}{2^y} = \frac{8.0}{16.0}$$

$$\frac{1}{2^y} = \frac{1}{2} \quad \therefore \quad y = 1$$

Alternatively, do the same thing holding $[Cl_2]$ constant.

$$\frac{\text{rate}^1}{\text{rate}^2} = \frac{8}{32} = \frac{1}{2^x} = \frac{1}{4} \quad \therefore \quad x = 2 \quad \therefore \quad \text{rate} = k[NO]^2[Cl_2]^1$$

The other three answers are incorrect because: (A) and (B) don't have any dependence on the $[Cl_2]$ which is easily seen from the experimental data. (C) doesn't account for the squared behavior of [NO] in the rate law.

110. **(D)**   is the correct answer. Simply choose 1 set of experimental data and solve the rate law for k.

$$k = \frac{\text{rate}}{[NO]^2} = \frac{(1.5 \, M/s)}{(.10 \, M)^2} = 1.5 \times 10^2 \, M^{-1}s^{-1}$$

The other three answers are incorrect because: (A) doesn't account for the correction due to the concentration of NO (it is the rate directly). (B) is obtained if you don't square the value for the concentration of NO (note units are wrong).

$$\frac{(1.5 \text{ M/s})}{(.10 \text{ M})} = 1.5 \times 10^1 \text{ s}^{-1}$$

(C) is obtained if you don't take a consistent row of data.

$$\frac{(1.5 \text{ M/s})}{(.20 \text{ M})^2} = 3.8 \times 10^1 \text{ M}^{-1}\text{s}^{-1}$$

111. **(A)** is the correct answer. Since it is a first order reaction half-life is given by the following equation:

$$t_{\frac{1}{2}} = \frac{\ln 2}{k} = \frac{.693}{k}$$

$$t_{\frac{1}{2}} = \frac{.693}{3.5 \times 10^{-2} s^{-1}} = 20 \text{ sec}$$

The other three answers are incorrect because: (B) is obtained by multiplying k by [NO] which gives the rate (note wrong units).

$$(.50 \text{ M})\ 3.5 \times 10^{-2}\text{s}^{-1}) = 1.2 \times 10^{-3} \text{ Ms}^{-1}$$

(C) is obtained by dividing k by [NO] (again wrong units).

$$\frac{(.50 \text{ M})}{(3.5 \times 10^{-2} s^{-1})} = 1.4 \times 10^1 \text{ Ms}$$

(D) is the inverse of choice (C).

$$\frac{1}{14 \text{ Ms}} = 7.1 \times 10^{-2} \text{ M}^{-1}\text{s}^{-1}$$

112. **(D)** is the correct answer. Using
$$t_{\frac{1}{2}} = \frac{1}{k[B]_0}$$

for the first half-life allows one to calculate this answer.

$$t_{\frac{1}{2}} = \frac{1}{(3.5 \times 10^{-2} \text{ M}^{-1}\text{s}^{-1})(.50 \text{ M})} = 5.7 \times 10^1 \text{ sec}$$

The other three answers are incorrect because: (A) is obtained if you simply take $1/k$ (note wrong units).

$$\frac{1}{3.5 \times 10^{-2} \text{ M}^{-1}\text{s}^{-1}} = 2.9 \times 10^2 \text{ s}^{-1}\text{M}^{-1}$$

(B) is obtained if you take $k[B]_0$ rather than the inverse (wrong units).

$$(3.5 \times 10^{-2} \text{ M-1s}^{-1})\ (.50 \text{ M}) = 1.7 \times 10^{-2} \text{ s}^{-1}$$

(C) is obtained if you take
$$t_{\frac{1}{2}} = \frac{\ln 2}{k[B]_0}.$$

$$t_{\frac{1}{2}} = \frac{.693}{(3.5 \times 10^{-2} \text{ M}^{-1}\text{s}^{-1})(.50 \text{ M})} = 4.0 \times 10^1 \text{ sec}$$

113. **(C)** is the correct answer. The rate law tells how many and which ones of the reactants are involved in the slowest step or rate determining step. The other three answers are incorrect because: (A) we do obtain some mechanistic information. (B) We not get all the information we need; only what is involved in the rate determining step. (D) The final step is not always the rate determining step.

114. **(D)** is the correct answer. The order of a reaction is defined as the sum of the exponents on the concentration terms.

For rate = $k[NO]^2 [Cl_2]^2$ $x = 2$ $y = 2$ ∴ order = 4

The other three answers are incorrect because: (A) The rate law says that there is a concentration dependence in the rate (zero infers concentration independence). (B) It has to be greater than 2 because both species concentration appear in the rate law. (C) Doesn't take into effect that there is a square dependence on the concentration.

115. **(A)** is the correct answer. Sulfur has 6 valence e⁻ and each fluorine will donate 1 e⁻ to pair with 1 e⁻ on the sulfur. 4 e⁻ on sulfur will form the bonds and there will be 1 e⁻ pair left over. The other three answers are incorrect because: (B) The extra 2 electrons are not shown. (C) An extra 2 electrons are shown which do not belong. (D) 2 extra electron pairs which do not belong are shown.

116. **(D)** is the correct answer. To put five electron pairs (4 bonding pairs and 1 lone pair) around sulfur we start with a trigonal bypyramid structure and place the lone pair of electrons in a more stable equatorial position. This yields the see-saw structure.

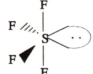

The other three answers are incorrect because: (A) The lone pair would push the other S-F bonds out of plane if square planar was exhibited. (B) Tetrahedral also doesn't take into account the lone pair of e⁻. (C) You can't see the lone pair of e⁻ so the one point in the trigonal plane would be observed.

117. **(D)** is the correct answer. Using the valence bond theory we observe that to get six uniform orbitals we must mix the s, all.

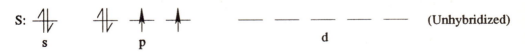

The other three answers are incorrect because: (A) This does not produce six uniform orbitals, only 4. (B) This hybridization infers using lower energy d orbitals rather than higher energy d orbitals which do not exist in sulfur. (C) This does not produce 6 uniform orbitals, only 5.

118. **(D)**   is the correct answer. Again employing Lewis structure we see that a trigonal bipyramid base structure for the electron pairs exists. The e⁻ pairs will be in the more stable equatorial positions which leads to a linear structure.

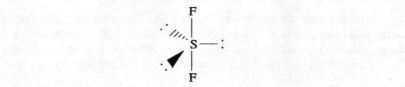

The other three answers are incorrect because: (A) Bent could only occur if 1 of the e⁻ pairs was located in a less stable axial position. (B) Trigonal bipyramid can be observed since the trigonal plane is made up of e⁻ pairs which we can't see. (C) Trigonal planar needs four atoms, we only have three.

119. **(C)**   is the correct answer. Using $PV = nRT$, you first find the number of moles and then using the molecular mass find the weight.

$$n = \frac{PV}{RT} = \frac{(.970 \text{ atm}) (250L)}{(.082L - \text{atm} / K - \text{mole})(298K)} = 9.92 \text{ moles}$$

wt. $= (\text{Mol. mass}) (n) = (26.04 \text{ g} / \text{mole}) (9.92 \text{ moles}) = 2.58 \times 10^2 \text{ g}$

The other three answers are incorrect because: (A) You've used T in degrees Celsius instead of K.

$$n = \frac{(.970 \text{ atm}) (250L)}{(.082L - \text{atm} / K - \text{mole})(25)} = 1.18 \times 10^2 \text{ moles}$$

wt. $= (26.04 \text{ g} / \text{mole}) (1.18 \times 10^2 \text{ moles}) = 3.08 \times 10^3 \text{ g}$

(B) is the number of moles not the weight of the gas. (C) is obtained if the molecular mass is divided by n (instead of multiplied) (units would be wrong).

$$\frac{26.04 \text{ g} / \text{mole}}{9.92 \text{ moles}} = 2.63 \text{ g} / \text{moles}^2$$

120. **(A)**   is the correct answer. Solve for the number of moles and then multiply by the molecular mass.

$(40.0 \text{ L}) (6.00 \text{ moles/L}) = 240 \text{ moles}$

$(36.46 \text{ g/mole}) (240 \text{ moles}) = 8.75 \times 10^3 \text{g}$

The other three answers are incorrect because: (B) is obtained if you assume only 6 moles.

(36.46 g/mole) (6 moles) $= 2.19 \times 10^2$ g

(C) is obtained if you divide the moles by the molecular mass (wrong units).

$$\frac{240 \text{ moles}}{36.46 \text{ g / mole}} = 6.58 \text{ moles}^2 / g$$

(D) if you divide the molecular units by the number of moles.

$$\frac{36.46 \text{ g / mole}}{240 \text{ moles}} = 1.52 \times 10^{-1} \text{ g}$$

121. **(B)**   is the correct answer. Solve for the number of moles and then correct for the stoichiometry of the rxn (1:1 in this case between reactants and products). Finally, multiply by the molecular mass of the product to obtain maximum yield.

$$\frac{41.0 \text{ g}}{26.04 \text{ g / mole}} = 1.57 \text{ moles of } C_2H_2$$

$$\frac{55.0 \text{ g}}{36.46 \text{ g / mole}} = 1.51 \text{ moles of HCl}$$

Since HCl is the limiting reagent there can only be 1.51 moles of product formed.

$$(1.51 \text{ moles HCl}) \left(\frac{1 \text{ mole } C_2H_2Cl}{1 \text{ mole HCl}} \right) (62.5 \text{ g / mole } C_2H_3CCl) = 94.4 \text{ g}$$

The other three answers are incorrect because: **(A)** assumes that you just totalled the weights of the two reacting species.

$$41.0 \text{ g} + 55.0 \text{ g} = 96.0 \text{ g}$$

(C) wrongly uses the number of moles of C_2H_2.

$$(1.57 \text{ moles } C_2H_2) \left(\frac{1 \text{ mole } C_2H_3Cl}{1 \text{ mole HCl}} \right) (62.5 \text{ g / mole } C_2H_3CCl) = 98.1 \text{ g}$$

(D) is obtained if you just say that the number of grams of HCl equals the maximum number of grams of product.

122. **(C)**   is the correct answer. % yield = (actual yield/theo. yield) $\times$ 100%.

$$\frac{49.8 \text{ g}}{66.6 \text{ g}} \times 100\% = 74.8\%$$

The other three answers are incorrect because: **(A)** This isn't multiplied by 100%. **(B)** This was

$$\frac{\text{theoretical yield - actual yield}}{\text{theoretical yield}} \times 100\%.$$

$$\frac{66.6 - 49.8}{66.6} \times 100\% = 25.2\%$$

(D) This is like choice (B); however you have not multiplied by 100%.

123. **(B)** is the correct answer. The new reaction equation is shown below.

$$C_2H_2 + \tfrac{1}{2} Cl_2 \longrightarrow C_2H_3Cl + \text{(non-Cl containing species)}$$

Solve for the number of moles of each reactant to determine limiting reagent. Correct for the stoichiometry to the number of moles and finally calculate the maximum amount.

$$\frac{25.6 \text{ g}}{26.04 \text{ g / mole}} = .984 \text{ moles } C_2H_2$$

$$\frac{10.1 \text{ g}}{70.9 \text{ g / mole}} = .142 \text{ moles } Cl_2$$

Even after correcting for the stoichiometry, Cl_2 is the limiting reagent. Solve for moles of product:

$$(.142 \text{ moles } Cl_2)\left(\frac{2 \text{ moles } C_2H_3Cl}{1 \text{ mole } Cl_2}\right) = .284 \text{ moles } C_2H_3Cl$$

Finally solve the maximal weight:

$$(.284 \text{ moles } C_2H_3Cl) \ (62.5 \text{ g/mole } C_2H_3Cl) = 17.75 \text{ g}$$

The other three answers are incorrect because: (A) is if you used moles of .984 from C_2H_2.

$$(.984 \text{ moles}) \ (62.5 \text{ g/mole}) = 61.5 \text{ g}$$

(C) Since Cl_2 is limiting you have wrongly assumed that it's only the weight of Cl_2 that is maximal. (D) is obtained if you use .142 moles of Cl_2 and do not correct for stoichiometry.

$$(.142 \text{ moles}) \ (62.5 \text{ g/mole}) = 8.88 \text{ g}$$

124. **(B)** is the correct answer. First calculate the mass of carbon and hydrogen knowing that all the carbon will be tied up in the carbon dioxide and the hydrogen will be held up in the water.

$$C_xH_yO_z + O_2 \rightarrow xCO_2 + \frac{y}{2} H_2O$$

$$9.55 \text{ g } CO_2 * \left(\frac{12.01 \text{ g C}}{44.01 \text{ g } CO_2}\right) = 2.61 \text{ g C}$$

$$5.86 \text{ g } H_2O * \left(\frac{2.016 \text{ g HC}}{18.02 \text{ g } H_2O}\right) = 0.6561 \text{ g H}$$

Mass of O: Total mass - (mass of C + mass of H)

$$5.00 \text{ g} - (2.61 \text{ g} + 0.656 \text{ g}) = 1.73 \text{ g O}$$

Next convert to moles:

$$\frac{(2.61 \text{ g C})}{12.01 \text{ g / mole C}} = .217 \text{ moles C}$$

$$\frac{(0.656 \text{ g H})}{1.008 \text{ g / mole H}} = .651 \text{ moles H}$$

$$\frac{(1.73 \text{ g O})}{16.00 \text{ g / mole O}} = .108 \text{ moles O}$$

This yields an empirical formula:

$$C_{.217}H_{.651}O_{.108} \text{ or } C_2H_6O$$

The other three answers are incorrect because: (A) uses 1.008 in the hydrogen calculation giving weights of .328 g for H and 2.06 g for O. This yields an empirical formula of C_2H_3O. (C) is obtained if you followed the mistake in choice (A) but doubled the values for C and H (1.69 and 2.52, respectively) prior to rounding as was done in (A). (D) is obtained if you use 32.00 g/mole in the oxygen moles calculation.

$$\frac{1.739 \text{ g}}{32.00 \text{ g / mole}} = .054 \text{ moles}$$

This yields an empirical formula of $C_4H_{12}O$.

125. **(A)**   is the correct answer. The formula weight of the empirical formula is:

$$\text{F.W.} = 2(12.01) + 3(1.008) + 16.00 = 43.04 \text{ g/mole}$$

To find the molecular formula, divide the formula weight into the molecular weight and use that integer to multiply the subscripts.

$$\frac{86.1 \text{ g / mole}}{43.04 \text{ g / mole}} = 2.0$$

$$(2.0)\,(C_2H_3O) = C_4H_6O_2$$

The other three answers are incorrect because: (B) is the empirical formula, but the molecular weight and formula weight are not equal. (C) has a molecular weight equal to 86.1 g/mole but has the wrong empirical formula (D) See choice (C).

126. **(D)**   is the correct answer. First solve for molality.

$$m = \frac{\Delta T_f}{k_f} = \frac{2.02°\text{C}}{1.86°\text{C / molal}} = 1.09 \text{ molal}$$

Find the number of moles:

$$(1.09 \text{ moles/kg } H_2O)\,(.1 \text{ kg } H_2O) = 1.09 \times 10^{-1} \text{ moles}$$

Calculate molecular weight:

$$\frac{5.00 \text{ g}}{1.09 \times 10^{-1} \text{ moles}} = 46.0 \text{ g / mole}$$

The other three answers are incorrect because: (A) is assuming you do not know $\Delta T_f = k_f m$. Otherwise, there is enough information to solve this problem. (B) is obtained by miscalculating m (inversion of

$$\frac{\Delta T_f}{k_f}$$

— note units would be wrong).

$$m = \frac{k_f}{\Delta T_f} = \frac{1.86°\text{C / molal}}{2.02°\text{C}} = .921°\text{C}^2 \text{ / molal}$$

$$\frac{5.00 \text{ g}}{(.921 \text{ molal}) \ (.1 \text{ kg})} = 54.3 \text{ g / mole}$$

(C) is obtained if you multiply by 1 kg instead of .1 kg.

127. **(D)**   is the correct answer. Osmotic Pressure $\pi = MRT$

$\pi = (1.00 \times 10^{-3} \text{ Molar}) \ (.0821 \text{ L-atm/K-mole}) \ (298 \text{ K}) = .024 \text{ atm.}$

The other three answers are incorrect because: (A) assumes you used $R = 8.314$ although units would be completely off.

$\pi = (1.00 \times 10^{-3} \text{ M}) \ (8.314 \text{ J/K-mole}) \ (298 \text{ K}) = 2.48 \text{ J/L}$

(B) is obtained if you do not convert to 298 K (again units are wrong).

$\pi = (1.00 \times 10^{-3} \text{ M}) \ (.0821 \text{ L-atm/K-mole}) \ (25°\text{C}) = 2.05 \times 10^{-3} \text{ atm } °\text{C/K}$

(C) is obtained if you do both mistakes in (A) and (B) (units are ridiculous).

$\pi = (1.00 \times 10^{-3} \text{ M}) \ (8.314 \text{ J/K-mole}) \ (25°\text{C}) = .021 \text{ J}°\text{C/LK}$

128. **(C)**   is the correct answer. Knowing $\Delta G°_f = \Delta H°_f - T\Delta S°_f$

$\Delta G°_f = -278 \text{ kJ/mole} - (298 \text{ K}) \ (-.346 \text{ kJ/mole K}) = -175 \text{ kJ/mole}$

The other three answers are incorrect because: (A) is obtained if you used $\Delta G°_f = \Delta H°_f + T\Delta S°_f$

$\Delta G°_f = -278 \text{ kJ/mole} + (298 \text{ K}) \ (-.346 \text{ kJ/mole}) = -381 \text{ kJ/mole}$

(B) is obtained if you do not change the units on $\Delta S°_f$

$\Delta G°_f = -278 \text{ kJ/mole} - (298 \text{ K}) \ (-.346 \text{ kJ/mole}) = 1.03 \times 10^5 \text{ kJ/mole}$

(D) is obtained if you made a similar sign error on the 278 kJ/mole for $\Delta H°_f$

$\Delta G°_f = 278 \text{ kJ/mole} - (298 \text{ K}) \ (-.346 \text{ kJ/mole K}) = 381 \text{ kJ /mole}$

129. **(D)**   is the correct answer. By definition the enthalpy of formation is a measure of the energy that is lost or gained when the reactants are the elements in their stable form at room temperature and pressure. Under these conditions all reactants have $\Delta H°_f = 0$ so the sum equals zero. The other three answers are incorrect because: (A) is the negative of the standard formation enthalpy. (B) is the standard enthalpy of formation and is equal to the ΔH of reaction only. (C) is obtained if you divide - 255 kK/mole by the number of unique atoms in the compound (3) = - 85.0 kJ/mole.

130. **(C)**   is the correct answer. The heat of reaction is the change of temperature multiplied by the heat capacity of the bomb calorimeter.

$(6.11 \times 10^4 \text{ J/}°\text{C}) \ (29.55 - 25.00°\text{C}) = 2.78 \times 10^2 \text{ kJ}$

The other three answers are incorrect because: (A) is obtained if you use 29.55 as the temperature difference.

$(6.11 \times 10^4 \text{ J/}°\text{C}) \ (29.55°\text{C}) = 1.81 \times 10^3 \text{ kJ}$

(B) is obtained if you change °C to K (note wrong units).

$$(6.11 \times 10^4 \text{ J/°C}) \, (277 \text{ K}) = 1.70 \times 10^4 \text{ k/°C}$$

(D) is obtained if you divide by the temperature difference (wrong units).

$$(6.11 \times 10^4 \text{ J/°C}) \, / \, 4.55°C = 1.34 \times 10^1 \text{ k/°C}^2$$

131. **(A)**   is the correct answer. In electrolytic cells the cathode, which is negatively charged, gains electrons from solution and shuttles them to the positively charged anode. The other three answers are incorrect because: (B) The salt bridge is often not found in an electrolytic cell but if present only provides ionic conduction through solution. (C) The ions in the solution do move towards the electrodes. However, electrons are not conducted through solution. (D) This answer is exactly opposite to the correct one.

132. **(C)**   is the correct answer. The reaction is $Cu^{2+} + 2e^- \rightarrow Cu^{\circ}_{(s)}$ and it is noted that 1 mole of $Cu_{(s)}$ is produced when 2 moles of e^- are gained.

$$(5.0 \text{ A}) \, (6.0 \text{ hrs}) \left(\frac{3600 \text{ s}}{1 \text{ hr}} \right) = 1.1 \times 10^5 \text{ A} \cdot \text{s} = 1.1 \times 10^5 \text{ C}$$

$$(1.1 \times 10^5 \text{ C}) \left(\frac{1 \text{ mole}^- e^-}{96.500 \text{ C}} \right) = 1.1 \text{ mole } e^-$$

$$(1.1 \text{ mole } e^-) \left(\frac{1 \text{ mole of Cu}}{2 \text{ mole of } e^-} \right) (63.55 \text{ g} / \text{mole Cu}) = 35 \text{ g Cu}$$

The other three answers are incorrect because: (A) is obtained if you assume 1 mole of Cu for 1 mole of e^-.

$$(1.1 \text{ mole } e^-) \left(\frac{1 \text{ mole of Cu}}{2 \text{ mole of } e^-} \right) (63.55 \text{ g} / \text{mole Cu}) = 70 \text{ g}$$

(B) is obtained if you do not correct from hr to sec (note units will be very wrong).

$$\frac{(30 \text{ C})}{96,500 \text{ C}} = 3.1 \times 10^{-4} \text{ mole } e^-$$

$$(3.1 \times 10^{-4} \text{ mole } e^-) \left(\frac{1 \text{ mole Cu}}{2 \text{ mole } e^-} \right) (63.55 \text{ g} / \text{mole Cu}) = 9.9 \times 10^{-3}$$

(D) is obtained if you do not correct using Faraday's Constant (96,500C/mole e^-) (units wrong).

$$(1.1 \times 10^5 \text{ C}) \left(\frac{1 \text{ mole of Cu}}{2 \text{ mole } e^-} \right) (63.55 \text{ g} / \text{mole}) = 3.5 \times 10^6 \text{ g}$$

133. **(D)**   is the correct answer. At the cathode, electrons are transferred into species in solution then leaving behind a (+) charge on the electrode. The opposite occurs on the anode. The other three answers are incorrect because: (A) are the charges that exist on the electrodes in electrolytic cells. (B) The cathode will be

positively charged but the other electrode must have the balancing charge. (C) the anode is never (+) charged and the cathode must have the balancing opposite charge.

134. **(B)** is the correct answer. You must remember that for a galvanic cell to work the sum of the reduction potentials must be positive. Since the concentrations in experiment 2 are 1M this is a standard cell and the cell potential will be the $\varepsilon°$ of the substance reduced - $\varepsilon°$ of the substance oxidized (using standard reduction potentials). The equation is $Cu^{2+} + Ni_{(s)} \rightarrow Cu_{(s)} + Ni^{2+}$.

$$\varepsilon°_{cell} = 0.34 \text{ V} - (- 0.25 \text{ V}) = ^+ 0.59 \text{ V}$$

The other three answers are incorrect because: (A) is obtained if you ignore the presence of the Ni. (C) is obtained if you just subtract the value of the standard reduction potential of Ni^{2+}.

$$\varepsilon°_{cell} = 0.34 \text{ V} - (0.25 \text{ V}) = 0.09 \text{ V}$$

(D) is obtained if you take the negative result outlined in (C).

135. **(C)** is the correct answer. Knowing $\Delta G° = - nF\varepsilon°_{cell}$ yields the correct answer using the values given in the problem.

$$\Delta G° = - (2.0) (96.500C) (0.11V) = - 2.1 \times 10^4 \text{ J}$$

$$= - 2.1 \times 10^1 \text{ kJ}$$

The other three answers are incorrect because: (A) makes a mistake by choosing $n = 1.0$.

$$\Delta G° = - (1.0) (96500C) (0.11V) = - 1.1 \times 10^4 \text{ J}$$

$$= - 1.1 \times 10^1 \text{ kJ}$$

(B) uses $n = 4.0$.

$$\Delta G° = - (4.0) (96500C) (0.11V) = - 4.2 \times 10^4 \text{ J}$$

$$= - 4.2 \times 10^1 \text{ kJ}$$

(D) uses $n = 1.0$ and $V = - 0.11 V$.

$$\Delta G° = - (1.0) (96500C) (-0.11V) = - 1.1 \times 10^4 \text{ J}$$

$$= - 1.1 \times 10^1 \text{ kJ}$$

136. **(D)** is the correct answer. If the galvanic cell reaction were written out it looks as follows:

$$Sn^{2+} + Ni_{(s)} \rightarrow Ni^{2+} + Sn_{(s)}$$

This yields a

$$Q = \frac{[Ni^{2+}]}{[Sn^{2+}]} .$$

The other three answers are incorrect because: (A) is the inverse of the correct answer. (B) includes the solid terms which do not belong in the expression for Q. (C) uses the solid terms, which is wrong since solids change their concentrations very little.

137. **(A)** is the correct answer. Using the Nernst equation yields the answer where

$$Q = \frac{[Ni^{2+}]}{[Sn^{2+}]} \ .$$

$$\varepsilon_{cell} = \varepsilon^{\circ}{}_{cell} -2.303 RT \, / \, nF \log Q$$

$$\varepsilon_{cell} = 0.11V - \frac{2.303(8.314 \text{ J} / \text{K - mole}) \ (298 \text{ K})}{(2) \ (96,500 \text{ C})} \log\!\left(\frac{.50}{.10}\right)$$

$$\varepsilon_{cell} = 0.09V$$

The other three answers are incorrect because: (B) uses $n = 1$, instead of 2, in the calculation.

$$\varepsilon_{cell} = 0.07 \text{ V}$$

(C) uses $T = 25°C$, rather than 298 K (note the wrong units).

$$\varepsilon_{cell} = 0.11 \text{ V}$$

(D) uses $1/Q$ rather than the correct Q.

$$\varepsilon_{cell} = 0.13 \text{ V}$$

138. **(B)** is the correct answer. $\Delta G^{\circ} = - RT \ln K_c$ is the operative equation and can be rearranged to solve for K_c.

$$K_c = e^{\frac{-\Delta G^{\circ}}{RT}} = e^{-\left(\frac{-2.3 \times 10^4 \text{ J/mole}}{8.314 \text{ J/K-mole} * 298\text{K}}\right)}$$

$$K_c = 1.1 \times 10^4$$

The other three answers are incorrect because: (A) is obtained if you use $R = 0.0821$, instead of $R = 8.314$ (note the wrong units), and use the negative value of ΔG°.

$$K_c = 0.0$$

(C) is obtained if you use the negative of the value for ΔG° (note wrong units in ΔG°).

$$e^{-\left(\frac{2.3 \times 10^1 \text{ kJ/mole}}{(8.314 \text{ J/K-mole})(298\text{K})}\right)} = 1.0$$

(D) is obtained if you use the negative of the value for ΔG° using correct units.

$$e^{-\left(\frac{2.3 \times 10^4 \text{ J/mole}}{(8.314 \text{ J/K-mole})(298\text{K})}\right)} = 9.3 \times 10^{-5}$$

139. **(C)** When the center of negative charge does not coincide with the center of positive charge in a molecule, it is said to be polar. The molecule constitutes a dipole: two equal and opposite charges separated in space. The molecule possesses a

dipole moment which is equal to the magnitude of the charge multiplied by the distance between the centers of charge.

In E-1, 2-dibromoethene,

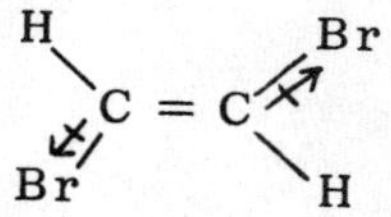

the dipole moment is zero; the individual bonds are polar but because of the symmetrical arrangement, they exactly cancel each other out. So, the dipole moment of a molecule depends not only upon the polarity of its individual bonds but also upon the way the bonds are directed, that is, upon the shape of the molecule. In carbon tetrachloride,

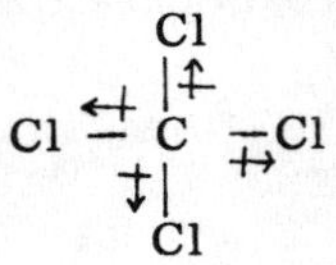

the individual bonds are also polar but they cancel each other out because of the symmetrical arrangement of the molecule.

In Z-1, 2-dichloroethene,

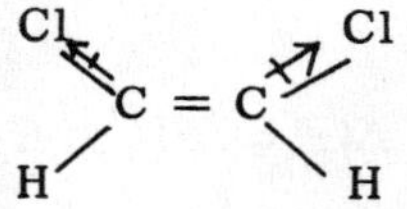

the individual bonds are polar and do not cancel each other out by the symmetrical arrangement of the dipoles. Therefore, Z-1, 2-dichloroethene has a net dipole moment.

140. **(D)** Power is defined as work divided by time,

$$P = \frac{W}{t}$$

and $W = Fs$ (where F and s are in the same direction, and are force and distance respectively). Then,

$$P = \frac{Fs}{t} \quad \text{and since} \quad \frac{s}{t} = v$$

$P = Fv$.

The force of friction can be calculated from $F = \mu N$, where μ is the coefficient of rolling friction and N is the normal force:

$$F = 0.005 \times (200 \text{ tons} \times 2000 \text{ lb/ton}) = 2000 \text{ lb}$$

Using $P = Fv$ from above, and the conversion factor $\left[\dfrac{550 \text{ ft} \cdot \text{lb} / \text{sec}}{1 \text{ hp}}\right]$ to convert 400 hp to power in units ft·lb/sec, we can find

$$400 \text{ hp } (550 \text{ ft·lb/sec/hp}) = 2000 \text{ lb} \times v$$

$$v = 110 \text{ ft/sec} = 75 \text{ mi/hr}.$$

141. **(A)** We know that 1 hp = 550 ft-lb/sec. In order to solve for horsepower in this problem we must get the units correct:

$$\left(45\,\frac{mi}{hr}\right)\left(\frac{1\ hr}{60\ min}\right)\left(\frac{1\ min}{60\ sec}\right)\left(\frac{5280\ ft}{1\ mi}\right)\times\left(\frac{200\ tons}{}\right)\left(\frac{2000\ lbs}{1\ ton}\right)\left(\frac{.005}{lb}\right)$$

$$132,000\,\frac{ft\text{-}lb}{sec}\left(\frac{1\ hp}{550\,\frac{ft\text{-}lb}{sec}}\right)=240\ hp$$

142. **(C)** Force can be calculated from the expression for power: $P = Fv$. Converting horsepower to ft-lb/sec, we have:

$$P = 240\ hp\times550\,\frac{ft\text{-}lb}{(sec)(hp)}=132,000\ ft\text{-}lb/sec$$

Since 60 mph = 88 ft/sec, 45 mph = 66 ft/sec. Then

$P = Fv$

132,000 ft-lb/sec = F(66 ft/sec)

F = 2,000 lbs.

Section 3 — Writing Sample

DEMONSTRATION ESSAY 1

At first glance, William James's observation about happiness, "One could not accept a happiness shared with millions if the condition of that happiness were the suffering of one lonely soul," sounds perfectly clear and agreeable. However, if one were to probe the statement at its limits, a few surprising thoughts appear. These thoughts suggest that while we may believe we act according to the statement, many of us derive happiness from the suffering of others.

Consider for a moment the statement's obvious meaning. No rational person would likely disagree with its premise. We prefer to think that any happiness we might receive from life should not be purchased at the expense of others. Most reasonable people try to live their lives without causing others to suffer. When we drive our automobiles, we try to take appropriate care so that we do not cause accidents that injure other people. In our work, we derive satisfaction, if not happiness, from a job well done and give credit, for help, to our colleagues who deserve it. When we go to a social event, we try to find happiness by enjoying the company of our friends or new acquaintances. In our personal relationships, we try to treat those we care about with concern, love, and dignity. All of these behaviors contribute to a sense of happiness in life that we gain through personal attributes, relationships with other people, and courteous and tactful treatment of others.

All well and good, but consider how each of the instances previously described could, in fact, involve "the suffering of one lonely soul" or of many other souls. Driving an automobile seems innocuous enough, but what happens if at that social event we imbibed too many mugs of beer? Perhaps we drive away drunk and smash another person's life to bits. Sure, we were happy at the party, even when we drove away. But we just didn't think we would cause such an "accident." Likewise, many of us feel we need to dominate other people in our personal relationships, which results in our own happiness. Doesn't it make us feel good (and happy?) when we beat our best friend at tennis? Or more darkly, we hear of, and perhaps know, people who derive their happiness from physical violence directed at a spouse or child. How about people at work? Don't we hear and perhaps know of people who gloat over their latest conquest? So what if one saves his six-figure a year income by crushing a union or by closing a plant and throwing workers into unemployment and suffering? So what if we work for a company we know is dumping toxic wastes that could cause people to suffer? That's not our problem. So what if these radioactive wastes from medical procedures end up in a dump in Mexico? We don't think we cause such things to happen, but we comply with them by not trying to stop such behavior.

So, what are we to do to live in a hostile, competitive world, one which may not allow us all that much opportunity to find happiness in the first place? We must first look to ourselves to discover our own identity so that we have a basis from which to act. We hope to find a humane self in various roles we play. We also can work toward particular outcomes. We can try to think ahead to look to the consequences of our actions. We can investigate both our own behavior and that of our work places and institutions to try to prevent inhumane acts from occurring. In short, we should discover our own ideals, form values from them that we can practice in an imperfect world, and be aware of the effects of our behavior.

From these basic and relatively simple steps we can derive a happiness based on a clear conscience. We can try to avoid a happiness purchased by the suffering of others. One embarking on such a task of self discovery and application of values will find the journey a difficult one. But, we can find true happiness only if we look for it and overcome the obstacles and temptations that cause—directly or indirectly—the sufferings of others.

EXPLANATION OF ESSAY

The paper as a whole focuses clearly on the topic defined by the statement and fully addresses each of the three writing tasks in the directions. The first paragraph announces the thesis or central idea of the whole piece quite clearly. Paragraph 2 responds to the first task ("Explain what you think the statement means"); Paragraph 3 responds to the second task ("Describe a specific situation in which people do accept happiness based on the suffering of others"); and Paragraphs 4 and 5 respond to the third task ("Discuss the criteria under which one could find happiness without causing the suffering of others").

The paper skates on relatively thin ice as it develops the topic and the implications of it in a reasonably thoughtful manner. Particularly toward the end, it almost edges into triteness or ignorant optimism. Nonetheless, the paper addresses the issues squarely and at a deep enough level (for a thirty-minute essay) to succeed. Notice how it develops a contrast between expected responses and how the expected sometimes is actually the unexpected. The development stays at a specific level, even though it drops to the very concrete level of example and illustration only once (the "dump in Mexico"). Even so, its development clearly addresses the topic on a level that explains the meanings needed. The last two paragraphs synthesize the apparent conflict with a discussion of the basis upon which one should try to achieve happiness without causing others to suffer.

One of the strengths of the essay is its unity and coherence. The essay never strays from the topic (and the tasks required) and connects the parts logically so that there is a smooth flow of thought. Each paragraph holds together around its topic, and each one also relates directly to the central idea. Transitions of various kinds (e.g., repetition of "consider" in Paragraphs 1 and 2; transitional words like "so") aid sentence-to-sentence and paragraph-to-paragraph coherence.

While the paper does not demonstrate flashes of brilliance in style and usage, it does use language appropriately and effectively. Sentence structures clarify and communicate, rather than obfuscate. Sentence variety makes the paper easy to read. A series of questions changes the pace of the essay (although this tactic can backfire, so be careful here). Occasional concrete word choices ("smash another person's life to bits") enliven the prose, as does the overall conversational tone. No significant grammar or mechanics (spelling, punctuation) errors appear.

DEMONSTRATION ESSAY 2

Good families seem to occur few and far between if we believe what we read and hear in the media and in sociological studies. Rapid changes occur in modern cultures, and the family, as an institution, has not escaped the ravages of change. Jane Howard's pithy observation in *Families* (1978), "Good families are much to all their members, but everything to none," sounds like an accurate description of a family as we approach the dawn of a new century.

Ms. Howard's comment, we should note, does limit itself to "good" families; but even so, it speaks volumes to us. Good families provide a host of things to each one of their members. People derive their basic values, their customs, their rituals, their hopes for the future from their parents, which they, in turn, derived from their parents, and so on, back to the earliest ancestors. The largest part of one's being—from the genetic and molecular level, to the social and cultural environment—devolves from the family. A family provides one with a beginning—a start in life, both biologically and socially. The parent derives satisfaction from passing on both genes and values to the next generation. So in that sense families, good or bad, "are much to all their members."

The corollary phrase, "but everything to none," sounds contradictory, but appropriate, and even necessary. All families should prepare their young to mature and strike out on their own. Good families take that process further by actively encouraging young people to discover their identities, to make decisions, to act appropriately in social settings, to find a vocation, and to find their own future relationships. At some point in the maturing process, all children need to declare independence from their parents. Eventually they begin their own families—in whatever shape or form.

We know, of course, that many people do not have good biological or foster families. At different times in life, all people turn outward from their family for certain things even good families cannot provide. At the extreme, we find youths joining gangs which become surrogate families. These surrogate families provide *everything* the member needs—at least to that individual. Security of a sort, love of a sort, stability of a sort, even income and sustenance of a sort (often illegally obtained), all come from the gang. To gang members, no doubt, it feels as though their surrogate families provide everything. One can argue that such members deceive themselves and that these surrogate families are anything but good, however, the members feel differently. Legitimate organizations often provide virtually the same surrogate feelings for children and adults. I can remember that the Boy Scouts and, later, the Explorers, provided such a surrogate family for me. My college dormitory floor also provided a sense of family and community that seemed everything I needed at the time.

To return to Ms. Howard's original point, however, we notice that these surrogate families really do not always provide all the needs of their members. Some surrogates even contribute to the destruction of the individual; this is especially true of gangs. These surrogates—like some biological families—may encourage role playing, immaturity, and allegiance to the group over all, rather than their opposites. So a "family"—surrogate or biological—does not necessarily constitute a "good" one. A good family recognizes and instills its values within its members, but it also recognizes the need for the individual to become independent. Hitler's Nazis and the Mafia both provided strong values for their members. But, they both also required absolute allegiance to the group (family). No inconveniences, such as conscience, can intervene with group allegiance. Good families, on the other hand, nurture their members without demanding absolute allegiance. They pass on humane values of love and respect for all, especially the family, and also for others. In that respect, the biblical Abraham may have failed his earthly family while attempting to obey his God. Likewise, when we read of families beating their children because of allegiance to another group's—often religious—values, we certainly have to question their notions of "family."

It remains, finally, not quite as easy a task, as originally thought, to decide what good families do. Many families ignore, or neglect, their duties even though they have the best of values at heart and the best of intentions in mind. Other activities—work, club, group—or duties interfere, perhaps. Unfortunately, this often results in a family providing little to all its members or nothing to some.

EXPLANATION OF ESSAY

The paper as a whole focuses clearly on the topic defined by the statement and fully addresses each of the three writing tasks in the directions. The first paragraph announces the thesis or central idea of the whole piece quite clearly. Paragraphs 2 and 3 respond to the first task ("Explain what you think the statement means"); Paragraph 4 responds to the second task ("Describe a specific situation in which the good family *may be* everything to its members"); and Paragraphs 4, 5, and 6 respond to the third task ("Discuss the criteria implied in the statement in order to have a 'good' family, and suggest how groups other than biological or foster families may be considered families").

The paper develops the topic, and the implications of it, in a reasonably thoughtful manner. Particularly toward the end, it almost seems to lose its direction because it mixes biological family and other groups in the same breath. Nonetheless, the paper addresses the issues squarely and at a deep enough level (for a thirty-minute essay) to succeed. Notice how it develops a contrast between biological families and surrogate families, such as gangs. The development stays at a specific level, even though it drops to the very concrete level of example and illustration twice: one, the personal experience of the writer (Scouts, dormitory); and two, near the end (Hitler, the Mafia, Abraham). Even so, its development clearly addresses the topic on a level that explains the meanings needed. The last two paragraphs synthesize the apparent differences as well as can reasonably be expected, within the time limit.

One of the strengths of the essay is its unity and coherence. The essay never strays from the topic (and the tasks required) and connects the parts logically so that there is a smooth flow of thought. Each paragraph holds together around its topic, and each one also relates directly to the central idea. Transitions of various kinds (e.g., repetition of "surrogate" and other phrases in Paragraphs 2 through 5; transitional words like "finally") aid sentence-to-sentence and paragraph-to-paragraph coherence.

The paper demonstrates some flashes of brilliance in style and usage ("pithy" in Paragraph 1, the last sentence of the essay), and it uses language appropriately and effectively throughout except that some of the repetitions mentioned, as transitions, actually seem unnecessarily repetitious. Sentence structures clarify and communicate, rather than obfuscate; however, the writer tends to overuse sentence interruptions, especially with the dash. Overall, sentence variety makes the paper easy to ready. Word choice in general seems appropriate to the tone and content level. No significant grammar or mechanics (spelling, punctuation) errors appear.

Section 4 — Biological Sciences

143. **(B)**   The correct answer is (B), as was stated early in the above paragraph. Active transport requires a fair amount of energy to be exerted by the cell, but passive transport still requires the molecules to have some minimal activation energy. Hence, choice (A) is wrong. Polar molecules pass through the lipoid layer without problem but require energy to leave it and enter the cytoplasm. Hence, (C) is incorrect. (D) is also wrong, since as was stated in the paragraph, even when going *with* a concentration gradient, a minimal activation energy is needed.

144. **(B)**   The correct answer is (B). Since this molecule is lipid soluble, it will be difficult to leave the lipoidal membrane and enter the aqueous cytoplasm. For the very reason (B) is correct, (A) is incorrect, as it will be easy for the molecule to leave an aqueous phase and enter a lipoidal one. (C) is incorrect since the molecule will have no trouble passing through the lipoidal layer. For this reason, (D) is also incorrect. Were the molecule of interest water soluble, the situation would be reversed.

145. **(D)**   The correct answer is (D), since propanol has half of the hydrogen bonds of the propandiols. These bonds must be broken before it can pass into the lipoidal membrane. (A) is wrong since all of these have -OH groups. (B) is wrong since these are all polar molecules, otherwise hydrogen bonding could not occur. (C) is wrong because all of the compounds in question have three carbons.

146. **(C)**   The correct answer is (C), decanol. (A) is wrong because water is very polar, and hence could not pass through the membrane easily. The remaining three choices are alcohols. Recall that the more carbons an alcohol has, the less it will behave as an alcohol, and the more it will resemble its analogous alkane. Hence, decanol, with ten carbons will behave much like decane, which is nonpolar, and therefore can easily pass through the lipoidal membrane.

147. **(A)**   The correct answer is (A). Thiourea is much more water soluble, hence it is more difficult for it to travel through the membrane. Although (B) is true, the difference in masses is so slight that it cannot explain this great of an energy difference. (C) might be true, but again the energy difference cannot be due totally to this. (D) is not correct because there is a possible explanation.

148. **(A)**   The correct answer is (A). KOH absorbs CO_2 and produces potassium bicarbonate ($KHCO_3$). (B) and (C) are wrong, as a high or low pH can be damaging

to living cells. Additionally (C) is also wrong since KOH cannot lower pH. (D) is wrong because, although potassium can be a nutrient, in the form of KOH, it is usually caustic.

149. **(C)**   The correct answer is (C). Changes in temperature will cause changes in the volume of the gases in the capillary tubing. Flask A will experience the same temperature changes. Hence, since they are on the other side of the bubble, they will cancel any temperature changes on the side of the cells. For this reason, the other choices are incorrect.

150. **(C)**   The correct answer is (C). As oxygen is consumed, carbon dioxide is produced, which is absorbed by the KOH, resulting in a decrease in volume. This will cause the bubble to move toward the cells. All other choices are true. (A) was covered in the above question. The fact that this apparatus has air-tight seals shows (B) to be true. (D) is simply taken from the volume of a cylinder.

151. **(A)**   The correct answer is (A). Yeast prefer to grow aerobically, and would require a great deal of oxygen if they were in rapid growth. The other choices would all require oxygen, but not nearly as much as choice (A).

152. **(B)**   The correct answer is (B). As the CO_2 is used, O_2 is produced, which when absorbed, results in a decrease in volume. (A) is wrong since photosynthesis cannot occur in the dark. (C) is wrong since the type of drop makes no difference (mercury is heavier, and not as sensitive to changes, as is kerosene). (D) is wrong for obvious reasons.

153. **(A)**   The correct answer is (A). The volume of a cylinder $= 1 \cdot \pi \cdot r^2$. The given diameter must be converted to radius ($\frac{1}{2}$ d = r). Converting the values in mm to cm, this gives a volume in cm^3, which is converted to liters by dividing by 1,000. If one forgets to convert to cm, one ends up with choice (B). Forgetting to change diameter to radius yields (C). (D) is wrong for a number of reasons.

154. **(C)**   The correct answer is (C). Many structures are mentioned as having borderline visibility with the resolving power of a light microscope. (A) is wrong, because although it is thought that spirochetes living symbiotically with other cells evolved into eukaryotic flagella, this is not brought up in the passage. (B) is wrong since bacteria lack nuclei and mitochondria. (D) is wrong because dark-field microscopy tells nothing of internal structures, although it is useful for sizing spirochetes.

155. **(D)**   The correct answer is (D). The axial filaments are mentioned in the passage, which also mentions at the beginning that they are non-photosynthetic and non-chemosynthetic, hence they must be heterotrophic. Answer (C) is wrong since many are free-living.

156. **(B)**   The correct answer is (B), as is mentioned in the text. All other choices are true, as is mentioned in the text.

157. **(D)**   The correct answer is (D). Look at the table to confirm this answer choice.

158. **(B)** The correct answer is (B). Look at the dimensions given in the chart. This genus is so large that it can easily be seen under the high power lens of a microscope.

159. **(D)** The genetic code is
(1) *commaless* because punctuation between nucleotides is unnecessary.
(2) *non-overlapping* because each nucleotide is part of only one codon.
(3) *degenerate* because an amino acid sequence may be specified by more than one codon.

160. **(B)** There is no centrosome present in a prophase chromosome.

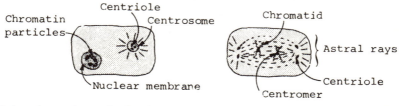

Interphase in animal mitosis   Prophase in animal mitosis without centrosome

161. **(D)** First, we must find the percentage of albinos in the population:

$^{18}/_{200} \times 100 = 9\%$

We know that albinism is the homozygous recessive trait (aa), so to find the frequency of the recessive allele, a, we take the square root of 9% (0.09) = $\sqrt{0.09}$ = 0.30. We also know that the frequency if the recessive allele (a) added to the frequency of the dominant allele (A) must equal 1. Thus, the frequency of the non-albino allele is 1 - 0.30 = 0.70. Squaring the frequency of the non-albino allele will give us the frequency of homozygous non-albinos (AA).

$(0.70)^2 = 0.49$ or 49%.

Then we multiply 0.49 × 200 and see that there are 98 homozygous dominant non-albinos (AA).

162. **(A)** The primitive atmosphere had essentially no free oxygen. All oxygen present was in the form of water and oxides.

163. **(B)** Ethers have the general formula R-O-R´, where R can be aryl and/or alkyl. Ethers can be formed by two alcohol molecules in the presence of a strong acid to release a water molecule. This is called acid-catalyzed dehydration of alcohols in the formation of ethers.
    The mechanism of this reaction resembles that of substitution. It involves the protonation of one alcohol and release of a water molecule to form a carbonium ion. A carbonium ion is a strong electrophile. It attacks the electron-rich oxygen of another alcohol, which releases a proton to form an ether:

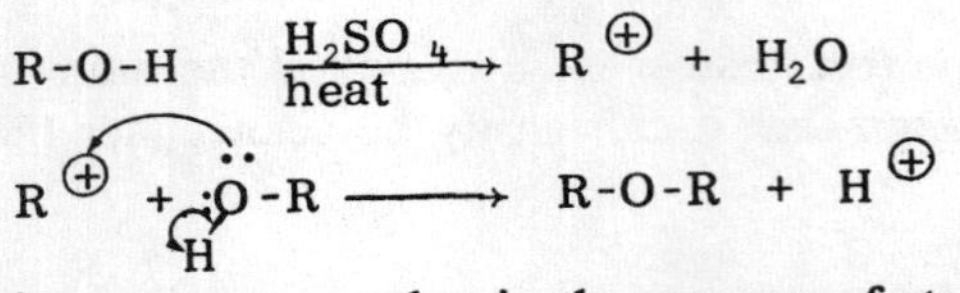

$$R-O-H \xrightarrow[\text{heat}]{H_2SO_4} R^{\oplus} + H_2O$$

$$R^{\oplus} + \overset{..}{\underset{H}{\overset{\frown\frown}{:O}}}-R \longrightarrow R-O-R + H^{\oplus}$$

Under closer scrunity, one can see that in the process of strong acid protonation of an alcohol, another reaction can occur instead of the substitution attack on another alcohol. A carbonium ion is a highly reactive species and can participate in a substitution reaction, as in ether formation, or undergo an elimination reaction to form an alkene. The latter reaction is most prominent for tertiary alcohols,

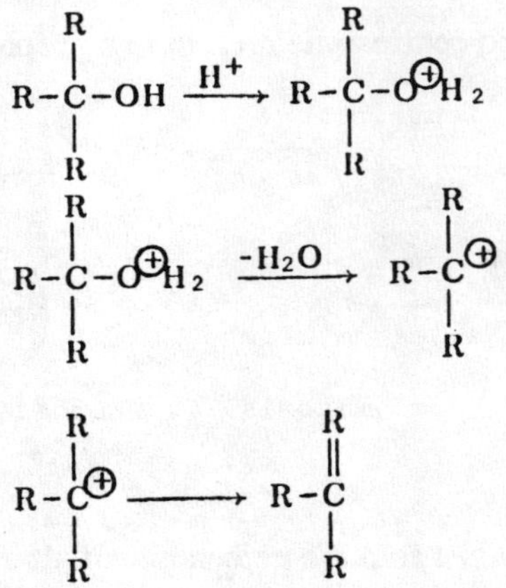

$$\underset{\overset{|}{R}}{\overset{\overset{R}{|}}{R-C-OH}} \xrightarrow{H^+} \underset{\overset{|}{R}}{\overset{\overset{R}{|}}{R-C-\overset{\oplus}{O}H_2}}$$

$$\underset{\overset{|}{R}}{\overset{\overset{R}{|}}{R-C-\overset{\oplus}{O}H_2}} \xrightarrow{-H_2O} \underset{\overset{|}{R}}{\overset{\overset{R}{|}}{R-\overset{\oplus}{C}}}$$

$$\underset{\overset{|}{R}}{\overset{\overset{R}{|}}{R-\overset{\oplus}{C}}} \longrightarrow \underset{\overset{|}{R}}{\overset{\overset{R}{||}}{R-C}}$$

164. **(C)**   Tertiary alcohols react most rapidly by the S_N1 mechanism because they form the relatively stable tertiary carbonium ion. The acid protonates the OH group of the alcohol thus making it a better leaving group. This leaves the iodide to react with the carbonium ion to produce the tertiary alkyl halide. The reaction mechanism (S_N1) involved is illustrated below.

$$(CH_3)_3COH \xrightarrow{H^+} (CH_3)_3CO^+H_2$$

$$(CH_3)_3CO^+H_2 \xrightarrow{-H_2O} (CH_3)_3C^+$$

$$(CH_3)_3C^+ \xrightarrow{I^-} (CH_3)_3CI$$

165. **(A)**   The correct answer is (A). Since both traits are recessive, the individual must be homozygous for both of them to display both of them. Choices (B) and (C) would appear as a totally unshaded figure.

166. **(B)**   The correct answer is (B). Because the figure is unshaded, it means this male individual has at least one dominant gene A and B. The fact that he has produced offspring showing traits a and b means that he must be heterozygous. The same holds true for A2.

167. **(D)**   The correct answer is (D). B2 could be AABB, AaBB, AABb, or AaBb. The fact that she has produced five offspring without either trait a or b, supports the probability that she is homozygous normal for both traits, but does not

prove it. Had her husband displayed one or both of the traits, it would have helped, but his genotype is unknown.

168. **(B)**   The correct answer is (B). This person displays no traits, yet has produced a son with traits a and b, and a daughter with trait a, hence he must be heterozygous for both traits.

169. **(A)**   The correct answer is (A). Since the individual displays trait b, he must be homozygous for it. Since trait a is not displayed, he can be either homo- or heterozygous normal, i.e., AAbb or Aabb. Since he has a son that has trait a, he must be heterozygous for that trait, i.e., Aabb.

170. **(C)**   The correct answer is (C). Since she displays trait a, she must be homozygous for it. She does not display trait b, so she could be homo- or heterozygous normal, i.e., aaBb or aaBB. However, she has produced a son with trait b, hence she must be heterozygous normal, i.e., aaBb.

171. **(D)**   The correct answer is (D). One can perform a variety of probability calculations, however, if one is logical and were C13 Aabb, he would display trait b. Since he does not, he cannot possibly be this genotype. There is a 67% chance of him being AaBb, and a 33% chance of his being AaBB.

172. **(B)**   The correct answer is (B). Only one of the parents have trait C/c, yet all of their children display it. With the cross between B1 and B2, half of the offspring show the trait, which would be expected of a homozygous mated with a heterozygous. The cross between B6 and B7 further supports this. The mating between B10 and B11, who both show the trait, produces children that do not have it, further supporting the idea that the normal condition is recessive. Hence CC or Cc will show trait C/c. cc will be normal.

173. **(A)**   The correct answer is (A). To show the trait, he can be either CC or Cc. Since he has produced normal children, he must be heterozygous, or Cc.

174. **(B)**   The correct answer is (B). Since this is a dominant trait, the fact that A2 is normal with respect to C/c indicates that he must be homozygous normal, or cc.

175. **(D)**   The correct answer is (D). A1 can be either CC or Cc. The fact that all of her children display trait C/c, even though her husband does not, indicates that she might be CC, but does not prove it. However, were she to only have one child without the trait, it would prove her to be Cc.

176. **(B)**   The correct answer is (B). This person is normal with respect to C/c, hence he must be cc, the recessive condition.

177. **(A)**   The correct answer is (A). It appears to be passed on from one male to all of his sons. Were it on the X chromosome, it would not show up this way, since a son receives his only X chromosome from his mother.

178. **(C)** The correct answer is (C). Since a male only has one Y chromosome, he can be neither homo- nor heterozygous for a gene found for it; thus he is called hemizygous. In this case, a person with one gene, D, would display trait D, a person with one gene, d, would be normal. A female, obviously, would have neither gene D nor d, since she would lack a Y chromosome.

179. **(C)** The correct answer is (C), for the same reason as in 178. Any male will be hemizygous for either D or d.

180. **(C)** The correct answer is (C). Since the person does not show the dominant trait C/c, he must be homozygous normal, i.e., cc. Since trait D is shown, and is on the Y chromosome, he is hemizygous for it, or D. This results in ccD.

181. **(C)** The correct answer is (C). Since B11 displays trait C/c, he could be either Cc or CC. However, since he has produced children without the dominant trait C/c, he must be heterozygous, i.e., Cc. He does not show the trait D, therefore his Y chromosome must have the normal gene, d. This results with Ccd.

182. **(A)** The correct answer is (A). Ozoneolysis will oxidize alkenes to aldehydes. In the case of a cyclic alkene, the ring structure is broken and two carbonyl groups are formed, one on each of the carbons that previously held the double-bond.

183. **(B)** The correct answer is (B). $KMnO_4$ will oxidize an alkene to a carboxylic acid. In the case of a cyclic alkene, the ring structure is broken and two carboxylic acid groups are formed, one on each of the carbons that previously held the double-bond. In this case, adipic acid (or by IUPAC, hexanedioic acid) is formed.

184. **(B)** The correct answer is (B). The solution above is known as *"Tollens Reagent"*, and is a test for aldehydes. The presence of aldehydes cause the silver to precipitate out of solution, and form a silver mirror, by the reaction: $RCHO + 2Ag(NH_3)_2OH \rightarrow 2Ag\downarrow + RCOONH_4 + H_2O + 3NH_3$.

185. **(B)** The correct answer is (B). Carboxylic acids are soluble in bases, and that one of the characteristic identity tests for that class of organic compounds.

186. **(A)** The correct answer is (A). $KMnO_4$ will further oxidize an aldehyde to a carboxylic acid.

187. **(C)** The correct answer is (C). Reacting a carboxylic acid with $SOCl_2$ and then with NH_3 produces an amide. (In this case the amide has the formula $H_2NOOC(CH_2)COONH_2$.) Amides are soluble in acidic solution.

188. **(A)** The correct answer is (A). All cells contain DNA. Neurons do not normally divide in adults, hence (B) is wrong, nor do they synthesize protein (which would require RNA, not DNA), hence (D) is also wrong. Memory is thought to be stored in RNA, not DNA, hence (C) is also wrong.

189. **(D)** The correct choice is (D). There are not enough other mammals on the graph to determine this.

190. **(C)**   The correct answer is (C). This is the point where the two lines diverge. If the logarithmic nature of the graph is neglected, (D) is obtained.

191. **(A)**   The correct answer is (A). Intracellular materials begin to change as soon as a cell dies. The shorter the time between cellular death and whatever experimental parameters are measured, the better. To a lesser extent diet (B), and to an even lesser extent temperature (C), might be able to influence DNA content, but these are slight enough to be neglected. RNA can readily be differentiated from DNA, so choice (D) is also incorrect.

192. **(C)**   The correct answer is (C). The graph contains data from fetal life through adulthood, hence the ratio of cells in the cerebrum (via DNA) can be measured against total body mass at any stage in development. For this reason all other choices are wrong.

193. **(B)**   Fats are triacyglycerols, that is, they are carboxylic esters derived from glycerol, $HOCH_2CHOHCH_2OH$. Fats have the general structure:

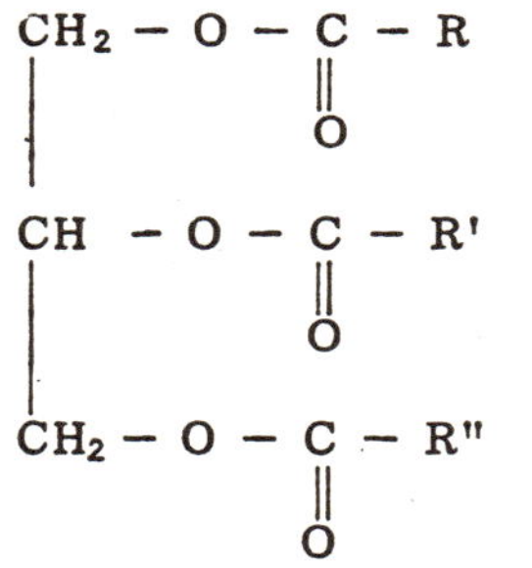

$$CH_2 - O - C - R$$
$$\qquad\qquad \| $$
$$\qquad\qquad O$$

$$CH \; - O - C - R'$$
$$\qquad\qquad \| $$
$$\qquad\qquad O$$

$$CH_2 - O - C - R''$$
$$\qquad\qquad \| $$
$$\qquad\qquad O$$

194. **(A)**   A racemic mixture is obtained by mixing equal quantities of each member of a pair of enantiomers. For a pair of enantiomers to exist, a compound must have a chiral carbon, that is, a carbon atom bonded to four different things. It must also have a non-superimposable mirror image, however, it can have neither a plane nor center of symmetry. Examining (A), we find that there are two chiral carbons in the molecule (labeled 1 and 2) depicted in the accompanying diagram, and that the molecule does have a non-superimposable mirror image. Also, the compound does not have a plane or center of symmetry:

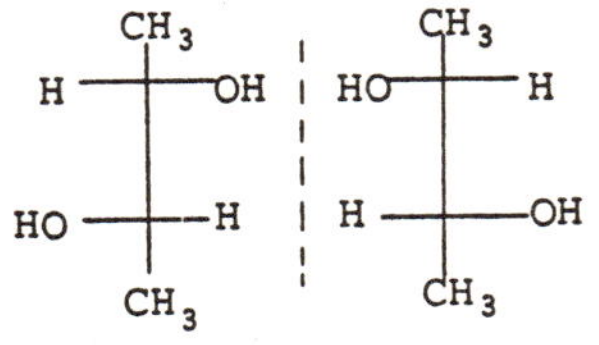

Therefore, this compound is capable of producing a racemic mixture. Choice (B) does not have a chiral carbon—two identical substituents are bonded to it. Therefore it is incapable of producing a racemic mixture. Choice (C) has a plane of symmetry, therefore it cannot comprise a racemate.

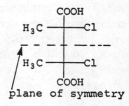

Choice (D) also has a plane of symmetry.

195. **(B)** Through the process of photosynthesis, which only green plants can perform, food can be made by reacting carbon dioxide and water to form carbohydrates.

$$6CO_2 + 12H_2O \xrightarrow[\text{chlorophyl, ATP, and enzymes}]{\text{red, blue, violet light}}$$

$C_6H_{12}O_6 + 6H_2O + 6O_2$
(carbohydrate)

Summary OF Photosynthesis

196. **(C)** Only the hyoid, which is a very small bone near the base of the tongue, is not a part of the human ear. The tectorial membrane is part of the cochlea which is in the inner ear. The oval window is a membrane which separates the middle ear and the inner ear. The malleus is one of the small bones in the middle ear which conducts sound.

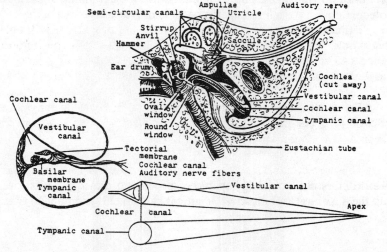

197. **(C)** The fovea consists of both rods which are used to detect objects in poor illumination and for night vision and cones, which are the photoreceptors for day vision and are used to perceive colors. There are more cones than rods because more vision in humans takes place in the daytime or in well lit environments.

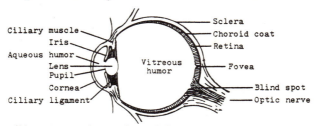

Diagrammatic section of the human eye.

198. **(D)** The correct response is (D). The response of the material to extreme temperatures and pH, as well as its specificity, indicate that it is an enzyme. An enzyme is a special type of catalyst made of protein; hence, all three choices are correct. In this case the enzyme is tyrosinase.

199. **(D)** The correct response is (D). Of the pH's tested, it worked best at pH 4. However, not enough data points were gathered to tell if this was optimum. It could work even better at a pH of 3, or 5, for example. However, it did work best within the acidic range.

200. **(A)** The correct response is (A). Boiling denatures proteins and is not reversible (one cannot unboil an egg!). An inorganic catalyst can be boiled without harm.

201. **(C)** The correct answer is (C). The phenylthiourea was binding with the tyrosinase (enzyme), so it could not interact with the pyrocathechol (substrate).

202. **(D)** The correct response is (D). Since the inhibitor locks onto the enzyme (phenylthiourea and tyrosinase (potato juice), respectively), adding more enzyme until the inhibitor is tied up will allow any additional enzyme added to react with the substrate. Adding more substrate (C) will do no good, since the enzyme is tied up. Adding more inhibitor (B) will certainly do no good, as would boiling (A).

203. **(B)** The correct response is (B). Remember that an enzyme will not cause a reaction that would not naturally occur. It simply helps it attain equilibrium faster. Hence, choice (A) is not correct. An enzyme does not chemically react with the substrate, and hence can be used over and over. This rules out choice (C).

204. **(B)** The correct answer is (B). Remember, a catalyst, or enzyme, will not cause a reaction to occur that would not occur on its own. The pyrocathechol will turn yellow on its own, but it will take a long, long time.

205. **(A)** The correct answer is (A). No more B cells for this group are shown after day 12. Mice could have been dying before this time (and probably were), but day 12 was the last day that there were any survivors. This graph does not show

mortality, but from the data it can be concluded that at least one mouse survived 12 days, and none survived any longer. Hence, the upper limit for survival is 12 days, and the lower limit is unknown.

206. **(C)**   The correct answer is (C). Remember that the graph is semi-logarithmic, and half of the pre-irradiated level was asked for. If one treats the plot as linear, choice (B) is the incorrect answer. If one looks for the pre-irradiation level, (D) is the incorrect answer. (D) results from many errors.

207. **(A)**   The correct choice is (A). Although this graph does not show mortality, it can be seen that there were mice still alive at the conclusion of the experiment at 9 weeks. How long they lived after that is unknown. Some of the treated mice could have died before the conclusion of the experiment, and that would not be shown on this graph.

208. **(B)**   The correct answer is (B). B cells, as well as other lymphocytes and erythroid and myeloid cells, arise from a common stem cell ancestor. A mouse fetus of the age used does not yet have B cells.

209. **(C)**   The correct answer is (C). Although B cells are important, other cells such as erythrocytes are even more necessary. Possibly, these are produced first from the stem cells that are injected. Only later, when conditions are less urgent, do some of these stem cells become B cells.

210. **(C)**   This reaction is a typical S_N1 reaction but also involves migration of a hydrogen atom.

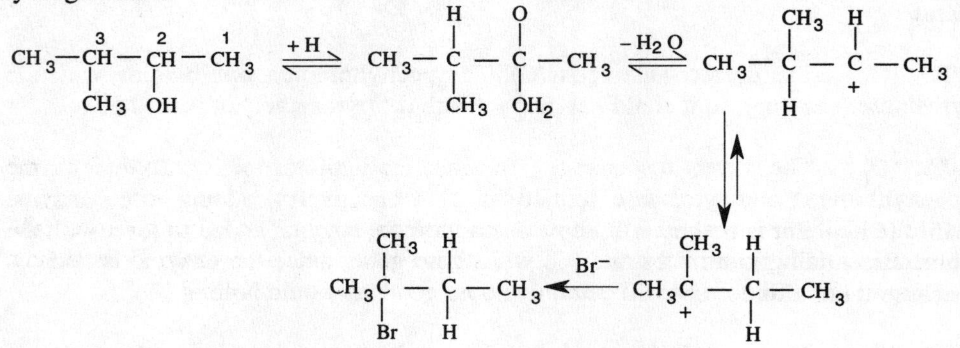

Because there is a carbocation intermediate which shifts to another carbon, this type of reaction is called a carbocation rearrangement.

211. **(C)**   As shown in the above illustration, the intermediate carbocation shifts from a secondary carbocation to the considerably more stable tertiary carbocation. Br⁻ reacts with this carbon, leading to 2-bromo-2-methylbutane instead of 2-bromo-3-methylbutane as essentially the sole product. (A) is false because, with carbanions, the order of stability is $1^O > 2^O > 3^O$ and there is no carbanion intermediate. (B) is a correct statement but it is false because the reaction does not involve a 1^O carbocation. (D) is wrong since this is not an SN2 reaction.

212. **(D)**   Since dectenium can be distinguished from H´ Hydrogen, and its posi-

tion on the carbon skeleton can be determined, it can be shown that the tertiary hydrogen moves to the secondary carbon after loss of H_2O. This has the effect of moving the carbocation from a secondary carbon to a tertiary one. Therefore choice (C) is correct. Choice (B) is also correct, because the rearrangements require an unstable intermediate. Because this is not an SN_2 reaction (due to the involvement of the carbocation intermediate), (A) is incorrect. Therefore (D) is the correct answer, for it allows one to choose both (C) and (B).

213. **(A)** The small amounts of 2-methyl-1-pentene require a carbocation intermediate at the tertiary carbon. Since much more 2-methyl-1-pentene is produced compared to 4-methyl-2-pentene, which can be produced only from a secondary carbocation in this case, one can assume the tertiary carbocation is more stable than the 2° carbocation. The major product, 2-methyl-2-pentene, could result from either carbocation intermediate, so this tells us nothing. While (B) is true, the experimental results do not apply to this question.

214. **(D)** Both reactions share the same intermediate, so the distribution of products should be similar.

215. **(B)** There is some carbocation rearrangement, but it does not go to equilibrium. Essentially no primary carbocation is generated, so III is wrong. IV is wrong, because it has a four-carbon skeleton.

216. **(B)** Through all five choices represent the development of an individual, the three primary germ layers first appear in the gastrula stage. The three germ layers are the endoderm, mesoderm and ectoderm. These layers will eventually differentiate to form the different organs and structures of the body.

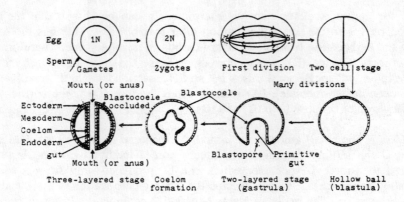

Early embryonic development in animals.

217. (A) Birds utilize celestial clues to guide them during migration. If a formerly caged bird is allowed to face the sun during the migration period, it will fly along its migratory route.

218. (D) The greatest similarity in structure occurs between members of the same species. In order of increasing specificity, the choices are: phylum-class-family-genus-species.

219. (A) Catalytic hydrogenation of an alkene is achieved by reacting the alkene with $H_2(g)$ on the surface of an appropriate catalyst such as Pt, Pd or Ni. Using D_2 instead of H2, the mechanism is probably described by the following diagram:

$$D_2 \quad CH_2=CH_2 \quad \xrightarrow{} \quad \overset{D \quad D}{\underset{/\!/\!/\!/\!/\!/\!/\!/}{|\qquad|}} \quad \xrightarrow{} \quad \overset{CH_2=CH_2}{\underset{/\!/\!/\!/\!/}{\overset{D \quad D}{|\quad|}}}$$

catalyst surface

$$\xrightarrow{} \quad \underset{/\!/\!/\!/\!/\!/\!/}{CH_2D-CH_2D}$$

As can be seen from the diagram, syn-addition is usually the result since only one side of the alkene is exposed to the catalyst surface. Keeping this in mind it can be seen that the hydrogenation of 2-methyl-2-pentene occurs in the following manner:

$$\underset{CH_3}{\overset{CH_3}{\underset{|}{C}}} \!\!\overset{D \quad D}{\underset{|\ \ \ |}{=}}\!\! \underset{H}{\overset{CH_2CH_3}{C}} \quad \longrightarrow \quad CH_3\overset{D}{\underset{CH_3}{\overset{|}{C}}} - \overset{D}{\underset{H}{\overset{|}{C}}}-CH_2CH_3$$

or in another form:

$$H_3C - \underset{\underset{CH_3}{|}}{\overset{\overset{D}{|}}{C}} - \underset{\underset{H}{|}}{\overset{\overset{D}{|}}{C}} - \underset{\underset{H}{|}}{\overset{\overset{H}{|}}{C}} - CH_3$$

Choice (B) is a product of anti-addition which does not occur with a platinum catalyst. Choice (C) is the catalytic hydrogenation product of 4-methyl-2-pentene. Choice (D) is also a product of anti-addition.

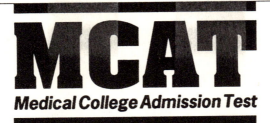

Test 3

MEDICAL COLLEGE ADMISSION TEST
TEST 3
ANSWER SHEET

Section 1:
Verbal Reasoning

1. Ⓐ Ⓑ Ⓒ Ⓓ
2. Ⓐ Ⓑ Ⓒ Ⓓ
3. Ⓐ Ⓑ Ⓒ Ⓓ
4. Ⓐ Ⓑ Ⓒ Ⓓ
5. Ⓐ Ⓑ Ⓒ Ⓓ
6. Ⓐ Ⓑ Ⓒ Ⓓ
7. Ⓐ Ⓑ Ⓒ Ⓓ
8. Ⓐ Ⓑ Ⓒ Ⓓ
9. Ⓐ Ⓑ Ⓒ Ⓓ
10. Ⓐ Ⓑ Ⓒ Ⓓ
11. Ⓐ Ⓑ Ⓒ Ⓓ
12. Ⓐ Ⓑ Ⓒ Ⓓ
13. Ⓐ Ⓑ Ⓒ Ⓓ
14. Ⓐ Ⓑ Ⓒ Ⓓ
15. Ⓐ Ⓑ Ⓒ Ⓓ
16. Ⓐ Ⓑ Ⓒ Ⓓ
17. Ⓐ Ⓑ Ⓒ Ⓓ
18. Ⓐ Ⓑ Ⓒ Ⓓ
19. Ⓐ Ⓑ Ⓒ Ⓓ
20. Ⓐ Ⓑ Ⓒ Ⓓ
21. Ⓐ Ⓑ Ⓒ Ⓓ
22. Ⓐ Ⓑ Ⓒ Ⓓ
23. Ⓐ Ⓑ Ⓒ Ⓓ
24. Ⓐ Ⓑ Ⓒ Ⓓ
25. Ⓐ Ⓑ Ⓒ Ⓓ
26. Ⓐ Ⓑ Ⓒ Ⓓ
27. Ⓐ Ⓑ Ⓒ Ⓓ
28. Ⓐ Ⓑ Ⓒ Ⓓ
29. Ⓐ Ⓑ Ⓒ Ⓓ
30. Ⓐ Ⓑ Ⓒ Ⓓ
31. Ⓐ Ⓑ Ⓒ Ⓓ

32. Ⓐ Ⓑ Ⓒ Ⓓ
33. Ⓐ Ⓑ Ⓒ Ⓓ
34. Ⓐ Ⓑ Ⓒ Ⓓ
35. Ⓐ Ⓑ Ⓒ Ⓓ
36. Ⓐ Ⓑ Ⓒ Ⓓ
37. Ⓐ Ⓑ Ⓒ Ⓓ
38. Ⓐ Ⓑ Ⓒ Ⓓ
39. Ⓐ Ⓑ Ⓒ Ⓓ
40. Ⓐ Ⓑ Ⓒ Ⓓ
41. Ⓐ Ⓑ Ⓒ Ⓓ
42. Ⓐ Ⓑ Ⓒ Ⓓ
43. Ⓐ Ⓑ Ⓒ Ⓓ
44. Ⓐ Ⓑ Ⓒ Ⓓ
45. Ⓐ Ⓑ Ⓒ Ⓓ
46. Ⓐ Ⓑ Ⓒ Ⓓ
47. Ⓐ Ⓑ Ⓒ Ⓓ
48. Ⓐ Ⓑ Ⓒ Ⓓ
49. Ⓐ Ⓑ Ⓒ Ⓓ
50. Ⓐ Ⓑ Ⓒ Ⓓ
51. Ⓐ Ⓑ Ⓒ Ⓓ
52. Ⓐ Ⓑ Ⓒ Ⓓ
53. Ⓐ Ⓑ Ⓒ Ⓓ
54. Ⓐ Ⓑ Ⓒ Ⓓ
55. Ⓐ Ⓑ Ⓒ Ⓓ
56. Ⓐ Ⓑ Ⓒ Ⓓ
57. Ⓐ Ⓑ Ⓒ Ⓓ
58. Ⓐ Ⓑ Ⓒ Ⓓ
59. Ⓐ Ⓑ Ⓒ Ⓓ
60. Ⓐ Ⓑ Ⓒ Ⓓ
61. Ⓐ Ⓑ Ⓒ Ⓓ
62. Ⓐ Ⓑ Ⓒ Ⓓ
63. Ⓐ Ⓑ Ⓒ Ⓓ
64. Ⓐ Ⓑ Ⓒ Ⓓ
65. Ⓐ Ⓑ Ⓒ Ⓓ

Section 2:
Physical Sciences

66. Ⓐ Ⓑ Ⓒ Ⓓ
67. Ⓐ Ⓑ Ⓒ Ⓓ
68. Ⓐ Ⓑ Ⓒ Ⓓ
69. Ⓐ Ⓑ Ⓒ Ⓓ
70. Ⓐ Ⓑ Ⓒ Ⓓ
71. Ⓐ Ⓑ Ⓒ Ⓓ
72. Ⓐ Ⓑ Ⓒ Ⓓ
73. Ⓐ Ⓑ Ⓒ Ⓓ
74. Ⓐ Ⓑ Ⓒ Ⓓ
75. Ⓐ Ⓑ Ⓒ Ⓓ
76. Ⓐ Ⓑ Ⓒ Ⓓ
77. Ⓐ Ⓑ Ⓒ Ⓓ
78. Ⓐ Ⓑ Ⓒ Ⓓ
79. Ⓐ Ⓑ Ⓒ Ⓓ
80. Ⓐ Ⓑ Ⓒ Ⓓ
81. Ⓐ Ⓑ Ⓒ Ⓓ
82. Ⓐ Ⓑ Ⓒ Ⓓ
83. Ⓐ Ⓑ Ⓒ Ⓓ
84. Ⓐ Ⓑ Ⓒ Ⓓ
85. Ⓐ Ⓑ Ⓒ Ⓓ
86. Ⓐ Ⓑ Ⓒ Ⓓ
87. Ⓐ Ⓑ Ⓒ Ⓓ
88. Ⓐ Ⓑ Ⓒ Ⓓ
89. Ⓐ Ⓑ Ⓒ Ⓓ
90. Ⓐ Ⓑ Ⓒ Ⓓ
91. Ⓐ Ⓑ Ⓒ Ⓓ
92. Ⓐ Ⓑ Ⓒ Ⓓ
93. Ⓐ Ⓑ Ⓒ Ⓓ
94. Ⓐ Ⓑ Ⓒ Ⓓ
95. Ⓐ Ⓑ Ⓒ Ⓓ
96. Ⓐ Ⓑ Ⓒ Ⓓ

97. Ⓐ Ⓑ Ⓒ Ⓓ
98. Ⓐ Ⓑ Ⓒ Ⓓ
99. Ⓐ Ⓑ Ⓒ Ⓓ
100. Ⓐ Ⓑ Ⓒ Ⓓ
101. Ⓐ Ⓑ Ⓒ Ⓓ
102. Ⓐ Ⓑ Ⓒ Ⓓ
103. Ⓐ Ⓑ Ⓒ Ⓓ
104. Ⓐ Ⓑ Ⓒ Ⓓ
105. Ⓐ Ⓑ Ⓒ Ⓓ
106. Ⓐ Ⓑ Ⓒ Ⓓ
107. Ⓐ Ⓑ Ⓒ Ⓓ
108. Ⓐ Ⓑ Ⓒ Ⓓ
109. Ⓐ Ⓑ Ⓒ Ⓓ
110. Ⓐ Ⓑ Ⓒ Ⓓ
111. Ⓐ Ⓑ Ⓒ Ⓓ
112. Ⓐ Ⓑ Ⓒ Ⓓ
113. Ⓐ Ⓑ Ⓒ Ⓓ
114. Ⓐ Ⓑ Ⓒ Ⓓ
115. Ⓐ Ⓑ Ⓒ Ⓓ
116. Ⓐ Ⓑ Ⓒ Ⓓ
117. Ⓐ Ⓑ Ⓒ Ⓓ
118. Ⓐ Ⓑ Ⓒ Ⓓ
119. Ⓐ Ⓑ Ⓒ Ⓓ
120. Ⓐ Ⓑ Ⓒ Ⓓ
121. Ⓐ Ⓑ Ⓒ Ⓓ
122. Ⓐ Ⓑ Ⓒ Ⓓ
123. Ⓐ Ⓑ Ⓒ Ⓓ
124. Ⓐ Ⓑ Ⓒ Ⓓ
125. Ⓐ Ⓑ Ⓒ Ⓓ
126. Ⓐ Ⓑ Ⓒ Ⓓ
127. Ⓐ Ⓑ Ⓒ Ⓓ
128. Ⓐ Ⓑ Ⓒ Ⓓ
129. Ⓐ Ⓑ Ⓒ Ⓓ
130. Ⓐ Ⓑ Ⓒ Ⓓ
131. Ⓐ Ⓑ Ⓒ Ⓓ
132. Ⓐ Ⓑ Ⓒ Ⓓ
133. Ⓐ Ⓑ Ⓒ Ⓓ
134. Ⓐ Ⓑ Ⓒ Ⓓ
135. Ⓐ Ⓑ Ⓒ Ⓓ
136. Ⓐ Ⓑ Ⓒ Ⓓ
137. Ⓐ Ⓑ Ⓒ Ⓓ
138. Ⓐ Ⓑ Ⓒ Ⓓ
139. Ⓐ Ⓑ Ⓒ Ⓓ

140. Ⓐ Ⓑ Ⓒ Ⓓ
141. Ⓐ Ⓑ Ⓒ Ⓓ
142. Ⓐ Ⓑ Ⓒ Ⓓ

Section 4:
Biological Sciences

143. Ⓐ Ⓑ Ⓒ Ⓓ
144. Ⓐ Ⓑ Ⓒ Ⓓ
145. Ⓐ Ⓑ Ⓒ Ⓓ
146. Ⓐ Ⓑ Ⓒ Ⓓ
147. Ⓐ Ⓑ Ⓒ Ⓓ
148. Ⓐ Ⓑ Ⓒ Ⓓ
149. Ⓐ Ⓑ Ⓒ Ⓓ
150. Ⓐ Ⓑ Ⓒ Ⓓ
151. Ⓐ Ⓑ Ⓒ Ⓓ
152. Ⓐ Ⓑ Ⓒ Ⓓ
153. Ⓐ Ⓑ Ⓒ Ⓓ
154. Ⓐ Ⓑ Ⓒ Ⓓ
155. Ⓐ Ⓑ Ⓒ Ⓓ
156. Ⓐ Ⓑ Ⓒ Ⓓ
157. Ⓐ Ⓑ Ⓒ Ⓓ
158. Ⓐ Ⓑ Ⓒ Ⓓ
159. Ⓐ Ⓑ Ⓒ Ⓓ
160. Ⓐ Ⓑ Ⓒ Ⓓ
161. Ⓐ Ⓑ Ⓒ Ⓓ
162. Ⓐ Ⓑ Ⓒ Ⓓ
163. Ⓐ Ⓑ Ⓒ Ⓓ
164. Ⓐ Ⓑ Ⓒ Ⓓ
165. Ⓐ Ⓑ Ⓒ Ⓓ
166. Ⓐ Ⓑ Ⓒ Ⓓ
167. Ⓐ Ⓑ Ⓒ Ⓓ
168. Ⓐ Ⓑ Ⓒ Ⓓ
169. Ⓐ Ⓑ Ⓒ Ⓓ
170. Ⓐ Ⓑ Ⓒ Ⓓ
171. Ⓐ Ⓑ Ⓒ Ⓓ
172. Ⓐ Ⓑ Ⓒ Ⓓ
173. Ⓐ Ⓑ Ⓒ Ⓓ
174. Ⓐ Ⓑ Ⓒ Ⓓ
175. Ⓐ Ⓑ Ⓒ Ⓓ
176. Ⓐ Ⓑ Ⓒ Ⓓ

177. Ⓐ Ⓑ Ⓒ Ⓓ
178. Ⓐ Ⓑ Ⓒ Ⓓ
179. Ⓐ Ⓑ Ⓒ Ⓓ
180. Ⓐ Ⓑ Ⓒ Ⓓ
181. Ⓐ Ⓑ Ⓒ Ⓓ
182. Ⓐ Ⓑ Ⓒ Ⓓ
183. Ⓐ Ⓑ Ⓒ Ⓓ
184. Ⓐ Ⓑ Ⓒ Ⓓ
185. Ⓐ Ⓑ Ⓒ Ⓓ
186. Ⓐ Ⓑ Ⓒ Ⓓ
187. Ⓐ Ⓑ Ⓒ Ⓓ
188. Ⓐ Ⓑ Ⓒ Ⓓ
189. Ⓐ Ⓑ Ⓒ Ⓓ
190. Ⓐ Ⓑ Ⓒ Ⓓ
191. Ⓐ Ⓑ Ⓒ Ⓓ
192. Ⓐ Ⓑ Ⓒ Ⓓ
193. Ⓐ Ⓑ Ⓒ Ⓓ
194. Ⓐ Ⓑ Ⓒ Ⓓ
195. Ⓐ Ⓑ Ⓒ Ⓓ
196. Ⓐ Ⓑ Ⓒ Ⓓ
197. Ⓐ Ⓑ Ⓒ Ⓓ
198. Ⓐ Ⓑ Ⓒ Ⓓ
199. Ⓐ Ⓑ Ⓒ Ⓓ
200. Ⓐ Ⓑ Ⓒ Ⓓ
201. Ⓐ Ⓑ Ⓒ Ⓓ
202. Ⓐ Ⓑ Ⓒ Ⓓ
203. Ⓐ Ⓑ Ⓒ Ⓓ
204. Ⓐ Ⓑ Ⓒ Ⓓ
205. Ⓐ Ⓑ Ⓒ Ⓓ
206. Ⓐ Ⓑ Ⓒ Ⓓ
207. Ⓐ Ⓑ Ⓒ Ⓓ
208. Ⓐ Ⓑ Ⓒ Ⓓ
209. Ⓐ Ⓑ Ⓒ Ⓓ
210. Ⓐ Ⓑ Ⓒ Ⓓ
211. Ⓐ Ⓑ Ⓒ Ⓓ
212. Ⓐ Ⓑ Ⓒ Ⓓ
213. Ⓐ Ⓑ Ⓒ Ⓓ
214. Ⓐ Ⓑ Ⓒ Ⓓ
215. Ⓐ Ⓑ Ⓒ Ⓓ
216. Ⓐ Ⓑ Ⓒ Ⓓ
217. Ⓐ Ⓑ Ⓒ Ⓓ
218. Ⓐ Ⓑ Ⓒ Ⓓ
219. Ⓐ Ⓑ Ⓒ Ⓓ

TEST 3

Section 1 — Verbal Reasoning

TIME: 85 Minutes
QUESTIONS: 1-65

DIRECTIONS: The verbal reasoning section contains seven passages, each followed by a series of questions. Based on the information given in a passage, choose the one best answer to each question. If you are not sure of an answer, eliminate those choices that you know are incorrect and choose an answer from among those remaining. Fill in the corresponding circle on the answer sheet to indicate your answer.

PASSAGE I (Questions 1-10)

In May 1774, in retaliation for the "Boston Tea Party," Parliament closed the port of Boston and virtually abolished provincial self-government in Massachusetts. These actions stimulated resistance across the land. That summer, the Massachusetts lower house, through the committees of correspondence, secretly invited all 13 Colonies to attend a convention. In response, on the fifth of September, 55 Delegates representing 12 Colonies, Georgia excepted, assembled at Philadelphia. They convened at Carpenters' Hall and organized the First Continental Congress.

Sharing though they did common complaints against the Crown, the Delegates propounded a wide variety of political opinions. Most of them agreed that Parliament had no right to control the internal affairs of the Colonies. Moderates, stressing trade benefits with the mother country, believed Parliament should continue to regulate commerce. Others questioned the extent of its authority. A handful of Delegates felt the answer to the problem lay in parliamentary representation. Most suggested legislative autonomy for the Colonies. Reluctant to sever ties of blood, language, trade, and cultural heritage, none yet openly entertained the idea of complete independence from Great Britain.

After weeks of debate and compromise, Congress adopted two significant measures. The first declared that the American colonists were entitled to the same rights as Englishmen everywhere and denounced any infringement of those rights. The second, the Continental Association, provided for an embargo on all trade with Britain. To enforce the embargo and punish violators, at the behest of Congress counties, cities and towns formed councils, or committees of safety—many of which later became wartime governing or administrative bodies. When Congress adjourned in late October, the Delegates resolved to reconvene in May 1775 if the Crown had not responded by then.

In a sense the Continental Congress acted with restraint, for while it was in session the situation in Massachusetts verged on war. In September, just before Congress met, British troops from Boston had seized ordnance supplies at Charlestown and Cambridge and almost clashed with the local militia. The next month, Massachusetts patriots, openly defying royal authority, organized a Revolutionary provincial assembly as well as a military defense committee. Whigs in three other colonies— Maryland, Virginia, and New Hampshire—had earlier that year formed governments. By the end of the year, all the Colonies except Georgia and New York had either set up new ones or taken control of those already in existence. During the winter of 1774-75, while Parliament mulled over conciliatory measures, colonial militia units prepared for war.

The crisis came in the spring of 1775, predictably in Massachusetts. Late on the night of April 18 the Royal Governor, Gen. Thomas Gage, alarmed at the militancy of the rebels, dispatched 600 troops from Boston to seize a major supply depot at Concord. Almost simultaneously the Boston council of safety, aware of Gage's intentions, directed Paul Revere and William Dawes to ride ahead to warn militia units and citizens along the way of the British approach, as well as John Hancock and Samuel Adams, who were staying at nearby Lexington. Forewarned, the two men went into hiding.

About 77 militiamen confronted the redcoats when they plodded into Lexington at dawn. After some tense moments, as the sorely outnumbered colonials were dispersing, blood was shed. More flowed at Concord and much more along the route of the British as they retreated to Boston, harassed most of the way by an aroused citizenry. What had once been merely protest had evolved into open warfare; the War for Independence had begun.

1.   Which of the following statements best summarizes the main theme of the passage?

    (A)   The Continental Congress was an assembly of reactionary Englishmen who ignited the War of Independence.

    (B)   The Revolutionary War was precipitated by the British elimination of colonial self-government in Massachusetts.

    (C)   The first Continental Congress was made up of like-minded men.

    (D)   The American Revolution was precipitated by a series of events that involved the first Continental Congress.

2.   "Common complaints against the Crown" included

    (A)   all restrictions against American colonists.

    (B)   those restrictions which deprived the colonists of representation and trade.

    (C)   only the closing of the Boston Harbor.

    (D)   only inadequate representation in Parliament.

3.   The idea of complete independence from Britain

    (A)   was never entertained by the colonists prior to 1775.

    (B)   was favored by the Moderates.

    (C)   was favored by all the Delegates to the Continental Congress.

    (D)   was never debated on the floor of the Continental Congress.

4. Parliament's retaliation for the "Boston Tea Party"

   (A) created reaction only in the state of Massachusetts.

   (B) almost completely stopped provincial self-government in Massachusetts.

   (C) immediately inspired the U.S. government to create the first military defense committee.

   (D) closed the meeting place of U.S. officials known as Carpenters' Hall.

5. It can be concluded that this passage

   (A) placed more significance on ideas than on men.

   (B) held Parliament responsible for the war.

   (C) attributed the start of the war to General Gage, Paul Revere and W. Dawes.

   (D) attributed the war to the Continental Congress.

6. One of the colonies which did NOT set up a revolutionary provisional assembly was

   (A) Virginia.   (B) Pennsylvania.

   (C) New Hampshire.   (D) Maryland.

7. "Whigs" refers to

   (A) military defense committees.

   (B) British troops.

   (C) British sympathizers.

   (D) patriots against kingly authority.

8. According to the passage, of the following men, who was not involved in the Battle of Concord?

   (A) William Dawes   (B) Thomas Gage

   (C) Paul Revere   (D) Samuel Adams

9. The Battle of Lexington may be said to be

   (A) the beginning of citizen protest.

   (B) the initial crisis of a larger war.

   (C) an insignificant skirmish.

   (D) another form of harassment of the British citizenry.

10. From the passage, the term "embargo" may be said to mean

   (A) opposition.   (B) protection.

   (C) prevention.   (D) proposition.

PASSAGE II (Questions 11-19)

The most serious threat to society from organized crime comes when criminal syndicates use vast sums of money gained from illicit enterprises to undermine legitimate business enterprises and political institutions. Organized crime has infiltrated labor unions, the entertainment business, manufacturing, real estate, and even the stock market. To measure its impact in terms of dollars would be a formidable, if not prohibitive, task.

In 1972 the stock brokerage industry alone estimated that stolen or missing securities of 1.2 billion dollars were being utilized in illegal operations around the world. The loss of income tax revenue from organized crime operations is incalculable. It has been estimated that illegal betting on horse racing, lotteries, and sporting events alone totals at least $20 billion a year with the syndicate taking about $6 to $7 billion as its share (this is about three times the amount of the annual budget for U.S. foreign aid). Loan sharks have been known to charge interest rates as high as 500 percent. Millions of dollars of cargo are pilfered from airports and piers by trucking companies and union locals working for a criminal group. Labor union pension funds have been used for loans to finance illegal or questionable enterprises, and construction companies have used shoddy materials and workmanship through kickback arrangements.

What this means, translated to the level of the everyday citizen, is higher prices through the monopolistic practices of organized crime, shoddy merchandise, poorly constructed and unsafe buildings, and higher taxes. More important is the threat to the free enterprise system. Organized crime operates on the local level as well, controlling businesses such as laundries, taxicab companies, paving-contract firms, travel agencies, insurance underwriting firms, vending machine companies, and restaurants.

The social costs of political corruption by organized crime are even more difficult to assess. Organized crime needs the involvement of the political system to profit from economic opportunities. The President's Commission concluded that "all available data indicate that organized crime flourishes only where it has corrupted local officials." Over and over again, investigations into criminal activities have turned up close connections with respectable persons in business and public officials at all levels of government. Corruption is achieved through bribes and contributions to political campaigns; a police officer is bribed or overlooks gambling and a state or Federal legislator's vote on a bill is bought by the criminal organization that contributed heavily to the person's campaign through a front organization. Hence, organized crime is, in part, a subversion of the democratic process which ultimately will produce a political system where the strong and powerful exist at the expense of the weak.

11.   Which of the following is the main theme of this passage?

   (A)   Organized crime is a tale of corruption.

   (B)   Free enterprise is threatened by organized crime.

   (C)   Organized crime is controlled by public officials and big business.

   (D)   The people will always pay the price of the loss of free enterprise.

12.   The passage states that organized crime has permeated so much of society that

I.   lotteries contribute to organized crime.

II.   bribes furnished by the syndicate are an inevitable part of the free enterprise system.

III.   it can flourish only with the support of public officials.

(A)   I only.   (B)   I and II only.

(C)   I and III only.   (D)   II and III only.

13.   Based on the passage, which of the following would not be suggested as having backing from organized crime?

     (A)   Political campaigns   (B)   Gambling

     (C)   Federal legislation   (D)   The democratic process

14.   Which of the following expressions fits the passage?

     (A)   The meek shall inherit the earth.

     (B)   Adaptation is the key to success.

     (C)   Might is right.

     (D)   "Survival of the fittest"

15.   Based on the passage, corruption

     (A)   means higher prices for every person.

     (B)   involves every working person.

     (C)   is the single cause of the loss of tax revenue.

     (D)   undermines the work of The President's Commission.

16.   On the basis of the information given in the passage,

     (A)   organized crime is an economic deterrent to foreign trade.

     (B)   organized crime fosters growth while diminishing profits.

     (C)   organized crime does not distinguish between big business and the person in the neighborhood.

     (D)   organized crime is allowed to thrive because gambling is a national pastime.

17.   From the passage it can be inferred that bribery

     (A)   involves only police officers.

     (B)   is but one form of corruption.

     (C)   is not connected to political campaigns.

     (D)   is an essential aspect of the operation of organized crime.

18.   Which of the following statements best describes organized crime's effect on the U.S. economy?

(A)   Laundered money contributes to overall loss of the country's capital as a result of organized criminal action.

(B)   Lotteries, loan sharks and missing securities account for a $20 billion dollar loss each year for the American people.

(C)   Pilfered cargo is the single source of the most lost capital.

(D)   Kickback arrangements are traceable to a fraudulent IRS.

19.   Based on the essay, which type of private enterprise might be immune from organized crime?

    (A)   The operation of freight carriers

    (B)   Bowling alley owners

    (C)   Organized religion

    (D)   Unionized postal workers

PASSAGE III (Questions 20-28)

In his celebrated essay *On Liberty,* John Stuart Mill argued that liberty of thought and expression were central and necessary elements of well-being for both individuals and societies. Mill argued that the only justification for the imposition of controls on self-expression would be if the means of self-expression posed a threat to the freedom of others. Conformity to the prevailing opinion or lifestyle cannot be forced for any reason other than that of preventing harm to the interests of others, where these interests are those which these others have a right or entitlement to enjoy. Mere displeasure or disagreeableness is not sufficient to warrant the stifling of thought and expression.

Mill argued for this liberty or expression in a two-pronged fashion, considering first the case where the stifled opinion is true and then in the case where the stifled opinion is false.

In the first case, where the opinion that is to be suppressed is true, we are in effect making an assumption of infallibility when we refuse to allow contrary opinions to be voiced. This assumption of infallibility does not exist in our assumption that our own beliefs are true. Rather, it exists in the undertaking to decide for others what is true, and a refusal to allow open debate about the truth of our own and these other doctrines. Certainly we should all have learned, both from our own experience and that of the entire human race, that we are all liable to error, even in those beliefs we hold most confidently to be true. For us to decide what will and will not be heard is to assume an unwarranted infallibility.

It has been claimed that there are some beliefs that are so dangerous that we are entitled to silence them for the health and safety of the society. However, the very claim that a belief is dangerous in itself is an opinion about which we may be in error, and so it too should be subject to open debate.

In refusing to allow opinion to be heard when it is true, though in our own belief false, we are not only assuming an unwarranted infallibility but are also eliminating our opportunity to rid ourselves of our false belief.

Conversely, suppose we are correct about the beliefs we hold, and the belief that we are silencing is the one that is false. In this case, we are eliminating the opportunity for our belief system to face the challenge of honest debate, establish its truth, and expose the error of the alternatives. The challenge of debate is what adds vitality to our beliefs; in the absence of such debate our beliefs deteriorate into dead dogmas and lose their energy. Constant challenge is not a harm to truth but a force that makes it a living faith rather than dogma; we see and feel its merit and force.

Normally, our beliefs are a mixture of these two cases. Some of our beliefs are true and some are false; some of the beliefs we would stifle are a mixture of the true and the false. It is for a combination of the above reasons that it is to our advantage not to stifle the free, forceful and open expression of opinion.

20. Mill argued that the silencing of opinion can be justified when

   (A)   the interests of others are threatened.

   (B)   harm to others is threatened.

   (C)   harm to the entitlements of others is threatened.

   (D)   these opinions are disagreeable to the majority.

21. In the passage given, an explanation of the concept of harm

   (A)   is given.

   (B)   is used in the arguments but not given.

   (C)   is not relevant to the argument.

   (D)   None of the above.

22. Mill accepted the idea that

   (A)   some restrictions on liberty of expression are warranted by the security needs of the society.

   (B)   no restrictions on liberty of expression are warranted by the security of the society.

   (C)   the security needs of the society are in themselves matters of opinion.

   (D)   the security needs of the society are not matters relating to the questions of freedom of expression.

23. Mill took infallibility to be the assumption that

   (A)   you are correct in your beliefs.

   (B)   you are not only correct in your beliefs but necessarily so, and there is no possibility of error.

   (C)   entitles you to control the expression of opinion.

   (D)   you may decide for others what beliefs are true.

24. According to Mill, where our beliefs are true and we know them for certain to be true, we

   (A)   should ensure that our beliefs are not threatened by false and seductive doctrines.

   (B)   should ensure that our beliefs are exposed by lively and free debate.

(C)   will see the error of opposing beliefs.

(D)   will have no need for contact with opposing doctrines.

25.   Mill argued that one of the benefits of open debate on all subjects is that

(A)   it will make for a healthier individual as well as a healthier society.

(B)   it will enable us to exchange our false beliefs for true beliefs.

(C)   it will avoid our acting on the unwarranted assumption of infallibility.

(D)   All of the above.

26.   Based on the passage, we could expect that Mill's argument would apply to

(A)   governmental strictures but not the censorship imposed by private individuals or organizations.

(B)   any kind of stricture from either government or private agents on the holding of beliefs but not on their expression.

(C)   strictures on both the expression of opinion and on one's choice of lifestyle.

(D)   opinions that are true and only those.

27.   According to the passage above, if some of our beliefs are true and some are false, we should

(A)   expose them all to open debate.

(B)   expose only the false ones to open debate.

(C)   examine them all carefully and determine which are true and which are false.

(D)   act on the true ones.

28.   Mill argued that debate may be expected to

(A)   publicize our beliefs.

(B)   enliven our beliefs.

(C)   weaken the social order.

(D)   weed out potential dictators.

PASSAGE IV (Questions 28-37)
The physical phenomenon responsible for converting light to electricity—the photovoltaic effect—was first observed in 1839 by a French physicist, Edmund Becquerel. Becquerel noted a voltage appeared when one of two identical electrodes in a weak conducting solution was illuminated. The PV effect was first studied in solids, such as selenium, in the 1870s. In the 1880s, selenium photovoltaic cells were built that exhibited 1%-2% efficiency in converting light to electricity. Selenium converts light in the visible part of the sun's spectrum; for this reason, it was quickly adopted by the then-emerging field of photography for photometric (light-measuring) devices. Even today, light-sensitive cells on cameras for adjusting shutter speed to match illumination are made of selenium.

Selenium cells have never become practical as energy converters because their cost is too high relative to the tiny amount of power they produce (at 1% efficiency). Meanwhile, work on the physics of PV phenomena has expanded. In the 1920s and 1930s, quantum mechanics laid the theoretical foundation for our present understanding of PV. A major step forward in solar-cell technology came in the 1940s and early 1950s when a method (called the Czochralski method) was developed for producing highly pure crystalline silicon. In 1954, work at Bell Telephone Laboratories resulted in a silicon photovoltaic cell with a 4% efficiency. Bell Labs soon bettered this to a 6% and then 11% efficiency, heralding an entirely new era of power-producing cells.

A few schemes were tried in the 1950s to use silicon PV cells commercially. Most were for cells in regions geographically isolated from electric utility lines. But an unexpected boom in PV technology came from a different quarter. In 1958, the U.S. Vanguard space satellite used a small (less than one-watt) array of cells to power its radio. The cells worked so well that space scientists soon realized the PV could be an effective power source for many space missions. Technology development of the solar cell has been a part of the space program ever since.

Today, photovoltaic systems are capable of transforming one kilowatt of solar energy falling on one square meter into about a hundred watts of electricity. One-hundred watts can power most household appliances: a television, a stereo, an electric typewriter, or a lamp. In fact, standard solar cells covering the sun-facing roof space of a typical home can provide about 8500-kilowatt-hours of electricity annually, which is about the average household's yearly electric consumption. By comparison, a modern, 200-ton electric-arc steel furnace, demanding 50,000 kilowatts of electricity, would require about a square kilometer of land for a PV power supply.

Certain factors make capturing solar energy difficult. Besides the sun's low illuminating power per square meter, sunlight is intermittent, affected by time of day, climate, pollution, and season. Power sources based on photovoltaics require either back-up from other sources or storage for times when the sun is obscured.

In addition, the cost of a photovoltaic system is far from negligible (electricity from PV systems in 1980 cost about 20 times that from conventional fossil-fuel-powered systems).

Thus, solar energy for photovoltaic conversion into electricity is abundant, inexhaustible, and clean; yet, it also requires special techniques to gather enough of it effectively.

29. Selenium PV cells, vis-à-vis silicon photovoltaic cells, exhibit

   (A)   less efficiency than silicon PV cells by at least 9%.

   (B)   more efficiency than silicon PV cells by 9%.

   (C)   greater cost than silicon PV cells by between 4% and 11%.

   (D)   less cost than silicon PV cells by between 6% and 11%.

30. The photovoltaic effect is the result of

   (A)   two identical negative electrodes.

   (B)   one weak solution and two negative electrodes.

   (C)   two positive electrodes of different qualities.

   (D)   positive electrodes interacting in a weak environment.

31. How long did it take before Bell Labs improved the power of the PV effect?

    (A) Approximately 30 years

    (B) Approximately 100 years

    (C) Approximately 4 years

    (D) Approximately 115 years

32. From this passage it can be concluded that

    (A) solar energy is still limited by problems of technological efficiency.

    (B) solar energy is the most efficient source of heat for most families.

    (C) solar energy represents the PV effect in its most complicated form.

    (D) solar energy is 20% cheaper than fossil-fuel powered systems.

33. The most appropriate title for this passage is

    (A) "Information on the Science of Edmund Becquerel."

    (B) "The History of the PV Effect."

    (C) "A Comparison of Selenium, Silicon and Solar PV Cells."

    (D) "The Adaptation of the PV Effect."

34. Commercially used PV cells power

    (A) car radios.   (B) space satellite radios.

    (C) telephones.   (D) electric utility lines.

35. Selenium was used for photometric devices because

    (A) selenium was the first solid to be observed to have the PV effect.

    (B) selenium is inexpensive.

    (C) selenium converts the visible part of the sun's spectrum.

    (C) selenium can adjust shutter speeds on cameras.

36. Two kilowatts of solar energy transformed by a PV system equal

    (A) 200 watts of electricity.

    (B) 100 watts of electricity.

    (C) no electricity.

    (D) two square meters.

37. Sunlight is difficult to procure for transformation into solar energy. Which of the following statements most accurately supports this belief derived from the passage?

    (A) Sunlight is erratic and subject to variables.

    (B) Sunlight is steady but never available.

(C)   Sunlight is not visible because of pollution.

(D)   Sunlight would have to be artificially produced.

PASSAGE V (Questions 38-46)

Old age—a difficult time for many people—can be especially so for blacks and members of other racial and ethnic minority groups. Compared to the majority of Americans, these individuals are likely to have less education and money, less adequate housing, poorer health, and fewer years of life.

Many minority groups—especially black, Hispanic, Asian, and Native Americans—bear the added burdens of racial prejudice, language barriers, suspicion of bureaucratic processes, and difficulty obtaining needed health and other services.

In addition, minority group members who have suffered racial discrimination all their lives are, in their later years, in double jeopardy because they may also be discriminated against for being old.

The number of individuals with ethnic affiliations is greater than the word "minority" might imply. According to a study supported by the National Institute on Aging (NIA), almost 40 percent of the entire U.S. population over age 65 in the 1980s will be black or first and second generation Americans belonging to various racial/ethnic subgroups.

Ethnic and racial affiliations are important in determining not only individual attitudes, problems, and needs, but the considerable strengths many minority members exhibit in adapting to old age. Yet society at large and the research community in particular seldom take these differences into account.

Among older blacks, for example, hypertension is twice as prevalent as among whites, and accidents are the leading cause of death for older Alaskan Natives and American Indians. The leading causes of death for Hispanics are not even known, because those statistics are just beginning to be collected.

Such diverse populations as Samoans, Chinese, Filipinos, Koreans, Hawaiians, Japanese, and Vietnamese are lumped together as Asian and Pacific Americans. Yet lifestyles, attitudes, and other differences exist among these populations. For example, food preferences and tastes vary among these groups and, in turn, have a great impact on the effectiveness of nutrition programs.

To add to our knowledge of aging minority group members, the NIA has funded a study of about 5,000 black Americans living in 100 communities across the Nation. This study, among the most extensive examinations ever conducted of these individuals, will focus on aging among blacks, and on the transmission of attitudes and values among generations. The study will explore regional differences among blacks in a number of important social and health-related areas, including work and retirement. Such efforts help law- and policymakers design programs that are genuinely helpful to minority groups.

For the future, the NIA is concerned with how different racial and ethnic minorities age in our society. Specifically, the research community, including investigators from minority groups, has been invited to study how family structure, social networks, occupations, lifestyles, environmental conditions, personality traits, attitudes, ways of coping, and health care practices of minority groups influence the way these individuals age.

It is clear that many concerns of the minority aged need further attention, not only in their own right, but because of their interrelationship with the problems of the elderly in general.

38.   The central idea of this passage is

   (A)   the American population is aging rapidly.

   (B)   the NIA should continue to be funded.

   (C)   we have inadequate knowledge of aging minorities in our country.

   (D)   studies are being done to assess the needs of our aging minorities.

39.   The author uses the information on Asian and Pacific Americans

   (A)   to discredit the value of these Americans for the study.

   (B)   to demonstrate the value of nutritional differences in some aging minori-
          ties.

   (C)   to compare blacks to other minorities.

   (D)   to increase the minority studies based on nutrition for the NIA.

40.   According to the passage, about 40% of the entire U.S. population over age 65
      in the 1980s will be minorities because

   (A)   "minority" has an expanded meaning according to the author.

   (B)   minorities will die or move away.

   (C)   whites have stopped reproducing.

   (D)   first and second generation Americans will be black only.

41.   It can be inferred from the passage that the NIA

   (A)   needs financial support from the private sector.

   (B)   utilizes minority studies as an essential way of determining the needs of
          all aged groups.

   (C)   has satisfactorily completed its studies.

   (D)   has singled out minority aging as their sole subject of research.

42.   Lawmakers and policymakers are assisted by NIA studies because

   (A)   they are unfamiliar with minority constituents.

   (B)   NIA studies are regional and demonstrate social needs.

   (C)   they do not know minority values.

   (D)   lawmakers and policymakers specifically fund the NIA studies.

43.   Compared to the majority of Americans, members of racial and ethnic groups
      may have

   I.   less education and money.

   II.   adequate housing.

   III.   poorer health but more years of life.

   (A)   I only.   (B)   I and II only.

   (C)   I and III only.   (D)   II and III only.

44. The above passage infers that studies reflecting differences among aging ethnic and social minorities

    (A) create a racist population.

    (B) determine the level of attention given to various needs of minorities.

    (C) allow other Americans to denigrate minorities.

    (D) determine the social status of minorities.

45. Among the leading causes of death among certain minorities, hypertension

    (A) is not present in older Alaskans.

    (B) is half as prevalent among older whites than blacks.

    (C) is not present in an older Hispanic population.

    (D) is more of a serious concern for all blacks than Alaskan natives.

46. The passage reveals that

    (A) many minorities have attitudes and values that exhibit graceful aging.

    (B) adaptation to old age is exclusively a minority problem.

    (C) many minorities exhibit explicit strengths in adapting to old age.

    (D) ethnic and racial affiliations are important.

PASSAGE VI (Questions 47-56)

It appears that it was Charles Darwin who first formulated the modern approach to the origins of life, with a view of the circumstances, not of today, but of the distant past when the first life was somehow formed. He wrote in a private letter in 1871: "If we could conceive in some warm little pond, with all sorts of ammonia and phosphoric salts, light, heat, electricity, etc., present, that a protein compound was chemically formed ready to undergo still more complex changes, at the present day such matter would be instantly devoured or absorbed which would not have been the case before living creatures were formed." In short, the logical needs for the *origin* of life include the *absence* of life: a sterile environment was exactly what was present then and what is utterly unknown in the biosphere today. But for 50 years such large ideas lay dormant. They were ahead of the state of biology and geology. The question was too grand. Pasteur's wonderful declaration is true for our geological epoch; the ancient epoch when life originated, which is not at all the present natural life-filled environment, was not brought under study.

In 1924, a young Russian biochemist published a preliminary account of his ideas on the chemical origins of life. In a booklet entitled *Proiskhozhdenie Zhizny,* he pointed out that the complex combination of manifestations and properties so characteristic of life must have arisen in the process of the evolution of matter. A. Oparin had learned Mendeleev's ideas on the possible origin of hydrocarbons from the carbides in the crust of the Earth, and injected into his own thinking a new notion concerning the reducing nature of the early atmosphere. To Oparin's great credit, this observation was made before the astrophysicists had realized that the stars were 90% hydrogen.

In 1928, J. B. S. Haldane, the British biologist, independently of Oparin, wrote a classic paper, "The Origin of Life." Haldane speculated on the early conditions suitable for the emergence of life. According to him, when UV light acted upon a mixture of water, carbon dioxide, and ammonia, a variety of organic substances were made, including sugars and apparently some of the materials from which proteins are built up. Before the origin of life they must have accumulated until the primitive oceans reached the constituency of a hot, dilute soup. Haldane gave us the concept of the "primordial soup."

Almost 20 years after Haldane's publication, J. D. Bernal of the University of London conjectured before the British Physical Society in a famous lecture entitled *The Physical Basis of Life* that clay surfaces were involved in the origin of life. He was looking for ways and means by which the primordial molecules in the hot, dilute soup could be brought together to give rise to polymers capable of replication. A physicist and crystallographer by training, Bernal was particularly attracted to the role of surface phenomena in the origin of life. He argued that favorable conditions for concentration, which may have taken place on a very large scale, were provided by the adsorption of organic molecules on the fine clay deposits. The role of clay in primordial organic synthesis is today a lively area of investigation.

47. Based on the information in the passage, Charles Darwin

    (A)   believed there was a time when life was dormant.

    (B)   wanted to create a simulation of the origin of life.

    (C)   believed the origin of life required an active environment.

    (D)   believed that without living creatures, complex compounds would continue to exist.

48. From the passage we can assume that A. Oparin, a Russian biochemist,

    (A)   utilized Mendeleev's idea that the stars were 90% hydrogen.

    (B)   discovered the principle that natural life contracts.

    (C)   conceived of the idea of the evolution of matter.

    (D)   believed that Charles Darwin's theory of the origin of life was wrong.

49. The concept of "primordial soup" refers to

    (A)   primitive oceans.

    (B)   water, carbon dioxide, sugars and the material of proteins.

    (C)   conditions suitable for the emergence of life.

    (D)   carbon dioxide and water.

50. Clay is important as an area of scientific investigation in the origin of life because

    (A)   clay, as a surface phenomenon, appears to contribute to our knowledge of organic synthesis.

    (B)   clay is a polymer.

    (C)   clay is an absorbed, organic molecule.

    (D)   clay replicates the origin of life.

51. From the passage it can be concluded that

    (A) only Darwin, Oparin and Haldane contributed to evolutionary theory.

    (B) Oparin, Haldane and Bernal disagreed with Darwin.

    (C) Darwin, Oparin, Haldane and Bernal were the only four significant contributors to evolutionary theory.

    (D) Darwin paved the way for the evolutionary theories of Oparin, Haldane and Bernal.

52. It can be inferred from this passage that life

    (A) began from pre-existent matter.

    (B) had no beginning.

    (C) is too complex to speculate on its beginnings.

    (D) and its absence are but two sides of the same coin.

53. An appropriate title for this passage would be "The Evolutionary Synthesis" because

    (A) "synthesis" is a synonym for "origin."

    (B) synthesis implies a contraction of matter.

    (C) all evolutionary theories are syntheses.

    (D) "synthesis" has similar meaning to "analysis."

54. Which description best interprets the sentence, "But for 50 years such large ideas lay dormant?"

    (A) Grand ideas are doomed to failure.

    (B) Time allows most ideas to die.

    (C) Important ideas usually lie in hiding for a time.

    (D) Ideas evolve slowly.

55. From the essay we may infer that the relation between the origin of life and the present study of matter

    (A) involves a direct cause-effect relationship to each other.

    (B) involves no cause-effect relationship to each other.

    (C) are equal.

    (D) are not equal.

56. From the work of the young Russian biochemist, A. Oparin, one can now

    (A) know the origin of life.

    (B) know the evolving complexity of life.

    (C) trace life forms and their point of origin.

    (D) dismiss the issue of the origin of life altogether.

PASSAGE VII (Questions 57-65)

Utilitarian moralists maintain that the moral value of an action depends upon the value of the consequences of that action. A person's motives in doing an action are not relevant in assessing the moral value of the action, although they may be considered in determining the moral character of the person who does the action. Thus, *consequences* determine the value of the action and *motives* are relevant only for determining the moral character of the person who does the action.

There are differences in how the consequences of an action are to be understood. There are those who take "consequences" in the sense of the results which come about from an action, regardless of whether or not these results were, or even could have been, foreseen. There are others who take consequences in the sense of the results that would normally come about or that should reasonably have been foreseen. Thus, utilitarian moralists will differ on their views of what kinds of consequences are relevant in assessing the moral character of an action: the actual consequences or the reasonably expected consequences.

There is yet a second way in which utilitarian moral theories will differ, and this is how they interpret the notion of an action. In one type of theory, an action will be thought of as a certain way of doing something, as an action of a certain type or kind. In the other type of theory, an action is thought of as a particular performance done by a person at some place and at some time. The key difference between these two ways of construing an action has to do with the concept of *repeatability*. Is the action thought of as something which is repeatable in principle? Can one person do this very same act a number of different times, or can many different people do this very same act either at the same time or at different times? If the answer is "yes," then the act may be said to be repeatable and is then thought of as a type or kind of action. On the other hand, if the answer to these questions is "no," then the action is thought of as a particular or concrete instance of an action.

These two different ways of thinking of an action will determine the type of utilitarian moral theory one holds. One stance maintains that the theory applies to types or kinds of action, while the other stance maintains that the theory applies to particular instances of types of actions. The first opinion, the one which considers actions as types, will then look to consequences as what normally results from doing a certain type of action. The actual consequences that do in fact result will not be considered relevant. The other type of theory will offer a choice of how the concept of consequences is to be conjoined with the concept of the action. We may look to either the reasonably expected consequences or to the actual consequences of a particular action in determining its moral worth.

57. Utilitarian theories evaluate the moral value of actions on the basis of

   (A) the motives a person has in doing the action.

   (B) a person's responsibility for the action.

   (C) the actual consequences of the type of action done.

   (D) the value of an action's consequences.

58. Whether or not an action is repeatable determines

   (A) whether or not it is considered by utilitarian theories.

   (B) whether or not it is a type of action or a particular action.

(C)   whether or not it has consequences.

(D)   All of the above.

59.   A utilitarian theory which understands "consequences" as actual occurrences

(A)   would be required to construe actions as types of actions.

(B)   would be required to construe actions as particular actions.

(C)   could construe actions as either types of or as particular actions.

(D)   could but would not be required to construe actions as types of actions.

60.   Suppose an action done by someone had an unexpectedly bad result. We can infer that utilitarian moralists would

(A)   differ about the moral appraisal of that action.

(B)   differ about the grounds for the moral appraisal of that action.

(C)   Both (A) and (B).

(D)   agree about the appraisal of that action.

61.   Utilitarian theories differ with respect to how they consider

(A)   the moral character of persons.

(B)   the relevance of a person's good intentions.

(C)   the action a person does.

(D)   what moral value depends on.

62.   Which of the following would be a legitimate excuse for all utilitarian moralists?

(A)   "I didn't mean to do it."

(B)   "Nobody got hurt."

(C)   "I didn't know that would happen, really."

(D)   None of the above.

63.   Based on the passage, utilitarian moralists

(A)   agree that consequences determine the moral value of an action.

(B)   agree on the moral values of actions.

(C)   agree on matters of responsibility.

(D)   agree on exactly what an action is.

64.   The actual results of an action would be considered

(A)   morally relevant by some but not all utilitarians.

(B)   morally relevant by all utilitarians.

    (C)   morally relevant only to those who construe actions as a form of responsibility.

    (D)   morally relevant by no utilitarians.

65.   If an action is thought of as repeatable, then

    (A)   one person can do this same action on many different occasions.

    (B)   many people can do this same action on one occasion.

    (C)   many people can do this same action on many different occasions.

    (D)   All of the above.

STOP

If time still remains, you may review work only in this section.
When the time allotted is up, you may go on to the next section.

Section 2 — Physical Sciences

TIME: 100 Minutes
QUESTIONS: 66-142

DIRECTIONS: Most of the questions in this section are arranged in groups, each corresponding to a descriptive passage. Based on the information given in a passage, choose the one best answer to each question in the group. Some questions are independent of a descriptive passage and of each other. Choose the one best answer to each of these questions. If you are not sure of an answer, eliminate those choices that you know are incorrect and choose an answer from among those remaining. Fill in the corresponding circle on the answer sheet to indicate your answer. You may refer to the periodic table at any time.

PASSAGE I (Questions 66-73)

A 10 mL sample of blood was drawn from a patient and several tests, as outlined below, were done on subsamples of this blood.

Test 1: The concentration of calcium in the blood was determined by adding oxalate ion to the blood subsample to precipitate calcium oxalate according to the equation:

$$Ca^{++} \text{ (in blood)} + C_2O_4^{=} \text{ (aq)} \longrightarrow CaC_2O_4 \text{ (s)}$$

The solid calcium oxalate was separated from the blood, dissolved in acid, and titrated with standardized potassium permanganate solution according to the equation:

$$2MnO_4^- \text{ (aq)} + 5H_2C_2O_4 \text{ (aq)} + 6H^+ \text{ (aq)} \longrightarrow 2Mn^{++} \text{ (aq)} + 10CO_2 \text{ (g)} + 8H_2O$$
(1)

The calcium in a 5.00 mL blood sample was precipitated as CaC_2O_4. After separation, the calcium oxalate was dissolved in 6.0 M HCl and titrated with 11.63 mL of 0.00100 M potassium permanganate solution.

Test 2: Using another blood subsample and a glass microelectrode, the pH of the blood was found to be pH = 7.45. The pH of blood is determined almost entirely by the carbonate species present in the blood. The Henderson-Hasselbach equation in the form below relates the pH to the concentrations of bicarbonate ion and carbonic acid (dissolved carbon dioxide):

$$pH = 6.1 + \log([HCO^-]/[H_2CO_3]$$

where 6.1 is the pKa of carbonic acid.

Test 3: The total carbonate species in the blood was determined by reacting the bicarbonate ion with acid, converting the carbonic acid to carbon dioxide gas, and collecting the resulting CO_2 gas. A microgasometer was used to collect the carbon dioxide from a 0.0300 mL sample of blood; it occupied a volume of 0.200 mL at 67.0 mm Hg pressure and 21° C.

66. What is the oxidation state (oxidation number) of carbon in calcium oxalate?

    (A) 0   (B) + 1

    (C) + 2   (D) + 3

67. The solubility product constant for calcium oxalate is 2.3×10^{-9}. What is the concentration of calcium ions in equilibrium with solid calcium oxalate in a solution that has an oxalate ion concentration of 0.115 M?

    (A) 2.6×10^{-10} M   (B) 2.0×10^{-8} M

    (C) 2.3×10^{-9} M   (D) 4.8×10^{-5} M

68. What hydrogen ion concentration corresponds to pH = 7.45?

    (A) 3.5×10^{-8} M   (B) 4.5×10^{-7} M

    (C) 6.3×10^{-6} M   (D) 1.2×10^{-5} M

69. According to the Henderson-Hasselbach equation for the bicarbonate equilibrium in blood, what is the ratio of the concentration of bicarbonate ion to that of carbonic acid in blood of pH = 7.45?

    (A) 0.14   (B) 0.84

    (C) 6.9   (D) 22.4

70. If a 5.00 mL blood sample required 11.63 mL of 0.00100 M potassium permanganate solution for titration of the calcium oxalate precipitated from it, what was the calcium ion concentration in the blood?

    (A) 0.00100 M   (B) 0.00233 M

    (C) 0.00581 M   (D) 0.00837 M

71. What volume would the sample of carbon dioxide gas (0.200 mL at 67.0 mm Hg. 21° C) occupy at STP (760 mm Hg, 0°C)?

    (A) 0.016 mL   (B) 0.019 mL

    (C) 2.11 mL   (D) 2.44 mL

72. What was the molar concentration of the carbon dioxide in the 0.0300 mL blood sample?

    (A) 0.010 M   (B) 0.024 M

    (C) 0.032 M   (D) 0.040 M

73. In aqueous solution, bicarbonate ion may react with water molecules. In this hydrolysis reaction, the bicarbonate ion may

    (A)   act as a Bronsted acid only.

    (B)   act as a Bronsted base only.

    (C)   act as either a Bronsted acid or Bronsted base.

    (D)   act as neither a Bronsted acid nor Bronsted base.

PASSAGE II (Questions 74-79)

A bag of white material, in the form of a fine white powder, was removed from the luggage of a passenger returning to the U.S. on an international flight. The white powder was discovered by a Customs Agent's dog, which had been trained to detect drugs. A rapid, preliminary, qualitative test indicated the presence of cocaine, $C_{17}H_{21}NO_4$, molar mass 303.15 g/mol. The bag of white powder was sent to a laboratory for more complete analysis.

An analysis of the white powder for nitrogen showed that it contained 1.43%, by mass, elemental nitrogen. Using suitable solvents, the white powder was found to be a mixture and was separated into two components, A and B. The sharpness of the melting points of each of the components indicated that each was a pure substance. Qualitative analysis confirmed that substance A was cocaine. Substance B was found to contain no nitrogen and to be readily soluble in water. Elemental analysis of B gave the following composition: 42.10% C, 6.48% H, and 51.42% O. A solution made by dissolving 1.00 g of substance B in 100.0 g of camphor had a freezing point of 178.58°C. The normal freezing point of pure camphor is 179.75°C and its molal freezing point lowering constant is 40.0°C/molal.

74. What percent, by mass, of cocaine is carbon?

    (A)   39.5%   (B)   67.3%

    (C)   82.1%   (D)   97.6%

75. What percent, by mass, of the white powder is cocaine?

    (A)   20.7%   (B)   31.0%

    (C)   47.8%   (D)   67.9%

76. What is the simplest, or empirical, formula of substance B?

    (A) CH_2O (B) $C_6H_{12}O_6$

    (C) CH_4O_2 (D) $C_{12}H_{22}O_{11}$

77. Using the freezing point lowering data, estimate the molar mass of substance B.

    (A)   60 g/mol   (B)   180 g/mol

    (C)   342 g/mol   (D)   684 g/mol

78. Which of the following would be the best solvent to dissolve the slightly polar cocaine from the mixture but not dissolve the very polar substance B?

    (A)   Water, H_2O (B)   Chloroform, $CHCl_3$

    (C)   Methanol, CH_3OH (D)   Acetone, CH_3COCH_3

79. If the chemical equation for the combustion of cocaine with excess oxygen gas to form carbon dioxide gas, water vapor, and nitrogen dioxide gas is balanced such that the coefficient of cocaine is four, what is the coefficient of oxygen gas?

(A)   10   (B)   42

(C)   68   (D)   85

PASSAGE III (Questions 80-84)

Table 1 below contains thermochemical data for two series of related compounds: the hydrogen halides (HF through HI) and four simple hydrocarbons. With the exception of hydrogen fluoride, there is a regular trend within each series of increasing enthalpy of vaporization, increasing normal boiling point and increasing critical temperature with increasing molecular weight. The diatomic molecules all have nearly the same Cp, whereas the Cp of the polyatomic molecules tends to increase with increasing number of atoms per molecule.

TABLE 1 — Thermodynamic Properties of Selected Substances

Substance	Enthalpy of Vaporization kJ/mole	Normal Boiling Point K	Critical Temperature K	Heat Capacity Cp J/mol K
HF	25.2	292.8	462.1	29.1
HCl	17.5	188.3	324.6	29.1
HBr	19.3	206.6	363.2	29.1
HI	21.2	238.1	423	29.2
CH_4, methane	8.9	111.6	191.0	35.3
C_2H_6, ethane	15.7	184.6	305.4	52.6
C_3H_8, propane	19.0	231.1	369.9	73.5
C_4H_{10}, n-butane	24.3	272.6	425.1	97.4

Table 2 below gives the standard enthalpies of combustion at 273.15 K and 1 bar pressure for three substances.

TABLE 2 — Standard Enthalpies of Combustion at 273.15 K.

Substance	kJ/mol
C (graphite)	- 393.5
H_2 (g)	- 285.8
CH_4 (g)	- 890.3

The combustion products consist of carbon dioxide gas and/or liquid water. The enthalpy of combustion of graphite is equivalent to the enthalpy of formation of carbon dioxide gas and the enthalpy of combustion of hydrogen gas is equivalent to the enthalpy of formation of liquid water. The standard enthalpy of formation of water in the gaseous state is - 241.8 kJ/mol at 25°C and 1 bar. The standard enthalpy of formation of water in the liquid state is - 285.8 kJ.mol at 25°C and 1 bar.

80.   With respect to the data in Table 1, hydrogen bonding can be used to explain which of the following?

(A)   The nearly constant molar heat capacities of the diatomic molecules

(B)   The unusually large molar enthalpy of vaporization of HF

(C)   The trend of increasing molar enthalpy of vaporization with increasing molar mass for the hydrocarbons

(D)   The trend of increasing molar heat capacity with increasing molar mass for the hydrocarbons

81.   How much heat energy is released when 32 g of HI gas condenses to liquid?

(A)   5.3 kJ   (B)   10.6 kJ

(C)   15.9 kJ   (D)   21.2 kJ

82.   How much heat energy is required to raise the temperature of two moles of ethane from 20°C to 30°C?

(A)   98 J   (B)   210 J

(C)   526 J   (D)   1052 J

83.   On the basis of the given enthalpies of formation of liquid water and gaseous water, calculate the enthalpy of vaporization of water at 25°C.

(A)   44.0 kJ/mol   (B)   127.2 kJ/mol

(C)   263.8 kJ/mol   (D)   527.6 kJ/mol

84.   On the basis of the data in Table 2, calculate the standard enthalpy for formation of methane at 25°C.

(A)   + 211.0 kJ/mol   (B)   - 1855.4 kJ/mol

(C)   - 74.8 kJ/mol   (D)   - 211.0 kJ/mol

QUESTIONS 85 - 90 are NOT based on a descriptive passage.

85.   The law which states that the relationship between volume and temperature of an ideal gas, where the pressure is kept constant, is such that the volume is proportional to the absolute temperature was propounded by

(A)   Charles.   (B)   Avogadro.

(C)   Boyle.   (D)   Newton.

86.   A ball is at the top of a hill. After a small amount of displacement, the ball moves to a new position. The ball was initially in

(A)   equilibrium.   (B)   neutral equilibrium.

(C)   unstable equilibrium.   (D)   natural equilibrium.

87.   An air column, whose length may be varied, is used to determine the speed of sound. This method of finding the speed makes use of

(A)   the Doppler effect.   (B)   Huygen's Principle.

(C)   resonance.   (D)   beats.

88. A mixture of oxygen and nitrogen is placed in a closed cylinder and a small hole is punched in the cylinder. What is the rate of effusion ratio of O_2 to N_2?

(A) $\sqrt{8/7}$

(B) $8/7$

(C) $\sqrt{7/8}$

(D) $7/8$

89. The change in enthalpy (ΔH) of a system is equal to the heat flow between the system and its surroundings (q) under which conditions?

(A) constant volume

(B) adiabatic conditions

(C) constant pressure

(D) constant temperature

90. A metal ball is dropped into a deep well with water on the very bottom. The time taken between dropping the ball from rest to hearing it splash the water is 6.83 s. Calculate the depth of the well assuming $c = 330$ m/s.

(A) 229 m

(B) 219 m

(C) 201 m

(D) 191 m

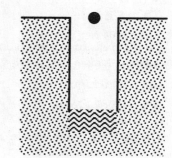

PASSAGE IV (Questions 91-96)

A common filling for tooth cavities is "dental amalgam," a solid solution made by dissolving tin and silver in mercury. Although amalgam fillings are inert and generally do not cause health problems, they can lead to quite a surprise if one bites on a piece of aluminum foil. The electrochemical reactions between the aluminum and the components of an amalgam, with saliva and gum tissue acting as the electrolyte, can "shock" the tooth's nerve by sending a small flow of electrons to it. Some half reactions involved, with standard reduction potentials at 25°C, include

		$E°$/V
Equation 1	Al^{3+} (aq) + 3e $\longrightarrow$ Al (s)	- 1.66
Equation 2	Sn^{2+} (aq) + 3Ag (s) + 2 e $\longrightarrow$ Ag_3Sn (s)	- 0.05
Equation 3	$3Hg_2^{2+}$ (aq) + 4Ag(s) + 6e $\longrightarrow$ $2Ag_2Hg_3$ (s)	+ 0.85

Aluminum is produced from its ore via an electrolytic method, the Hall-Heroult process. Aluminum oxide, Al_2O_3, is extracted from the ore, dissolved in molten cryolite, Na_3AlF_6, maintained at 980°C, and electrolized at low voltage but very high current, for example, 5.0 V and 10,000 A. In actual practice, about 7 kilowatt-hours of electric energy (excluding the energy needed to heat the furnace) is required to produce one pound of aluminum by electrolysis. This is equivalent to about 55.5 kJ/g Al.

91. What is the standard cell potential for the spontaneous reaction obtained by combining the half reactions of equation 1 and equation 2?

    (A) + 1.61 V   (B) - 1.61 V

    (C) + 1.71 V   (D) - 1.71 V

92. If a Galvanic or Voltaic cell were constructed in which the overall, spontaneous reaction obtained by combining the half reactions of equation 2 and equation 3 takes place

    (A) Ag_3Sn (s) is the anode and electrons flow from Ag (s) to Ag_3Sn (s).

    (B) Ag_3Sn (s) is the cathode and electrons flow from Ag_3 Sn (s) to Ag (s).

    (C) Ag_3Sn (s) is the anode and electrons flow from Ag_3Sn(s) to Ag(s).

    (D) Ag_3Sn(s) is the cathode and electrons flow from Ag(s) to Ag_3Sn(s).

93. If the half reactions for equations 2 and 3 are combined to obtain an overall, net ionic equation for a spontaneous cell reaction, the minimum coefficient of Ag(s) in the balanced equation is

    (A) 1.   (B) 4.

    (C) 5.   (D) 9.

94. How much energy is used in one minute in the electrolysis of aluminum oxide at 5.0 V with a current of 10,000 A?

    (A) 0.5 MJ   (B) 1.0 MJ

    (C) 2.0 MJ   (D) 3.0 MJ

95. If the half reactions for equations 1 and 3 are combined to form a Galvanic cell with standard cell potential + 2.51 V, what is the equilibrium constant for the resulting reaction (for which the balanced equation contains two moles of Al)? The gas constant is 8.31 j/K mol and the Faraday constant is 96,500 C.

    (A) 10^{255} (B) 10^{59}

    (C) 10^{-19} (D) 10^{-126}

96. If the electrolytic production of aluminum were carried out with 100% efficiency at 5.0 V, what energy would be required per gram of Al produced?

    (A) 46.8 kJ/g   (B) 51.7 kJ/g

    (C) 53.6 kJ/g   (D) 55.5 kJ/g

PASSAGE V (Questions 97-102)

The kinetics of the hydrolysis of methyl acetate, in the presence of hydrogen ion, was studied in a series of experiments. The overall reaction is:

$$CH_3OOCCH_3 + H_2O + H^+ \longrightarrow CH_3OH + HOOCCH_3 + H^+$$

In the first set of experiments, the temperature was held constant at 25°C and the initial concentrations of methyl acetate and hydrogen ion were varied. The initial reaction rate was measured. The results are summarized in Table 1.

TABLE 1 - Initial Reaction Rate at 25°C

[methyl acetate]	[HCL]	Initial Rate (relative units)
0.1 M	0.1 M	1
0.2 M	0.1 M	2
0.3 M	0.1 M	3
0.2 M	0.5 M	10
0.2 M	1.0 M	20

In the second experiment, the concentration of methyl acetate as a function of time was measured at 25°C:

Time/min.	0.00	1.75	4.76
[methyl acetate]/M	0.30	0.20	0.10

In a third set of experiments, the half time for the hydrolysis was measured for the same initial concentrations of methyl acetate and HCl at different temperatures.

Temperature/°C	0	10	20	30
half time/min	18.8	8.68	4.23	2.16

97. The hydrolosis of methyl acetate is first order with respect to methyl acetate and what order with respect to hydrogen ion?

   (A) Zeroth   (B) First

   (C) Second   (D) Third

98. The most likely first step in the mechanism of the hydrolysis of methyl acetate in the presence of hydrogen ion is

   (A) $C_3H_6O_2 \longrightarrow CH_3^+ + CH_3COO^-$.

   (B) $C_3H_6O_2 + H_2O \longrightarrow C_3H_8O_3$.

   (C) $C_3H_6O_2 + H_2O \longrightarrow C_3H_7O_3^- + H^+$.

   (D) $C_3H_6O_2 + H^+ \longrightarrow C_3H_7O_2^+$.

99. If a reaction were half order with respect to a reactant, by what factor would the initial rate of reaction increase if the concentration of the reactant were doubled?

   (A) 0.50   (B) 0.71

   (C) 1.4   (D) 2.0

100. The hydrolysis of methyl acetate can be followed by titrating the acetic acid produced. Which graph below best represents the change in acetic acid concentration with time?

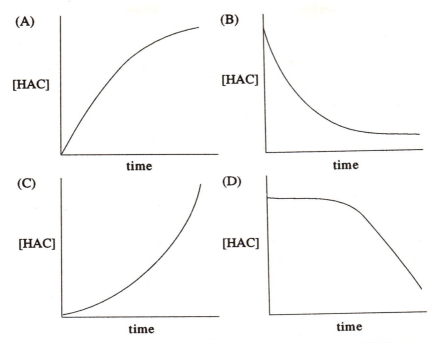

(A) [HAC] vs time

(B) [HAC] vs time

(C) [HAC] vs time

(D) [HAC] vs time

101. What is the half time for the hydrolysis of methyl acetate at 25°C?

(A) 2.8 min

(B) 3.0 min

(C) 3.2 min

(D) 3.4 min

102. What is the Arrhenius activation energy for the hydrolysis of methyl acetate?

(A) 30 kJ/mol

(B) 40 kJ/mol

(C) 50 kJ/mol

(D) 60 kJ/mol

PASSAGE VI (Questions 103-107)

A compound microscope consists of an objective lens mounted at the bottom of the barrel and an eye lens mounted at the top of the barrel, as illustrated here. In many microscopes, the tube length, the distance from the objective lens to the real image that it forms, is 16 cm.

The magnification of a lens is defined as the ratio of the image size to the object size. It can be shown that the magnification, M, for an image distance of 16 cm from a lens of focal length f (in cm) is:

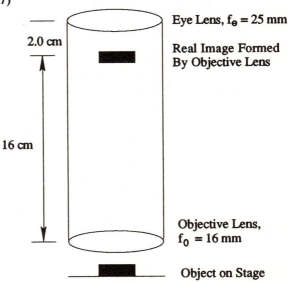

Eye Lens, f_e = 25 mm

Real Image Formed By Objective Lens

2.0 cm

16 cm

Objective Lens, f_0 = 16 mm

Object on Stage

$$M = (16 \text{ cm}/f) - 1.$$

Magnifying power is defined as the ratio of the image size as viewed with the lens to the object size as viewed at 25 cm without the lens. It can be shown that the magnifying power, MP, of a lens of focal length f (in cm) is:

$$MP = (25 \text{ cm}/f) + 1.$$

The magnifying power of a compound microscope is the product of the magnification of the objective lens times the magnifying power of the eye lens:

$$MP_c = [(16 \text{ cm}/f_o) - 1] [(25 \text{ cm}/f_e) + 1] \qquad \text{Equation (1)}$$

It is useful to express the magnifying power without the "ones;"

$$MP_c = (16 \text{ cm}/f_o) (25 \text{ cm}/f_e) \qquad \text{Equation (2)}$$

103. When a microscope with an objective lens focal length of $f_o = 16$ mm is focused such that the real image is at 16 cm, what is the distance from the lens to the object?

    (A)   14 mm

    (B)   16 mm

    (C)   18 mm

    (D)   20 mm

104. In the illustration, the focal length of the eye lens is 25 mm. The object for the eye lens is the image formed by the objective lens. What type of image (with respect to the image of the objective lens, not with respect to the object below the objective lens) is formed by the eye lens for the dimensions shown in the illustration?

    (A)   Virtual, erect

    (B)   Virtual, inverted

    (C)   Real, erect

    (D)   Real, inverted

105. For focal lengths $f_o = 16$ mm and $f_e = 25$ mm, what percent error is made by using Equation 2 in place of Equation 1?

    (A)   1%

    (B)   2%

    (C)   3%

    (D)   4%

106. The object to be viewed through a microscope is usually covered with a thin glass "cover slip." If the cover slip is not completely uniform in thickness, the variation in the divergence of the light when it leaves the cover slip and travels through the air to the objective lens will lead to a reduction in quality of the final image. To reduce this problem the space between the cover slip and the objective lens is sometimes filled with oil. The oil should be chosen with an index of refraction that is

    (A)   nearly equal to the index of refraction of air.

    (B)   nearly equal to the index of refraction of the glass.

    (C)   much smaller than the index of refraction of air.

    (D)   much smaller than the index of refraction of the glass.

107. A scale or graticule is placed 16 cm above the objective lens in the microscope illustrated to measure the length of the image. An image appears to be 0.15 mm long when viewed using lenses with the focal lengths shown in the illustration. What is the actual length of the object on the microscope stage?

(A)   14 μm   (B)   15 μm

(C)   16 μm   (D)   17 μm

QUESTIONS 108-112 are NOT based on a descriptive passage.

---

108. Phosgene, molecular formula $COCl_2$, is a poisonous gas used in World War I. The gas causes rapid, painful death by

(A)   complexing with hemoglobin faster than oxygen.

(B)   causing coagulation of the blood.

(C)   reacting with water to produce hydrochloric acid.

(D)   disrupting hydrogen bonding.

109. In human digestion, fats are hydrolized to

(A)   glucagon and glucose.   (B)   glycerol and glucagon.

(C)   xylenol and fatty acids.   (D)   glycerol and fatty acids.

110. A triose may be defined by all of the following except as being

(A)   a sugar.

(B)   a three-carbon organic compound.

(C)   a hydroxyaldehyde.

(D)   a trisaccharide.

111. Which of the following is not true for all waves?

(A)   Their speed depends on the temperature of the transmitting medium.

(B) $v = f\lambda$

(C)   They can produce interference.

(D)   They can be diffracted.

112. An inclined plane is 15 m long and 3 m high. The force required to prevent a box weighing 120 N from sliding down this frictionless plane is

(A)   8N.   (B)   24N.

(C)   40N.   (D)   45N.

PASSAGE VII (Questions 113-120)

An automobile of mass 2,000 kg is parked on a steep hill. The coefficient of static friction between the tires and the road surface is 1.00 and the coefficient of sliding friction is independent of speed. A second car, while attempting to park behind the first car, gives the first car a slight bump which starts it sliding down the hill. At the bottom of the hill the road makes a sharp turn, with radius of curvature 50 m. The first car slides straight down the hill and collides with a solid stone wall at the edge of the road near the foot of the hill. The car slid 200 m along the road surface while descending a vertical distance of 100 m. The car had reached a speed of 20 m/s (~45 mph) just before it reached the stone wall and came to rest 0.50 s after striking the wall.

The driver of the second car saw that there was a public telephone just beyond the curve at the bottom of the hill. The second car drove down the hill, past the wreckage of the first car, rounding the curve with a speed of 13.4 m/s (~30 mph). The driver of the second car applied the brakes and came to a stop by the telephone booth over a distance of 100 m. When it started, the second car accelerated from rest to 13.4 m/s in the first 100 m, continued at constant speed for another 200 m down the hill and around the curve before starting to decelerate.

The incident happened at a place where the acceleration due to gravity is 9.80 m/s^2.

113. What is the maximum angle the road surface could make with respect to the horizontal and still allow the first car to park without sliding?

   (A)   15°   (B)   30°

   (C)   45°   (D)   60°

114. Assuming the first car starts from rest and slides down the hill with constant acceleration, what is the coefficient of sliding friction between its tires and the road surface?

   (A)   ≅0.118   (B)   ≅0.314

   (C)   ≅0.408   (D)   ≅0.502

115. What is the deceleration of the first car when it strikes the wall?

   (A)   10 m/s^2 (B)   20 m/s^2

   (C)   30 m/s^2 (D)   40 m/s^2

116. What is the first car's potential energy, with respect to the bottom of the hill, when it is at the top of the hill?

   (A)   1.9 MJ   (B)   3.1 MJ

   (C)   3.5 MJ   (D)   4.0 MJ

117. What is the first car's kinetic energy just before it strikes the wall?

   (A)   0.2 MJ   (B)   0.3 MJ

   (C)   0.4 MJ   (D)   0.5 MJ

118. What is the magnitude of the first car's momentum just before it strikes the wall?

(A)   10 Mg m/s   (B)   20 Mg m/s

(C)   30 Mg m/s   (D)   40 Mg m/s

119.   What apparent outward central acceleration (expressed as a fraction of the acceleration due to gravity) does the driver of the second car experience when rounding the curve?

(A)   0.25   (B)   0.37

(C)   0.52   (D)   0.75

120.   Assuming constant acceleration and deceleration, how long did it take for the second car to travel from the top of the hill to the telephone booth?

(A)   15 s   (B)   30 s

(C)   45 s   (D)   60 s

PASSAGE VIII (Questions 121-126)

Human blood varies substantially from person to person, with state of health, etc. Typical values of the density of blood plasma and blood cells are 1025 kg/m^3 and 1125 kg/m^3, respectively. The viscosity of blood at 37°C is about 2.7 centipoise, much greater than the viscosity of water at the same temperature (~0.7 centipoise). The flow of blood in the human circulatory system, which consists of nearly circular cross section blood vessels, can be described quite well using Poiseuille's equation:

$$\frac{V}{t} = \frac{\pi(P_1 - P_2)R^4}{8L\mu}$$

V/T is the volume of blood flow per unit time. P_1 - P_2 is the pressure difference between the ends of a tube of radius R and length L. μ is the fluid's coefficient of viscosity, or more simply just the viscosity.

121.   What is the mass of 500 mL of blood plasma which has a density of 1025 kg/m^3?

(A)   205 g   (B)   488 g

(C)   512 g   (D)   762 g

122.   What is the apparent weight (i.e., net downward force) on a blood cell of volume 150 μm^3 and density 1125 kg/m^3 suspended in plasma of density 1025 kg/m^3? (g = 9.8 m/s^2)

(A)   0.15 pN   (B)   0.30 pN

(C)   0.45 pN   (D)   0.60 pN

123.   The viscosity of a fluid can be determined by measuring the time taken for a given volume of the fluid to flow through a fixed length of capillary tube of fixed radius. The pressure difference is the fluid static pressure difference over the height of the tube. According to Poiseuille's equation, the relative flow time for a liquid of density d in this type of viscometer is directly proportional to

(A)   the viscosity.

(B)   the viscosity divided by the density.

(C)   the viscosity times the density.

(D)   the density divided by the viscosity.

124. When blood moves from a blood vessel with diameter 5.0 mm to a blood vessel of diameter 3.0 mm, the speed of flow increases by a factor of

(A)   1.3   (B)   1.7

(C)   2.0   (D)   2.8

125. According to Bernoulli's law, the concentration of blood cells is greater near the center than near the wall of a blood vessel because

(A)   both the fluid speed and pressure are lower near the center.

(B)   the speed is greater but the pressure is lower near the center.

(C)   the speed is smaller but the pressure is greater near the center.

(D)   both the fluid speed and pressure are greater near the center.

126. According to Poiseuille's equation, the volume of blood flow per unit time is reduced to what percent of the initial value when blood that was flowing in a 5.0 mm diameter blood vessel enters a 3.0 mm diameter blood vessel, the pressure difference per unit length remaining constant?

(A)   13%   (B)   22%

(C)   36%   (D)   60%

PASSAGE IX (Questions 127-132)
    A basketball player of mass 70 kg (weight 686 N) raises on the ball of one foot to take a shot. To do this, the gastrocnemius muscle pulls on the heel through the Achilles tendon with force F and the tibia pushes down on the ankle joint with P. The floor pushes up on the ball of the foot with force mg, equal to the player's weight. The situation is diagrammed in Figure 1.

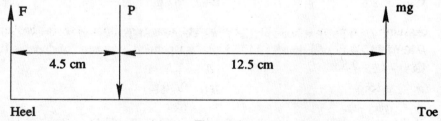

Figure 1

The player shoots the basketball (mass 1.50 kg) from a height of 2.00 m above the floor, at an angle of 45° above the horizontal and with an initial speed of 10.0 m/s. The ball does not reach the basket. During the scuffle under the basket, the ball is thrown violently back toward the player who took the shot and strikes him in the thigh. The ball, moving horizontally with a speed of 15.0 m/s, strikes the vertical thigh and rebounds horizontally with a speed of 10.0 m/s. This situation is diagrammed in Figure 2.

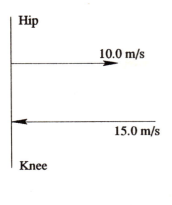

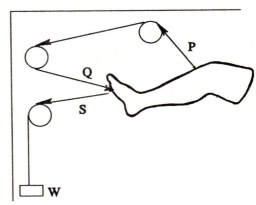

Figure 2   Figure 3

The force of the blow is so great that the player's femur is broken. The player is required to spend some time in traction. The Russell system of traction, which was used, is diagrammed in Figure 3.

The forces S, Q, and P are all equal in magnitude and equal in magnitude to the tension in the cord (i.e., the weight, W, hanging from the cord). The vector sum or resultant of the forces S, Q, and P is the force pulling on the femur. With respect to the horizontal, S makes an angle of 20° below (sin 20° = 0.342/cos 20° = 0.940), Q an angle of 30° above and P an angle of 45° above.

127. When the player raises on the ball of his foot, what force, F, is exerted on the heel by the Achilles' tendon?

(A) 0.69 kN   (B)   1.9 kN

(C) 2.6 kN   (D)   4.7 kN

128. When the player raises on the ball of his foot, what force, P, is exerted on the ankle joint?

(A) 0.69 kN   (B)   1.9 kN

(C) 2.6 kN   (D)   4.7 kN

129. Assuming no air resistance, to what height above the floor does the basketball rise when the player shoots?

(A) 1.55 m   (B)   2.55 m

(C) 3.55 m   (D)   4.55 m

130. If the ball were not intercepted, at what horizontal distance from the shooter would it strike the floor? (Neglect air resistance.)

(A) 6 m   (B)   8 m

(C) 10 m   (D)   12 m

131. If the force of the impact of the ball with the player's thigh were 3.75 kN, how long was the ball in contact with the thigh?

(A)   10 ms   (B)   25 ms

(C)   33 ms   (D)   50 ms

132. What is the magnitude of the resultant force on the femur when the player's broken leg is in traction? Express the result as a multiple of the weight, W.

(A)   1.4 W (B)   2.7 W

(C)   4.2 W (D)   5.1 W

PASSAGE X (Questions 133-138)

A tandem van de Graaff accelerator can be used to produce low to medium energy charged particles for nuclear reaction and nuclear structure studies. A tandem van de Graaff consists of a high voltage terminal, a negative ion source, evacuated beam tube running from the ion source through the high voltage terminal, and magnets to bend the beam of charged particles. The high voltage terminal is charged by the terminal by a charging belt. When the whole system is enclosed within a tank containing an inert gas, e.g., sulfur hexafluoride, potentials of more than 20 MV may be achieved. In operation, negative ions, e.g., H^-, He^-, etc. are produced at the negative ion source. These negative ions are attracted to the positive high voltage terminal. When the ions enter the zero electric field region within the hollow terminal they continue to move at constant speed and are allowed to collide with an electron stripper (very thin metal foil or low density stream of gas) where they are converted to positive ions, e.g., H^+, He^{++}, etc. When the positive ions move out of the terminal, they are repelled by it. The accelerated beam of positive ions is then directed to a target by magnets. Nuclear reactions and the energy levels of the protons and neutrons within the nucleus can be studied with very high energy resolution using the beam from a van de Graaff accelerator.

133. If the current resulting from the loss of charge when the high voltage terminal is maintained at 20 MV is 50 mA, what is the effective resistance between the terminal and ground?

(A)   1 $M\Omega$ (B)   70 $M\Omega$

(C)   250 $M\Omega$ (D)   400 $M\Omega$

134. To a first approximation at a given temperature, the speed of sound in a gas is inversely proportional to the square root of the molecular weight of the gas. When there is an electric discharge between the high voltage terminal and the tank wall ("tank spark"), a "boom," similar to thunder, is heard. How fast does the speed of a tank spark travel in SF_6 as compared to the speed of sound in air at the same temperature? The average molecular weight of air is about 29.

(A)   0.20   (B)   0.45

(C)   2.2   (D)   5.0

135. If an He^- ion is accelerated from ground to +20 MV, stripped of all of its electrons to form a He^{++} ion, and then accelerated from + 20 MV to ground, what is its final kinetic energy?

(A)   20 MeV   (B)   40 MeV

(C)   60 MeV   (D)   80 MeV

136. What must be the strength of a magnetic field if it is to bend an alpha particle
      ($_2^4$He^{++}) through a radius of curvature of 1.00 m if it has an energy of 25 MeV,
      i.e., speed of 3.5×10^7 m/s? The electron charge is $- 1.6 \times 10^{-19}$ C and one
      atomic mass unit is 1.66×10^{-27} kg.

      (A)   0.73 T   (B)   1.96 T

      (C)   2.84 T   (D)   3.92 T

137. If a 32 MeV $_2^4$He^{++} ion collides with and sticks to a $_6^{12}$C target nucleus, what is
      the recoil kinetic energy of the resulting $_8^{16}$O nucleus?

      (A)   4 MeV   (B)   6 MeV

      (C)   8 MeV   (D)   10 MeV

138. If a 32 MeV alpha particle ($_2^4$He^{++}) is incident on a $_{13}^{27}$Al target nucleus and one
      reaction product is a neutron, what is the other reaction product?

      (A) $_{14}^{30}$Si   (B) $_{14}^{31}$Si

      (C) $_{15}^{30}$P   (D) $_{15}^{31}$P

QUESTIONS 139-142 are NOT based on a descriptive passage.

---

139. An aldol is the product of

      (A)   the reaction of two moles of alcohol with one mole of ketone.

      (B)   the self-condensation of two moles of aldehyde.

      (C)   the mixed-condensation of one mole of ketone and one mole of ester.

      (D)   the self-condensation of two moles of ester.

140. A car traveling on level ground at a speed of 15 meters per second stops 10
      seconds after a braking force of 3000 newtons is applied. What is the mass of
      the car?

      (A)   1,500 kg   (B)   2,000 kg

      (C)   2,500 kg   (D)   3,000 kg

Two satellites, M_1 and M_2, are in a circular orbit at
a distance (s) of 6.7×10^6 meters from the center
of the earth as indicated. The mass of satellite
M_2 is 100 kg and the mass of the earth is
6.0×10^{24} kg. The speed of satellite M_1 is
7.7×10^3 m/s. $G = 6.67 \times 10^{-11}$ N-m²/kg².

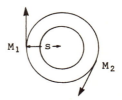

141. Which vector indicates the direction of the centripetal acceleration of M_1 in its present position?

    (A) ↑

    (B) →

    (C) ↗

    (D) ←

142. If M_2 has a mass twice as great as M_1, the orbit speed of M_2, as compared to M_1, is

    (A) $^1/_2$ as great.

    (B) the same.

    (C) twice as great.

    (D) 4 times as great.

STOP

If time still remains, you may review work only in this section.

When the time allotted is up, you may go on to the next section.

Section 3 — Writing Sample

TIME: 60 minutes
2 essays, separately timed
30 minutes each

DIRECTIONS: This section tests your writing skills by asking you to write two essays. You will have 30 minutes to write each one.

During the first 30 minutes, work only on the first essay. If you finish it in less than 30 minutes, you may review what you have written, but do not begin the second essay. During the second 30 minutes, work only on the second essay. If you finish it in less than 30 minutes, you may review what you have written for that essay only. Do not go back to the first essay.

Read each assigned topic carefully. Make sure your essays respond to the topics as they are assigned.

Make sure your essays are written in complete sentences and paragraphs, and are as clear as you can make them. Make any corrections or additions between the lines of your essays. Do not write in the margins.

On the day of the test, you are given three pages to write each essay. You are not required to use all of the space provided, but do not skip lines so you will not waste space. Illegible essays cannot be scored.

Part 1

Consider this statement:

> In a world of potentially conflicting self-interests, no one can really say that one value system is better than another.
>
> Robert N. Bellah from *Habits of the Heart*

Write a comprehensive essay in which you accomplish the following objectives: (1) Explain what you think the statement means. (2) Describe a current situation which might exemplify potentially conflicting self-interests. (3) Discuss a resolution to this dilemma.

STOP

If time still remains, you may review work only in this section.

When the time allotted is up, you may go on to the next section.

Part 2

Consider this statement:

> I am pessimistic about the human race because it is too ingenious for its own good. Our approach to nature is to beat it into submission. We would stand a better chance of survival if we accommodated ourselves to this planet and viewed it appreciatively instead of skeptically and dictatorially.

E.B. White

Write a comprehensive essay in which you accomplish the following objectives: (1) Describe the conflict alluded to in this statement. (2) Take the opposite perspective and defend it. (3) Respond to whether or not you believe the two positions are reconcilable.

STOP

If time still remains, you may review work only in this section.

When the time allotted is up, you may go on to the next section.

Section 4 — Biological Sciences

TIME: 100 Minutes
QUESTIONS: 143-219

> **DIRECTIONS:** Most of the questions in this section are arranged in groups, each corresponding to a descriptive passage. Based on the information given in a passage, choose the one best answer to each question in the group. Some questions are independent of a descriptive passage and of each other. Choose the one best answer to each of these questions. If you are not sure of an answer, eliminate those choices that you know are incorrect and choose an answer from among those remaining. Fill in the corresponding circle on the answer sheet to indicate your answer. You may refer to the periodic table at any time.

PASSAGE I (Questions 143-148)

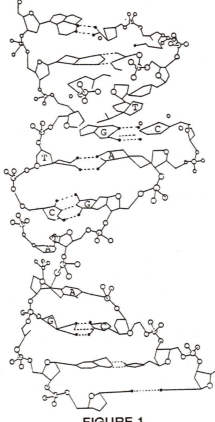

FIGURE 1.

A version of the modern molecular model of DNA structure, which is a modification of the one first proposed by Francis Crick and James Watson in 1953, is depicted in Figure 1 in a flat, or uncoiled, form. In this view, the only atoms identified are those of oxygen and phosphorous. Using this limited information, supplemented by your knowledge of the Watson-Crick model of DNA structure, answer the following questions.

143. Which of the following statements regarding DNA is NOT correct?

    (A) DNA is the nucleic acid with the greatest molecular weight.

    (B) DNA is a double-stranded molecule.

    (C) DNA contains the five-carbon sugar ribose.

    (D) DNA can be found outside the nucleus of a eukaryotic cell.

144. The polarity of a single chain of nucleic acid is such that the end known as 5´ is the end with a free

    (A) adenine base.   (B) guanine base.

    (C) phosphate.   (D) pentose sugar.

145. Which of the following nucleic acid bases are known as purines?

    (A) Adenine and guanine   (B) Adenine and thymine

    (C) Cytosine and guanine   (D) Thymine and uracil

146. Which element is found in BOTH nucleic acids and proteins?

    (A) Nitrogen   (B) Phosphorus

    (C) Iodine   (D) Sulfur

147. According to a rule of base-pairing known as Chargaff's Principle, regardless of the source of DNA the amounts of _____ and _____ nucleotides are always equal.

    (A) adenine - guanine   (B) guanine - cytosine

    (C) cytosine - thymine   (D) thymine - uracil

148. A DNA nucleotide might consist of _____, _____, and a phosphate.

    (A) uracil - deoxyribose   (B) thymine - ribose

    (C) guanine - ribose   (D) cytosine - deoxyribose

PASSAGE II (Questions 149-156)

Embryological development of vertebrates is initiated by fusion of sperm and egg. This fusion of gametic cells, known as plasmogamy, establishes the polarity of the future embryo (with the exception of certain groups of animals, including mammals) and is followed by karyogamy in normal development of vertebrates. The resultant zygote undergoes cleavages that begin a well described and predictable series of major developmental events of embryology. The triggering mechanism of embryonic development is usually the fusion of egg and sperm membranes, although this can be experimentally replaced by a variety of other stimuli. Initiation of cleavage, therefore, does not depend on fertilization and certain animals regularly utilize such parthenogenetic development in their life cycles.

The amount of yolk present in vertebrate eggs determines, in large part, the mechanics of cleavage and subsequent events. In the extreme case of telolecithal eggs of birds and reptiles, for example, the huge amount of yolk results in meroblastic cleavages and development of the embryo proceeds as a blastodisc lying on the surface of the yolk. Amphibian eggs, which contain yolk, but in much smaller amounts, show cleavages through the yolk material of the vegetal hemisphere. Much modern embryology is based on classic experiments that described amphibian development and the controlling influence of its immediate cellular and chemical environment on developmental patterns.

All adult structures of vertebrates, as well as the extraembryonic membranes of amniotes, develop from one or more of three germinal layers in the embryo — ectoderm, mesoderm, and endoderm. The fates of these germ layers are known from early studies and are consistent throughout the vertebrate subphylum.

149. Fertilization of a frog egg sets up the polarity of the adult organism. Accordingly, the point of penetration of the sperm will be the future _____ of the frog.

    (A)   dorsal surface   (B)   left side

    (C)   ventral surface   (D)   anterior end

150. The following is a correct, but not necessarily complete, sequence of stages in the development of a frog embryo:

    (A)   zygote, gastrula, blastula, neural plate.

    (B)   blastula, gastrula, neural tube, neural groove.

    (C)   gastrula, morula, blastula, neural tube.

    (D)   morula, blastula, neural plate, neural tube.

151. Formation of ectoderm, mesoderm, and endoderm is accomplished during which of the following stages of amphibian embryological development?

    (A)   Neurula   (B)   Gastrula

    (C)   Morula   (D)   Blastula

152. The spinal cord of vertebrates is derived from

    (A)   ectoderm only .   (B)   mesoderm only.

    (C)   endoderm only.   (D)   mesoderm and ectoderm.

153. All of the following adult vertebrate structures are derived from ectoderm, EXCEPT

    (A)   epidermis.   (B)   lining of the mouth.

    (C)   vertebrae.   (D)   scales, hair, and feathers.

154. The limb buds of a human embryo are formed during the

    (A) first week.   (B) fifth week.

    (C) eighth week.   (D) tenth week.

155. The influence of one group of cells on the development of another group is known as

    (A) induction.   (B) determination.

    (C) transformation.   (D) differentiation.

156. Primordial germ cells, which give rise to spermatogonia and oogonia in adult gonads, are formed in which extraembryonic membrane of mammals?

    (A) Amnion   (B) Yolk sac

    (C) Allantois   (D) Chorion

PASSAGE III (Questions 157-162)

Carbohydrates may undergo several reactions to lengthen their chains, to shorten their chains, or to modify the functional groups present.

The Kiliani-Fischer synthesis extends the chain by one carbon and creates a new chiral center.

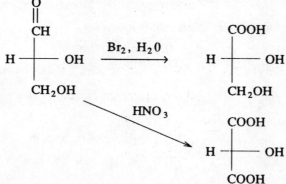

The Ruff degradation shortens the chain by one carbon at the CHO end.

Oxidation reactions can convert carbohydrates into carboxylic acids or dicarboxylic acids.

Note that chiral centers are represented as Fischer projections, where

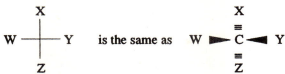

Consider the carbohydrates shown (the D - aldoses) and answer Questions 157- 162.

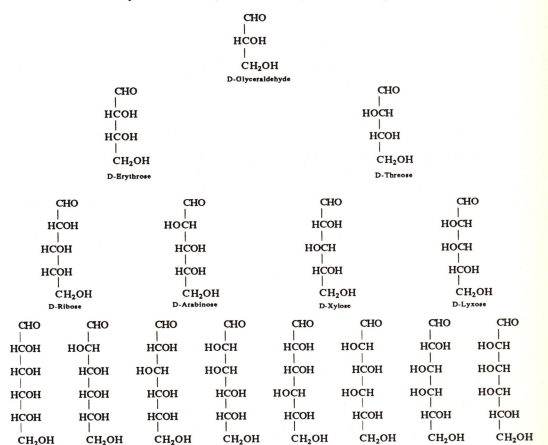

157. Which of the aldopentoses will give a meso compound when reacted with HNO$_3$?

    (A) Ribose only   (B) Lyxose only

    (C) Lyxose and arabinose   (D) Ribose and xylose

158. How many of the aldohexoses will form meso compounds when reacted with HNO$_3$?

    (A) One   (B) Two

    (C) Three   (D) Four

159. Arabinose subjected to the Ruff degradation will form

    (A) erythrose.   (B) erythrose and threose.

    (C) glyceraldehyde.   (D) threose.

160. Xylose extended by the Kiliani-Fischer synthesis will form

    (A) gulose and idiose.   (B) galactose and talose.

    (C) allose and altrose.   (D) glucose and mannose.

151. Which of the aldotetroses will form an optically inactive compound when treated with Br_2/H_2O?

    (A) Erythrose   (B) Threose

    (C) Both of them.   (D) Neither of them.

162. The aldose shown below is drawn with Fischer projection, but unconventionally.

$$\begin{array}{c}
\quad OH \quad O \\
\quad \quad \quad \parallel \\
H \longrightarrow CH \\
HOCH_2 \longrightarrow H \\
\quad OH
\end{array}$$

M

Which conventional figure below is identical to *M*?

(A)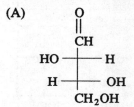

(B)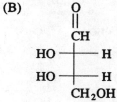

(C)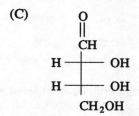

(D)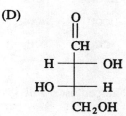

PASSAGE IV (Questions 163-168)

Ventilation of the lungs of humans and other mammals depends on changing pressure differentials between the atmosphere and the thoracic cavity of the animal. This is accomplished by contractions of the intercostal muscles of the chest and the diaphragm. Atmospheric air then moves into or out of the lungs in response to subsequent changes in intrapulmonary pressures. Figure 1 is a spirogram showing respiratory air volumes during quiet, resting breathing. Pulmonary disease may reduce vital capacity of the lungs or significantly increase the time required for expiration.

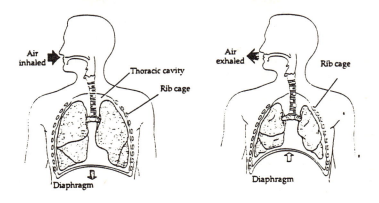

Figure 1

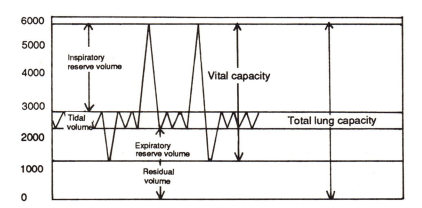

Figure 2

Actual gas exchange occurs across the moist membranes of air sacs known as alveoli. No active transport of gases occurs: rather, oxygen (and other gases) first dissolves in the moist film covering the alveolar epithelium and then diffuses across the epithelium. Similarly, gases carried in the blood of the capillaries serving the alveoli diffuse across the epithelium into the lobed alveoli. Since diffusion rates are a function of the differences in partial pressures of the gases involved, carbon dioxide moves from the blood into the alveoli and oxygen moves from the alveoli into the blood. Changes in partial pressures of atmospheric gases (due to changes in altitude, for example) or changes in the partial pressures of gases in the blood thus will affect gas exchange rates and amounts.

163. The partial pressure of O_2 at one atmosphere is approximately

    (A) 21 mm Hg.   (B) 78 mm Hg.
    (C) 159 mm Hg.   (D) 760 mm Hg.

164. As seen in the spirogram given as Figure 2, the maximum amount of air that can be expired after a maximum inspiration is known as

    (A) inspiratory reserve volume.

    (B) tidal volume.

    (C) total lung capacity.

    (D) vital capacity.

165. Which of the following is a correct, but not necessarily complete, sequence of structures through which air flows during inhalation by a mammal?

    (A) Pharynx, trachea, bronchus, bronchioles

    (B) Nares, pharynx, bronchus, trachea

    (C) Trachea, bronchus, pharynx, alveoli

    (D) Nasal cavity, bronchus, bronchioles, trachea

166. Normal inspiration in mammals involves

    (A) contraction of external intercostal muscles and relaxation of the diaphragm.

    (B) relaxation of internal intercostal muscles and contraction of the diaphragm.

    (C) relaxation of external intercostal muscles and relaxation of the diaphragm.

    (D) contraction of external intercostal muscles and contraction of the diaphragm.

167. The majority of the carbon dioxide in the blood of mammals is carried as

    (A) carboxyhemoglobin.

    (B) bicarbonate.

    (C) dissolved carbon dioxide gas.

    (D) carbonic anhydrase.

168. Referring to Figure 2, the volume of the air this patient expires in each breath during quiet breathing is about

    (A) 6000 cc.   (B) 4800 cc.
    (C) 500 cc.   (D) 3500 cc.

QUESTIONS 169-174 are NOT based on a descriptive passage.

---

169. The expected product of the reaction shown below would be

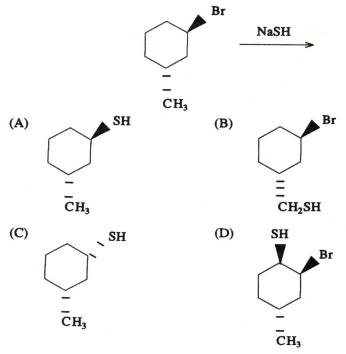

(A) SH ... CH₃

(B) Br ... CH₂SH

(C) SH ... CH₃

(D) SH ... Br ... CH₃

170. Protozoans can reproduce in a variety of ways; however, they are incapable of

(A) sporulation.

(B) binary fission.

(C) sexual reproduction.

(D) viviparity.

171. Vitamin deficiency can lead to disease. All of the following are vitamin deficiency diseases except

(A) scurvy.

(B) beriberi.

(C) phenylketonuria.

(D) rickets.

172. The main factor that determines the uptake and dissociation of oxygen and carbon dioxide in the blood is

(A) the partial pressure of oxygen.

(B) the partial pressure of carbon dioxide.

(C) the level of carbonic anhydrase.

(D) Both (A) and (B).

173. The event necessary for the implantation of a fertilized human egg in the uterus is

(A) the disintegration of the zona pellucida.

(B) the formation of the placenta.

    (C)   the involution of the corpus luteum.

    (D)   a fall in the progestrone level.

174.   The initiation of the heartbeat normally originates from the

    (A)   atrio-ventricular (A-V) node of the heart.

    (B)   sino-atrial (S-A) node of the heart.

    (C)   central nervous system.

    (D)   thyroid gland.

PASSAGE V (QUESTIONS 175-177)

α-Amino acids, the building blocks of proteins, have properties that suggest they are much more polar then their structural formula, as Formula 1 indicates. In fact, their properties are attributed to their preference for existing as zwitterions (inner salts), Formula 2.

$$R — CH— CO_2H \qquad\qquad R — CH— CO_2{}^+$$
$$\qquad\quad | \qquad\qquad\qquad\qquad\qquad\quad |$$
$$\qquad\quad NH_2 \qquad\qquad\qquad\qquad\quad NH_3{}^+$$

Formula 1   **Formula 2**

The side chains, R, may also be ionized if they contain acidic (COOH) or basic (NH$_2$) groups. The ionization of all groups will depend on the pH of the surroundings.

Consider the following amino acids and answer questions 175-177.

$$H_2N — CH_2 — COOH \qquad\qquad H_2N — CH — COOH$$
$$\qquad\qquad\qquad\qquad\qquad\qquad\qquad\qquad\qquad\qquad |$$
$$\qquad\qquad\qquad\qquad\qquad\qquad\qquad\qquad\qquad (CH_2)_4NH_2$$

        glycine   lysine

$$H_2N — CH — COOH \qquad\qquad H_2N — CH — COOH$$
$$\qquad\qquad | \qquad\qquad\qquad\qquad\qquad\qquad\qquad\qquad |$$
$$\qquad\quad CH_2OH \qquad\qquad\qquad\qquad\qquad CH_2COOH$$

        serine   aspartic acid

175.   Which will have the greatest negative charge at pH 10.0?

    (A)   Aspartic acid   (B)   Glycine

    (C)   Lysine   (D)   Serine

176.   Which structure is an accurate representation of lysine at pH 1.0?

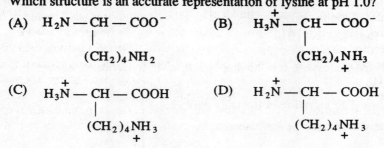

    (A) $H_2N — CH — COO^-$ (B) $\overset{+}{H_3N} — CH — COO^-$

                  $(CH_2)_4NH_2$ $(CH_2)_4\overset{+}{NH_3}$

    (C) $\overset{+}{H_3N} — CH — COOH$ (D) $H_2N — CH — COOH$

                  $(CH_2)_4\overset{+}{NH_3}$ $(CH_2)_4\overset{+}{NH_3}$

177. Which of the amino acids cannot be resolved into enantiomers?

(A) Aspartic acid   (B) Glycine

(C) Lysine   (D) Serine

PASSAGE VI (Questions 178-184)

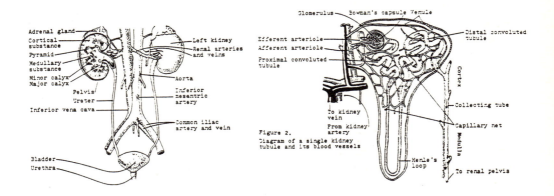

Figure 1   Figure 2

    The excretory system of a vertebrate is comprised of a pair of kidneys, each connected by a ureter to the urinary bladder which is connected to a urethra through which the stored urine is eliminated. The excretory system functions to maintain homeostasis of the body through regulation of the composition and volume of blood. Consequently, the kidneys are highly vascularized. Solutes are selectively removed from blood by filtration and secretion, and carried from the body in varying amounts of water as urine.

    The functional unit of a kidney is the nephron. Collectively, the nephrons of an adult human produce about 175 liters of filtrate daily. This is accomplished by forcing fluid out of glomerular capillaries and into glomerular (Bowman's) capsules using the hydrostatic pressure of the arterial system. The vast majority (99%) of this filtrate is returned to the circulatory system and the remaining small volume of fluid containing concentrated solute is continuously delivered to the urinary bladder.

    Concentration of glomerular filtrate into a hypertonic urine involves establishment of an osmotic gradient within the tissues of the kidney. This is accomplished by active pumping of ions (sodium and/or chloride) through the wall of certain portions of the nephron. As filtrate flows through the collecting tubules on its way into the renal pelvis, it encounters increasingly hypertonic tissue fluids in the medulla of the kidney. Water osmotically moves through the walls of collecting tubules into this surrounding tissue fluid and the filtrate thus becomes concentrated into urine. Capillaries associated with the tubules of the nephron reabsorb water, as well as some ions and small molecules, to return it to the circulatory system. The urine formed by this process travels to the urinary bladder through the ureter.

178. The ion pumps for Na⁺ (or Cl⁻) that establish the countercurrent multiplier system in the medulla of a vertebrate kidney are located in the cell membranes of the

    (A) proximal convoluted tubules.

    (B) distal convoluted tubules.

    (C) collecting tubules.

    (D) ascending loops of Henle.

179. Which of the following is a correct, but not necessarily complete, sequence of structures through which glomerular filtrate passes in a human kidney?

    (A) Collecting tubule, proximal convoluted tubule, ascending loop of Henle

    (B) Proximal convoluted tubule, collecting tubule, distal convoluted tubule

    (C) Ascending loop of Henle, distal convoluted tubule, collecting tubule

    (D) Bowman's capsule, descending loop of Henle, proximal convoluted tubule

180. The process whereby urea is removed from blood in the glomerulus is known as

    (A) tubular secretion.　　(B) reabsorption.

    (C) ultrafiltration.　　(D) osmosis.

181. Which of the following would be LEAST likely to be present in glomerular filtrate entering the proximal convoluted tubule?

    (A) Glucose　　(B) Platelets

    (C) Amino acids　　(D) Urea

182. Which one of the following processes that occur in the kidney does NOT require active transport?

    (A) Reabsorption of salts in the tubules

    (B) Reabsorption of amino acids in the tubules

    (C) Tubular secretion of chemicals from the blood into the urine

    (D) Movement of water out of the collecting tubules

183. Which of the following correctly traces the removal of nitrogenous wastes from the human body?

    (A) Conversion to urea in the liver - filtration in the kidney

    (B) Conversion to ammonia in the liver - tubular secretion by the kidney

(C)   Conversion to urea in the kidney - tubular secretion by the kidney

(D)   Conversion to ammonia in the kidney - filtration in the kidney

184.   Abnormally low blood pressure in a human causes a decrease in the production of urine because there would also be a(n)

(A)   decrease in the osmotic concentration of the blood plasma.

(B)   decrease in hydrostatic pressure in the glomerulus.

(C)   increase in osmotic concentration of the blood plasma.

(D)   decrease in the concentration of urea in the blood plasma.

PASSAGE VII (Questions 182-186)

The Hardy-Weinberg Law of population genetics predicts if certain conditions of stability are met, that the frequencies of genotypes will remain constant from generation to generation in populations of sexually reproducing organisms. The Hardy-Weinberg formula is used to determine allelic frequencies.

The conventional algebraic expression of Hardy-Weinberg equilibria assumes Mendelian inheritance (i.e., segregation of alleles and independent assortment of genes for different characters — Mendel's so-called "Laws") and assigns the symbols "p" and "q" to the dominant and recessive alleles, respectively. Since these are, by definition, the only two alleles for a given gene in a population under study, the sum of the frequencies of "p" and "q" is always 1. Expansion of the binomial $(p + q)^2$ therefore yields the formula for Hardy-Weinberg equilibria.

185.   If 70% of the alleles of a given human gene are dominant and the only other known allele is recessive, what percentage of the population is heterozygous for this characteristic?

(A)   30%   (B)   42%

(C)   49%   (D)   70%

186.   According to the Hardy-Weinberg equilibrium, $p^2 =$

(A) $1 - 2pq - q^2$.   (B) $2pq + 2^2$.

(C) q^2.   (D) $2pq$.

187.   In a population that is in Hardy-Weinberg equilibrium, the frequency of homozygous recessive individuals is 36%. What is the frequency of homozygous dominant individuals in the population?

(A)   6%   (B)   48%

(C)   13%   (D)   16%

188.   Which of the following is NOT one of the conditions that must be met for genetic equilibrium in the gene pool of a population?

(A)   Mating among genotypes must be random.

(B)   No alteration of allelic frequencies must occur from immigration or emigration.

(C)   The population must be small.

(D)   There must be no mutations that alter allelic frequencies.

189. According to Mendel's "Laws," a dihybrid cross between two heterozygotic pea plants, each producing tall plants with red flowers, would result in the classic 9:3:3:1 phenotypic ratio. In this ratio, the total number of plants showing the red flower phenotype would be

(A)   1.   (B)   3.

(C)   4.   (D)   12.

PASSAGE VIII (Questions 190-192)
    The acidity of carboxylic acids may be expressed as an acidity constant, Ka.

$$RCOOH + H_2O \longleftrightarrow RCOO^- + H_3O^+$$

$$Ka = \frac{[RCOO^-][H_3O^+]}{[RCOOH]}$$

pKa is defined as a negative log of Ka; pKa = - log Ka. Therefore, an acid with Ka = 1×10^{-5} will have pKa = 5.
    The acidity of some para-substituted benzoic acids is given below.

$$Y-\!\!\left\langle\!\!\bigcirc\!\!\right\rangle\!\!- COOH$$

Y	pKa
H	4.19
OH	4.55
Cl	3.96
CN	3.55

190. The strongest acid listed has Y =

(A)   H.   (B)   OH.

(C)   Cl.   (D)   CN.

191. If Y were CH_3, you would expect its pKa to be

(A)   between 3.55 and 3.96.   (B)   between 3.96 and 4.19.

(C)   between 4.19 and 4.55.   (D)   greater than 4.55.

192. We can make predictions about other reactions from acidity data. Which of the following substituted benzenes, Y-Ph, would you expect to be LEAST reactive toward electrophilic substitution on the ring?

(A)   Y = H   (B)   Y = OH

(C)   Y = Cl   (D)   Y = CN

QUESTIONS 193-198 are NOT based on a descriptive passage.

193. DNA does not contain

   (A) thymine.   (B) adenine.

   (C) uracil.   (D) cytosine.

194. All of the following enzymes are involved in the digestion of food except

   (A) pepsin.   (B) trypsin.

   (C) ribonuclease.   (D) ligase.

195. The physiological response of an organism to cycles of light and dark is called

   (A) photoperiodism.   (B) phototropism.

   (C) The light cycle.   (D) thigmotropism.

196. The peptide bond proteins is best represented as a resonance hybrid.

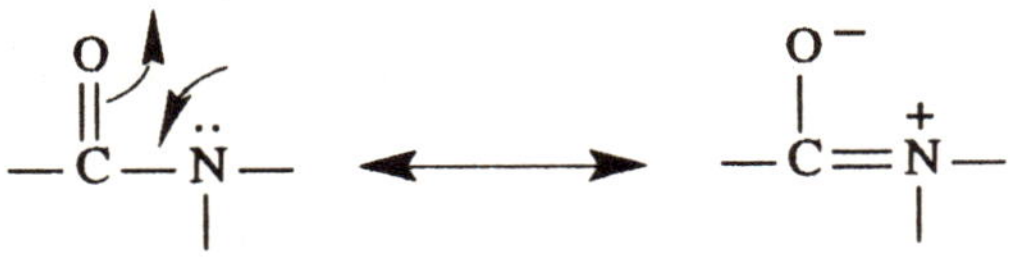

   Which of the following properties is not attributable to the electron delocalization in the hybrid?

   (A) C-N bond planarity in the peptide bond

   (B) The optical activity of the peptide

   (C) Decreased basicity of the nitrogen atom in the peptide bond

   (D) C-N bond length in the peptide bond

197. The axon of a neuron

   (A) is involved in contraction.

   (B) contains the nucleus.

   (C) conducts impulses away from the cell body.

   (D) synthesizes neural transmitters.

198. A female zygote will develop when the sperm cell carries

   (A) an X-chromosome.   (B) a Y-chromosome.

   (C) two X-chromosomes.   (D) two Y-chromosomes

PASSAGE IX (Questions 199-201)

   Amines react with p-toluenesulfonyl chloride (tosyl chloride) to give solid sulfonamide derivatives.

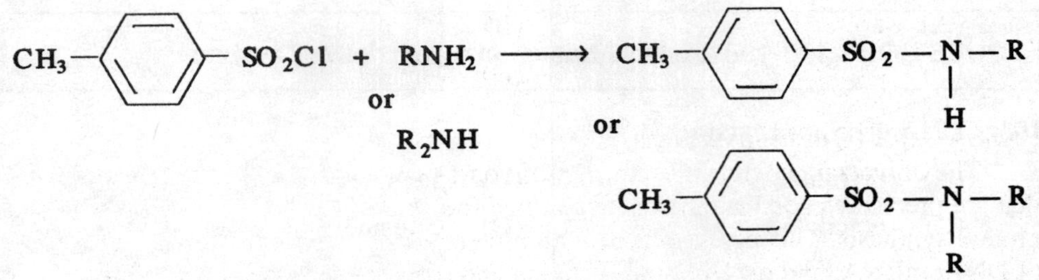

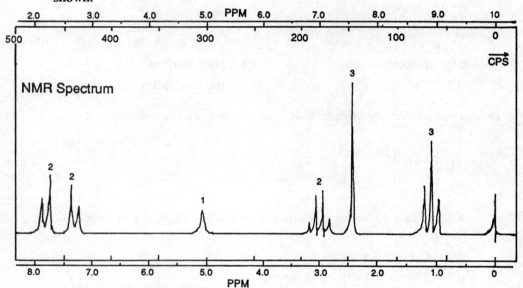

199. An amine reacts with tosyl chloride to give a solid with the NMR spectrum shown.

The structure of the amine is

(A) $CH_3CH_2NH_2$

(B) $CH_3NHCH_2CH_3$

(C) $(CH_3)_2NH$

(D) CH_3NH_2

200. Which class of amines will NOT react with sulfonyl chlorides?

(A)   Primary

(B)   Secondary

(C)   Tertiary

(D)   All will react.

201. Sulfonamides with the structure shown will undergo an acid-base reaction with aqueous NaOH. Which hydrogen is the OH⁻ removing from the sulfonamide?

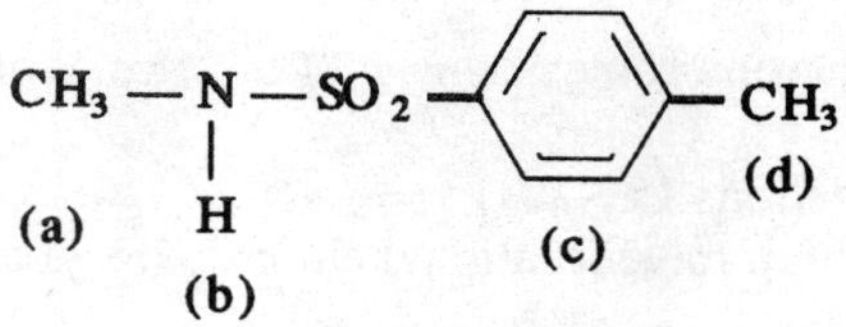

$$CH_3 - N - SO_2 - \underset{(c)}{\bigcirc} - CH_3$$

(a)   H   (d)

(b)

(A) a   (B) b

(C) c   (D) d

PASSAGE X (Questions 202-207)

The universal genetic code consists of non-overlapping triplets of nucleotides that are precisely coded and translated in the processes of nucleic acid replication and protein synthesis. This passage deals with protein synthesis — specifically the roles of DNA, mRNA, and tRNA in transcription and translation of the genetic code.

DNA differs from the three types of RNA in molecular size as well as in the specific nucleic acid bases and pentose sugars found in each molecule. The sequence of bases in DNA indirectly determines the sequence of amino acids that are peptide-bonded during protein synthesis by specifying the sequence of ribonucleic acid bases that make up individual mRNA molecules.

Using this information, the genetic code found in Figure A, and your general knowledge of molecular genetics, answer the following questions.

Second letter

First letter (5′ end)		U	C	A	G	Third letter (3′ end)
	U	UUU UUC } phe / UUA UUG } leu	UCU UCC UCA UCG } ser	UAU UAC } tyr / UAA stop / UAG stop	UGU UGC } cys / UGA stop / UGG trp	U C A G
	C	CUU CUC CUA CUG } leu	CCU CCC CCA CCG } pro	CAU CAC } pro / CAA CAG } gln	CGU CGC CGA CGG } arg	U C A G
	A	AUU AUC } ile / AUA / AUG met	ACU ACC ACA ACG } thr	AAU AAC } asn / AAA AAG } lyx	AGU AGC } ser / AGA AGG } arg	U C A G
	G	GUU GUC GUA GUG } val	GCU GCC GCA GCG } ala	GAU GAC } pro / GAA GAG } gln	GGU GGC GGA GGG } gly	U C A G

Figure 1

202. The three-base sequence of nucleotides known as an anticodon is found on molecules of

    (A) DNA.   (B) tRNA.

    (C) rRNA.   (D) mRNA.

203. The process of synthesizing a polypeptide according to the sequence of bases on mRNA is called

   (A)   transcription.   (B)   translation.

   (C)   transformation.   (D)   translocation.

204. If a tRNA molecule specialized for transfer of the amino acid alanine has the anticodon CGA, with what *codon* on mRNA will it bind?

   (A)   CAG   (B)   GAC

   (C)   GTC   (D)   GCU

205. Which of the following statements regarding the genetic code is correct?

   (A)   Each of the 64 possible codons has a function in protein synthesis.

   (B)   Some, but not all, codons code for more than one amino acid.

   (C)   Every possible codon codes for an amino acid.

   (D)   There is a single codon for each of the 20 naturally-occurring amino acids.

206. The following is a hypothetical, short mRNA sequence:

   (5′) CAGGUAAAAGCGUAA (3′)

   The sequence of bases in DNA that codes for this mRNA sequence is

   (A)   (5′) CAGGUAAAAGCGUAA (3′).

   (B)   (5′) GTCCATTTTCGCATT (3′).

   (C)   (5′) TTACGCTTTTACCTG (3′).

   (D)   (5′) UAAGCGAAAAUGGAC (3′).

207. The "one-gene-one-enzyme" principal was discovered by Beadle and Tatum. A modern and more accurate interpretation of this would be

   (A)   one codon codes for one enzyme.

   (B)   one nucleic acid base codes for one protein.

   (C)   one nucleotide codes for one enzyme.

   (D)   one gene codes for one polypeptide.

PASSAGE XI (Questions 208-211)

   Animal fats and vegetable oils are tricylglycerols, triesters of glycerols with three long-chain carboxylic acids. Generally, at room temperature fats are solid and oils are liquid. Both may be converted to glycerol and the carboxylic acids by basic hydrolosis, a reaction called saponification.

   The fatty acids obtained by hydrolysis of natural triacyglycerols are unbranched, contain an even number of carbon atoms, and may be either saturated or unsaturated. The table below contains data regarding some common fatty acids.

$$CH_2OCR^1 \quad \quad \quad CH_2OH \quad \quad \quad R^1CO_2H$$

$$\begin{array}{c} O \\ \| \\ CH_2OCR^1 \\ | \quad O \\ CHOCR^2 \\ | \\ CH_2OCR^3 \\ \| \\ O \end{array} \xrightarrow[\text{2) } H_3O^+]{\text{1) } OH^-, \Delta} \begin{array}{c} CH_2OH \\ | \\ CHOH \\ | \\ CH_2OH \end{array} + \begin{array}{c} R^1CO_2H \\ R^2CO_2H \\ R^3CO_2H \end{array}$$

Structures of Some Common Fatty Acids

Name	Carbons	Structure	Melting point (°C)
Saturated			
Lauric	12	$CH_3(CH_2)_{10}COOH$	44
Myrustuc	14	$CH_3(CH_2)_{12}COOH$	58
Palmitic	16	$CH_3(CH_2)_{14}COOH$	63
Stearic	18	$CH_3(CH_2)_{16}COOH$	70
Arachidic	20	$CH_3(CH_2)_{18}COOH$	78
Unsaturated			
Palmitoleic	16	$CH_3(CH_2)_5CH{=\!=}CH(CH_2)_7COOH$ (cis)	32
Oleic	18	$CH_3(CH_2)_7CH{=\!=}CH(CH_2)_7COOH$ (cis)	4
Ricinoleic	18	$CH_3(CH_2)_5CH(OH)CH_2CH{=\!=}CH(CH_2)_7COOH$ (cis)	5
Linoleic	18	$CH_3(CH_2)_4CH{=\!=}CHCH_2CH{=\!=}CH(CH_2)_7COOH$ (cis, cis)	-5
Arachidonic	20	$CH_3(CH_2)_4(CH{=\!=}CHCH_2)_4CH_2CH_2COOH$ (all cis)	- 50

Fatty acids are susceptible to oxidation by dioxygen. Since dioxygen has unpaired electrons, it can abstract a hydrogen atom, forming a free radical. This radical can react further with dioxygen and degrade the fats by forming odoriferious low-molecluar weight acids and aldehydes. The more unsaturated the fatty acid, the more susceptible it is to attack by dioxygen.

$$O_2 + R\text{-}CH_2\text{-}CH_2\text{-}CO_2H \longrightarrow HOO^{\cdot} + R\text{-}\overset{\cdot}{C}H\text{-}CH_2\text{-}CO_2H$$
$$\downarrow$$
further reaction and degradation

208. Assuming that melting tendencies of fatty acids are conferred on their triacylglycerols, which of the following will have the *lowest* melting point?

(A) Glyceryl trioleate

(B) Glyceryl tripalmitate

(C) Glyceryl - 1 - palmitate - 2, 3 - distearate

(D) Glyceryl - 1 - oleate - 2, 3 - dilinoleate

209. A fat containing a high proportion of which of these acids would be *most* susceptible to attack by dioxygen?

(A) Linoleic　　　　(B) Palmitoleic

(C) Oleic　　　　(D) Stearic

210. A triacylglycerol containing which of these acids would exhibit a peak at about 330 cm^{-1} in the infrared spectrum?

(A) Palmitic (B) Lineoleic

(C) Ricinoleic (D) Oleic

211. Margarine (an emulsion of water or skim milk in fats) and solid cooking shortening are produced from vegetable oils. What chemical reaction is used for the conversion of vegetable oils to solids?

(A) Saponification of the triester

(B) Catalytic hydrogenation of unsaturated bonds

(C) Transesterification of the triester

(D) Oxidation of the saturated acids

PASSAGE XII (Questions 212-216)

Epithelial tissue makes up the covering of internal and external body surfaces and is usually divided into simple and stratified types. The stratified types consist of two or more cell layers. Epithelial tissue is usually separated from tissues beneath it by a basement membrane. Simple types occasionally appear stratified because of irregular cell shape but, since each cell of the single layer contacts the basement membrane, this pseudostratified type is technically simple epithelium. The cells of epithelial tissues are packed very tightly and provide a boundary through which materials must pass as they leave or enter the body. Epithelial cells may be specialized in structure, having cilia, cellular processes, or glandular structures. They may also be specialized for functions such as protection from injury and invasive agents, secretion of a variety of extracellular products, absorption of nutrients, or filtration of certain substances. The permeabilities of epithelial cell membranes play an important role in regulating the movement of materials within the body and between the body and its external environment.

Connective tissues are characterized by an extensive extracellular matrix in which the cells are embedded. This matrix ranges from liquid to solid and constitutes a large amount of the total tissue volume. The only connective tissues with a liquid matrix are blood and lymph. The major supportive tissues of the vertebrate body are classified as connective tissue. These supportive tissues are further divided into the categories of connective tissue proper, cartilage, and bone. The matrix of connective tissue proper always contains fibers. Cartilage has a matrix with a rubberlike consistency and contains relatively few cells, which are located in cavities of the matrix. The matrix of bone is hard and the most rigid of all connective tissue. The bone matrix may have collagen fibers and contains large amounts of inorganic salts, especially calcium carbonate and calcium phosphate.

212. The epithelial tissue typically found in walls of the urinary bladder is

(A) squamous. (B) transitional.

(C) columnar. (D) cuboidal.

213. Which of the following fibers is NOT found in connective tissue proper?

    (A) Elastic
    (B) Reticular
    (C) Projection
    (D) Collagenous

214. Normal human blood contains about _____ erythrocytes per mm³.

    (A) 10,000
    (B) 50,000
    (C) 100,000
    (D) 5,000,000

215. Mast cells are specialized for the production of heparin and are found in _____ tissue.

    (A) areolar connective
    (B) epithelial
    (C) dense connective
    (D) elastic cartilage

216. A "haversian system" would be found in which of the following tissues?

    (A) Hyaline cartilage
    (B) Fibrocartilage
    (C) Bone
    (D) Elastic cartilage

QUESTIONS 217-219 are NOT based on a descriptive passage.

---

217. Nitrogeneous wastes are excreted by different species of animals in all of the following forms except

    (A) creatinine.
    (B) uracil.
    (C) ammonia.
    (D) urea.

218. How many ATPs are derived from one molecule of pyruvate via the Krebs cycle and the electron transport system?

    (A) 12
    (B) 14
    (C) 15
    (D) 18

219. β-D-glucopyranose, the closed chair form of D-glucose, can be depicted by a Haworth projection as shown in the figure. A more accurate spatial representation uses the chair form. The chair form of β-D-glucopyranose is

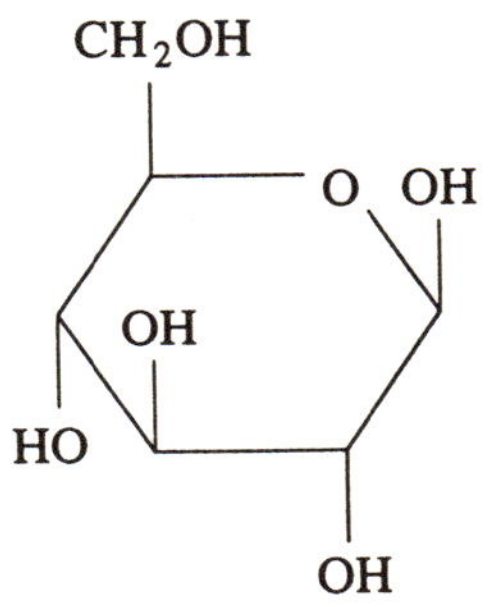

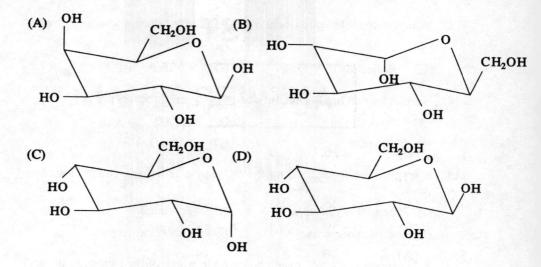

STOP

If time still remains, you may review work only in this section.

TEST 3

ANSWER KEY

1.	(D)	26.	(C)	51.	(D)	76.	(D)
2.	(B)	27.	(A)	52.	(A)	77.	(C)
3.	(A)	28.	(B)	53.	(B)	78.	(B)
4.	(B)	29.	(A)	54.	(C)	79.	(D)
5.	(A)	30.	(D)	55.	(B)	80.	(B)
6.	(B)	31.	(D)	56.	(B)	81.	(A)
7.	(D)	32.	(A)	57.	(D)	82.	(D)
8.	(B)	33.	(D)	58.	(B)	83.	(A)
9.	(B)	34.	(B)	59.	(B)	84.	(C)
10.	(C)	35.	(C)	60.	(B)	85.	(A)
11.	(B)	36.	(A)	61.	(C)	86.	(C)
12.	(B)	37.	(A)	62.	(D)	87.	(C)
13.	(D)	38.	(D)	63.	(A)	88.	(A)
14.	(C)	39.	(B)	64.	(A)	89.	(C)
15.	(A)	40.	(A)	65.	(D)	90.	(D)
16.	(C)	41.	(B)	66.	(D)	91.	(A)
17.	(B)	42.	(B)	67.	(B)	92.	(C)
18.	(A)	43.	(A)	68.	(A)	93.	(C)
19.	(C)	44.	(B)	69.	(D)	94.	(D)
20.	(C)	45.	(B)	70.	(C)	95.	(A)
21.	(B)	46.	(C)	71.	(A)	96.	(C)
22.	(C)	47.	(D)	72.	(B)	97.	(B)
23.	(D)	48.	(B)	73.	(C)	98.	(D)
24.	(B)	49.	(B)	74.	(B)	99.	(C)
25.	(D)	50.	(A)	75.	(B)	100.	(A)

101.	(B)	131.	(A)	161.	(D)	191.	(C)
102.	(C)	132.	(B)	162.	(A)	192.	(D)
103.	(C)	133.	(D)	163.	(C)	193.	(C)
104.	(A)	134.	(B)	164.	(D)	194.	(D)
105.	(A)	135.	(C)	165.	(A)	195.	(A)
106.	(B)	136.	(A)	166.	(D)	196.	(B)
107.	(D)	137.	(C)	167.	(B)	197.	(C)
108.	(C)	138.	(C)	168.	(C)	198.	(A)
109.	(D)	139.	(B)	169.	(C)	199.	(A)
110.	(D)	140.	(B)	170.	(D)	200.	(C)
111.	(A)	141.	(B)	171.	(C)	201.	(B)
112.	(B)	142.	(B)	172.	(D)	202.	(B)
113.	(C)	143.	(C)	173.	(A)	203.	(B)
114.	(A)	144.	(C)	174.	(B)	204.	(D)
115.	(D)	145.	(A)	175.	(A)	205.	(A)
116.	(A)	146.	(A)	176.	(C)	206.	(C)
117.	(C)	147.	(B)	177.	(B)	207.	(D)
118.	(D)	148.	(D)	178.	(D)	208.	(D)
119.	(B)	149.	(D)	179.	(C)	209.	(A)
120.	(C)	150.	(D)	180.	(C)	210.	(C)
121.	(C)	151.	(B)	181.	(B)	211.	(B)
122.	(A)	152.	(A)	182.	(D)	212.	(B)
123.	(B)	153.	(C)	183.	(A)	213.	(C)
124.	(D)	154.	(B)	184.	(B)	214.	(D)
125.	(B)	155.	(A)	185.	(B)	215.	(A)
126.	(A)	156.	(B)	186.	(A)	216.	(C)
127.	(B)	157.	(D)	187.	(A)	217.	(B)
128.	(C)	158.	(B)	188.	(C)	218.	(C)
129.	(D)	159.	(B)	189.	(D)	219.	(D)
130.	(D)	160.	(A)	190.	(D)		

DETAILED EXPLANATIONS
OF ANSWERS

Section 1 — Verbal Reasoning

1. **(D)** (D) is the correct answer because it represents a complete overview of the passage. (A) focuses on the Continental Congress only. (B) focuses only on the cause of the Revolutionary War. The passage explicitly states that the delegates held a wide variety of political opinions, so (C) is incorrect.

2. **(B)** (B) is correct because it employs neither "all" nor "only," thereby giving a clue that exclusions or further inclusions might be possible. (A), (C), and (D) each asks to cautiously examine such statements.

3. **(A)** (A) is correct because it is true as stated. (B) is false because moderates wanted Parliament's intervention, not exclusion, in U.S. trade. (C) is inclusive and thereby false. (D) contradicts the purpose of the Continental Congress.

4. **(B)** In retaliation for the "Boston Tea Party," Parliament virtually abolished provincial self-government in Massachusetts, so (B) is correct. These actions stimulated resistance across the land, not just within Massachusetts, so (A) is incorrect. Massachusetts patriots, not the U.S. government, who openly defied royal authority organized a military defense committee several weeks after the retaliatory actions, not immediately, so (C) is incorrect. Parliament closed the Boston port in retaliation, not Carpenters' Hall where the First Continental Congress met, so (D) is incorrect.

5. **(A)** (A) is correct because it represents an overview of the whole passage. (B), (C), and (D) each takes a particular and specific true idea, but each is not complete in itself when considering the other ideas within the passage.

6. **(B)** This is a purely factual question testing reading ability. The passage does not mention Pennsylvania's involvement in setting up an assembly, but it does note the other states' involvement.

7. **(D)** (D) is the correct description by inference from the description within the passage. (A), (B) and (C) are incorrect, because those groups are never referred to as Whigs, although they are mentioned.

8. **(B)** General T. Gage orders men to go to Concord to secure a depot. (A), (C) and (D) are all men who fled the scene or who warned the citizenry that the British were coming, and are therefore incorrect.

9. **(B)** (B) is the correct answer because the passage notes the onset of the War of Independence as a result of this battle. (A) is incorrect because citizen protest

had occurred in the past. (C) minimizes the importance of the battle. (D) trivializes the importance of the battle.

10.   **(C)**   An embargo prevents trade goods from leaving or entering a country. An embargo is not opposing viewpoints or extra security or a proposal, like (A), (B), (D) suggest, respectively.

11.   **(B)**   The question asks for the main theme of the passage. (A), (C) and (D) may each be claimed to be contained in the passage, but only (B) contains the ideas collectively. The theme must be broader than any one point emphasized in the essay.

12.   **(B)**   Because the syndicate takes a substantial share of the profit made from lotteries, option I is correct. Option II is also correct because the passage notes organized crime's infiltration into both business and politics, which includes the offering of bribes. Both options are right, so (B) is correct. (A) is incorrect because it only presents option I. (C) and (D) are incorrect because option III is presented, which is an incorrect statement because of the word "only" which makes the statement exclusive and universal in how it defines organized crime.

13.   **(D)**   This demands knowledge of a definition that can be inferred and is not directly addressed in the passage. "The democratic process" transcends the specific issue of the essay, which clearly notes organized crime's involvement in gambling (B), and politics (A) and (C).

14.   **(C)**   "Might is right" is a stoic, ethical principle that attributes mortal strength to influential power and persuasion. Organized crime reflects power and persuasion and gives the appearance of "right." (A) implies the opposite of what the essay states. (B) and (D) have little to do with power and crime and are instead biological theories.

15.   **(A)**   (A) is clearly the correct answer as stated in the passage. (B) assumes every working person is involved in crime, while not everyone is. In (C), the word "single" is misleading. (D) assumes organized crime has also infiltrated that specific federal commission. This is a misreading of the work of the Presidential Commission in the passage.

16.   **(C)**   (A) is incorrect because foreign trade isn't alluded to in the passage. (B) deceives the reader by asking about the growth rate of an unknown source. While gambling is a national pastime, one cannot conclude that gambling is an exclusive cause of organized crime. The passage gives many causes and consequences of organized crime, therefore (D) is incorrect.

17.   **(B)**   (A) is incorrect because it excludes bribes offered to others. (C) negates an essential locus of bribes. (D) negates the importance of organized crime and the total intent of the passage. (B) is the only true statement.

18.   **(A)**   (A) correctly summarizes the paragraph. A key to understanding the passage is the definition of "laundered money." Even if you do not know the term, (B), (C) and (D) are either partially true (B) and (D) or too exclusive (C).

19. **(C)** There isn't a hint in the essay that organized religion is implicated in the workings of organized crime. Freight carrier operators and postal workers are unionized, so (A) and (D) are incorrect. Bowling alley owners represent small business and by inference from the passage may be implicated in organized crime, therefore (B) is incorrect.

20. **(C)** (C) is correct. It is not harm to others, but harm to the "rightful interests" or entitlements of others that warrants the silencing of opinion, and so both (A) and (B) are false. There is no basis at all for (D).

21. **(B)** (B) is correct. The passage does not contain an explanation of the concept of harm, so (A) is false, but it does employ the concept of harm. Thus, (B) is true and (C) false.

22. **(C)** (C) is correct. The passage does not state that (A) is true, so it is left an open question, as is (B). However, the question is raised, so (D) is false. Going by the information provided in the passage given, (C) is the best answer we are warranted in giving.

23. **(D)** (D) is correct. The description of infallibility does not fit with (A) - (C), as given in the passage.

24. **(B)** (B) is correct. Mill urges that lively debate is a help to us in the way in which we hold our beliefs and should be welcomed, so we would reject both (A) and (D). There is no guarantee that (C) alone, in the absence of lively debate, will be true.

25. **(D)** (D) is correct. The passage claims each of these merits of free and open debate.

26. **(C)** (C) is true. Nothing in the passage restricts these principles to government, so there is no reason for (A). Line 2 shows that Mill is concerned with both thought and expression, so (B) is false, the argument applies to dealing with false opinions as well as true ones, and so we should reject (D).

27. **(A)** (A) is correct. The speaker rules out (B), and (A) is itself the means by which we would bring about (C), so (C) is not independent of (A). The argument does not warrant (D).

28. **(B)** (B) is correct. The passage claims that debate "adds vitality" to our beliefs. While open debate may be conducted in public, this is not necessary to make it "free and open," and so (A) is incorrect. (C) is incorrect because, clearly, the speaker believes that open debate is good for society. The passage makes no claim as stated in (D).

29. **(A)** (A) is the correct response by comparing the practical results of silicon PV cells with selenium PV cells. The passage states that "Selenium cells have never become practical as energy converts because their cost is too high relative to the tiny amount of power they produce (at 1% efficiency)." The last part of the paragraph

tells us the range of silicon PV cells from 4% to 11% efficiency. Take the top level of efficiency at 11% and the lowest level at 1% and subtract.

30.   **(D)**   (D) is correct because it cites the correct interaction of electrodes in the correct solution. (A), (B) and (C) incorrectly identify the electrodes or do not stipulate the correct kind of environment.

31.   **(D)**   To arrive at this answer, it is necessary to figure the years between 1839, the year the PV effect was discovered, and 1954, the year Bell Labs made the improvement.

32.   **(A)**   Solar energy is not the most efficient (B). Solar energy is relatively simple but difficult to capture (C). Solar energy is not cheaper than fossil-fuel powered energy (D).

33.   **(D)**   (D) is the most appropriate title from those given because (A) is limited to the initial work of Becquerel. (B) assumes all that could be said historically has been said and that may or may not be true. (C) does capture much of the sense of the passage, but it does not include by inference the details of solar energy and its limitations.

34.   **(B)**   (B) is the correct answer based on the part of the passage that states, "In 1958, the U.S. Vanguard space satellite used a small ... amount of cells (solar) to power its radio." (A) is not addressed. (C) and (D) might be inferred from the passage, but telephones and electric utility lines are discussed in conjunction with potential effects of solar energy and not in the context of actual use.

35.   **(C)**   Although (A) is a true statement, it does not reflect why selenium is used for photometric devices. (B) is false. (D) is a misreading of the sentence, "Even today, light sensitive cells on cameras for adjusting shutter speed to match illumination are made of selenium."

36.   **(A)**   This answer is arrived at by doubling the amounts in the sentence, "Today, photovoltaic systems are capable of transforming one kilowatt of solar energy falling on one square meter into about a hundred watts of electricity."

37.   **(A)**   (A) captures the sense of both the difficulty and the availability of sunlight as a source of solar energy. (B) negates any availability of the sun. (C) reflects only one of the variables that impacts the invisibility of the sun. (D) does not address the question.

38.   **(D)**   (D) is most inclusive of the overall content of the essay. (A) is partially true, but neglects to state anything about minorities. Funding is never addressed in the article, so (B) is incorrect. (C) simply repeats a partially true statement, but the article is more about general knowledge than of aging minorities.

39.   **(B)**   (B) is most clearly the correct answer to a question meant to distract the reader. (A) and (C) are wrong because there is no information to confirm those statements. (D) gives an unsubstantiated motive for including the information.

40. **(A)** (A) is the only correct answer because there isn't any information such as (B) suggests. Also, there is no comment in the passage on reproduction, thereby excluding (C). The passage also states that various racial and ethnic subgroups, not just blacks, will comprise first and second generation Americans, so (D) is incorrect.

41. **(B)** Many concerns of the minority aged need further attention and study because of their interrelationship with the problems of the elderly in general, so (B) is correct. (A) is incorrect because the NIA gives financial support, it does not receive it. (C) is incorrect because the passage states that the studies are ongoing. Because the passage does not state that the minority aging is the only issue studied by the NIA, (D) is incorrect.

42. **(B)** There is nothing mentioned in the passage concerning the familiarity of law and policymakers with minority constituents and values, therefore (A) and (C) are incorrect. (D) is a positive statement, but the passage clearly demonstrates financial support from the NIA. The only answer addressing the issue of assistance is (B).

43. **(A)** Members of racial and ethnic minority groups are likely to have less education and money, less adequate housing, poorer health and therefore fewer years of life. Option I is the only answer that truly represents this idea, so (A) is correct. Option II is incorrect because the less than adequate housing conditions are not mentioned, so the answers which mention option II are incorrect, (B) and (D). Option III is incorrect because it states that more years of life are the result of poorer health, so (C) is incorrect.

44. **(B)** (B) is the correct answer because it conveys an overview of the essay. (A) and (D) talk about racist intentions, but a discussion of racism is not the purpose of the essay. (C) asks the student to interpret the vocabulary word "denigrate," which is a perjorative term irrelevant to the essay.

45. **(B)** (B) is the correct answer. It is another way of saying, "Among older blacks … hypertension is twice as prevalent as among whites …" (A), (C), and (D) cannot be known from the content of this passage.

46. **(C)** (C) The fact that many minorities have the strength to adapt to old age is clearly articulated in the passage, more so than (D) which is close, but not the most explicit belief of those listed. (B) has no basis in the essay. The essay doesn't talk about "graceful" aging, therefore, (A) is incorrect.

47. **(D)** A careful reading of this passage unveils Darwin's belief that "a protein compound… would be instantly devoured or absorbed which would not have been the case before living creatures were formed." Therefore, (D) is the correct answer. (A) is misleading because the word "dormant" does not mean "absent," a belief of Darwin. (B) assumes the concept was an attempted simulation and the passage doesn't articulate that. (C) is incorrect because a sterile environment is the opposite of an active environment.

48. **(B)** The passage doesn't tell us who hypothesized that the stars were 90% hydrogen (A). The passage does state that Oparin had the new "notion concerning the

reducing nature of the early atmosphere" Therefore (B) is correct. (C) is incorrect because, while Oparin contributed to the idea of the evolution of matter, the passage does not attribute the concept to him. The information in (D) is not given in the passage and there is information in the passage to suggest the opposite.

49. **(B)** (A) is a synonym for "primordial soup," but does not explain the contents of the "primordial soup," like (B) which is the correct answer. (C) refers to conditions of the primordial soup, rather than the elements of it. (D) is not inclusive of all elements of the organic substances which make up the "primordial soup."

50. **(A)** (A) is the only correct answer because clay is a surface phenomenon which is still under investigation. The passage does not specifically state that clay is a polymer (B). Absorbed, organic molecules are found *on* clay (C). Clay is a surface phenomenon and can't replicate the origin of life (D).

51. **(D)** The passage only discusses Oparin, Darwin, Bernal and Haldane. Others may have contributed to evolutionary theory. (A) and (C) are incorrect, therefore, due to the inclusion of "only." Others may have contributed to evolutionary science but are simply not discussed here. In addition, the passage does not indicate any disagreement among the scientists, so (B) is incorrect.

52. **(A)** (A) is incorrect since "primordial soup" is pre-existent matter. (B) is blatantly refuted in the passage. (C) would render the passage unnecessary or moot. (D) is an answer that may seem correct, but evolution implies linear progress, not a cyclical perspective.

53. **(B)** Synthesis means bringing elements together, weaving a single thread. It is not a synonym for "origin" (A). (D) is incorrect because the opposite of "synthesis" is "analysis," pulling apart ideas to make conclusions. The passage speaks only of four theories, not about all theories (C).

54. **(C)** Interpreting the meaning of this sentence involves knowing the meaning of "dormant" in the context of the paragraph. Obviously, (A) and (B) translate "dormant" incorrectly. (D) may be true, but that evidence is not contained in the sentence.

55. **(B)** (B) is clearly the answer and found explicitly in the first paragraph twice: 1) "A sterile environment was exactly what was present then and what is utterly unknown in the biosphere today." 2) "The ancient epoch when life originated, which is not at all the present life-filled environment, was not brought under study." In addition, this answer calls for an understanding of the cause-effect relationship when used in a sentence. (C) and (D) refer to "equality." Nothing is inferred from or directly mentioned about the issue.

56. **(B)** (B) is clearly indicated in the passage. (A) is the antithesis of the intent of the essay, as is (C). (D) may be a possibility except that while the way of matter is known, it is not dismissed as an issue.

57. **(D)** (B) is correct. (A) is wrong because a person's motives are not important in assessing the moral value of the action. (B) is mistaken in that responsibility is

not mentioned as a reason for evaluating actions. (C) is incorrect, because not all utilitarians take the actual consequences to be decisive.

58.　**(B)**　(B) is correct. For (A), whether or not an action is repeatable does not determine whether or not it is considered, but how it is considered, as is explained in (B). (C) is incorrect because the repeatability of an action does not determine if it has consequences but rather the type of consequences considered.

59.　**(B)**　(B) is correct. The passage explains that consequences in the sense of actual results can only be associated with actions thought of as particular or concrete. Types of actions will not have actual consequences but only consequences that normally occur.

60.　**(B)**　(B) is correct. The result was unexpected, which would matter to some, but not all, utilitarians. While the resulting evaluation may not differ, thus making (A) false, it need not be the same, thus making (D) false. All we can say is that the grounds for the evaluation will differ.

61.　**(C)**　(C) is correct. Utilitarians agree that motives are not relevant to evaluating actions but they are relevant to evaluating persons, and that evaluations of actions do depend on considering consequences. These points of agreement thus rule out all but (C).

62.　**(D)**　(D) is correct. For a utilitarian who takes the reasonably expected consequences to be important, both (A) and (B) would be beside the point, since what matters is what could have been foreseen. Other utilitarians who take actual consequences to be important would not regard (C) as changing the moral value of the action.

63.　**(A)**　(A) is correct. The passage does not talk about responsibility, so (C) is incorrect. Because of the different methods of assessing morality, both (B) and (D) are false.

64.　**(A)**　(A) is correct. Since not all utilitarians agree on how to determine moral relevance, (B) is false. Actual results are not considered by those who take actions as types of kinds. (C) is false since responsibility is not mentioned. Utilitarians do consider consequences relevant, so (D) is false.

65.　**(D)**　(D) is correct. All of these are true when the action is thought of as respectable.

Section 2 — Physical Sciences

66.　**(D)**　Calcium, a group two element, has an oxidation state of +2 in its compounds and oxygen (except in peroxides and super oxides) is -2. For the neutral compound, the sum of the oxidation states must be zero. If x = oxidation state of carbon, then

$$+2 + 2x + 4(-2) = 0$$

$$x = (8 - 2) / 2 = +3$$

67. **(B)**

$$Ksp = 2.3 \times 10^{-9} = [Ca^{++}] [C_2O_4^{=}]$$

$$[C_2O_4^{=}] = 0.115 \text{ M}$$

$$[Ca^{++}] = Ksp / [C_2O_4^{=}] = 2.3 \times 10^{-9} / 0.115$$

$$[Ca^{++}] = 2.0 \times 10^{-8} \text{ M}$$

68. **(A)**

$$pH = -\log[H^+]$$

$$[H^+] = 10^{-pH} = 10^{-7.45} = 3.5 \times 10^{-8} \text{ M}$$

69. **(D)**

$$pH = 6.1 + \log([HCO_3^-] / [H_2CO_3])$$

$$\log([HCO_3^-] / [H_2CO_3]) = pH - 6.1 = 7.45 - 6.1 = 1.35$$

$$[HCO_3^-] / [H_2CO_3] = 10^{1.35} = 22.4$$

70. **(C)**   From the volume of titrant, its concentration, and the mole ratios, find the millimoles of calcium which can then be divided by the 5.00 mL volume of blood.

$$(11.63 \text{ mL}) (0.00100 \text{ mmol KMnO}_4 / \text{mL})$$

$$\left(\frac{5 \text{ mmol H}_2\text{C}_2\text{O}_4}{2 \text{ mmol KMnO}_4} \right) \left(\frac{1 \text{ mmol Ca}^{++}}{1 \text{ mmol H}_2\text{C}_2\text{O}_4} \right)$$

$$= 0.0291 \text{ mmol Ca}^{++}$$

$$\frac{0.0291 \text{ mmol Ca}^{++}}{5.00 \text{ mL}} = 5.81 \times 10^{-3} \text{ M}$$

71. **(A)**   Convert the temperature from Celsius to Kelvin and apply the combined gas laws.

$$0.200 \text{ mL} \times \frac{67.0 \text{ mm Hg}}{760 \text{ mm Hg}} \times \frac{273 \text{ K}}{294 \text{ K}} = 0.016 \text{ mL}$$

72. **(B)**   Use the ideal gas law to find the moles of carbon dioxide, then divide by the volume of blood.

$$pV = nRT$$

$$n = \frac{pV}{RT} = \frac{\left(\frac{67.0}{760} \text{ atm}\right)(0.200 \times 10^{-3} \text{ L})}{\left(0.08206 \, \frac{\text{L atm}}{\text{mol K}}\right)(294 \text{ K})} = 7.31 \times 10^{-7} \text{ mol}$$

$$\frac{7.31 \times 10^{-7} \text{ mol}}{0.0300 \times 10^{-3} \text{ L}} = 0.024 \text{ mol } CO_2 \, / \, L \text{ blood}$$

73. **(C)** Bicarbonate ion may either act as an acid by donating a proton to water or as a base by accepting a proton from water.

$$HCO_3^- + H_2O \longrightarrow H_2CO_3 + OH^-$$

$$HCO_3^- + H_2O \longrightarrow CO_3^= + H_3O^+$$

74. **(B)** The formula of cocaine shows 17 moles of carbon per mole of cocaine. That is, (17 mol) 12.0 g/mol = 204 g C per 303.15 g cocaine. The percent carbon is then (204/303) × 100 = 67.3%.

75. **(B)** Since the white powder is 1.43% N, 100 g of it would contain 1.43 g N. The mass of cocaine that contains 1.43 g nitrogen is:

$$1.43 \text{ gN} \times \frac{1 \text{ mol N}}{14.0 \text{ gN}} \times \frac{1 \text{ mol } C_{17}H_{21}NO_4}{1 \text{ mol N}} \times \frac{303.15 \text{ g } C_{17}H_{21}NO_4}{1 \text{ mol } C_{17}H_{21}NO_4}$$

$$= 31.0 \text{ g } C_{17}H_{21}NO_4 \text{ per } 100 \text{ g white powder, i.e. } 31\%$$

Since 100 g white powder must contain the 31.0 g cocaine, the white powder is 31.0% cocaine.

76. **(D)** For 100 g of compound, the percent of each element corresponds to its mass in grams. Convert these masses to moles and reduce the mole ratio to a small whole number ratio.

$$\frac{42.10 \text{ g L}}{12.011 \text{ g / mol}} = 3.505 \text{ mol C}$$

$$\frac{6.48 \text{ g H}}{1.0079 \text{ g / mol}} = 6.479 \text{ mol H}$$

$$\frac{51.42 \text{ g O}}{15.9994 \text{ g / mol}} = 3.214 \text{ mol O}$$

Divide each by the smallest

$$\frac{3.505}{3.214} = 1.091; \quad \frac{6.429}{3.214} = 2.000; \quad \frac{3.214}{3.214} = 1.000$$

A little trial and error experimentation will show that multiplying each by 11 yields integers:

$$1.091 \times 11 = 12.00$$
$$2.000 \times 11 = 22.00 \quad \Big\} \quad C_{12}H_{22}O_{11}$$
$$1.000 \times 11 = 11.00$$

77. **(C)**   The lowering of the freezing point for the solution made by dissolving 1.00 g of B in 100 g of camphor is proportional to the molal concentration, c, of the solution. Calculate the molality (mol/kg), find the grams of B dissolved per kg camphor, and combine these two results to obtain the molar mass.

$$\Delta T_f = K_f C$$

$$C = \frac{\Delta T_f}{K_f} = \frac{(179.75 - 178.58)^\circ C}{(40.0^\circ C \,/\, \text{molal})}$$

$$= \frac{1.17}{40.0} \text{ mol} \,/\, \text{kg} = 0.0292 \text{ mol} \,/\, \text{kg}$$

$$\frac{1.00 \text{ g B}}{0.100 \text{ kg Camphor}} = 10.0 \text{ g} \,/\, \text{kg}$$

$$\frac{10.0 \text{g} \,/\, \text{kg}}{0.0292 \text{ mol} \,/\, \text{kg}} = 342 \text{ g} \,/\, \text{mol}$$

78. **(B)**   The general rule for solubility is "like dissolves like"; that is, polar solvents dissolve polar and ionic solutes well and nonpolar solvents dissolve nonpolar solutes well. To dissolve the slightly polar substance B, choose the least polar solvent listed, i.e., chloroform. The other three choices are all solvents of moderate to high polarity. Since cocaine contains many carbon atoms and relatively few oxygen and nitrogen atoms to make it polar, it would be expected to have relatively small polarity and to be relatively insoluble in polar solvents.

79. **(D)**   If four cocaine molecules are used, then $4 \times 17 = 68$ carbon dioxide, $4 \times 21 / 2 = 42$ water, and four nitrogen dioxide must appear in the products.

$$4C_{17}H_{21}NO_4 + 85O_2 \longrightarrow 68CO_2 + 42H_2O + 4NO_2$$

80. **(B)**   Hydrogen bonding is a result of very polar bonds involving hydrogen and a very electronegative atom such as oxygen, nitrogen or fluorine. Because fluorine is the most electronegative element, HF would have the strongest hydrogen bonding of the compounds listed in Table 1. The attraction among the HF molecules, due to hydrogen bonding, results in an increase in the energy needed to separate molecules from the liquid to form a gas, and hence an unusually large molar enthalpy of vaporization. The nearly constant Cp's for the HX molecules may be explained by the fact that only translational and nearly the same rotational energy must be changed to change their temperature. The increase in molar enthalpy of vaporization and increase in Cp for the hydrocarbons are associated with their increase in molar mass and increase in vibrational energy, respectively.

81.   **(A)**   The same amount of heat is released when a substance condenses as is absorbed when it vaporizes. Thus, multiply the molar enthalpy of vaporization (which has the same magnitude of the molar enthalpy of condensation) by the number of moles condensed.

HI: $1 + 127 = 128$ g/mol.

32 g $\times 1$ mol/128 g $= 0.25$ mol

$(0.25$ mol$) (21.2$ kJ/mol$) = 5.3$ kJ

82.   **(D)**   The total heat transferred can be calculated as the mass times the specific heat times the temperature change or as the amount (moles) times the molar heat capacity times the temperature change.

$$\Delta T = 30°C - 20°C = 10°C = 10 \text{ K}$$

$$q = nC_p \Delta T = (2 \text{ mol}) (52.6 \text{ J/mol K}) (10 \text{ K})$$

$$q = 1052 \text{ J}$$

83.   **(A)**   Apply Hess' Law by reversing the reaction for the formation of liquid water and adding it to the reaction for the formation of gaseous water.

H_2O (l) $\longrightarrow H_2$ (g) $+ \frac{1}{2} O_2$ (g)	$-(- 285.8$ kJ/mol$)$
H_2 (g) $+ \frac{1}{2} O_2$ (g) $\longrightarrow H_2O$ (g)	$(- 241.8$ kJ/mol$)$
H_2O (l) $\longrightarrow H_2O_2$ (g)	$+ 44.0$ kJ/mol

84.   **(C)**   The enthalpy of combustion can be calculated from the enthalpies of formation. The expression can be solved for the enthalpy of formation of methane.

$$CH_4 \text{ (g)} + 2O_2 \text{ (g)} \longrightarrow CO_2 \text{ (g)} + 2H_2O \text{ (l)}$$

$$\Delta H\text{comb} = \Delta H_f (CO_2) + 2\Delta H_f (H_2O) - \Delta H_f (CH_4)$$

$$\Delta H_f (CH_4) = \Delta H_f (CO_2) + 2\Delta H_f (H_2O) - \Delta H_{comb}$$

$$\Delta H_f (CH_4) = -393.5 + (2) (- 285.8) - (- 890.3)$$

$$\Delta H_f (CH_4) = -74.8 \text{ kJ/mol}$$

85.   **(A)**   The relationship between volume of a gas and its temperature was first announced by the French scientist Jacques Charles in 1787. The law states that, at constant pressure, the volume of a gas varies directly with the Kelvin temperature.

$$\frac{V_1}{T_1} = \frac{V_2}{T_2}$$

86.   **(C)**   A body is said to be in unstable equilibrium when it does not return to

its original equilibrium position after moving a small distance; rather it moves to another position.

87. **(C)** When a vibrating tuning fork is held over the mouth of the air column, a sudden increase in the volume of the sound can be heard if the column is adjusted to the correct length. At this point, standing waves are set up and the air column is vibrating with the same frequency as the tuning fork; the two are in resonance. The shortest length of the air column for which resonance occurs is a quarter wavelength $\lambda/4$. By measuring this length and multiplying it by 4, we get the wavelength of the sound. Since the frequency of the tuning fork is known, we can compute the velocity of the sound in air at room temperature by using $v = f\lambda$.

88. **(A)** By Graham's law of effusion:

$$\frac{M_y}{M_x} = \left[\frac{R_x}{R_y}\right]^2$$

where M_x and M_y are the molecular weights of gases X and Y and R_x and R_y are the rates of effusion of gases X and Y. From this, the ratio of their effusion rates is

$$\frac{R_x}{R_y} = \sqrt{\frac{M_y}{M_x}} = \sqrt{\frac{32}{28}} = \sqrt{\frac{8}{7}}$$

89. **(C)** Enthalpy is defined as the constant-pressure heat of reaction. The constant-volume heat of reaction is the internal energy (E or U). The two are related as shown below:

$$H = E + PV$$

$$\Delta H = \Delta E + P\Delta V + V\Delta P \tag{1}$$

Taking the constant pressure case ($\Delta P = 0$), and substituting $\Delta E = q - P_{(opposing)} \Delta V$ into (1):

$$\Delta H = q - P_{opp} \Delta V + P_{sys} \Delta V + 0$$

At constant pressure, the pressure of the system is equal to the pressure opposing the system throughout the reaction, that is , $P_{opp} = P_{sys}$. Therefore:

$$\Delta H = q \text{ at constant pressure}$$

90. **(D)** The total time is a combination of the fall time plus the time for the sound wave to propagate.

$$t = \sqrt{2h / g} + h / c$$

$$h + c\sqrt{2 / g}\sqrt{h} - ct = 0$$

$$h + 149.08\sqrt{h} - 2253.90 = 0$$

Completing the square

$$(\sqrt{h} + 74.54)^2 = 2253.90 + 5556.12$$

$$\sqrt{h} = -74.54 + 88.37$$

thus $h = 191m.$

91.   **(A)**   For a spontaneous reaction, the overall cell potential must be positive. Equation 1 must be reversed and added to Equation 2. The overall cell potential is then the potential for Equation 1 minus that for Equation 2.

$E°$ cell $= -.050 - (-1.66) = +1.61$ V

92.   **(C)**   To obtain a positive cell potential, reverse Equation 2 and add to Equation 3:

Ag_3Sn (s) $\longrightarrow Sn^{2+}$ (aq) $+ 3Ag$ (s) $+ 2e$ (oxidation)

$3Hg_2^{2+}$ (aq) $+ 4Ag$ (s) $+ 6e \longrightarrow 2Ag_2 Hg_3$(s)   (reduction)

In any cell oxidation takes place at the anode. Tin changes oxidation state from 0 to +2 when Ag_3Sn reacts in this cell. Thus Ag_3Sn is the anode. As the half reaction shows, electrons are produced at the Ag_3Sn anode and flow to the Ag cathode.

93.   **(C)**   Multiply the reverse of Equation 2 by three (so that the electrons will cancel) and add to Equation 3.

$3Ag_3Sn$ (s) $\longrightarrow 3Sn^{2+}$ (aq) $+ 9Ag$ (s) $+ 6e$

$3Hg_2^{2+}$ (aq) $+ 4Ag$ (s) $+ 6e \longrightarrow 2Ag_2 Hg_3$(s)

$3Ag_3Sn$ (s) $+ 3Hg_2^{2+}$ (aq) $+ 4Ag$ (s) $\longrightarrow 3Sn^{2+}$ (aq) $+ 9Ag$ (s) $+ 2Ag_2Sn_3$ (s)

Cancel excess Ag (s) to obtain the net ionic equation

$3Ag_3Sn$ (s) $+ 3Hg_2^{2+}$ (aq) $\longrightarrow 3Sn^{2+}$ (aq) $+ 5Ag$ (s) $+ 2Ag_2Sn_3$ (s)

94.   **(D)**   Electrical potential is energy per unit charge (1 V = 1 J/C) and electric current is charge per unit time (1 A = 1 C/s). Electric power is then the product of current times voltage: $P = IV$. The total energy can then be obtained by multiplying the power by the time:

$E = Pt = IVt.$

Electric energy = (10000 C/s) (5.0 J/C) (60 s) = 3.0×10^6 J = 3.0 MJ

95.   **(A)**   The equilibrium constant is related to the standard cell potential through the standard Gibbs function.

$\Delta G° - nFE° = -RT/nK$

$\ln K = nFE° / RT$

	E°
$2Al(s) \longrightarrow 2Al^{3+}$ (aq) + 6e	+ 1.66 V
$3Hg_2^{2+}$ (aq) + 4Aq(s) + 6e $\longrightarrow 2Ag_2\,Hg_3(s)$	+ 0.85 V
	+ 2.51 V

$$\ln K = \frac{(6)\,(96500)\,(2.51)}{(8.31)\,(298)} = 587$$

$$K = e^{587} = 10^{587/2.303} = 10^{255}$$

Many calculators will not display exponents greater than 99. It may be necessary to use the fact that $e^{2.303} = 20$ or $2.303 \ln (x) = \log(x)$ to convert to a power of ten.

96. **(C)** Note that three moles of electrons are required per mole of Al (Equation 1). Find the total charge to produce one gram of Al and then multiply by the voltage to obtain the energy.

$$(1 \text{ g Al})\left(\frac{1 \text{ mol Al}}{27 \text{ g Al}}\right)\left(\frac{3 \text{ mol e}}{1, \text{mol Al}}\right)\left(\frac{96500 \text{ C}}{1 \text{ mol e}}\right)(5.0 \text{ J}/\text{C})$$

$$= 5.36 \times 10^4 \text{ J} = 53.6 \text{ kJ}$$

97. **(B)** Inspection of the data in Table 1 shows that the initial rate is proportional to [HCl] (to the first power) for constant methyl acetate concentration of 0.2 M (lines 2, 4, and 5). That is, Rate = k[HCl], which is the rate law for a first order reaction.

98. **(D)** The data of Table 1 shows that the reaction depends on the concentrations of both methyl acetate and HCl. It is most likely that the first step of the mechanism involves both methyl acetate and H.

99. **(C)** "Half order" means that

$$\text{Rate} = k[A]^{\frac{1}{2}} = k\sqrt{[A]}.$$

If [A] changes by a factor of 2, then the rate must change by a factor of $\sqrt{2} = 1.4$.

100. **(A)** At the start (time zero) there is no acetic acid present, so eliminate (B) and (D). The concentration of acetic acid must increase with time, but as the methyl acetate is used up the rate of acetic acid production must decrease (eliminate (C)) as shown in (A).

101. **(B)** Use the data for the concentration of methyl acetate as a function of time at 25°C. The half time is the time for the concentration to change from any value to one half that value, for example from 0.20 M to 0.10 M; 4.76 - 1.75 = 3.01 min.

102. **(C)**   According to the Arrhenius rate theory, the rate constant

$$k = Ae^{-E/RT}$$

where E is the activation energy, T the absolute temperature, R the gas constant, and A is a constant which depends on the geometry of the rectangle. Taking the natural logarithm and subtracting the resulting equation at one temperature, T_1 from the corresponding equation at a second temperature, T_2 leads to:

$$k \ = \ Ae^{-E/RT}$$

$$\ln k \ = \ \ln A - E/RT$$

$$\ln k_2 \ = \ \ln A - E/RT_2$$

$$-(\ln k_1) \ = \ \ln A - E/RT_1$$

$$\overline{\ln k_2 - \ln k_1 \ = \ -E/RT_2 + E/RT_1}$$

$$\ln \frac{K_2}{K_1} = \frac{E}{R}\left(\frac{1}{T_1} - \frac{1}{T_2}\right)$$

Since the half time (t) is inversely proportional to the rate constant:

$$\ln \frac{t_1}{t_2} = \frac{E}{R}\left(\frac{1}{T_1} - \frac{1}{T_2}\right)$$

Using any pair of points from the temperature dependence of the half time data yields:

$$\ln \frac{18.8}{8.68} = \frac{E}{R}\left(\frac{1}{273} - \frac{1}{283}\right)$$

$$0.773 = \frac{E}{R}(1.294 \times 10^{-4})$$

$$E = \frac{0.773R}{1.294 \times 10^{-4}} = \frac{(0.773)(8.31)}{(1.294 \times 10^{-4})}$$

$$E = 5.0 \times 10^4 \text{ J} = 50 \text{ kJ}$$

103. **(C)**   Use the lens equation

$$1/p + 1/q = 1/f$$

where p is the image distance, q is the object distance, and f is the focal length.

$$1/160 \text{ mm} + 1/q = 1/16 \text{ mm}$$

$$1/q = 1/16 - 1/160 = (160 - 16)/(16)(160)$$

$$q = (16)(160)/(144) = 18 \text{ mm}$$

104. **(A)** A ray diagram shows that the image is virtual and erect.

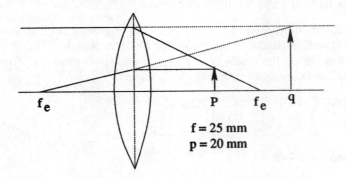

f_e 　　　　　　　P 　 f_e 　 q

$$f = 25 \text{ mm}$$
$$p = 20 \text{ mm}$$

105. **(A)** Equation 1:

$$MP_c = (16/1.6 - 1)\,(25/2.5 - 1) = 99$$

Equation 2:

$$MP_c = (16/1.6)\,(25/2.5) = 100$$

% error: $[(100 - 99)/99]100 = 1\%$

106. **(B)** The purpose of the oil is to reduce the divergence when the light leaves the glass. The angles of the rays when light travels from one medium to another are related to the indices of refraction of the media by Snell's law:

$$n_1 / n_2 = \sin (A_2) / \sin (A_1).$$

To have the angles A_1 and A_2 be the same, the indices of refraction, n_1 and n_2, must be equal. If the index of refraction of the oil equals that of the glass, there will be no divergence.

107. **(D)** The magnification of the objective lens is $(16/1.6) - 1 = 9$. The real image formed on the scale is 9 times larger than the object or the object is 1/9 as large as the image. $(1/9)\,(0.15 \text{ mm}) = 0.017 \text{ mm} = 17\ \mu\text{m}$.

108. **(C)** Phosgene reacts with water in the lungs to produce hydrochloric acid in the following manner:

$$COCL_2 + H_2O \longrightarrow 2HCl + CO_2$$

109. **(D)** In human digestion, fats are hydrolized to glycerol and fatty acids. Fats are triacylglycerols; they are carboxylic esters derived from glycerol, $HOCH_2CHOHCH_2OH$. Fats have the general structure:

$$
\begin{array}{l}
CH_2 - O - C - R \\
\qquad\qquad\ \parallel \\
\qquad\qquad\ O \\[4pt]
CH - O - C - R' \\
\qquad\quad\ \parallel \\
\qquad\quad\ O \\[4pt]
CH_2 - O - C - R'' \\
\qquad\qquad\ \parallel \\
\qquad\qquad\ O
\end{array}
$$

where R, R' and R'' may represent either one, two or three different radical groups. Hydrolysis of a fat will yield the three corresponding fatty acids and a molecule of gylcerol:

$$
\begin{array}{c}
CH_2-O-C-R \\
\quad\quad\quad\; || \\
\quad\quad\quad\; O \\
| \\
CH-O-C-R' \quad\xrightarrow[\;(H_2O)\;]{\text{hydrolysis}} \\
\quad\quad\quad\; || \\
\quad\quad\quad\; O \\
| \\
CH_2-O-C-R'' \\
\quad\quad\quad\quad\; || \\
\quad\quad\quad\quad\; O
\end{array}
\quad
\begin{array}{c}
CH_2-OH \\
| \\
CH-OH \quad + \\
| \\
CH_2-OH \\
\text{glycerol}
\end{array}
\quad
\begin{array}{c}
O \\
|| \\
RC-OH \\
\text{fatty acid} \\[6pt]
O \\
|| \\
R'\;C-OH \\
\text{fatty acid} \\[6pt]
O \\
|| \\
R''\;C-OH \\
\text{fatty acid}
\end{array}
$$

110. **(D)**   A triose is a three-carbon sugar. It may be referred to as a hydroxyaldehyde since it contains both a hydroxyl (OH) group and an aldehyde group (HC = O). It is not a trisaccharide, which consists of three bonded monosaccharide units. An example of a triose is given by:

$$
\begin{array}{c}
HC{=}O \\
| \\
HO-C-H \\
| \\
CH_2OH
\end{array}
$$

111. **(A)**   The speed of light is not temperature-dependent unlike the speed of sound.

112. **(B)**   The effort required depends on the ratio of the length of the plane (15 m) to the height (3 m).

$$\frac{\text{resistance}}{\text{effort}} = \frac{\text{length}}{\text{height}}$$

$$\frac{120\ N}{x} = \frac{15\ m}{3\ m}$$

x = effort required.

$$360\ N \cdot m = 15\ mx$$

$$x = 24\ N$$

113. **(C)**   By definition, coefficient of static friction, the ratio of the component of the car's weight along the slope to the component of its weight normal to the slope

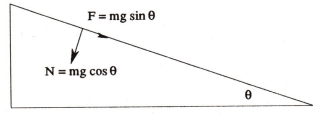

is equal to the tangent of the critical angle for which the car will just start to slide.

$$\mu = 1 = \frac{F}{N} = \frac{mg \sin \theta}{mg \cos \theta} = \frac{\sin \theta}{\cos \theta} = \tan \theta$$

$$\theta = \tan^{-1}(\mu) = \tan^{-1}(1) = 45°$$

114. **(A)**   The car reached a speed of 20 m/s after moving a distance of 200 m. Its (constant) acceleration is

$a = v^2 / 2x.$

$a = (20 \text{ m/s})^2 / (2) (200) = 1.0 \text{ m/s}^2.$

The angle of the slope is given by $\sin(100 \text{ m} / 200 \text{ m}) = 30°$. The coefficient of sliding friction is the ratio of the force in the direction of the motion to the normal force:

$(2000 \text{ kg}) (1.0 \text{ m/s}^2) / (2000 \text{ kg}) (9.80 \text{ m/s}^2) (\cos 30°) \cong 0.118$

115. **(D)**   The car's velocity changed from 20 m/s to zero in 0.5 s, thus the deceleration is (20 m/s) / (0.5 s) = 40 m/s².

116. **(A)**   The potential energy is given by

$PE = mgh$

$PE = (2000 \text{ kg}) (9.80 \text{ m/s}^2) (100 \text{ m}) = 1.96 \times 10^6 \text{ J} = 1.9 \text{ MJ}.$

117. **(C)**   The kinetic energy is given by

$KE = \frac{1}{2} mv^2.$

$KE = \frac{1}{2} (2000 \text{ kg}) (20 \text{ m/s})^2 = 4.0 \times 10^5 = 0.4 \text{ MJ}.$

118. **(D)**   The momentum is given by

$p = mv.$

$p = (2000 \text{ kg}) (20 \text{ m/s}) = 4.0 \times 10^4 \text{ kg m/s} = 40 \text{ Mg m/s}.$

119. **(B)**   The central acceleration is given by

$a = v^2/r.$

$a = (13.4 \text{ m/s})^2 / (50 \text{ m}) = 3.59 \text{ m/s}^2.$

Expressed as a fraction of the acceleration due to gravity,

$a/g = 3.59/9.80 = 0.37.$

Note: The driver experiences an apparent outward acceleration, but the acceleration causing him and the car to travel around the curve is directed toward the center of the curved path.

120. **(C)**   For constant acceleration, starting from rest, the average speed is one half the final speed. The time to travel distance x is

$t = x / (v/2) = 2x/v.$

The same expression applies to constant deceleration to rest. For the first 100 m, the time is

$2(100\ \text{m}) / (13.4\ \text{m/s}) = 15\ \text{s}.$

For the last 100 m, the time is also 15 s. The time to travel 200 m at a constant speed of 13.4 m/s is

$(200\ \text{m}) / (13.4\ \text{m/s}) = 15\ \text{s}.$

The total time is $15\ \text{s} + 15\ \text{s} + 15\ \text{s} = 45\ \text{s}.$

121. **(C)**   Since the choices are given in grams and the volume in milliliters, it is convenient to convert the density from kg/m^3 to g/mL, and then multiply density by volume.

$$(1025\ \text{kg} / \text{m}^3)\left(\frac{1\ \text{m}}{10^2\ \text{cm}}\right)^3\left(\frac{1\ \text{cm}^3}{1\ \text{mL}}\right)\left(\frac{10^3\text{g}}{1\ \text{kg}}\right) = 1.025\ \text{g} / \text{mL}$$

$(1.025\ \text{g} / \text{mL}) (500\ \text{mL}) = 512\ \text{g}$

122. **(A)**   The difference in densities gives the apparent mass per unit volume, which when multiplied by the volume and acceleration due to gravity gives the apparent weight.

$(1125 - 1025) = 100\ \text{kg} / \text{m}^3$

$$(100\ \text{kg} / \text{m}^3)\left(\frac{1\ \text{m}}{10^6\ \mu\text{m}}\right)(150\ \mu\text{m}^3)\ (9.8\ \text{m} / \text{s}^2) = 1.5 \times 10^{-13}\text{N} = 0.15\,p\text{N}$$

123. **(B)**   For constant V, R, and L, Poiseuille's equation reduces to the reciprocal of the flow time and is proportional to the pressure difference divided by the viscosity. For a fixed, vertical flow length, the pressure difference is proportional to the density of the fluid. Thus the reciprocal of the flow time is proportional to the density divided by the viscosity or the flow time is directly proportional to the viscosity divided by the density.

124. **(D)**   Since the volume of blood flowing per unit time must remain the same, the cross-sectional area times the flow speed must be constant. The cross-sectional area is proportional to the square of the diameter, which leads to:

$d_1^2 v_1 = d_2^2 v_2$ or $v_2/v_1 = d_1^2/d_2^2 = (d_1/d_2)^2 = (5/3)^2 = 2.8.$

125. **(B)**   One consequence of Bernoulli's law (the sum of the pressure, kinetic energy per unit volume and potential energy per unit volume is constant) is that the pressure near the wall of a blood vessel is higher than near the center of the blood

vessel because the flow speed, and hence kinetic energy per unit volume, is lower near the wall due to the frictional forces between the wall and blood. This pressure gradient, higher near the wall to lower near the center, pushes the blood cells toward the center.

126. **(A)** For $(P_1 - P_2)/L$ constant, Poisuille's equation reduces to:

$$\frac{V}{t} \quad \alpha \quad R^4 \quad (\text{Diameter})^4$$

$$\left(\frac{3.0 \text{ mm}}{5.0 \text{ mm}}\right)^4 (100) = 13\%$$

127. **(B)** For rotational equilibrium, equate the moments about the ankle joint.

$$F(4.5 \text{ cm}) = (686 \text{ N})(12.5 \text{ cm})$$

$$F = \frac{(686)(12.5)}{(4.5)} = 1906 \text{ N} = 1.9 \text{ kN}$$

128. **(C)** For rotational equilibrium, equate the moments about the heel:

$$P(4.5 \text{ cm}) = (686 \text{ N})(17.0 \text{ cm})$$

$$P = \frac{(686)(17.0)}{(4.5)} = 2592 \text{ N} = 2.6 \text{ kN}$$

Another approach is to use the result of Question 127 with the condition for translational equilibrium:

$$P = F + mg$$

$$P = 1.9 + 0.7 = 2.6 \text{ kN}$$

129. **(D)** The vertical component of the ball's velocity is

$$(10 \text{ m/s}) \sin(45°) = 7.07 \text{ m/s}.$$

The final speed is zero. The initial height is $y_0 = 2.00$ m and the acceleration is due to gravity. The rate of change of velocity equals the acceleration:

$$(v - v_0)/t = a,$$

which rearranges to

$$t = (v - v_0)/a,$$

the time to reach the maximum height.

$$t = (0 - 7.7)/(-9.8) = 0.72 \text{ s}.$$

The distance may then be calculated:

$$y = \tfrac{1}{2} at^2 + v_0 t + y_0 = \tfrac{1}{2}(-9.8)(0.72)^2 + (7.07)(0.72) + 2.00 = 4.55 \text{ m}.$$

130. **(D)** The horizontal motion is at constant velocity. The total distance is the product of the horizontal component of the initial velocity, $(10 \text{ m/s}) \sin 45° = 7.07$ m/s, times the total time of flight. The total time is the sum of the time to rise to the maximum height, fall back to 2.00 m (which must be the same as the rise time), and the time to fall 2.00 m starting with an initial downward speed which is the same as the initial upward speed.

$$t = \frac{V'' - V_0''}{-g} + \frac{V' - V_0'}{g} + \frac{-V_0' + \sqrt{V_0^2 + 2gy}}{g}$$

$$t = \frac{0 - 7.07}{-9.8} + \frac{7.07 - 0}{9.8} + \frac{-7.07 + \sqrt{(7.07)^2 + 2(9.8)(2.00)}}{9.8}$$

$$t = 0.72\text{s} + 0.72\text{s} + 0.24\text{s} = 1.68\text{s}$$

$$x = (7.07 \text{ m/s})(1.68 \text{ s}) = 12 \text{ m}$$

131. **(A)** Force equals the rate of change of momentum:

$$F = m(v_2 - v_1)/t$$

$$t = m(v_2 - v_1)/F = (1.5 \text{ kg})[(15.0 \text{ m/s}) - (-10.0 \text{ m/s})]/(3.75 \text{ kN}) = 10 \text{ ms}.$$

132. **(B)** Resolve the forces into components, add the components, and calculate the magnitude of the resultant. Since each force has magnitude W, the magnitudes will equal unity in units of W.

$S_x = \cos(-20°)$	$= 0.940$	$S_y = \sin(-20°)$	$= -0.342$
$Q_x = \cos(30°)$	$= 0.866$	$Q_y = \sin(30°)$	$= 0.500$
$P_x = \cos(45°)$	$= 0.707$	$P_y = \sin(45°)$	$= 0.707$
R_x	$= 2.513$	R_y	$= 0.865$

$$R = R_x^2 + R_y^2 = 2.513^2 + 0.865^2 = 2.66 \text{ (times } W)$$

133. **(D)** Apply Ohm's law:

$$V = IR.$$

$$R = V/I = (20 \times 10^6 \text{ V})/(50 \times 10^{-3} \text{ A})$$

$$R = 0.4 \times 10^9 \ \Omega = 400 \text{ M}\Omega.$$

134. **(B)** Molecular weight of SF_6:

$$32 + 6(19) = 146$$

The speed of sound in a gas is inversely proportional to the density of the gas. Note: volume in this case is constant.

$$\text{speed } SF_6 \text{ / speed air } = \sqrt{29/146} = 0.45$$

135. **(C)** The product of the charge, in units of the electron charge, times the terminal voltage, in megavolts, is the energy, in megaelectronvolts, acquired.

For the singly negative ion (1) (20) = 20 MeV

For the doubly positive ion (2) (20) = 40 MeV

Total energy = 20 + 40 = 60 MeV

136. **(A)** The force on a moving charge is

$$F = Bqv = mv^2/r$$

where B is the magnetic field strength, q the charge, v the speed, m the mass, and r the radius of curvature. For this case,

$q = 2(1.6 \times 10^{-19} \text{ C})$, $m = 4(1.66 \times 10^{-27} \text{ kg})$, $v = 3.5 \times 10^7$ m/s, and $r = 1.00$ m.

Solving for B and substituting:

$$B = \frac{mv}{qr} = \frac{(4)(1.66 \times 10^{-27})(2.5 \times 10^7)}{(2)(1.60 \times 10^{-19})(1.00)} = 0.73\ T$$

137. **(C)** Use conservation of momentum: momentum of projectile equals moment of recoil:

$$mv = MV.$$

Square both sides, divide by 2, and rearrange:

$$\frac{m^2 v^2}{2} = \frac{M^2 V^2}{2}$$

$$m(\tfrac{1}{2} mv^2) = M(\tfrac{1}{2} MV^2)$$

$$mE_{\text{projectile}} = ME_{\text{recoil}}$$

$$E_{\text{recoil}} = \frac{m}{M} E_{\text{projectile}} = \frac{4}{16}(32\text{ MeV}) = 8\text{ MeV}$$

138. **(C)** Balance the nuclear equation by requiring conservation of mass number and conservation of atomic number.

$$^{27}_{13}\text{Al} + {}^{4}_{2}\text{He} \longrightarrow {}^{1}_{0}\text{n} + {}^{30}_{15}\text{P}$$

139. **(B)** An aldol is produced by the self-condensation of two moles of aldehyde in the following manner:

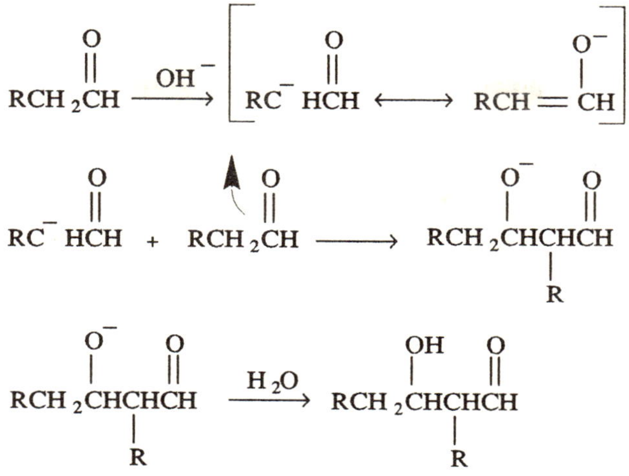

$$\underset{RCH_2CH}{\overset{\overset{O}{\|}}{}} \xrightarrow{OH^-} \left[\underset{RC^-\ HCH}{\overset{\overset{O}{\|}}{}} \longleftrightarrow \underset{RCH=CH}{\overset{\overset{O^-}{|}}{}} \right]$$

$$\underset{RC^-\ HCH}{\overset{\overset{O}{\|}}{}} + \underset{RCH_2CH}{\overset{\overset{O}{\|}}{}} \longrightarrow \underset{R}{\underset{|}{\underset{RCH_2CHCHCH}{\overset{\overset{O^-}{|}\quad\overset{O}{\|}}{}}}}$$

$$\underset{R}{\underset{|}{\underset{RCH_2CHCHCH}{\overset{\overset{O^-}{|}\quad\overset{O}{\|}}{}}}} \xrightarrow{H_2O} \underset{R}{\underset{|}{\underset{RCH_2CHCHCH}{\overset{\overset{OH}{|}\quad\overset{O}{\|}}{}}}}$$

140. **(B)**   Using Newton's second law, in terms of momentum, we obtain

momentum $= mv$

Since mass is a scalar quantity and velocity is a vector quantity (momentum), the product of the two is a scalar quantity.

Since acceleration is defined as

$$a = \frac{v_f - v_i}{t}$$

Expressing a in the equation $F = ma$ as above, we obtain

$$F = m\frac{v_f - v_i}{t}$$

This equation states that the rate of change of momentum of a body is equal to the unbalanced force acting upon the body and is in the direction of the force.

Breaking force $= -3000$ N

$$-3000\text{ N} = m\ \frac{0 - 15\text{ m/sec}}{10\text{ sec}}$$

$$-3000\text{ N} = m\frac{-15\text{ m/sec}}{10\text{ sec}}$$

$$-3000\text{ kg}\cdot\text{m/sec}^2 = m(-1.5\text{ m/sec}^2)$$

$$2000\text{ kg} = m$$

141. **(B)**   According to Newton's law of inertia, a body in motion tends to move in a straight line. To change straight-line motion into circular motion, an outside force must constantly pull the body toward the center of rotation. Such a central force is called a centripetal force.

142. **(B)** If a satellite is to remain in a circular orbit, the centripetal force required to keep it in its orbit is provided by the gravitational attraction between the satellite and the earth. Thus, we arrive at the following equation:

$$\frac{m_s v_s^2}{r} = G \frac{m_s m_e}{r^2}$$

where

m_s = mass of satellite

v_s = velocity of the satellite

m_e = mass of the earth

r = distance between satellite and center of earth

Solving, we obtain

$$v_s^2 r = G m_e$$

Since G and m_e are constants

$$v_s^2 r = \text{Constant}$$

Since the mass of the satellite has cancelled out, this shows that a light satellite and a heavy satellite, both having the same orbital speed, will occupy the same orbit. Since M_2 and M_2 are in the same orbit, they have the same speed.

Section 3 — Writing Sample

DEMONSTRATION ESSAY 1

The world is getting smaller and smaller, yet the understanding which one might assume would result from a smaller world seems farther and farther away. As each nation wrestles with survival and development, as in the third world countries, or with progress and growth, as in the economically powerful nations of the world, the preoccupation of each is with its own people. Each particular people, with its history, culture, and pride will always prize its values above those of other nations. Self-interest is the law of survival. It is the will-to-live that perpetuates values, whether those values complement other cultures or not.

Of course, it would be erroneous to assume that this very same law of survival will not create national, and often international, conflict over individual groups' rights. The heated conflict in the Middle East, though it ostensibly represents an economic conflict, is fundamentally a difference of values. This difference is so basic that it is difficult to realize an easy solution, other than one which asks one or the other value systems to compromise. Although compromise may appear to be the American way of negotiation, compromise often suggests weakness and a "soft will" to those who pride themselves on their ability to maintain control and dominance.

Conflicting value systems have coexisted peacefully at various times in history. In the Arab world, during the time of Mohammed, Jews, Christians, and Arabs coexisted because they shared a common basis for belief: they each had a holy book. Though each read it differently and interpreted it through different holy persons, each was elected to share in the truth. The vastness of the world demands the same spirit of cooperation now.

When the needs of a people are satisfied, harmony is possible; when those needs are unmet, conflicting values will emerge to test the mettle of a people. Such is the dilemma the world faces in the clash of wills in the Middle East.

DEMONSTRATION ESSAY EXPLANATION

The essay focuses clearly on the topic defined by the statement and fully addresses each of the three writing tasks. The first paragraph shows that the student understands the problem. It responds to the request to discuss the meaning of the statement. The next paragraph illustrates the student's interpretation of the meaning of the statement by referring to a current international example. The last paragraph shows both the difficulty in resolving the dilemma, and the potential for doing so.

This is a particularly good essay because it is a thoughtful and simple approach to the idea posed in the given quote. The essay does not force the point; neither does it avoid dealing with the issue.

The writing in this essay is clear and controlled. The essay responds to the tasks at hand. One feels that the student understands the question and the breadth of its importance. Also helpful to the argument is the way the student draws on an historical point that is germane to the illustration selected.

DEMONSTRATION ESSAY 2

We are a technologically literate people. Some might argue that we have forgotten "the nature of things" in achieving this status. The ingenious among us have advanced industry, both for the production of the necessities of life and for the efficient use of resources. Both of these motives appear innocent enough. After all, they represent the best of "the American Way!" Efficiency, however, has often meant the disregard of the disposal of waste materials. It has also often meant the violation of human dignity, as the work that was once honorable has become dangerous, repetitive and unrewarding. American ingenuity is the curious creator and benefactor of the consequences to the environment with which we are left. Consequences such as pollution, death to wildlife, and disease, are the result of a lack of conscience and a refusal to recognize the negative results of the so-called progress of the American way of life. For most of us, these results are regarded as too far into the future to be concerned about. Making the earth do what we want in the name of the progress of humankind shows that we do not understand the law of entropy and how it is closing in on us.

It would be possible, I suppose, to see the positive contributions of technology by looking at the small picture. Home life is made more efficient; entertainment is conveniently at our fingertips; space is being conquered; military tactics are made more complex and, paradoxically, more accurate in locating and defeating the enemy. Progress, power, and the quality of life are enhanced by the control of the environment made possible by technology. This argument is prevalent among those who also favor the free enterprise of big business. Corporations, real estate developers, and profitable scientific ventures all benefit from this way of thinking.

It would be easy to believe that the choice of one or the other of these positions is the legacy we will be forced to leave to the next generation. Actually both choices are too extreme. The earth is to be both nurtured and nurturing; humanity can both use and respectfully replenish the earth. For every progressive effort there must be a cautious limit or protection. For every tree cut, one must be planted; for every human being displaced there must be a new job created. It is not an either/or proposition; it is an "all or nothing" proposition.

While pessimism about the human race is justified at this time in our history, despair is premature. With small voices, groups are creating an environment that is forcing legislators and communities to respond to the needs of nature by recycling, using biodegradeable products and, in general, becoming aware of the enormous task before us.

DEMONSTRATION ESSAY EXPLANATION

The first paragraph lends assistance to the author's point of view by providing a rationale for what might prompt the author to make such a declaration. The second paragraph offers the counter-position and defends the use of technology and the progress that results from that use. Finally, the student specifically suggests the nominal, but real, efforts underway to foster a new consciousness, thus alleviating some of the ultimate "gloom and doom" of the author.

Writing an essay that is a response to a value judgment creates a very specific task for the student. It demands that the student clarify the meaning of the position, understand its implications, and then respond with a counter value statement. As simply and as much to the point as possible, the essay attends to the reader's sense of judgment and provides sufficient information that allows the reader to acknowledge the value orientation of the essay.

The essay provides a coherent and clear statement that responds to the statement without pretense. Straightforward sentences express the perspective advocated by the writer in response to the three tasks.

Section 4 — Biological Sciences

143. **(C)** Both DNA and RNA contain five-carbon (pentose) sugars in the component nucleotides. However, since DNA contains deoxyribose (while RNA contains ribose) this is not a correct statement regarding DNA. The other three choices describe valid attributes of DNA — it is far larger than any of the three types of RNA; it is almost always a double-stranded molecule; and DNA *can* be found outside the nucleus (most notably in chloroplasts and mitochondria).

144. **(C)** The 5' and 3' notations refer to two specific carbon atoms in the ring forms of the pentose sugars deoxyribose and ribose. The inorganic phosphate molecule that is a part of each DNA and RNA nucleotide is covalently bonded to the 5' carbon of the pentose. Therefore, the end of a nucleic acid molecule that has a "free" phosphate is referred to as the 5' end. Adenine and guanine, choices (A) and (C) respectively, are purine bases found in both DNA and RNA and have nothing to do with polarity of the molecules. The pentose sugar end of a nucleic acid molecule has nothing bonded to the 3' position and is therefore described as the 3' end of the molecule. You should notice therefore, in Figure 1, that each of the two strands of DNA has a 5' end and a 3' end, but that the two strands run in opposite directions with respect to this polarity.

145. **(A)** Adenine and guanine are the two nitrogenous nucleic acid bases resembling the organic molecule purine, with a double-ring structure, and are given that generic name; they are found in both DNA and RNA. The other three nitrogenous bases (cytosine, thymine, and uracil) found in DNA and RNA are similar to the

molecule pyrimidine, which has a single-ring structure, and are therefore described as pyrimidines. Cytosine is found in both DNA and RNA nucleotides. However, thymine is unique to DNA while uracil is unique to RNA and, in a sense, "replaces" thymine in RNA. Among the four choices for this item, the only one in which *both* bases are purines is choice (A).

146. **(A)** All nucleic acid bases contain at least two atoms of nitrogen and each amino acid contains at least one. The macromolecules known as nucleic acids and proteins therefore both contain considerable amounts of nitrogen. The other choices are incorrect: phosphorous is found in nucleic acids (as phosphate in nucleotides), but not in proteins; iodine is found in neither nucleic acids nor proteins; and sulfur is found in protein (as part of the amino acids methionine and cysteine).

147. **(B)** Looking at Figure 1, or simply recalling knowledge of base-pairs in double-stranded DNA, you should be able to determine that purines base-pair with pyrimidines. Choice (B) gives the only correct pairing of a purine (guanine) and a pyrimidine (cytosine). Since each molecule of guanine in a given double-stranded molecule of DNA would be paired with a molecule of cytosine, the total amounts of each would be equal. (The observation that DNA always contained equal amounts of guanine and cytosine, as well as equal amounts of adenine and thymine, was made by Erwin Chargaff prior to the Watson-Crick model.) Choices (A), (C), and (D) offer impossible pairings between two purines or two pyrimidines and are, therefore, incorrect.

148. **(D)** This item tests your understanding of composition of DNA nucleotides. Choice (A) is not correct because uracil is a pyrimidine base found in RNA, not DNA, while choices (B) and (C) are incorrect because the pentose sugar in DNA nucleotides is deoxyribose, not ribose. The correct choice, (D), matches one of the four possible DNA nucleic acid bases (in this case, cytosine) with deoxyribose, the pentose sugar found in DNA.

149. **(D)** The fusion of an egg and sperm sets into motion the events of embryonic development beginning with a rapid change in egg membrane potential that prevents fusion with additional sperm. Unlike mammals, where there is no apparent polarity of the embryo until the blastocyst stage, embryonic axes are already determined in the zygotes of amphibians. The point of sperm penetration will be the anterior end of the developing embryo, so choice (D) is correct. The gray crescent, which forms opposite the penetration point of the sperm, marks the site of the future blastopore and, eventually, the anus. The first cleavage is parallel to the dorsiventral axis, bisecting the gray crescent and, thus, dividing the two-celled embryo into left and right halves.

150. **(D)** Following fertilization of the egg, the major developmental stages of an amphibian embryo, in correct sequence, are: morula, blastula, gastrula, neural plate, neural groove (or fold), neural tube, tail bud, and tadpole. The only choice that presents a correct sequence of stages is (D); other choices have stages out of proper sequence. You will need to be familiar with this sequence and the major developmental events that occur in embryology of vertebrates to answer other questions about animal development.

151. **(B)**   The three primary germ layers of triploblastic animals are formed during gastrulation. The correct choice for this question is, therefore, (B). Organogenesis — the development of these germ layers into rudimentary organs — follows formation of the germ layers.

152. **(A)**   To answer this question, you must be familiar with the adult tissue and organ derivatives of the primary germ layers. Choice (A) correctly identifies ectoderm as the germ layer precursor of the nervous system, including the spinal cord and brain. The other choices are incorrect because the spinal cord is derived from ectoderm (as the embryonic neural groove or primitive streak) exclusively.

153. **(C)**   The question also tests your knowledge of adult derivatives of the primary germ layers, in this case the derivatives of ectoderm. Choice (C) correctly identifies the vertebrae as not being ectodermally derived. All other choices present tissues and structures that are developed from ectoderm. The vertebrae (along with the notochord, circulatory system, skeletal muscles, excretory and reproductive systems, and the lining of the coelom) are among the adult tissues derived from mesoderm.

154. **(B)**   To answer this question you must be familiar with the events of human embryonic development, specifically the development of the appendicular skeleton. By the fifth week, bud-like rudiments of both anterior and posterior extremities (i.e., arms and legs) have appeared. Arm buds precede leg buds by several days. Choice (B) correctly identifies the time frame of their appearance. You should also be familiar with the timing of appearance of other structures in human development.

155. **(A)**   Dorsal ectoderm is induced into forming the neural tube by the underlying notochord and is one example of the general phenomenon of induction. The choice that correctly identifies this term is (A). The other choices give incorrect terms for this question, although you should be familiar with their definitions: determination refers to the fates of each cell in a developing embryo (the potential developmental fates of these cells become increasingly restricted); biologically, transformation refers to the incorporation of extrinsic genetic material into a cell's genome, especially as it occurs in bacteria; and, differentiation is the term that describes the progressive specialization in the form and/or function of cells and tissues throughout development.

156. **(B)**   Spermatogonia and oogonia are the cells from which sperm and ova, respectively, are produced by meiosis and cytokinesis in animals. They are derived from primordial germ cells that form in the yolk sac of mammalian embryos and migrate to the site of future gonads during the fourth week of development. The yolk sac has no yolk in mammals, and production of the germ cells (along with early production of blood) is one of the few functions of this extraembryonic membrane. You need to be familiar with the other three extraembryonic membranes (given in the three incorrect choices) and their roles in embryonic development.

157. **(D)**   Meso compounds contain chiral centers, but are optically inactive because of some symmetry element in the molecule. Both ribose and xylose will give diacids which have a plane of symmetry when reacted with HNO_3. (A) is only par-

tially correct; (B) and (C) are incorrect, since neither Lyxose nor arabinose will give meso diacids.

158. **(B)**   Of the aldohexoses, only allose and galactose will form diacids with a plane of symmetry when reacted with HNO_3.

159. **(B)**   Since the Ruff degradation destroys the chiral center at the number 2 carbon (by converting it to an aldehyde), the configuration of the remaining chiral centers determines which new aldose will form. The configurations of carbons 3 and 4 of arabinose match the configuration of erythrose. None of the other answers is reasonable.

160. **(A)**   Since the Kiliani-Fischer synthesis adds a new chiral center non-stereoselectively, two new aldoses will form, differing only in the configuration at the new chiral center. Both gulose and idose are identical to xylose at carbons 3, 4, and 5. None of the other pairs meets this criterion.

161. **(D)**   Bromine water is a very mild oxidizing agent; it will convert aldehydes to acids, but will not oxidize the terminal alcohol as nitric acid will. Consequently, the monoacid formed has no symmetry element and remains an optically active compound.

162. **(A)**   In order to see the rotation needed to change this projection to the conventional form, it is probably easiest to rewrite it using dashed lines and wedges to indicate stereochemistry.

The other answers are various perturbations of incorrect rotations around the chiral centers.

163. **(C)**   To answer this question you must apply Dalton's Law. The total pressure of a gas is the sum of the pressures that the individual gases in the mixture

would exert independently (Dalton's Law). Accordingly, atmospheric pressure is the sum of the pressures of its constituent gases. Atmospheric pressure at sea level (i.e., one atmosphere) is 760 mm Hg. Since our atmosphere is approximately 21% oxygen, the partial pressure of oxygen (i.e., that part of atmospheric pressure contributed by oxygen) equals 760 mm × .21, or 159 mm Hg. The correct choice is (C). The actual partial pressure of oxygen entering the lungs is reduced to about 150 mm Hg because of the fact that the inspired air is saturated with water vapor (which has a partial pressure of about 47 mm Hg at body temperature).

164. **(D)** This question deals with the terms used to describe various capacities of pulmonary function. That part of the total lung capacity that can be forcefully expired after a maximum inspiration is known as the vital capacity of the lungs (choice (D)). Note from reading the spirogram in Figure 2, there remains a certain amount of gas, the residual volume, that cannot be expired. The lungs, therefore, cannot be normally emptied of gas. The other choices are incorrect: inspiratory reserve volume is the amount of air that can be inspired after a tidal inspiration; tidal volume is the amount of air expired during each cycle of quiet breathing; and, vital capacity of the lungs is the maximum amount of air that can be expired after a maximum inspiration (i.e., the maximum volume of air that can be exchanged with the environment, as can be seen from the spirogram).

165. **(A)** To answer this question, you must be familiar with the pathway of airflow through the mammalian respiratory system. Choice (A) is the only correct sequence. From the pharynx, air travels through the glottis, larynx, trachea, bronchii (there are two), bronchioles, and into the sac-like alveoli. You should note that air can enter the respiratory tract either through the mouth or nares, and that the pharynx is a structure common to the respiratory and digestive systems (the glottis must be covered by the epiglottis to prevent aspiration of material from the digestive tract during swallowing).

166. **(D)** Referring to Figure 1, and being familiar with the mechanics of mammalian pulmonary ventilation, you should know that increase in the volume of the thoracic cavity is accomplished by contraction of both the external intercostal muscles *and* the diaphragm (choice (D)). The other choices are incorrect. In fact, contraction of the internal intercostals is used during forced expiration, not inhalation.

167. **(B)** About 70% of the carbon dioxide in mammalian blood is in the form of bicarbonate anions, so choice (B) is correct. When carbon dioxide dissolves in aqueous solution, it forms carbonic acid which quickly dissociates into hydrogen ions and bicarbonate ions. The hydrogen ions (protons) combine with deoxyhemoglobin of red blood cells and their acidic influence is effectively buffered out. This bicarbonate buffering system is important in maintaining normal blood pH of 7.4, in addition to serving to transport carbon dioxide. The other choices are incorrect: carboxyhemoglobin is the combination of hemoglobin and carbon monoxide; dissolved carbon dioxide gas comprises only about 10% of the carbon dioxide carried by the blood; and carbonic anhydrase is the enzyme that catalyzes the conversion of carbonic acid to carbon dioxide and water in the pulmonary capillaries.

168. **(C)** By reading the spirogram in Figure 2 and knowing that the amount of air exchanged during quiet breathing is known as the tidal volume, you can determine that this patient's tidal volume is about 500 cc. The other choices are incorrect: 6000 cc is the total lung capacity as read from the spirogram; 4800 cc is the approximate vital capacity of this individual; and, 3500 cc is the sum of the tidal and inspiratory reserve volumes.

169. **(C)** The SH⁻ ion would displace the bromine atom from the backside of the carbon in a nucleophilic displacement reaction (S_N2), leading to a product with inverted configuration at that carbon. (A) would be formed if the reaction proceeded with retention of configuration. (B) and (D) are not chemically feasible reactions.

170. **(D)** Protozoans are single-celled animals whose cells are often highly specialized, containing many organelles. They can reproduce both asexually and sexually. However, they cannot give birth to live progeny, viviparity, in the way that mammals can.

171. **(C)** Vitamins are usually coenzymes or parts of coenzymes. They are organic molecules that cannot be synthesized by an organism and hence must be supplied in the diet. The deprivation of vitamins in the diet can lead to many diseases. Scurvy is a result of vitamin C deficiency; beriberi is caused by a lack of vitamin B_1; rickets is a result of vitamin D deficiency in children; and xerophthalmia, which can lead to permanent blindness, is caused by insufficient vitamin A. Phenylketonuria, however, is a genetically transmitted disease in which an individual cannot convert phenylalanine to tyrosine because the enzyme phenylalanine H-monooxygenase is absent.

172. **(D)** The partial pressures of oxygen and carbon dioxide are the main determinants of whether oxygen will be picked up or released by hemoglobin. When there is a large amount of oxygen (a high partial pressure) and a low partial pressure of carbon dioxide, hemoglobin picks up oxygen. This is the case in the alveoli of the lungs. Oxyhemoglobin dissociates oxygen when the partial pressure of carbon dioxide is high and that of oxygen is low. This occurs in the tissues that are serviced by the systemic circulation.

173. **(A)** The disintegration of the zona pellucida begins when the sperm penetrates the egg. The zona pellucida is one of the membranous layers that surrounds the unfertilized egg which must be totally disintegrated by the time the zygote reaches the uterus. Its disintegration frees the trophoblast layer of cells, which then adheres to the uterine wall.

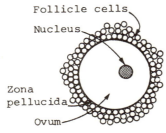

Fig. (a) Ovum before ovulation and fertilization

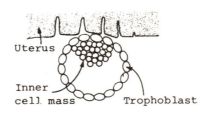

(b) After fertilization and implantation

174. **(B)** The sino-atrial (S-A) node is a small strip of specialized muscle in the wall of the heart's right atrium. This node has the contractile properties of muscle and can transmit impulses like a nerve. The S-A node generates the rhythmic self-excitatory impulse which causes a wave of contraction across the walls of the atria. This wave reaches a second mass of nodal tissue, the atrio-ventricular (A-V) node, which is then stimulated to contract. This contraction is transmitted to all parts of the ventricles causing them to contract as a unit.

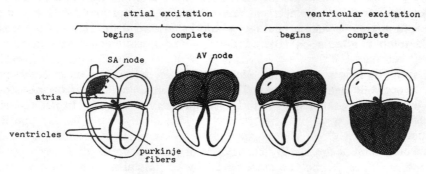

Sequence of cardiac excitation.

175. **(A)** At pH 10.0, which is a very alkaline system, all acidic protons will be removed. Since aspartic acid has a carboxylic acid side chain, it will have a net charge of -2 at high pH. All of the others will have a net charge of -1 at high pH.

176. **(C)** At pH 1.0, all basic groups will be protonated. Since Lysine has a basic side chain, the side chain and the alpha amino group will both be protonated, giving Lysine a net charge of +2 at pH 1.0.

177. **(B)** The only amino acid without a chiral alpha carbon is glycine, which contains two hydrogens attached to this carbon. Therefore, it has no optical activity and cannot be resolved into enantiomers.

178. **(D)** Choice (D) correctly identifies the location of the ion pumps in the nephron. The ion pumps located in the ascending limb of the loop of Henle, and maybe only in the thick segments of that limb, are directly involved in establishing an increasingly high osmolality from renal cortex to renal medulla. Active transport of Na^+ and/or Cl^- across the epithelial walls of the ascending limb seems to be occurring. In the process, the filtrate within the tubule becomes hypotonic to the surrounding fluid. There is reabsorption of Na^+, Cl^-, amino acids, and glucose across the proximal convoluted tubule (choice (A)) and distal tubule (choice (B)) walls; in both cases, the solute uptake is back into the blood and is not involved in the countercurrent multiplier system. The wall of collecting tubule (choice (C)) is permeable to water, but not salt, and as filtrate passes through the collecting tubule it becomes increasingly concentrated in urea and other remaining solutes. Some of the urea diffuses into the surrounding tissue and, along with the salt present there, helps account for the steep osmotic gradient encountered as the collecting tubule passes farther into the medulla.

179. **(C)**   By referring to Figure 1, or through your familiarity with the structure and function of a nephron, you should be able to identify choice (C) as the only correct sequence of structures through which glomerular filtrate flows. Each of the other three choices has a portion of the nephron listed out of sequence.

180. **(C)**   This question requires that you know the three processes through which the vertebrate nephron controls the composition of blood solutes. Hydrostatic pressure of the arterial portion of the circulatory system forces fluid out of the glomerular capillaries and into the lumen of the nephron. Among the solutes in this fluid is urea, the principal nitrogenous waste of humans and other mammals. Hence, the mechanism for removal of urea from the blood is the ultrafiltration that occurs in Bowman's capsules (the correct choice is (C)). While ultrafiltration is a non-selective process, secretion (choice (A)) and reabsorption (choice (B)) are very selective processes that occur through active transport across the epithelial walls of various portions of the nephron. Osmosis (choice (D)) is the diffusion of water across differentially permeable membranes in response to concentration gradients. While osmosis is very important in making the urine concentrated, it is not directly involved in removing urea from the blood.

181. **(B)**   The ultrafiltration of blood should force fluid and small solute molecules from glomerular capillaries into the nephron. No large molecules, like blood proteins, or cellular components, should enter the lumen of the nephron. Choice (B) is correct because it identifies a blood component that is too large to pass through the capillary pores of the glomerulus under normal circumstances. Choices (A), (C), and (D) identify molecules that are small enough to pass through the pores and are normally found in glomerular filtrate.

182. **(D)**   The question requires that you understand that water movement across the walls of the collecting tubule is by osmosis and therefore does not involve active transport. Choice (D) correctly identifies this passive process. Both reabsorption choices (A) and (B) and tubular secretion (choice (C) are ATP-dependent, active transport processes.

183. **(A)**   To correctly answer this question, you must know that: 1) urea is the principal nitrogenous waste produced by humans; 2) urea is produced in the liver; and, 3) urea is removed from the blood by ultrafiltration in the kidney. Choice (A) includes the correct information on all three points. The other three choices have incorrect information regarding at least one of the three points.

184. **(B)**   A decrease in blood pressure would mean a decrease in the hydrostatic pressure that drives ultrafiltration through glomerular capillaries. Urine production would slow down because of the decreased glomerular filtration rate that would accompany low blood pressure, so choice (B) is correct. Neither osmotic concentration of blood plasma (choices (A) and (C)) nor concentration of blood urea should be affected by changes in blood pressure.

185. **(B)**   This item requires that you be able to expand the binomial $(p + q)^2$ and then solve for $2pq$, which is the frequency of heterozygotes. If "p" represents the frequency of the dominant allele in a population and "q" the recessive, then in this item

p equals 70% or 0.7. Since $p + q = 1$, then $q = 1 - .7 = .3$. Substituting these values in the expanded binomial expression $p^2 + 2pq + q^2 = 1$, you should find that the value for "$2pq$" is .42 or 42%. The correct choice for this item is, therefore, (B). The other choices present values that represent other frequencies in this problem, so you need to be careful: the frequency of the recessive gene "q" in the population is 30%; the frequency of homozygous dominant individuals (p^2) is 49%; and, the given frequency of the dominant allele is 70%, obviously not the same as the frequency of heterozygotes.

186. **(A)**   This item asks you to do a simple manipulation of the Hardy-Weinberg formula $p^2 + 2pq + q^2 = 1$. Solving for p^2 yields $1 - 2pq - q^2$, so choice (A) is correct.

187. **(A)**   This item requires that you be able to expand the binomial $(p + q)^2$ and then solve for p^2, which represents the frequency of homozygous dominant individuals. That value can be derived by taking the square root of .36 (or, q^2, the given value for the frequency of homozygous recessive individuals). This yields .6, or q. Since $p + q = 1$, then $p = 1 - q$, or .4. Squaring .4 yields .16 (or, p^2). The correct answer is found in choice (D).

188. **(C)**   There are five general conditions that must be met if the gene pool of a population is to be in Hardy-Weinberg equilibrium: 1) the population must be sufficiently large (at least 500 individuals is a commonly accepted value); 2) there must be no mutations; 3) there must be no emigration or immigration that will change allelic frequencies; 4) mating within the population must be completely random; and, 5) there cannot be selective survival and reproductive success rates of offspring with respect to genotype. Three of these conditions are correctly stated in choices (A), (B), and (D). Choice (C), which says the population must be small, is not a correct statement of a condition necessary for equilibrium and, therefore, is the correct choice for this item.

189. **(D)**   For this item, you must be able to work the classic Mendelian dihybrid cross. The information given in the item tells you the dominant phenotypes — tall and red — for two different genes. You don't need to know the recessive phenotypes, but you may recall that they were short and white, respectively, in Mendel's original work. The conventional ratio of 9:3:3:1 must be correctly understood to mean nine dominant/dominant: 3 dominant/recessive: 3 recessive/dominant: 1 recessive/recessive with respect to the two characters. Knowing this, you can easily see that there will be $9 + 3 = 12$ dominant (red) phenotypes for *every* sixteen offspring. Choice (D) is correct; the others offer numbers that can be obtained from the numbers in the ratio, but obviously none of these is correct.

190. **(D)**   To answer this question, you must recognize that the lower the pKa, the stronger the acid, since you are dealing with a negative logarithm. This means that the electron-withdrawing CN^- group confers the greatest acidity on the carboxylic acid of any of these groups.

191. **(C)**   You must know that CH_3 is more electron-donating than H but less so than OH to answer this question. This means the pKa of $Y = CH_3$ will be between 4.19 and 4.55.

192. **(D)** Electrophilic substitution occurs when electrophiles are attracted to the pi electrons on the benzene ring. An electron-withdrawing group makes these electrons less available for reaction. The acidity data shows that CN^- is the most strongly electron-withdrawing group of those shown.

193. **(C)** The nitrogenous bases found in DNA are adenine, guanine, cytosine, and thymine. The nitrogenous bases present in RNA are adenine, guanine, cytosine, and uracil. Thus, the pyrimidine base uracil is found in RNA instead of the pyrimidine base thymine found in DNA.

194. **(D)** Many enzymes are involved in the breakdown of foods into the macromolecular components needed by the body. Of the enzymes listed, all are involved in digestion except for ligase. Ligase is the enzyme that seals nicks in DNA.

195. **(A)** Photoperiodism is a biological response to changes in light and dark in periodic cycles. Many biological activities are controlled by this response such as the induction of flowering in some plants, stimulation of the germination of some seeds, and the initiation of mating in some insects, birds, fish and mammals.

196. **(B)** There is no chiral center as part of the peptide bond, so resonance delocalization does not affect optical activity. All of the other answers are properties that can be attributed to the electron delocalization in the peptide bond.

197. **(C)** The axon usually, but not always, conducts impulses from the cell body. Axons can send impulses to other cells. In some neurons, they may be several feet long. In vertebrate cells, axons are usually ensheathed by Schwann cells which provide nutrition to the axon. These Schwann cells may then be enveloped by myelin.

198. **(A)** In humans, the female genotype is always XX, and the male genotype is always XY. Of these two sex-determining chromosomes, only one may vary. This is due to the female parent only being able to donate an X chromosome. The only variable factor is whether the father will donate an X or a Y chromosome. For a female zygote to form, he must donate an X chromosome.

199. **(A)** Solving this problem requires you to recognize which signals in the nmr spectrum are due to the p-toluenesulfonyl moiety, subtract these from the spectrum, and deduce the structure from the remaining signals. The parasubstituted ring is responsible for the peaks in the aromatic region centered at 7.5, while the singlet at 2.5 can only be attributed to the methyl group attached to the ring. This leaves the characteristic peaks for an ethyl group at 1.1 and 3.1 and a 1 H singlet at 5.0. The only compound shown which would react with tosyl chloride to give these nmr signals is ethylamine, (A).

200. **(C)** Since the passage shows reaction with primary and secondary amines, you must only know the difference between the classes of amines and that tertiary amines have the structure R_3N to answer this question.

201. **(B)** A proton reacting with NaOH must be adjacent to a strongly electron-

withdrawing group which will stabilize the negative charge on the product anion. The SO_2 group is very electron-withdrawing and so the proton attached to the nitrogen is acidic.

202. **(B)** An anticodon is a three-base sequence that is complementary to a specific codon. The translation part of protein synthesis uses this complementarity to "match" codons on mRNA with their respective anticodons on tRNA, thereby assuring that the appropriate amino acid is inserted in the primary structure of the polypeptide being constructed. With respect to the three incorrect responses, there is no term to describe the three-base sequence on DNA from which a codon is transcribed; the nucleotides of rRNA carry no specific information regarding the amino acid sequence in a polypeptide; mRNA contains codons as already described.

203. **(B)** The process of building a polypeptide chain with the precise sequence of amino acids occurs on ribosomes and can be compared to translating one language into another (the language of nucleic acids into the language of proteins, for example). Hence, the terms "translation" has been applied. The other choices are incorrect because the terms legitimately apply to other biological or biochemical processes — transcription is the process of copying a segment of DNA, usually the cistron, to form a molecule of mRNA; transformation refers to the incorporation of DNA fragments into bacterial cells; translocation describes the interchange of segments of non-homologous chromosomes (or the movement of substances through the phloem of a plant).

204. **(D)** Anticodons on tRNA and codons on mRNA bind by base pairing between purine and pyrimidine bases in those respective molecules. It is well known that guanine base pairs with cytosine and that adenine base pairs with uracil (or with thymine in the case of DNA). The correct response can therefore be deduced with this knowledge — cytosine with guanine, guanine with cytosine, and adenine with uracil. Choice (D) is the only one that presents the appropriate codon for the anticodon CGA.

205. **(A)** Of the sixty four possible triplets in the genetic code, sixty one code for amino acids (from one to six amino acids for each codon) and three are "nonsense" triplets that do not code for amino acids but appear to function as punctuation in the translation (again using the language metaphor). Therefore, each codon has a function in protein synthesis. The remaining choices incorrectly describe the code — every possible codon does not code for an amino acid, since three are punctuation codons; and, most amino acids have more than one codon (in fact only methionine and tryptophan have single codons).

206. **(C)** Transcription moves from the 3' end of DNA to the 5' end of the molecule and synthesizes a strand of mRNA having the opposite polarity (i.e., 5' to 3'). Therefore, the complementary bases must be read in an anti-parallel fashion. That is, the base at the 5' end of the DNA molecule sequence will be the complement of the base at the 3' end of the mRNA molecule. By carefully proceeding from the 3' end of the hypothetical sequence of DNA presented in this item and remembering that thymine "replaces" uracil in DNA, the appropriate mRNA sequence can be constructed. Choices other than (C) are incorrect — choice (A) is identical to the

mRNA sequence given and is not possible, because it contains uracil among other reasons; (B) contains correct sequence of complementary bases, but is constructed in a parallel fashion, not anti-parallel; and (D) is anti-parallel, but only with respect to *entire codons,* not individual bases.

207. **(D)** George Beadle and Edward Tatum's classic work with the mold *Neurospora crassa* showed that specific mutant colonies of the mold were deficient in a single enzyme and that the mutation could be inherited through a single gene. Enzymes are made of, or contain, proteins, while genes (in the biochemical sense) consist of a specific sequence of DNA bases. However, since it is also known that many proteins consist of two or more polypeptides, the modern interpretation of the "one-gene-one-enzyme" principle is correctly stated in choice (D). The remaining choices are incorrect because one codon does not code for an enzyme or a polypeptide, only one amino acid; a nucleic acid base is only part of a nucleotide; a nucleotide is only one "letter" in a codon.

208. **(D)** Since linoleic acid has the lowest melting point of the fatty acids mentioned, (D) which has two of these and one oleic acid, will have the lowest point of the fats shown. (A) would be the next lowest since it has three of the monounsaturated oleate groups. (B) and (C) contain only saturated acids, which have higher melting points.

209. **(A)** The correct answer to this question requires you to know that free radicals are stabilized by adjacent double bonds (*cf.* allyl and benzyl free radicals). The free radical intermediate that is the product of reaction with dioxygen with linoleic acid can be stabilized by two adjacent double bonds.

$$R—CH=CH—CH—\overset{\bullet}{CH}=CH—R$$

Oleic acid, (C), and palmitoleic, (B), are also susceptible to oxidation, but less so than linoleic. (D), stearic acid, will be least reactive with dioxygen.

210. **(C)** The region around 3300 cm^{-1} in the infrared is where the OH group absorbs. The only one of the fatty acids that contains an OH group is ricinoleic.

211. **(B)** To answer this question, you need to know that catalytic hydrogenation adds hydrogens across carbon-carbon double bonds, converting unsaturated compounds to saturated compounds. Since the conversion of oils to fats involves raising the melting points, converting the unsaturated bonds to saturated bonds is the only feasible way to accomplish this.

212. **(B)** This item tests your knowledge of the types and distribution of epithelial tissues. Choice (B) correctly identifies the epithelial tissue unique to the luminal surfaces of the urinary bladder (and ureters) as transitional. Transitional epithelium is a type of stratified epithelium and its multiple layers of rounded cells allow for considerable distension. The other three choices identify types of simple epithelia found as coverings elsewhere in the body.

213. **(C)** Connective tissue proper is characterized by three types of fibers that are produced by fibroblasts: elastic, reticular, and collagenous fibers. Choice (C) is

correct because the fiber identified by this choice, projection fibers, are actually part of the nervous system that transmit impulses from the cerebrum to other parts of the brain and are, therefore, not part of connective tissue at all.

214. **(D)**   Blood is a type of connective tissue with a liquid matrix. There are two types of blood cells: erythrocytes and leukocytes. This item tests your knowledge of the relative number of erythrocytes in human blood with the correct number, about five million per cubic millimeter, given in choice (D). There are slightly more in human males and slightly less in females.

215. **(A)**   Areolar (loose) connective tissue functions primarily as binding and packing for skin, muscle, and blood vessels. The areolar tissue surrounding blood vessels contains mast cells that are specialized for the production of the anticoagulant heparin, which prevents blood from clotting within the vessels. Choice (A) correctly identifies the location of these unique cells.

216. **(C)**   Haversian canals contain vascular and nerve tissues that serve bone cells (osteocytes). The haversian canal along with the spaces containing osteocytes and the radiating canals called canaliculi are known as haversian systems. Choice (C) correctly identifies bone as the tissue characterized by these systems.

217. **(B)**   Of all the choices, only uracil is not a nitrogenous, excretory component. It is, however, a nitrogenous base found in RNA.

218. **(C)**   The electron transport system yields 6 ATPs and the Krebs cycle yields 9 ATPs for a total of 15 ATPs.

219. **(D)**   The Haworth projection indicates that all of the bulky groups (OH⁻ and CH_2OH) in glucose are *trans* to each other. This means that in the chair form all of the groups must be in either the axial positions or all in the equatorial positions. Since the equatorial positions are less hindered than axial, (D) is the preferred structure. None of the other answers has the groups all *trans* to each other.

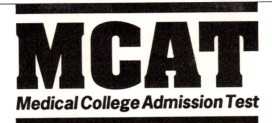

Test 4

MEDICAL COLLEGE ADMISSION TEST
TEST 4
ANSWER SHEET

Section 1:
Verbal Reasoning

1. Ⓐ Ⓑ Ⓒ Ⓓ
2. Ⓐ Ⓑ Ⓒ Ⓓ
3. Ⓐ Ⓑ Ⓒ Ⓓ
4. Ⓐ Ⓑ Ⓒ Ⓓ
5. Ⓐ Ⓑ Ⓒ Ⓓ
6. Ⓐ Ⓑ Ⓒ Ⓓ
7. Ⓐ Ⓑ Ⓒ Ⓓ
8. Ⓐ Ⓑ Ⓒ Ⓓ
9. Ⓐ Ⓑ Ⓒ Ⓓ
10. Ⓐ Ⓑ Ⓒ Ⓓ
11. Ⓐ Ⓑ Ⓒ Ⓓ
12. Ⓐ Ⓑ Ⓒ Ⓓ
13. Ⓐ Ⓑ Ⓒ Ⓓ
14. Ⓐ Ⓑ Ⓒ Ⓓ
15. Ⓐ Ⓑ Ⓒ Ⓓ
16. Ⓐ Ⓑ Ⓒ Ⓓ
17. Ⓐ Ⓑ Ⓒ Ⓓ
18. Ⓐ Ⓑ Ⓒ Ⓓ
19. Ⓐ Ⓑ Ⓒ Ⓓ
20. Ⓐ Ⓑ Ⓒ Ⓓ
21. Ⓐ Ⓑ Ⓒ Ⓓ
22. Ⓐ Ⓑ Ⓒ Ⓓ
23. Ⓐ Ⓑ Ⓒ Ⓓ
24. Ⓐ Ⓑ Ⓒ Ⓓ
25. Ⓐ Ⓑ Ⓒ Ⓓ
26. Ⓐ Ⓑ Ⓒ Ⓓ
27. Ⓐ Ⓑ Ⓒ Ⓓ
28. Ⓐ Ⓑ Ⓒ Ⓓ
29. Ⓐ Ⓑ Ⓒ Ⓓ
30. Ⓐ Ⓑ Ⓒ Ⓓ
31. Ⓐ Ⓑ Ⓒ Ⓓ

32. Ⓐ Ⓑ Ⓒ Ⓓ
33. Ⓐ Ⓑ Ⓒ Ⓓ
34. Ⓐ Ⓑ Ⓒ Ⓓ
35. Ⓐ Ⓑ Ⓒ Ⓓ
36. Ⓐ Ⓑ Ⓒ Ⓓ
37. Ⓐ Ⓑ Ⓒ Ⓓ
38. Ⓐ Ⓑ Ⓒ Ⓓ
39. Ⓐ Ⓑ Ⓒ Ⓓ
40. Ⓐ Ⓑ Ⓒ Ⓓ
41. Ⓐ Ⓑ Ⓒ Ⓓ
42. Ⓐ Ⓑ Ⓒ Ⓓ
43. Ⓐ Ⓑ Ⓒ Ⓓ
44. Ⓐ Ⓑ Ⓒ Ⓓ
45. Ⓐ Ⓑ Ⓒ Ⓓ
46. Ⓐ Ⓑ Ⓒ Ⓓ
47. Ⓐ Ⓑ Ⓒ Ⓓ
48. Ⓐ Ⓑ Ⓒ Ⓓ
49. Ⓐ Ⓑ Ⓒ Ⓓ
50. Ⓐ Ⓑ Ⓒ Ⓓ
51. Ⓐ Ⓑ Ⓒ Ⓓ
52. Ⓐ Ⓑ Ⓒ Ⓓ
53. Ⓐ Ⓑ Ⓒ Ⓓ
54. Ⓐ Ⓑ Ⓒ Ⓓ
55. Ⓐ Ⓑ Ⓒ Ⓓ
56. Ⓐ Ⓑ Ⓒ Ⓓ
57. Ⓐ Ⓑ Ⓒ Ⓓ
58. Ⓐ Ⓑ Ⓒ Ⓓ
59. Ⓐ Ⓑ Ⓒ Ⓓ
60. Ⓐ Ⓑ Ⓒ Ⓓ
61. Ⓐ Ⓑ Ⓒ Ⓓ
62. Ⓐ Ⓑ Ⓒ Ⓓ
63. Ⓐ Ⓑ Ⓒ Ⓓ
64. Ⓐ Ⓑ Ⓒ Ⓓ
65. Ⓐ Ⓑ Ⓒ Ⓓ

Section 2:
Physical Sciences

66. Ⓐ Ⓑ Ⓒ Ⓓ
67. Ⓐ Ⓑ Ⓒ Ⓓ
68. Ⓐ Ⓑ Ⓒ Ⓓ
69. Ⓐ Ⓑ Ⓒ Ⓓ
70. Ⓐ Ⓑ Ⓒ Ⓓ
71. Ⓐ Ⓑ Ⓒ Ⓓ
72. Ⓐ Ⓑ Ⓒ Ⓓ
73. Ⓐ Ⓑ Ⓒ Ⓓ
74. Ⓐ Ⓑ Ⓒ Ⓓ
75. Ⓐ Ⓑ Ⓒ Ⓓ
76. Ⓐ Ⓑ Ⓒ Ⓓ
77. Ⓐ Ⓑ Ⓒ Ⓓ
78. Ⓐ Ⓑ Ⓒ Ⓓ
79. Ⓐ Ⓑ Ⓒ Ⓓ
80. Ⓐ Ⓑ Ⓒ Ⓓ
81. Ⓐ Ⓑ Ⓒ Ⓓ
82. Ⓐ Ⓑ Ⓒ Ⓓ
83. Ⓐ Ⓑ Ⓒ Ⓓ
84. Ⓐ Ⓑ Ⓒ Ⓓ
85. Ⓐ Ⓑ Ⓒ Ⓓ
86. Ⓐ Ⓑ Ⓒ Ⓓ
87. Ⓐ Ⓑ Ⓒ Ⓓ
88. Ⓐ Ⓑ Ⓒ Ⓓ
89. Ⓐ Ⓑ Ⓒ Ⓓ
90. Ⓐ Ⓑ Ⓒ Ⓓ
91. Ⓐ Ⓑ Ⓒ Ⓓ
92. Ⓐ Ⓑ Ⓒ Ⓓ
93. Ⓐ Ⓑ Ⓒ Ⓓ
94. Ⓐ Ⓑ Ⓒ Ⓓ
95. Ⓐ Ⓑ Ⓒ Ⓓ
96. Ⓐ Ⓑ Ⓒ Ⓓ

97. Ⓐ Ⓑ Ⓒ Ⓓ	140. Ⓐ Ⓑ Ⓒ Ⓓ	177. Ⓐ Ⓑ Ⓒ Ⓓ
98. Ⓐ Ⓑ Ⓒ Ⓓ	141. Ⓐ Ⓑ Ⓒ Ⓓ	178. Ⓐ Ⓑ Ⓒ Ⓓ
99. Ⓐ Ⓑ Ⓒ Ⓓ	142. Ⓐ Ⓑ Ⓒ Ⓓ	179. Ⓐ Ⓑ Ⓒ Ⓓ
100. Ⓐ Ⓑ Ⓒ Ⓓ		180. Ⓐ Ⓑ Ⓒ Ⓓ
101. Ⓐ Ⓑ Ⓒ Ⓓ		181. Ⓐ Ⓑ Ⓒ Ⓓ
102. Ⓐ Ⓑ Ⓒ Ⓓ		182. Ⓐ Ⓑ Ⓒ Ⓓ
103. Ⓐ Ⓑ Ⓒ Ⓓ	**Section 4:**	183. Ⓐ Ⓑ Ⓒ Ⓓ
104. Ⓐ Ⓑ Ⓒ Ⓓ	**Biological Sciences**	184. Ⓐ Ⓑ Ⓒ Ⓓ
105. Ⓐ Ⓑ Ⓒ Ⓓ		185. Ⓐ Ⓑ Ⓒ Ⓓ
106. Ⓐ Ⓑ Ⓒ Ⓓ	143. Ⓐ Ⓑ Ⓒ Ⓓ	186. Ⓐ Ⓑ Ⓒ Ⓓ
107. Ⓐ Ⓑ Ⓒ Ⓓ	144. Ⓐ Ⓑ Ⓒ Ⓓ	187. Ⓐ Ⓑ Ⓒ Ⓓ
108. Ⓐ Ⓑ Ⓒ Ⓓ	145. Ⓐ Ⓑ Ⓒ Ⓓ	188. Ⓐ Ⓑ Ⓒ Ⓓ
109. Ⓐ Ⓑ Ⓒ Ⓓ	146. Ⓐ Ⓑ Ⓒ Ⓓ	189. Ⓐ Ⓑ Ⓒ Ⓓ
110. Ⓐ Ⓑ Ⓒ Ⓓ	147. Ⓐ Ⓑ Ⓒ Ⓓ	190. Ⓐ Ⓑ Ⓒ Ⓓ
111. Ⓐ Ⓑ Ⓒ Ⓓ	148. Ⓐ Ⓑ Ⓒ Ⓓ	191. Ⓐ Ⓑ Ⓒ Ⓓ
112. Ⓐ Ⓑ Ⓒ Ⓓ	149. Ⓐ Ⓑ Ⓒ Ⓓ	192. Ⓐ Ⓑ Ⓒ Ⓓ
113. Ⓐ Ⓑ Ⓒ Ⓓ	150. Ⓐ Ⓑ Ⓒ Ⓓ	193. Ⓐ Ⓑ Ⓒ Ⓓ
114. Ⓐ Ⓑ Ⓒ Ⓓ	151. Ⓐ Ⓑ Ⓒ Ⓓ	194. Ⓐ Ⓑ Ⓒ Ⓓ
115. Ⓐ Ⓑ Ⓒ Ⓓ	152. Ⓐ Ⓑ Ⓒ Ⓓ	195. Ⓐ Ⓑ Ⓒ Ⓓ
116. Ⓐ Ⓑ Ⓒ Ⓓ	153. Ⓐ Ⓑ Ⓒ Ⓓ	196. Ⓐ Ⓑ Ⓒ Ⓓ
117. Ⓐ Ⓑ Ⓒ Ⓓ	154. Ⓐ Ⓑ Ⓒ Ⓓ	197. Ⓐ Ⓑ Ⓒ Ⓓ
118. Ⓐ Ⓑ Ⓒ Ⓓ	155. Ⓐ Ⓑ Ⓒ Ⓓ	198. Ⓐ Ⓑ Ⓒ Ⓓ
119. Ⓐ Ⓑ Ⓒ Ⓓ	156. Ⓐ Ⓑ Ⓒ Ⓓ	199. Ⓐ Ⓑ Ⓒ Ⓓ
120. Ⓐ Ⓑ Ⓒ Ⓓ	157. Ⓐ Ⓑ Ⓒ Ⓓ	200. Ⓐ Ⓑ Ⓒ Ⓓ
121. Ⓐ Ⓑ Ⓒ Ⓓ	158. Ⓐ Ⓑ Ⓒ Ⓓ	201. Ⓐ Ⓑ Ⓒ Ⓓ
122. Ⓐ Ⓑ Ⓒ Ⓓ	159. Ⓐ Ⓑ Ⓒ Ⓓ	202. Ⓐ Ⓑ Ⓒ Ⓓ
123. Ⓐ Ⓑ Ⓒ Ⓓ	160. Ⓐ Ⓑ Ⓒ Ⓓ	203. Ⓐ Ⓑ Ⓒ Ⓓ
124. Ⓐ Ⓑ Ⓒ Ⓓ	161. Ⓐ Ⓑ Ⓒ Ⓓ	204. Ⓐ Ⓑ Ⓒ Ⓓ
125. Ⓐ Ⓑ Ⓒ Ⓓ	162. Ⓐ Ⓑ Ⓒ Ⓓ	205. Ⓐ Ⓑ Ⓒ Ⓓ
126. Ⓐ Ⓑ Ⓒ Ⓓ	163. Ⓐ Ⓑ Ⓒ Ⓓ	206. Ⓐ Ⓑ Ⓒ Ⓓ
127. Ⓐ Ⓑ Ⓒ Ⓓ	164. Ⓐ Ⓑ Ⓒ Ⓓ	207. Ⓐ Ⓑ Ⓒ Ⓓ
128. Ⓐ Ⓑ Ⓒ Ⓓ	165. Ⓐ Ⓑ Ⓒ Ⓓ	208. Ⓐ Ⓑ Ⓒ Ⓓ
129. Ⓐ Ⓑ Ⓒ Ⓓ	166. Ⓐ Ⓑ Ⓒ Ⓓ	209. Ⓐ Ⓑ Ⓒ Ⓓ
130. Ⓐ Ⓑ Ⓒ Ⓓ	167. Ⓐ Ⓑ Ⓒ Ⓓ	210. Ⓐ Ⓑ Ⓒ Ⓓ
131. Ⓐ Ⓑ Ⓒ Ⓓ	168. Ⓐ Ⓑ Ⓒ Ⓓ	211. Ⓐ Ⓑ Ⓒ Ⓓ
132. Ⓐ Ⓑ Ⓒ Ⓓ	169. Ⓐ Ⓑ Ⓒ Ⓓ	212. Ⓐ Ⓑ Ⓒ Ⓓ
133. Ⓐ Ⓑ Ⓒ Ⓓ	170. Ⓐ Ⓑ Ⓒ Ⓓ	213. Ⓐ Ⓑ Ⓒ Ⓓ
134. Ⓐ Ⓑ Ⓒ Ⓓ	171. Ⓐ Ⓑ Ⓒ Ⓓ	214. Ⓐ Ⓑ Ⓒ Ⓓ
135. Ⓐ Ⓑ Ⓒ Ⓓ	172. Ⓐ Ⓑ Ⓒ Ⓓ	215. Ⓐ Ⓑ Ⓒ Ⓓ
136. Ⓐ Ⓑ Ⓒ Ⓓ	173. Ⓐ Ⓑ Ⓒ Ⓓ	216. Ⓐ Ⓑ Ⓒ Ⓓ
137. Ⓐ Ⓑ Ⓒ Ⓓ	174. Ⓐ Ⓑ Ⓒ Ⓓ	217. Ⓐ Ⓑ Ⓒ Ⓓ
138. Ⓐ Ⓑ Ⓒ Ⓓ	175. Ⓐ Ⓑ Ⓒ Ⓓ	218. Ⓐ Ⓑ Ⓒ Ⓓ
139. Ⓐ Ⓑ Ⓒ Ⓓ	176. Ⓐ Ⓑ Ⓒ Ⓓ	219. Ⓐ Ⓑ Ⓒ Ⓓ

TEST 4

Section 1 — Verbal Reasoning

TIME: 85 Minutes
QUESTIONS: 1-65

> **DIRECTIONS:** The verbal reasoning section contains seven passages, each followed by a series of questions. Based on the information given in a passage, choose the one best answer to each question. If you are not sure of an answer, eliminate those choices that you know are incorrect and choose an answer from among those remaining. Fill in the corresponding circle on the answer sheet to indicate your answer.

PASSAGE I (Questions 1-9)

John Hancock, born in 1737 at Braintree (presently Quincy), Mass., lost his father, a Congregational pastor, at the age of seven. He spent the next six years with his grandparents at Lexington before joining his guardian, Thomas Hancock, a childless uncle who was one of the richest merchant-shippers in Boston. After studying at Boston Latin School and graduating from Harvard College in 1754, John began working as a clerk in his uncle's business and learned it rapidly. In 1760-61, while visiting London to observe the English side of the business, he attended the funeral of George II and the coronation of George III, who apparently granted him an audience. In 1763 he became a partner of his uncle, who died the next year and willed him the firm, a fortune that was probably the greatest in New England, and a luxurious house on Beacon Street.

Hancock allied with other merchants in protesting the Stamp Act (1765), and the next year inaugurated a long legislative career, but he did not strongly identify with the patriots until two years later. At that time, British customs officials, their courage bolstered by the arrival of a warship in Boston Harbor, charged him with smuggling and seized one of his ships. During the ensuing riots, the terrified customs officials fled to an island in the harbor. A few months later, the first major contingent of British troops sailed into port and created a tense situation that resulted in the Boston Massacre (1770). John Adams ably defended Hancock in court until the British dropped the smuggling charge, but the episode made him a hero throughout the colonies.

Other factors tied Hancock to the patriots. Samuel and John Adams, shrewdly perceiving the advantages of a rich and well-known affiliate, welcomed him into their ranks, encouraged his idolatry by the populace, and pushed him upward in the Revolutionary hierarchy. When the first provincial congress met at Salem and Concord in 1774, he acted as its president as well as chairman of the vital council of safety. The second provincial congress, convening the next year at Cambridge and Concord, elected him to the Continental Congress.

On April 18, only three days after the provincial congress adjourned, British troops marched from Boston to seize rebel stores at Concord. Warned of their approach during the night by Paul Revere, Hancock and Samuel Adams, who were visiting at nearby Lexington, escaped. But the British-American clashes at Lexington and Concord marked the outbreak of war.

From 1775 until 1777 Hancock presided over the Continental Congress. The very first year, his egotism, which regularly aroused the antipathy of many Members, created personal embitterment as well. Blind to his own limitations, particularly his lack of military experience, he unrealistically entertained the hope that he, instead of Washington, would be appointed as commander in chief of the Continental Army.

Only Hancock and Charles Thompson, the President and Secretary of Congress, signed the broadside copy of the Declaration, printed the night of its adoption, July 4, 1776, and disseminated to the public the following day. At the formal signing of the parchment copy on August 2, tradition holds that Hancock wrote his name in large letters so that the King would not need spectacles to recognize him as a "traitor." After resigning as presiding officer in 1777, he remained a Member of Congress until 1780, though he spent much of his time in Boston and the for the rest of his life solidified his political position in Massachusetts. In 1788, as a major general in the militia, he commanded an expedition that failed to recapture Newport, R.I., from the British. He made a more tangible contribution to the war by accepting Continental currency from his debtors, even though his fortune had already been dented by wartime-induced reverses.

In 1780, the same year Hancock gave up his seat in Congress and attended his Commonwealth's constitutional convention, he was overwhelmingly elected as first Governor (1780-85). He won reelection in 1787-93. In the interim (1785-86), he once again sat in Congress. In 1788 he chaired the Massachusetts convention that ratified the U.S. Constitution, which he favored.

While still Governor, in 1793 at the age of 56, Hancock died at Boston. His funeral, one of the most impressive ever held in New England, culminated in burial at Old Granary Burying Ground.

1. Which of the following factors is not given as associating Hancock with the patriots?

   (A) His wealth

   (B) His being charged with smuggling

   (C) His status as a hero

   (D) His acquaintance with King George

2. The author points out John Hancock's early ties to England and King George in order to

   (A) show the impetus for the Stamp Act resistance.

   (B) demonstrate Hancock's fluctuating loyalty.

   (C) establish Hancock's privileged childhood.

   (D) show that America's freedom took precedence over wealth and important political connections for Hancock.

3. Hancock's wealth, mind for business and lack of military experience caused Hancock to

    I.   be elected as commander in chief of the Continental Army.

    II.   win his battle at Newport, Rhode Island.

    III.   overestimate his political abilities.

    (A)   I only.   (B)   III only.

    (C)   I and II only.   (D)   II and III only.

4. The passage supports the view that John Hancock

    (A)   greatly profited financially from the Revolutionary War.

    (B)   was a strong egotistical person.

    (C)   was a smuggler.

    (D)   was a reclusive personality.

5. The passage on John Hancock gives evidence primarily based on

    (A)   public historical records.

    (B)   eyewitness accounts.

    (C)   private letters.

    (D)   autobiographical revelations.

6. The war between America and England affected Hancock by making him

    I.   more humble.

    II.   more politically successful.

    III.   more wealthy.

    (A)   II only.   (B)   III only.

    (C)   I and II only.   (D)   I and III only.

7. The passage suggests that despite his wealth and conceit, Hancock

    (A)   lost re-election as Governor.

    (B)   was popular and well liked by American citizens.

    (C)   was not eligible to chair the Massachusetts convention to ratify the U.S. constitution.

    (D)   was voted out of his seat in Congress.

8. From this passage, it is reasonable to assume that the Boston Massacre could have been prevented if

    (A)   Hancock had supported the Stamp Act.

    (B)   John Adams had not defended Hancock in court.

    (C)   the British had not seized one of Hancock's ships.

    (D)   Hancock had not smuggled goods.

9.   For the last thirteen years of his life, John Hancock

    (A)   concentrated on his political position in Massachusetts.

    (B)   concentrated on his business.

    (C)   served in Congress.

    (D)   served as Governor of Massachusetts.

PASSAGE II (Questions 10-18)

John Adams and Thomas Jefferson were the first two occupants of the White House, official residence of our Nation's Presidents since 1800. It is a national shrine that symbolizes the honor and dignity of the highest office in the land, and has been the scene of many historic events and brilliant social affairs. Like the Nation itself, it bears the influence of successive Chief Executives. Although rebuilt and modernized, it retains the simplicity and charm of its original appearance.

President George Washington approved the plans for the White House, drawn by Irish-born James Hoban, winner of the prize competition. Maj. Pierre Charles L'Enfant, the French artist-engineer, located the mansion in his plan of the Federal City, in which it and the Capitol were the first public buildings erected. The cornerstone was laid on October 13, 1792. Workmen used light gray sandstone from the Aquia Creek Quarries, in Virginia, for the exterior walls. During the course of construction or soon thereafter, they apparently were painted white. The building was thus unofficially termed the "White House" from an early date, but for many years it was usually referred to as the "President's House" or the "President's Palace."

In the Palladian style of architecture, the main facade resembles the Duke of Leinster's mansion in Dublin. Hoban probably derived the details of other faces and the interior arrangement from other contemporary European mansions. He supervised the original construction; the rebuilding after the burning by British forces, in 1814; and the erection of the north and south porticoes, some years later. Over the course of time, however, various architects modified Hoban's original plans, notably Benjamin H. Latrobe during and after the Jefferson administration.

President and Mrs. John Adams were the first occupants, in November 1800 when the Government moved from Philadelphia to Washington. The interior had not yet been completed, and Mrs. Adams used the unfinished East Room to dry the family's wash. During Jefferson's administration the east and west terraces, or pavilions, were built. Jefferson, who practiced democratic simplicity in his social life, opened the mansion each morning to all arrivals.

During the War of 1812, British forces captured the city and set the torch to the White House, the Capitol, and other Government buildings in retaliation for the destruction by U.S. troops of some public buildings in Canada. Only the partially damaged exterior walls and interior brickwork of the White House remained in the spring of 1815 when reconstruction began. In 1817 the recently elected President, James Monroe, was able to occupy the structure. In 1824 builders erected the south portico; and in 1829, the large north portico over the entrance and driveway. The west wing, including the President's oval office, was added during the first decade of the 20th century. The east wing was built in 1942.

Over the years, the White House proper has been extensively renovated and modernized on various occasions. The old sandstone walls have been retained, however. The aim has been to keep the historical atmosphere while providing a more livable home for the President and his family.

Located on the first floor of the main building are the East Room, Green Room, Blue Room, Red Room, State Dining Room, and Family Dining Room. These richly furnished rooms are open to the public on a special schedule. The ground and second floors are restricted to the use of the presidential family and guests. On the ground floor are the Diplomatic Reception Room, Curator's Office, Vermeil Room, China Room, and Library. The second floor contains the Lincoln Bedroom, Lincoln Sitting Room, Queen's Bedroom (Rose Guest Room), Treaty Room, Yellow Oval Room, and Empire Guest Room. Neither of the wings, reserved for the President and his staff, are ordinarily accessible to the public.

The simple dignity of the White House is enhanced by the natural beauty of its informal but carefully landscaped grounds.

10. The passage states that the White House in its first few years of existence was

   (A)   actually grey in color.

   (B)   fully furnished with many spare rooms.

   (C)   first occupied by President John Adams and his wife.

   (D)   located in Philadelphia.

11. The passage suggests that the original plans for the White House reflect the influence of which of the following countries?

   I.   Ireland

   II.   England

   III.   France

   (A)   I only   (B)   II only

   (C)   I and III only   (D)   II and III only

12. The time required for originally building the White House was

   (A)   8 years.   (B)   15 months.

   (C)   2 years.   (D)   36 months.

13. Throughout the history of the White House the building has

   (A)   been fully reconstructed twice.

   (B)   retained its original sandstone walls.

   (C)   undergone moderate renovation.

   (D)   been noted for its intricate architecture.

14. Which of the following concerning public accessibility of the White House is NOT true?

   I.   The first and ground floors are open to the public.

   II.   The top floor is reserved for the President's family and guests.

   III.   All wings are open to the general public.

(A)   I only.   (B)   II only.

(C)   III only.   (D)   I and III only.

15.   The first floor of the main building of the White House contains

(A)   13 rooms.   (B)   6 rooms.

(C)   9 rooms.   (D)   23 rooms.

16.   According to the author, the White House is a symbol of

I.   the power of the United States.

II.   the wealth and youth of the United States.

III.   the honor and dignity of the Presidency.

(A)   I only.   (B)   II only.

(C)   III only.   (D)   I and III only.

17.   Which of the following is NOT a repercussion of the U.S. troops' destruction of some public buildings in Canada?

(A)   British troops captured the city of Washington.

(B)   The French helped remodel the burned White House in the fashion of those buildings destroyed.

(C)   Only the walls and some brickwork of the White House remained after foreign troops set fire to it.

(D)   The White House couldn't be occupied until 1817.

18.   Based on information in the article, after how many presidents are rooms in the White House named?

(A)   One   (B)   Two

(C)   Three   (D)   Five

PASSAGE III (Questions 19-28)

Alcohols are members of a group of chemicals identified by their unique combination of carbon, hydrogen, and oxygen atoms. Alcohols range from methanol, which has only one carbon atom, to ethanol with two, to the higher alcohols, with progressive additions of carbon atoms.

Because alcohols can be burned with oxygen to give off large amounts of heat, they have a significant potential value as liquid fuels. In general, the higher alcohols, those with the most carbon atoms, have the highest heating value. This is because more carbon-hydrogen bonds can be broken to form carbon dioxide and water, releasing more energy. However, it is more difficult and expensive to produce the higher alcohols. Therefore, the simpler alcohols — methanol and ethanol — are favored for use as alcohol fuels.

Methanol, the simplest alcohol, has a chemical formula of CH_3OH. It is most commonly produced by gasification of coal, a nonrenewable resource. Methanol-production techniques acceptable in terms of environmental standards and resource availability are not cost-effective at this time. However, methanol can also be produced from environmentally safe biomass feedstocks, and much research is focused on this area.

Since ethanol, also called grain alcohol, is the intoxicant in alcoholic beverages, its production, use, distribution, and marketing are regulated by the Bureau of Alcohol, Tobacco and Firearms (BATF) of the U.S. Department of the Treasury.

Ethanol is legally measured in proof gallons. Each number of proof represents the ethanol content in increments of one-half percent by volume. Therefore a mixture of 50% ethanol by volume is referred to as 100 proof, while pure ethanol, which is anhydrous, or water free, is 200 proof.

Methanol and ethanol can be used alone as fuels for spark-ignited internal combustion engines. However, because methanol has less than half the heat content of gasoline, and ethanol has less than two-thirds, engine modifications must be made in order to achieve satisfactory performance. On the other hand, blends up to about 10% of either of these two alcohols with gasoline have been successfully used in vehicles without engine modifications, although other components such as fuel lines may require exchanging.

The term "gasohol" was coined and registered as a trademark in 1973 by the Nebraska Agricultural Products Industrial Utilization Committee. By its definition, gasohol is a blend of 10% anhydrous, agriculturally derived ethanol and 90% unleaded gasoline. Through popular usage it has become the generic term for all ethanol or methanol and gasoline blends. For the sake of accuracy, however, it is best to identify other ethanol-gasoline blends with a number identifying the percentage of ethanol used, as in fuel blend E20. Similarly, for methanol-gasoline blends, fuel blend M10 identifies a 10% mix in methanol gasoline. Gasohol made from its component, fermentation ethanol is the most widely used alcohol fuel in the United States today.

19.   Methanol and ethanol are favored over the higher alcohols for use as alcohol fuels because

    (A)   they have fewer carbon atoms.

    (B)   they release more energy.

    (C)   they are more common.

    (D)   they are simpler and cheaper to produce.

20.   Researchers focus upon methanol as a fuel because

    (A)   coal, the major source of methanol, is an ample resource.

    (B)   it is a complex fuel which meets environmental standards.

    (C)   it can be produced from biomass feedstocks that are safe for the environment.

    (D)   coal, the major source of methanol, is cost-efficient.

21.   Which is NOT an aspect of anhydrous ethanol?

    I.   it is water-free.

    II.   it is an ethanol mixture.

    III.   it is measured in proof gallons.

(A)   I only.   (B)   II only.

(C)   III only.   (D)   I and II only.

22.   The main thrust of this passage is

(A)   ethanol and methanol are just two types of simple alcohol fuels which scientists believe will soon become common cost-efficient, environmentally safe fuels.

(B)   alcohols are measured chemically by their additions of carbon atoms, ethanol and methanol having a low measurement, making them unable to supply power to fuel engines.

(C)   methanol and ethanol are gasoline substitutes.

(D)   gasohol, a blend of alcohol fuels, is the fuel of the future.

23.   Used alone as a fuel for spark-ignited internal combustion engines,

(A)   methanol and ethanol yield equal energy.

(B)   methanol yields less energy than ethanol.

(C)   methanol yields more energy than ethanol.

(D)   neither methanol nor ethanol is a possible fuel.

24.   An ethanol-gasoline blend of E30 would be

(A)   30% gasoline.   (B)   70% gasoline.

(C)   70% ethanol.   (D)   30% methanol.

25.   The most widely used alcohol fuel in the United States today is

(A)   gasohol made from fermentation ethanol.

(B)   coal-derived methanol.

(C)   unleaded gasoline.

(D)   anhydrous ethanol.

26.   Which of the following is a factor for why alcohols have a significant potential value as liquid fuels?

(A)   They are cheap to produce.

(B)   They can be produced from renewable resources.

(C)   They can be burned to give off large amounts of heat.

(D)   They are non-polluting.

27.   Grain alcohol has

(A)   one carbon atom.   (B)   two carbon atoms.

(C)   three carbon atoms.   (D)   no carbon atoms.

28.   The Department of the Treasury regulates ethanol because

   (A)   ethanol is an alcohol.

   (B)   ethanol is subject to taxation.

   (C)   ethanol is a grain product.

   (D)   ethanol is the intoxicant in alcoholic beverages.

PASSAGE IV (Questions 29-38)

   A long-standing problem of philosophical theology is the problem of evil. The problem may be stated as follows:

(1)   Either God cannot prevent evil or God will not prevent evil.

(2)   If God cannot prevent evil, then God is not all-powerful.

(3)   If God will not prevent evil, then God is not all-loving.

(4)   Hence, either God is not all-powerful or God is not all-loving.

   The response to this problem has taken many forms. One response has been to claim that (2) is false. The argument here is that God has endowed human beings with a free will, a will to choose freely between good and evil. Therefore, God could not give human beings the ability to freely choose between good and evil and then intervene so as to make the choice of evil impossible. That would have been a negation of the gift of free will. When we talk about God's ultimate power, we mean God's ability to do any logically possible thing, but it would not be a logically possible thing for God to give genuine free will to humans and then so arrange things that this freedom could not be exercised in the choice between good and evil.

   A second response has been to deny the truth of (3). The argument here is that there are some virtues which require the prior existence of evil in order to be themselves exercised, such as sympathy or compassion. We see only a very small part of the total picture and so we do not see the roles that evil plays in the grand scheme of things. If we did, we might understand that those evils that God allows make for a better world than there would be if those evils did not exist. Those evils may make possible the existence of virtues.

   Still another response to the problem has been to point out that an underlying assumption of the problem is that there is such a thing as evil, and this has been called into question. Certainly there is what to us appears to be evil, but our perspective is only that of the very limited part of existence that we inhabit, evil is, like beauty, in the eye of the beholder, and who are we to say that evil exists from the perspective of God? All of God's creation is good, even if some parts of it from our limited perspective appear problematical. These problematical parts we deem "evil." However, if we had the perspective of the whole creation before us, we would see, as does God, that the whole of creation is perfectly good, and evil is nowhere to be found in it. What we call "evil" is really just a perceived lack of goodness, and everything that exists is good.

   Finally, there have been those who found the initial argument persuasive and concluded that either God's power or God's goodness is limited. Of these two options, most have tended to infer that it is God's power that is limited. It has even been argued that this limitation of God's power invests us with a purposeful moral responsibility for the way things are. We cannot just sit back and leave it all to God, for the nature of things depends on us and our actions.

29. Based on this passage, the problem of evil shows that

    (A) there is a problem with our conception of God.

    (B) there is a problem with how to eliminate evil.

    (C) there is a problem with whether evil exists.

    (D) there is a problem with freedom of the will.

30. The passage poses a problem about

    (A) evil.   (B) God.

    (C) our conception of evil.   (D) our conception of God.

31. One response to the problem has been to affirm that

    (A) God intervenes in human affairs.

    (B) evil does not exist.

    (C) God can do any logically possible thing.

    (D) if God will not prevent evil, then God is not all-loving.

32. According to the passage, those who deny that evil exists hold that

    (A) we think evil exists because of our limited perspective.

    (B) God's power is limited.

    (C) evil is necessary for goodness.

    (D) evil is really goodness.

33. In the passage's presentation of the problem of evil, justifying reasons are given for:

    (A) all of the statements.   (B) none of the statements.

    (C) one of the statements.   (D) two of the statements.

34. The problem of evil claims to show

    (A) God does not exist.

    (B) an all-powerful God does not exist.

    (C) an all-good God does not exist.

    (D) an all-good and all-powerful God does not exist.

35. One response to the problem has involved the claim that

    (A) human beings have a free will.

    (B) God could not choose between good and evil.

    (C) good will overcome evil.

    (D) human beings are evil.

36. The passage presents and describes

    (A) four responses to the problem of evil.

    (B) three responses to the problem of evil.

    (C) two responses to the problem of evil.

    (D) no response to the problem of evil.

37. The passage notes that the problem of evil, as presented, has as an unstated premise that

    (A) evil exists.   (B) God exists.

    (C) God knows that evil exists.   (D) God is unable to destroy evil.

38. Which of the following would be a satisfactory response to the problem of evil:

    (A) to resolve to do good.

    (B) to have faith in God.

    (C) to actively participate in doing God's work.

    (D) to show that evil is an illusion.

PASSAGE V (Questions 39-47)
    There are some properties which things have as inherent or necessary parts of their very make-up, properties which we might call primary or necessary properties. These are properties or qualities which the thing cannot be without and still remain what it is. There are other properties which things may have but which are not primary properties. These are properties which they may or may not have without affecting their essential nature. These we may call secondary or contingent properties. For example, the property of "having three sides" would be a primary property of a triangle, while the property of "being inscribed in a circle" would not be. For a basketball, properties of circumference and weight would be primary, while those of color would be secondary.
    This distinction between primary and secondary properties underlies one of the most ancient arguments for the existence of God, the so called "Ontological Argument."
    One version of this argument notes that the term "God" signifies a supremely perfect being. The question is whether such a being exists in actuality or only as a figment of our imaginations. There can be no doubt that we have a conception of God; there is only the question as to whether or not there is anything in reality corresponding to our conception.
    Now if the concept of God is that of a perfect being, then we must assume that in conceiving of God we are conceiving of God with whatever properties a perfect being would have as primary properties, as properties which are essential to its nature. Surely existence is just such a property, for a being which was perfect but which lacked existence would be "less perfect" than a being which had those same properties and also had existence as well. But this would then mean that such a being which lacked existence would not be the most perfect being possible, since another being could be conceived as "more perfect" than it. Hence, this most perfect conceivable

being would have to have as one of its essential properties the property of existence. But this means that the property of existence could not be separated from the nature of that being.

There may seem to be an element of magic about this, even a kind of sophistry. Why may we not just make the same argument for any object? The answer is that this argument holds only for a being described as "a supremely perfect being" or "a being more perfect than any other." Only of such a being may it be affirmed that the property of existence is one of its primary or essential properties.

39.   The ontological argument claims that

   (A)   whatever we conceive exists in the actual world.

   (B)   whatever we conceive we must conceive as having whatever primary properties it has.

   (C)   whatever we conceive must have whatever secondary properties it has.

   (D)   All of the above

40.   An underlying assumption of the ontological argument is that

   (A)   existence is a property.

   (B)   God exists.

   (C)   God necessarily exists.

   (D)   whatever we conceive of exists.

41.   Primary properties are properties which things

   (A)   must have.

   (B)   must have if they exist.

   (C)   are known to have.

   (D)   may have or not have as part of their nature.

42.   The essential nature of a thing is determined by

   (A)   its secondary properties.

   (B)   its primary properties.

   (C)   Both (A) and (B)

   (D)   Our concept of both (A) and (B).

43.   The argument claims that if God is the most perfect being possible, then

   (A)   God would have existence as a primary property.

   (B)   God would have existence as a secondary property.

   (C)   we would have a concept of God.

   (D)   something more perfect than God would exist.

44. The reason the ontological argument does not hold for things other than God is that

    (A) existence is a necessary property of God.

    (B) existence is a necessary property only of a supremely perfect being.

    (C) existence is a secondary property.

    (D) None of the above

45. The property of "being a sister"

    (A) might be a primary property of a woman.

    (B) might be a secondary property of a woman.

    (C) would be a primary property of a woman.

    (D) would be a secondary property of a woman.

46. If two objects had the same primary properties in common, then

    (A) they would be identical.

    (B) they would have the same secondary properties in common.

    (C) both (A) and (B)

    (D) None of the above

47. According to the ontological argument

    (A) if God exists, then God exists.

    (B) it is necessarily true that God exists.

    (C) whatever we conceive of exists.

    (D) a being even more perfect than God exists.

PASSAGE VI (Questions 48-58)

Music's power to affect moods and stir emotions has been well known for as long as music has existed. Stories about the music of ancient Greece tell of the healing powers of Greek music. Leopold Mozart, the father of Wolfgang, wrote that if the Greeks' music could heal the sick, then our music should be able to bring the dead back to life. Unfortunately, today's music cannot do quite that much.

The healing power of music, taken for granted by ancient man and by many primitive societies, is only recently becoming accepted by medical professionals as a new way of healing the emotionally ill.

Using musical activities involving patients, the music therapist seeks to restore mental and physical health. Music therapists usually work with emotionally disturbed patients as part of a team of therapists and doctors. Music therapists work together with: physicians, psychiatrists, psychologists, physical therapists, nurses, teachers, recreation leaders, family of patients.

The therapy that a music therapist gives to patients can be in the form of listening, performing, lessons on an instrument or even composing. A therapist may help a patient regain lost coordination by teaching the patient how to play an instrument. Speech defects can sometimes be helped by singing activities. Some patients need the social awareness of group activities, but others may need individual attention to build self-confidence. The music therapist must learn what kinds of activities are best for each patient.

In addition to working with patients, the music therapist has to attend meetings with other therapists and doctors to work with the same patients to discuss progress and plan new activities. Written reports to doctors about patients' responses to treatment are another facet of the music therapist's work.

Hospitals, schools, retirement homes, and community agencies and clinics are some of the sites where music therapists work. Some music therapists work in private studies with patients sent to them by medical doctors, psychologists, and psychiatrists. Music therapy can be done in studios, recreation rooms, hospital wards, or classrooms depending on the type of activity and needs of the patients.

Qualified music therapists have followed a four-year course with a major emphasis in music plus courses in biological science, anthropology, sociology, psychology, and music therapy. General studies in English, history, speech, and government complete the requirements for a Bachelor of Music Therapy. After college training, a music therapist must participate in a six-month training internship under the guidance of a registered music therapist.

Students who have completed college courses and have demonstrated their ability during the six-month internship can become registered music therapists by applying to the National Association for Music Therapy, Inc. New methods and techniques of music therapy are always being developed, so the trained therapist must continue to study new articles, books, and reports throughout his/her career.

48.   Which statement best summarizes the central idea of this passage?

(A)   Music therapy is a multi-faceted area of professional life.

(B)   The healing power of music therapy is extensive and intensive.

(C)   Music therapy is complex and always involves the teaching of songs and instruments.

(D)   A music therapist is a medical person.

49.   Mozart's statement that music can bring the dead back to life implies that

(A)   the dead can hear music.

(B)   music is powerfully therapeutic.

(C)   music appeals to a dead mind.

(D)   one's health cannot be maintained without music.

50.   The passage suggests that music therapists

(A)   take the place of psychiatrists.

(B)   are licensed medical practitioners.

(C)   work with speech pathologists, psychiatrists and teachers.

(D)   are hired to write reports for a team of doctors.

51.   Some ancient cultures believed that music

(A) affected moods thereby healing emotional pain.

(B) quelched emotions.

(C) was useful only for the emotionally ill.

(D) is nature's way of signaling pain.

52. Which one of the following would not be listed as a therapeutic aspect of music?

(A) Performing music before a live audience

(B) Listening to music at work

(C) Criticizing musical theory

(D) Creating musical arrangements for a community group

53. The qualifications for becoming a licensed music therapist consist of all but which of the following?

(A) Working with a registered therapist

(B) Training on one's own

(C) A sustained internship

(D) The ability to utilize current therapeutic techniques

54. It can be reasonably inferred from this passage that music therapists

(A) have high-paying jobs.

(B) must have extensively studied music and psychiatry.

(C) have an education that draws on academic knowledge and practiced training.

(D) must return to formal schooling every academic year.

55. Self-confidence can be rebuilt through music. Which of the following reasons supports this statement?

I. A skill can strengthen the will to succeed.

II. All persons have musical ability.

III. All persons may enjoy music.

(A) I only.   (B) II only.

(C) I and III only.   (D) II and III only.

56. In this essay the term "patient" specifically refers to

(A) a person in need of the services of medical personnel.

(B) a person in need of resocialization.

(C) a person in psychoanalysis.

(D) a person disabled by loss of coordination, hearing or speech.

57. Which one of the following is the only place not conducive to doing music therapy?

   (A) A church   (B) A dance studio

   (C) A concert hall   (D) A dormitory

58. On the basis of the essay, the relationship of healing to music therapy is one of

   (A) cause and effect.   (B) symptom and treatment.

   (C) process and consequence.   (D) health and disease.

PASSAGE VII (Questions 59-65)

The official birth date of American naval aviation, (sometimes referred to as the U.S. Navy's air arm) has been set as May 8, 1911. This is the date on which the United States Navy bought its first aircraft. This flimsy little craft, which was offered for sale to the Navy by Glenn Curtis, cost the Navy $5,500. Despite the simple and fragile construction and the relative high unit cost of this little craft, the date of the sale was an important one, for it marked the birth of what has come to be the greatest and most effective naval air arm of any nation.

In 1890, Captain A.T. Mahan, USN, pointed out in his writings that the nation which controls the seas also controls the lands and thereby wins the wars. Despite the advancement of naval aviation, his doctrine is still very much in effect. However, a qualification to this doctrine must be added today — in order to control the seas, one must first control the air over the seas. In order to control the seas and the air over them, the Navy's air, surface, and undersea forces work as a team to accomplish the task at hand.

The U.S. Navy has never separated its aviation branch from the other forces. This is due mainly to the foresight of those senior officers that were in positions of great responsibility over the past 60 years or more. Great Britain tried such a separation of its air and surface forces after World War I. This experiment did not work. As a result, the air arm was brought back into the Royal Navy only a short time before World War II. The British Admiral of the Fleet, Lord Keys (Retired), stated in 1944 that the success of the U.S. Navy in the Battle of the Philippines was only made possible because the United States Navy had been free to develop its own naval aviation. He stated further that in the complex business of waging war on the seas, no one factor or force can win alone. All forces must work together as a team. Fortunately, the Navy tends its air, surface, and undersea forces with motherly devotion and fairness, thereby creating a unified force that is unparalleled in history.

The mission of the Navy is to insure open sealanes in the oceans of the world in time of war, and to deny their use to the enemy. The continuous appearance of new and modern sophisticated weapons changes the techniques of naval aviation. This also adds to the Navy's capabilities. However, the command of the seas is still the primary mission of the Navy. Naval aviation, regardless of the sophistication of its present arms and of those to come, still has as its primary function close coordination with other forces of the Navy in order to maintain command of the seas.

59. It can be inferred from this passage that the U.S. Navy

   I. is the oldest of the Armed Forces.

   II. shares its command of the seas.

III.   highly parallels the thought and development of the British Navy.

(A)   I only   (B)   II only

(C)   III only   (D)   I and III only

60.   May 8, 1911, is significant because

(A)   it is the date of the addition of a new craft to the Navy.

(B)   it represents the first effort to join air and sea.

(C)   it was the most money ever spent on an aircraft.

(D)   it is the recorded date for the beginning of naval aviation.

61.   According to this passage the Navy is

(A)   the seafaring arm of the armed forces.

(B)   the undersea, air and seafaring arm of U.S. defense.

(C)   comparable to the Navy of Great Britain.

(D)   the idea of Captain A.T. Mahan.

62.   It can be concluded from this passage that naval aviation has played a significant role in United States history because

(A)   war is an essential part of any nation's history.

(B)   a navy represents the nation with superior strength.

(C)   air and sea forces must cooperate in a united effort.

(D)   naval authorities had the vision to provide a cooperative effort in significant events.

63.   From the facts in this passage, it may be concluded that

(A)   the navy has not changed its techniques since 1911.

(B)   the navy commands the seas without assistance.

(C)   command of the navy reflects the maternal care of the U.S. government.

(D)   the future is in the hands of those leaders who have vision in matters of defense.

64.   It can be reasonably inferred from this passage that war is

I.   a complex effort.

II.   necessary for peace.

III.   a necessary evil.

(A)   I only   (B)   III only

(C)   I and II only   (D)   II and III only

65.   From the passage one may conclude that weapons

   (A)   are standard and only aviation can really handle the tactics of war.

   (B)   are unimportant in the naval operation.

   (C)   alter the state of naval training.

   (D)   are only used to insure open sealanes in the oceans of the world.

STOP

If time still remains, you may review work only in this section.

When the time allotted is up, you may go on to the next section.

Section 2 — Physical Sciences

TIME: 100 Minutes
QUESTIONS: 66-142

DIRECTIONS: Most of the questions in this section are arranged in groups, each corresponding to a descriptive passage. Based on the information given in a passage, choose the one best answer to each question in the group. Some questions are independent of a descriptive passage and of each other. Choose the one best answer to each of these questions. If you are not sure of an answer, eliminate those choices that you know are incorrect and choose an answer from among those remaining. Fill in the corresponding circle on the answer sheet to indicate your answer. You may refer to the periodic table at any time.

PASSAGE I (Questions 66-72)

A chemist determined the solubility of KNO_3 in water at a given temperature by measuring the mass of a saturated solution at that temperature and then measuring the mass of solute that remained after all the water had been removed. After determining the solubility at a variety of temperatures, the chemist plotted the solubility as a function of temperature, as shown below:

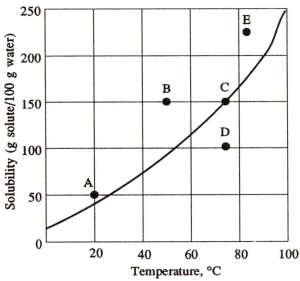

Points A, B, C, D and E represent various aqueous solutions of KNO_3.

66. Which solution(s) is (are) unsaturated?

(A) A, B, and E

(B) A, B, C, and E

(C) C only

(D) D only

67. Which solution(s) can become saturated as a result of an increase in temperature?

   (A) A, B, and E (B) A, B, C, and E

   (C) C only   (D) D only

68. Addition of a tiny crystal of KNO_3 can initiate crystallization in solution(s)

   (A) A, B, and E (B) A, B, C, and E

   (C) C only   (D) D only

69. Which solution is the most concentrated?

   (A) B (B) D

   (C) A (D) E

70. At 80°C, a solution contains 100 g of KNO_3 in 100 g of water. This solution is

   (A)   unstaturated.

   (B)   saturated.

   (C)   supersaturated.

   (D)   either unsaturated or saturated.

71. Estimate the mass (g) of water required to dissolve 85 g of KNO_3 at 80°C.

   (A)   13   (B)   22

   (C)   50   (D)   77

72. Estimate the mass (g) of KNO_3 that can dissolve in 60 g of water at 20°C.

   (A)   7   (B)   18

   (C)   37   (D)   62

PASSAGE II (Questions 73-80)

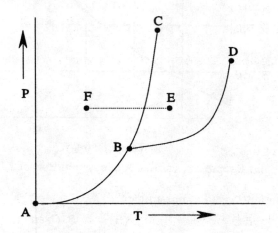

A chemist studied the response of solid, liquid, and vapor phases of CO_2 to changes in pressure and temperature by measuring the sublimation, freezing, and boiling temperatures of CO_2 at various pressures. The chemist also determined the temperature above which CO_2 vapor cannot be liquefied no matter how high a pressure is applied. These data are plotted on the curve on the previous page.

Points A, B, C, D, E, and F represent CO_2 at various conditions of pressure and temperature.

73. At all temperatures along the lines connecting points A and B

    (A)   the rate at which liquid boils to form a vapor equals the rate at which vapor condenses to form a liquid.

    (B)   the rate at which solid melts to form a liquid equals the rate at which liquid freezes to form a solid.

    (C)   the rate at which solid melts to form a liquid exceeds the rate at which liquid freezes to form a solid.

    (D)   the rate at which solid sublimes to form a vapor equals the rate at which vapor condenses to form a solid.

74. How many variables (degrees of freedom) must be specified in order to define point E?

    (A)   0   (B)   1

    (C)   2   (D)   3

75. If one heated CO_2 at a constant pressure starting at point F until point E is reached, what phase change would occur?

    (A)   melting   (B)   boiling

    (C)   sublimation   (D)   condensation

76. If one decreased the external pressure on CO_2 at point E, while keeping the temperature constant, what conversion would occur?

    (A)   solid to vapor   (B)   liquid to vapor

    (C)   solid to liquid   (D)   liquid to solid

77. The triple point for CO_2 occurs at 5.11 atm and 216.6 K. When CO_2 solid is heated at 1.00 atm, it

    (A)   melts.   (B)   boils.

    (C)   sublimes.   (D)   freezes.

78. The slope of line BC indicates that the melting point of CO_2

    (A)   increases with increasing pressure.

    (B)   increases with decreasing pressure.

    (C)   is not affected by changes in pressure.

    (D)   decreases with increasing pressure.

79. The slope of line BC also indicates that

    (A) CO_2 solid is less dense than CO_2 liquid.

    (B) CO_2 solid is more dense than CO_2 liquid.

    (C) CO_2 solid is less dense than CO_2 vapor.

    (D) CO_2 vapor is more dense than CO_2 liquid.

80. Liquid CO_2 can exist at all of the following locations except:

    (A) point E (B) point F

    (C) point B (D) along line BC

PASSAGE III (Questions 81-86)

"Fixed" nitrogen is nitrogen that has been combined chemically with other elements. In the Haber process, atmospheric nitrogen is fixed by allowing it to react with hydrogen to form ammonia:

$$N_2 \text{ (g)} + 3H_2 \text{ (g)} \rightleftharpoons 2 NH_3 \text{ (g)}$$

The enthalpy change, $\Delta H°$, for this reacton is - 92 kJ.

In a quantitative study of this process, a chemist mixed the two reactants together so that the initial concentrations of nitrogen and hydrogen inside a container were 0.500 M and 0.800 M, respectively. When the mixture reached equilibrium, the concentration of ammonia became 0.150 M.

81. Calculate the concentration of N_2 in the equilibrium mixture.

    (A) 0   (B) 0.725 M

    (C) 0.425 M   (D) 0.500 M

82. The equilibrium constant for this reaction is expressed as

    (A) $\dfrac{[N_2][3H_2]^3}{[2 NH_3]^2}$ (B) $\dfrac{[N_2][H_2]^3}{[NH_3]^2}$

    (C) $\dfrac{[2 NH_3]^2}{[N_2][3 H_2]^3}$ (D) $\dfrac{[NH_3]^2}{[N_2][H_2]^3}$

83. An increase in pressure caused by decreasing the volume of this system at equilibrium would result in

    (A) an increase in the number of N_2 molecules.

    (B) an increase in the number of H_2 molecules.

    (C) a decrease in the number of NH_3 molecules.

    (D) an increase in the concentration of NH_3.

84. An increase in the temperature of this system at equilibrium would result in

    (A) an increase in the concentration of N_2.

(B)   an increase in the number of NH_3 molecules.

(C)   a decrease in the number of H_2 molecules.

(D)   a decrease in the number of N_2 molecules.

85.   At constant temperature, addition of N_2 gas to the system at equilibrium would result in

(A)   an increase in the equilibrium constant.

(B)   a decrease in the equilibrium constant.

(C)   an increase in the concentration of NH_3.

(D)   an increase in the concentration of H_2.

86.   Addition of a catalyst to the system at equilibrium will

(A)   increase the equilibrium constant.

(B)   decrease the equilibrium constant.

(C)   increase the rate of the forward reaction and decrease the rate of the reverse reaction.

(D)   increase the rate of the forward and reverse reactions.

QUESTIONS 87-93 are NOT based on a descriptive passage.

---

87.   A 10 g bullet is fired into a 2 kg ballistic pendulum as shown in the figure. The bullet remains in the block after the collision and the system rises to a maximum height of 20 cm. Find the initial speed of the bullet.

(A)   28.0 m/s

(B)   23.8 m/s

(C)   719 m/s

(D)   398 m/s

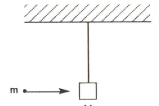

88.   Isotopes of the same element have the same atomic number and a different mass number. Which statement is true?

(A)   Isotopes have more protons and electrons than their element.

(B)   Isotopes have fewer protons and electrons than their element.

(C)   Isotopes have a different number of neutrons.

(D)   Isotopes have a different number of neutrons and protons.

89.   The density of a steel alloy is 7.8 gm/cm^3. What would be the mass of a 2 meter × 3 meter × 5 meter block constructed out of this alloy?

(A)   2.34 gm   (B) 2.34×10^8 gm

(C)   234 gm   (D)   3900 gm

90. This neurotransmitter is found at neuromuscular junctions in the brain and at junctions in the internal organs.

    (A) Norepinephrine   (B) Serotonin

    (C) Dopamine   (D) Acetylcholine

91. Which of the following is a naturally occurring wax?

    (A) $CH_2OCOC_{15}H_{31}$

    $CHOCOC_{15}H_{31}$

    $CH_2OCOC_{15}H_{31}$

    (B) $\overset{+}{N}H_3 CH_2 CH_2 CHO-\overset{\overset{\displaystyle O}{\|}}{\underset{\underset{\displaystyle O^-}{|}}{P}}-O-\overset{|}{\underset{\underset{\displaystyle CH_2OCOC_{15}H_{31}}{|}}{\underset{\displaystyle CHOCOC_{15}H_{31}}{CH_2}}}$

    (C) $CH_2 OHCHOHCH_2 OH$

    (D) $CH_{15}H_{31}\overset{\overset{\displaystyle O}{\|}}{C}OC_{16}H_{33}$

92. A cold, dilute solution of $KMnO_4$ will oxidize

    I. $CH_3CH{=}CH_2$

    II. $CH_3CH_2OCH_3$

    III. $CH_3\overset{\overset{\displaystyle CH}{\|}}{\underset{\displaystyle O}{}}$

    IV. $ClH_2\overset{\overset{\displaystyle C}{}}{C}COH$ with $\overset{\|}{O}$

    (A) I only.   (B) II only.

    (C) I and III only.   (D) II and IV only.

93. What does X represent in the following radioactive decay?

    $$^{238}_{92}Y \rightarrow {}^{238}_{93}Z + X$$

    (A) a proton   (B) an electron

    (C) a neutron   (D) an α-particle.

PASSAGE IV (Questions 94-99)

In order to determine the rate law for the decomposition of substance X, a chemist carried out two experiments. In each the initial rate was determined at given initial concentrations of X at a temperature of 20°C. Following is a summary of the results of those experiments:

Experiment	Initial conc X (M)	Rate (mol/L·s)
1	0.10	0.12
2	0.20	0.48

After using these data to determine the rate law, the chemist used that expression to predict the rate of decomposition of X at a new initial concentration and also to predict the initial concentration required to produce a given initial rate.

94. Determine the order of the reaction.

    (A) 0   (B) 2

    (C) 3/2   (D) 1

95. Determine the rate constant for the decomposition.

    (A) 1.2   (B) 1200

    (C) 120   (D) 12

96. Use the rate law to predict the initial rate of decomposition of X for an initial concentration of 0.30 M.

    (A) 3.6 mol/L·s   (B) 2.4 mol/L·s

    (C) 0.90 mol/L·s   (D) 1.1 mol/L·s

97. Use the rate law to predict the initial concentration of X required to produce an initial rate of 1.08 mol/L ·s.

    (A) 0.25 M   (B) 0.30 M

    (C) 0.35 M   (D) 0.40 M

98. The half-life of this reaction is

    (A) directly proportional to the initial concentration.

    (B) directly proportional to the square of the initial concentration.

    (C) independent of the initial concentration.

    (D) inversely proportional to the initial concentration.

99. If Experiment 1 had been carried out at 30°C instead of 20°C,

    (A) the rate constant would be higher.

    (B) the rate constant would be lower.

    (C) the order would be higher.

    (D) the order would be lower.

PASSAGE V (Questions 100–106)

In order to evaluate the thermodynamic aspects of the reaction at 25°C between methane gas, CH_4, and excess oxygen:

$$CH_4 \text{ (g)} + 2O_2 \text{ (g)} \longrightarrow CO_2 \text{ (g)} + 2H_2O \text{ (l)}$$

a chemist used a Table of Heats of Formation to calculate the enthalpy change, $\Delta H°$, and a Table of Standard Entropies to calculate the entropy change, $\Delta S°$. Using these values in the Gibbs-Helmholtz equation, the chemist calculated the free energy change, $\Delta G°$. These values are:

$$\Delta H° = -890.3 \text{ kJ}$$

$$\Delta S° = -0.2428 \text{ kJ/K}$$

$$\Delta G° = -817.9 \text{ kJ}$$

The molar masses of reactants and products are:

$$CH_4 = 16, \quad O_2 = 32, \quad CO_2 = 44, \quad H_2O = 18.$$

100. The value of $\Delta H°$ indicates that this reaction is

   (A) rapid.   (B) slow.

   (C) endothermic.   (D) exothermic.

101. The value of $\Delta S°$ indicates that

   (A) the entropy of the products is less than the entropy of the reactants.

   (B) the entropy of the reactants is less than the entropy of the products.

   (C) the reaction is rapid.

   (D) the reaction is slow.

102. The value of $\Delta G°$ indicates that the reaction is

   (A) rapid.   (B) slow.

   (C) spontaneous.   (D) nonspontaneous.

103. Since the sign of $\Delta H°$ for this reaction is negative and the sign of $\Delta S°$ is also negative, this reaction is

   (A) spontaneous only at high temperatures.

   (B) spontaneous only at low temperatures.

   (C) always spontaneous.

   (D) never spontaneous.

104. Calculate $\Delta H°$ for the formation of 8 moles of H_2O.

   (A) -3561.2 kJ   (B) -7122.4 kJ

   (C) -222.6 kJ   (D) $+3721.1$ kJ

105. Calculate the number of grams of CH_4 required to produce 445.2 kJ.

(A) 8.6   (B) 6.1

(C) 8.0   (D) 2.4

106. Calculate $\Delta H°$ for the reaction:

$$CO_2 \text{ (g)} + 2H_2O \text{ (l)} \longrightarrow CH_4 \text{ (g)} + 2\,O_2 \text{ (g)}$$

(A) − 890.3 kJ   (B) − 732.6 kJ

(C) + 732.6 kJ   (D) + 890.3 kJ

QUESTIONS 107-111 are NOT based on a descriptive passage.

---

107. If a 25 kg object is raised 10 meters, what is the work being done?

(A) 1250 J   (B) 2400 J

(C) 2450 J   (D) 250 J

108. The phenomenon which occurs when a wave spreads into the region behind an obstruction is known as

(A) refraction.   (B) diffraction.

(C) dispersion.   (D) superposition.

109. During the human menstrual cycle, peak levels of estrogen and luteinizing hormone are associated with

(A) the early part of the follicular phase.

(B) the latter part of the follicular phase.

(C) the early part of the luteal phase.

(D) the latter part of the luteal phase.

110. Which of the following statements is not always true?

(A) A neutral solution has a pH of 7.

(B) The atomic number is equal to the number of protons in the nucleus.

(C) An ion possesses a positive or negative charge.

(D) The anode is the oxidation site.

111. The major constituent of gallstones is (are)

(A) calcium salts.   (B) silicate.

(C) cholesterol.   (D) cholecystokinin.

PASSAGE VI (Questions 112-117)

A chemist added a piece of tin metal to an aqueous solution containing silver ions. The chemist observed the formation of crystalline silver in the solution. The equation for this reaction is:

$$Sn + 2\,Ag^+ \longrightarrow Sn^{2+} + 2\,Ag$$

The chemist was able to design a voltaic cell in which this reaction was used to produce electrical energy.

Standard reduction potentials at 25°C are:

$$Sn^{2+} + 2e^- \longrightarrow Sn; \quad E° = -0.14\ V$$

$$Ag^+ + e^- \longrightarrow Ag; \quad E° = 0.80\ V$$

112. Which species is the oxidizing agent in this cell?

   (A) Sn
   (B) Ag^+
   (C) Sn^{2+}
   (D) Ag

113. What is the half-reaction that takes place at the anode?

   (A) $Sn \longrightarrow Sn^{2+}$
   (B) $Sn^{2+} \longrightarrow Sn$
   (C) $Ag^+ \longrightarrow Ag$
   (D) $2\,Ag^+ \longrightarrow 2\,Ag$

114. Calculate E° for the cell.

   (A) 0.66 V
   (B) – 0.66 V
   (C) 0.28 V
   (D) 0.94 V

115. The cell can be abbreviated

   (A) $Sn/2\,Ag^+ \parallel Sn^{2+}/2\,Ag$
   (B) $Sn/Ag^+ \parallel Sn^{2+}/Ag$
   (C) $Ag^+/Ag \parallel Sn/Sn^{2+}$
   (D) $Sn/Sn^{2+} \parallel Ag^+/Ag$

116. The chemical reaction in this cell

   (A) is irreversible.
   (B) has a negative E°.
   (C) is spontaneous.
   (D) is rapid.

117. In this cell the electron flow between electrodes is from

   (A) Sn to Ag
   (B) Sn^{2+} to Sn
   (C) Ag^+ to Ag
   (D) Ag to Ag^+

PASSAGE VII (Questions 118-123)

   In a study of the conditions for static equilibrium in a body acted upon by concurrent forces, a physicist suspended a 100 kg ball using two ropes, as shown in the following figure.

   (sin 30° = 0.500; cos 30° = 0.866)

   The physicist was able to calculate the various forces acting on the ball. These values were then determined experimentally using spring balances inserted along the ropes.

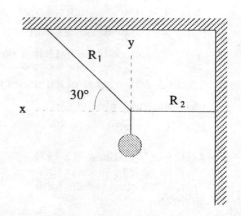

118. The gravitational force on the ball is

    (A)   50 kg up.
    (B)   50 kg down.
    (C)   100 kg up.
    (D)   100 kg down.

119. the sum of the forces exerted in the y direction by ropes R_1 and R_2 at the junction is equal to

    (A)   0 kg.
    (B)   50 kg up.
    (C)   50 kg down.
    (D)   100 kg up.

120. The sum of all the forces acting in the x direction is equal to

    (A)   0 kg.
    (B)   50 kg up.
    (C)   50 kg down.
    (D)   100 kg up.

121. The force exerted in the y direction by ropes R_1 and R_2 is

    (A) $R_1 \sin 30° + R_2$.
    (B) $R_1 \cos 30° + R_2$.
    (C) $R_1 \sin 30°$.
    (D) $R_1 \cos 30°$.

122. The force exerted on the ball by rope 1 is

    (A)   100 kg.
    (B)   200 kg.
    (C)   50 kg.
    (D)   87 kg.

123. The force exerted on the ball by rope 2 is

    (A)   173 kg.
    (B)   421 kg.
    (C)   201 kg.
    (D)   0 kg.

PASSAGE VIII (Questions 124-129)

In a study of Ohm's law as applied to circuit components, a physicist set up an electrical circuit that contained several resistors in series, a pair of resistors in parallel, and a single voltage source. A diagram of the circuit is shown below:

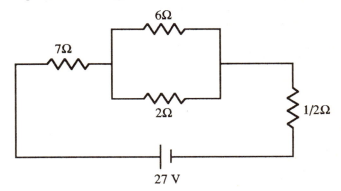

Amperages and voltages across the resistors were calculated using Ohm's law. These values were then determined experimentally using an ammeter and a voltmeter.

124. Calculate the equivalent resistance of the 6Ω and 2Ω resistors.

    (A) 1/8Ω   (B) 3/2Ω
    (C) 2Ω   (D) 3Ω

125. Calculate the total resistance of the entire network of resistors.

    (A) 3Ω   (B) 5Ω
    (C) 7Ω   (D) 9Ω

126. Calculate the current through the 7Ω resistor.

    (A) 1 amp   (B) 3 amp
    (C) 5 amp   (D) 7 amp

127. Calculate the voltage drop across the 7Ω resistor.

    (A) 3 volts   (B) 7 volts
    (C) 21 volts   (D) 24 volts

128. Calculate the voltage drop across the 6Ω resistor.

    (A) 4.5 volts   (B) 6.0 volts
    (C) 8.0 volts   (D) 1.5 volts

129. Calculate the current in the 6Ω resistor.

    (A) 0 amp   (B) 0.25 amp
    (C) 0.50 amp   (D) 0.75 amp

PASSAGE IX (Questions 130-134)
    In order to study some of the properties of spherical mirrors, a physicist inserted a convex mirror having a radius of curvature of 50 cm in a mirror holder and placed it at the 0 cm mark of an optical bench. The physicist made sure that the convex surface of the mirror faced the object to be placed on the optical bench. A 60 cm tall lamp was placed at the 100 cm mark on the optical bench. The physicist made sure that the axes of the lamp and mirror were aligned.

130. Calculate the focal length of the mirror.

    (A) 10 cm   (B) 20 cm
    (C) 25 cm   (D) 40 cm

131. Calculate the distance from the mirror to the image of the lamp.

    (A) 55 cm behind the mirror

    (B) 40 cm behind the mirror

    (C) 40 cm in front of the mirror

    (D) 20 cm behind the mirror

132. How tall is the image of the lamp?

    (A)   24 cm   (B)   28 cm

    (C)   16 cm   (D)   12 cm

133. Which one of the following statements about convex mirrors is false?

    (A)   The focal length is negative.

    (B)   The image is always erect.

    (C)   The image is always virtual.

    (D)   The image is always in front of the mirror.

134. If the convex mirror was replaced by a plane mirror and the lamp was moved to 200 cm from that mirror, how tall would the image of the lamp be?

    (A)   20 cm   (B)   40 cm

    (C)   60 cm   (D)   140 cm

PASSAGE X (Questions 135-139)

In order to determine the characteristics of simple harmonic waves in stretched strings, a physicist studied various guitar strings. One of these strings was stretched (tuned) so that when it was plucked, the transverse wave produced corresponded to a note of A at a frequency of 110 Hz. This note was played at a loudness of 20 decibels (dB). The note made by this instrument interfered with a note of A made by a second instrument. The beat frequency was 5 beats per second.

The speed of these sound in air can be calculated from the formula:

$$v = 331 + 0.6\,T$$

in which T is in °C and v in meters/ second.

135. What is the frequency of this note when played one octave higher?

    (A)   55 Hz   (B)   110 Hz

    (C)   111 Hz   (D)   220 Hz

136. The energy of this sound is _____ times the loudness of the softest audible sound.

    (A)   0.20   (B)   100

    (C)   200   (D)   220

137. What are the possible frequencies of the note made by the second instrument?

    (A)   105 Hz only   (B)   115 Hz only

    (C)   110 Hz or 115 Hz   (D)   105 Hz or 115 Hz

138. Calculate the speed of this sound in air at 10°C.

    (A)   110 m/s   (B)   220 m/s

    (C)   330 m/s   (D)   337 m/s

139. This sound wave will travel fastest in

    (A) pure water.   (B) salt water.

    (C) elastic solids.   (D) air.

QUESTIONS 140-142 are NOT based on a descriptive passage.

---

140. A 55 year old woman has a near point of 100 cm. What lens should be used to see clearly an object at the normal near point of 25 cm? (Find the focal length of the required lens.)

    (A) 20.0 cm   (B) − 33.3 cm

    (C) 33.3 cm   (D) − 25.0 cm

141. The resistance of a piece of copper wire is 10 ohms. The resistance, in ohms, of a piece of copper wire of the same diameter but twice as long is

    (A) 5 Ω.   (B) 10 Ω.

    (C) 20 Ω.   (D) 80 Ω.

142. In the photoelectric effect, electromagnetic radiation is incident upon the surface of a metal. Which of the following is not a true statement about the photoelectric effect?

    (A) The stopping potential V_0 is proportional to v^2.

    (B) v_0 is characteristic of the cathode material.

    (C) The stopping potential is independent of the intensity.

    (D) There is no photocurrent unless $v > v_0$.

STOP

If time still remains, you may review work only in this section.

When the time allotted is up, you may go on to the next section.

Section 3 — Writing Sample

TIME: 60 minutes
2 Essays, separately timed
30 minutes each

DIRECTIONS: This section tests your writing skills by asking you to write two essays. You will have 30 minutes to write each one.

During the first 30 minutes, work only on the first essay. If you finish it in less than 30 minutes, you may review what you have written, but do not begin the second essay. During the second 30 minutes, work only on the second essay. If you finish it in less than 30 minutes, you may review what you have written for that essay only. Do not go back to the first essay.

Read each assigned topic carefully. Make sure your essays respond to the topics as they are assigned.

Make sure your essays are written in complete sentences and paragraphs, and are as clear as you can make them. Make any corrections or additions between the lines of your essays. Do not write in the margins.

On the day of the test, you are given three pages to write each essay. You are not required to use all of the space provided, but do not skip lines so you will not waste space. Illegible essays cannot be scored.

Part 1

Consider this statement:

> Layer upon layer, past times preserve themselves in the city until life itself is finally threatened with suffocation; then, in sheer defense, modern man invents the museum.

> Lewis Mumford

Write a comprehensive essay in which you accomplish the following objectives. Explain what you think the statement means. Describe specifically in what ways the city encourages rather than stultifies life. Discuss the place of the city in the life of modern man.

STOP

If time still remains, you may review work only in this section.

When the time allotted is up, you may go on to the next section.

Part 2

Consider this statement:

> A nation built on the idea that all men are of equal worth and equal rights summons every one of its citizens to a life-long commitment to put that idea into practical effect.

Bruce Catton

Write a comprehensive essay in which you accomplish the following objectives. Explain what you think the statement means. Describe specific situations which set up an opposition to the statement. Discuss how citizens might work toward "equal worth and equal rights."

STOP

If time still remains, you may review work only in this section.

When the time allotted is up, you may go on to the next section.

Section 4 — Biological Sciences

TIME: 100 Minutes
QUESTIONS: 143-219

> **DIRECTIONS:** Most of the questions in this section are arranged in groups, each corresponding to a descriptive passage. Based on the information given in a passage, choose the one best answer to each question in the group. Some questions are independent of a descriptive passage and of each other. Choose the one best answer to each of these questions. If you are not sure of an answer, eliminate those choices that you know are incorrect and choose an answer from among those remaining. Fill in the corresponding circle on the answer sheet to indicate your answer. You may refer to the periodic table at any time.

PASSAGE I (Questions 143-150)

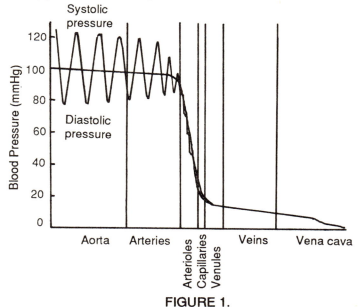

FIGURE 1.

Mammalian circulatory systems are closed systems in which blood is pumped by a four-chambered heart. It is often described as a "double" circulatory system becaue of its pulmonary and systemic circuits. Because cardiac muscle tends to contract as a unit, blood is driven through the vessels of the body by pulses of pressure. As blood moves farther away from the heart, the overall pressure in the system decreases. The difference in pressure caused by contraction and relaxation of the heart also decreases.

Rates of blood flow fluctuate according to changes in heart rate, stroke volume, and cross-sectional area of the vessels through which blood flows. Water is forced out of blood by hydrostatic pressure as the blood enters capillary beds from arterioles and is taken back into venules by osmotic pressure as blood leaves capillary beds. Most (about 99 percent) of this water is thus reabsorbed, but a small amount of fluid remains in the tissues of the capillary bed. This fluid is ultimately returned to the blood circulatory through lymph capillaries and veins.

Use the information given in this passage, your general knowledge of circulatory, and the graph of systemic circulation that appears as Figure 1, to answer the following questions.

143. In a mammal, blood pressure is lowest in the

   (A) aorta.
   (B) vena cavae.
   (C) capillaries of the arm.
   (D) veins of the leg.

144. If the blood pressure of a person is 140/85, then

   (A) pulse pressure is 55 mm Hg.
   (B) diastolic pressure is 140 mm Hg.
   (C) systolic pressure is the sum of 140 and 85 mm Hg.
   (D) diastolic pressure is the sum of 140 and 85 mm Hg.

145. Lymph is returned to the blood circulatory system through large lymph ducts that empty into the

   (A) subclavian veins.
   (B) hepatic portal system.
   (C) abdominal aorta.
   (D) inferior vena cava.

146. The connection between the aorta and pulmonary artery of a mammalian fetus is known as the

   (A) foramen ovale.
   (B) foramen magnum.
   (C) ductus ateriosus.
   (D) ligamentum arteriosum.

147. In an adult mammallian heart, the pulmonary artery is carrying

   (A) oxygen-rich blood to the lungs.
   (B) oxygen-rich blood from the lungs.
   (C) oxygen-poor blood from the lungs
   (D) oxygen-poor blood to the lungs.

148. All of the following statements about the mammalian circulatory system are correct, EXCEPT

   (A) blood pressure is lower in a capillary bed than in the arteriole leading to it.
   (B) water content of blood is regulated by concentration of blood protein.
   (C) osmotic pressure across capillary walls is regulated by active transport of water.
   (D) blood flows faster in the arteriole than in the capillary bed.

149. The pulmonary circuit of a mammalian circulatory system connects which chambers of the heart?

    (A) Right ventricle to left atrium

    (B) Left ventricle to right atrium

    (C) Left atrium to left ventricle

    (D) Right atrium to right ventricle

150. The normal pH of human blood is

    (A) 7.0.   (B) 6.5.

    (C) 7.8.   (D) 7.4.

PASSAGE II (Questions 151-154)

Sodium dissolved in deuterium oxide (D_2O) gives a solution that will replace exchangeable hydrogen atoms in organic compounds with deuterium atoms. Exchangeable hydrogens are defined as those that are acidic because of their proximity to electron-withdrawing groups. The sodium dissolves to give deuterium gas (D_2) and the strong base, NaOD. The OD⁻ will react with protons on carbons adjacent to groups which stabilize the negative charge by induction or by resonance.

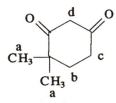

Y is an electron-withdrawing group.

151. Which of the following compounds would undergo hydrogen-deuterium exchange when reacted with $NaOD/D_2O$?

    (A) Hexane   (B) Nitromethane

    (C) Trimethylamine   (D) Formaldehyde

152. For the compound below, which of the labelled hydrogens will react fastest with $NaOD/D_2O$?

    (A) a   (B) b

    (C) c   (D) d

153. The product of the reaction of $NaOD/D_2O$ and the optically active ketone shown below would be:

$$\text{(+) Ph} - \underset{O}{\overset{CH_3}{\underset{\|}{C}}} - CH \overset{CH_3}{\underset{CH_2CH_3}{<}} \xrightarrow{\text{NaOD / D}_2\text{O}}$$

(A) (+) Ph—C(=O)—CH(CH$_2$D)(CH$_2$CH$_3$)

(B) (−) Ph—C(=O)—CD(CH$_3$)(CH$_2$CH$_3$)

(C) (+) Ph—C(=O)—CD(CH$_3$)(CH$_2$CH$_3$)

(D) (±) Ph—C(=O)—CD(CH$_3$)(CH$_2$CH$_3$)

154. In describing the mechanism of the reaction in Questions 152 and 153, the intermediate would be called

(A) an enolate.

(B) a carbocation.

(C) a free racical.

(D) an enol.

PASSAGE III (Questions 155-159)

Encochondral bone formation is essentially a process of replacing a cartilaginous model with osseus tissue. The developing bone, which is highly vascularized, is formed by deposition of calcium salts of phosphate and carbonate within the intercellular matrix already defined by the chondrocytes of the cartilaginous model. Hypertrophication of chondrocytes in the shaft of the bone occurs as the model grows and calcification follows as minerals are deposited within the matrix.

As calcification causes chondrocytes to die because of nutrient starvation, selected cells of the perichondrium are giving rise to osteoblasts. An uncalcified bone matrix known as osteoid is produced by the osteoblasts. Calcification of the periochondrium follows to form the periosteal bone collar. In the center of the developing bond, a primary ossification center is formed as cartilage is invaded by osteoblasts and vascular tissue. Two secondary ossification centers are similarly formed at the ends of the bone.

Elongation of the bone is now essentially a function of chondrocyte production in the epiphyseal plates, which are located between the primary ossification activity in the middle of the bone and the two secondary centers at each end. As long as cell division continues in the epiphyseal plates, bone growth will proceed. Eventually, the epiphyseal plates ossify and the bone will no longer increase in length.

Remodeling of bone tissue already formed occurs throughout the life of a vertebrate. Osteoblasts in the periosteum secrete osteoid as the bone is physically stressed and additional bone is deposited. Simultaneously, bone cells next to the medullary cavity are reabsorbed by osteoclasts thereby keeping the size of the cavity proportional to the size of the bone.

Use the information given in this passage and your knowledge of the bone structure to answer the following questions.

155. Compact bone would most likely be found

    (A)   directly underneath the periosteum.

    (B)   in the medullary cavity of a long bone.

    (C)   on either side of the epiphyseal line of adult bone.

    (D)   in the secondary ossification centers of fetal bone.

156. The proximal epiphyseal plate of a human humerus would be closest to which of the following?

    (A)   The ulna

    (B)   The insertion of the triceps brachii

    (C)   The scapula

    (D)   The insertion of the biceps brachii

157. Knee and elbow joints are examples of bone articulations known as

    (A)   synarthroses.   (B)   synchondroses.

    (C)   amphiarthroses.   (D)   diarthroses.

158. The shaft of a long bone is properly known as the

    (A)   diaphysis.   (B)   ephphysis.

    (C)   amphiarthrosis.   (D)   symphysis.

159. A band of connective tissue that binds bone to bone is known as a

    (A)   tendon.   (B)   chorda tendinea.

    (C)   ligament.   (D)   choroid plexus.

QUESTIONS 160–161 are NOT based on a descriptive passage

---

160. The correct name, using the Cahn-Ingold-Prelog designation of absolute configuration, for the compound below is

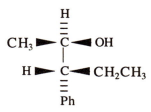

    (A)   (2R, 3S)-3-Phenyl-2-pentanol.

    (B)   (2R, 3R)-3-Phenyl-2-pentanol.

    (C)   (2S, 3S)-3-Phenyl-2-pentanol.

    (D)   (2S, 3R)-3-Phenyl-2-pentanol.

161. The correct IUPAC name for the compound shown is

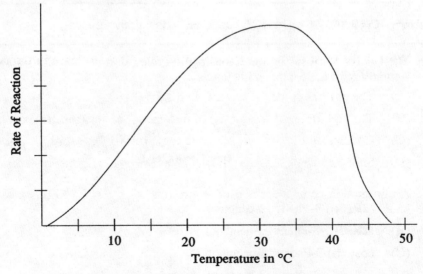

$$CH_3-C=C-H$$
$$CH_3CH_2 \quad CH_2-CH-CH=CH_2$$
$$CH_3$$

(A)   (E)-3, 6-dimethyl-1, 5-octadiene.

(B)   (Z)-3, 6-dimethyl-1, 5-octadiene.

(C)   (Z)-3, 6-dimethyl-3, 7-octadiene.

(D)   (E)-3, 6-dimethyl-3, 7-octadiene.

PASSAGE IV (Questions 162-168)

Enzymes are highly specialized proteinaceous, organic catalysts that, like all catalysts, lower the energy of activation necessary for a chemical reaction to occur. The molecule on which an enzyme acts is known as a substrate. An enzyme greatly speeds up the specific reaction it catalyzes to the extent that one enzyme molecule can cause thousands of substrate molecules to be converted into product each second. Some enzymes contain a non-protein component that is essential to the activity of the enzyme; others require a brief, loose bonding with metal ions or nonproteinaceous organic compounds called cofactors to catalyze the reaction.

Like inorganic catalysts, enzymes are not themselves changed during the reaction and can function repeatedly. The specificity of enzyme activity depends on steric compatibility between substrate and the surface of the enzyme, or more precisely certain areas on the surface of the enzyme known as active sites. The activity of an enzyme requires that the conformation of the active site fits, or can be induced to fit, the shape of the substrate molecule. Anything that disrupts this precise fit will reduce enzyme activity or inhibit it entirely.

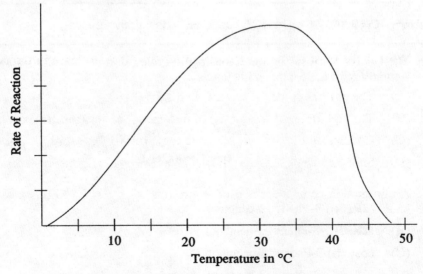

Figure 1 — Hand-drawn curve — rate vs. temp.

Suppose an enzyme catalyzes the conversion of molecule X to molecule Y. A third molecule A, which has no seric resemblance to X, binds with the surface of the enzyme at some distance from the active site and has the effect of increasing the reaction rate. A fourth molecule, B, which is quite similar to X, binds with the enzyme at the active site and has the effect of reducing the reaction rate. Adding more of molecule X to the reaction mixture reverses the effect of molecule B and the reaction rate again increases.

Figure 1 plots the rate of this enzyme-catalyzed reaction against temperature. You will have to refer to this plot, the information given above, and draw on your knowledge of enzymes in general to answer the questions in this passage.

162. In the reaction described in this passage, the substrate is

(A) molecule X.   (B) molecule Y.

(C) molecule A.   (D) molecule B.

163. In this reaction, molecule A is

(A) the substrate.   (B) a competitive inhibitor.

(C) a cofactor.   (D) an allosteric modulator.

164. In this reaction, moledule B is

(A) a cofactor.

(B) an allosteric modulator.

(C) a noncompetitive inhibitor.

(D) a competitive inhibitor.

165. The optimum temperature for the reaction plotted in Figure 1 is approximately _____ °C.

(A) 5   (B) 25

(C) 35   (D) 45

166. What is the most probable explanation for the sharp decrease in the curve at about 40°C?

(A) The enzyme starts to denature at this temperature

(B) The equilibrium constant (K) of the reaction is changed at this point

(C) Competitive inhibition of the enzyme is occurring

(D) Substrate molecules are not available at higher temperatures

167. A non-protein component part of an enzyme, as described in this passage, is known as a(n)

(A) allosteric modulator.   (B) prosthetic group.

(C) coenzyme.   (D) secondary structure.

168. Enzymes have, as do all proteins, well defined levels of structure. Disulfide bridges between cysteine molecules *within* a single polypeptide chain in the enzyme molecule are important in maintaining the _____ level of its structure.

    (A) primary

    (B) secondary

    (C) tertiary

    (D) quaternary

PASSAGE V (Questions 169-172)

Steroids are defined as derivatives of perhydrocyclopentano-phenanthrene.

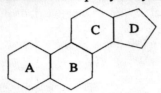

The most common steroid, cholesterol, is also a precursor of many other steroids that greatly influence biological activity. Shown below are several important steroids.

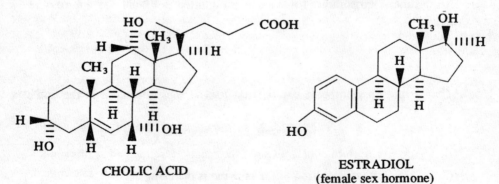

169. The most water soluble of the steroids shown is

    (A) androsterone.

    (B) estradiol.

    (C) cholic acid.

    (D) cholesterol.

170. The number of chiral centers in androsterone is

    (A) 1.

    (B) 3.

    (C) 5.

    (D) 7.

171. The only one of these compounds that will show absorption in the 6.5-7.5 δ region of the nmr spectrum is

    (A) estradiol.
    (B) androsterone.
    (C) cholic acid.
    (D) cholesterol.

172. The ring junction in cholic acid that is *cis* fused is

    (A) A, B.
    (B) B, C.
    (C) C, D.
    (D) None of them

QUESTIONS 173-177 are NOT based on a descriptive passage.

---

173. In preparing tissues for light microscopy, the sample must be fixed in order to

    (A) have a firm support.
    (B) distinguish subcellular regions from each other.
    (C) afford an unimpeded view of deep layers.
    (D) prevent autolysis.

174. The placenta originates from

    (A) embryonic cells.
    (B) maternal cells.
    (C) paternal cells.
    (D) Both (A) and (B).

175. The Golgi apparatus primarily functions in

    (A) packaging protein for secretion.
    (B) synthesizing protein for secretion.
    (C) packaging protein for hydrolysis.
    (D) synthesizing protein for hydrolysis.

176. For the protons in methyl propanoate, what is the order of *increasing* distance downfield from TMS in the NMR spectrum?

$$\overset{a}{C}H_3\overset{b}{C}H_2\overset{O}{\overset{\|}{C}}O\overset{c}{C}H_3$$

    (A) c, a, b
    (B) a, b, c
    (C) b, c, a
    (D) a, c, b

177. What is the major product of the following sequence of reactions?

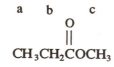

(A) COOH

NO_2

(B) CH_2CH_3

NO_2

(C) COOH

NO_2

(D) $CH=CH_2$

NO_2

PASSAGE VI (Questions 178-183)

Irrespective of the organism or tissues involved, the liberation of energy from carbohydrates involves the same fundamental biochemical reactions at the cellular level. The reactions can be divided into three basic groups — glycolysis, the Krebs (or citric acid) cycle, and the electron transport chain. Each occurs in a specific region or structure within the cell and each consists of numerous reactions. Collectively, these three groups of reactions can be referred to as cellular respiration.

Glycolysis is essentially an anaerobic process that breaks glucose into pyruvic acid, producing some ATP and reduced coenzymes (specifically, NADH+H⁺). Under certain conditions, some cells are capable of converting pyruvic acid into ethanol and carbon dioxide or into lactic acid. In these cases, the overall process is known as fermentation and the entire breakdown of glucose to these products occurs without requiring oxygen. Under appropriate conditions, the pyruvic acid is then converted into acetyl-Coenzyme A by oxidative decarboxylation in preparation for the Krebs cycle.

The Krebs cycle is a complex series of coupled reactions that yields carbon dioxide, reduced coenzymes, and some GTP (the energy of which can then be used to synthesize ATP). The electrons carried by these reduced coenzymes are shunted to the electron transport chain where the majority of the ATP from cellular respiration is produced by chemiosmotic synthesis. Ultimately, at their lowest energy level, these electrons are donated to oxygen and, with the addition of hydrogen ions, leave respiration as water.

178. Glycolysis takes place in the

    (A) ribosome.
    (B) nucleus.
    (C) mitochondrion.
    (D) cytosol.

179. The process by which ATP is synthesized as electrons from NADH+H⁺ and are moved along the electron transport chain is called

    (A) photophosphorylation .
    (B) dephosphorylation.
    (C) oxidative phosphorylation.
    (D) substrate-level phosphorylation.

180. It is generally accepted that the number of ATP molecules that can be synthesized by fermentation of one glucose molecule is

(A) 2.

(B) 18.

(C) 36.

(D) 42.

181. In eukaryotes, the electron transport chain is located in the

(A) cytosol.

(B) outer compartment of the mitochondrion.

(C) inner membrane of the mitochondrion.

(D) plasma membrane.

182. An acetyl group from acetyl-CoA enters the Krebs cycle by combining with

(A) citric acid.

(B) succinic acid.

(C) pyruvic acid.

(D) oxaloacetic acid.

183. Which of the following verterbrate tissues or organs is BEST adapted for anaerobic respiration?

(A) Skeletal muscle

(B) Brain

(C) Cardiac muscle

(D) Smooth muscle

PASSAGE VII (Questions 182-187)

In 1931, Erich Hückel applied the principles of molecular orbital theory to aromatic compounds. He formulated the $4n + 2$ rule, which states that *planar, cyclic fully conjugated polyenes possessing $4n + 2\pi$ electrions will have special aromatic stability* (n is 0 or an integer). This stability leads to decreased heats of combustion and reduced reactivity with many reagents, among other properties. Hückel also recognized that certain cyclic charged intermediates could have aromatic properties and that non-bonding electrons on heterocyclic atoms could be conjugated with the π electrons in a ring.

Consider the following structures and answer questions 184 –187.

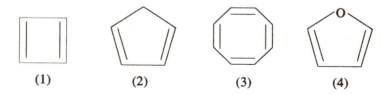

(1)   (2)   (3)   (4)

184. Which of these compounds is aromatic?

(A) 1

(B) 2

(C) 3

(D) 4

185. Which compound can form an aromatic entity by reacting with the strong base NaNH$_2$?

(A) 1   (B) 2

(C) 3   (D) 4

186. Which of these compounds would show absorption peaks 6-8 ppm downfield from TMS in the NMR spectrum?

(A) 1   (B) 2

(C) 3   (D) 4

187. Which of the following compounds would react most readily with (aq) AgNO₃?

(A) 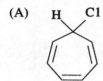   (B)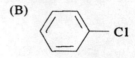

(C) 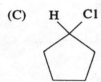   (D) H   Cl

PASSAGE VIII (Questions 188-194)

One of the unifying principles of modern biology is the concept of evolutionary change. Evidence for evolutionary change existed before Darwin, but he was the first to present evidence that natural selection was the agent for such change. Among the observations that Darwin made to support the role of natural selection were morphological similarities among adults of related species. Comparative anatomy of the limbs of vertebrates suggested common origins of many of these structures, leading to the contemporary concepts of evolutionary homology and evolutionary analogy.

Additional evidence for evolutionary change was seen in comparative embryology of both invertebrate and vertebrate animals. Haeckel's conclusion of ontogenic recapitulation of phylogeny, while not literally correct, provided an intellectual framework for interpreting the developmental similarities among related taxonomic groups of organisms.

The well known ability of plant and animal breeders to make changes in characteristics of domesticated species was interpreted by Darwin as further confirmation that variation could be selected and retained. He perceived that the only difference between natural selection and this artificial selection was that humans were acting as the agents of selection. Given the geological time frame involved in natural changes of species, he reasoned that the same mechanisms were clearly involved. The only differences were, therefore, the intensity of the selective pressures and the concomitant modification in the rate of change.

188. All of the following are homologous structures EXCEPT

(A) the foreleg of a horse and the wing of a bat.

(B) the wing of an insect and the wing of a bird.

(C)   the arm of a human and the flipper of a seal.

(D)   the wing of a penguin and the foreleg of a turtle.

189.   Genetic variation is acted upon by natural selection to cause evolutionary change. Which of the following conditions would NOT be susceptible to natural selection?

(A)   A recessive allele in the homozygous condition

(B)   A dominant allele in the heterozygous condition

(C)   A recessive allele in the heterozygous condition

(D)   A dominant allele in the homozygous condition

190.   Contemporary models of Earth's primordial atmosphere predict the presence of little or no free

(A)   hydrogen.   (B)   nitrogen.

(C)   oxygen.   (D)   carbon dioxide.

191.   Which of the following intrinsic isolation mechanisms would act to prevent production of interspecific hybrids AFTER mating of the parents?

(A)   Behavioral isolation

(B)   Mechanical isolation

(C)   Ecogeographic isolation

(D)   Developmental isolation

192.   Which of the following is NOT a general characteristic of chordates?

(A)   Pharyngeal gill slits

(B)   Vertebral column

(C)   Dorsal hollow nerve cord

(D)   Notochord

193.   The best definition of an organism's "fitness" in the evolutionary sense is its

(A)   ability to perform optimally in its environment.

(B)   chances of survival.

(C)   probable genetic contribution to future generations.

(D)   physical condition at reproductive maturity.

194.   Which of the following is NOT a distinguishing characteristic of a species as it is understood in modern biology?

(A)   Ability to mate within the group

(B)   Sharing of a common gene pool

(C)   A genetically distinct group of natural populations

(D)   Reproductive isolation from all other similar groups

QUESTIONS 195-196 are NOT based on a descriptive passage.

---

195.   The aldol condensation of two molecules of acetaldehyde gives the product

$$2 \text{ CH}_3\overset{\overset{\displaystyle O}{\|}}{\text{CH}} \xrightarrow[\text{H}_2\text{O}]{\text{OH}^- \text{ or H}^+}$$

(A) $\text{CH}_3\overset{\overset{\displaystyle O}{\|}}{\text{C}}-\overset{\overset{\displaystyle O}{\|}}{\text{C}}\text{CH}_3$

(B) $\text{CH}_3-\underset{\underset{\displaystyle \text{CH}_3}{|}}{\text{CH}}-\overset{\overset{\displaystyle O}{\|}}{\text{CH}}$

(C) $\text{CH}_3\underset{\underset{\displaystyle \text{OH}}{|}}{\text{CH}}\text{CH}_2\overset{\overset{\displaystyle O}{\|}}{\text{CH}}$

(D) $\text{CH}_3\overset{\overset{\displaystyle O}{\|}}{\text{C}}\text{CH}_2\overset{\overset{\displaystyle O}{\|}}{\text{CH}}$

196.   The interconversion of glyceraldehyde (1) and dihydroxyacetone (2) involves the intermediate

$$\underset{\underset{\displaystyle \text{OH} \ \ \text{OH}}{| \ \ \ |}}{\text{CH}_2\text{CH}\overset{\overset{\displaystyle O}{\|}}{\text{CH}}} \rightleftharpoons \underset{\underset{\displaystyle \text{OH} \ \ \text{OH}}{| \ \ \ |}}{\text{CH}_2\overset{\overset{\displaystyle O}{\|}}{\text{C}}\text{CH}_2}$$

(A) $\text{CH}_2{=}\text{CH}\overset{\overset{\displaystyle O}{\|}}{\text{CH}}$

(B) $\underset{\underset{\displaystyle \text{OH} \ \text{OH} \ \text{OH}}{| \ \ \ | \ \ \ |}}{\text{CH}_2\text{C}{=}\text{CH}}$

(C) $\underset{\underset{\displaystyle \text{OH}}{|}}{\text{CH}_2\text{CHCH}}\overset{+ \ \overset{\displaystyle O}{\|}}{}$

(D) $\underset{\underset{\displaystyle \text{OH}}{|}}{\text{CH}_2\text{CHCH}}\overset{- \ \overset{\displaystyle O}{\|}}{}$

PASSAGE IX (Questions 197-204)

There are generally considered to be four major tissue types in vertebrates — epithelial, connective, muscle, and nerve. Within each category can be found subcategories with specialized cell types and/or intercellular matrices.

While many cells have some contractile properties, muscle tissues exhibit the characteristic to a much greater extent. The three principal types of muscle tissue are known as skeletal, smooth, and cardiac. The ability to generate and propagate electrochemical membrane potentials is critical to the function of these tissues. The functional unit of skeletal and cardiac muscle is known as a sarcomere and is visible us-

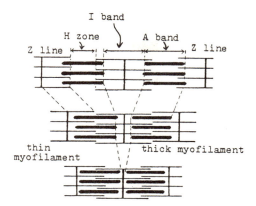

Figure. Changes in banding pattern resulting from the movements of thick and thin filaments past each other during contraction.

Figure 1

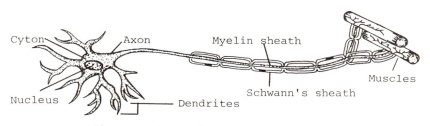

The structure of a neuron.

Figure 2

ing electron microscopy. A diagram of a sarcomere is given in Figure 1.

Nerve cells are specialized for response to a variety of stimuli and for the rapid transmission of changes in electrochemical membrane potentials (i.e., action potentials or nerve impulses). The extensions of nerve cells, known as fibers, can be quite long thereby distinguishing certain neurons as the longest cells in the body. A drawing of a myelinated motor neuron is given in Figure 2.

The establishment of an initial (resting) electrostatic potential depends largely on a differential "leakage" of potassium and, to a lesser extent, sodium ions across the membrane of the neuron. Propagation of a nerve impulse is accomplished by a series of momentary ion-specific changes in membrane permeability that first allow sodium ions to rush into the cell and then allow potassium ions to rush out of the cell, thereby reversing polarity of the membrane briefly. The resting potential is regenerated by local diffusion of ions away from the membrane surface while a sodium-potassium pump aids in maintaining the sodium and potassium ion concentration gradients across the membrane. Transmission of an impulse between neurons or between a neuron and an effector occurs at synapses. These synapses may involve a direct coupling of cells (through gap junctions) or, more commonly, a narrow space known as a synaptic cleft. Where synaptic clefts are involved, transmission depends on chemical neurotransmitters released by the presynaptic membrane that diffuse across the cleft. The neurotransmitters may have an excitatory or inhibitory effect on the postsynaptic membrane.

197. Which of the following statements correctly describes a fully contracted sarcomere compared to one that is relaxed?

    (A)   The A-band remains the same length.

    (B)   The H-zone remains the same length.

    (C)   The I-bands remain the same length.

    (D)   The Z-lines remain equidistant from each other.

198. Striations and multiple nuclei are characteristic of _____ muscle.

    (A)   smooth   (B)   skeletal

    (C)   cardiac   (D)   skeletal and cardiac

199. The normal resting potential of a neuron is about _____ millivolts.

    (A)   120   (B)   12

    (C)   -45   (D)   -70

200. Which of the following sensory or motor tissues would most likely have electrical synapses?

    (A)   Cardiac muscle   (B)   Skeletal muscle

    (C)   Retina   (D)   Pressure receptors

201. When an action potential moves along skeletal muscle fibers, calcium ions are released from the sarcoplasmic reticulum. The calcium ions bind with what molecular component of the thin filaments?

    (A)   Actin   (B)   Troponin complex

    (C)   Myosin   (D)   Tropomyosln

202. The openings through which sodium and potassium ions move to create an action potential are known as _____ channels.

    (A)   potential   (B)   electrochemical

    (C)   ion   (D)   voltage-gated

203. Many neurons outside the central nervous system are enveloped by neuroglial cells called Schwann cells, which give rise to myelin sheaths. Compared to the speed of other nerve impulses, those moving along axons with myelinated sheaths travel

    (A)   much faster.   (B)   slightly faster.

    (C)   slightly slower.   (D)   much slower.

204. As the sodium-potassium pump functions in a neuron membrane, _____ Na^+ is/are pumped out for every _____ k^+ pumped in.

(A) 1 ... 2   (B) 2 ... 3

(C) 3 ... 2   (D) 2 ... 1

PASSAGE X (Questions 205-208)

Nucleophilic substitution reactions involve the displacement of a leaving gorup by a nucleophile.

$$Nu: \quad + \quad C—X \longrightarrow Nu—C \quad + \quad X:$$

If this occurs in a one-step reaction, it is called an S_N2 mechanism. S_N2 reactions proceed with inversion of configuration at chiral centers and echibit second-order kinetics:

Rate = k[Nu][R - X].

A one-step reaction, S_N1, involves a reactive intermediate, (1), and exhibits first-order kinetics:

Rate = k[R - X].

Because the intermediate can react with the nucleophile to give both enantiomers, a racemate is formed.

$$C—X \xrightarrow{\text{slow}} (1) \quad + \quad X^-$$

$$(1) \quad + \quad Nu: \xrightarrow{\text{fast}} Nu—C \quad + \quad C—Nu$$

205. What kind of intermediate is (1)?

(A) A carbanion   (B) A carbocation

(C) An enolate   (D) A free radical

206. For the reaction

$$\underset{(2)}{NaOC_2H_5} \quad + \quad \underset{(3)}{(R)-PhCHBr} \xrightarrow{C_2H_5OH} PhCHOC_2H_5 \quad + \quad NaBr$$

with CH_3 groups on the PhCHBr and PhCHOC₂H₅ carbons

What is the mechanism and expected rate equation if the product is found to be devoid of optical activity?

(A) S_n2, Rate = k[2][3]   (B) S_n2, Rate = k[3]

(C) S_n1, Rate = k[2]   (D) S_n1, Rate = k[3]

207. Elimination reactions compete with substitution reactions. What is the major elimination product of the following reaction?

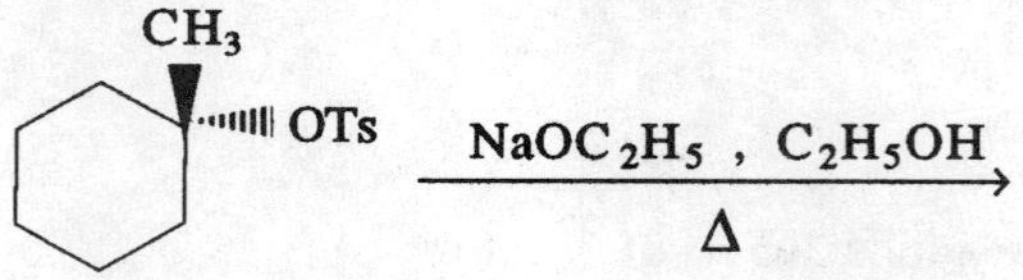

(A) 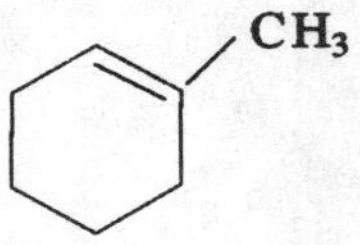 CH_3

(B) 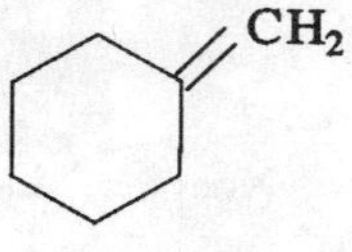 CH_2

(C) 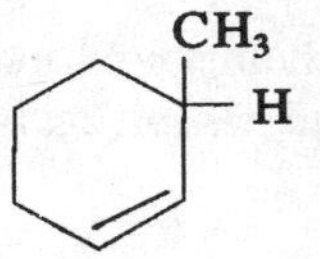 CH_3 — H

(D) 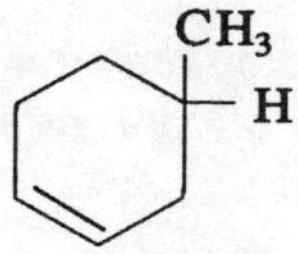 CH_3 — H

208. Acid-catalyzed elimination of alcohols can produce alkenes with rearranged carbon atoms, e.g.,

$$Ph-\underset{\underset{CH_3}{|}}{CH}-CH_2OH \xrightarrow[\Delta]{H+} Ph-\underset{\underset{CH_3}{|}}{C}=CH_2 + Ph-CH=CH-CH_3$$

Which of the following alcohols will not produce rearranged product when heated with acid?

(A) $CH_3CH_2-\underset{\underset{HO}{|}}{CH}-\underset{\underset{H}{|}}{\overset{\overset{CH_3}{|}}{C}}-CH_3$

(B) $(CH_3)_3COH$

(C) $CH_3CH_2CH_2CH_2OH$

(D) $(CH_3)_2CH-\underset{\underset{OH}{|}}{CH}-CH_3$

PASSAGE XI (Questions 209-213)

Many diseases are the result of pathogenic microorganisms that have become sufficiently numerous in an animal to directly affect their normal metabolism and bodily functions. Following the acceptance of Pasteur's Germ Theory of Disease in the late 1800s, many such pathogens were identified and found to be the cause of common diseases. Bacteria and viruses, as well as some eucaryotic microorganisms, were among the pathogens discovered.

Experiment 1:

An animal was brought into a diagnostic laboratory suffering from an unknown ailment and was placed in an isolation area. Since the body temperature of the sick animal was elevated, the diagnostician suspected a pathogen was involved, but the symptoms did not match those caused by any known microorganism. Blood work in the pathology lab indicated that a bacillus bacterium was present and that this bacillus was also present in blood samples of other afflicted animals from the same population.

Experiment 2:

After trying a variety of culture protocols and growth media, technicians found they could aerobically maintain a pure culture of the bacillus on blood agar at 37 degrees Celsius. Sufficient cultures of the presumed pathogenic bacillus were produced to test its virulence on laboratory animals.

Experiment 3:

Healthy animals that had never shown characteristics similar to the ailments of the original animal were inoculated with pure cultures of the bacillus. They developed the same symptoms as the original animal that had been brought into the lab. They were also placed in isolation. The disease progressed in these test animals just as it had in the one first brought into the lab.

Experiment 4:

Subsequent blood work showed an identical bacillus was now widespread in the systems of the test animals. When these bacillus were cultured by the same protocol, they showed the same morphological and metabolic characteristics as the bacterial bacillus isolate.

209. The diagnosticians concluded that the bacterial bacillus isolate they had initially found was indeed the cause of the animal's disease. They could draw this conclusion from the results of

   (A)   Experiment 1 only.

   (B)   Experiments 1 and 2 only.

   (C)   Experiments 1, 2, and 3 only.

   (D)   The results of all four experiments were necessary for this conclusion.

210. Viruses attack bacterial cells as well as eucaryotic cells. The protein coat, or capsid, of a virus encloses a core of

   (A)   RNA or DNA.   (B)   RNA only

   (C)   DNA only.   (D)   RNA and DNA.

211. Which of the following cytological structures are NOT found in any bacteria?

   (A)   Polysaccharide cell wall   (B)   Ribosomes

   (C)   Mitochondria   (D)   Cell membrane

212. The procedures described in the passage were used by Robert Koch to discover the cause of which disease in humans?

   (A)   Bubonic plague   (B)   Tuberculosis

   (C)   Cholera   (D)   Leprosy

213. A particular bacterium requires about 45 minutes to divide by fission into 2 cells. If 10 bacteria are originally inoculated into a fresh culture medium and you assume all cells survive, approximately how many bacteria will exist after 12 hours of culture?

(A) 75,000   (B) 225,000

(C) 475,000   (D) 650,000

QUESTIONS 214-219 are NOT based on a descriptive passage.

---

214. The autonomic nervous system is involved when you

(A) sight a deer and turn your head to see it more clearly.

(B) run to catch the bus and develop a rapid heart rate, an increase in respiration rate, and an increase in blood pressure.

(C) are hit by a hammer on your knee and your knee jerks.

(D) walk barefoot, step on a thorn and immediately raise your foot.

215. _____ are not examples of homologous structures.

(A) The flippers of whales and the wings of bats

(B) The wings of bats and the wings of birds

(C) The wings of birds and the wings of butterflies

(D) The forelegs of cats and the arms and hands of humans

216. When two long-winged flies are mated, their progeny consist of 77 flies with long wings and 24 flies with short wings. The parental geontypes are

(A) LI × LI.   (B) LL × LL

(C) II × II.   (D) LL × LI.

217. Which of the following is mismatched?

(A) Lymphatic system-regulation of body temperature, depot for glycogen, cholesterol and water

(B) Nervous system-reception, conduction, integration

(C) Skeletal system-posture, locomoation, blood cell production

(D) Gastrointestinal system-absorption, secretion, digestion, egestion

218. The somatic nervous system controls

(A) heart (cardiac) muscle.

(B) smooth muscle.

(C) skeletal (striated) muscle.

(D) the arrector pili.

219. A plant with no meristematic tissue will be unable to

    (A)   photosynthesize.   (B)   transport water.

    (C)   transport nutrients.   (D)   produce fruits.

STOP

If time still remains, you may review work only in this section.

TEST 4

ANSWER KEY

1.	(D)	26.	(C)	51.	(A)	76.	(B)
2.	(D)	27.	(B)	52.	(C)	77.	(C)
3.	(B)	28.	(D)	53.	(B)	78.	(A)
4.	(B)	29.	(A)	54.	(C)	79.	(B)
5.	(A)	30.	(D)	55.	(C)	80.	(B)
6.	(A)	31.	(B)	56.	(D)	81.	(C)
7.	(B)	32.	(A)	57.	(D)	82.	(D)
8.	(C)	33.	(C)	58.	(C)	83.	(D)
9.	(A)	34.	(D)	59.	(B)	84.	(A)
10.	(C)	35.	(A)	60.	(D)	85.	(C)
11.	(A)	36.	(A)	61.	(B)	86.	(D)
12.	(A)	37.	(A)	62.	(D)	87.	(D)
13.	(B)	38.	(D)	63.	(D)	88.	(C)
14.	(D)	39.	(B)	64.	(A)	89.	(B)
15.	(B)	40.	(A)	65.	(C)	90.	(D)
16.	(C)	41.	(B)	66.	(D)	91.	(D)
17.	(B)	42.	(B)	67.	(A)	92.	(C)
18.	(A)	43.	(A)	68.	(A)	93.	(B)
19.	(D)	44.	(B)	69.	(D)	94.	(B)
20.	(C)	45.	(B)	70.	(A)	95.	(D)
21.	(B)	46.	(D)	71.	(C)	96.	(D)
22.	(A)	47.	(B)	72.	(B)	97.	(B)
23.	(B)	48.	(A)	73.	(D)	98.	(D)
24.	(B)	49.	(B)	74.	(C)	99.	(A)
25.	(A)	50.	(C)	75.	(A)	100.	(D)

101.	(A)	131.	(D)	161.	(B)	191.	(D)
102.	(C)	132.	(D)	162.	(A)	192.	(B)
103.	(B)	133.	(D)	163.	(D)	193.	(C)
104.	(A)	134.	(C)	164.	(D)	194.	(A)
105.	(C)	135.	(D)	165.	(C)	195.	(C)
106.	(D)	136.	(B)	166.	(A)	196.	(B)
107.	(C)	137.	(D)	167.	(B)	197.	(A)
108.	(B)	138.	(D)	168.	(C)	198.	(B)
109.	(B)	139.	(C)	169.	(C)	199.	(D)
110.	(A)	140.	(C)	170.	(D)	200.	(A)
111.	(C)	141.	(C)	171.	(A)	201.	(B)
112.	(B)	142.	(A)	172.	(A)	202.	(D)
113.	(A)	143.	(B)	173.	(A)	203.	(A)
114.	(D)	144.	(A)	174.	(D)	204.	(C)
115.	(D)	145.	(A)	175.	(A)	205.	(B)
116.	(C)	146.	(C)	176.	(B)	206.	(D)
117.	(A)	147.	(D)	177.	(C)	207.	(A)
118.	(D)	148.	(C)	178.	(D)	208.	(B)
119.	(D)	149.	(A)	179.	(C)	209.	(D)
120.	(A)	150.	(D)	180.	(A)	210.	(A)
121.	(C)	151.	(B)	181.	(C)	211.	(C)
122.	(B)	152.	(D)	182.	(D)	212.	(B)
123.	(A)	153.	(D)	183.	(A)	213.	(D)
124.	(B)	154.	(A)	184.	(D)	214.	(B)
125.	(D)	155.	(A)	185.	(B)	215.	(C)
126.	(B)	156.	(C)	186.	(D)	216.	(A)
127.	(C)	157.	(D)	187.	(A)	217.	(A)
128.	(A)	158.	(A)	188.	(B)	218.	(C)
129.	(D)	159.	(C)	189.	(C)	219.	(D)
130.	(C)	160.	(B)	190.	(C)		

DETAILED EXPLANATIONS
OF ANSWERS

Section 1 — Verbal Reasoning

PASSAGE I (Questions 1-9)

1. **(D)** is correct. In the second paragraph, (B) and (C) are listed as factors identifying Hancock with the patriots. (A) is given as an additional factor at the start of the third paragraph. (D) is not given as a factor which tied Hancock to the patriots.

2. **(D)** While it is important to note Hancock's wealth (C), it is more important to show Hancock's loyalty to America (D) by losing money during a war which he supported and helped direct. Hancock's devotion to America is never questioned (B), and Hancock's connection with England, a purely business relation, in no way influenced the large American resistance to the Stamp Act.

3. **(B)** Hancock did not have the military experience to run an army like George Washington, the man elected as commander-in-chief (I), nevertheless, Hancock was a major general in 1778. His expedition failed, however, making Option II incorrect. Because of this loss, one may assume that Hancock overestimated his political abilities, Option III.

4. **(B)** is correct. In the fifth paragraph, mention is made of his egotism, which "regularly aroused the antipathy of many Members." Regarding (A), the passage states that Hancock's fortune was dented by wartime financial reverses. (C) is false, for Hancock was accused of smuggling, but the charges were dropped. His political activity and egotism show that (D) is false.

5. **(A)** is the best answer. The narrative reports matters of public record and does not purport to give elements from the other kinds of sources listed.

6. **(A)** Although Hancock lost the one military action which he led, Hancock was highly involved in American politics and elected to many political seats. The passage states that Hancock remained very egotistical (I), even though he lost a great deal of his wealth (III) during the war.

7. **(B)** Hancock remained popular and idolized by Americans throughout a great part of his political career. Because of this, Hancock held many political positions, including re-election as Governor (A), a chair at the Massachusetts convention (C), and seats in Congress (D).

8. **(C)** British customs officials, bolstered by the presence of a warship in the Boston harbor, seized one of Hancock's ships after accusing him of smuggling. Repercussions of this action resulted in the Boston Massacre. Hancock *did* support

the Stamp Act (A), and was falsely accused of smuggling (D). Adams successfully defended Hancock in court *after* the Boston Massacre (B).

9.   **(A)**   is correct. In the sixth paragraph, we learn that Hancock remained a member of Congress until 1780 and for the rest of his life (13 years) "solidified his political position in Massachusetts." During this period, he did serve in Congress for a time and he did serve as Governor for a time, but he did neither for the whole thirteen year period, therefore, (C) and (D) are not entirely correct. There is no evidence for (B).

PASSAGE II (Questions 10-18)

10.   **(C)**   President Adams and his wife were the first occupants of the White House in November 1800. This is right after the government moved to Washington (D). The interior had not yet been completed (B). The passage also states that during construction or very soon after, the White House was painted white, therefore (A) is incorrect because the grey color was immediately painted over, not left unpainted for the first years of the building's existence like the question poses.

11.   **(A)**   The original architect of the White House, James Hoban, was Irish and most likely fashioned the White House after a duke's mansion in Dublin. French architects *later* helped design additions (Option II), and the British had no part in the building's construction (Option III).

12.   **(A)**   is correct. The passage states that cornerstone was laid in October of 1792 and we have that the first occupancy took place in November of 1800, so there was an eight year period of construction.

13.   **(B)**   During the War of 1812 when the British captured the city and burned the White House, only the building's exterior walls and interior brickwork remained. The White House was only rebuilt once after this 1812 fire, not twice (A). It has, however, undergone extensive renovations, making (C) incorrect. The building has retained its simple design, nevertheless, making (D) also incorrect.

14.   **(D)**   Only the first floor of the White House is opened to the public on a special schedule. The ground floor is for the Presidential family and guests, so Option I is not true. Also, none of the wings are open to the public, so Option III is also not true, therefore, I and III are the answers.

15.   **(B)**   is the best answer. In the next to last paragraph, there are six rooms listed on the first floor of the main building. We are not told that there are any more.

16.   **(C)**   is correct. This point is made in the opening paragraph, and no claim is made about the elements listed in the other choices.

17.   **(B)**   When U.S. troops destroyed some Canadian buildings, the British in retaliation captured Washington (A) and burned the White House leaving only walls and brickwork unharmed (C). Reconstruction of the building caused it to be unfit and unfinished for living until 1817 when President Monroe moved in (D). The French

did not offer any assistance in reconstructing the White House, although two French architects, L'Enfant and Latrobe, worked on designs for additions for the buildings before and after the 1812 reconstruction. Therefore, (C) is not true, and is the answer.

18.   **(A)**   is the answer. In the next to last paragraph, we are given a listing of rooms, and only one President's name is attached to any of these rooms, the name of Lincoln. Notice that the question is not about how many rooms are named after presidents (2 are given), but rather after how many presidents rooms are named.

PASSAGE III (Questions 19-28)

19.   **(D)**   is correct. This point is made at the end of the second paragraph. Notice that they are not favored fuels because they are more common, as (C) claims; if they are more common, it is because they are favored and simpler and cheaper to produce.

20.   **(C)**   Methanol is the simplest, not the most complex (D), alcohol and is most commonly produced by coal, a non-renewable source, not in ample supply (A), that is costly to use (B). Research focuses on environmentally safe production of methanol (C).

21.   **(B)**   Anhydrous ethanol is pure ethanol, not an ethanol mixture (Option II). Because it is a type of ethanol, it, too, is measured in proof gallons, so Option III is an aspect of anhydrous ethanol. The word anhydrous means without water, or water-free, so Option I is another aspect of it.

22.   **(A)**   More research is needed, but ethanol and methanol are simple, cost-efficient, environmentally positive fuels that can be blended to power engines. (D) is incorrect because gasohol is a blend of alcohol fuels and gasoline. (B) is incorrect because ethanol and methanol can be used alone to ignite some engines, although not all which also makes (C) incorrect.

23.   **(B)**   is correct. In the next to last paragraph, note that methanol has less than half the energy value of gasoline, while ethanol has less than two thirds the energy value. This means that ethanol can rise to a higher energy level than methanol, to all but a third the value of gasoline as compared with to all but half of methanol. In this same paragraph, we learn that both methanol and ethanol can be used as fuels, making (D) false.

24.   **(B)**   is correct. In the last paragraph, we learn that the number in an "E" blend identifies the percentage of ethanol used. Thus, a blend of E30 would contain 30% ethanol, and 70% gasoline.

25.   **(A)**   is correct. This is taken directly from the very last sentence of the passage.

26.   **(C)**   is correct. This reason is given at the start of the second paragraph. Notice that not all alcohol fuels are cheap to produce and not all come from renew-

able resources. Nothing is said about questions of pollution as a factor in making alcohols valuable fuels.

27. **(B)** is correct. In the fourth paragraph, we learn that ethanol is also called grain alcohol, and we learn in the first paragraph that ethanol has two carbon atoms.

28. **(D)** is correct. This reason is given in the fourth paragraph. The other factors are not relevant by themselves; they do not explain control by the Treasury Department.

PASSAGE IV (Questions 29-38)

29. **(A)** is correct. Notice Lines 8-9 specify the problem as one of how we specify God's attributes. (B) is suggested as associated with one of the responses to the problem (Lines 46-53) and (C) with yet another of the responses (Lines 32-45). (D) is mentioned as involved in still another response, in Lines 10-21.

30. **(D)** is correct. The reasoning here is similar to that in question 1.

31. **(B)** is correct, see Lines 32-45. Neither (A) nor (C) are suggested as responses to the problems and (D) is simply one of the premises of the problem, but not a response to the problem.

32. **(A)** is correct, see Lines 32-45. Both (B) and (C) are suggested as parts of different responses to the problem than that which denies the existence of evil. (D) is wrong because since the existence of evil is denied, it therefore cannot be goodness.

33. **(C)** is correct. The passage presents the problem in Lines 2-9. Statement (4) in Lines 8-9 is represented as following from, and so justified by, statements (1)-(3) in Lines 3-7. No support or justification for any of the other statements comprising the problem is presented.

34. **(D)** is correct, see Lines 8-9. The problem presented is not that God does not exist (A), and neither of (B) nor (C) taken singly. The problem is that God is not both all-good and all-powerful, which is (D).

35. **(A)** is correct, see Lines 10-21. None of the other choices are discussed in the passages as parts of a proposed solution.

36. **(A)** is correct. The first response is in Lines 10-21, the second in Lines 22-31, the third in Lines 32-45, and the fourth in Lines 46-53.

37. **(A)** is correct. Lines 32-34 point out this underlying assumption is noted in the passage. (D) is not an unstated premise of the problem but a part of one of the responses to the problem (Lines 48-53). Choices (B) and (C) are not noted in the passage as assumptions of the problem.

38. **(D)** is correct, see Lines 32-45. The other choices would represent re-

sponses to how we should deal with the existence of evil, but these would not be responses to the problem as posed in Lines 3-9.

PASSAGE V (Questions 39-47)

39. **(B)** is correct, see Lines 3-5 and 23-27. Neither of (A) nor (C) is affirmed in the passage.

40. **(A)** is the answer. Lines 27-37 make clear that existence is assumed to be a property and the argument is that it must be a property of a supremely perfect being. (B), (C) and (D) are not assumptions of the argument. The argument tries to establish (C), from which (B) then follows, and no claim is made in support of (D).

41. **(B)** is correct, see Lines 1-5. (A) is incorrect, since if a thing does not exist, it will not have any properties, including its primary properties. (C) is incorrect because primary properties do not depend on their being known, and (D) is incorrect because an object cannot exist as what it is without its primary properties.

42. **(B)** is correct, see Lines 1-8. Lines 5-8 rule out (A), and consequently both (C) and (D).

43. **(A)** is correct, see Lines 23-30. This rules out (B), and (C) is an independent premise of the argument, not dependent upon God being the most perfect being possible. The argument does not take (D) as following from the stated assumption.

44. **(B)** is the answer, see Lines 38-44. (A) gives no answer to the question of why the argument would not apply to other things and (C) is denied by Lines 23-30 in connection with God.

45. **(B)** is correct. In order to be a woman, it is not necessary that she be a sister, so (A) and (C) are false. (D) is false because there are some women who in fact are not sisters.

46. **(D)** is correct. Individual human beings have, as humans, the same primary properties, but they are not identical so (A) is false, and they do not have the same secondary properties, so (B) is false.

47. **(B)** is correct, see lines 36-37. (A) is true but not what the ontological argument claims and (C) is also not the claim of the argument. The argument does not support (D).

PASSAGE VI (Questions 48-58)

48. **(A)** is correct because it includes the broad spectrum of the discussion of music therapy in the passage. (B) is too narrow in its response. (C) contains an error in isolating teaching from a variety of options. (D) is plainly untrue because it is too vague to be true without qualification.

49. **(B)** Being able to identify (B) as the correct answer means being able to

identify the meaning of the power of music. In the context of Greek music healing the sick, (B) entends the power of healing. (A) is absurd. (D) may be true, but is not so stated in the passage. (C) negates the power of music and therefore the thrust behind the passage.

50. **(C)** (A) is wrong because it states that music therapy replaces an entire profession. (B) puts the word "medical" in the response and that needs clarification. (D) represents one fact about the work of the music therapist. (C) is the most extensive answer and is therefore true.

51. **(A)** (B) implies the opposite meaning of the purpose of music therapy. (C) conveys an exclusive use of music therapy and is not complete according to the information in the passage. (D) may be true, but is not conveyed in the passage.

52. **(C)** (C) is the only possible answer because it refers to an academic purpose, not a healing purpose, of music. (A), (B) and (D) are each positive results of music therapy.

53. **(B)** The passage alludes to (A), (C) and (D) as needed to qualify as a music therapist. (B) refers to self-training while the passage indicates training under supervision.

54. **(C)** (C) is inclusive of the two educational aspects of the preparation to become a music therapist. (A) may be true, but the passage does not suggest this. (B) is too exclusive and fails to include other academic preparation. (D) turns the continuing education of the music therapist into formal requirements of classes. That kind of schooling may be the form continual learning takes, but not necessarily.

55. **(C)** Because a person's will to succeed may vary as much as a person's enjoyment of music, options I and III have the potential to rebuild self-confidence. Therefore, (C) is correct. (A) only represents Option I. Answers (B) and (D) represent option II which is incorrect. Option II states that all people have musical ability, which is false.

56. **(D)** (D) is the only answer that clarifies the fact that music therapists relate to persons with disabilities, rather than to persons either under the care of a physician or nurse, or simply in need of a social worker, like in answers (A), (B) and (C) which are incorrect.

57. **(D)** A dormitory is a place for sleeping and therefore silence is required. Any one of the other places cited may be useful for music in one form or another.

58. **(C)** This answer requires the student to be aware of the simple logic in relating the process of music therapy to the consequences of healing while not inferring any more than this from the passage. Cause and effect might be a logical choice, but that implies a completed fact. In most cases, it is not known that music therapy will indeed heal. It is known that a probable consequence of music therapy is healing. (B) indicates a relationship between symptom and treatment, as (D) indicates a

relationship between disease and health. In both cases a medical model is implied. Both (B) and (D) are too medically specific.

PASSAGE VII (Questions 59-65)

59.   **(B)**   An important aspect of the U.S. Navy fleet is its kinship to its air force, which enables both to protect the skies and seas at the same time; therefore option II is correct. There is not enough information in the passage to know if the U.S. Navy is the oldest of the Armed Forces, so (A) and (D) are incorrect because they offer option I. Option III suggests that the U.S. Navy is similar to the British Navy, when in fact, the failure of the early British Navy was due to its lack of development between itself and its air force — a key aspect of the U.S. Navy; therefore (C) is incorrect because option III is presented.

60.   **(D)**   The key word in this question is "significant." Although a new craft joined the Navy on that day, (A) doesn't account for its impact on the U.S. (B) is an assumption one cannot make on the basis of the information given. (C) is deceptive because of the qualifier "most."

61.   **(B)**   This answer is correct because it is the most thorough and complete answer. (A) is exclusive. (C) is incorrect because there is not enough information in this passage to determine this. Though the idea of a navy was important to Capt. Mahan, it cannot be concluded that the Navy was the idea of one individual, therefore (D) is incorrect.

62.   **(D)**   (A) presumes a cause-effect relationship among war, Navy and history. While they are related, the causal connection is not suggested in this passage. (B) is an unfounded statement. (C) avoids the question. (D) is the only complete and accurate answer based on the information in the passage.

63.   **(D)**   (A) is a negative statement refuted by the essay. (B) undermines the joint efforts of Air Force and Army. (C) is restrictive in its focus and leaves "maternal care" unclear. (D) focuses on the theme of the essay and captures the essence of it; therefore it is correct.

64.   **(A)**   Because the passage emphasizes the complexity of need for development and cooperation between the many facets of the Armed Forces, option I is correct. Options II and III are incorrect because peace is never mentioned in the article, just history of the Navy, and no judgments are made as to the ramifications of having a navy. Because (A) offers option I, it is correct. Because (B), (C), (D) offer options II and III, they are incorrect.

65.   **(C)**   (C) is the appropriate answer since it goes no further than the essay suggests. (A) and (B) read "only" and that eliminates other possibilities. (D) is incorrect because based on the information in the passage, there is no cause-effect relationship between weapons and open sea lanes unless war is assumed to have been declared.

Section 2 — Physical Sciences

PASSAGE I (Questions 66-72)

66. **(D)**   Solution D is the only solution that has a concentration lower than that of a saturated solution at the same temperature. Solution C is saturated (and at the same temperature as solution D); solutions A, B, and E are supersaturated.

67. **(A)**   Solutions A, B and E are supersaturated (contain an excess of solute at the temperature shown). At higher temperatures, the amount of solute will become that required for saturation. (B) and (C) are incorrect because solution C is already saturated. (D) is incorrect because solution D is unsaturated.

68. **(A)**   Supersaturated solutions A, B, and E contain more solute than allowed by equilibrium considerations; they are unstable to addition of solute. (B) and (C) are incorrect because solution C is saturated. (D) is incorrect because solution D is unsaturated.

69. **(D)**   Solution E has a higher value on the solubility axis than solutions A, B, and D, i.e., it has the highest number of grams of solute/100 grams of water.

70. **(A)**   This solution contains less solute than that required for saturation at 80°C (170 g KNO_3/100 g water), therefore it must be unsaturated. (B) and (D) are incorrect because the solution does not contain enough solute to be saturated. (C) is incorrect because the solution does not contain a higher concentration of solute than that required for saturation.

71. **(C)**   The solubility of KNO_3 at 80°C is about 170 k KNO_3/100 g water.

$$? \text{ g water} = 85 \text{ g } KNO_3 \times \frac{100 \text{ g water}}{170 \text{ g } KNO_3} = 50 \text{ g water}$$

Incorrect answers can result from misreading the solubility and/or setting up an equation in which the units do not cancel out to produce units of g of water.

72. **(B)**   The solubility of KNO_3 at 20°C is about 30 k KNO_3/100 g water.

$$? \text{ } KNO_3 = 60 \text{g water} \times \frac{30 \text{ g } KNO_3}{100 \text{ g water}} = 18 \text{ g } KNO_3$$

Incorrect answers can result from misreading the solubility and/or setting up an equation in which the units do not cancel out to produce units of g of KNO_3.

PASSAGE II (Questions 73-80)

73. **(D)**   The region to the left of line *AB* is the solid region. The region to the right is the vapor region. All points along the line represent temperatures and pressures at which the solid is in equilibrium with the vapor.

74. **(C)**   The two variables that must be specified are temperature and pressure.

75. **(A)** Point F is in the solid region. Point E is in the liquid region. The phase change when a solid changes to liquid is melting. (B) is incorrect because boiling is a change from liquid to vapor. (C) is incorrect because sublimation is a change from solid to vapor. (D) is incorrect because condensation is a change from vapor to liquid.

76. **(B)** Point E is in the liquid region. Lowering the pressure will cause the substance to enter the vapor region (below line *BD*). Thus the liquid will become a vapor.

77. **(C)** Because the pressure at the triple point, the point at which solid, liquid, and vapor coexist in equilibrium, is greater than 1.00 atm, CO_2 solid will not melt. Instead it is converted directly into a vapor, i.e., it sublimes.

78. **(A)** Line *BC* is the melting point curve. For CO_2, as for most substances, this line has a positive slope. The higher the pressure along this curve, the higher the corresponding melting point.

79. **(B)** An increase in pressure favors the formation of the more dense phase. Since an increase in pressure on CO_2 results in the conversion of liquid to solid, the solid phase is the more dense one.

80. **(B)** Point F is in the solid region. (A) is incorrect because point *E* is in the liquid region. (C) is incorrect because point B represents equilibrium between solid, liquid, and vapor. (D) is incorrect because this line represents equilibrium between solid and liquid.

PASSAGE III (Questions 81-86)

81. **(C)** The quantity of N_2 required to produce the NH_3 is calculated from a knowledge of the stoichiometric coefficients of the balanced equation:

$$? \frac{\text{mole } N_2}{L} = 0.150 \frac{\text{mol } NH_3}{L} \times \frac{1 \text{ mol } N_2}{2 \text{ mol } NH_3}$$

$$= 0.075 \frac{\text{mol } N_2}{L}$$

Subtracting this quantity from the initial N_2 concentration gives the remaining N_2 concentration:

$$[N_2] = 0.500 \text{ M} - 0.075 \text{ M} = 0.425 \text{ M}$$

(A) is incorrect because some N_2 must remain at equilibrium. (B) is incorrect because the N_2 concentration must decrease rather than increase. (D) is incorrect because the N_2 concentration must decrease from its initial value.

82. **(D)** The equilibrium constant is equal to the product of the molar concentrations at equilibrium of the products, each raised to the stoichiometric coefficient in the balanced equation, divided by the product of the molar concentrations at equilibrium of the reactants, each raised to the stoichometric coefficient in the balanced

equation. (A) and (B) are incorrect becuase they show reactant concentrations in the numerator and product concentrations in the denominator. (C) is incorrect because the molar concentrations should not be multiplied by the stoichiometric coefficients.

83.　**(D)**　When the volume is decreased, the concentrations of all substances is increased. (A) and (B) are incorrect because the equilibrium would shift to the right, resulting in fewer H_2 and N_2 molecules. (C) is incorrect becuase the equilibrium shift to the right would result in more NH_3 molecules.

84.　**(A)**　Since $\Delta H°$ is negative, this reaction is exothermic and the heat term is on the right-hand side of the equation. An increase in temperature (added heat) shifts the equilibrium position to the left to remove some of the excess heat. As a result, N_2 molecules are formed. (B) is incorrect because the number of NH_3 molecules decreases. (C) and (D) are incorrect because the number of H_2 and of N_2 molecules increases.

85.　**(C)**　The equilibrium will shift to the right to use up some of the added N_2. This will result in the production of additional NH_3 molecules. (A) and (B) are incorrect because the equilibrium constant is unchanged at constant temperature. (D) is incorrect because H_2 molecules react with the added N_2 molecules.

86.　**(D)**　The presence of a catalyst speeds the reverse reaction as well as the forward reaction. (C) is incorrect because the rate of the reverse reaction increases. (A) and (B) are incorrect because the equilibrium constant is unchanged.

87.　**(D)**　If v' is the velocity of the combined system of the pendulum and the bullet right after the collision, then according to the conservation of linear momentum

$$mv = (m + M)v'$$

From the conservation of energy

$$\tfrac{1}{2}(m + M)v'^2 = (m + M)\, gy$$

m ● ⟶
　　v
　　M
initially

finally

↕ y

Some energy has been lost during the collision and converted to heat.

$$v = \frac{M + m}{m} v' = \frac{M + m}{m} \sqrt{2gy}$$

$$= \frac{2.010}{.010} \sqrt{2(9.8)(.20)}$$

$$= 398 \ m/s$$

88. **(C)** Although all the atoms of a given element have exactly the same chemical properties (the same atomic number, Z), they do not always have the same mass. Atoms which are chemically alike but which differ in mass are called isotopes. All isotopes of a given element have the same number of electrons and protons, but have different numbers of neutrons.

89. **(B)** Using the equation

$$Density = \frac{Mass}{Volume}$$

we obtain

Mass = (Density) (Volume).

Since density is in gm/cm^3 let us use the CGS system. Hence, we must convert the measurements of the block into centimeters.

2 meters = 200 centimeters
3 meters = 300 centimeters
5 meters = 500 centimeters

Now, finding the volume of the block

$$V = l \times w \times h = 200 \times 300 \times 500$$

Finally, we can find the mass:

Mass = $(7.8 \ gm/cm^3) (3.0 \times 10^7 \ cm^3)$

Mass = 2.34×10^8 gm

90. **(D)** Acetylcholine is the neurotransmitter which is found at neuromuscular junctions in the brain and at junctions in the internal organs.

91. **(D)** Waxes are esters of long-chain carboxylic acids with long-chain acids. (A) is a glyceride or fat, (B) is a phosphoglyceride, and (C) is glycerol.

92. **(C)** Mild oxidative conditions such as dilute $KMnO_4$ at 0°C serve to oxidize alkenes to diols and aldehydes to carboxylic acids. Ethers and carboxylic acids, however, are resistant to oxidation to mild conditions.

93. **(B)** Balancing the reaction we obtain

$$^{238}_{92}Y \rightarrow {}^{238}_{93}Z + {}^{0}_{-1}X.$$

Since there is no change in mass number and the charge on the emitted particle is - 1, X must be an electron. In this case, a neutron has been split, producing a proton and an electron. The electron is emitted and the proton is retained, resulting in an increase of nuclear charge with no loss of nuclear mass.

94. **(B)** Comparing Experiments 1 and 2: doubling the concentration of X quadruples the rate. This is characteristic of a second order reaction, in which rate depends on concentration to the second power.

95. **(D)**   Since the decomposition is second order in X:

$$\text{rate} = k(X)^2$$

$$k = \frac{\text{rate}}{(X)^2}$$

Using the data from Experiment 1:

$$k = \frac{0.12}{(0.10)^2} = 12$$

96. **(D)**

$$\text{rate} = k(X)^2 = 12(0.30)^2 = 1.1 \text{ mol/L·s}$$

97. **(B)**

$$(X)^2 = \frac{\text{rate}}{k} = \frac{1.08}{12} = 0.090 \quad (X) = \sqrt{0.090} = 0.30 \text{ M}$$

98. **(D)**   For a second order reaction, the half-life is equal to $1/kX_0$.

99. **(A)**

$$\text{rate} = k(X)^2$$

An increase in temperature results in an increase in rate. Both concentration and the order of reaction are unchanged, thus the $(X)^2$ term is unchanged. k must increase to increase the value of the expression on the right-hand side of the rate law equation.

PASSAGE V (Questions 100-106)

100. **(D)**   A negative $\Delta H°$ indicates an exothermic reaction. (C) is incorrect because an endothermic reaction is indicated by a positive ΔH^8. (A) and (B) are incorrect because the value of $\Delta H°$ gives no information about reaction rate.

101. **(A)**

$$\Delta S = S_{\text{products}} - S_{\text{reactants}}$$

Since the value $\Delta S°$ for this reaction is negative, this difference must result from subtracting a larger reactant entropy from a smaller product entropy. (B) is incorrect because subtracting a smaller reactant entropy from a larger entropy results in a positive value of $\Delta S°$. (C) and (D) are incorrect because the value of $\Delta S°$ gives no indication of the rate of reaction.

102. **(C)** $\Delta G°$ has a negative value in this reaction. if $\Delta G°$ is negative, the reaction is spontaneous. (D) is incorrect because a reaction is nonspontaneous only if $\Delta G°$ is positive. (A) and (B) are incorrect because the value of $\Delta G°$ gives no indication of the rate of reaction.

103. **(B)**

$$\Delta G° = \Delta H° - T\Delta S°$$

The reaction will be spontaneous when $\Delta G°$ is negative. Since $\Delta H°$ is negative, this term will tend to make $\Delta G°$ negative. Since $\Delta S°$ is negative, the $-T\Delta S°$ term is positive and will tend to make $\Delta G°$ positive. If T is small enough (at low temperatures), the positive $-T\Delta S°$ term will be smaller than the negative $\Delta H°$ term, and the resulting $\Delta G°$ will be negative.

104. **(A)**

$$? \text{ kJ } = 8 \text{ mol } H_2O \times \frac{-890.3 \text{ kJ}}{2 \text{ mol } H_2O} = -3561.2 \text{ kJ}$$

Incorrect answers can result from setting up an equation in which the units do not cancel out to produce units of kJ.

105. **(C)**

$$? \text{ g } CH_4 = 445.2 \text{ kJ} \times \frac{16 \text{ g } CH_4}{890.3 \text{ kJ}} = 8.0 \text{ g } CH_4$$

Incorrect answers can result from setting up an equation in which the units do not cancel out to produce units of g of CH_4.

106. **(D)**　　$\Delta H°$ for a reaction is equal in magnitude but opposite in sign to $\Delta H°$ for the reverse reaction. The reaction given in this equation is the reverse of the reaction for which the data are given.

$$\Delta H°_{reverse} = -(\Delta H°_{forward})$$

$$= -(-890.3 \text{ kJ})$$

$$= +890.3 \text{ kJ}$$

107. **(C)**

$$\text{Work} = \text{Force} \times \text{distance}$$

We know the distance is 10 meters. We must, however, find F. We use the relationship

$$F = \text{mass} \times \text{acceleration}$$

$$a = 9.8 \text{ m/sec}^2$$

$$m = 25 \text{ kg}$$

$$F = (25 \text{ kg}) (9.8 \text{ m/sec}^2)$$

$$F = 245.0 \text{ kg·m/sec}^2 = 245.0 \text{ newtons}$$

Now, we can substitute into the first equation:

$$\text{Work} = F \times d = (245 \text{ N}) (10 \text{ m}) = 2450 \text{ J}$$

108. **(B)** Diffraction is the tendency of a wave to spread into a region behind an obstruction. This also includes the tendency of a wave to spread out when passing through a small aperture.

109. **(B)** As follicles grow they release increasing amounts of estrogen. The high estrogen levels (or possibly the slowdown in estrogen buildup as the peak is reached) elicit a sharp, spiked surge of luteinizing hormone from the pituitary. This, in turn, triggers the opening of the follicle and ovulation.

110. **(A)** A solution is defined as neutral when the hydronium ion and hydroxide ion concentrations are equal. At 25°C,

$$[H^+] [OH^-] = 10^{-14}$$

and the pH of a neutral solution is 7 when $[H^+] = [OH^-]$. However, just as other equilibrium constants vary with temperatures, $[H^+] [OH^-]$ is not 10^{-14} at other temperatures. This difference allows the pH of a neutral solution to have different values at different temperatures.

111. **(C)** Gallstones are composed of approximately 80% cholesterol.

PASSAGE VI (Questions 112-117)

112. **(B)** An oxidizing agent causes the oxidation of another species. In the process, the oxidizing agent is reduced. Reduction is the gain of electrons. In this reaction, Ag^+ gains electrons and is therefore the oxidizing agent. (D) is incorrect because Ag is the end-product of the reduction. (A) is incorrect becuase Sn is the reducing agent. (C) is incorrect because Sn^{2+} is the end-product of the oxidation of Sn.

113. **(A)** The anode is the electrode where oxidation takes place. Oxidation is the loss of electrons. At the anode:

$$Sn \rightarrow Sn^{2+} + 2e^-.$$

(B), (C), and (D) are incorrect because they are reduction half-reactions.

114. **(D)** Reversing the equation for the standard reduction potential changes the sign of E°:

$$Sn \longrightarrow Sn^{2+} + 2e^- ; \qquad E°_{ox} = + 0.14 \text{ V}$$

Doubling each quantity in the standard reduction potential does not affect E°:

$$2e^- + 2 Ag^+ \longrightarrow 2 Ag; \qquad E°_{red} = + 0.80 \text{ V}$$

Adding the two half-reactions

$$Sn \longrightarrow Sn^{2+} + 2e^- ; \qquad E°_{ox} = + 0.14 \text{ V}$$

$$2e^- + 2 Ag^+ \longrightarrow 2 Ag; \qquad E°_{red} = + 0.80 \text{ V}$$

$$\overline{Sn + 2 Ag^+ \longrightarrow Sn^{2+} + 2 Ag; \quad E°_{tot} = + 0.94 \text{ V}}$$

115. **(D)** In this notation, the anode reactant and product are shown on the left side of the double line; the cathode reactant and product are shown on the right side of the double line; the double line represents a salt bridge. (A) and (B) are incorrect because they show oxidizing and reducing agents together at the anode. (C) is incorrect because the anode and cathode half-reactions are each on the wrong side of the double lines.

116. **(C)** The driving force for voltaic cells is the spontaneity of their reactions. (A) is incorrect because the reaction is reversible. (B) is incorrect because voltaic cells have a positve E°. (D) is incorrect because the reaction takes place at a controlled rate.

117. **(A)** At the anode (Sn) electrons are produced:

$$Sn \longrightarrow Sn^{2+} + 2e^-$$

These electrons travel to the cathode (Ag) where they are picked up by the Ag^+ ions:

$$e^- + At^+ \longrightarrow Ag$$

(B), (C), and (D) are incorrect because they indicate electron flow between forms of the same element.

PASSAGE VII (Questions 118–123)

118. **(D)** The weight of the ball, 100 kg, is the downward-acting gravitational force on the ball.

119. **(D)** The upward forces exerted by the ropes must equal the downward force exerted by the ball, i.e., 100 kg.

120. **(A)** Since the ball does not move, the sum of the forces must be zero.

121. **(C)** $R_1 \sin 30°$ is the y-axis component of the force exerted by rope 1. Rope 2 does not exert a force in the y direction, because the force exerted by rope 2 is normal to the y direction.

122. **(B)** The upward force exerted in the y direction by rope 1, $R_1 \sin 30°$ must equal the downward force exerted by the ball, i.e., 100 kg.

$$R_1 \sin 30° = 100 \text{ kg}$$

$$R_1 = \frac{100 \text{ kg}}{0.500} = 200 \text{ kg}$$

123. **(A)** The sum of the forces acting in the x direction is equal to zero. These forces are provided by rope 2 and the x-component of the force exerted by rope 1.

$$R_2 - R_1 \cos 30° = 0$$

$$R_2 = R_1 \cos 30°$$

$$= (200)\,0.866$$

$$= 173 \text{ kg}$$

PASSAGE VIII (Questions 124-129)

124. **(B)**   For the resistors in parallel:

$$\frac{1}{R_{\text{parallel}}} = \frac{1}{R_1} + \frac{1}{R_2} = \frac{1}{6} + \frac{1}{2}$$

$$R_{\text{parallel}} = \frac{3}{2}\,\Omega$$

125. **(D)**   For the resistors in series:

$$R_{\text{total}} = R_3 + R_p + R_5$$

$$= 7 + \frac{3}{2} + \frac{1}{2} = 9\,\Omega$$

126. **(B)**   Current is the same throughout a series network. Therefore, the current through the 7Ω resistor is the same as the current through the total of the resistors in series given in Question 125.

$$I = \frac{V}{R} = \frac{27}{9} = 3 \text{ amps}$$

127. **(C)**   Now that the current is known the voltage drop is just found by Ohm's Law.

$$V = IR = 3 \times 7 = 21 \text{ volts}$$

128. **(A)**   The voltage drop across the 6Ω resistor is the same as the voltage drop across the equivalent resistance. (R_{parallel} as in Question 124).

$$V = IR = 3 \times \frac{3}{2} = 4.5 \text{ volts}$$

129. **(D)**   The voltage drop across the 6Ω resistor is known from Problem 128 so the current is again found by Ohm's Law.

$$I = \frac{V}{R} = \frac{4.5}{6} = 0.75 \text{ amps}$$

Note: The current in the 2Ω resistor will be 2.25 amps. When this current is added to the .75 amps it will produce the total 3 amps that entered the two parallel resistor network.

PASSAGE IX (Questions 130-134)

130. **(C)** The focal length is half the radius of curvature:

$^1/_2 \times 50$ cm $= 25$ cm.

131. **(D)** The image distance obeys the rule:

$$\frac{1}{f} = \frac{1}{D_0} + \frac{1}{D_i}$$

where f is the focal length (which is negative in a convex mirror), D_0 is the object distance, and D_i is the image distance.

$$\frac{1}{-25 \text{ cm}} = \frac{1}{100 \text{ cm}} + \frac{1}{D_i}$$

$$\frac{1}{D_i} = \frac{-25 \text{ cm} - 100 \text{ cm}}{(25 \text{ cm})(100 \text{ cm})}$$

$$D_i = -20 \text{ cm}$$

The negative sign indicates that the image is behind the mirror.

132. **(D)** The sizes of the object, S_0, and the image, S_i, are in the same ratio as their respective distances.

$$\frac{S_i}{S_0} = \frac{D_i}{D_0}$$

$$S_i = S_0 \left(\frac{D_i}{D_0} \right) = 60 \text{ cm} \left(\frac{-20 \text{ cm}}{100 \text{ cm}} \right) = -12 \text{ cm}$$

133. **(D)** In convex mirrors, the image is always behind the mirror.

134. **(C)** In a plane mirror, the size of the image is always the same as the size of the object.

PASSAGE X (Questions 135-139)

135. **(D)** An increase of one octave represents doubling the frequency:

2×110 Hz $= 220$ Hz

136. **(B)** Since each 10 decibels have 10 times the energy of the softest audible sound, this sound has 10×10 or 100 times the loudness of the softest audible sound.

137. **(D)**   Beats result from alternating constructive and destructive interference. The beat frequency is the difference between the frequencies of the two notes, thus the frequency of the second note is 110 ± 5 Hz.

138. **(D)**   Using the formula given in the problem:

$v = 331 + 0.6(10) = 337$ m/s.

139. **(C)**   The speed of a sound wave depends on the medium in which it travels. It travels faster in elastic solids than in water or air. (A), (B), and (D) are incorrect because sound travels more slowly in water or air than in elastic solids.

140. **(C)**   We would like a lens that brings objects from 25 cm to 100 cm. Note that s' is negative because the image is supposed to be located on the same side of the lens as the object.

$$s = +25 \text{ cm}, \quad s' = -100 \text{ cm}$$

$$\frac{1}{f} = \frac{1}{s} + \frac{1}{s'} = \frac{1}{25} - \frac{1}{100}$$

$$f = 33.3 \text{ cm}$$

141. **(C)**   When the length of a conductor is increased, the number of collisions between free electrons and vibrating atoms is increased. Doubling the length of a conductor doubles the average number of collisions. In general, the resistance is directly proportional to the length of the conductor. Hence, if a piece of wire is doubled in length then its resistance is doubled.

142. **(A)**

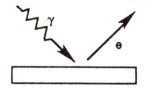

In the photoelectric effect, by conservation of energy

$$h\upsilon = \tfrac{1}{2} mv^2 + \phi$$

where ϕ is the work function of the metal. Furthermore,

$$eV_0 = \tfrac{1}{2} mv^2.$$

Thus the stopping potential V_0 is directly proportional to the incident light frequency υ:

$$eV_0 = hv - \phi \quad \text{or} \quad V_0 = \frac{h}{e} v - \frac{\phi}{e}$$

In fact, this is one way of determining Planck's constant.

Section 3 — Writing Sample

DEMONSTRATION ESSAY 1

Commuters trapped in their cars on a jammed freeway, or those wedged into crammed buses or trains entering or leaving a city, would agree with the statement that in the city "life itself is finally threatened with suffocation." Outsiders who have fought the masses and pollution to reach the city find themselves overwhelmed in vast tracts of glass-faced skyscrapers which honor money and greed. Workers, like drones, live out an existence of depressing sameness, scurrying from appointment to appointment, driven by machines meant to serve them but which often appear to enslave them. Once people have returned to the suburbs — real estate costing so much in cities that few can afford to live there — the cities become desolate wastelands of crime and disease. The homeless and poor sleep on the warm air vents in the doorways of skyscrapers or on station benches which commuters will once again stream by heedlessly the following morning.

Cities, built for man's ease, entertainment, safety, and business have become unlivable, Mumford suggests, because of the accretion of layers of the past. When the Industrial Revolution herded people into cities there was no forethought, little planning as to how such cities could accommodate the millions of people that would eventually attempt city-life. Hence the "city" is built upon the errors of the past and is doomed to repeat them. For example, the water and sewage systems very often belong to the nineteenth century; to repair or replace them would not only bankrupt the city but also disrupt its business life. The mass transport systems designed to carry the labor force into the city are either totally dismantled because of obsolescence, with no funds to resurrect them, or operate on antiquated methods that waste rather than save time and money. The judicial system and police force are strained to the limit, laboring in buildings that belong to another century, or in streets that form a warren in which criminals can escape or turn back upon the enforcer. The very infrastructure of the city seems tottering, ready to fall with the next crime-wave.

No wonder modern man "in sheer defense" invents the museum. How much easier to gaze longingly at the past achievements of man in the Smithsonian than to contemplate the soaring murder rate in the city of Washington, D.C.? Mumford's statement suggests that we cannot survive in the city but we can erect monuments to it.

The museum then becomes a testament to the fact that men once did live in cities and led lives both full and satisfying . Modern man invents the museum as a haven of rest and peace from the modern city life, where people in Florence escape the screech of traffic to wonder at medieval art, and people in New York escape pressure and marvel at the ruins of ancient Egypt. Modern man mulls over the past life of the "city" and perhaps yearns for those places so carefully chosen by our forefathers.

Admittedly Mumford's view is gloomy, seeing only one side of the darkened city. After a period of "urban blight" in the seventies, cities have begun to recapture the magic if not the calm of past city life. Areas that were architecturally stunning but fallen into neglect have been resurrected into art galleries or antique malls bringing more commerce to flagging city coffers. Cynics may scoff at the quality of life in such areas but the city will come to life again if the projects are well conceived. One such project, Faneuil Hall in Boston, exemplifies the aims of a city (which itself was turning into a museum) determined to revitalize its existence.

Similarly, New York, for all its rapidly decaying infrastructure, managed to revive the Seaport area which brings more acclaim with each new development of the project. "The city that never sleeps" offers the best in drama, ballet and music for those who can afford it. If, like Boston, New York would serve the people with improved travel and housing, the city could live again as the civilized metropolis it once was.

In other words, city life can be resurrected. The seemingly out-of-grasp civility of past eras can be relived outside of the museum. There is a place for the city in the life of modern man — we simply have to be more careful and thoughtful about the *quality* of life we choose for the city. Culture should be available for everyone. Parks should be safe for joggers at midnight. Riverfronts should be populated by thriving businesses. The displaced poor must be offered humane living conditions. We should preserve the life of the city within the city and not simply within the museum.

EXPLANATION OF ESSAY 1

The essay deals with all three tasks fully, paying particular attention to the key words of the tasks, *explain*, *describe* and *discuss*. Paragraphs one through four explain thoroughly each part of the statement: the suffocating life of the modern city; the reason for this being the accretions of the past; the invention of the museum as a defense. The opening paragraph involves the reader in the explanation because most people have suffered city commutes. It also introduces the notion of city dwellers as drones, an idea which plays as a useful motif.

Paragraph two deals with the "layer upon layer of past times" showing how the past has caused problems in the present, using specific examples from the life of the city. Paragraphs three and four extend the explanation into the concept of the museum becoming a monument to the city, a testament that men could once survive happily within a city.

Paragraph five sets up an argument against the statement that cities are indeed livable for the modern man, giving specific examples of cities that have revitalized themselves. Paragraph six then discusses the place of the modern city, picking up details from the previous paragraphs to bring the essay to a satisfying "wrapped up" ending.

Each paragraph is clearly structured with a topic sentence, limiting sentence, and evidence to back up the topic. For example paragraph two sets up the topic sentence about cities being unlivable. Two limiting sentences focus on past lack of planning and present living with errors. The next sentence gives examples to "prove" the central point. The last sentence gives a dramatic conclusion suggesting that cities are about to crumble. The entire paragraph reads like a miniature essay, as it should.

Each sentence in each paragraph relates to another, often by giving very simple "signals" to the reader. Time links or transitions like" *Once* people have returned to the suburbs ..." (paragraph one), introductory phrases such as *"For example ..."* (paragraph two), and comparison links such as *"Similarly ..."* (paragraph three) are several examples. All such linking devices make for unity within the paragraph and push the meaning forward.

Beside sentence links within the paragraphs, strong links or transitions *between* the paragraphs hold the essay together: "No wonder modern man ..." (paragraph two into three) simply picks up on all the negatives of the previous paragraph and moves to the point of the museum smoothly ... "As a result" would also have worked but is not so forceful. "The museum *then* becomes a testament ..."(paragraph three into four) is both a time transition and a consequence transition ..." Thus would have also worked but is more formal than the voice of the essay requires. "In other words, city life can be resurrected." (last paragraph) gathers together all the previous points and moves the reader to the conclusion.

Overall the writing is clear and to the point. The sentence structure is varied, mixing long sentences with multiple subordinate clauses: "Outsiders who have fought the masses" ... (paragraph one), with short simple sentences: "Culture should be available for everyone ..." (last paragraph). Vocabulary is apt "Commuters *trapped ... wedged ... crammed* ..." (paragraph one). The mechanics of the paper: spelling, punctuation, syntax are sound, all working together to provide an unimpeded piece of prose for the reader.

DEMONSTRATION ESSAY 2

Ideally, in the "best of all possible worlds," the concept of all men being created equal, with "equal worth and equal rights" should indeed work. No matter what race, gender, class or religion people are born into, they should have equality if the nation into which they are born has committed itself to such a belief. It should not matter what color people are born with because all colors should be equal, one not having more positive connotation over the others. When a nation like America committed itself to equality, a certain idealism was at play. The men making the commitment of belief, signing the belief into law, were automatically superior to those for whom they were making the commitment: the masses, many illiterate, many incapable of signing, never mind reading the document pledging equality. However, having made such a pledge, every member of the nation should set aside personal ambition and preferences to promote equal worth and equal rights. All people should be entitled to housing and the safety of the family home. All people should live in neighborhoods where it is safe to walk after dark. Jobs and education should be available to all, each person receiving equal not elitist treatment. Expert health care should be available for everyone at the same cost, at the same level of excellence. Lastly, each person within the nation should be accorded equal worth, human dignity, owning a name and identity that all respect, equally. There should be race harmony within a nation made up of a "salad bowl" of peoples; no class system because class suggests a caste system of "higher" and "lower"; and a melding of different religions because no one religious choice is "better" than another.

Of course in the real world, George Orwell's statement holds more validity than Catton's: "All{men} are born equal but some are more equal than others." A child born into the "Nob Hill" area of a city in America will definitely be "more equal" than one born in an inner-city ghetto. A Nob Hill child is entitled to have a safe home and environment; the ghetto child may not have a permanent home and the environment will be dangerous. The Nob Hill child will automatically inherit an education pattern; private school with first-class teachers and state-of-the-art equipment, followed by Ivy League universities. If the child is a girl she may encounter problems with certain schools not welcoming her in certain disciplines and certain jobs not in her province, but money and status can usually overcome such barriers. The ghetto child meanwhile inherits no pattern of education; he or she is not "entitled" to private schools and universities, nor a choice of equal jobs. The ghetto girl-child can look forward to a life on welfare or menial jobs where she will not be paid equally for the same job performed by males. Inequality in health will have already demonstrated itself, even before the birth of each child, in pre-natal care; the birth itself in totally different hospitals (if indeed the ghetto birth takes place in a hospital) will underline the inequality. Finally, human dignity will not be afforded the ghetto child even if she or he makes it out of the ghetto and makes it into the life on Nob Hill — the gap lessens but the identity remains, the label cannot be removed.

Within such structures how can every citizen make a life-long commitment to put equality into practice? Given that absolute equality is impossible — we are all different in all kinds of ways from birth — citizens must make a conscious effort to practice the original concept of our forefathers. There must be made available the means for all people to achieve equality. Education is the obvious means to raise everyone to a suitable standard of living, affording the poorest of its citizens the highest level of learning. No nation committed to equality should lower its standards to the lowest common denominator. The recent upheaval in communist countries proves that abject equality is not the answer (and within such equality some definitely were "more equal" than others as the leaders of Romania demonstrated). A structure should exist, however, in which all people have access to forms of education to help those who so wish to move across race, gender, religion, class and color barriers.

EXPLANATION OF ESSAY 2

The essay immediately sets up the thesis that equality is possible only in an ideal world. It explains the concept behind the statement in terms of what should happen in a nation built on the belief of equality for all men. The first two paragraphs set up the pattern for the rest of the essay, within the explanation of the statement. The next long paragraph takes each one of the points in the previous paragraph as an argument against the statement, that in America it is not feasible for equal worth and equal rights because of an entrenched hierarchial society. The last paragraph deals with the possible solution for an "acceptable equality" — that everyone can agree on and work toward, based on improved education levels.

The essay fulfills the tasks demanded by tapping into the notion of the founding fathers, as well as Orwell's statement on "equality," and the recent events in communist countries. The essay is structured on a contrast basis using the two classes of children as examples. Each point in the first two paragraphs is dealt with in the next, with a repetition in the conclusion of the categories used in the opening lines, (race, gender, religion and color) bringing the essay full circle, giving cohesion.

The paragraphs develop from a clearly stated topic sentence, limiting sentences, and examples. Simple sentences cue the reader to the structure of the paragraph: "Lastly" (paragraph two); "Finally" (paragraph three). The rhetorical question in the last paragraph sets up the topic for the last paragraph, the paragraph attempting to answer that question. Each paragraph flows smoothly into the next with the use of simple transitional phrases or words: "However ..." (paragraph one into two); "Of course in the real world ... " (paragraph two into three, pushing the readers forward yet reminding them of the contrast between the "ideal" and "real"); "Within such structures ..." (paragraph three into four, pulling together the ideas of the last paragraph but pushing forward to an answer for the problem).

The sentences are suitably varied and often rely on parallel structure or repetition to stress certain points: "All people should be entitled ..."; "All people should live in neighborhoods ..." The use of punctuation is appropriate, as is the vocabulary. Words to be stressed are often "lifted" into quotation marks: "salad bowl," "entitled." The awkwardness of the he/she pronoun has been avoided through the use of the plural or "the child." Overall the language skills and techniques work well, never impeding or making the reader stumble over clumsy sentences, poor spelling or weak punctuation.

Section 4 — Biological Sciences

PASSAGE I (Questions 143-150)

143. **(B)**   As can be seen from the graph of blood pressure in a human circulatory system (Figure 1), the lowest blood pressure exists just before blood is returned to the heart from systemic circulation. Pressure is highest in the aorta and then decreases through arterial, capillary, and venous circulation.

144. **(A)**   Two values (in mm of Hg) are typically given for blood pressure. Systolic pressure is generated by contraction of the ventricles and diastolic pressure is that which exists in the circulatory system during relaxation of the ventricles. By convention, blood pressure is presented as the systolic value over the diastolic value. The difference between the two values is known as pulse pressure and, therefore, the correct response to this item is (A). The correct diastolic pressure in this example is 55 mm Hg and the correct systolic pressure is 140 mm Hg.

145. **(A)**   There are two principal ducts that return lymph to the circulatory system — the thoracic duct and the right lymphatic duct. The thoracic duct is the larger of the two and empties into the left subclavian vein while the right lymphatic duct empties into the right subclavian vein. None of the other choices describe vessels that participate in the return of lymph to the circulatory system.

146. **(C)**   This item tests your understanding of fetal circulation in mammals. Choice (C) gives the correct name of the connection between the aorta and the pulmonary artery. Choice (A) is the name of the opening between the atria of a fetal heart, while choice (D) gives the name of the adult derivative of the ductus arteriosus. Choice (B) is the name of the large opening in the occipital bone of the cranium through which the spinal cord passes.

147. **(D)**   This item tests your understanding of the definition of arteries and veins as well as the role of the pulmonary artery. Since arteries always carry blood away from the heart and the blood going *to* the lungs from the heart is oxygen-poor, choice (D) is the correct one. Blood returning to the heart from the lungs will be carried in veins and will be oxygen-rich.

148. **(C)**   Osmotic pressure of any solution is determined by the concentration of solute. Active transport of water does not occur, either across the walls of capillaries or through any other membranes; only solute can be actively transported. The other statements in this item correctly state facts regarding mammalian circulation.

149. **(A)**   This item tests your understanding of the connection between pulmonary circulation and the heart of mammals. The right ventricle pumps oxygen-poor blood to the lungs via the pulmonary artery and the left atrium receives oxygen-rich blood from the lungs via the pulmonary veins. Choice (A) is therefore correct. The left ventricle to right atrium connection is made via the systemic component of mammalian circulation, so choice (B) is incorrect. The other two choices describe

two correct sequences of heart chambers in normal circulation, but neither sequence includes pulmonary circulation.

150. **(D)** This is a very straight-forward test of your knowledge of the normal pH of human blood with choice (D) being the correct one. The other values offered as choices are not within normal range of blood pH and are, therefore, incorrect.

PASSAGE II (Questions 151-154)

151. **(B)** This question tests your knowledge of functional groups; a knowledge of nomenclature is also necessary. The nitro group, NO_2, is very electron-withdrawing and will therefore make nitromethane, CH_3NO_2, acidic. Hexane, C_6H_{14}, *A*, has no functional group to confer acidity. Trimethyl amine, $(CH_3)_3N$, *C*, has a nitrogen atom, but it is not electronegative enough to make the adjacent hydrogen acidic. Formaldehyde, *D*, has two hydrogens connected to the carbonyl group ($H_2C == O$); these are not acidic.

152. **(D)** These two protons are *between* two electron-withdrawing carbonyl groups and are therefore very acidic. The c protons are acidic, but much less so than *d*. Protons *a* and *b* are not adjacent to electron-withdrawing groups and are not acidic at all.

153. **(D)** The acidic proton alpha to the carbonyl group is on the chiral carbon. When the base removes this proton, an achiral enolate ion is formed. Addition of a deuterium thus will produce a mixture of the two enantiomers. Therefore, neither (B) nor (C) is correct; a mixture of these is formed. (A) would not be formed; the methyl group is not acidic.

154. **(A)** The removal of a proton leaves a negative charge that resides largely on the electronegative oxygen atom.

$$R - \overset{-}{C}H - \overset{\overset{\displaystyle O}{\|}}{C} - R \; \rightleftharpoons \; R - CH = \overset{\overset{\displaystyle O^-}{|}}{C} - R$$

(D) would be correct in acidic solution, but not in basic solution. Neither a positive ion, (B), nor a free radical, (C), are involved in the reaction.

PASSAGE III (Questions 155-159)

155. **(A)** The outermost ossified region of a bone is known as compact, or dense, bone and lies directly beneath the periosteum. Choice (A) correctly identifies the location of compact bone. The other three choices are incorrect: the medullary cavity, which contains marrow, is the hollow core of the diaphysis of long bones; the bone tissue on either side of the epiphyseal bone is known as cancellous, or spongy, bone; and, secondary ossification centers of long bones, which first appear during fetal development, contain no compact bone.

156. **(C)**   This question requires a knowledge of skeletal anatomy and the directional terminology used in anatomy. The term "proximal" means "toward the main mass of the body" (as opposed to distal) so the proximal epiphyseal plate of the humerus would be in the head of that bone. Among the choices given, choice (C) is correct because the scapula is closest to the head of humerus. The other choices are incorrect, since they all identify anatomical features found near the distal end of the humerus.

157. **(D)**   The classification of articulations, based on degree of movement permitted, recognizes three types: synarthroses (immovable), amphiarthroses (slightly movable), and diarthroses (freely movable). The knee and elbow joints are classic examples of diarthroses, so choice (D) is correct. You should be familiar with other examples of diarthroses — shoulder and hip joints, intercarpal and intertarsal joints, etc. You may also need to be familiar with examples of synarthroses (choice (A) and amphiarthroses (choice (C)). Choice (B), which is incorrect for this question, gives the term "synchondrosis," which refers to the epiphyseal plates of long bones, a subtype of synarthrotic joint.

158. **(A)**   This question is another test of your knowledge of bone nomenclature. The proper name for the shaft of a long bone is "diaphysis," so choice (A) is correct. An epiphysis (choice (B)) is the end segment of a long bone, which during growth of the individual was separated from the diaphysis by the epiphyseal plate. Choice (C) is incorrect because it gives the term used to refer to the type of bone joint that is slightly movable (i.e., an amphiarthrosis). A symphysis (choice (D)) is a type of amphiarthrosis, examples of which are seen in intervertebral joints and in the sacro-iliac.

159. **(C)**   Bones are joined to other bones across articulations (especially diarthroses) by bands of dense connective tissue known as ligaments, hence choice (C) is correct. A tendon (choice (A)) is also made of dense connective tissue, but attaches muscle to bone. Choice (B), chorda tendinea, gives the term that refers to one of the tendinous bands that connect papillary muscles within ventricles of the heart to the atrio-ventricular valves and is, therefore, incorrect.

160. **(B)**   The Cahn-Ingold-Prelog system of nomenclature uses priorities to establish the R or S designation. With the lowest priority group oriented away from the observer, the R designation is given if movement from the highest to next highest priority is clockwise. If it is counterclockwise, the atom is designated S. Manipulation of the structure shown will allow easy designation of the absolute configuration, if you know how to assign priorities.

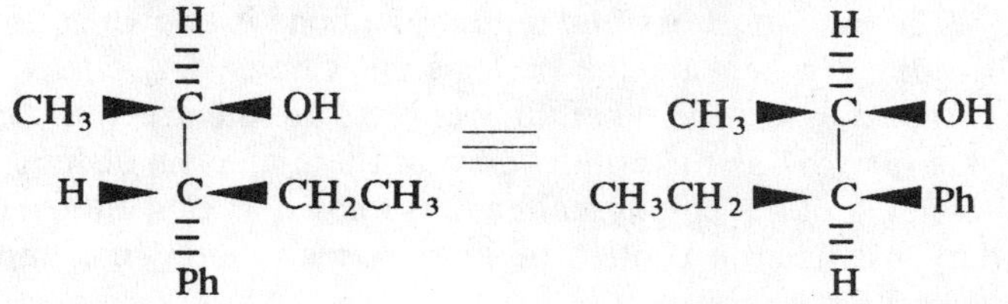

161. **(B)** The 1, 5-octadiene describes the longest chain containing the diene, using the lowest possible numbers to locate the double bonds (following the 1 and 5 carbons). Once these numbers are assigned, the 3, 6-dimethyl follows. Assignment of stereochemistry at the 5,6 double bond is made by assigning priorities to the groups attached to each carbon of the double bond. Since the higher priority groups are on the same side of the double bond, the Z (zusammen) designation is given. E (entgegen) indicates that the higher priority groups are on opposite sides of the double bond. The 1,2 double bond has no stereochemistry (two hydrogens are on one carbon), so no designation is necessary. (C) would allow you to draw the correct structure for the molecule, but it is incorrect nomenclature since the numbers are larger. (A) and (B) have the wrong stereochemistry for the double bond.

PASSAGE IV (Questions 162-168)

162. **(A)** The substrate is the molecule on which an enzyme acts, so choice (A) is the correct one for this question. Molecule Y would be a product molecule, molecule A is the modulator that binds on the enzyme away from the active site (i.e., it's allosteric), and molecule B competes with the substrate because its binds with the enzyme at the active site. Choices (B), (C), and (D) are therefore incorrect.

163. **(D)** This question requires that you know about enzyme kinetics. Because molecule A affects the rate of enzyme activity and does so by binding with the enzyme at a site physically distinct from the active site, it must be an allosteric modulator, or regulator. Choice (D) is, therefore, correct. It should be noted that allosteric inhibitors may themselves be products of a series of enzyme reactions that regulate one of the previous enzymes (often the first of the series) through feedback inhibition. The other choices are incorrect: molecule A is obviously not the substrate because it is not changed by the reaction; a competitive inhibitor reduces enzyme activity by binding with the enzyme at the active site; and, a cofactor is usually a small inorganic or metal ion that is required for catalytic activity.

164. **(D)** Since molecule B reduces the rate of this reaction by binding at the active site, it is acting as a competitive inhibitor of the enzyme and choice (D) is the correct answer. The effect of competitive inhibitors is reversible by increasing the substrate concentration. The other choices are incorrect because: cofactors bind with the enzyme loosely, if at all, and do not inhibit the reaction (actually, they may be required for activity); allosteric modulators can inhibit enzyme reactions (e.g., through feedback inhibition) but they do not bind at the active site: and, noncompetitive inhibitors are reversible inhibitors of enzyme activity that bind away from the active site.

165. **(C)** By simply reading the plot seen in Figure 1, you can determine that the optimum temperature (i.e., the one at which the reaction proceeds fastest) is about 35 degrees C (choice (C)). At 5 and 25 degrees C, the reaction is occurring, but more slowly than at 35 degrees. At 45 degrees C, the reaction has almost entirely ceased most likely because the enzyme has been denatured.

166. **(A)** As can be seen in Figure 1, the reaction rate reaches its optimum at about 35 degrees C and then quickly decreases. To correctly answer this question, you must recall that most proteins begin to denature at about 40 degrees C and reason that, since enzymes are proteinaceous, the enzyme catalyst of this reaction is most probably being denatured. Competitive inhibition could not explain the precipitous decline in enzyme activity at a specific temperature, so choice (B) is not correct. Choices (C) and (D) are also incorrect: the energy of activation is less at higher temperatures, but that should speed up the reaction not slow it down; and, the availability of substrate molecules is unlikely to be affected by increased temperatures.

167. **(B)** The non-protein structural component described in the passage is called a prosthetic group, correctly given by choice (B). An allosteric modulator (choice (A)) is a molecule, often a product of a subsequent enzyme reaction in a series, that regulates enzyme activity by binding with the enzyme away from the active site. Coenzymes (choice (C)) are often required for enzyme activity, but they are separate molecules, usually organic, and are not part of the structure of enzymes.

168. **(C)** To correctly answer this question, you must know about the four levels of protein structure. The level of structure determined by disulfide bridges within a single polypeptide chain is the tertiary level, so choice (C) is correct (hydrogen and ionic bonds are also important in tertiary structure). The other three choices are incorrect because: primary protein structure is simply the linear sequence of amino acids in the polypeptide(s) that make up the protein; secondary structure involves three-dimensional structure (alpha helices and pleated sheets) of a polypeptide, but does not involve disulfide bonds between cysteine molecules; and, quaternary structure describes the conformation of a protein that results from the relationship between two or more polypeptides (disulfide bridges are also important here).

169. **(C)** Cholic acid, which emulsifies dietary fats in the small intestine, has three OH groups and one COOH group. These are polar, hydrogen-bonding groups which enhance water solubility. None of the other three would exhibit any water solubility, since they are largely non-polar and hydrophobic.

170. **(D)** Chiral centers have four different groups bound to a carbon atom. Androsterone has seven such carbons.

171. **(A)** The 6.5 - 7.5 δ area of the nmr spectrum is where aromatic protons appear. The only one of the steroids with an aromatic ring, ring A, is estradiol.

172. **(A)** The stereochemistry of a fused ring junction is indicated by the stereochemistry of the attached groups. In cholic acid, the CH_3 group and the H of the A, B, junction are *cis* to each other. This means the rings are also *cis*. The other two ring junctions are *trans*, as indicated by the stereochemistry of attached hydrogen and methyl groups.

173. **(A)** The preparation of tissues for light microscopy involves mounting them on a slide to provide a firm support.

174. **(D)**   The placenta is a region where a portion of the embryonic chorion and the maternal uterine wall join. It functions in the exchange of nutrients, wastes and gases between the mother and the fetus.

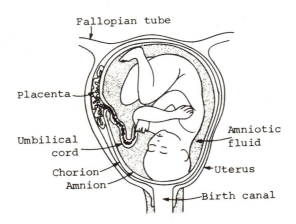

175. **(A)**   The Golgi apparatus is an organelle that is responsible only for the packaging of protein for secretion.

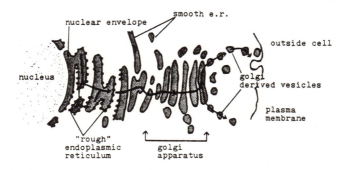

Schematic representation of the secretion of a protein in a typical animal cell. The solid arrow represents the probable route of secreted proteins.

176. **(B)**   This question requires a knowledge of nmr chemical shifts. Alkyl protons, *a*, are not deshielded and appear close to TMS (ca. 1.0 δ). Protons on a carbon adjacent to a carbonyl group can be found in the 2.0 - 2.5 δ region. Protons on a carbon attached to an oxygen usually occur in the 3.5 - 4.0 δ region. The other answers are perturbations of the correct answer.

177. **(C)**   Your knowledge of several chemical reactions is tested by this question. The reactions would yield the following products:

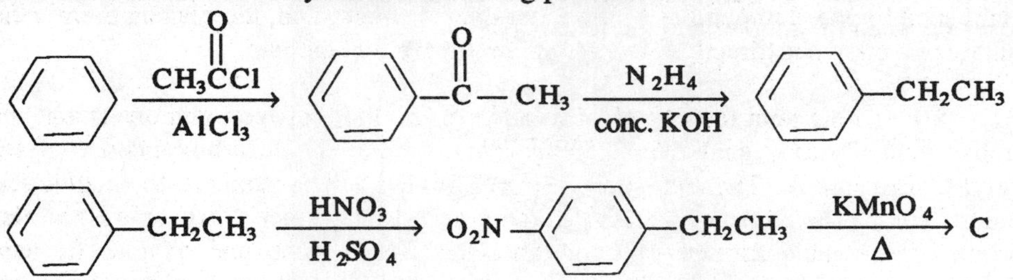

The first reaction is a Friedel-Crafts acylation. It is followed by a Wolff-Kishner reduction, which produces an ortho-para directing ethyl group. Nitration then produces para-nitroethylbenzene (and some ortho), which can be oxidized to *p*-nitrobensoic acid, (C). (A) would be the product if the ethyl group was meta direction. (B) would be the product if no oxidation of the ethyl group took place. (D) is not a feasible answer since no reaction shown would lead to the vinyl group.

PASSAGE VI (Questions 178-183)

178. **(D)**   The enzymes that catalyze the reactions known as glycolysis are soluble proteins found in the cytosol, or cytoplasm. The end result of this process is pyruvic acid, ATP, and NADH+H$^+$. Ribosomes are the site of protein synthesis (i.e., translation of mRNA) and the nucleus contains chromosomal DNA and is the site of transcription. Mitochondria have catabolic enzymes, specifically those of the Krebs cycle and the electron transport chain, but are not involved in glycolysis.

179. **(C)**   This item tests your ability to distinguish among the three principal types of phosphorylation — the addition of an inorganic phosphate to ADP to form ATP. Photophosphorylation is the process that forms ATP in the light reactions of photosynthesis that occur in the thylakoids of chloroplasts. Substrate-level phosphorylation is the name given to the direct addition of inorganic phosphate to ADP as in the formation of ATP in glycolysis. Dephosphorylation describes the loss of a high-energy phosphate from ATP, not the addition. The correct choice is (C); oxidative phosphorylation occurs in the electron transport chain in the inner membrane of mitochondria.

180. **(A)**   Fermentation of glucose is an anaerobic process that produces either lactic acid (as in skeletal muscle) or ethanol and carbon dioxide (as in yeast cells). There is a direct yield of two molecules of ATP per glucose molecule fermented in this process, so (A) is the correct choice. Complete aerobic metabolism of one glucose molecule yield thirty-six (thirty-eight in procaryotes) molecules of ATP, the number given in Choice (C). Choices (B) and (D) do not reflect the number of ATP molecules produced by either aerobic or anaerobic breakdown of glucose and are, therefore, incorrect.

181. **(C)**   The carrier molecules (Co-enzyme Q, cytochromes, and other proteinaceous molecules acting as enzymes) of the electron transport chain are located within the inner membrane of mitochondria, therefore choice (C) is correct. The other

choices are incorrect: the cytosol is the location of the enzymes of glycolysis; the outer compartment of the mitochondrion is the site of the electrochemical gradient established by H+ pumped out of the inner compartment; and, the plasma membrane contains no enzymes directly related to intermediary metabolism.

182. **(D)**   This item tests your knowledge of the link between glycolysis and the Krebs cycle. Pyruvic acid from glycolysis is oxidatively decarboxylated to form acetyl-CoEnzyme-A. The two-carbon acetyl group then is donated to oxaloacetic acid to "begin" the Krebs cycle. Choice (D) is therefore correct. Citric acid is the six-carbon organic acid formed by combining the acetyl group and oxaloacetic acid while succinic acid is a four-carbon intermediate of the Krebs cycle, so these choices are obviously incorrect.

183. **(A)**   While all the tissues identified by the choices for this item can techni-cally carry out anaerobic respiration, skeletal muscle is the best adapted for this process and can function for some time under very low oxygen tensions (building so-called "oxygen debt"). Brain cells are among the most sensitive to lack of oxygen while cardiac and smooth muscle are less so, but still not as well adapted as skeletal muscle.

PASSAGE VII (Questions 184-187)

184. **(D)**   To answer this and succeeding questions, you must know that each carbon-carbon dioxide bond has two π electrons that can be delocalized if they are conjugated with other double bonds.

185. **(B)**   Sodium amide, NaNH$_2$, will react with acidic protons in a neutraliza-tion reaction.

$$NaNH_2 + RH \longrightarrow NH_3 + Na^+R^-$$

Ordinary hydrocarbons are not acidic, but cyclopentadiene, (B), will react to form an aromatic entity, where the electrons of the carbonion conjugate with the 4 π electrons of the double bonds. None of the other compounds can react with a base to form an aromatic entity.

186. **(D)**   This question tests your knowledge of nmr spectrometry. The area described is the aromatic region of the spectrum, thus only the aromatic compound 4 will show peaks there. The other compounds will absorb in the alkene region.

187. **(A)**   Silver nitrate reacts with halides to give a precipitate of sliver halide. Ordinarily, one must destroy the organic molecule by a sodium fusion reaction to yield NaX before getting a reaction with silver nitrate. (A), however, will react readily with silver nitrate to yield a trophylium cation.

The tropylium ion has 6π electrons and these can form different resonance structures by delocalization of the positive charge and π electrons. The stability of this aromatic species enhances the reactivity of its precursor. (B) is an aromatic compound and the C—Cl bond is very strong. Breaking the bond would actually disrupt an aromatic species. (D) would yield a cation where delocalization is theoretically possible, but the 4π electrons would not be aromatic. (C) is an ordinary alkyl halide which would not be reactive.

188. **(B)**　This item tests your understanding of homologous and analogous structures. Homologous structures have evolved from a common ancestral form. Of the choices presented, all but (B) represent structures that are homologous as vertebrate forelimbs since they have common bone structures. The wing of an insect is *analogous* to the wing of a bird because it has a common function, but because it evolved independently from the bird wing it is not homologous.

189. **(C)**　In order for an allele to be subject to selective pressures, it must be expressed (i.e., there must be a phenotype). A heterozygote expresses the dominant phenotype while the recessive allele is masked from selective pressure. Choice (C) describes this situation; the other three choices all indicate alleles that would be expressed and, therefore, would be susceptible to positive and negative selective pressures.

190. **(C)**　This item tests your knowledge of the conditions on earth between the time of its formation and the appearance of the first life forms (from approximately 4.5 billion years ago to about 3 billion years ago). While it is not possible to directly measure atmospheric composition from that time period, it can be deduced that the primordial atmosphere must have been a chemically reducing atmosphere. One model suggests large amounts of elemental hydrogen and reduced forms of nitrogen and carbon — NH_3 and CH_4, respectively. Another model hypothesizes other gases, similar to those found coming from modern volcanos. Both models suggest water vapor was present, but neither model allows for any free, or molecular, oxygen because of the reductive nature of the atmosphere. Choice (C) is, therefore, correct.

191. **(D)**　All four choices in this item identify mechanisms that act to prevent interspecific hybridization. However, choices (A), (B), and (C) describe mechanisms that act to *prevent* mating between species. In those cases where interspecific mating can occur, developmental isolation (as well as gametic isolation) prevent the formation of viable offspring. Choice (D) correctly identifies this situation. In some instances, viable hybrid offspring can develop but they may be subject to other isolating mechanisms such as hybrid sterility (e.g., a mule).

192. **(B)**　The classic characteristics of the phylum Chordata are the occurrence of pharyngeal gill slits, a notochord, and a dorsal hollow nerve cord at some time in the animal's development. A cartilaginous or bony vertebral column is found only in the subphylum Vertebrata and is, therefore, *not* a general phylum characteristic.

193. **(C)**　This item tests your understanding of the Darwinian concept of "fitness," probably the most misunderstood part of natural selection. Evolutionary fitness is not necessarily measured by an animal's ability to survive or compete with

other members of its species in the environment. Rather, fitness is determined by the degree to which an organism is able to pass on its genes to future generations as identified in choice (C).

194. **(A)**   This item tests your ability to understand subtleties in the definition of a species. While individuals of a species certainly have the ability to mate within the group, they often can mate with members of other species. If the mating pair are from different species, there will normally be no viable or fertile offspring under natural conditions. Choice (A), therefore, is not a species characteristic. The other three choices give commonly held characteristics of a species.

195. **(C)**   The aldol condensation is a reaction between an enolate ion and an uncharged aldehyde. The product is an aldehyde with an alcohol functional group (aldol). (D) would require the displacement of a hydride ion. Neither (A) nor (B) are feasible products of an aldol condensation.

196. **(B)**   The interconversion occurs through a symmetrical ene-diol intermediate that involves keto-enol tautomerism. None of the other possibilities is feasible.

PASSAGE IX (Questions 197-204)

197. **(A)**   This item tests your knowledge of the sliding-filament theory of skeletal and cardiac muscle contraction. The functional unit of a muscle known as a sarcomere is diagrammed in Figure 1 at the beginning of this passage. The sarcomere contracts as the thick myosin slide by the thin actin filaments. This is accomplished as cross bridges from the myosin "pull" the actin filaments. During the contraction of a sarcomere, the Z lines move closer to each other, the I bands of each sarcomere shorten, and the H zone gradually disappears. The A band remains virtually the same length since it corresponds to the length of the myosin filaments. Choice (A) is a correct description of this fact.

198. **(B)**   Smooth muscle has no cross striations, but both cardiac and skeletal muscle show striations due to the arrangement of actin and myosin into sarcomeres. Unlike cardiac muscle, however, skeletal muscle is multinucleate. Choice (B) correctly identifies skeletal muscle as the only striated, multinucleate muscle.

199. **(D)**   The inside of a neuron is about 70 millivolts negative compared to the outside (the actual value may range from - 65mv to - 85mv in neurons and muscle cells). This potential difference is referred to as the resting membrane potential, or simply resting potential, of the neuron. The only correct value for a neuron resting potential is given in choice (D).

200. **(A)**   This item tests your knowledge of types of synapses. Synapses are of two types: electrical and chemical. Electrical synapses occur between cells that are joined by gap Junctions, which are found in both cardiac and smooth muscle. The only correct choice for this item is, therefore, (A).

201. **(B)**   In this item, your understanding of the complex process of muscle fiber contraction is tested. As an action potential moves along a muscle cell, calcium ions

released from the sarcoplasmic reticulum bind with one of two regulatory proteins found as part of the thin filaments. The protein with which calcium binds is known as the troponin complex, so the correct choice is (B). This binding causes a slight conformational change in the other regulatory protein known as tropomyosin. Because of this change, the myosin cross bridges can then attach to specific sites on the actin and the contraction process can proceed.

202. **(D)** An action potential is generated by rapid, differential diffusion of ions across membranes, thereby temporarily reversing polarity across the membrane. The channels through which first sodium and then potassium move during this process are regulated by changes in membrane voltage, hence the name "voltage-gated." Choice (D) gives the correct name of these channels, while the terms found in other choices have no reference to membrane channels.

203. **(A)** Neurons that are enveloped by Schwann cells have action potentials only at the nodes of Ranvier (see Figure 2 at the beginning of this passage). These neurons, therefore, transmit impulses by the "jumping" of action potentials from node to node. The type of conduction is known as saltatory conduction and is much more rapid than conduction in neurons without Schwann cells, so the correct choice for this item is (A).

204. **(C)** The sodium-potassium pump moves sodium ions from the inside of a cell to the outside and potassium ions from the outside to the inside. The "pump" is actually a protein embedded in the cell membrane that resembles a rocker switch as it changes from one conformation to another. These conformational changes (or at least one of them) require energy in the form of ATP and result in sodium ions being pumped out and potassium ions being pumped into the cell in a ratio of approximately three-to-two during each cycle. This ratio is correctly given in choice (C).

PASSAGE X (Questions 205-208)

205. **(B)** The step leading to (1) involves heterolysis of the C-X bond. Since X⁻ is formed, the carbon is left with a positive charge. (D), a free radical, would form if bond homolysis occurred. (A) or (D) would be formed if an acid-base reaction removed a proton.

206. **(D)** Loss of optical activity means that an S_N1 reaction is the likely mechanism; since ionization of the alkyl halide is the rate-determining (slow) step, the rate is dependent on the concentration of alkyl halide. (C) would imply that sodium ethoxide was involved in the rate-determining step; it is not. The loss of optical activity rules out (A) and (B).

207. **(A)** Reaction of the base with a hydrogen beta to the leaving group (OTs) is required for elimination. Only answers (A) and (B) show products of such a reaction. (B) is not correct since it is a less substituted alkene than (A) (Saytzeff's rule).

208. **(B)** t-Butyl alcohol will react via a tertiary carbocation that will not rearrange.

$$(CH_3)_3COH \xrightarrow{\ H+\ } (CH_3)_3 \overset{H}{\underset{+}{C}}OH$$

$$\Big\downarrow -H_2O$$

$$CH_2 {=} C \Big\langle {}^{CH_3}_{CH_3} \quad \longleftarrow \quad (CH_3)_3C^+$$

Protonation and dehydration of (A) and (D) will yield secondary cations that can rearrange by a hydride shift to a more stable tertiary cation. (C) will yield a primary cation that can rearrange to a more stable secondary cation.

209. **(D)** The four "experiments" described in the passage are actually descriptions of the application of the rules of procedure known as "Koch's Postulates." Only after successfully completing all four steps, as described in the passage or in analogous situations, can it be concluded that a suspected pathogen is actually the cause of a disease.

210. **(A)** This item tests your knowledge of the molecular components of virus particles. Irrespective of the specific structure of the protein coat, all viruses *have* such a coat or capsid. Similarly, every virus has a nucleic acid core of *either* DNA or RNA. Viruses that attack bacteria are known as bacteriophage, or simply "phage", and their structure can be quite elegant. The first phage to be chemically elucidated had DNA cores. It is now known, however, that some phage have RNA cores, so the correct choice is (A). Some phage have DNA, some have RNA, but none has *both* DNA and RNA.

211. **(C)** In this item you must recall the components of a bacterial cell. Bacteria have cell walls, not made of cellulose like plant cell walls, but of a related polysaccharide. While bacteria are prokaryotic, they do have ribosomes, which are not membrane-bound organelles. Bacterial ribosomes are, however, different from those of eukaryotes in several aspects. All bacterial cells are enclosed in a cell membrane that exists just inside the cell wall. Given this information, choice (C) is the only one possible. You should also be able make this selection by recalling that only eukaryotes have mitochondria and they are not found in bacteria.

212. **(B)** The passage describes the application of Koch's postulates to verify the pathogen of a hypothetical disease. Robert Koch first used this procedure to find the cause of anthrax in cattle, horses, sheep, and humans. Subsequently, he discovered that tuberculosis (choice (B)) in humans was also caused by a bacillus. These were the first diseases for which the cause was proven to be bacterial and are therefore of historical note to epidemiologists.

213. **(D)** This item requires you to calculate the approximate number of bacterial cells that will be produced after a given time period. Given the replication time of forty-five minutes, you should be able to determine that a single bacterium will go through sixteen divisions in twelve hours to produce 2^{16}, or approximately 65,000,

cells. Since there were ten bacterial cells initially placed inoculated into the medium there will be approximately $10 \times 65,000 = 650,000$ cells at the end of twelve hours.

214. (B) The autonomic nervous system innervates the heart, some glands, the smooth muscles of the digestive tract, the respiratory system, the reproductive system and the blood vessels. Only (B) describes processes innervated by the autonomic pathways. The other choices are all parts of the somatic pathways of the nervous system which usually innervate skeletal muscle.

215. (C) Homologous structures have a similar evolutionary origin. They may have diverged in their functions and phenotypic appearances, but their relationships to adjacent structures and their embryonic development are similar. The wings of birds and butterflies are not homologous structures; they are analogous structures. They are similar in function and outward appearance but have different evolutionary origins.

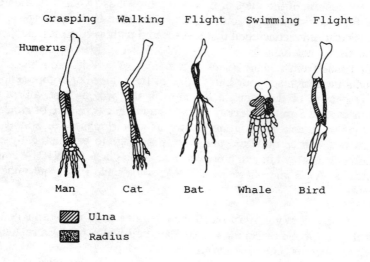

216. (A) By dividing one group of progeny by the other, 77/24, the Mandelian ratio of approximately 3:1, is obtained. This suggests that the long-winged phenotype is dominant to the short-winged phenotype. This implies that neither of the parents were homozygous because that situation would have not produced any short-winged flies:

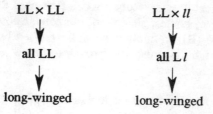

Since some recessive flies are the result of the cross, both parents must have had a recessive, *l*, allele. Constructing a punnet square, we find:

	L	*l*
L	LL	L*l*
l	L*l*	*ll*

75% – phenotypically long

25% – phenotypically short

217. **(A)**   The lymphatic system is responsible for filtration, transportation of proteins lost from the blood, fat absorption and the production of some white blood cells. The functions listed in (A) are functions of the epidermis.

218. **(C)**   The somatic nervous system innervates skeletal muscles which are under voluntary control. The other muscles are controlled by the autonomic nervous system.

219. **(D)**   Fruit production requires active cell division. In plants, only regions of meristematic tissue are capable of active cell division. The removal of all of the meristematic tissue from a plant leaves it incapable of cell division; therefore, incapable of producing fruits.

MCAT
Medical College Admission Test

Test 5

Test 5 is also on CD-ROM in our special interactive MCAT TEST*ware*®. It is highly recommended that you take this exam on computer first. You will then have the additional study features and benefits of enforced timed conditions, individual diagnostic analysis, and instant scoring. See page 2 for guidance on how to get the most out of our MCAT book and software.

MEDICAL COLLEGE ADMISSION TEST
TEST 5
ANSWER SHEET

Section 1:
Verbal Reasoning

1. Ⓐ Ⓑ Ⓒ Ⓓ
2. Ⓐ Ⓑ Ⓒ Ⓓ
3. Ⓐ Ⓑ Ⓒ Ⓓ
4. Ⓐ Ⓑ Ⓒ Ⓓ
5. Ⓐ Ⓑ Ⓒ Ⓓ
6. Ⓐ Ⓑ Ⓒ Ⓓ
7. Ⓐ Ⓑ Ⓒ Ⓓ
8. Ⓐ Ⓑ Ⓒ Ⓓ
9. Ⓐ Ⓑ Ⓒ Ⓓ
10. Ⓐ Ⓑ Ⓒ Ⓓ
11. Ⓐ Ⓑ Ⓒ Ⓓ
12. Ⓐ Ⓑ Ⓒ Ⓓ
13. Ⓐ Ⓑ Ⓒ Ⓓ
14. Ⓐ Ⓑ Ⓒ Ⓓ
15. Ⓐ Ⓑ Ⓒ Ⓓ
16. Ⓐ Ⓑ Ⓒ Ⓓ
17. Ⓐ Ⓑ Ⓒ Ⓓ
18. Ⓐ Ⓑ Ⓒ Ⓓ
19. Ⓐ Ⓑ Ⓒ Ⓓ
20. Ⓐ Ⓑ Ⓒ Ⓓ
21. Ⓐ Ⓑ Ⓒ Ⓓ
22. Ⓐ Ⓑ Ⓒ Ⓓ
23. Ⓐ Ⓑ Ⓒ Ⓓ
24. Ⓐ Ⓑ Ⓒ Ⓓ
25. Ⓐ Ⓑ Ⓒ Ⓓ
26. Ⓐ Ⓑ Ⓒ Ⓓ
27. Ⓐ Ⓑ Ⓒ Ⓓ
28. Ⓐ Ⓑ Ⓒ Ⓓ
29. Ⓐ Ⓑ Ⓒ Ⓓ
30. Ⓐ Ⓑ Ⓒ Ⓓ
31. Ⓐ Ⓑ Ⓒ Ⓓ

32. Ⓐ Ⓑ Ⓒ Ⓓ
33. Ⓐ Ⓑ Ⓒ Ⓓ
34. Ⓐ Ⓑ Ⓒ Ⓓ
35. Ⓐ Ⓑ Ⓒ Ⓓ
36. Ⓐ Ⓑ Ⓒ Ⓓ
37. Ⓐ Ⓑ Ⓒ Ⓓ
38. Ⓐ Ⓑ Ⓒ Ⓓ
39. Ⓐ Ⓑ Ⓒ Ⓓ
40. Ⓐ Ⓑ Ⓒ Ⓓ
41. Ⓐ Ⓑ Ⓒ Ⓓ
42. Ⓐ Ⓑ Ⓒ Ⓓ
43. Ⓐ Ⓑ Ⓒ Ⓓ
44. Ⓐ Ⓑ Ⓒ Ⓓ
45. Ⓐ Ⓑ Ⓒ Ⓓ
46. Ⓐ Ⓑ Ⓒ Ⓓ
47. Ⓐ Ⓑ Ⓒ Ⓓ
48. Ⓐ Ⓑ Ⓒ Ⓓ
49. Ⓐ Ⓑ Ⓒ Ⓓ
50. Ⓐ Ⓑ Ⓒ Ⓓ
51. Ⓐ Ⓑ Ⓒ Ⓓ
52. Ⓐ Ⓑ Ⓒ Ⓓ
53. Ⓐ Ⓑ Ⓒ Ⓓ
54. Ⓐ Ⓑ Ⓒ Ⓓ
55. Ⓐ Ⓑ Ⓒ Ⓓ
56. Ⓐ Ⓑ Ⓒ Ⓓ
57. Ⓐ Ⓑ Ⓒ Ⓓ
58. Ⓐ Ⓑ Ⓒ Ⓓ
59. Ⓐ Ⓑ Ⓒ Ⓓ
60. Ⓐ Ⓑ Ⓒ Ⓓ
61. Ⓐ Ⓑ Ⓒ Ⓓ
62. Ⓐ Ⓑ Ⓒ Ⓓ
63. Ⓐ Ⓑ Ⓒ Ⓓ
64. Ⓐ Ⓑ Ⓒ Ⓓ
65. Ⓐ Ⓑ Ⓒ Ⓓ

Section 2:
Physical Sciences

66. Ⓐ Ⓑ Ⓒ Ⓓ
67. Ⓐ Ⓑ Ⓒ Ⓓ
68. Ⓐ Ⓑ Ⓒ Ⓓ
69. Ⓐ Ⓑ Ⓒ Ⓓ
70. Ⓐ Ⓑ Ⓒ Ⓓ
71. Ⓐ Ⓑ Ⓒ Ⓓ
72. Ⓐ Ⓑ Ⓒ Ⓓ
73. Ⓐ Ⓑ Ⓒ Ⓓ
74. Ⓐ Ⓑ Ⓒ Ⓓ
75. Ⓐ Ⓑ Ⓒ Ⓓ
76. Ⓐ Ⓑ Ⓒ Ⓓ
77. Ⓐ Ⓑ Ⓒ Ⓓ
78. Ⓐ Ⓑ Ⓒ Ⓓ
79. Ⓐ Ⓑ Ⓒ Ⓓ
80. Ⓐ Ⓑ Ⓒ Ⓓ
81. Ⓐ Ⓑ Ⓒ Ⓓ
82. Ⓐ Ⓑ Ⓒ Ⓓ
83. Ⓐ Ⓑ Ⓒ Ⓓ
84. Ⓐ Ⓑ Ⓒ Ⓓ
85. Ⓐ Ⓑ Ⓒ Ⓓ
86. Ⓐ Ⓑ Ⓒ Ⓓ
87. Ⓐ Ⓑ Ⓒ Ⓓ
88. Ⓐ Ⓑ Ⓒ Ⓓ
89. Ⓐ Ⓑ Ⓒ Ⓓ
90. Ⓐ Ⓑ Ⓒ Ⓓ
91. Ⓐ Ⓑ Ⓒ Ⓓ
92. Ⓐ Ⓑ Ⓒ Ⓓ
93. Ⓐ Ⓑ Ⓒ Ⓓ
94. Ⓐ Ⓑ Ⓒ Ⓓ
95. Ⓐ Ⓑ Ⓒ Ⓓ
96. Ⓐ Ⓑ Ⓒ Ⓓ

97. Ⓐ Ⓑ Ⓒ Ⓓ
98. Ⓐ Ⓑ Ⓒ Ⓓ
99. Ⓐ Ⓑ Ⓒ Ⓓ
100. Ⓐ Ⓑ Ⓒ Ⓓ
101. Ⓐ Ⓑ Ⓒ Ⓓ
102. Ⓐ Ⓑ Ⓒ Ⓓ
103. Ⓐ Ⓑ Ⓒ Ⓓ
104. Ⓐ Ⓑ Ⓒ Ⓓ
105. Ⓐ Ⓑ Ⓒ Ⓓ
106. Ⓐ Ⓑ Ⓒ Ⓓ
107. Ⓐ Ⓑ Ⓒ Ⓓ
108. Ⓐ Ⓑ Ⓒ Ⓓ
109. Ⓐ Ⓑ Ⓒ Ⓓ
110. Ⓐ Ⓑ Ⓒ Ⓓ
111. Ⓐ Ⓑ Ⓒ Ⓓ
112. Ⓐ Ⓑ Ⓒ Ⓓ
113. Ⓐ Ⓑ Ⓒ Ⓓ
114. Ⓐ Ⓑ Ⓒ Ⓓ
115. Ⓐ Ⓑ Ⓒ Ⓓ
116. Ⓐ Ⓑ Ⓒ Ⓓ
117. Ⓐ Ⓑ Ⓒ Ⓓ
118. Ⓐ Ⓑ Ⓒ Ⓓ
119. Ⓐ Ⓑ Ⓒ Ⓓ
120. Ⓐ Ⓑ Ⓒ Ⓓ
121. Ⓐ Ⓑ Ⓒ Ⓓ
122. Ⓐ Ⓑ Ⓒ Ⓓ
123. Ⓐ Ⓑ Ⓒ Ⓓ
124. Ⓐ Ⓑ Ⓒ Ⓓ
125. Ⓐ Ⓑ Ⓒ Ⓓ
126. Ⓐ Ⓑ Ⓒ Ⓓ
127. Ⓐ Ⓑ Ⓒ Ⓓ
128. Ⓐ Ⓑ Ⓒ Ⓓ
129. Ⓐ Ⓑ Ⓒ Ⓓ
130. Ⓐ Ⓑ Ⓒ Ⓓ
131. Ⓐ Ⓑ Ⓒ Ⓓ
132. Ⓐ Ⓑ Ⓒ Ⓓ
133. Ⓐ Ⓑ Ⓒ Ⓓ
134. Ⓐ Ⓑ Ⓒ Ⓓ
135. Ⓐ Ⓑ Ⓒ Ⓓ
136. Ⓐ Ⓑ Ⓒ Ⓓ
137. Ⓐ Ⓑ Ⓒ Ⓓ
138. Ⓐ Ⓑ Ⓒ Ⓓ
139. Ⓐ Ⓑ Ⓒ Ⓓ

140. Ⓐ Ⓑ Ⓒ Ⓓ
141. Ⓐ Ⓑ Ⓒ Ⓓ
142. Ⓐ Ⓑ Ⓒ Ⓓ

Section 4:
Biological Sciences

143. Ⓐ Ⓑ Ⓒ Ⓓ
144. Ⓐ Ⓑ Ⓒ Ⓓ
145. Ⓐ Ⓑ Ⓒ Ⓓ
146. Ⓐ Ⓑ Ⓒ Ⓓ
147. Ⓐ Ⓑ Ⓒ Ⓓ
148. Ⓐ Ⓑ Ⓒ Ⓓ
149. Ⓐ Ⓑ Ⓒ Ⓓ
150. Ⓐ Ⓑ Ⓒ Ⓓ
151. Ⓐ Ⓑ Ⓒ Ⓓ
152. Ⓐ Ⓑ Ⓒ Ⓓ
153. Ⓐ Ⓑ Ⓒ Ⓓ
154. Ⓐ Ⓑ Ⓒ Ⓓ
155. Ⓐ Ⓑ Ⓒ Ⓓ
156. Ⓐ Ⓑ Ⓒ Ⓓ
157. Ⓐ Ⓑ Ⓒ Ⓓ
158. Ⓐ Ⓑ Ⓒ Ⓓ
159. Ⓐ Ⓑ Ⓒ Ⓓ
160. Ⓐ Ⓑ Ⓒ Ⓓ
161. Ⓐ Ⓑ Ⓒ Ⓓ
162. Ⓐ Ⓑ Ⓒ Ⓓ
163. Ⓐ Ⓑ Ⓒ Ⓓ
164. Ⓐ Ⓑ Ⓒ Ⓓ
165. Ⓐ Ⓑ Ⓒ Ⓓ
166. Ⓐ Ⓑ Ⓒ Ⓓ
167. Ⓐ Ⓑ Ⓒ Ⓓ
168. Ⓐ Ⓑ Ⓒ Ⓓ
169. Ⓐ Ⓑ Ⓒ Ⓓ
170. Ⓐ Ⓑ Ⓒ Ⓓ
171. Ⓐ Ⓑ Ⓒ Ⓓ
172. Ⓐ Ⓑ Ⓒ Ⓓ
173. Ⓐ Ⓑ Ⓒ Ⓓ
174. Ⓐ Ⓑ Ⓒ Ⓓ
175. Ⓐ Ⓑ Ⓒ Ⓓ
176. Ⓐ Ⓑ Ⓒ Ⓓ

177. Ⓐ Ⓑ Ⓒ Ⓓ
178. Ⓐ Ⓑ Ⓒ Ⓓ
179. Ⓐ Ⓑ Ⓒ Ⓓ
180. Ⓐ Ⓑ Ⓒ Ⓓ
181. Ⓐ Ⓑ Ⓒ Ⓓ
182. Ⓐ Ⓑ Ⓒ Ⓓ
183. Ⓐ Ⓑ Ⓒ Ⓓ
184. Ⓐ Ⓑ Ⓒ Ⓓ
185. Ⓐ Ⓑ Ⓒ Ⓓ
186. Ⓐ Ⓑ Ⓒ Ⓓ
187. Ⓐ Ⓑ Ⓒ Ⓓ
188. Ⓐ Ⓑ Ⓒ Ⓓ
189. Ⓐ Ⓑ Ⓒ Ⓓ
190. Ⓐ Ⓑ Ⓒ Ⓓ
191. Ⓐ Ⓑ Ⓒ Ⓓ
192. Ⓐ Ⓑ Ⓒ Ⓓ
193. Ⓐ Ⓑ Ⓒ Ⓓ
194. Ⓐ Ⓑ Ⓒ Ⓓ
195. Ⓐ Ⓑ Ⓒ Ⓓ
196. Ⓐ Ⓑ Ⓒ Ⓓ
197. Ⓐ Ⓑ Ⓒ Ⓓ
198. Ⓐ Ⓑ Ⓒ Ⓓ
199. Ⓐ Ⓑ Ⓒ Ⓓ
200. Ⓐ Ⓑ Ⓒ Ⓓ
201. Ⓐ Ⓑ Ⓒ Ⓓ
202. Ⓐ Ⓑ Ⓒ Ⓓ
203. Ⓐ Ⓑ Ⓒ Ⓓ
204. Ⓐ Ⓑ Ⓒ Ⓓ
205. Ⓐ Ⓑ Ⓒ Ⓓ
206. Ⓐ Ⓑ Ⓒ Ⓓ
207. Ⓐ Ⓑ Ⓒ Ⓓ
208. Ⓐ Ⓑ Ⓒ Ⓓ
209. Ⓐ Ⓑ Ⓒ Ⓓ
210. Ⓐ Ⓑ Ⓒ Ⓓ
211. Ⓐ Ⓑ Ⓒ Ⓓ
212. Ⓐ Ⓑ Ⓒ Ⓓ
213. Ⓐ Ⓑ Ⓒ Ⓓ
214. Ⓐ Ⓑ Ⓒ Ⓓ
215. Ⓐ Ⓑ Ⓒ Ⓓ
216. Ⓐ Ⓑ Ⓒ Ⓓ
217. Ⓐ Ⓑ Ⓒ Ⓓ
218. Ⓐ Ⓑ Ⓒ Ⓓ
219. Ⓐ Ⓑ Ⓒ Ⓓ

TEST 5

Section 1 — Verbal Reasoning

TIME: 85 Minutes
QUESTIONS: 1-65

DIRECTIONS: The verbal reasoning section contains seven passages, each followed by a series of questions. Based on the information given in a passage, choose the one best answer to each question. If you are not sure of an answer, eliminate those choices that you know are incorrect and choose an answer from among those remaining. Fill in the corresponding circle on the answer sheet to indicate your answer.

PASSAGE I (Questions 1-9)

Granting that computer literacy consists in knowing what sorts of skills and what levels of skills can and should be taught using computers, where should the literate educator stand on the question?

Computers are marvelous tools which, when used as electronic blackboards, interactive simulators, and conjecture testers, greatly improve sociality and intuition in the classroom. Provided one does not narrow one's goal to forcing the student to think procedurally like a computerized problem-solver, there is no limit to the level of skill that imaginative new learning environments may be able to foster. Computers are also useful as rule-following, literal-minded tutees, as long as one limits oneself to teaching elementary math and programming, as most LOGO users now do.

But the outlook for the computer as tutor is less bright. If one accepts our skill model, one is forced to conclude that the level of skill appropriately taught using the computer is quite limited. At the beginning level the computer can be useful for drill and practice in subjects requiring nothing more than the memorization of facts, rules, and procedures such as spelling and subtraction. In restricted areas, where trained competence, not educated expertise, is the goal, computers and interactive media like videodisks may indeed prove useful. However, one should not attempt to tutor any higher level of skill, for that would require giving logic machines skills that have proved to be beyond their capacities.

We have seen that the advocates of computers as tutors and tutees think, like Socrates and Plato, that we cannot teach what we do not understand and that we only understand what we can formulate in the sorts of rules and procedures used by a logic machine. If that were true, teachers could be gradually replaced by computers. But teachers are no doubt aware, and parents must become aware, that expertise in teaching does not consist in knowing complicated rules about their discipline and about coaching — what tips to give, when to keep silent, when to intervene — although teachers may have learned such rules in graduate school. What an expert teacher gains from experience is not more facts about some field plus rules of coaching of the sort he or she once explicitly followed as a beginner; rather, the teacher learns intuitively and spontaneously to draw on the commonsense knowledge and experience he or she shares with the student in order to provide the tips and examples needed by the advanced beginner. The teacher also learns how to motivate the involved practice by which a student gains experience in any domain .

From Hubert L. Dreyfus and Stuart E. Dreyfus, *Mind over Machine*, 1986.

1.   The primary subject of the passage is

   (A)   what constitutes computer literacy.

   (B)   the qualities good teachers must have.

   (C)   appropriate uses of computers in education.

   (D)   limitations of computers as educational tools.

2.   Which of the following statements is LEAST accurate? The authors believe that intuition

   (A)   can be fostered by computers used as educational tools.

   (B)   is compatible with expertise.

   (C)   plays an important role in expert teaching.

   (D)   is less essential than logic in education.

3.   The authors believe that computers as educational tools can be effective in developing

   I.   logical skills.

   II.   procedural problem-solving skills.

   III.   classroom sociality.

   (A)   I only.   (B)   I and II only.

   (C)   II and III only.   (D)   I, II, and III.

4.   One can infer from the passage that the authors believe that the acquisition of expertise derives chiefly from

   (A)   experience and intuition.

   (B)   mastery of the facts in a given discipline.

   (C)   careful coaching and problem-solving.

   (D)   logic combined with informed advice.

5.   One can infer from the passage that the authors believe that the greatest danger in using computers as educational tools is

   (A)   enforcing rigid modes of thought.

   (B)   expecting students to master skills for which they are temperamentally unsuited.

(C)   the fostering of anti-social behavior.

(D)   demanding that computers perform tasks they are unable to perform.

6.   A study that proved that computers can be useful in fostering educated expertise would force the authors to change

(A)   their discussion of computers as tools.

(B)   their discussion of computers as tutees.

(C)   their discussion of computers as tutors.

(D)   none of their essay.

7   With which of the following statements would the authors most likely agree?

(A)   One can teach what one does not understand.

(B)   Expert teachers derive their expertise largely from rules learned in graduate school.

(C)   Teachers can be replaced by computers.

(D)   We only understand what we can formulate in logical rules and procedures.

8.   Based on the authors' distinction between trained competence and educated expertise, which of the following would they classify as trained competence?

I.   a champion race-car driver.

II.   a computerized defense system such as "Star Wars."

III.   a chess grandmaster.

(A)   I only.   (B)   II only.

(C)   III only.   (D)   I and III only.

9.   Which of the following statements best summarizes the authors' view of the use of computers in education?

(A)   Their uses are virtually unlimited.

(B)   They can be very useful educational tools as long as their limitations are recognized.

(C)   They can be valuable, but are generally abused because people fail to realize that they can only be used as tools, not as tutors or tutees.

(D)   They are greatly overrated and should seldom be used.

PASSAGE II (Questions 10-19)

   In both oral and typographic cultures, information derives its importance from the possibilities of action. Of course, in any communication environment, input (what one is informed about) always exceeds output (the possibilities of action based on information). But the situation created by telegraphy, and then exacerbated by later technologies, made the relationship between information and action both abstract and remote. For the first time in human history, people were faced with the problem of information glut, which means that simultaneously they were faced with the problem of a diminished social and political potency.

You may get a sense of what this means by asking yourself another series of questions: What steps do you plan to take to reduce the conflict in the Middle East; or the rates of inflation, crime and unemployment? I shall take the liberty of answering for you: You plan to do nothing about them. You may, of course, cast a ballot for someone who claims to have some plans, as well as the power to act. But this you can do only once every two or four years by giving one hour of your time, hardly a satisfying means of expressing the broad range of opinions you hold. Voting, we might say, is next to the last refuge of the politically impotent. The last refuge is, of course, giving your opinion to a pollster, who will get a version of it through a desiccated question, and then will submerge it in a Niagara of similar opinions, and convert them into — what else?— another piece of news. Thus, we have here a great loop of impotence: The news elicits from you a variety of opinions about which you can do nothing except to offer opinions as more news, about which you can equally do nothing.

Prior to the age of telegraphy, the information-action ratio was sufficiently close so that most people had a sense of being able to control some of the contingencies in their lives. What people knew about had action-value. In the information world created by telegraphy, this sense of potency was lost, precisely because the whole world became the context for news. Everything became everyone's business. For the first time, we were sent information which answered no question we had asked, and which, in any case, did not permit the right to reply.

We may say then that the contribution of the telegraph to public discourse was to dignify irrelevance and amplify impotence. But this was not all: telegraphy also made public discourse essentially incoherent. It brought into being a world "of broken time and broken attention," to use Lewis Mumford's phrase. The principal strength of the telegraph lay in its capacity to move information, not collect it, explain it or analyze it. In this respect, telegraphy was the exact opposite of typography. Books, for example, are an excellent container for the accumulation, quiet scrutiny and organized analysis of information and ideas. A book is an attempt to make thought permanent and to contribute to the great conversation conducted by authors of the past. Therefore, civilized people everywhere consider the burning of a book a vile form of anti-intellectualism. But the telegraph demands that we burn its contents. The value of telegraphy is undermined by applying the tests of permanence, continuity or coherence. The telegraph is suited only to the flashing of messages, each to be quickly replaced by a more up-to-date message.

Adapted from Neil Postman, *Amusing Ourselves to Death*, 1985.

10. According to the author, most Americans plan to do nothing to reduce conflict in the Middle East because

    (A) they lack information about the area.

    (B) they are socially irresponsible.

    (C) they feel politically impotent.

    (D) they are preoccupied with personal economic success.

11. The author regards voting chiefly as

(A) a satisfying way of expressing an individual's various political beliefs.

(B) a way of directly contributing to the solution of important national and international problems.

(C) the crucial act upon which democracy depends.

(D) a relatively ineffective expression of powerlessness.

12. From the passage, it is clear that the author regards polls chiefly as

(A) a means of manufacturing news.

(B) an effective way of influencing public opinion.

(C) an attempt to shape foreign and domestic policy.

(D) part of a system of political checks and balances.

13. "Information-action ratio" refers to

(A) the relationship between accurate information and government policies based on accurate information.

(B) the degree to which people can take meaningful action on the basis of information they receive.

(C) the individual's need to have global and not merely local news.

(D) the relationship between historical facts and current events.

14. According to the author, technological advances in conveying information have

(A) led to a more responsible electorate.

(B) increased the individual's sense of social helplessness.

(C) made public discourse more thoughtful.

(D) made people more responsive to the problems of people in other cultures.

15. According to the author, people in pre-telegraphic cultures had a greater sense of being able to control some of the contingencies in their lives than people in telegraphic cultures because

(A) the context of their news was less global.

(B) they derived their news chiefly from oral sources.

(C) their news had less action-value.

(D) there was greater personal contact between individuals.

16. According to the author, telegraphy has

I.   made public discourse more incoherent.

II.   increased the flow of irrelevant information.

III. given individuals a greater sense of social responsibility.

(A)   I only.   (B)   I and II only.

(C)   I and III only.   (D)   I, II, and III.

17.   The author's statement that the "telegraph is suited only to the flashing of messages" is designed to support his contention that telegraphy

(A)   dignifies irrelevance.

(B)   increases the individual's sense of political impotence.

(C)   created a world of broken time and broken attention.

(D)   makes the relationship between information and action abstract.

18.   Based on information in the passage, with which of the following statements would the author most likely agree?

(A)   All news contributes to the individual's social or political well-being.

(B)   Technological advances in communication have contributed significantly to the analysis of news.

(C)   Public discourse is enhanced by telegraphic achievements.

(D)   Typography is better able to withstand tests of continuity than is telegraphy.

19.   The author would probably consider which of the following cultures most intellectual?

(A)   oral   (B)   typographic

(C)   telegraphic   (D)   post-telegraphic

PASSAGE III (Questions 20-28)

We base our expectations of the future on what we have observed about the past, both in our daily lives and in our professions. It was the great philosopher David Hume who called to our attention the problem we face as we do this.

Hume pointed out that no matter how many observations we have made of a correlation between events, we can never be sure that this correlation will be repeated in the future. There is no way for us to know whether the future will resemble the past that we have observed. Furthermore, there is no observation we can make about any particular object or event that will necessarily reveal to us its future nature, or how it will be related to other objects or events in the future, or even if there will be a future at all. An examination of the present and past, no matter how detailed and complete, will not suffice as proof that the future will be one way rather than another.

It might be thought that, although we cannot know the future with certainty, we can at least have some assurance of probability about the resemblance of the future to the past. But even here, Hume raised questions about the validity of this assumption. How can we say that the past makes a particular future more likely, except by appealing to the fact that this is the way things have always been, so that we project this expectation into the future? The projection of either probability or certainty into the future, however, is the very point at issue.

Thus, there is a critical problem involving the conceptual basis on which we conduct our lives, the justification for the extrapolation of past observations to future expectations. This is a problem for which we have as yet no satisfactory solution. Still, we continue to shape and fashion our lives as if this problem did not exist.

Hume observed that this disposition to fashion expectations of the future based on the past is a part of our human nature. He did not urge us to try to reshape our human nature as we form these expectations. What must be considered is not what we do but rather the nature of our justification for what we do.

20. The main problem considered in the passage concerns

   (A)   the truth of our judgments about the future.

   (B)   the justification of our judgments about the future.

   (C)   the probability of our judgments about the future.

   (D)   the existence of the future.

21. Based on this passage, we should conclude that

   (A)   the future will not resemble the past.

   (B)   the future may not resemble the past.

   (C)   the future will probably not resemble the past.

   (D)   None of the above.

22. According to the passage, the philosopher David Hume would be most likely to say that

   (A)   we should live only for today and take no care for tomorrow.

   (B)   we should predict the future in terms of probability rather than certainty.

   (C)   we should be aware that our knowledge of the future rests on an uncertain foundation.

   (D)   we should not make predictions about the future.

23. Justification in the form of good evidence for a belief proves that

   (A)   our belief is true.

   (B)   we know why the belief is true.

   (C)   Both (A) and (B).

   (D)   Neither (A) nor (B).

24. The problem raised in this passage is really a problem about

   (A)   our projection of belief about the past into the future.

   (B)   the resemblance of the future to the past.

   (C)   the nature of the future.

   (D)   our human nature.

25. According to the passage, our assurance about how the future will be

    (A) rests on no foundation at all.

    (B) rests on no justified foundation at all.

    (C) rests on no justified foundation that we can prove.

    (D) All of the above.

26. The problem identified in the passage could be solved by

    (A) gathering more data.

    (B) being more precise in analyzing our data.

    (C) both gathering more data and being more precise in analyzing the data.

    (D) None of the above.

27. Hume would say that judgments of probability are no better than judgments of certainty because

    (A) either one of them may turn out to be false.

    (B) each requires a presumption of the relevance of past information to future expectations.

    (C) each requires a presumption of the effect of the past on the future.

    (D) our human nature is such that no knowledge is possible for us.

29. According to Hume's description, which of the following would be an example of human nature in operation?

    (A) Guessing the outcome of a coin toss

    (B) Tossing a coin to make a decision about the future

    (C) Carrying an umbrella on a cloudy day

    (D) Getting wet when it rains

PASSAGE IV (Questions 29-37)

The literature on elderly drug use indicates that the elderly are at high risk for drug misuse and that they may also be at considerable risk for drug abuse involving legal drugs. In addition, a small group of elderly opiate addicts exists. There are findings that some addicts do mature out of their addiction, but the majority adapt and conceal their habits by using other drugs, such as hydromorphone hydrochloride; by decreasing their daily usage; and by substituting more legally available substances such as alcohol or barbiturates. The abusive use of drugs by the elderly may be associated with coping problems related to retirement, physical problems, loss of family and friends, dependence, and feelings of depression and low self-esteem.

Elderly alcohol abuse is a more widely acknowledged and more thoroughly researched problem than elderly drug abuse. One-third of the alcoholics developed their problems after entering their elderly years. Their drinking seems to be related more to attempts to cope with the stresses and problems of old age than to more deeply rooted psychological difficulties. Elderly alcohol abusers are likely to drink more often but in smaller quantities than younger alcohol abusers. Elderly alcohol abusers also have fewer severe and obvious social or physical problems or impairments than do younger alcohol abusers. Hiding, denial, or lack of awareness of the problem is common among the elderly. As the environmental stresses of the growing elderly population increases and as increasing proportions of the elderly become non-abstainers, the number of elderly alcoholics may increase dramatically over the next ten to fifteen years.

Drug abuse among the elderly may follow a pattern comparable to that for alcohol abuse. Neither elderly alcohol abusers nor elderly drug abusers seem to mature out to the extent previously believed. An aging of both abuser populations is likely, along with reductions, adaptations, and concealment of abuse as old age is reached. Both forms of abuse may either begin or recur during old age. Elderly alcoholism and elderly drug abuse appear mainly to involve small but frequent doses of legal substances. For many elderly persons, alcohol abuse and other drug abuse may be part of a single pattern.

Adolescence and old age have many similarities that may relate to drug abuse. Both involve uncertain and changing roles and self-concepts, lower social status, disadvantages with respect to employment and income, shifting and uncertain social supports, and other characteristics. Both groups are limited in their ability to become self-reliant and assert their independence and have limited resources for coping. Both groups find drugs readily available, although from different sources. This, and the elderly's regard for lawfulness and social conformity, result primarily in illicit drug use among adolescents and licit drug use among the elderly.

The stepping-stone theory, in which initial use of alcohol and tobacco is said to lead gradually to marijuana use and then to hard drug use among adolescents, may have a parallel in the use of licit drugs by the elderly. Psychological characteristics of the aged, including reduced intellectual and problem-solving abilities, may also increase the tendency among some elderly persons to return to the use of more primitive defense mechanisms such as somatization and, thus, to drug use. In addition, psychoactive drug use may reflect the more passive copying styles of many older adults.

29. Elderly drug abuse involves primarily

    (A) marijuana.   (B) opium.

    (C) legal substances.   (D) All of the above.

30. The passage predicts that the number of elderly alcoholics may increase dramatically in the near future due to

    (A) the longer life expectancy that will be achieved during this time.

    (B) greater environmental stresses on a larger elderly population.

    (C) the decreasing availability of illicit drugs.

    (D) the increasing expense of licit drugs.

31. The purpose of this passage is to

    (A) suggest methods for preventing substance abuse among the elderly.

    (B) suggest methods for treating substance abuse among the elderly.

(C)   explain why certain adolescent substance abusers become elderly substance abusers.

(D)   identify the causes of certain kinds of substance abuse among the elderly.

32.   According to information contained in the passage, it can be concluded that

    (A)   one-third of all alcoholics are elderly.

    (B)   one-third of all elderly alcoholics had not developed their problems before entering their elderly years.

    (C)   one-third of persons entering their elderly years have become alcoholics.

    (D)   None of the above.

33.   Elderly alcohol abusers are likely to

    (A)   drink more often but in smaller quantities than younger alcohol abusers.

    (B)   drink more often and in greater quantities than younger alcohol abusers.

    (C)   drink less often but in greater quantities than younger alcohol abusers.

    (D)   drink about the same amount with the same frequency as younger alcohol abusers.

34.   Which of the following is not suggested as a possible factor in elderly substance abuse?

    (A)   Lower social status

    (B)   Limited self-reliance

    (C)   Depression

    (D)   The use of sophisticated defense mechanisms

35.   According to the stepping-stone theory, which of the following would be most likely to occur?

    (A)   An adolescent who uses cocaine later becomes an alcoholic.

    (B)   An adolescent who drinks begins to smoke cigarettes.

    (C)   An adolescent who is a cocaine addict becomes an opium addict when elderly.

    (D)   An elderly person who abuses over-the-counter sleeping medication becomes dependent on barbiturates.

36.   The passage suggests that the elderly's regard for lawfulness and social conformity

    (A)   helps to explain the low incidence of drug abuse among the elderly.

    (B)   helps to explain which substances are most likely to be abused by the elderly.

    (C)   decreases once the elderly person begins to abuse drugs.

    (D)   None of the above.

37.   Elderly alcohol abusers are more likely than younger alcohol abusers to

(A)   have severe and obvious physical problems.

(B)   have severe and obvious social problems.

(C)   also abuse licit drugs.

(D)   abstain from alcohol for long periods of time.

PASSAGE V (Questions 38-47)

The submarine first became a major component in naval warfare during World War I, when Germany demonstrated its full potentialities. Wholesale sinking of Allied shipping by the German U-boats almost swung the war in favor of the Central Powers. Then, as now, the submarine's greatest advantage was that it could operate beneath the ocean surface where detection was difficult. Sinking a submarine was comparatively easy, once it was found — but finding it before it could attack was another matter

During the closing months of World War I, the Allied Submarine Devices Investigation Committee was formed to obtain from science and technology more effective underwater detection equipment. The committee developed a reasonably accurate device for locating a submerged submarine. This device was a trainable hydrophone, which was attached to the bottom of the ASW ship, and used to detect screw noises and other sounds that came from a submarine. Although the committee disbanded after World War I, the British made improvements on the locating device between that time and World War II and named the device after the committee.

American scientists further improved on the device, calling it sonar, a name derived from the underlined initials of the words sound navigation and ranging.

At the end of World War II, the United States improved the snorkel (a device for bringing air to the crew and engines when operating on submerged diesels) and developed the Guppy (short for greater underwater propulsion power), a conversion of the fleet-type submarine of World War II fame. The superstructure was changed by reducing the surface area, streamlining every protruding object, and enclosing the periscope shears in a streamlined metal fairing. Performance increased greatly with improved electronic equipment, additional battery capacity, and the addition of the snorkel.

Since World War II, the submerged endurance of the submarine has improved sufficiently to make submarine detection difficult. The problem increases as the submarine goes faster and deeper and stays down longer. To cope with the modern submarine, we now have better detection devices, more modern weapons, and newer ships, but the battle for supremacy is a never-ending one.

During World War II, submarines sent millions of tons of shipping to the bottom. Early in the war, England's lifelines were nearly strangled by German submarines. American submarines played a large role in the defeat of Japan by sinking nearly all her merchant marine. Obviously, the submarine is a potent weapon, requiring equally effective countermeasures. The United States and Great Britain were successful in developing equipment, weapons, and tactics that enabled the destruction of the German submarine force. Japan was never able to develop an effective defense against our submarines.

38.   American submarines played a large role in the defeat of Japan in World War II by

    (A)   sinking almost all of Japan's merchant marine.

    (B)   sinking almost all of Japan's aircraft carriers.

    (C)   developing the Guppy.

    (D)   threatening Japanese home ports.

39.   The purpose of this passage is

    (A)   to explain why the Allies won World War II.

    (B)   to identify the major improvements in submarine technology since World War I.

    (C)   to explain why submarines will not be important in future wars.

    (D)   to compare Allied and German submarine technology.

40.   The result of the formation of the Allied Submarine Devices Investigation Committee was an improvement in submarine

    (A)   navigation.   (B)   stealth.

    (C)   location.   (D)   construction.

41.   The nation that first developed the effective use of submarines as a part of naval strategy was

    (A)   the United States.   (B)   Great Britain.

    (C)   Japan.   (D)   Germany.

42.   The greatest difficulty in anti-submarine warfare is

    (A)   finding the enemy submarine.

    (B)   sinking the enemy submarine once it is found.

    (C)   drawing the enemy submarine to the surface.

    (D)   escaping the enemy submarine once contact is made.

43.   The snorkel is a device for

    (A)   increasing underwater propulsion power.

    (B)   viewing surface objects from a submerged submarine.

    (C)   bringing air to a submerged submarine.

    (D)   navigation.

44.   During World War II, the primary means of submarine detection was based on

    (A)   surface sightings.   (B)   intelligence reports.

    (C)   satellite surveillance.   (D)   sound reports.

45.   Which of the following countries did not participate in the development of the submarine detection device that was eventually known as sonar?

(A) Germany   (B) Great Britain

(C) The United States   (D) France

46. Which of the following is not mentioned as an element contributing to the difficulty of locating a submarine?

(A) The submarine's speed

(B) The submarine's depth

(C) The submarine's size

(D) The length of time the submarine remains submerged

47. The author of the passage says that, in the early part of World War II,

(A) American submarines almost destroyed Japanese shipping.

(B) German submarines almost destroyed shipping to England.

(C) English submarines almost destroyed shipping to Germany.

(D) Japanese submarines almost destroyed American shipping.

PASSAGE VI (Questions 48-56)

Americans know of Hebrew as the language of the Old Testament. Hebrew had been a living language, that is, it was spoken as a native language by a community of people, at least until the First Century, B.C., and possibly for several centuries after that. But even though it ceased to be a living language in this sense, a large and important body of literature has remained in constant daily use for prayer and study.

During the Middle Ages and into the Renaissance, Hebrew served as a *lingua franca* for Jews throughout the world, and the literature was expanded by scholars and poets. Hebrew thus remained familiar, and in the last century successful efforts were begun to revive it as a modern language.

Today Hebrew is the official language of the state of Israel. It is taught to immigrants who speak a wide variety of native languages, with the goal of having all of Israel's inhabitants able to speak it.

To be sure, modern Hebrew is different from the Biblical languages. The phonology (sound system) has been simplified, and new syntactic patterns and vocabulary have been developed to express concepts not dreamed of two thousand years ago. But the modern language is unmistakably the descendant of the language of the Psalms and the prophets.

Modern Hebrew is a living language and as such it is changing daily. Slang expression, coinages, variant pronunciations, and grammatical innovations are characteristic of any living language. Furthermore, Hebrew is spoken and written in a variety of styles. These vary from highly formal to highly informal.

Formal spoken style is very similar to the literary style and is more like the traditional Hebrew that is taught. Formal style is used, as the name implies, for public speaking, official meetings, radio news broadcasts, or on other occasions where the speaker would use deferential or deliberate speech.

Informal spoken style is that used by native speakers in ordinary, relaxed conversation. It is often more rapid than the formal style and is the speech which seems most "natural" to native Israelis.

There is a highly informal style which contains much slang, contractions and dropping of sounds, and is fairly rapid. The student should not attempt to learn it until he or she is fairly fluent in the ordinary informal style.

The goal of studying a language is performance. One "knows" Hebrew in the same sense that one "knows" how to drive a car. It is not necessary to be an automotive engineer or to know the technical terms for the parts of a car in order to be a good driver. Many excellent drivers even have wrong notions about the mechanical aspects of an automobile. Similarly, it is not necessary to be able to discuss accurately and comprehensively the grammar of a language in order to speak it fluently and correctly. Intensive drilling will produce the proper habits. When one is able to participate in conversation easily and fluently with a minimum of either "accent" or conscious effort, then one has achieved the goal of studying a language.

48. Modern Hebrew and Biblical Hebrew are identical in

    (A)   phonology.   (B)   syntax.

    (C)   vocabulary.   (D)   None of the above.

49. A living language is identified as one that

    (A)   has a long history.

    (B)   is richly expressive.

    (C)   is spoken as a native language by a community of people.

    (D)   has both written and oral forms.

50. Ancient Hebrew

    (A)   ceased to be a living language at approximately the first century, B.C.

    (B)   existed only as an oral language.

    (C)   became a forgotten language during the Middle Ages.

    (D)   is now the official language of Israel.

51. The passage represents the goal of studying a language as

    (A)   knowing the grammar of the language.

    (B)   conversational ease in using the language.

    (C)   broadening one's cultural heritage.

    (D)   learning the vocabulary of the language.

52. Modern Hebrew is spoken in

    (A)   only a formal style.

    (B)   only an informal style.

    (C)   both formal and informal styles.

    (D)   None of the above.

53. Ancient Hebrew was the language of

(A)   the Prophets.   (B)   the Old Testament.

(C)   the Psalms.   (D)   All of the above.

54. The passage states that the state of Israel has the goal of

(A)   having all its inhabitants learn to speak Hebrew.

(B)   having all its inhabitants speak only Hebrew.

(C)   having all its inhabitants learn Biblical Hebrew.

(D)   having all its inhabitants learn both Biblical and modern Hebrew.

55. The passage represents knowing a language as

(A)   knowing how to do something.

(B)   knowing why something is the way it is.

(C)   being able to explain how something works.

(D)   None of the above.

56. The formal spoken style of Hebrew is said to be

(A)   more rapid than the informal style.

(B)   more natural to native Israelis than the informal style.

(C)   more similar to traditional Hebrew than the informal style.

(D)   used more often by native Israelis than the informal style.

PASSAGE VII (Questions 57-65)

Perhaps the most remarkable trauma seen by the paleopathologist is trephination or the surgical removal of a portion of the skull. The earliest written accounts of trephination are found in the Hippocracic writings (460-377 B.C.). However, the evidence of trephining goes back at least to the Neolithic period (10,000 B.C.).

It is clear that the identification of the cause of holes in the skull cannot always be made. However, there are some criteria that will be important in any analysis. The first question to be resolved is whether the hole is the result of mechanical intervention. Evidence for curing or scraping may still exist even if healing has taken place. The next problem to be clarified is if the cutting was done before or after death. The significant question here is whether we are seeing the product of a surgical procedure or the result of some postmorten ritual. Any evidence of healing or inflammatory reaction to the cutting is indicative of trephination. However, it is possible that a patient can die during the trephination or so soon after it that no reaction takes place. Such a situation in an archaeological example of trephination may be indistinguishable from postmortem ritual removal. In such situations the demonstration of unambiguous trephination in the same geographical area would certainly be significant in interpreting the equivocal cases. Another important criterion is the presence of fracture in association with evidence of cutting. Many, if not most trephinations occur in association with skull fracture. As with most other problems in paleopathology careful observation combined with a comprehensive knowledge of the options is the most important prerequisite in determining the presence of trephination.

In trephination, four basic responses can occur. First, in those cases where trauma preceded the trephination procedure, death may be due to the initial trauma. Second, the surgical procedure itself may cause death. Third, the surgical procedure may not directly cause death but may introduce disease organisms that cause infection and possibly death. Fourth, there may be no complications resulting from surgery, in which case the individual survives with varying degrees of repair to the surgically induced defect. If there is no healing, as evidenced by the lack of remodeling of the cut edges or fill in of exposed spaces, the reasonable assumption is that death occurred at the time of, or shortly after, surgery. A zone of porous, reactive bond surrounding the surgical area suggests survival for some time after surgery, but with the possibility of infection complicating the healing process and causing death. Partial to complete refill of the surgical defect is indicative of recovery and long-term survival after surgery.

57. Trephination is a surgical procedure involving the removal of a portion of the skull in

  (A)   a living patient.

  (B)   a corpse.

  (C)   either a living patient or a corpse.

  (D)   a postmortem ritual.

58. Evidence of healing or inflammation is a sign of

  (A)   a fracture in the skull.

  (B)   trephination.

  (C)   postmortem ritual removal.

  (D)   None of the above.

59. The lack of evidence of healing

  (A)   is proof of trephination.

  (B)   is proof of postmortem ritual removal.

  (C)   is proof of inflammation.

  (D)   is inconclusive in determining whether trephination or postmortem ritual removal occurred.

60. The passages specifies that many trephinations

  (A)   cause skull fractures.

  (B)   result from skull fractures.

  (C)   are associated with skull fractures.

  (D)   None of the above.

61. The passage specified that four basic responses to trephination can occur. Three of these four involve the death of the patient. Therefore,

    (A)   75% of the patients die during this procedure.

    (B)   75% of the patients die after this procedure.

    (C)   25% of the patients die from this procedure.

    (D)   None of the above.

62. Trephination is a surgical procedure dating from

    (A)   the discovery of anesthesia in the 19th century.

    (B)   the time of Hippocrates.

    (C)   the Neolithic period.

    (D)   the fourth century B.C.

63. The passage describes

    (A)   some of the reasons for trephination.

    (B)   some of the problems in differentiating trephination from postmorten cutting of the skull.

    (C)   some of the surgical procedures use in trephination.

    (D)   some of the tools used in trephination.

64. In this passage, the word "trauma" should be taken to mean

    (A)   a painful emotional response to something.

    (B)   a frightful or fearful condition.

    (C)   a bodily wound or injury or shock.

    (D)   All of the above.

65. Which of the following would be the best evidence for long-term survival after trephination?

    (A)   Partial refilling of the damaged skull

    (B)   Exposed spaces in the skull

    (C)   Signs of an inflammatory reaction

    (D)   Absence of reshaping or the cut edges of the skull

STOP

If time still remains, you may review work only in this section.

When the time allotted is up, you may go on to the next section.

Section 2 — Physical Sciences

TIME: 100 Minutes
QUESTIONS: 66-142

DIRECTIONS: Most of the questions in this section are arranged in groups, each corresponding to a descriptive passage. Based on the information given in a passage, choose the one best answer to each question in the group. Some questions are independent of a descriptive passage and of each other. Choose the one best answer to each of these questions. If you are not sure of an answer, eliminate those choices that you know are incorrect and choose an answer from among those remaining. Fill in the corresponding circle on the answer sheet to indicate your answer. You may refer to the periodic table at any time.

PASSAGE I (Questions 66-74)

A bullet of mass $m_1 = 0.01$ kg is fired with a muzzle speed of 100 m/sec to the RIGHT along the horizontal. The gun recoils with a speed of 1 m/sec. The bullet encounters an approximately constant force of air resistance equal to its weight as it heads towards a block of mass $m_2 = 1$ kg which is initially at rest on a rough horizontal surface a distance of 10 m from where the bullet was fired. The bullet imbeds itself in the block, a process that takes 0.01 sec from the initial time of contact. The combination bullet-in-block then slides 2 m before coming to rest. Use $g = 10$ m/sec^2.

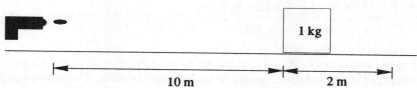

66. The mass of the gun is

    (A)   1 g

    (B)   100 g

    (C)   0.01 kg

    (D)   1 kg

67. The horizontal acceleration of the bullet due to air resistance was

    (A)   10 m/s^2 to the LEFT

    (B)   0.1 m/s^2 to the LEFT

    (C)   0.1 m/s^2 to the RIGHT

    (D)   1 m/s^2 to the RIGHT

68. The speed of the bullet as it impacted the block was

    (A)   100 m/s

    (B)   101 m/s

    (C)   99 m/s

    (D)   0 m/s

69. The impulse received by the earth during the bullet's flight was

   (A)   0.01 kgm/s LEFT
   (B)   0.01 kgm/s RIGHT
   (C)   1 kgm/s RIGHT
   (D)   1 kgm/s LEFT

70. The speed of the bullet-in-block combinations just after impact was

   (A)   0.98 m/s
   (B)   98 m/s
   (C)   99 m/s
   (D)   9.9 m/s

71. The impulse received by the block due to the impact was

   (A)   98 kgm/s
   (B)   100 kgm/s
   (C)   9.9 kgm/s
   (D)   0.98 kgm/s

72. The average force experienced by the bullet during impact was

   (A)   10,000 N
   (B)   9800 N
   (C)   9900 N
   (D)   98 N

73. The acceleration of the combination over the 2 m slide was

   (A)   0.24 m/s^2 LEFT
   (B)   9.8 m/s^2 LEFT
   (C)   49 m/s^2 RIGHT
   (D)   1 m/s^2 LEFT

74. The force of friction which stopped the combination was

   (A)   1.01 N
   (B)   0.24 N
   (C)   9.9 N
   (D)   49.5 N

PASSAGE II (Questions 75-84)

Sulfur dioxide is produced by burning sulfur-containing substances in air:

$$S\ (s) + O_2\ (g) \longrightarrow SO_2\ (g)$$

Most of the atmospheric SO_2 comes from electrical power plants, smelting plants, sulfuric acid plants, and burning coal or oil for home heating. The average sulfur content of all coal mined in the United States is about 2.0%. In 1984, 91.8% of the 890 million short tons of coal produced in the United States were burned in the United States.

Sulfur dioxide is a primary pollutant that is oxidized in air to a secondary pollutant, SO_3, according to the following **unbalanced** equation:

$$SO_2 + O_2 \longrightarrow SO_3$$

which dissolves in water to form sulfuric acid.

$$SO_3 + H_2O \longrightarrow H_2SO_4$$

The SO_2 formed during the combustion of coal also reacts with $CaCO_3$ (limestone) and water to produce Calcium sulfite dihydrate and a gas as shown in the (unbalanced) equation below:

$$CaCO_3 + SO_2 + H_2O \longrightarrow CaSO_3 \cdot 2H_2O + \underline{\hspace{1cm}}$$

This reaction is responsible for the disintegration of marble statues and buildings.

The reaction of an acid with a hydroxide-containing base yields a salt and water as shown by the following reaction:

$$2\,NaOH + H_2SO_4 \longrightarrow Na_2SO_4 + 2\,H_2O$$

This is an example of a neutralization reaction, which can be used to destroy strong acids such as the sulfuric acid produced during this pollution process.

75. Consider the reaction between SO_2 and oxygen to form SO_3. How many moles of oxygen are required to produce 10.0 moles of SO_3 if there is sufficient SO_2 in the air?

(A)   10.0   (B)   20.0

(C)   5.00   (D)   None of the above.

76. Using the same equation as in Question 75 find the number of grams of SO_3 that would be formed when 10.0 grams of SO_2 react with 10.0 grams of oxygen.

(A)   50.0   (B)   25.0

(C)   12.5   (D)   40.0

77. If 10.0 moles of SO_3 are produced during the reaction, what volume will this gas occupy at 23°C and 380 torr?

(A)   486 liters   (B)   0.640 liters

(C)   1.56 liters   (D)   0.050 liters

78. What is the density (g/liter) of the SO_2 produced in this reaction at 300°C and 380 torr?

(A)   1.5   (B)   517

(C)   0.68   (D)   987

79. How many grams of sulfur would be required to react with sufficient oxygen to produce 29.8 liters of SO_2 at 25°C and 380 torr assuming 100% yield?

(A) 1.5×10^4 (B)   19

(C)   232   (D)   53

80. Considering the information provided in the passage, how many kilograms of sulfur dioxide would be produced when 500 lbs of coal is combusted in air

(A)   9.08   (B)   908

(C) 9.80×10^6 (D)   0.102

81. SO_3 is called a(n)

(A)   basic oxide.   (B)   basic anhydride.

(C)   amphoteric oxide.   (D)   acidic anhydride.

82. If 640 grams of SO_3 are produced at STP, how many liters of oxygen reacted

with excess SO_2 according to the equation used in Question 75?

(A)   224

(B)   448

(C)   112

(D)   0.0022

83.   Complete and balance the equation for the reaction between sulfur dioxide and calcium carbonate that was given in the passage. Give the coefficient of water, the gas formed, and the number of grams of $CaCO_3$ dissolved when it reacts with 64 grams of SO_2 and excess water.

(A) $1 \ldots CO_2 \ldots 100$

(B) $2 \ldots CO_2 \ldots 100$

(C) $2 \ldots CO_2 \ldots 0.01$

(D) $1 \ldots O_2 \ldots \ 100$

84.   According to the reaction presented in the passage, adding sodium hydroxide to the sulfuric acid formed by the reaction of SO_3 with water will neutralize the acid. How much 0.2000 N NaOH will be needed to react with 25.00 ml of 0.1000 N H_2SO_4?

(A)   12.50

(B)   25.00

(C)   0.08000

(D)   0.04000

PASSAGE III (Questions 85-93)

NASA wishes to launch a military satellite consisting of a payload of mass $m = 500$ kg. As launched from Cape Canaveral, the initial horizontal speed of the rocket is determined from the known latitude of 28.4°. The satellite is deployed in a roughly circular orbit at a distance of 10,000 km from the center of the earth. The satellite will require 3 complete revolutions around the earth to complete each mission of photographing certain key military installations around the globe. The radius of the earth is 6400 km, the mass of the earth is 6×10^{24} kg, the universal gravitational constant is $G = 6.67 \times 10^{-11}$ Nm^2/kg^2, and the constant of proportionality in Kepler's third law for the earth is $K = 9.86 \times 10^{-14}$ s^2/m^3.

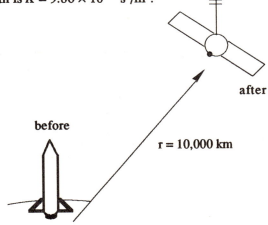

85.   What is the tangential speed of the satellite as it rests on the launch pad prior to launch?

(A)   409 m/s

(B)   0 m/s

(C)   465 m/s

(D)   110 m/s

86. How long does it take the satellite to make one complete revolution about the center of rotation when it is on the launch pad?

    (A) 1 day
    (B) 24 hours
    (C) 1440 min
    (D) all of these

87. What is the kinetic energy of the satellite as it rests on earth prior to launch?

    (A) 0 J
    (B) 4.18×10^7 J
    (C) 5.41×10^7 J
    (D) 1.21×10^7 J

88. What is the gravitational potential energy of the satellite as it rests on the launch pad as measured relative to the point at $r = \infty$?

    (A) 0 J
    (B) $+3.14 \times 10^{10}$ J
    (C) -3.13×10^{10} J
    (D) -1.42×10^{10} J

89. What is the period of the satellite in its deployed orbit?

    (A) 1 day
    (B) 48 hours
    (C) 4.3×10^3 s
    (D) 166 min

90. How far does the satellite travel in completing each mission of photographing key military installations?

    (A) 6.28×10^7 m
    (B) 1.89×10^8 m
    (C) 0 m
    (D) 4.21×10^{10} m

91. What is the kinetic energy of the satellite in its stable orbit?

    (A) 1×10^{10} J
    (B) 0 J
    (C) 5.34×10^{10} J
    (D) 1.67×10^5 J

92. What is the gravitational potential energy of the satellite in its stable orbit?

    (A) 4.9×10^{10} J
    (B) 2.45×10^{10} J
    (C) -3.13×10^{10} J
    (D) -2.00×10^{10} J

93. How much energy was expended in putting the satellite into orbit?

    (A) 0 J
    (B) -1.05×10^{10} J
    (C) $+2.13 \times 10^{10}$ J
    (D) $+1.05 \times 10^{10}$ J

QUESTIONS 94-101 are NOT based on a descriptive passage.

---

94. What is the total resistance of the circuit on the following page?

    (A) 12 Ω
    (B) 4.7 Ω
    (C) 8/3 Ω
    (D) 2 Ω

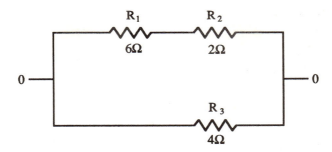

95. Find the resistance of an electric blender if it uses a current of 5 amperes when connected to a 120-volt circuit.

    (A) 540 ohms   (B) 115 ohms

    (C) 30 ohms   (D) 24 ohms

96. If white light is dispersed by a prism, which colors will have the greatest angle of deviation and the smallest angle of deviation?

    (A) orange-blue   (B) red-violet

    (C) green-yellow   (D) violet-red

97. A 15 volt battery is attached to a circuit containing resistances of 2 ohms, 3 ohms, and 5 ohms connected in series. The current in the circuit is

    (A) 1.5 amperes.   (B) 3 amperes.

    (C) 5 amperes.   (D) 0.5 amperes.

98. Two forces of 10 newtons and 6 newtons act on an object. In order to produce a resultant force of 4 newtons, how many degrees apart must they be oriented with respect to each other?

    (A) 45°   (B) 60°

    (C) 90°   (D) 180°

99. A 25 lb cannonball is shot from a cannon horizontally situated 3 ft above the ground. The muzzle velocity is 550 ft/sec. At the same time, an identical 25 lb cannonball is dropped from the same 3 ft height. Assuming ideal conditions, the dropped cannonball will

    (A) strike the ground before the one which was shot.

    (B) strike the ground with a lesser vertical velocity than the shot cannonball.

    (C) strike the ground with greater vertical velocity than the shot cannonball.

    (D) strike the ground at the same time as the one which was shot.

100. A 100 gram marble strikes a 25 gram marble lying on a smooth horizontal surface squarely. In the impact, the speed of the larger marble is reduced from 100 cm/sec to 60 cm/sec. What is the speed of the smaller marble immediately after impact?

(A)	60 cm/sec	(B)	100 cm/sec
(C)	40 cm/sec	(D)	160 cm/sec

101. A cart of mass 5 kg moves horizontally across a frictionless table with a speed of 1 m/sec. When a brick of mass 5 kg is dropped on the cart, what is the change in velocity of the cart?

(A)	- 0.5 m/sec	(B)	0.5 m/sec
(C)	No change	(D)	1.5 m /sec

PASSAGE IV (Questions 102-112)

The laws of thermodynamics are especially relevant in today's society considering the problems that we face in supplying the nation with energy. Are we really running out of energy? How long will it take? What are the consequences of using various types of energy? These questions involve many of the principles of thermodynamics. You should be familiar with terms such as state function, energy, entropy, enthalpy and free energy and the equations associated with the laws. The following is some useful information for working problems in this section.

Bond Energies (kcal/mole)

H – H	104	C – O	83
H – F	135	C = O	178
H – O	111	O = O	118
H – Cl	103	Cl – Cl	58
C – Cl	79	C = C	146
H – C	87	C – C	83

Heats of Formation (kcal/mole)

CO (g)	– 26.4	Fe_3O_4 (s)	– 267
CO_2 (g)	– 94.1	FeO (s)	– 63.7
Fe_2O_3 (s)	– 197	SO_2 (g)	– 71.0

Free Energy of Reaction (kJ/mole)

$$CO (g) \; {}^1/_2 \, O_2 (g) \longrightarrow CO_2 (g) \qquad - 257.2$$

	$G°_f$ (kJ/mo)	$H°_f$ (kJ/mol)	$S°_f$ (J/mol K)
Fe_3O_4 (s)	– 1018	– 1121	145.3
FeO (s)	NA	– 272.0	60.75
Fe_2O_3 (s)	– 743.6	– 825.5	87.40
CH_3CH_2OH (l)	– 174.8	– 277.6	161
CH_3CHO (g)	– 133.7	– 166	266
H_2O (g)		– 242	188.7
H_2O (l)		– 286	—

Experiment 1

This experiment was designed to study the vaporization of water.

$$H_2O \text{ (l)} \longleftrightarrow H_2O \text{ (g)}$$

Experiment 2

In this experiment the change in entropy involved in the vaporization of one mole of freon, CCl_2F_2 (coolant used in refrigeration and air conditioning), at 25° was found to be 57.7 J/(mol K). These chloro-floro-hydrocarbons are believed to be responsible for the depletion occurring in the ozone layer above the earth.

Experiment 3

It has been found that alkenes undergo addition reactions in the presence of halogens rather than the substitution reactions observed with alkanes (catalyst needed for alkanes). The following is an example of an addition reaction using ethene (ethylene):

$$C_2H_4 + Cl_2 \longrightarrow C_2H_4Cl_2$$

Experiment 4

The most desirable iron ores contain hematite, Fe_2O_3, or magnetite, Fe_3O_4. The oxide is reduced in blast furnaces by carbon monoxide:

$$Fe_2O_3 \text{ (s)} + 3CO \text{ (g)} \longrightarrow 2Fe \text{ (s)} + 3CO_2 \text{ (g)}$$

Most of the oxide is reduced to molton iron by the carbon monoxide, although some is reduced directly by coke (carbon):

$$Fe_2O_3 \text{ (s)} + 3C \text{ (s)} \longrightarrow 2Fe \text{ (l)} + 3CO \text{ (g)}$$

Experiment 5

In another oxidation-reduction reaction iron is oxidized to form magnetite, While the carbon in carbon dioxide is reduced to form carbon monoxide:

$$3FeO \text{ (s)} + CO_2 \text{ (g)} \longrightarrow Fe_3O_4 \text{ (s)} + CO \text{ (g)}$$

Experiment 6

The first reaction is simply a condensation reaction:

$$H_2O \text{ (g)} \longrightarrow H_2O \text{ (l)} \tag{1}$$

The following reaction is a decomposition reaction involving limestone:

$$CaCO_3 \text{ (s)} \longrightarrow CaO \text{ (s)} + CO_2 \text{ (g)} \tag{2}$$

In the blast furnace used in Experiment 5, coke is mixed with limestone and crushed iron ore is admitted at the top of the furnace as the "charge." A blast of hot air from the bottom burns the coke to carbon monoxide with the evolution of more heat:

$$2C \text{ (s)} + O_2 \text{ (g)} \longrightarrow 2CO \text{ (g)} + \text{heat}$$

The limestone, called a flux, is added to react with the silica gangue in the ore to form a molten slag of calcium silicate.

$$CaO \text{ (s)} + SiO_2 \text{ (s)} \text{ (gangue)} \longrightarrow CaSiO_3 \text{ (l)} \text{ (slag)}$$

Experiment 7

Ethanol, or ethyl alcohol, was first prepared by fermentation a long time ago — the most ancient literature contains references to beverages that were obviously alcoholic! The fermentation of blackstrap molasses, the residue from the purification of cane sugar, sucrose, is one important source of ethanol:

$$C_{12}H_{22}O_{11} + H_2O \xrightarrow{\text{yeast}} 4CH_3CH_2OH + 4CO_2$$

In one experiment the oxidation of ethanol results in the formation of ethanol and hydrogen. Many different reagents can be used to oxidize ethanol.

$$CH_3CH_2OH \text{ (l)} \longrightarrow CH_3CHO \text{ (g)} + H_2 \text{ (g)}$$

Experiment 8

The internal energy, E, of a specific amount of a substance represents all the energy contained within the substance. It includes all kinds of energy. The difference between the internal energy of the products and the internal energy of the reactants of a chemical reaction of physical change is related to the heat lost or gained and the work done on or by the system.

In this experiment a gas is heated up and gains 65 J of heat from the surroundings. As the gas heats up, it does work on the surroundings equal to 22 J.

Experiment 9

The following reaction involves the oxidation of iron in ferrous oxide to form hematite. Fe_2O_3, but it can also be classified as a combination reaction:

$$4FeO \text{ (s)} + O_2 \text{ (g)} \longrightarrow 2 Fe_2O_3 \text{ (s)}$$

102. Consider the reaction under consideration in Experiment 1. What is the entropy of formation of liquid water at its normal boiling point?

    (A)   70.7   (B)   27.5

    (C)   306.7   (D)   118

103. Use the data in Experiment 2 to determine the heat that will be evolved when 100 grams of liquid freon vaporizes at 25°C?

    (A)   - 14.2 kJ   (B)   14.2 kJ

    (C)   - 17.2 kJ   (D)   17.2 kJ

104. Which of the following processes involves a positive change in entropy?

    (A) $2 C \text{ (s)} + O_2 \text{ (g)} \longrightarrow 2 CO \text{ (g)}$

    (B)   Condensation of water

    (C) $CO_2 \text{ (g)} + CaO \text{ (s)} \longrightarrow CaCO_3 \text{ (s)}$

    (D)   None of the above.

105. Given the bond energies in the passage and the reaction studied in Experiment 3, calculate the energy change in the following reaction.

    (A)   42   (B)   - 37

    (C)   + 37   (D)   None of the above.

106. Find the heat (enthalpy) of reaction for the reduction of hematite with carbon monoxide as discussed in Experiment 4.

    (A) − 28

    (B) 28

    (C) 486.4

    (D) − 486.4

107. Determine the heat (enthalpy) of reaction for equation under study in Experiment 5.

    (A) − 8.2

    (B) 8.2

    (C) 136.5

    (D) − 135.6

108. Consider the reactions under study in Experiment 6. Increasing the temperature in these reactions would

    (A) make both more spontaneous.

    (B) make both less spontaneous.

    (C) make (1) more spontaneous and (2) less spontaneous.

    (D) make (2) more spontaneous and (1) less spontaneous.

109. Find the approximate value for the equilibrium constant for the oxidation of ethanol in Experiment 7.

    (A) 10^7

    (B) 10^{-8}

    (C) 10^{16}

    (D) 10^{-17}

110. What are q, w, and the change in internal energy for the conditions described in Experiment 8?

    1) $q = + 65$

    5) $E = 87$

    2) $q = - 65$

    6) $E = 43$

    3) $w = + 22$

    7) $E = - 87$

    4) $w = - 22$

    8) $E = - 43$

    (A) 1, 3 and 6

    (B) 1, 4 and 5

    (C) 2, 4 and 5

    (D) 2, 3 and 7

111. Consider the reaction discussed in Experiment 9. Which of the following sets of answers will be the correct signs for each of the quantities?

    1) $H = +$

    5) $G = -$

    2) $H = -$

    6) $G = +$

    3) $S = +$

    7) $G = ?$

    4) $S = -$

    (A) 1, 3 and 7

    (B) 2, 4 and 7

    (C) 1, 4 and 6

    (D) 2, 3 and 5

112. Consider the following phase diagram. The point *B* on this diagram represents

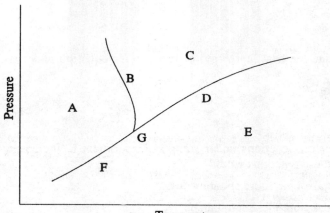

1)	solid	3)	gas
2)	liquid	4)	equilibrium
(A)	1, 2 and 4	(B)	2, 3 and 4
(C)	1, 3 and 4	(D)	1, 2, 3 and 4

PASSAGE V (Questions 113-117)

The solenoid which is connected to the starter in your automobile may look something like the one pictured below. S is your ignition switch which allows the solenoid to draw current from your 12 Volt battery. This energizes the solenoid so that it produces a magnetic field in opposition to that of the permanent magnet in its core. The permanent magnet is thus pushed upwards, closing the contact of a spring switch which connects the starter to your battery, allowing it to draw sufficient current to start your car. The solenoid has resistance $R = 3\Omega$ and is wound about a core with a permeability of $\mu = 25 \times 10^{-7}$ H/m. When the ignition switch is closed, the magnetic field (B) at the center of the solenoid is measured to be 0.1 T.

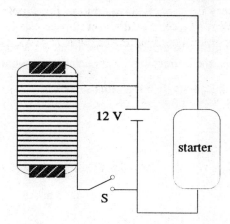

113. What current will flow in the solenoid when the ignition switch is closed?

    (A) 0.25 A   (B) 4 A

    (C) 36 A   (D) 120 A

114. What is the number of turns per unit length of coil which comprises this solenoid?

    (A) 10,000   (B) 160,000

    (C) 1,100   (D) 500

115. The quantity which is computed as the product of the magnetic field strength (B) times the cross-sectional area (A) of the solenoid is called

    (A) Magnetic flux   (B) Magnetic field

    (C) Electromagnetic Radiation (D) A Faraday

116. The process by which the permanent magnet reacts to be pushed upwards from the solenoid is called

    (A) Magnetic induction   (B) Magnetic deduction

    (C) Magnetic invasion   (D) Magnetic repulsion

117. Solenoids are generally stationed so that the permanent magnet operates vertically because

    (A) the earth's magnetic field is always horizontal.

    (B) the car develops a horizontal magnetic field as it moves.

    (C) a horizontal placement would interfere with the car radio.

    (D) None of the above.

PASSAGE VI (Questions 118-128)

The attractive forces between ions and molecules are largely responsible for many of the observed physical properties of compounds and elements, such as solubility, boiling points, melting points, and vapor pressure. These attractive forces, such as coulombic forces of attraction between ions, ion-dipole attractions, hydrogen bonding, and Van der Waals forces of attraction (dipole-dipole interactions, and London forces) are also important in explaining colligative properties.

Experiment 1

In this experiment the molal freezing point depression constant for water was determined to be $1.86°C/m$ and the molal boiling point elevation constant for water was $0.51°C/m$.

Experiment 2

The solubility of CO_2 was determined experimentally and found to be 0.68 g/100 g H_2O at 4.0 atm.

Experiment 3

During another laboratory experiment a mixture of 10.0 g of urea, $CO (NH_2)_2$, and 40.0 g of methanol, CH_3OH, was found to form an ideal solution. The vapor pressure of pure methanol at 20°C was determined to be 90 torr Hg. The vapor pressure of pure CS_2 and pure $C_4H_8O_2$ were also determined at 28°C and found to be 400 torr and 110 torr respectively..

Experiment 4

This experiment was used to determine the boiling point of a solution composed of 9.81 grams of an unknown non-volatile molecular compound and 90.0 g of water. At 760 torr the boiling point of the solution was found to be 100.37°C.

Experiment 5

In this experiment a 0.20 gram sample of a small protein was dissolved in 100 ml of water and the osmotic pressure was observed to be 9.8 torr at 25°C.

Experiment 6

During this experiment a semipermeable membrane was used to separate compartment A, which contains 0.10 m $BaCl_2$, from compartment B. Several different solutions were placed in compartment B and the level of the water in the two compartments was observed.

Experiment 7

In this experiment a solution made by dissolving 1.00 g of $CHCl_3$ in 750 ml of solution. The density of the solution was determined to be 1.023 g/ml.

118. Which of the following compounds has the lowest vapor pressure under the same conditions?

(A) CH_3NH_2 (B) CH_3OCH_3

(C) CH_3SH (D) CH_3Cl

119. Which of the following compounds would exhibit the lowest boiling point under the same conditions?

(A) $CH_3CH_2CH_3$

(B) CH_3OCH_3

(C) CH_3CH_2OH

(D) Impossible to answer since (A), (B) and (C) have very close boiling points, they would all boil at about the same temperature.

120. Which of the following compounds should be most soluble in water?

(A) $CH_3CH_2CH_2CH_2CH_2CH_3$

(B) CCl_4

(C) CH_3OH

(D) CH_3Cl

121. Consider the solubility of CO_2 determined in Experiment 2, what would be the solubility of the CO_2 if the partial pressure of CO_2 is 0.0025 atm?

(A) 1.088×10^3 g/100 g H_2O

(B) 4.25×10^{-4} g/100 g H_2O

(C)   0.015 g/100 g H_2O

(D)   None of the above.

122. Use the results obtained in Experiment 3 to determine the vapor pressure of the methanol solution?

(A)   12.0   (B)   102

(C)   10.6   (D)   None of the above.

123. Considering the results of Experiment 3, what is the vapor pressure of an ideal solution containing 50.0 g of CS_2, carbon disulfide, and 50.0 g of $C_4H_8O_2$ at 28°C?

(A)   255   (B)   244

(C)   266   (D)   None of the above.

124. Use the results obtained in Experiment 1 to calculate the freezing point of a 0.020 m solution of NaCl in water.

(A)   - .037   (B)   - .074

(C)   - .019   (D)   - .020

125. Consider the result of Experiment 4. What is the approximate molecular weight of the substance?

(A) 1.26×10^4 (B) 46.6×10^1

(C)   150   (D)   79

126. Using the results from Experiment 5, determine the approximate molecular weight of the protein?

(A)   318   (B) 6.09×10^3

(C) 3.79×10^3 (D)   None of the above.

127. Considering the data presented in Experiment 6, which of the following solutions, when placed in compartment B, will cause the water to rise in compartment B?

(A)   0.10 m NaCL   (B)   0.20 m CH_3CO_2H

(C)   0.10 m $MgCl_2$ (D)   0.10 m $Al_2(SO_4)_3$

128. What is the molality of a solution prepared and studied in Experiment 7?

(A)   - 0.0110   (B)   - 0.618

(C)   - 0.161   (D)   - 0.0274

PASSAGE VII (Questions 129-135)

A robot used to deliver parts along an assembly line is programmed so that its time at each station is minimized and correlated with the work being done on the line. Its motion has been modelled with the use of simple linear fitting so that its accelerations are assumed constant over different time intervals. A portion of this modelling over an eight-second interval is shown in the graph below.

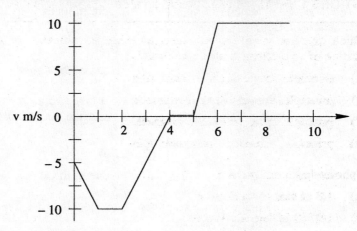

129. What is the robot's speed at $t = 1.5$ seconds?

    (A)   0 m/s   (B)   10 m/s
    (C)   5 m/s   (D)   10 m/sec^2

130. What is the robot's average speed between $t = 2$ and $t = 5$ seconds?

    (A)   0 m/s   (B)   5 m/s
    (C)   3.33 m/s   (D)   10 m/s

131. The robot is at rest at

    (A)   4.5 s.   (B)   1.5 s.
    (C)   6.5 sec.   (D)   7 sec.

132. What is the robot's average acceleration between $t = 4$ and $t = 7$ seconds?

    (A)   0 m/s^2 (B)   5 m/s^2
    (C)   10 m/s^2 (D)   3.33 m/s^2

133. What is the robot's acceleration at $t = 7$ seconds?

    (A)   10 m/s^2 (B)   5 m/s^2
    (C)   0 m/s^2 (D)   - 5 m/s^2

134. How much distance does the robot cover between $t = 2$ and $t = 4$ seconds?

    (A)   10 m   (B)   30 m
    (C)   0 m   (D)   20 m

135. How far from its position at $t = 0$ seconds will the robot be after 8 seconds?

    (A)   2.5 m   (B)   0 m

    (C)   25 m   (D)   52.5 m

QUESTIONS 136-142 are NOT based on a descriptive passage.

---

136. Which quantum numbers, in order, are required uniquely to determine the location of an electron around a nucleus?

    (A)   principle, magnetic, azimuthal, spin

    (B)   principle, azimuthal, spin, magnetic

    (C)   principle, spin, azimuthal, magnetic

    (D)   principle, azimuthal, magnetic, spin

137. A photon has a rest mass of

    (A)   1/8 of that of an electron.

    (B)   1/1760 of that of a proton.

    (C)   Zero.

    (D)   None of the above.

138. How many coulombs of charge are required to plate out 127 g of Cu (molecular weight of Cu = 63.5 g/mole)?

    (A)   2 C   (B)   3 C

    (C)   4 C   (D)   5 C

139. Consider a covalent bond between hydrogen and arsenic, with the atomic radii given by 0.37 Å and 1.21 Å, respectively. What is the approximate length of the hydrogen-arsenic bond ($1 Å = 10^{-8}$ cm; the molecular formula is AsH_3)?

    (A)   2.32 Å   (B)   0.45 Å

    (C) 15.8×10^{-8} cm   (D) 1.58×10^{-8} cm

140. If the average adult inhales 300 l of air a day, how much oxygen would be inhaled in that length of time? (Air is composed of 78% N_2, 20% O_2, and 2% other elements.)

    (A)   60 l (B)   15 l

    (C)   600 l (D)   6 l

141. Compound X has an atomic number of 25. It forms an ion with the electronic configuration,

    $1s^2\, 2s^2\, 2p^6\, 3s^2\, 3p^6\, 3d^5$.

    What is the proper ionic symbol for X?

(A) X^+ (B) X^{2+}

(C) X^{3+} (D) None of the above.

142. A spaceship traveling at 1.50×10^8 m/s leaves the Earth in the year 2050 with John on board. John leaves his twin brother James behind on Earth and goes off to a star 25 light-years away. Upon arrival, he immediately returns. On return, what is the difference in their ages?

(A) 3.3 years   (B) 6.7 years

(C) 12.5 years   (D) 10.0 years

STOP

If time still remains, you may review work only in this section.

When the time allotted is up, you may go on to the next section.

Section 3 — Writing Sample

TIME: 60 minutes
2 essays, separately timed
30 minutes each

DIRECTIONS: This section tests your writing skills by asking you to write two essays. You will have 30 minutes to write each one.

During the first 30 minutes, work only on the first essay. If you finish it in less than 30 minutes, you may review what you have written, but do not begin the second essay. During the second 30 minutes, work only on the second essay. If you finish it in less than 30 minutes, you may review what you have written for that essay only. Do not go back to the first essay.

Read each assigned topic carefully. Make sure your essays respond to the topics as they are assigned.

Make sure your essays are written in complete sentences and paragraphs, and are as clear as you can make them. Make any corrections or additions between the lines of your essays. Do not write in the margins.

On the day of the test, you are given three pages to write each essay. You are not required to use all of the space provided, but do not skip lines so you will not waste space. Illegible essays cannot be scored.

Part 1

Consider this statement:

"The tree of humanity forgets the labour of the silent gardeners who sheltered it from the cold, watered it in time of drought, shielded it against wild animals; but preserves faithfully the names mercilessly cut into its bark."

Heine, *The Romantic School*, 1833

Write a comprehensive essay in which you accomplish the following objectives. Explain what you think the statement means. Discuss what you think Heine meant by "silent gardeners." Whose names do you think are "mercilessly cut" on the tree? Be sure to include examples.

STOP

If time still remains, you may review work only in this section.

When the time allotted is up, you may go on to the next section.

Part 2

Consider this statement:

"As soon as any part of a person's conduct affects prejudicially the interests of others, society has jurisdiction over it, and the question whether the general welfare will or will not be promoted by interfering with it, becomes open to discussion. But there is no room for entertaining any such question when a person's conduct affects the interests of no persons besides himself,..."

John Stuart Mill, *On Liberty*

Write a comprehensive essay in which you accomplish the following objectives. Explain the meaning of Mill's statement. Consider Mill's idea in relation to a specific situation that might contradict or limit this idea. Discuss the possibility of resolving this contradiction.

STOP

If time still remains, you may review work only in this section.
When the time allotted is up, you may go on to the next section.

Section 4 — Biological Sciences

TIME: 100 Minutes
QUESTIONS: 143-219

DIRECTIONS: Most of the questions in this section are arranged in groups, each corresponding to a descriptive passage. Based on the information given in a passage, choose the one best answer to each question in the group. Some questions are independent of a descriptive passage and of each other. Choose the one best answer to each of these questions. If you are not sure of an answer, eliminate those choices that you know are incorrect and choose an answer from among those remaining. Fill in the corresponding circle on the answer sheet to indicate your answer. You may refer to the periodic table at any time.

PASSAGE I (Questions 143-149)

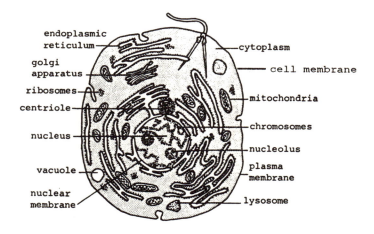

FIGURE 1.

A diagram of a "typical" animal cell is presented in Figure 1. In reality, there are many kinds, sizes, and shapes of animal cells depending on their position and function within body tissues. However, the basic roles of the organelles depicted in Figure 1 here remain the same irrespective of tissue type. The presence of membrane-bound organellea distinguishes eukaryotic from procaryotic cells.

The plasma membrane that delimits a cell from its surrounding medium is basically a bilayer of phospholipids into which are inserted a variety of extrinsic and intrinsic proteins. Movement of substances through the plasma membrane and within the cell can occur passively or actively. The membrane contains a variety of channels and pumps to regulate this movement, although it remains subject to external factors such as the osmotic pressure of the surrounding fluids.

Nuclear division (karyokinesis) is usually followed by cell division (cytokinesis) in animal cells. Somatic cells of animals undergo a type of karyokinesia known as mitosis, which proceeds in a series of stages as part of an overall cell cycle. This cycle usually approximates a twenty-four hour period, but may occur in less than an hour or take several days to complete.

143. The plasma membrane described above is best described in contemporary terms as the _____ model.

    (A) unit-membrane
    (B) plasmalemma
    (C) Davson-Danielli
    (D) fluid-mosaic

144. The enzyme for the Krebs Cycle and electron transport chain are found within

    (A) mitochondria.
    (B) the Golgi apparatus.
    (C) smooth endoplasmic reticulum.
    (D) the cytoplasm.

145. The following stages of the cell cycle occur directly after mitosis

    (A) S, G_1, G_2.
    (B) G_1, G_2, S.
    (C) G_1, S, G_2.
    (D) S, G_2, G_1.

146. The stage of mitosis in which separation of chromatids at the centromere occurs is

    (A) metaphase.
    (B) anaphase.
    (C) telophase.
    (D) prophase.

147. Celery sticks that are left in a dish of freshwater for several hours become stiff and hard. Similar sticks left in a salt solution become limp and soft. From this we can deduce that the cells of the celery sticks are

    (A) hypotonic to both freshwater and the salt solution.
    (B) hypertonic to both freshwater and the salt solution.
    (C) hypertonic to freshwater but hypotonic to the salt solution.
    (D) hypotonic to freshwater but hypertonic to the salt solution.

148. Lysosomes contain

    (A) hydrolytic enzymes.
    (B) the enzymes to carry out glycolysis.
    (C) various chemical products to be secreted out of the cell.
    (D) their own DNA.

149. Protein synthesis occurs on or in

    (A) the nucleus.

    (B) rough endoplasmic reticulum.

    (C) the Golgi apparatus.

    (D) mitochondria.

PASSAGE II (Questions 150-154)

The external sex organs of male and female mammals are homologous structures, having developed from an embryonic bisexual primordium called the genital
tubercle. Differentiation of human genitalia occurs during the eighth week of development. Production of testosterone and a polysaccharide called mullerian inhibition
factor (MIF) by the newly differentiated testes causes masculinization of the genital
tubercle and associated structures. In the absence of MIF and testosterone, these
structures develop into female genitalia.

Gametogenesis in mammals, as in other animals, is by meiosis. Both spermatogenesis and oogenesis are initiated during embryonic development and both are arrested in the first meiotic division, not to resume until puberty. Germ cells that migrate from the yolk sac early in embryological development are the source of the
spermatogonia and oogonia from which sperm and eggs develop. Spermatogonia
reproduce themselves mitotically so that sperm production is continuous throughout
the adult life of males, while the number of oogonia remains fixed after embryogen-
esis.

Spermatogenesis produces four functional spermatozoa, but the unequal cleavages of oogenesis result in only one functional ovum. Furthermore, the second meiotic division of oogenesis only occurs if the secondary oocyte is fertilized. Because
of unequal cleavages, virtually all of the cytoplasm of the oogonium is preserved in
the ovum and, therefore, the zygote. The other products of oogenesis, the polar bodies, degenerate and have no known function in reproduction.

A further difference between male and female gamete production in mammals
can be seen in the cyclic nature of ovulation. While sperm are produced continuously
by males, females release an egg or eggs periodically during menstrual cycles (in
humans and some other primates) or estrous cycles. These cyclic ovulations are under complex hormonal control and cease during the middle to late stages of adult life.
In humans, this phenomenon is known as menopause and usually occurs between the
ages of forty and fifty years.

150. Which of the following is a correct, but not necessarily complete, sequence of
     cells formed during spermatogenesis in animals?

    (A) Primary spermatocyte, secondary spermatocyte, spermatogonium

    (B) Secondary spermatocyte, spermatid, spermatozoan

    (C) Spermatogonium, spermatid, primary spermatocyte

    (D) Spermatozoan, spermatid, secondary spermatocyte

151. A diploid cell with a chromosome number of 12 undergoing meiosis and
     cytokinesis would ultimately produce

(A) two cells each with 12 chromosomes.

(B) two cells each with 6 chromosomes.

(C) four cells each with 12 chromosomes.

(D) four cells each with 6 chromosomes.

152. The structure in which oogenesis occurs in mammalian ovaries is known as a(n)

(A) follicle.   (B) oocyte.

(C) corpus luteum.   (D) endometrium.

153. Spermatogenesis occurs in the _____ of mammals.

(A) epididymis   (B) prostate gland

(C) seminiferous tubules   (D) vas deferens

154. The external female genital structure that is homologous to (i.e., arose from the same embryonic tissue as) the penis is the

(A) vagina.   (B) cervix.

(C) labia major.   (D) clitoris.

PASSAGE III (Questions 155-161)

Collection of the mechanical, thermal, chemical, electromagnetic or other forms of stimulus energy from the environment and its conversion into the electrochemical energy of nerve impulses is the function of various sensory receptors found in animals. These receptors vary in complexity from single-neuron mechanoreceptors of the skin to the large, multi-receptor eyes and ears of vertebrates.

The process converting stimulus energy into nerve impulses is known as transduction. The senses of vision and hearing represent two different mechanisms of transduction, each with varying degrees of integration.

In the vertebrate eye, transduction of light energy involves a cis-trans isomerization of photo-sensitive molecules located in receptor cells of the retina. The light-induced conformational changes ultimately lead to action potentials in sensory neurons of the retina through changes in permeability of the neuron membranes. The original photo-sensitive form of the receptor molecules is re-established by an enzymatic, energy-dependent conversion. Qualitative and quantitative differences in light are perceived by integration of the action potentials of the two kinds of photoreceptor cells, the rods and cones. In this way, humans and certain other vertebrates can detect changes in wavelength and light intensity as color and brightness.

Hearing involves the transduction of pressure waves in the atmosphere into action potentials. This process involves mechanical movements of membranes and the ossicles of the middle ear which then induce pressure waves in the fluids of the cochlea. Displacement of the cilia of sensory hair cells located on the basilar membrane of the organ of Corti cause action potentials to form in sensory neurons of the cochlear nerve. Different frequency sounds cause different portions of the basilar membrane to vibrate and the hair cells of those portions are thereby stimulated. The cochlear nerve carries impulses from different parts of the basilar membrane to correspondingly different parts of the cerebral cortex. The brain then perceives differences in volume and pitch of sound, respectively, by the number of action potentials received and the particular region of the cerebral cortex which receives them. That is, high amplitude sound causes more sensory neurons to fire and the cerebral cortex is mapped to recognize impulses from specific regions of the basilar membrane.

Use the information presented in this passage and your general knowledge of vision and hearing in mammals to answer the following questions.

155. The following is a correct, but not necessarily complete, sequence of structures through which sound waves act in mammalian hearing.

(A) Malleus, stapes, round-window, vestibular canal

(B) Stapes, oval windows, round window, tympanic canal

(C) Tympanic membrane, malleus, round-window, vestibular canal

(D) Oval window, vestibular canal, tympanic canal, round window

156. The visual pigment found in the rods of vertebrate eyes is

(A) hemoglobin.   (B) phytochrome.

(C) rhodopsin.   (D) rhabdom.

157. Compared to the cones of a human eye, rods are

(A) less sensitive to light intensity.

(B) more numerous.

(C) concentrated in the center of the retina.

(D) capable of detecting color.

158. Clear focusing of the light waves falling on the retina when viewing close objects is accomplished by adjusting the

(A) shape of the lens.   (B) length of the eyeball.

(C) position of the retina. (D) diameter of the pupil.

159. The cilia of sensory hairs on the basilar membrane are embedded in the

(A) round window.   (B) tectorial membrane.

(C) oval window.   (D) vestibular canal.

160. There is a certain region of the vertebrate eye known as the "blind spot." This region is actually the

(A) edge of the lens.

(B) fovea centralis.

(C) exit point of the optic nerve.

(D) macula lutea.

161. The inner ear of mammals also contains the apparatus for balance and equilibrium. Changes of the position of the head with respect to gravity, as in bending forward, are detected by hair cells in chambers known as the

(A) semicircular canals.

(B) vestibular canal.

(C) statocyst.

(D) utricle and saccule.

QUESTIONS 162-167 are NOT based on a descriptive passage.

---

162. A molecule passing from the nucleus to the cytoplasm must pass through two membranes. Which other organelle has a double membrane?

(A) Mitochondrion

(B) Golgi apparatus

(C) Ribosome

(D) Endoplasmic reticulum

163. Most nutrient absorption occurs in the

(A) mouth.

(B) stomach.

(C) small intestine.

(D) large intestine.

164. Secretory proteins that are synthesized on the _____ are destined for packaging in the _____ before they are released by exocytosis.

(A) rough endoplasmic reticulum ... nucleus

(B) rough endoplasmic reticulum ... Golgi apparatus

(C) smooth endoplasmic reticulum ... rough endoplasmic reticulum

(D) Golgi apparatus ... rough endoplasmic reticulum

165. Colchicine inhibits the formation of microtubules. Which cellular process would be disrupted by colchicine?

(A) growth

(B) respiration

(C) cytokinesis

(D) meiosis

166. The developmental homologue (homologues) to the front flipper of the seal is (are)

(A) a bird's wing.

(B) a cat's paw.

(C) a butterfly's wing.

(D) (A) and (B) only.

167. An undifferentiated cell can be induced to follow the developmental patterns of a different species by

(A) replacing the original nucleus with one from another (chosen) species.

(B) introducing cytoplasm from another species.

(C) removing the native nucleus.

(D) no known means.

168. Alleles

   (A)   are always expressed.

   (B)   can cross-over.

   (C)   are variations of genes on homologous chromosomes.

   (D)   are always sex-linked.

PASSAGE IV (Questions 169-173)

Figure 1 — Characteristics of Red, Intermediate, and White Muscle Fibers.

	Red (Type I)	Intermediate (Type IIA)	White (Type IIB)
Diameter	Small	Intermediate	Large
Z-line thickness	Wide	Intermediate	Narrow
Glycogen content	Low	Intermediate	High
Resistance to fatigue	High	Intermediate	Low
Capillaries	Many	Many	Few
Myoglobin content	High	High	Low
Respiration type	Aerobic	Aerobic	Anaerobic
Twitch rate	Slow	Fast	Fast
Myosin ATPase content	Low	High	High

The muscle fibers of skeletal muscles can be categorized into two fundamental groups based on the time required to reach maximum tension following stimulation. These two muscle fiber types are known as slow-twitch and fast-twitch; muscles containing a predominance of slow-twitch fibers may require as much as 100 msec to reach maximum tension while a muscle made up primarily of fast-twitch fibers may reach maximum tension in as little as 10 msec. Because of differences in myoglobin content, these fibers are also identified as red (slow-twitch) and white (fast-twitch) fibers.

As can be seen from Figure 1, fast-twitch and slow-twitch fibers differ in a variety of ways. Figure 1 also characterizes a special type of fast-twitch fiber, an intermediate form, that has a greater capacity for aerobic production of ATP than the classic fast-twitch type.

Use the information from the table in Figure 1 and your knowledge of muscle fiber characteristics in general to answer the questions following this passage.

169. Muscles involved in maintaining posture would be expected to contain predominantly

   (A)   white muscle fibers. (B)   red muscle fibers.

   (C)   intermediate muscle fibers. (D)   anaerobically respiring muscle fibers.

170. From the information in Figure 1, it can be deduced that the muscle fiber type(s) with large numbers of mitochondria is (are)

    (A)   Type I.

    (B)   Type IIA.

    (C)   Type IIB.

    (D)   Type I and Type IIA would both have many mitochrondia.

171. Fatigue from lactic acid production would be most likely in

    (A)   white muscle fibers.

    (B)   intermediate muscle fibers.

    (C)   red muscle fibers.

    (D)   aerobically respiring muscle fibers.

172. The three muscle fiber types described in this passage are all found in skeletal muscle. Skeletal muscle fibers are similar to smooth muscle fibers in which of the following ways?

    (A)   Both are multinucleate

    (B)   Both have sarcomeres

    (C)   Both have electrical synapses

    (D)   Both contract in response to Ca^{++}

173. The most common neurotransmitter of vertebrate neuromuscular synapses is

    (A)   epinephrine.   (B)   acetycholine.

    (C)   norepinephrine.   (D)   serotonin.

PASSAGE V (Questions 174-179)

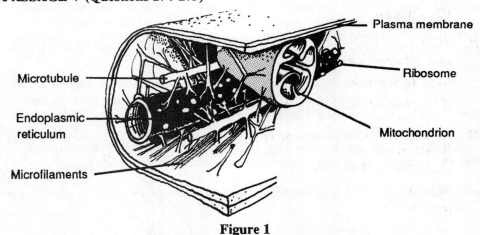

Figure 1

    Quite unlike the way it was perceived before the development of electron microscopy, a eukaryotic cell is now known to have an internal supporting meshwork called the cytoskeleton (see Figure 1). The fibers making up the cytoskeleton (microfilaments, microtubules, and intermediate filaments) may be assembled and reassembled in a variety of ways, thus enabling a cell to change morphology. These fibers are also associated with a cell's ability to move, by their involvement with muscle cell contraction, activity of flagella and cilia, and formation of pseudopodia during amoeboid movement. Materials are transported within a cell by moving along pathways determined by the arrangement of these fibers. Cellular import and export of materials can involve vacuole formation by cytoskeleton-induced changes in the cell membrane. There are many methods of cellular import/export of materials. Cytoskeleton-induced changes do account for vacule formation.

Microtubules are particularly important in the structure and motion of flagella and cilia. The arrangement of paired tubules, and the mechanism of movement, seen in cross-sections of flagella and cilia is identical for all eukaryotes. The proteins in these paired tubules slide past one another in a way that is similar to the sliding-filament contraction of skeletal muscle.

In a similar comparison, centrioles and the basal bodies to which flagella and cilia are anchored have common structures involving microtubules. Basal bodies serve as the template from which cilia and flagella are initially patterned. Centrioles are virtually identical to basal bodies and they seem to have a role in the organization of microtubule structure during cell growth. Centrioles are not present in cells of vascular plants (with the exception of flagellated gametes).

174.   Of the fibers that make up the cytoskeleton, the largest is known as

   (A)   a microfilament.   (B)   a microtubule.

   (C)   an endoplasmic reticulum.   (D)   an intermediate filament.

175.   Microfilaments are involved in muscle contraction as well as being structural components of the cytoskeleton. The globular protein that makes up microfilaments is

   (A)   actin.   (B)   dynein.

   (C)   tubulin.   (D)   myosin.

176.   The type of intercellular junction that connects cardiac muscle fibers and allows for direct, electrical synapsing is known as a

   (A)   tight junction.   (B)   desmosome.

   (C)   plasmodesmata.   (D)   gap junction.

177.   As seen with electron microscopy, a cross section of a eukaryotic cilium or flagellum consists of _____ pairs of microtubules surrounding a central core of _____ pair(s) of microtubules.

   (A)   6 ... 1   (B)   7 ... 2

   (C)   9 ... 2   (D)   9 ... 3

178.   The spindle fibers that appear during prophase of mitosis consist of

   (A)   microfilaments.   (B)   kinetochores.

   (C)   intermediate filaments.   (D)   microtubules.

179. Which of the following events of cytokinesis is most likely to involve microfilaments?

    (A) Centripetal cell wall formation in fungi

    (B) Centrifugal cell wall formation in plants

    (C) Cleavage furrow formation in animals

    (D) Cell plate formation in plants.

PASSAGE VI (Questions 180-185)

The numerous enzymatic processes involved in all of the different aspects of cellular metabolism are regulated in a variety of ways. One of the most common regulatory mechanisms is that of feedback inhibition. This occurs when an end product of the enzymatic process accumulates in a sufficiently high enough concentration to inhibit a crucial enzyme, which is usually involved in the beginning of the pathway. The flow of substances through the enzymatic pathway is prevented and as a result there is no further end product formation.

For example, the amino acid isoleucine is produced in the following manner:

$$\text{threonine} \xrightarrow{\text{threonine deaminase}} \alpha\text{-ketobutyrate} \to \to \to \to \text{isoleucine}$$

As isoleucine accumulates, it will inhibit the enzyme threonine deaminase which will prevent the further production of isoleucine. Conversely, as the concentration of isoleucine decreases, threonine deaminase will become active once again and the production of isoleucine will increase. In this way, the amount of end product generated by an enzymatic pathway can be matched precisely to the metabolic need for that product.

180. In a metabolic pathway regulated by feedback inhibition, the rate of the entire reaction is determined by

    (A) the activity of the last enzyme in the pathway.

    (B) end product concentration.

    (C) substrate concentration.

    (D) activator concentration.

181. Feedback inhibition serves a useful purpose in cellular metabolism because it

    (A) speeds up the rate at which enzymatic reactions occur.

    (B) reduces the availability of substrates.

    (C) regulates the flux through an enzymatic pathway, matching product supply to demand.

    (D) provides a means for genetic regulation of metabolic processes.

182. An increase in the concentration of which of the following would inhibit the enzyme threonine deaminase?

    (A) α-ketobutyrate   (B) leucine

    (C) threonine   (D) isoleucine

183. A researcher wants to know if feedback inhibition is operative in the reaction below. Using five different concentrations of substance B, he measures the activity of enzyme 1 and finds that it is the same in all cases. What conclusion can be drawn from these results?

$$A \xrightarrow{\text{enzyme 1}} B$$

   (A) There is no feedback inhibition by substance B within the range of concentrations tested.

   (B) Feedback inhibition caused the activity of enzyme 1 to remain constant.

   (C) Feedback inhibition by substance A occurred to limit the activity of enzyme 1.

   (D) The data are inconclusive in regard to feedback inhibition.

184. The opposite of feedback inhibition is

   (A) positive feedback, in which an increase in end product increases enzyme activity.

   (B) negative feedback, in which an increase in end product decreases enzyme activity.

   (C) competitive inhibition, in which a molecule similar in structure to the substrate blocks the active site of the enzyme.

   (D) positive modulation, in which a decrease in substrate increases enzyme activity.

185. When a high concentration of isoleucine is present, what effect would increasing the threonine concentration have on threonine deaminase activity?

   (A) Enzyme activity would increase, resulting in the production of isoleucine.

   (B) Enzyme activity would decrease due to a threonine-induced conformational change in the enzyme's structure.

   (C) There would be no effect on enzyme activity because the high concentration of isoleucine would inhabit threonine deaminase.

   (D) There would be no effect on enzyme activity because the high concentration of threonine would inhibit threonine deaminase.

QUESTIONS 186-189 are NOT based on a descriptive passage.

---

186. Which of the following is not one of the vitamin B-complex?

   (A) Thiamine   (B) Ecdysone

   (C) Riboflavin   (D) Biotin

187. A mammalian heart has _____ chamber(s).

    (A) one
    (B) two
    (C) three
    (D) four

188. Nitrous acid converts cytosine to uracil by deamination. This type of conversion in one DNA strand would lead to a change in the complementary base in the other strand to

    (A) adenine.
    (B) cytosine.
    (C) thymine.
    (D) guanine.

189. Messenger RNA does not contain

    (A) adenine.
    (B) uracil.
    (C) guanine.
    (D) thymine.

PASSAGE VII (Questions 190-196)

Carboxylic acids can be modified to form several useful derivatives, shown below:

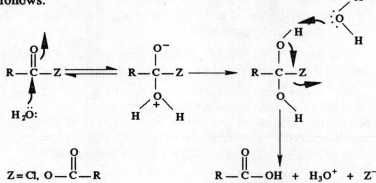

All of these may be hydrolized by aqueous acid or base. Acid chlorides and anhydrides may be reactive enough to be hydrolyzed by water alone. Amides are the most stable of the derivatives toward hydrolysis. The mechanism of hydrolysis may be written as follows:

190. Acid anhydrides react with water more slowly than acid chlorides because

    (A) the chloride ion is a better leaving group than the carboxylate ion.

    (B) the electronegative chlorine atom makes the carbonyl carbon more susceptible to attack by water.

(C)   Both (A) and (B) are correct.

(D)   None of the above.

191.   Acid added to the water increases the rate of hydrolysis because

(A)   it protonates the carbonyl oxygen.

(B)   it protonates the carbonyl carbon.

(C)   it protonates the leaving group.

(D)   it stabilizes the product.

192.   The hydrochloric acid hydrolysis of ethyl benzoate in water labelled with oxygen-18 yields the following labeled product

(A)   Benzoic acid   (B)   Benzoyl chloride

(C)   Benzoic anhydride   (D)   Ethanol

193.   Which of the following reactions is suitable for preparing benzamide?

(A) $\underset{\displaystyle PhCCl}{\overset{\displaystyle O}{\|}}$ + NH$_3$ (B) $Ph - \underset{\displaystyle }{\overset{\displaystyle O}{\|}}C - O - \underset{\displaystyle }{\overset{\displaystyle O}{\|}}C - Ph$ + NH$_3$

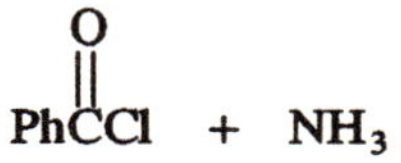

(C) $Ph - \underset{\displaystyle }{\overset{\displaystyle O}{\|}}C - O - Ph$ + NH$_3$ (D)   All of the above.

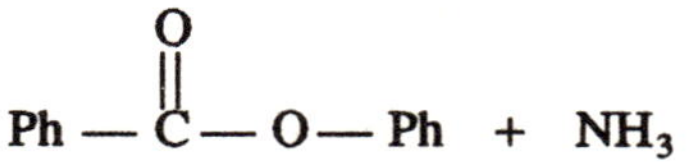

194.   Biological reactions frequently involve the phosphate ion as a leaving group. 1,3-bisphosphoglycerate has the structure shown:

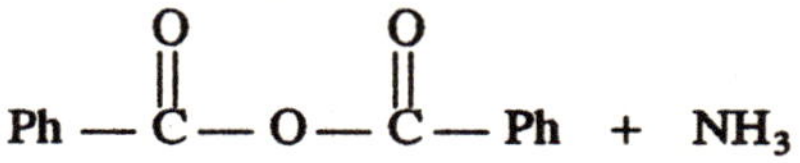

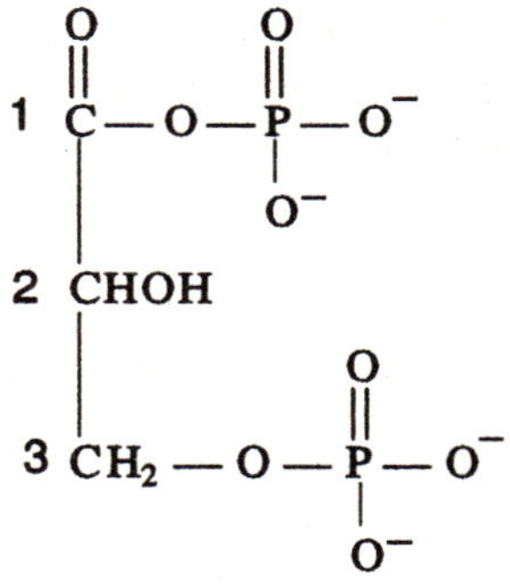

$$1 \ \ C - O - P - O^- $$

with carbonyl O on C and two =O on P, O$^-$ below P

$$2 \ \ CHOH$$

$$3 \ \ CH_2 - O - P - O^-$$

with =O on P and O$^-$ below P

Which product will result from the hydrolysis of 1,3-bisphosphoglycerate under conditions that remove only *one* of the phosphate groups?

(A)   2-phosphoglycerate

(B)   1-phosphoglycerate

(C)   3-phosphoglycerate

(D)   A mixture of all three will be formed.

195.   Which of the following amines will be *least* reactive toward an acid chloride or acid anhydride?

(A)

$O_2N-\!\!\!\!<\!\!\bigcirc\!\!>\!\!-NH_2$

(B)

$CH_3O-\!\!\!\!<\!\!\bigcirc\!\!>\!\!-NH_2$ with OCH_3

(C)

$O_2N-\!\!\!\!<\!\!\bigcirc\!\!>\!\!-NH_2$ with NO_2

(D)

$CH_3O-\!\!\!\!<\!\!\bigcirc\!\!>\!\!-NH_2$

196. The following sequence of reactions would produce which product?

$$\bigcirc\!\!-\!\!\overset{\overset{\displaystyle O}{\|}}{C}\!\!-OH \xrightarrow{1)\ SOCl_2} \xrightarrow{2)\ (CH_3)_2NH}$$

(A)

CO_2H / $N(CH_3)_2$

(B)

$\overset{\overset{\displaystyle O}{\|}}{C}\!\!-N(CH_3)_2$ / Cl

(C)

$\overset{\overset{\displaystyle O}{\|}}{C}\!\!-N(CH_3)_2$

(D)

$\overset{\overset{\displaystyle O}{\|}}{C}\!\!-Cl$ / $N(CH_3)_2$

PASSAGE VIII (Questions 197-204)

Vertebrates, like all other heterotrophic organisms, must obtain their energy-rich molecules from food sources outside their bodies. This food is taken into a two-ended digestive tract that allows one-way transport and processing of these ingested substances. The fundamental processes that occur in the vertebrate digestive system are ingestion, digestion, absorption, and elimination (defecation) of indigestible materials. The organic molecules ingested are usually in the form of large polymers that are then mechanically and chemically broken down into the monomeric constituents at various points within the system.

Digestion begins in the buccal cavity and involves both mechanical and enzymatic activity. The majority of digestive activity, however, occurs in the stomach and small intestine. The gastric juice produced by the stomach consists of hydrochloric acid and digestive enzymes, produced in the form of inactive precursors known as zymogens. After leaving the stomach, the partially digested food is acted upon by a variety of other enzymes secreted into the lumen of the digestive tract by the pancreas, liver, and the wall of the small intestine itself. Most absorption of the digested food molecules occurs in the small intestine. The large intestine functions primarily in the reabsorption of water from the digestive tract, the excretion of certain salts from the circulatory system, and the reabsorption of bile salts for return to the liver.

Once food has entered the esophagus, its movement is accomplished by peristaltic contractions of the digestive tract. At certain points along the tract, rings of muscle called sphincters regulate the movement of the material within the tract. Not all food molecules ingested can be broken down the action of the human digestive tract. Cellulose, for example, cannot be enzymatically digested and is passed through the tract essentially untouched. Such undigestible material is considered necessary to provide bulk for the stimulation of peristalsis.

197. The principal digestive function of bile is in the breakdown of

(A)   fats.   (B)   starches.

(C)   protein.   (D)   carbohydrates.

198. The following is a correct, but not necessarily complete, sequence of structures through which food passes in a human digestive tract

(A)   esophagus, duodenum, large intestine, small intestine.

(B)   duodenum, small intestine, transverse colon, ascending colon.

(C)   pyloric sphincter, duodenum, small intestine, transverse colon.

(D)   pharynx, esophagus, pyloric sphincter, stomach.

199. All of the following enzymes are produced by the pancreas EXCEPT

(A)   trypsin.   (B)   lipase.

(C)   chymotrypsin.   (D)   pepsin.

200. Which of the following does NOT correctly pair an enzyme with its function?

(A)   Amylase - hydrolysis of starch

(B)   Pepsin - hydrolysis of sucrose

(C)   Trypsin - hydrolysis of protein

(D)   Lipase - hydrolysis of fats

201. Villi and microvilli are found lining the inside of a mammal's

(A)   small intestine.   (B)   stomach.

(C)   esophagus.   (D)   large intestine.

202. The movement of the tongue during chewing forms food in the buccal cavity into a mass known as a

(A)   chyme.   (B)   pylorus.

(C)   bolus.   (D)   caecum.

203. Enzymes to digest starch are produced by both the

(A)   salivary glands and stomach.

(B)   pancreas and salivary glands.

(C)   stomach and small intestine.

(D)   small intestine and pancreas.

204.   The human digestive and respiratory tracts share usage of one structure, which
       is the

(A)   nasal cavity.   (B)   esophagus.

(C)   trachea.   (D)   pharynx.

PASSAGE IX (Questions 205-208)

Compound (1), $C_{10}H_{10}O$, exhibits a strong peak at 1680 cm^{-1} in the infrared
spectrum, indicating that it is an aldehyde or ketone. Reaction with I_2/OH^- gives a
yellow precipitate. Acidification and ether extraction of the supernatunt gave compound (2). The nmr spectrum of (2) shows the following absorptions:

   4.7 - 5.5 δ, multiplet, 2H;

   7.2 δ, multiplet, 5H;

   12.0 δ, singlet, 1H.

205.   The structure of (2) is

(A)   ⬡— CH = CH – CO_2H

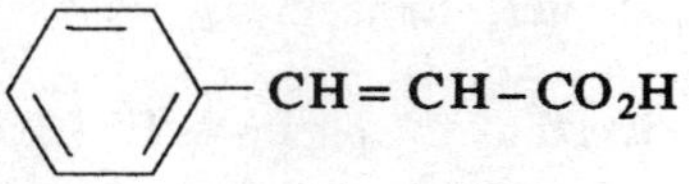

(B)   ⬡— $\overset{\overset{\displaystyle O}{||}}{C}$ – CH_2 – $\overset{\overset{\displaystyle O}{||}}{C}$ – H

(C)   H – $\overset{\overset{\displaystyle O}{||}}{C}$ —⬡— CH_2 – $\overset{\overset{\displaystyle O}{||}}{C}$ – H

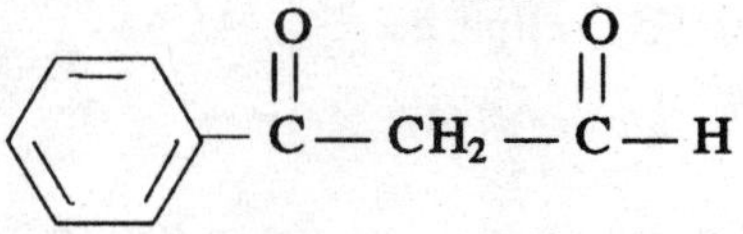

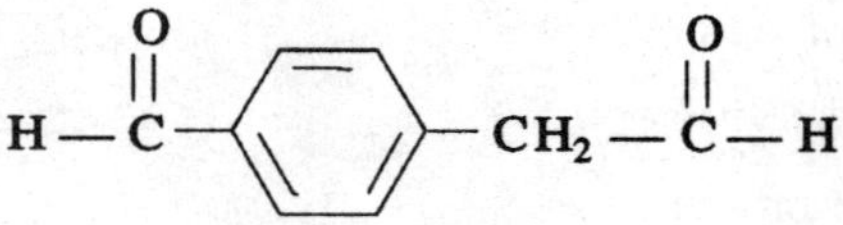

(D) CH_2 = CH —⬡— CO_2H

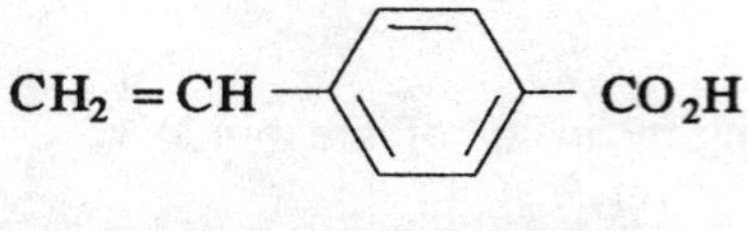

206.   The reaction of (1) with I_2/OH^- to give (2) and a yellow precipitate showed
       that (1) was

(A)   a methyl ester.   (B)   an aldehyde.

(C)   an ether.   (D)   a methyl ketone.

207.   In addition to I_2/OH^-, compound (1) would react with which of the following
       test solutions?

(A) Br_2 inCCl_4 (B)   Tollen's reagent

(C)   aq. $NaHCO_3$ (D)   aq. $AgNO_3$

208. Compound (1) will react with $NaBH_4$ to give a compound that will have a new peak in the infrared spectrum at about

(A) 2750 cm^{-1}.　　　　　　　　(B) 3300 cm^{-1}

(C) 2200 cm^{-1}　　　　　　　　(D) 1350 cm^{-1}

QUESTIONS 208-211 are NOT based on a descriptive passage.

---

209. The hybridization of carbons a, b, and c in the following compound is

$$\underset{\text{a}}{CH_2} = \underset{}{CH} - \underset{\text{b}}{\overset{\overset{\displaystyle O}{\|}}{C}} - \underset{\text{c}}{CH_3}$$

(A) $a = sp^2$ $b = sp$ $c = sp^3$　　(B) $a = sp$ $b = sp$ $c = sp^3$

(C) $a = sp^2$ $b = sp^2$ $c = sp$　　(D) $a = sp^2$ $b = sp^2$ $c = sp^3$

210. All of the following are reasonable resonance contributors to the structure of N,N-dimethyl formamide, EXCEPT

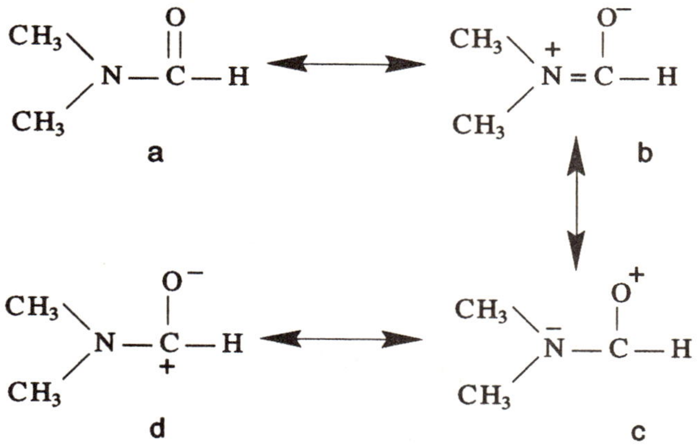

(A) a　　　　　　　　　　　(B) b

(C) c　　　　　　　　　　　(D) d

211. What sequence of reactions would be used to carry out the following synthesis?

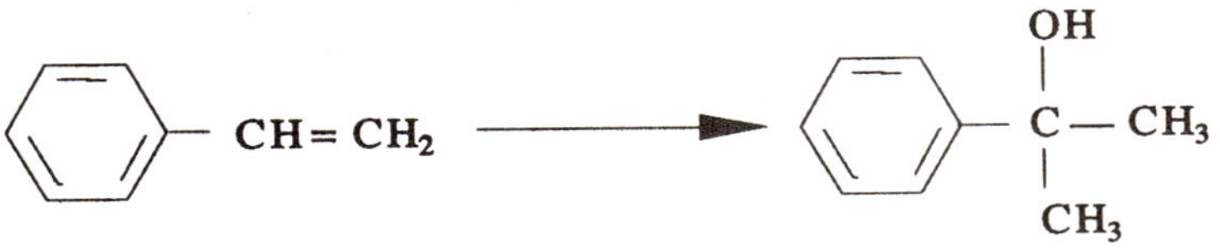

(A) 1) CH_3MgI 2) Cr_2O_3 3) H_3O+, Δ

(B) 1) Br_2/CCl_4 2) KOH/CH_3CH_2OH 3) CH_3MgL 4) H_3O+

(C) 1) H_2O, H+ 2) Cr_2O_3 3) CH_3MgI 4) H_3O+

(D) 1) CH_3MgI 2) Cr_2O_3 3) $LiAIH_4$

212. Which will be the shortest carbon-carbon bond in the structure shown?

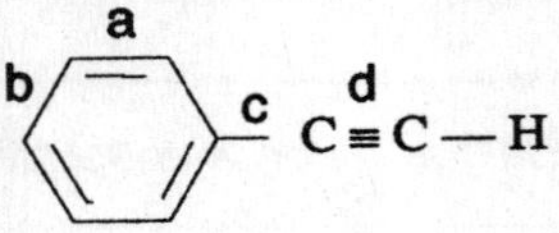

(A) a   (B) b

(C) c   (D) d

PASSAGE X (Questions 213-216)

Newman projections are a convenient way of indicating spatial arrangements and interactions for many compounds. Shown below are Newman representations of conformational states of ethane, C_2H_6, viewed along the C-C bond.

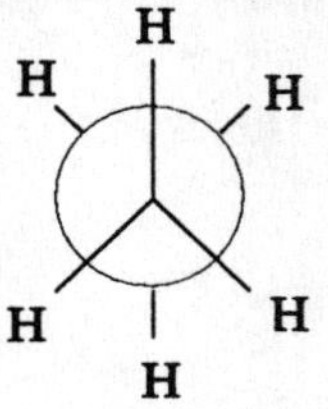

staggered 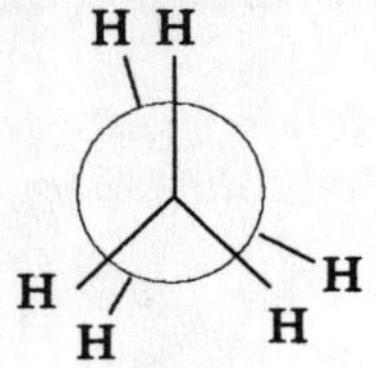   eclipsed

The conformation states of n-butane, C_4H_{10}, viewed along the C_2-C_3 bond, may be represented as

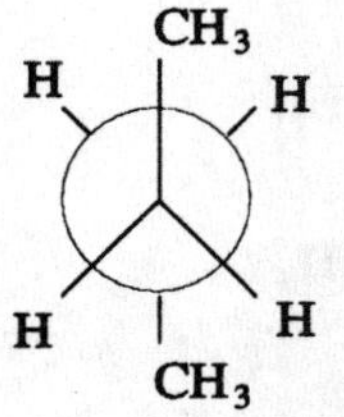

anti 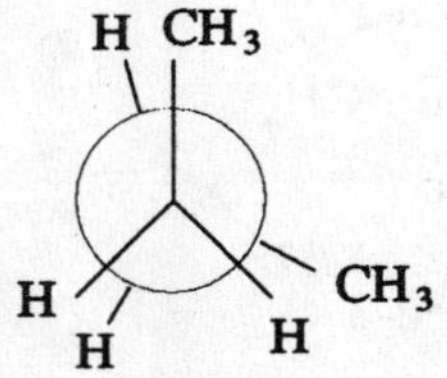   eclipsed-1

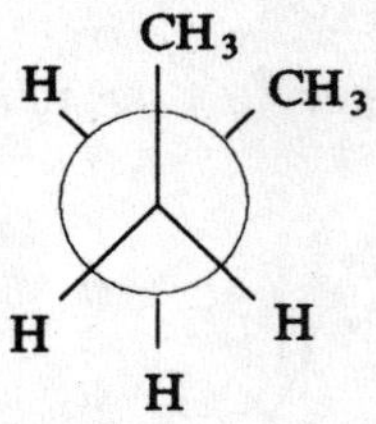

gauche 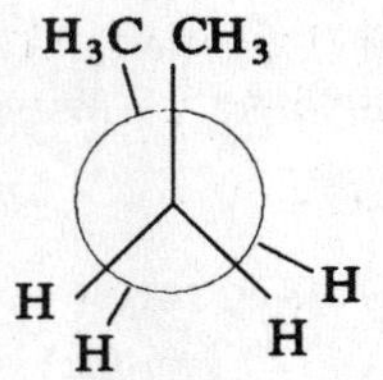   eclipsed-2

Successive rotations of 60° around the C_2-C_3 bond gives the plot of potential energy vs. conformational states of n-butane:

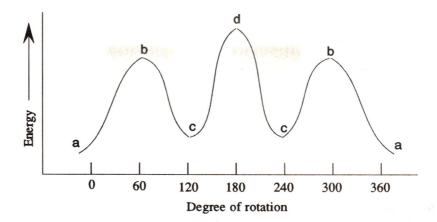

Degree of rotation

For Questions 213-216, match the position on the energy diagram that corresponds to the conformation shown above.

213. Anti

    (A)   a   (B)   b

    (C)   c   (D)   d

214. Gauche

    (A)   a   (B)   b

    (C)   c   (D)   d

215. Eclipsed-1

    (A)   a   (B)   b

    (C)   c   (D)   d

216. Eclipsed-2

    (A)   a   (B)   b

    (C)   c   (D)   d

PASSAGE XI (Questions 217-219)

Carboxylate ions are formed by the reaction of carboxylic acids with bases.

$$RCO_2H + B^- \longrightarrow RCO_2^- + BH$$

Phenolate ions are formed by the reaction of phenols with bases.

$$ArOH + B^- \longrightarrow ArO^- + BH$$

In general, carboxylic acids will react with aqueous $NaHCO_3$, while the stronger base NaOH must be used for reaction with phenols. Such phenols as 2,4-dinitrophenol, however, will react with $NaHCO_3$.

$$O_2N - \langle \bigcirc \rangle - OH$$
$$NO_2$$

217. In general, carboxylic acids are stronger acids than phenols because

    (A) they form strong hydrogen bonds to each other.

    (B) they have lower boiling points than phenols.

    (C) the carboxylate ion is stabilized by charge delocalization.

    (D) the carboxylate ion is destabilized by charge delocalization.

218. 2,4-Dinitrophenol is very acidic because

    (A) the electron-withdrawing nitro groups stabilize the phenolate ion.

    (B) the electron-donating nitro groups stabilize the phenolate ion.

    (C) the nitro groups increase the melting point of the compound.

    (D) the nitro groups change the conformation of the ring.

219. Consider the following carboxylate ions:

$$CH_3CH_2CH_2 - \overset{O}{\overset{||}{C}} - O^- \qquad CH_3CH_2\underset{Br}{CH} - \overset{O}{\overset{||}{C}} - O^- \qquad CH_3\underset{Br}{CH}CH_2 - \overset{O}{\overset{||}{C}} - O^-$$

$$(1) \qquad\qquad\qquad (2) \qquad\qquad\qquad (3)$$

How would they be ranked in DECREASING order of basicity?

    (A) 1, 2, 3   (B) 1, 3, 2

    (C) 2, 1, 3   (D) 2, 3, 1

STOP

If time still remains, you may review work only in this section.

TEST 5

ANSWER KEY

1.	(C)	26.	(D)	51.	(B)	76.	(C)
2.	(D)	27.	(B)	52.	(C)	77.	(A)
3.	(D)	28.	(C)	53.	(D)	78.	(C)
4.	(A)	29.	(C)	54.	(A)	79.	(B)
5.	(A)	30.	(B)	55.	(A)	80.	(A)
6.	(C)	31.	(D)	56.	(C)	81.	(D)
7.	(A)	32.	(B)	57.	(A)	82.	(C)
8.	(B)	33.	(A)	58.	(B)	83.	(B)
9.	(B)	34.	(D)	59.	(D)	84.	(A)
10.	(C)	35.	(D)	60.	(C)	85.	(A)
11.	(D)	36.	(B)	61.	(D)	86.	(D)
12.	(A)	37.	(C)	62.	(C)	87.	(B)
13.	(B)	38.	(A)	63.	(B)	88.	(C)
14.	(B)	39.	(B)	64.	(C)	89.	(D)
15.	(A)	40.	(C)	65.	(A)	90.	(B)
16.	(B)	41.	(D)	66.	(D)	91.	(A)
17.	(C)	42.	(A)	67.	(A)	92.	(D)
18.	(D)	43.	(C)	68.	(C)	93.	(C)
19.	(B)	44.	(D)	69.	(B)	94.	(C)
20.	(B)	45.	(A)	70.	(A)	95.	(D)
21.	(D)	46.	(C)	71.	(D)	96.	(D)
22.	(C)	47.	(B)	72.	(D)	97.	(A)
23.	(D)	48.	(D)	73.	(A)	98.	(D)
24.	(A)	49.	(C)	74.	(B)	99.	(D)
25.	(C)	50.	(A)	75.	(C)	100.	(D)

101.	(A)	131.	(A)	161.	(D)	191.	(A)
102.	(A)	132.	(D)	162.	(A)	192.	(A)
103.	(B)	133.	(C)	163.	(C)	193.	(D)
104.	(A)	134.	(A)	164.	(B)	194.	(C)
105.	(B)	135.	(A)	165.	(D)	195.	(A)
106.	(A)	136.	(D)	166.	(D)	196.	(C)
107.	(A)	137.	(C)	167.	(A)	197.	(A)
108.	(D)	138.	(C)	168.	(C)	198.	(C)
109.	(A)	139.	(D)	169.	(B)	199.	(D)
110.	(A)	140.	(A)	170.	(D)	200.	(B)
111.	(D)	141.	(B)	171.	(A)	201.	(A)
112.	(A)	142.	(B)	172.	(D)	202.	(C)
113.	(B)	143.	(D)	173.	(B)	203.	(B)
114.	(A)	144.	(A)	174.	(B)	204.	(D)
115.	(A)	145.	(C)	175.	(A)	205.	(A)
116.	(D)	146.	(B)	176.	(D)	206.	(D)
117.	(D)	147.	(C)	177.	(C)	207.	(A)
118.	(A)	148.	(A)	178.	(D)	208.	(B)
119.	(A)	149.	(B)	179.	(C)	209.	(D)
120.	(C)	150.	(B)	180.	(B)	210.	(C)
121.	(B)	151.	(D)	181.	(C)	211.	(C)
122.	(D)	152.	(A)	182.	(D)	212.	(D)
123.	(C)	153.	(C)	183.	(A)	213.	(A)
124.	(B)	154.	(D)	184.	(A)	214.	(C)
125.	(C)	155.	(D)	185.	(C)	215.	(B)
126.	(C)	156.	(C)	186.	(B)	216.	(D)
127.	(D)	157.	(B)	187.	(D)	217.	(C)
128.	(A)	158.	(A)	188.	(A)	218.	(A)
129.	(B)	159.	(B)	189.	(D)	219.	(B)
130.	(B)	160.	(C)	190.	(C)		

DETAILED EXPLANATIONS
OF ANSWERS

Section 1 — Verbal Reasoning

1.   **(C)**   The passage is concerned chiefly with the proper uses of computers in education — i.e., what they can and cannot do, and what some of the potential dangers are in using them. (A), (B), and (D) are included in the passage, but do not constitute its chief subject matter.

2.   **(D)**   The authors believe that the development of expertise depends on intuition (hence not (B)) and experience. As educational tools, computers can foster intuition in the classroom (hence not (A)). Further, the expert teacher learns intuitively (paragraph four) to draw on commonsense knowledge (hence not (C)). Hence intuition plays an essential role in education from the point of view of both teacher and student.

3.   **(D)**   Paragraph two asserts that computers as educational tools can foster logical skills, classroom sociality, and procedural problem-solving skills. The authors also warn against making logical skills and procedural problem-solving skills the only goals of computer use in education.

4.   **(A)**   Although mastery of facts (B), careful coaching (C), and logic (D) are important in early stages, expertise derives from intuition and experience (see paragraph four).

5.   **(A)**   The greatest danger is the temptation to "narrow one's goal to forcing the student to think procedurally like a computerized problem-solver." Computers can encourage classroom sociality (hence not (C)). The authors do not address the issue contained in (B). (D) does present a danger, but the author defines computer literacy as knowing what levels of skills can be taught using computers; presumably those using computers in education are expected to be computer literate.

6.   **(C)**   The authors say that computers can be used as tutors where trained competence, not educated expertise, is the goal, and that one should not try to tutor a higher level of skill because such levels are beyond the capacity of logic machines. If it were proved that computers can teach such skills, the authors would have to revise their discussion of computers as tutors. Computers as tools and as tutees do not seek to teach educated expertise, so these discussions would not be affected.

7.   **(A)**   Rules learned in graduate school are a first step in teaching, but expertise derives from intuition and experience (hence not (B)). Since computers do not function on the basis of experience and intuition, they cannot replace teachers (hence not (C)). The authors disagree with the assumptions made by advocates of computers

as tutors that we cannot teach what we do not understand and that we only understand what we can formulate in logical rules and procedures (hence not (D)).

8.   **(B)**   A champion race-car driver and a chess grandmaster both develop skill through experience and intuition, whereas a computerized defense system depends on neither.

9.   **(B)**   The authors believe computers can teach a wide range of skills and can be used as tools, tutors, and tutees, but they cannot teach educated expertise (that is, their uses as tutors are quite limited). Hence (B) best summarizes the authors' view of the use of computers in education.

10.   **(C)**   Postman's point is that telegraphic means of transmitting news have created an information glut, in the sense that people receive information about people and events they are powerless to influence. Americans receive sufficient information about the Middle East (hence (A) is incorrect), but feel politically impotent. Americans may be preoccupied with economic gain and may also be socially irresponsible, but these are not the reasons Postman assigns for inaction.

11.   **(D)**   Postman says that the last refuge of the politically impotent is to give one's opinion to a pollster. Next to the last refuge is voting; hence (D) is the correct choice. (A) and (B) are in conflict with the author's main thesis; the author does not discuss voting as a crucial democratic act.

12.   **(A)**   The second paragraph makes clear that the author regards polls chiefly as instruments for gathering opinions, which are then compiled and presented as news, thus completing a "loop of impotence" (i.e., information about which the public can do nothing). Polls may or may not influence foreign policy and public opinion and may or may not play a role in a system of checks and balances, but the author's interest is in polls as part of a telegraphic information system that contributes to the public's sense of helplessness.

13.   **(B)**   The information-action ratio involves input (what one is informed about) and output (the possibilities of action based on information). The possibility of meaningful action based on received information was relatively high in pre-telegraphic cultures, but technological advances have made the relationship abstract and remote. The ratio does not involve accuracy of information or the relationship between history and current events. Local news may be more relevant for meaningful action than global news, but the ratio refers to all forms of news.

14.   **(B)**   Rather than making people more responsive to the problems of others, technological advances have made people feel increasingly helpless as they know more about matters, including social problems, that they are unable to influence. The author also says that telegraphy has made public discourse more incoherent, not more thoughtful. In his view, the electorate has become more frustrated than responsible.

15.   **(A)**   Because the context of news for people in pre-telegraphic cultures was more local than global, they received more "relevant" news (i.e., news that could result in meaningful action). Some pre-telegraphic cultures were oral, but some were

not (hence not (A)). The author does not discuss degrees of personal contact among individuals in various types of culture (hence not (D)). News of course had more, not less, action-value (not (C)).

16. **(B)**   Telegraphy has made public discourse more incoherent (see paragraph four) and has provided information upon which no meaningful action can be based. However, it has not increased the public sense of social responsibility even though it has provided more information (see paragraph two).

17. **(C)**   The author's statement occurs in the context of his discussion of the ways in which telegraphy has made public discourse essentially incoherent. Telegraphy had indeed dignified irrelevance (A), increased a sense of political impotence (B), and made the information-action relationship more abstract (D), but this particular statement (C) supports his argument in paragraph four about incoherent public discousre (Mumford's "broken time and broken attention").

18. **(D)**   Books (typography) make permanent contributions to continuing dialogues with the past whereas the contents of telegraphs are momentary and isolated, demanding to be burned. (A) and (C) conflict with the author's chief contentions. (B) may be true, but is not addressed by the author.

19. **(B)**   Typographic culture is the only one that the author discusses in relation to intellectualism (burning books is anti-intellectual; books encourage analysis and explanation). Telegraphy is contrasted with typography's intellectualism. The intellectual content of oral cultures is not discussed.

20. **(B)**   is correct. This problem, discussed throughout the passage, is summarized in the fourth paragraph.

21. **(D)**   is correct. Based on the points made in the third paragraph of this passage, there are no grounds for saying what might or will happen in the future.

22. **(C)**   is correct. Nothing in the passage relates to an acceptance of (A). Since, according to paragraph 3, projections of probable future events are no more justified than projections of certainty, (B) is also not a good choice. The final paragraph gives reasons for rejecting (D). This leaves (C), which is supported by the cautions made in the first and fourth paragraphs.

23. **(D)**   is correct. Our evidence may be good and our belief justified, yet this belief may still be false. Even if our belief does correspond to the truth, our reasons for belief may have nothing to do with why it is true. Thus, neither (A) nor (B) is correct.

24. **(A)**   is correct. The first paragraph suggests that this is the problem to be considered, and paragraph 4 restates this problem.

25. **(C)**   is correct. We do have a foundation (our observations of the past and present), so (A) is false, and we do not claim to know that our foundation is not justified, so (B) is false. The problem is that we cannot prove the justification of our foundation.

26. **(D)** is correct. The second paragraph indicates that none of the procedures mentioned here would solve the problem, since the problem is not in the amount of data or our analysis of this data, but in how we justify the relevance of this data to our judgments about the future.

27. **(B)** is correct. Paragraphs 2 and 3 consider this issue. Since Hume's concern is with belief and not actuality — in particular, with the basis for our belief, not the truth of our belief — (A) is irrelevant. The effect of the past on the future, choice (C), is also not Hume's concern. There is no claim in this passage to support (D).

28. **(C)** is correct. According to the last paragraph, Hume believes it is part of our human nature to use past experiences to predict the future. Since clouds have been associated with rain in the past, predicting rain on a cloudy day and carrying an umbrella to avoid getting wet would be human nature. Since a coin toss is a random event, past experience could not be used to predict the outcome, so (A) is incorrect. Items (B) and (D) are irrelevant to Hume's definition of human nature.

29. **(C)** is correct. The final sentence of paragraph 4 points to this and makes (A) incorrect. Because the question asks for the primary substance abused by the elderly, answer (B) is incorrect; only a small number of elderly opiate addicts exists, according to paragraph 1.

30. **(B)** is correct. The final sentence of paragraph 2 gives these reasons for the predicted increase in the number of elderly alcoholics. No mention is made of changes in the life expectancy, in the availability of illicit drugs, or in the expense of licit drugs, so these answers are incorrect.

31. **(D)** is correct. The author links coping problems among the elderly to substance abuse, but no recommendation is made about how to prevent or treat substance abuse. While similarities and differences between adolescent and elderly substance abuse are identified, no causal relationship between them is expressed.

32. **(B)** is correct. Since paragraph 2 states that one-third of alcoholics developed their problems after entering their elderly years, it can be concluded that this population had not developed their problems before entering their elderly years. No information is given in this passage about the percentage of the alcoholic population that is elderly or about the percentage of the elderly population that is alcoholic, so both (A) and (C) are incorrect.

33. **(A)** is correct. This point is made in the middle of the second paragraph.

34. **(D)** is correct. Both (A) and (B) are listed as factors relating to elderly substance abuse in paragraph 4, and (C) is listed as a factor at the end of the first paragraph. At the end of the final paragraph, a return to primitive defense mechanisms (as opposed to sophisticated ones) is cited as a possible factor in elderly drug abuse, so (D) is not a factor.

35. **(D)** is correct. The trend among adolescents, described in the last paragraph, begins with both alcohol and cigarettes and leads first to marijuana and then to

hard drugs, so both (A) and (B) are incorrect. Choice (C) is not relevant to the theory. Since the trend predicted by the theory goes from "weaker" to "stronger" drugs, (D) is the best choice.

36.　**(B)**　is correct. In paragraph 4, this connection is suggested. The relative incidence of drug abuse among the elderly is not discussed in this passage, so (A) is incorrect. In the first paragraph, the desire among elderly addicts to conceal their habits is mentioned, so (C) is also incorrect.

37.　**(C)**　is correct. This claim is made in the third paragraph, which also eliminates (D), since the pattern of small but frequent usage by the elderly is described. The information contained in paragraph 2 eliminates (A) and (B) as answers.

38.　**(A)**　is correct. This claim is made in the fourth paragraph.

39.　**(B)**　is correct. The passage considers only the naval aspect of World War II, not its overall outcome, so (A) is incorrect. The final paragraph mentions the continuing competition between ship and submarine technology, which suggests that submarines will continue to be important, so (C) is incorrect. German submarine technology is not compared to Allied technology, so (D) is also incorrect.

40.　**(C)**　is correct. Paragraph 2 describes the purpose and outcome of the formation of this committee, which developed the trainable hydrophone for detecting submarines.

41.　**(D)**　is correct. In the first paragraph, it is noted that Germany first demonstrated the full potentiality of the submarine as a weapon during World War I.

42.　**(A)**　is correct. This point is made in the first paragraph.

43.　**(C)**　is correct. The purpose of the snorkel is identified in the fifth paragraph.

44.　**(D)**　is correct. The passage describes the development of asdic and sonar technologies for the detection of submarines, and both of these were based on detecting the sound from submarines. The other elements were not described as methods for locating submarines in this passage.

45.　**(A)**　is correct. Paragraphs 2 and 3 describe the development of the hydrophone by the Allies, its improvement and renaming as asdic by the British, and its further refinement and renaming as sonar by the Americans. The only possible correct answers are Germany and France, and since Germany is not a member of the Allied Powers (as paragraph 1 indicates), it is the correct choice.

46.　**(C)**　is correct. The other three elements are all mentioned in the last paragraph as factors that contribute to the difficulty of locating a submarine.

47.　**(B)**　is correct. In the fourth paragraph, this claim is made. Notice that (A) is not correct because, while American submarines nearly destroyed the Japanese merchant marine, this is not mentioned as occurring early in the war.

48. **(D)** is correct. In the fourth paragraph, modern Hebrew is said to be unmistakably the descendent of Biblical Hebrew, but in none of these ways are the two identical.

49. **(C)** is correct. This point is made in the opening paragraph.

50. **(A)** is the best answer. This claim is made in the first paragraph. Since this paragraph also mentions the survival of written texts from this period, (B) is incorrect. Paragraph 2 makes (C) incorrect. Regarding (D), note that modern Hebrew, not ancient Hebrew, is the official language of the state of Israel.

51. **(B)** is correct. This point is discussed in the last paragraph of the passage.

52. **(C)** is correct. In the fifth paragraph, it is noted that both the written and spoken forms of modern Hebrew occur in a range of styles, from the highly formal to the highly informal.

53. **(D)** is correct. In paragraphs one and four, (A), (B), and (C) are mentioned, and thus (D) is the correct response.

54. **(A)** is correct. This point is made in the third paragraph. Note that the claim is not made that the state of Israel is attempting to have only Hebrew spoken, and so (B) is false.

55. **(A)** is the best answer. In the last paragraph, the comparison is made between knowing a language and knowing how to drive a car. The stress is on performance (knowing how) rather than explanation (knowing why).

56. **(C)** is correct. This point is made on the sixth paragraph. Points (A) and (B) are negated by the information in paragraph 7. Since these two paragraphs describe the limited use of formal Hebrew and the naturalness of informal Hebrew to native Israelis, (D) is incorrect.

57. **(A)** is correct. In the second paragraph, evidence that would differentiate between cutting of a skull before death (during trephination of a living patient) and after death (as part of a postmortem ritual) is described.

58. **(B)** is correct. In the second paragraph, it is noted that evidence of either healing or inflammation around a hole in the skull is indicative of trephination.

59. **(D)** is correct. As the second paragraph indicates, the absence of healing, like the absence of inflammation, is compatible with death during the surgical procedure or soon thereafter, so this lack of evidence is inconclusive.

60. **(C)** is correct. In the second paragraph, we are told that "many, if not most, trephinations occur in association with skull fracture." We cannot draw from this any conclusion as to whether the surgical procedure causes or results from fracture, and so neither (A) nor (B) is a valid assumption.

61.   **(D)**   is correct. We are told nothing about the relative frequencies of the various outcomes, and so we cannot make any assessment of the validity of the survival rates given in (A), (B), and (C).

62.   **(C)**   is correct. This point is stated in the first paragraph.

63.   **(B)**   is correct. The passage discusses ways of getting around the difficulty of distinguishing between the surgical procedure and operations performed on a corpse. Reasons for this surgical procedure are not offered, and procedures and tools used in trephination are not described, so (A), (C), and (D) are incorrect.

64.   **(C)**   is correct. The passage does not deal with trauma as a psychological condition, and the first and third paragraphs refer to the physical trauma associated with trephination.

65.   **(A)**   is correct. The final paragraph mentions this as an indication of long-term survival. This paragraph also mentions (B) and (D) as evidence for death during or shortly after surgery, since no healing has had time to occur. (C) may be associated with short-term or long-term survival, since the inflammatory reaction indicates that death was not immediate, but this does not eliminate infection as a complicating factor that might have prevented a complete recovery.

Section 2 — Physical Sciences

66.   **(D)**   By the conservation of momentum, the product of the mass of the bullet times its speed must equal the product of the mass of the gun times its recoil speed, or:

$$m_b v_b = m_g v_g$$

$$(0.01 \text{ kg}) (100 \text{ m/s}) = m_g (1 \text{ m/s})$$

$$1 \text{ kg} = m_g$$

67.   **(A)**   Using Newton's second law ($F_{net} = ma$) we find

$$F = \text{Weight}$$

$$ma = mg$$

$$a = g = 10 \text{ m/s}^2$$

The direction of a is the LEFT because the bullet is slowing down as it travels to the block … the air friction causes this deceleration.

68.   **(C)**   Using the kinematic formula for constant acceleration we obtain the following:

$$v^2 = 2ad \ v_0^2$$

$$v^2 = 2\,(\text{- }10 \text{ m/s}^2)\,(10 \text{ m}) + (100 \text{ m/s})^2$$

$$v^2 = 9800$$

$$v = 99 \text{ m/s}$$

Even without having calculated the acceleration above, one should realize that all other answers are unreasonable in this question.

69. **(B)** An impulse is defined as the change in the momentum of an object. Thus, the bullet experienced an impulse, having slowed down due to the air resistance. The impulse is thus:

$$I = \Delta p = p_f - p_i = m(v_f - v_i)$$

$$= (0.01 \text{ kg})\,(99 \text{ m/s - } 100 \text{ m/s})$$

$$= \text{ - } 0.01 \text{ kgm/s}$$

But, by the conservation of momentum, the earth must experience an equal but opposite impulse. Thus, the correct response is to the RIGHT, or the NEGATIVE of the impulse experienced by the bullet.

70. **(A)** By the conservation of linear momentum, the perfectly inelastic collision requires that the bullet and the block have the same final speed. Since the block was originally stationary the result is:

$$m_b v_{bi} = (m_b + m_{b1})v_f$$

$$(0.01 \text{ kg})\,(99 \text{ m/s}) = (0.01 \text{ kg} + 1 \text{ kg})v_f$$

$$v_f = 0.98 \text{ m/s}$$

Note here how reasonable this is compared with the recoil speed of the gun ... the block and the gun have the same mass, but the bullet has lost some speed due to air friction. Thus, even without correct computations above, the only reasonable answer is (A). Also note that answer (D) is obtainable by the incorrect use of the conservation of kinetic energy, not applicable here.

71. **(D)** As in Question 69, the impulse experienced by the block is simply its change in momentum:

$$I = \Delta p = p_f - p_i = m(v_f - v_i)$$

$$= (1 \text{ kg})\,(0.98 \text{ m/s - 0 m/s})$$

$$= 0.98 \text{ kgm/s}$$

Since this is POSITIVE the direction is to the RIGHT for the block.

72. **(D)** The other definition of impulse is through Newton's second law as the product of the average force experienced by the object times the amount of time the force acts on the object, or:

$$I = F\Delta t$$

$$F = I/\Delta t$$

$$= (0.98 \text{ kgm/s}) / (0.01 \text{ sec})$$

$$= 98 \text{ N}$$

73.   **(A)**   We use the same kinematic equation as in Question 68, but this time we'll find the acceleration given the initial and final speeds of the combination and the distance over which it travels:

$$\frac{v^2 - v_0{}^2}{2d} = a$$

$$(0^2 - (0.98 \text{ m/s})^2) / (2(2)) = a = -0.24 \text{ m/s}^2$$

The NEGATIVE sign, once again, reminds us of the direction of the acceleration as it slows the combination down along the rough surface.

74.   **(B)**   Getting back to Newton's second law we find:

$$F = ma = (1.01 \text{ kg}) (0.24 \text{ m/s}^2) = 0.24 \text{ N}$$

In order to understand Questions 75-84, you must understand stoichiometric relationships, gas laws, and basic acid base definitions and normality.

75.   **(C)**   Using the factor method the problem is solved in one step:

$$? \text{ mole } O_2 = 10.0 \text{ mole } SO_3 \times \frac{1 \text{ mole } O_2}{2 \text{ mole } SO_3} = 5.00 \text{ moles } O_2$$

Answer (A) is obtained if the equation is not balanced so that the factor is a 1:1 ratio. Answer (B) is obtained if the ratio is inverted.

76.   **(C)**   This problem is a limiting reagent problem. One way to solve the problem is to simply work the problem twice and choose the smaller answer since the reagent producing the smaller amount of product will be used up when this amount of product is formed.
     The factor method requires three factors in this case:

$$? \text{ g } SO_3 = 10.0 \text{ g } SO_2 \times \frac{1 \text{ mole } SO_2}{64.0 \text{ g } SO_2} \times \frac{2 \text{ mole } SO_3}{2 \text{ mole } SO_2} \times \frac{80.0 \text{ g } SO_3}{1 \text{ mole } SO_3}$$

$$= 12.5 \text{ g}$$

$$? \text{ g } SO_3 = 10.0 \text{ g } O_2 \times \frac{1 \text{ mole } O_2}{32.0 \text{ g } O_2} \times \frac{2 \text{ mole } SO_3}{1 \text{ mole } O_2} \times \frac{80.0 \text{ g } SO_3}{1 \text{ mole } SO_3}$$

$$= 50.0 \text{ g}$$

The answer is 12.5 since all of the SO_2 will be used up at this point. Even though there is sufficient oxygen to form 50.0 g of product only 12.5 grams can be produced.
     An alternative to working this problem is to find the limiting reagent first.

$$? \text{ mole } SO_3 = 10.0 \text{ g } SO_2 \times \frac{1 \text{ mole } SO_2}{64.0 \text{ g } SO_2} \times \frac{2 \text{ mole } SO_3}{2 \text{ mole } SO_2} = 0.156$$

$$? \text{ mole } SO_3 = 10.0 \text{ g } O_2 \times \frac{1 \text{ mole } O_2}{32.0 \text{ g } O_2} \times \frac{2 \text{ mole } SO_3}{2 \text{ mole } SO_2} = 0.31$$

Since only 0.156 mole of SO_3 from 10.0 g of SO_2, the limiting reagent is SO_2. Therefore,

$$? \text{ g } SO_3 = 0.16 \text{ mole } SO_3 \times \frac{80.0 \text{ g } SO_3}{1 \text{ mole } SO_3} = 12.5 \text{ g}$$

Answer (A) uses the wrong reagent. Answer (B) may have used a 2:1 ratio of moles. Answer (D) may have used the wrong molecular weight.

77. **(A)**   This is an ideal gas law problem:

$n = 10.0$ moles,

$T = 23 + 273 = 296$ K,

$P = 380$ torr $\times$ 1 atm/760 torr $= 0.5$ atm and

$R = 0.821$ (1 atm) / (K mole)

$P_V = nRT$

$V = nRT/P$

$\quad = (10.0 \text{ moles}) (0.0821 \text{ 1 atm}) (\text{K mol})^{-1} (296 \text{ K}) /)0.5 \text{ atm}$

$\quad = 486$ liters

Answer (B) you forgot to convert torr to atm. Answer (C) you inverted (B) — i.e., you set up the problem upside down. Answer (D) you forgot to convert both torr to atm and °C to K.

78. **(C)**   Another gas law problem:

$T = 300 + 273 = 573$ K;

$P = 380$ torr $\times$ 1 atm/760 torr $= .500$ atm

You need to use $PV = gRT/MM$; however, the equation must be rearranged to solve for density:

$PVMM = gRT$

$d = g/V = PMM/RT$

$d = (0.500 \text{ atm}) (64.0 \text{ g/mol}) / (0.0821 \text{ 1 atm/mol K}) (573 \text{ K})$

$\quad = 0.68$ g/liter

Answer (A), you turned the problem upside down. Answer (B), you forgot to change torr to atm. Answer (D), you forgot to convert both °C and torr.

79. **(B)**   You must work this problem in two steps: If both substances had been gases, you could have simply used the stoichiometric relationship from the equations, for example,

$$? \text{ liters } O_2 = 25.0 \text{ liters } SO_2 \times \frac{1 \text{ liter } O_2}{2 \text{ liters } SO_2} = 12.5 \text{ liters}$$

However, in this case, you must first find the moles of oxygen from the ideal gas law equation and then convert moles of oxygen into grams of sulfur using the stoichiometric relationships:

$$n = PV/RT$$

$$= (0.500 \text{ atm}) (29.8 \text{ l}) / (0.0821 \text{ l atm/mol K}) (298 \text{ K})$$

$$= 0.609 \text{ moles } SO_2$$

$$gS = 0.609 \text{ moles } SO_2 \times 1 \text{ mole S}/1 \text{ mole } SO_2 \times 32 \text{ g S}/1 \text{ mole S}$$

$$= 19 \text{ } gS$$

Answer (A), you forgot to convert 380 torr into 0.5 atm. Answer (C), you forgot to convert °C into K. Answer (D), you inverted the problem when you were finding moles of SO_2.

80. **(A)**   This problem may be worked using the factor method:

$$? \text{ kg } SO_2 = 500 \text{ lb coal} \times \frac{454 \text{ g coal}}{1 \text{ lb coal}} \times \frac{2 \text{ grams S}}{100 \text{ g coal}} \times \frac{1 \text{ mole S}}{32.0 \text{ g S}}$$

$$\times \frac{1 \text{ mole } SO_2}{1 \text{ mole S}} \times \frac{64.0 \text{ g } SO_2}{1 \text{ mole } SO_2} \times \frac{1.0 \text{ kg } SO_2}{1000 \text{ g } SO_2} = 9.08 \text{ kg}$$

Answer (B), you put in 2 grams without 100 grams coal in the denominator. Answer (C), you multiplied by 1000 instead of dividing. Answer (D), you worked the problem upside down.

81. **(D)**   Metal oxides are called basic oxides, while nonmetal oxides are called acidic oxides. Nonmetal oxides are also called acidic anhydrides since they form acids when added to water. Since S is a nonmetal, this is an acidic oxide or an acidic anhydride.

82. **(C)**   This problem can be worked using the factor method or the ideal gas law:

$$? \text{ liters } O_2 = 640 \text{ g } SO_2 \times \frac{1 \text{ mole } SO_2}{64.0 \text{ g } SO_2} \times \frac{1 \text{ mole } O_2}{2 \text{ mole } SO_2} \times \frac{22.41 O_2}{1 \text{ mole } O_2}$$

$$= 112 \text{ liters}$$

$$PV = gRT/MM$$

$$V = gRT/PMM$$

$$= \left[\frac{640 \text{ g SO}_2 \times 0.0821 \text{ l atm} / (\text{mole K}) \, 273 \text{ K}}{1 \text{ atm} \times 64.0 \text{ g} / \text{mole}} \right] = 224 \text{ l}$$

$$? \text{ O}_2 = 224 \text{ liters SO}_2 \times \frac{1 \text{ liter O}_2}{2 \text{ liters SO}_2} = 112 \text{ liters O}_2$$

Answer (A), you forgot to use the 1:2 ratio of moles. Answer (B), you inverted the mole:mole ratio. Answer (D), you worked the problem upside down.

83. **(B)** The balanced equation requires a 2 in front of the water and that the gas be CO_2 in order to balance the number of atoms of reactants and products:

$$CaCO_3 + SO_2 + 2H_2O \longrightarrow CaSO_3 * 2H_2O + CO_2$$

1 Ca	1 Ca
1 C	1 C
7 O	7 O
4 H	4 H
1 S	1 S

Finding the grams of $CaCO_3$ can be done using the factor method:

$$? \text{ CaCO}_3 = 64 \text{ g SO}_2 \times \frac{1 \text{ mole SO}_2}{64 \text{ g SO}_2} \times \frac{1 \text{ mole CaCO}_3}{1 \text{ mole SO}_2} \times \frac{100 \text{ g CaCO}_3}{1 \text{ mole CaCO}_3}$$

$$= 1.0 \times 10^2 \text{ grams CaCO}_3$$

Answer (A), you didn't balance the equation. Answer (C), you worked the problem upside down. Answer (D), you didn't balance the equation.

84. **(A)** You really do not need a balanced equation to work this problem since equivalents of acid must equal equivalents of base at the equivalence point in any titration. Consequently, the simplest way to work this problem is to use the following relationship:

$$\text{Vol} \times N = \text{Vol} \times N$$

$$\text{ml NaOH} = 25.00 \text{ ml H}_2\text{SO}_4 \times \frac{0.1000 \text{ eq H}_2\text{SO}_4}{1000 \text{ ml H}_2\text{SO}_4} \times \frac{1 \text{ eg NaOH}}{1 \text{ eq H}_2\text{SO}_4}$$

$$= \frac{1000 \text{ ml NaOH}}{0.2000 \text{ N NaOH}} = 12.50 \text{ ml}$$

Answer (B), you probably used the mole to mole ratio from the equation. Answer (C), you worked the problem upside down. Answer (D), you turned the set-up in Answer (B) upside down.

85.   **(A)**   At the equator, the tangential speed is determined by the simple relationship

Circumference/Time = $2\pi R_e$ / 24 hrs.

At any latitude (θ), the relationship must be through cos θ, such that at the poles (θ = 90°) there will be ZERO tangential speed. Thus:

$v = (2\pi R_e)$ cos θ/ T

$v = 2\pi(6.4 \times 10^6)$ cos (28.4°) / (24 hrs) (3600 s/hr)

$v = 409$ m/s

Answer (B) is assumed by those who refuse to believe that the earth rotates while answer (C) is correct at the equator only.

86.   **(D)**   All points which rotate on the surface of the earth have the same period of 1 day = 24 hrs = 1440 min. Thus, ALL answers are correct.

87.   **(B)**   Kinetic energy is found to be:

$KE = \frac{1}{2} mv^2 = \frac{1}{2}$ (500 kg) (409 m/s)^2 = 4.18 $\times 10^7$ J

Answer (C) would be the result only at the equator. Answer (A) parallels the same response to the previous question.

88.   **(C)**   Gravitational potential energy is found to be not from the center of the earth, but from the point at $r = \infty$:

$U = - GM_e m / r$

$U = - (6.67 \times 10^{-11}$ Nm^2 / kg^2) (6 $\times 10^{24}$ kg) (5000 kg) / (6.4 $\times 10^6$ m)

$U = - 3.13 \times 10^{10}$ J

Answer (A) is correct only if the earth's surface was the zero reference point. Answer (B) is computed as if the center of the earth was the zero reference point.

89.   **(D)**   Kepler's third law states that the square of the period is proportional to the cube of the radius: Thus:

$T^2 = kr^3 = (9.8 \times 10^{-14}$ s^2/m^3) (1 $\times 10^7$ m)^3

$T = 9930$ sec = 166 min

Both answers (A) and (B) are wrong by inspection, as the satellite speed must become very rapid so that it does not fall back to earth under the influence of the pull of gravity.

90.   **(B)**   For the circular orbit assumed, the circumference is simply

$C = 2 \pi r = 2\pi(1 \times 10^7$ m) = 6.28 $\times 10^7$ m.

But, it takes the satellite 3 complete revolutions for each mission and thus the correct answer is

$d = 3C = 1.89 \times 10^8$ m.

91. **(A)**   Having computed the period T and circumference C of its orbit, we now compute the satellite's kinetic energy as:

$$KE = \frac{1}{2} mv^2 = \frac{1}{2} m(C/T)^2 = \frac{1}{2} \ (500 \text{ kg}) \ ((6.28 \times 10^7 \text{ m}) \ / \ (9930 \text{ s}))^2$$

$$KE = 1 \times 10^{10} \text{ J}$$

92. **(D)**   As above, the gravitational potential energy is given by the expression:

$$U = - GM_e m \ / \ r$$

$$U = - \ (6.67 \times 10^{-11} \text{ Nm}^2 / \text{kg}^2) \ (6 \times 10^{24} \text{ kg}) \ (500 \text{ kg}) \ / \ (1 \times 10^7 \text{ m})$$

$$U = - 2 \times 10^{10} \text{ J}$$

Answer (A) is computed as if $g = 9.8 \text{ m/s}^2$ were a constant to this radius of 10,000 km. Answer (B) is exactly half of the value given in (A) as if an average $g = 4.9 \text{ m/s}^2$ is used. Answer (C) is the value obtained on the surface of the earth and must be incorrect at this altitude.

93. **(C)**   The energy expended is the work done in getting the satellite into orbit and is just the difference between the total energies:

$$W \ = \ E_f - E_i = (KE + U)_f - (KE + U)_i$$

$$W \ = \ (1 \times 10^{10} \text{ J} - 2 \times 10^{10} \text{ J}) - (4.18 \times 10^7 \text{ J} - 3.13 \times 10^{10} \text{ J})$$

$$W \ = \ + 2.13 \times 10^{10} \text{ J}$$

Answers (A) and (B) are absurd, as witnessed by the tremendous expense of putting satellites into orbit about the earth.

94. **(C)**   Resistances R_1 and R_2 are in series, so we can use the following formula to combine them.

$$R_{Total} = R_1 + R_2 + R_3 + \ ... \ R_n$$

Therefore

$$8\Omega = 6\Omega + 2 \ \Omega$$

Now, we have simplified the circuit to

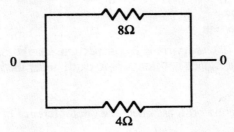

which has two resistors connected in parallel. We therefore use the following

$$\frac{1}{R_{Total}} = \frac{1}{R_1} + \frac{1}{R_2} + \frac{1}{R_3} + ... + \frac{1}{R_n}$$

Therefore

$$\frac{1}{R_{Total}} = \frac{1}{8\Omega} + \frac{1}{4\Omega} = \frac{3}{8}\ \Omega\ ;\ \text{and}\ R_{Total} = \frac{8}{3}\ \Omega$$

95.　**(D)**　To answer this question, we must apply Ohm's law, in the form

$$R = \frac{V}{I}$$

$V = 120$ volts　$I = 5$ amps

Therefore

$$R = \frac{120\ \text{volts}}{5\ \text{amps}} = 24\ \text{ohms.}$$

96.　**(D)**　When light is sent through a prism, the refraction at the two surfaces is dependent upon the index of refraction. The index is larger for small wavelengths than for longer wavelengths. Therefore, violet (which has the shortest wavelength) will be deviated the most, and red (which has the longest wavelength) will be deviated the least.

97.　**(A)**　First, we must find the total resistance of the circuit.

$$R_{Total} = 2\Omega + 3\Omega + 5\Omega = 10\Omega$$

Then, applying Ohm's law we get

$$I = \frac{V}{R} = \frac{15\ \text{volts}}{10\Omega} = 1.5\ \text{amps}$$

98.　**(D)**　Since the resultant force is the difference between the two forces, the forces must be oriented exactly opposite to each other.

99.　**(D)**　Gravitational acceleration on a body is unaffected by the horizontal velocity if ideal conditions are assumed, i.e., no wind resistance. The two cannonballs, therefore, strike the ground simultaneously.

100.　**(D)**　The law of conservation of momentum is applicable here, as it is in all collision problems. Therefore,

Momentum after impact = Momentum before impact.

Momentum before impact $= M_{B_1} \times V_{B_1}$

$$= 100\ \text{gm} \times 100\ \text{cm} / \text{sec}$$

$$= 10,000\ \text{gm - cm} / \text{sec}$$

Momentum after impact $= M_{A_1} \times V_{A_1} + M_{A_2} \times V_{A_2}$

$$= 100\ \text{gm} \times 60\ \text{cm} / \text{sec} + 25\ \text{gm} \times V_{A_2}\ \text{cm} / \text{sec}$$

Then

$$10,000 \text{ gm-cm/sec} = 6000 \text{ gm-cm/sec} + 25 \text{ g} \times V_{A_2}$$

whence

$$V_{A_2} = 160 \text{ sm/sec.}$$

101. (A) Assume that the brick has no horizontal velocity when it is dropped on the cart. Its initial horizontal momentum is therefore zero. Since no external horizontal forces act on the system of cart and brick, horizontal momentum must be conserved. We can thus say for the horizontal direction,

$$m_c v_{ci} + m_b v_{bi} = m_c v_{cf} + m_b v_{bf}$$

Since the final velocities of the brick and cart are the same,

$$m_c v_{ci} = (m_c + m_b) v_f$$

Substituting values,

$$v_f = \frac{m_c v_{ci}}{m_c + m_b} = \frac{(5 \text{ kg}) (1 \text{ m / sec})}{(5 \text{ kg} + 5 \text{ kg})} = .5 \text{ m / sec}$$

The change in velocity of the cart is

$$v_f - v_{ci} = (0.5 - 1.0) \text{ m/sec} = -0.5 \text{ m/sec.}$$

This section, (Questions 102-112) requires an understanding of the laws of thermodynamics — both concepts and problem-solving. Also some knowledge of various phases (phase diagrams) is required.

102. (A) First, you must recognize that this system is at equilibrium. Therefore, the change in Gibbs free energy is zero. Next, calculate the change in enthalpy:

$$\Delta H = -242 - (-286) = 44 \text{ kJ/mole}$$

$$\Delta G = \Delta H - T\Delta S$$

$$0 = 44 \times 10^3 \text{ J/mol} - 373 (\Delta S)$$

$$\Delta S = 118 \text{ J/mol K}$$

$$118 = 188.7 - x$$

$$x = 70.7 \text{ J/mol K}$$

Answer (B), you used 273 K instead of the normal boiling point 373 K. Answer (C), you subtracted products from reactants instead of reactants from products. Therefore, the change in enthalpy was negative instead of positive. Answer (D), you stopped when you found the change in entropy, not the entropy of the liquid water.

103. (B) The equation for working this problem is

$$\Delta G° = \Delta H° - T\Delta S°$$

which gives the relationship between free energy, enthalpy and entropy. The change in free energy is a measure of the spontaneity of the reaction. If the change in free energy is negative, the reaction is spontaneous, if it is positive, the reaction is nonspontaneous, and if it is 0, the reaction is at equilibrium. In this case, the reaction is at equilibrium — true for any phase occurring at the boiling point, melting point, or sublimation point.

$$0 = \Delta H° - T\Delta S°$$

$$0 = \Delta H° - 298 \text{ K } (57.7 \text{ J/mole K})$$

$$\Delta H° = 1.72 \times 10^4 \text{ J/mole} = 17.2 \text{ kJ/mol} \times 1 \text{ mole}/121 \text{ g} \times 100\text{g}$$

$$= 14.2 \text{ kJ}$$

This is the amount of heat required for 100 grams which is less than one mole.

Answer (A), you forgot to change the sign. Answer (C), you used 25°C instead of 298 K. Answer (D), you assume one mole instead of 100 grams.

104. (A)   A positive change in entropy accompanies an increase in the number of gas molecules during the reaction because the entropy of a solid is less than that of a liquid which is less than that of a gas. (A) 1 mole of gas reactants - 2 moles of gas products. (B) 1 mole of gas reactants - 0 moles of gas products. (C) 1 mole of gas reactants - 0 moles of gas products.

105. (B)   Energy is released when a bond is broken so the sign is negative. On the other hand, energy is absorbed when a bond is broken, so the sign is positive. In order to calculate the change in energy for the reaction, we need only add up the energy of the bonds formed (-) and subtract from the energy required for the bonds broken.

4 C-H bonds + 1 C=C bond + 1 Cl-Cl bond   Reactants

4(87) + 1 (146) + 1(58) = 552

4 C-H bonds + 1 C-C bond + 2 Cl-Cl bonds   Products

4(87) + 1 (83) + 2(79) = -589

Change in energy = 552 - 589 = - 37. (A) You didn't multiply the C-Cl bond energy by 2. (C) You reversed the signs.

106. (A)   The heat of formation of Fe_2O_3 (s) is given so you may write the equation for the formation of a compound from its elements

$$2Fe \text{ (s)} + 3/2O_2 \text{ (g)} \longrightarrow Fe_2O_3 \text{ (s)} \text{ H° - 743.6}$$

This equation must be reversed so that Fe_2O_3 appears on the left-hand side of the equation because that is where it appears in the equation that we are evaluating. When you reverse an equation, you must also change the sign of the enthalpy change. Use this equation with the one given in the passage to find the equation that you want.

$$Fe_2O_3 \text{ (s)} \longrightarrow 2Fe \text{ (s)} + 3/2O_2 \text{ (g)} + 743.6$$

$$3CO \text{ (g)} + 3(1/2)O_2 \text{ (g)} \longrightarrow 3CO_2 \text{ (g)} \quad 3(-257.2)$$

The second equation must be multiplied by 3 in order to eliminate the oxygen and also because there are 3 CO and 3 CO_2 in the equation required. When an equation is multiplied by a number, the change in enthalpy must also be multiplied by the same number.

Adding the two equations together cancels the oxygen and gives the required equation:

$$Fe_2O_3 \text{ (s)} + 3CO \text{ (g)} \longrightarrow 2Fe \text{ (s)} + 3CO_2 \text{ (g)} - 28 \text{ kJ}$$

Answer (B), you reversed the equations. Answer (C), you didn't multiply the change in enthalpy for the second equation by 3. Answer (D), you didn't multiply by 3 and you reversed the equations.

107. **(A)**   You must use Hess' Law. Look up the heats of formation for all of the reactants and products. If a reactant or product has a coefficient, multiply the enthalpy by the coefficient. Add up the enthalpies for all of the products and add up the enthalpies for the reactants. Subtract the sum of the enthalpies of the reactants from the sum of the enthalpies for the products. This is the change in enthalpy for the reaction or the heat of reaction.

$$\Delta H = [1(-267) + 1(-26.4)] - [3(-63.7) + 1(-94.1)]$$

$$\Delta H = -8.2 \text{ kJ} / \text{mole}$$

(A) You subtracted reactants - products. (C) You didn't multiply the enthalpy for FeO by 3. (D) You didn't multiply by 3 and you subtracted products from reactants.

108. **(D)**   Use the equation

$$\Delta G = \Delta H - T\Delta S$$

If ΔH is + and ΔS is +, increasing the temperature will make the reaction more spontaneous. However, if ΔH is - and ΔS is -, increasing the temperature will make the reaction less spontaneous.

$\Delta H = -$ and $\Delta S = -$ Equation (1)

$\Delta H = +$ and $\Delta S = +$ Equation (2)

Therefore, (D) is the correct answer.

109. **(A)**   First find the change in energy for the reaction from the given data (Products - Reactants):

$$\Delta G = -174.8 - 133.7 = -41.1$$

Use the equation:

$$\Delta G = -RT \ln K$$

to find the equilibrium constant.

$$-41.1 \text{ kJ} = -(8.314 \times 10^{-3} \text{ kJ/mole K}) (298 \text{ } K) \ln K$$

$$\ln K = (41.1) / [8.314 \times 10^{-3} (298)]$$

$$= 16.59$$

$$K = 1.60 \times 10^7$$

Answer (B), you forgot to cancel the negative sign. Answer (C), you used log instead of ln. Answer (D), you used log instead of ln and didn't cancel the sign.

110. **(A)**   Any process in which heat is absorbed has a positive q. Endothermic process ($q = +$), exothermic process ($q = -$). When the system does work, it loses energy so $w = +$. If work is done on the system, the system gains energy so $w = -$. Use the equation

$$\Delta E = q - w$$

Therefore, if $q = +$ and $w = +$, then $\Delta E = + 65 - (22) = 43$.

Answer (B), you used the wrong sign for w. Answer (C), you sued the wrong sign for q and w. Answer (D), you used the wrong sign for q.

111. **(D)**   First, find the change in enthalpy for the reaction:

$$\Delta H = 2(- 1121) - 4(-272.0) = - 1154 \text{ kJ/mole}$$

Then, find the change in entropy for the reaction:

$$\Delta S = 2(145.3) - 4(60.75) = 47.6 \text{ J/mole K}$$

Since ΔH is negative and ΔS is positive, the change in free energy will always be negative and the reaction is spontaneous at any temperature.

Answer (A), you obtained the wrong sign for ΔH. Answer (B), you obtained the wrong sign for ΔS. Answer (C), you obtained the wrong sign for ΔH *and* ΔS.

112. **(A)**   In the phase diagram A = solid, C = liquid and E = gas;

B = equilibrium between solid and liquid - melting point

D = equilibrium between liquid and gas - boiling point

F = equilibrium between solid and gas - sublimation point

G = equilibrium between all three - triple point.

113. **(B)**   Ohm's law gives the relationship between the voltage V, the resistance R, and current I as

$$V = IR$$

or:

$$I = V/R = (12 \text{ V}) / (3\Omega) = 4A$$

Answer (A) is the mathematical inverse sometimes achieved by incorrect algebra, while answer (C) is the product of V times R, an incorrect statement of Ohm's law.

114. **(A)**   The relationship for the magnetic field (B) at the center of a long solenoid is:

$$B = \mu n I$$

where n is the number of turns per unit length of core and I is the current in the windings. Thus:

$$n = B/\mu I = (0.1 \ T) \ / \ (25 \times 10^{-7} \ \text{H/m}) \ (4 \ \text{A})$$

$$n = 10,000$$

115. **(A)**   Magnetic flux through a solenoid is found to be the product of the constant field times the cross-sectional area. Answer (C) (electromagnetic radiation) results from oscillatory fields, not steady fields while answer (D) (the Faraday) is the unit of capacitance, not magnetic flux.

116. **(D)**   The repulsive nature of like magnetic poles is the cause of the motion of the permanent magnet here. Answer (A) involves changing magnetic fields through secondary coils, not the interaction between fields and magnets.

117. **(D)**   The correct answer would be so that gravity helps prevent the solenoid from sticking, a phenomenon known to kill automobile batteries. Just as with a lock cylinder, the gravitational aid to recovering the initial conditions is most desirable. Answer (A) is only correct at the equator, while it is actually a small electric field that is produced along your car as you drive, not a magnetic field as answer (B) would have you think.

This problem set (Questions 118-128) requires an understanding of the polarity of molecules in determining the attractive forces between molecules. You must know that the strongest attractive forces exist between ions and that these attractive forces decrease as the polarity of the molecule decreases. In general, the stronger the attractive forces between the molecules, the lower the vapor pressure and the higher the boiling point. Increasing the attractive forces in the solution will, therefore, lower the vapor pressure and increase the boiling point of the solution. If the attractive forces are all alike, then the molecular weight will control the vapor pressure and boiling point.

118. **(A)**   The stronger the attractive forces between the molecules the lower the vapor pressure and the higher the boiling point. The vapor pressure is simply the pressure exerted by the molecules above the surface of the liquid. The stronger the attractive forces between the molecules in the liquid, the more energy is required to break these attractive forces and free the molecules to go to the vapor state. Attractive forces decrease in the following order:

ion-ion > ion-dipole > H-bonding > dipole-dipole > London

The strength of ion-ion attractive forces is evidenced by the extremely high melting points of ionic compounds. Ion-dipole attractive forces are formed when ionic compounds dissolve in polar solvents (like dissolves like). H-bonding is only possible if one of the molecule contains a N-H, O-H, or F-H bond and the other molecule contains O, N, or F. Since polar molecules exhibit dipole moments, dipole-dipole attractive forces are simply the attractive forces between polar molecules. The weakest forces of attraction are between nonpolar molecules - London force. The molecule in answer (A) exhibits H-bonding, while the remaining molecules are polar (review molecular geometries) but are not capable of H-bonding since none of them possess O-H, N-H or F-H bonds.

119. **(A)** Since all of these compounds have similar molecular weights, the distinguishing feature in determining the boiling point will be the attractive forces between the molecules. The compound in (A) is nonpolar while the compound in (B) is polar and the compound in (C) exhibits H-bonding. Consequently the boiling points will increase in that order:

$$A < B < C$$

because the attractive forces increase in this order. The weakest attractive forces (London forces) exist in solutions of nonpolar molecules such as those in (A).

120. **(C)** Just as attractive forces determining the vapor pressure boiling point of a compound or solution, they are also responsible for solubility. The rule — like dissolves like — refers to the polarity of the solution. Polar substances tend to be soluble in other polar substances and nonpolar substances are more likely to dissolve in other nonpolar substances. You must be able to determine the polarity of the molecules involved in order to predict their solubility. Review molecular geometries and their effect on the polarity of the molecule. If H-bonding is possible between the solute (the smaller amount of compound) and the solvent (the larger amount of compound in the solution), it will cause a molecule to be even more soluble. In this problem H-bonding is possible between the compound in C (CH_3O-H) and water (H-O-H). Therefore, this compound will be more soluble in water. The compounds in (A) and (B) are both nonpolar and will NOT be soluble in water. They are more likely to be soluble in each other or some other nonpolar compound. The compound in (C) (CH_3Cl) is somewhat polar and may be slightly soluble in water.

121. **(B)** Henry's law states that the solubility of a gas is directly proportional to its partial pressure ($S = kP$). Therefore, a ratio of solubilities to partial pressures can be set up:

$$S_1/P_1 = S_2/P_2$$

In Answer (B) this ratio gives

(0.68 g/100 g) / 4.0 atm = x/0.0025 atm.

$x = 4.25 \times 10^{-4}$ g/100 g.

Answer (A)

4 atm / 0.0025 atm = x (0.68 g/100 g)

$x = 1.088 \times 10^3$ g/100 g.

You substituted incorrectly. The answer is unreasonable since you know that decreasing the pressure should decrease the solubility. Answer (C)

4 atm / (0.68 g/100 g) = x / 0.0025 atm

$x = 0.015$ atm^2 (100 g/g).

You substituted incorrectly. If you look at the units you can see that the answer must be wrong.

122. (D) Raoult's law states that the partial pressure above a solution will be directly proportional to the product of the mole fraction of the solvent and its vapor pressure when pure:

$$P_a = X_a P^\circ_a$$

The mole fraction is the moles of one substance divided by the total moles:

$$X_a = \text{moles } A \,/\, \text{total moles}$$

In this problem you must first find the moles of each compound, then find the mole fraction and finally use Raoult's law to find the partial pressure:

$$\text{moles CO(NH}_2)_2 = 10.0 \text{ g} \times \frac{1 \text{ mole}}{60.0 \text{ g}} = 0.1667 \text{ moles}$$

$$\text{moles CH}_3\text{OH} = 40.0 \text{ g} \times \frac{1 \text{ mole}}{32 \text{ g}} = 1.25 \text{ moles}$$

$$X_{\text{CH}_3\text{OH}} = 1.25 \text{ moles} \,/\, (1.25 \text{ moles} + 0.167 \text{ moles}) = 0.882$$

$$P_{\text{CH}_3\text{OH}} = 0.882 \,(90 \text{ torr}) = 79.4 \text{ torr}$$

This is a reasonable answer since the vapor pressure should decrease because of the H-bonding that results for example, from the attraction of the H in the O-H bond in CH_3OH for the O in the C=O bond of $CO(NH_2)_2$ and the H-bonds possible between the H of the N-H bond with the O of the O-H bond, etc. There are several possibilities of H-bonding between these two substances.

Answer (A), you used 0.167/1.25 for the mole fraction. This is simply a ratio of the moles — not the mole fraction. The pressure is much too low to be a reasonable answer. Answer (B), you inverted the mole fraction (1.417/0.167) (90). The answer is unreasonable — the partial pressure cannot be greater than the pure vapor pressure if this is an ideal solution. answer (C), you used the mole fraction of the solute rather than the mole fraction of the solvent: (.167/1.417) (90). Again, the answer is unreasonable because we should observe a small decrease in pressure not a change that is this great.

123. (C) Since both substances are volatile, you must find the partial pressure of both and add them together as dictated by Dalton's Law of Partial Pressures (the total pressure is equal to the sum of the partial pressures). First, you must find the moles of each substance, then, find the mole fractions and the partial pressures, and finally add them together:

$$\text{moles CS}_2 = 50.0 \text{ g} \times \frac{1 \text{ mole}}{76 \text{ g}} = 0.658 \text{ moles}$$

$$\text{moles C}_4\text{H}_8\text{O}_2 = 50.0 \text{ g} \times \frac{1 \text{ mole}}{88.1} = 0.568 \text{ moles}$$

$$X_{\text{CS}_2} = 0.658 \,/\, (0.658 + 0.568) = 0.537$$

$$X_{\text{C}_4\text{H}_8\text{O}_2} = 0.568 \,/\, (0.658 + 0.568) = 0.463$$

Notice the sum of the mole fractions must be equal to 1.

$$P_{CS_2} = 0.537 \times 400 \text{ torr} = 215 \text{ torr}$$

$$P_{C_4H_8O_2} = 0.463 \times 110 \text{ torr} = 51 \text{ torr}$$

$$P_T = 215 + 51 = 266$$

Answer (A), you used the weight fraction instead of the mole fraction:

$$50/(50 + 50) = 0.5$$

$$P_T = 0.5 \, (400 \text{ torr}) + 0.5 \, (110 \text{ torr}) = 255 \text{ torr}$$

Answer (B), you switched the pure vapor pressures:

$$P_T = .537 \times 110 \text{ torr} + .463 \times 400 \text{ torr} = 244 \text{ torr}$$

124. **(B)** Freezing point depression is one of four collective properties (depends upon number of particles in solution and not the kind of particle). The lowering of the freezing point is directly proportional to the molality of the solution and the van Hoff factor (i = number of particles formed per mole).

$$T = K_f(m) \, (i)$$

In this case NaCl forms 2 moles of particles per mole. Actually the number of particles is never exactly 2. However, i approaches the whole number as the solution becomes more dilute. Therefore, in this case i will approach 2.

$$T = 1.86°C/m \, (0.020 \, m) \, (2) = 0.0744°C$$

The freezing point of pure water is 0.0°C. Adding a solute to the water lowers the freezing point. Therefore, the freezing point of the solution must be 0 - 0.074 = - 0.074°C. Think about why you must add salt to the ice water in order to make homemade ice cream.

Answer (A), you used $i = 1$ instead of 2. Answer (C), you divided by 2 instead of multiplying by 2. Answer (D), you used K_b instead of K_f.

125. **(C)** You may work this problem using the factor method

$$? \, g \, x \, / \, \text{mole} \, x = \frac{9.81 \, g \, x}{90.0 \, g \, H_2O} \times \frac{0.51°C \, \text{kg} \, H_2O}{0.37°C \, \text{mole} \, x} \times \frac{10^3 \, g \, H_2O}{1 \, \text{kg} \, H_2O}$$

$$= 150 \, g \, / \, \text{mole}$$

The 0.37 in the denominator of the second term is the change in the boiling point.

Another way to work the problem is to solve

$$T = K_b \, (m) \, (i)$$

for m:

$$m = 0.37/0.51 = .725 \, m$$

Then use the factor method to find the moles of x:

$$\text{moles} \times \frac{0.725 \, \text{mole}}{1 \, \text{kg} \, H_2O} \times \frac{1 \, \text{kg} \, H_2O}{10^3 \, g \, H_2O} \times 90.0 \, g \, H_2O = 0.0653$$

Then divide the grams given in the problem by the moles to find the molecular weight:

$$\text{mol wt} = 9.81 \text{ g} x / 0.0653 \text{ mole } x = 150 \text{ g/mole}$$

Answer (A), you divided grams of water by grams of x instead of grams of x by grams of water — inverted the first factor. Answer (B), you inverted the first factor and used 100.37 instead of the change in temperature. Answer (D), you inverted the second factor. In other words, you divided the change in temperature by K_b instead of dividing K_b by the change in temperature.

126. **(C)** The formula for finding osmotic pressure (another colligative property) is:

$$ii = MRT$$

The osmotic pressure ii must be in atmospheres since R is 0.0821 l atm/ (mole K).

$$ii = 9.8/760 = 0.01289 \text{ atm}$$

First, find the molarity, M.

$$M = \frac{ii}{RT} = \frac{0.01289 \text{ atm}}{\left(0.0821 \dfrac{1 \text{ atm}}{\text{K mole}}\right)(298 \text{ K})} = 5.27 \times 10^{-4}$$

Then find the moles:

$$\frac{5.27 \times 10^{-4} \text{ mole}}{\text{liter}} \times 100 \text{ ml} \times \frac{1 \text{ liter}}{10^3 \text{ ml}} = 5.27 \times 10^{-5} \text{ moles}$$

Divide the grams given by the moles to obtain the molecular weight:

$$\text{g/mol} = 0.2 \text{ g} / 5.27 \times 10^{-5} = 3.79 \times 10^3$$

Answer (A), you didn't change the temperature to Kelvin. Answer (B), you multiplied the pressure by 760 instead of dividing and you didn't change the volume to liters.

127. **(D)** You must find the osmolality of each of the solutions in order to determine which way the water molecules will flow through the semipermeable membrane. The solution in compartment A is 0.10 m $BaCl_2$. Its osmolality is 0.10 m $\times$ 3 particle/mole = 0.30 Os

(A) $0.10 \times 2 = 0.20$ Os

(B) $0.20 \times 1 = 0.20$ Os

(C) $0.10 \times 3 = 0.30$ Os

(D) $0.10 \times 5 = 0.50$ Os

Therefore, since (A) and (B) have the same osmolality which is less than that in compartment A, the water will flow into compartment A causing the water level to rise. Since answer (C) has the same osmolality as the solution in compartment A, the water will not flow in this case.

Solution (D) has a higher osmolality than the solution in compartment A; therefore the water will flow from A into B causing the water level to rise.

128. **(A)** You may work this problem by using the factor method:

$$\frac{\text{mole CHCl}_3}{\text{kg H}_2\text{O}} = \frac{1.00 \text{ g CHCl}_3}{750 \text{ ml H}_2\text{O}} \times \frac{1 \text{ ml H}_2\text{O}}{1.023 \text{ g H}_2\text{O}} \times \frac{1 \text{ mole CHCl}_3}{118.5 \text{ g CHCl}_3}$$

$$\times \frac{10^3 \text{ g H}_2\text{O}}{1 \text{ kg H}_2\text{O}} = 0.011 \text{ m}$$

Answer (B), you inverted the first factor — the units won't work and the answer is unreasonable! Answer (C), you inverted the second and third factor and did not include the factor for converting grams to kg. This is not only an unreasonable answer, but the units still do not work. Answer (D), the molecular weight is incorrect.

129. **(B)** The speed, or more precisely, the instantaneous speed of an object is determined from the graph on the v-axis as the magnitude of the velocity. Thus, at 1.5 s, the velocity is shown to be - 10 m/s so that the speed must be 10 m/s. Answer (A) is the value of the slope of the graph at that point and is the acceleration, not the speed of the object. The units are incorrect in answer (D).

130. **(B)** The average speed of an object is found as the mathematical average of $^1/_2$ the sum of the initial and final values and is thus:

$$s = {}^1/_2 \, (s_i + s_f) = {}^1/_2 \, (10 \text{ m/s} + 0) = 5 \text{ m/s}$$

131. **(A)** To be at rest is to have zero speed. When the object has zero velocity, it has zero speed. This occurs throughout the time interval between 4 s and 5 s. Answer (A) is thus the only answer that fits within this range. All other answers are within range where the slopes are zero and thus the accelerations are zero, not necessarily the speeds.

132. **(D)** The average acceleration of an object is defined as the ratio of the change in the velocity to the time interval over which it changes. It is thus found to be:

$$a = \frac{v_f - v_i}{t} = \frac{(10 \text{ m/s}) - (0 \text{ m/s})}{(3 \text{ s})} = 3.33 \text{ m/s}$$

133. **(C)** The instantaneous acceleration at any point is the slope of the v vs t graph at that point. This is commonly computed as the "rise over the run" to be:

$$a = \Delta v / \Delta t = 0$$

134. **(A)** To obtain distance (or more accurately displacement) from the v vs t graph, we compute the area under the curve. Here, the area is a simple triangle of base $b = 2$ s and height $h = 10$ m/s to give:

$$d = \text{Area} = {}^1/_2 \, bh = {}^1/_2 \, (2 \text{ s}) (10 \text{ m/s}) = 10 \text{ m}$$

Answer (D) is incorrectly obtained by failing to account for the change in speed over the time interval.

135. **(A)** Again, the displacement is here found as the area under the curve. The extra complication here is that some of the motion is along the NEGATIVE direction (when v is negative) and some is POSITIVE (when v is positive). We must not only compute the magnitudes of the areas, but account for the direction by taking the area below the $v = 0$ axis to be NEGATIVE. The graph is reproduced below with the areas of rectangles and triangles segmented. Their evaluations are:

$a = (1) (- 5) = - 5$ m $d = \frac{1}{2} (2) (- 10) = - 10$ m

$b = \frac{1}{2} (1) (- 5) = - 2.5$ m $e = \frac{1}{2} (1) (10) = 5$ m

$c = (1) (- 10) = - 10$ m $f = (2) (10) = 20$ m

The magnitude of the sum of the values is thus the correct answer. Answer (D) is obtained if all magnitudes are added instead.

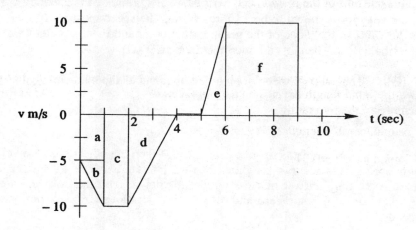

136. **(D)** In the wave mechanical theory, four quantum numbers are needed to describe the electrons of an atom. The first or principal quantum number, n, designates the main energy level of the electron and has integral values of 1, 2, 3, ... n. The second or azimuthal quantum number, l, designates the energy sublevel within the main energy level. The values of l depend upon the value of n and range from zero to $n - 1$. The third or magnetic-quantum number, m_l, designates the particular orbital within the energy sublevel. The number of orbitals of a given kind per energy sublevel is equal to the number of m_l values $(2l + 1)$. The quantum number m_l can have any integral value from $+ l$ to $- l$ including zero. The fourth or spin quantum number, s, describes the two ways in which an electron may be aligned with a magnetic field $(+\frac{1}{2}$ or $- \frac{1}{2})$.

The states of the electrons within atoms are described by the four quantum numbers in the order: n (principal), l (azimuthal), m_l (magnetic) and s(spin).

137. **(C)** The rest mass of a photon is given to be zero.

138. **(C)** In this question, you are dealing with the phenomenon of electrolysis. When an electric current is applied to a solution containing ions, the ions will either be reduced or oxidized to their electronically neutral state.

To answer this question, you must realize that Cu^{2+} ions exist in solution. To plate out copper, 2 electrons must be added to obtain the copper atom, Cu. Since the Cu^{2+} must gain electrons, it must be reduced. The amount of electricity that produces a specific amount of reduction (or oxidation) is related by $q = nF$ (Faraday's Law). Where q = the quantity of electricity in coulombs, n = number of equivalents oxidized or reduced and F = Faradays. The number of equivalents equals the weight of material oxidized or reduced (m) divided by the gram-equivalent weight of the material (M_{eq}) i.e.,

$$N = \frac{M}{M_{eq}}.$$

A faraday = 96,490 coulombs or one mole of electrons.

Since copper ion requires two electrons for reduction, the gram-equivalent weight is one half of the atomic weight or 31.75g-equiv. You have, therefore

$$q = \frac{127}{31.75} F = 4F$$

139. **(D)** One may assume that the two atoms are spheres. Thus, as in the figure shown, the bond length defined as the distance between the two nuclei is the sum of the lengths of the two radii;

bond length = length of H radius + length of As radius.

bond length = 0.37Å + 1.21Å = 1.58Å.

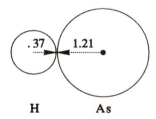

H   As

140. **(A)** If a person inhales 300*l* of air a day, which contains 20% O_2, he would inhale:

20% × 300*l*

of oxygen per day. This is equal to

0.20 × 300 *l* = 60 *l*.

141. **(B)** The ionic symbol of an atom is equal to the charge on the atom. This charge is determined by comparing the atomic number Z to the number of electrons as shown in the electronic configuration. The atomic number corresponds to the net positive charge on the nucleus and the number of electrons indicates the magnitude of the negative charge of the electron cloud.

One writes the electronic configuation of hydrogen as 1s¹. "1s" indicates the atomic orbital, and the superscript 1 indicates that there is one electron in the orbital. Thus, one can determine the number of electrons present by taking the sum of the superscripts. The net charge of an atom is found by adding the net negative charge (the sum of the electrons) and the net positive charge (the atomic number, which is equal to the number of protons). For hydrogen, $(Z = 1)$ $1s^1$, the net negative charge is -1 and the net positive charge is $+1$. Thus, the atom is neutral and no ionic symbol is used. One uses this method to determine the ionic symbols for the atoms described in the problem.

142. **(B)**   This is the standard twin paradox problem. We are given $v = 1.50 \times 10^8$ m/s. Hence

$$\beta = \frac{v}{c} = \frac{1}{2} \text{ and } \gamma = \frac{1}{\sqrt{1-\beta^2}} = \frac{2}{\sqrt{3}}.$$

The time dilation equation is $t = t_0\gamma$ where t_0 is spaceship time and t is Earth time.

$$t_0 = \frac{t}{\gamma}$$

$$= \frac{50}{(2/\sqrt{3})}$$

$$= 25\sqrt{3}$$

$$= 43.3 \text{ years}$$

$$\Delta t = t - t_0 = 50 - 43.3 = 6.7 \text{ years.}$$

Section 3 — Writing Sample

DEMONSTRATION ESSAY 1

History is a form of social memory. Just as individuals remember some experiences and forget others, so the human race selects some events and records these events in history books. In this way, a few events are considered important and a few individuals are considered famous, while most of human experience and those who experienced it are forgotten.

Heine makes a clear distinction between those who are forgotten by history and those who are remembered. Who are the "silent gardeners" who, according to Heine, are forgotten? The phrase is a metaphor. It implies that humanity lives and grows like a plant or tree in a garden. It implies that some individuals are nurturing like gardeners. They help to meet the needs of fellow humans just as a gardener provides care for the plants in a garden. They help to protect fellow humans just as a gardener protects plants from the cold and from wild animals. According to Heine, these gardeners are "silent." They do not call attention to themselves. Their achievements are not recorded in history books and they are forgotten.

Many different people might serve as examples. Parents who spend time with their children and raise them into good adults would be examples of nurturers who are not famous. A teacher, whose efforts go unheralded, might also be an example. In fact, anyone who simply does a good job and thereby provides for the needs of others might be tending to at least a part of the garden. Perhaps one reason the "silent gardeners" are forgotten is that they are just doing what we expect everyone to do ideally.

In contrast to these "silent gardeners" are those whose names are "mercilessly cut" in the bark of humanity. Now the image is that of a tree. The action is a violent one. The metaphor implies that to be remembered in history, an individual must do something to hurt others. There are many obvious examples. History books are full of outrageous dictators, from Nero to Hitler, who are famous for their cruelty.

One might argue with Heine that some of the nurturers are in fact remembered. One could point to such famous examples as Gandhi, Socrates, Martin Luther King, and Mother Theresa. A more basic argument, however, could be directed at the metaphor itself. While humans tame animals and raise crops, humans themselves are not raised to serve the needs of some other species. Heine's metaphor separates the nurturers from the nurtured. At this point the metaphor breaks down. If humans are viewed as animals in nature just like other wild animals, then the destructive humans may be a part of nature. As much as we might detest these violent individuals when they threaten us personally, they may have a role in the scheme of things. Heine may misrepresent the human condition as tame, separating it from the natural context of other wildlife.

EXPLANATION OF DEMONSTRATION ESSAY 1

The essay explains what Heine means by "silent gardeners." It is essential that the essay accomplish the specific tasks assigned in the directions. In the first paragraph, the writer sets up an intellectual framework in terms of which the quote will be interpreted. In this framework, history is viewed as "social memory." The general assignment, to explain what the whole statement means, is broken down into several more manageable tasks. The first of these is to explain what Heine means by "silent gardeners." The writer explains the term by the method of expansive paraphrase. The terms are put in his or her own words, expanding upon the phrase in order to explore all of its implications. First considerations go to the implications of "gardeners" as a metaphor since the noun establishing the underlying meaning of the noun phrase. The writer then discusses the implications of "silent" since the adjective modifies the meaning of the noun. By paraphrasing Heine's phrase, an understanding of the quote is demonstrated.

The essay explains whose names are "mercilessly cut" on the tree. In the fourth paragraph, the writer tackles the second of the assigned tasks. Since Heine's statement makes a distinction, the sides of that distinction must, to a certain extent, be defined in terms of each other. The writer shows an awareness of this relationship by beginning the fourth paragraph, "In contrast to these 'silent gardeners'..." This opening phrase serves as a signpost, guiding the reader from one paragraph to the next. Signposts of this sort are essential to expressing the logical structure of the essay.

The essay includes specific examples of both of the above groups. The directions conclude with the explicit admonition: "Be sure to include examples." When directions are so explicit, it is imperative to follow them in order to do well on the assignment. Those evaluating the essays are sure to look for specific examples in determining whether the writer has accomplished the assigned tasks. After explaining in the second paragraph what Heine means by "silent gardeners," the writer immediately illustrates this explanation with specific examples: parents, teachers, and others. After explaining in the fourth paragraph what Heine means by those whose names are "mercilessly cut" on the tree, the writer concludes the paragraph with specific examples: Nero and Hitler. In choosing appropriate examples, the writer demonstrates an ability to move intellectually from the general to the specific, to understand the general in terms of the specific and the specific in terms of the general. Perhaps most important, however, the writer demonstrates, by providing specific examples, the ability to follow directions and the ability to accomplish the assigned task.

Note that the assigned tasks need not be accomplished in the essay in exactly the same order in which they are presented in the directions. Different strategies may all be successful. The important thing is not following a particular sequence, but rather making sure that *all* of the assigned tasks have been accomplished. If the directions had explicitly requested a sequence, then the writer should follow that sequence. In general, however, a variety of set-ups may be successful as long as every assigned task is accomplished.

The essay not only demonstrates an understanding of the quote, but goes beyond this to a criticism of Heine's point of view. The directions ask the writer to "discuss what you think Heine meant by 'silent gardeners.'" The phrase, "Discuss what you think," opens the essay up for some interpretation. The directions do not specifically ask, however, for any discussion of the issues beyond this interpretation of what Heine meant. Therefore, before the writer launches into a discussion of personal views on the topic, it is essential that the writer should have already accomplished all of the tasks assigned in the directions. In this case, this means giving an interpretation of the quote (specifically, the two sides of the distinction) and citing examples to illustrate that interpretation. This having been accomplished, the writer may still enhance the essay by going beyond the limitations of a paraphrase.

The grammar is correct according to accepted standards. The sentences are well constructed. The paragraphs are unified and coherent. There are no sentence fragments. There are no run-on sentences. There are no errors in subject-verb agreement, parallel syntax, pronoun case or verb inflection. The syntax is clear and unambiguous. The language is not wordy or repetitious. Each paragraph addresses a particular topic. Within each paragraph, the sentences move easily and naturally through the logic of the discussion. There are not abrupt transitions. Finally, punctuation and style conform to accepted standards.

DEMONSTRATION ESSAY 2

Mill makes a distinction between those actions that harm another person and those actions that have no effect on anyone else. According to Mill, only actions of the first type should be subject to legal regulations.

Examples of the first type of action are obvious enough. It is generally assumed that there should be laws to protect the individual from the harmful actions of others. Murder, rape, and robbery are all punishable because they are actions against members of society.

It is not so obvious however, to determine when, in Mill's words, "a person's conduct affects the interests of no persons besides himself." The law forbids suicide, for example, but apparently Mill would argue that society is not warranted in interfering with suicide because the harmful action is not directed at someone else. By the same token the law should not interfere with risky activities such as tightrope walking, mountain climbing, or skydiving. The same argument might be extended to narcotics addiction and gambling.

One difficulty with this sort of argument is that the consequences of an action are seldom limited so as to affect no one else. A suicide, a drug addict, or a gambler may hurt his or her immediate family. Even if there is no immediate family, there are neighbors and others in the vicinity who suffer because of the suicide's action. No one lives in total independence of everyone else. Every individual is necessarily a part of society. A drug addict, for example, becomes a problem for society because hr or she causes a drain on the health and law enforcement resources of the community.

What Mill sees as the proper concern of law might be more applicable to civil law. In civil law, one individual can sue another for an amount equal to damages or harm incurred as a result of the actions of the other individual. In criminal law, on the other hand, it is not actually the harmed individual who is a party to the case, but the state. A criminal is arrested, tried, and punished by the society — the state, as a whole. Criminal law might then be said not merely to protect one individual from another, but to enforce the moral values of society. The criminal has transgressed, not necessarily against an individual, but against society. In the case of civil law, a transgression against moral values which cannot be properly deemed as the values of society could not be considered a valid legal argument.

EXPLANATION OF DEMONSTRATION ESSAY

The first sentence is about the main topic: the distinction made by Mill. The writer does not discuss the essay itself or writing the essay. The writer does not refer to himself or herself. Instead, the writer directs the reader's attention to the topic.

The writer follows the directions for writing the essay and demonstrates an understanding of the quote. The writer does this by explaining the distinction that Mill has made. The writer demonstrates understanding by *paraphrasing* the quotation, restating Mill's idea in his or her own words. Thus Mill's reference to an individual's conduct that "affects prejudicially the interests of others," is paraphrased as "actions that harm another person." Similarly, Mill's reference to an individual's conduct that "affects the interests of no persons besides himself" is paraphrased as "actions that have no effect on anyone else." By putting Mill's ideas in his or her own words, the writer demonstrates an understanding of those ideas.

The writer also follows the directions for writing the essay and demonstrates an understanding of the quote by choosing appropriate examples. As examples of "actions that harm another person," the writer lists "murder, rape, and robbery." As examples of actions that might be considered to "have no effect on anyone else," the writer discusses suicide, tightrope walking, mountain climbing, drug addiction, and gambling. The writer recognizes that some of these actions might in fact be harmful to others. The writer shows understanding by exploring the issue in relation to these concrete examples. By choosing appropriate examples, the writer demonstrates an understanding of the abstract terms in Mill's statement.

In the last two paragraphs, the writer extends the discussion beyond a simple restatement of Mill's idea. The point is not whether Mill is right or wrong. Nor is the point whether you agree with the writer's opinion or not. Judge the essay solely on how well the writer argues his or her point, whatever that point may be. The writer could just as well agree or disagree with Mill, but he or she follows the directions for writing the essay by presenting an example that contradicts or limits Mill's thesis and by considering how this contradiction might be resolved.

They essay is organized in a series of unified and coherent paragraphs. Each paragraph has a particular function in the development of the argument. The first paragraph is an introduction. The second and third paragraphs present the two sides of Mill's distinction. The fourth and fifth paragraphs extend the discussion beyond this restatement and explanation of Mill's idea. The unity, coherence, and logical sequence of the paragraphs gives the essay the appearance of being carefully planned. In this way, the writer presents himself or herself as someone who has considered the topic in some detail and who is not just writing down whatever he or she happens to think of next.

A consistent style is maintained that is neither so casual as to seem careless nor so formal as to seem pretentious. The writer avoids clichés. In this way, the style does not become a distinction, but instead directs the attention of the reader to the topic.

The writer uses correct spelling, correct word-usage, and standard idioms. The writer observes the generally accepted grammar rules concerning subject-verb agreement, verb forms, and sentence punctuation. The writer avoids constructions with ambiguous modifiers or ambiguous pronouns. In this way, the writing does not call attention to itself, but rather allows the reader to focus on the topic.

Section 4 — Biological Sciences

143. **(D)**   Early models (ca. 1930-1970) of cell membranes assumed a homogeneous, or unit, structure. The work of Danielli and Davson was recognized by naming a model membrane structure in their honor. Electron microscopy seemed to confirm this unit-membrane morphology and it was generally accepted until 1972 when a new model was proposed that recognized the ability of proteins to move around within the phospholipid matrix of a cell membrane. The term "fluid-mosaic," choice (D) is the correct name of this modern model. The term "plasmalemma" is simply an alternative name for the cell membrane.

144. **(A)**   This item tests your knowledge of the location of some important metabolic activities of eukaryotic cells. The oxidation of pyruvic acid into carbon dioxide and water is accomplished by the enzymes of the Krebs cycle and the Electron transport chain. The enzymes that catalyzed these reactions are membrane-bound in the mitochondria and choice (A) is therefore correct. The other choices are incorrect: the Golgi are active in packaging secretory products of a cell; smooth endoplasmic reticulum serves as a pathway for movement of mRNA and other molecules throughout the cell; and, the cytoplasm, or cytosol, is the location of the reactions of glycolysis (among many other functions).

145. **(C)**   This item tests your ability to identify the stages of the cell cycle. The accompanying diagram gives the names, approximate times (based on a 24-hour rhythm), and events of the cell cycle. Choice (C) gives the correct sequence of stages that immediately follow mitosis (and cytokinesis in most cases).

146. **(B)**   The four stages of mitosis are presented as possible choices for this item, which tests your knowledge of the events of these stages. Pairs of sister chromatids (the "diad") appear during mitosis, line up independently at the cells' equatorial plate during metaphase, and separate at the centromeres during anaphase. Telophase features the uncoiling of chromatids, appearance of new nuclear membranes, and usually marks the time of cytokinesis. Based on this information, choice (B) is the correct one.

147. **(C)**   In this item, you are asked to recall osmotic relationships that exist between the cytoplasm of living cells and certain solutions. Osmosis is the diffusion of water across cell (or other differentially permeable) membranes in response to concentration gradients. A solution that is hypertonic to a reference solution will tend to gain water across a membrane; one that is hypotonic will tend to lose water. Choice (C) correctly identifies the relationships between the living cells and the two solutions in which they were placed.

148. **(A)**   Lysosomes are unique to animal cells and contain hydrolytic enzymes that will, when released, digest the contents of a cell. Choice (A) correctly identifies this fact. Other choices are incorrect: the enzymes of glycolysis are distributed as soluble proteins throughout the cytosol; secretory products are packaged by Golgi bodies; and lysosomes do not contain any DNA.

149. **(B)**   mRNA synthesized in the nucleus is translated by ribosomes located throughout the cytosol. Of the organelles given as choices for this item, however, the only one that is a site for protein synthesis is rough endoplasmic reticulum, or rough ER, so choice (B) is correct. Proteins made by the ribosomes of rough ER are released into the lumen of the ER and usually are packaged by Golgi for secretion.

150. **(B)**   To answer this question you must recall the events of spermatogenesis in animals. Spermatogonia, located in the outer region of seminiferous tubules, developed from primordial germ cells that migrated to this region during the fourth week of embryonic development. The spermatogonia undergo mitotic and cytokinetic divisions to form a primary spermatocyte and another spermatogonium, thereby perpetuating themselves. Meiosis begins with the primary spermatocyte and produces secondary spermatocytes, and then haploid spermatids. The spermatids mature into spermatozoa (with the help of Sertoli, or nurse cells). Choice (B) offers the only correct sequence of cells formed during spermatogenesis. You should also be familiar with the corresponding, but significantly different, process of oogenesis.

151. **(D)**   To answer this question you must have an understanding of meiosis. Meiosis is the nuclear division, or karyokinesis, that produces four nuclei from one; each of the resultant nuclei will have half the chromosome number of the original nucleus (in animals, the original nucleus is usually diploid and the resultant nuclei are usually haploid). Cytokinesis partitions these nuclei into cells; cleavages may be equal or unequal depending on where meiosis is occurring. Knowing this, the only correct choice for this item is (D).

152. **(A)**   Oogonia begin meiosis in ovarian structures called primordial follicles. Primordial follicles then become primary and secondary follicles as meiosis proceeds. By the time it is ready for ovulation, the structure is known as a vesicular ovarian, or graafian, follicle and contains a secondary oocyte. Choice (A) gives the correct term for this structure. The other choices are incorrect: an oocyte (primary and then secondary) follows the oogonium in the sequence of cells produced during oogenesis; the endometrium is the highly vascularized inner lining of the uterus.

153. **(C)** In mammals, spermatogenesis occurs in the seminiferous tubules of the testes. Choice (C) correctly identifies the location of spermatogenesis. In the epididymis, choice (A), spermatozoa acquire motility and are stored prior to ejaculation. The prostate gland, choice (B), surrounds the urethra of the male and adds an alkaline secretion to the semen during ejaculation. Choice (D), the vas deferens, is incorrect; the vas deferens is the tube that carries sperm from the epididymis to the ejaculatory duct.

154. **(D)** As described in the passage, male and female genitalia are homologous; the female homologue of the penis is the clitoris, having also developed from a genital tubercle. Choice (D) correctly identifies this structure. The other choices are incorrect: the vagina, which is not part of the external female genitalia, is the tubular opening between the uterus and the vestibule of the female reproductive tract; the cervix, also not part of the external genitalia, is the opening of the uterus into the vagina; the labia major, which are external genitalia, develop from the labioscrotal folds (they are homologous to the scrotum of male genitalia).

155. **(D)** To answer this question, you must recall the structures of the outer, middle, and inner ear in the sequence of their involvement in detecting sound. Sound waves collected by the external ear (pinna) cause small vibrations of the tympanic membrane. These vibrations, in turn, cause movement in the following structures or fluids in sequence: malleus, incus, states, oval window, fluid of vestibular canal, fluid of tympanic canal, and the round window. The malleus, incus, and stapes are bones (ossicles) of the middle ear, while the remaining structures are part of the cochlea of the inner ear. Given this information, the only correct choice is (D).

156. **(C)** Transduction of light waves begins with a conformational change in special light-sensitive molecules. The conversion is actually a photochemical conversion of 11-cis-retinaldehyde to all-trans-retinaldehyde. In its photosensitive form, retinaldehyde in rod cells is associated with a protein called opsin to form a pigmented molecule known as rhodopsin. Choice (C) correctly identifies this molecule. The light-induced change in conformation of retinaldehyde causes it to dissociate from opsin; an enzyme catalyzed reaction combines retinaldehyde and opsin again to regenerate rhodopsin. Similar reactions occur in cones but with a different protein for each of three types of cones. The other three choices are incorrect: hemoglobin is the pigment of red blood cells that is responsible for carrying oxygen and carbon dioxide; phytochrome is a photo-sensitive pigment (it has a similar photochemical-enzyme conformational conversion) found in the membranes of plant cells that is responsible for detecting changes in day length; and, a rhabdom is a tiny, translucent cylinder found in the center of an ommatidium in an arthropod compound eye.

157. **(B)** Rods and cones differ in several ways; you need to recall those differences to answer this question. Choice (B) correctly indicates that rods are more numerous than cones. Choice (A) is incorrect because rods are actually more sensitive to light, not less. Rods are most numerous at the periphery of the retina, not in the center (the fovea centralis has none), so choice (C) is incorrect. Choice (D) is also incorrect; rods are not color-sensitive, they only provide quantitative information about light. In addition to these differences, you should know that cones provide

greater visual acuity, principally because ganglion cells receive information from individual cones in the fovea (the ratio of rods-to-ganglia in the periphery of the retina is much higher).

158. **(A)**   The principal focusing element of the vertebrate eye is the cornea; final adjustment of the focus is accomplished through a change in the shape of the lens by the ciliary muscles. This phenomenon is known as accommodation; choice (A) correctly describes the action. The other three choices are incorrect: length of the eyeball cannot be adjusted; the position of the retina does not change; and, adjustment of the diameter of the pupil by circular muscles of the iris controls the amount of light entering the eye, but has no role in focusing.

159. **(B)**   The cilia of sensory hair cells located on the basilar membrane of the cochlea are embedded in the tectorial membrane, so choice (B) is correct. Distortion of these sensory hairs causes nerve impulses to be sent to specific regions of the cerebral cortex where they are interpreted as sound of a Particular frequency. The structures indicated by the other three choices for this question are involved in hearing but are not in direct contact with the sensory hair cilia.

160. **(C)**   To correctly answer this question, you must be familiar with the anatomy of the retina of the vertebrate eye. The axons of the ganglion neurons transmitting information from photoreceptor cells (i.e., rods and cones) are in the vitreous chamber and exit the eye through the retina. The area where they come together to form the optic nerve as they leave the vitreous chamber is known as the optic disc, or blind spot (because there are no photoreceptors in this region). Choice (C) correctly identifies the blind spot as the optic nerve's exit point. The other choices are incorrect: the edge of the eye is rich in rods and very sensitive to dim light; the fovea centralis is the area of sharpest vision, with a dense population of cones, near the center of the retina; and, the macula lutea, also rich in cones, is the area immediately surrounding the fovea.

161. **(D)**   Of the three areas of the inner ear, or labyrinth, — vestibule, semicircular canals, and cochlea — the vestibule has two interconnected sacs called the utricle and saccule. These sacs have receptors that are sensitive to straight-line movements of the head and to gravity. Choice (D) correctly identifies these chambers. The other three choices are incorrect: the three semicircular canals are also located in the labyrinth, but they respond to rotational movements of the head; the vestibular canal, or scala vestibuli, is the fluid-filled upper chamber in the cochlea, separated from the lower chamber (scala tympani) except for a narrow connection at the apex called the helicotrema; and, a statocyst is a mechanoreceptor of invertebrates, containing sand or other granular substances, that functions as an organ of equilibrium.

162. **(A)**   Mitochondria generate energy in the form of ATP. They are enclosed by two membranes: the outer membrane is a continuous covering while the inner membrane is thrown into many folds that extend to the interior of the organelle. These folds, called cristae, greatly increase the surface area of the inner membrane. This increases the metabolic efficiency of the confined space of the mitochrondia for it allows for may more enzymes of the respiratory process to be inserted.

163. **(C)**   Pancreatic and intestinal enzymes are released into the small intestine when the partially digested food arrives from the stomach. These enzymes can digest carbohydrates, fats, proteins and nucleic acids. The products of digestion are absorbed by the walls of the small intestine. The intestine has a very large surface area due to its length, its numerous folds and the villi and microvilli that cover the surface of the intenstine's lining.

164. **(B)**   The protein to be secreted is synthesized on the rough endoplasmic reticulum. Vesicles containing small quantities of the synthesized protein bud off from the endoplasmic reticulum. These vesicles carry the proteins to the Golgi apparatus. There, the protein is concentrated by the removal of water, and it is released in the form of secretory granules. These granules containing the protein are separated from the cytoplasm by a membrane that can fuse with the plasma membrane. When the secretory granule fuses with the plasma membrane, its contents are expelled from the cell by exocytosis.

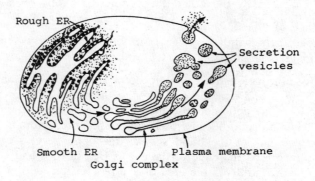

165. **(D)**   Centrioles are made by microtubules. Thus, their activity will be blocked by colchicine because they participate in the formation of spindle fibers. If spindle formation is blocked, meiosis (and mitosis) will not proceed beyond metaphase.

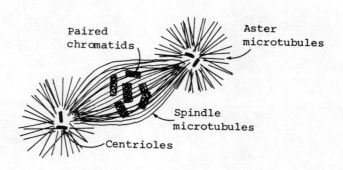

166. **(D)**   Homologous structures have similar evolutionary origins. They may have diverged in their functions and phenotypic apparance, but their relationships to adjacent structures and embryonic development are essentially the same. The bonds of seal flippers, bird wings, and cat paws are very similar; this reveals their common ancestry.

167. **(A)**   The nucleus is the control center of the cell. Experiments have successfully demonstrated that the replacement of one nucleus with that of another species is sufficient for that cell to develop as if it were the other species. Thus, all of the necessary hereditary information is contained in the nucleus.

168. **(C)**   Alleles are variations of genes. They occupy the same loci on homologous chromosomes and they are responsible for the variety that appears in the phenotypes of all organisms.

169. **(B)**   Since postural muscles are skeletal muscles that must sustain contractions over long periods of time, it would be advantageous for them to have the characteristics of red muscle fibers listed in Figure 1. These muscles, in fact, have a predominance of type I, or red muscle, fibers so choice (B) is correct. Type IIB, white muscle fibers, with anaerobically adapted fast-twitch characteristics would not be found in great numbers in postural muscles. Nor would intermediate type IIA fibers be found in postural muscles, despite their increased capacity for aerobic respiration. Anaerobically respiring muscle fibers (i.e., type IIB) would not be expected in postural muscles for reasons already presented. Choices (A), (C), and (D) are, therefore not correct.

170. **(D)**   High aerobic capacity implies large numbers of mitochondria because of the need for utilization of the electron transport chain contained there. Hence, both type I and type IIA (also known as fast-twitch red fibers because they have a lot of myoglobin) would be expected to have large numbers of mitochondria. Choice (D) correctly identifies this information and is, therefore, the best answer. Type IIB fibers, which are adapted for anaerobic production of ATP have significantly fewer mitochondria, so choice (C) is obviously incorrect.

171. **(A)**   To correctly answer this question, you must recall that anaerobic production of ATP in skeletal muscle is essentially a fermentation process in which pyruvic acid (from glycolysis) is converted to lactic acid. Thus, the muscle fibers with the greatest adaptation for anaerobic production of ATP would also produce the greatest amount of lactic acid. White muscle fibers (A) have the greatest adaptation for anaerobic production of ATP, therefore it is the correct choice.

172. **(D)**   In this question, you must be aware of similarities and differences between skeletal and smooth muscle fibers. One of the similarities is that contraction in muscle fibers (cardiac, skeletal, and smooth) is induced by calcium ions. In the case of cardiac and skeletal muscle fibers, the calcium comes from the sarcoplasmic reticulum; for smooth muscle fibers calcium comes from extracellular fluids. However, both skeletal and smooth fibers contract in response to calcium, so choice (D) is the correct one. The other choices are incorrect: skeletal muscle fibers are multinucleate, but smooth fibers are uninucleate; smooth muscle fibers do not have sar-

comeres; and, neither skeletal nor smooth muscle fibers have electrical synapses (cardiac muscle does, however).

173. **(B)** All of the choices listed for this question identify known neurotransmitters. Acetylcholine is used at parasympathetic nerve endings, some neurons of the central nervous system, and at the neuromuscular junction (synapse) of somatic motor neurons. The correct choice is, therefore, (B). Epinephrine, norepinephrine (both are catecholamines), and serotonin all serve as neurotransmitters in the peripheral and/or the central nervous systems. However, the predominant neurotransmitter at neuromuscular junctions is acetylcholine.

174. **(B)** This question requires that you understand that the cytoplasm of a cell is infiltrated by a network of fibers. Figure 1 gives one interpretation of this network. known as the cytoskeleton. Of the three types of "fibers" making up the cytoskeleton, the largest is the microtubule (choice (B)). A microtubule is actually hollow, having a diameter of approximately 25 nm, and consists of two globular proteins called tubulins. The microtubule is constructed by joining dimers of the tubulins in a linear fashion to form the coiled microtubule. Microfilaments (choice (A)) are small (7 nm) rods of the globular protein actin arranged in a helix. Intermediate filaments (choice (D)) are not well described and consist of a variety of fibers that range in size between that of microtubules and microfilaments. Choice (C) is incorrect because endoplasmic reticulum is part of the endomembrane system of a cell that includes the nuclear envelope, Golgi, lysosomes, and other membranous components.

175. **(A)** The protein that makes up microfilaments is known as actin (choice (A)). The best known occurrence of actin microfilaments is in muscle where they are interdigitated with myosin and participate in sliding-filament contraction. Choice (B) is wrong because dynein is the protein that forms the connections between microtubule pairs in eukaryotic cilia and flagella (dynein forms the cross-bridges that cause adjacent microtubule pairs to slide past one another, thereby effecting movement in the cilia and flagella). Tubulin (choice (C)) is a protein found in microtubules and myosin (choice (D)) makes up the "thick" filaments of muscle fibers.

176. **(D)** This question requires a knowledge of intercellular junctions. Gap junctions (choice (D)) are circular interconnections between adjacent cells large enough to allow small molecules to move from cell to cell. They also allow action potentials to pass directly from one cell to another as in the so-called electrical synapses of cardiac muscle (intercalated discs are essentially gap junctions) so (D) is the correct choice. Tight junctions (choice (A)) and desmosomes (choice (B)) are two other intercellular junctions of animal cells; plasmodesmata (choice (C)) are membrane-lined channels through cell walls of adjacent plant cells.

177. **(C)** All cilia and flagella of eukaryotic cells have the same cross-sectional ultrastructure that consists of two central pairs of microtubules surrounded by nine additional pairs, so choice (C) is the correct choice. This structure runs the length of the cilium or flagellum and connects with a basal body having a ring of nine triplets of microtubules (the same structure as a centriole). Adjacent pairs of microtubules slide past one another due to dynein cross-arms attaching and reattaching.

178. **(D)** Microtubules have a variety of functions, among them is the separation of chromatids in mitosis and meiosis where they form the spindle fibers; choice (D) is, therefore, correct. Choices (A) and (C) identify two other fibers found as part of the structure of the cytoskeleton, but microfilaments and intermediate filaments are not involved in spindle fiber architecture. Choice (B) identifies the region of the centromere of a chromatid to which spindle fibers attach, but is an incorrect choice because it is part of the chromatic not the spindle fiber.

179. **(C)** This question requires that you can distinguish among the three principal types of cytokinesis. Choice (C) is the correct answer because cleavage (of animal cells) involves a contractile ring of actin microfilaments that pinch off the cytoplasm into two units (myosin is probably involved also, although it has not been directly seen). Cytokinesis in plants and fungi (and some protists) involves the formation of new cell walls, either from the center outward (choice (B)) in plants, or from the periphery inward (choice (A)). The cell plate (choice (D)), or phragmoplast, is the precursor of the centrifugally-formed cell wall of plants.

180. **(B)** This questions requires an understanding of the process of feedback inhibition in which the concentration of end product determines the degree of enzyme inhibition and thus determines the overall rate of reaction. Answer (A) is incorrect because the activity of the last enzyme of a pathway depends upon the amount of substrate reaching it, which in turn depends upon the activity of the enzymes preceding it. Answer (C) is incorrect because substrate concentration has little affect on reaction rate if enzyme inhibition is present. Answer (D) is wrong because the rate is determined by inhibitor, not activator, concentraiton.

181. **(C)** Feedback inhibition is important in metabolic processes because it offers a mechanism whereby the production of a substance can be matched precisely to the demand that exists for that substance, minimizing the waste of both materials and energy. Answer (A) is incorrect because feedback inhibition slows down enzymatic reactions. Answer (B) is wrong because the availability of substrate is unaffected by enzyme inhibition. Answer (D) is wrong because feedback inhibition is not a form of genetic regulation.

182. **(D)** Isoleucine is the end product of the pathway and therefore is most liekly to be responsible for feedback inhibition. Answer (A) is incorrect because α-keotbutyrate is an intermediate product, not an end product. Answer (B) is incorrect because leucine is not involved in this particular pathway. Answer (C) is wrong because threonine is the initial substrate in the pathway.

183. **(A)** If feedback inhibition were operative, an increase in the concentration of substance B would have decreased the activity of enzyme 1. Since enzyme activity was unaffected, the only conclusion is that feedback inhibition by substance B was not present. Answer (B) is incorrect because feedback inhibition would have caused enzyme activity to decrease. Answer (C) is wrong because the substrate, substance A, would not have been involved in feedback inhibition. Answer (D) is incorrect because a conclusion can be drawn from the data given.

184. **(A)** The opposite of feedback inhibition occurs when an increase in end product concentration increases enzyme activity instead of decreasing it. Answer (B)

is incorrect because negative feedback is the same as feedback inhibition. Answer (C) is incorrect because competitive inhibition will also decrease enzyme activity. Answer (D) is wrong because a change in substrate concentration is not involved in positive modulation.

185. **(C)**   Since feedback inhibition by isoleucine decreases threonine deaminase activity, increasing the availability of substrate would have little if any effect on enzyme activity. Answer (A) is wrong because enzyme activity would remain depressed. Answer (B) is incorrect because isoleucine, not threonine, induces the conformational change leading to decreased enzyme activity. Answer (D) is wrong because threonine does not inhibit the enzyme.

186. **(B)**   The vitamin B complex are a group of vitamins that function as parts coenzymes used in the oxidation of glucose to form ATP. A deficiency in the B vitamins can lead to listlessness and a lack of energy for normal activities. Ecdysone, however, is the hormone that induces molting in insects.

187. **(D)**   The four chambers of the mammalian heart are the upper left and right atrium and the lower left and right ventricles. The atria serve as entryways to the ventricles and the ventricles supply the main force that propels blood to the lungs and throughout the body.

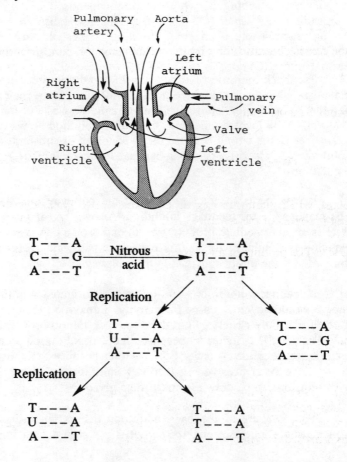

188. **(A)**   Cytosine normally binds to guanine and uracil normally binds to adenine. A conversion of cytosine to uracil would lead to a conversion of guanine to adenine in the complementary strand. Thus a CG to AU (or AT) event has occurred.

189. **(D)**   RNA contains uracil where DNA contains thymine. Uracil is the base partner of adenine in RNA. One way of distinguishing between RNA and DNA is to check for the presence of uracil.

190. **(C)**   Attack by the nucleophile on a carbonyl carbon is enhanced by the electronegative Cl attached to it, since electron withdrawal makes the carbonyl carbon more electron deficient. But it is also true that the chloride ion is a better leaving group than carboxylate ion, so both (A) and (B) are correct. To understand why the chloride ion is a better leaving group, you need some understanding of relative acidities of carboxylic acids and hydrochloric acid, as well as solvation of ionic species.

191. **(A)**   To answer this question, you must recognize that the non-binding electron-pairs of oxygen will be protonated by acid. Protonation of the carbonyl oxygen greatly diminishes the electron density on the carbonyl carbon.

$$\ddot{O}: \quad :\overset{+}{O}{\diagup}^{H} \quad :\ddot{O}{\diagup}^{H}$$
$$R-\overset{\|}{C}-Z \xrightarrow{H+} R-\overset{\|}{C}-Z \longleftrightarrow R-\underset{+}{\overset{\|}{C}}-Z$$

(A) is not correct because the proton will not be attracted to the electron-deficient carbon atom. Neither (C) nor (D) can account for the ehnahced reactivity.

192. **(A)**   References to the mechanism shows that the oxygen of the attacking water becomes incorporated into the product acid.

$$Ph-\overset{O}{\overset{\|}{C}}-OEt \xrightarrow[\substack{18 \\ H_2O}]{HCl} Ph-\overset{O}{\overset{\|}{C}}{}^{18}-OH + EtOH$$

(D), ethanol, will contain the oxygen to which it was attached in the ester. (B) and (C) are not products of the reaction.

193. **(D)**   The product of all of these reactions is a stable amide.

$$Ph-\overset{O}{\overset{\|}{C}}-Z \xrightarrow{NH_3} Ph-\overset{O}{\overset{\|}{C}}-NH_2 + ZH$$

$$Z = Cl, OOCPh, OPh$$

The acid chloride will react most readily, but the anhydride and ester can also be used in the preparation.

194. **(C)**   Since we are looking for the *product* of the reaction, we must realize that the most easily removed phosphate is on carbon 1. This is an anhydride; carbon 3 has a phosphate ester. Since anhydrides are more labile than esters, the anhydride will be hydrolyzed, leaving the ester on carbon 3.

195. **(A)**   Any of these will theoretically react with an acid chloride or anhydride in the manner of NH_3, except that a substituted amide will be formed. Since the reaction depends on nucleophilic attack of the carbonyl group by the unshared pair of electrons on the nitrogen atom, any substituents which are electron-withdrawing will slow the reaction. The methoxy groups are electron-donating, therefore neither (B) nor (D) is correct. The nitro group is electron-withdrawing; since (A) has *two* of these to (C)'s one, (A) will be the slower reacting.

196. **(C)**   The reaction with thionyl chloride, $SOCl_2$, will produce the acid chloride. This will react with the amine to give N,N-dimethylbenzamide. The other answers involve reaction with the ring, which would not occur.

197. **(A)**   Bile is produced by the liver, stored in the gallbladder, and released into the doudenum through the bile duct. Pigments and cholesterol are essential waste product components of bile, while its digestive function is accomplished by the salts it contains. These bile salts serve to emulsify fats, thereby making them appropriate substrates for lipase enzymes produced by the pancreas. Choice (A) correctly identifies the function of bile; the other organic compounds listed are not affected by bile.

198. **(C)**   This item tests your knowledge of the structures found in the human digestive tract. While all of the choices contain structures found in the tract (none of the choices is a complete list) only choice (C) lists a correct *sequence* of structures and is therefore the proper choice.

199. **(D)**   This item tests your knowledge of the enzymes secreted into the digestive tract. The pancreas is one of two principal sources of enzymes, the other being the glands of the small intestine. Trypsin, lipase, and chymotrypsin (in addition to amylase) are produced by the pancreas. Pepsin is produced as pepsinogen by the stomach, *not* by the pancreas, and is the correct choice.

200. **(B)**   This item asks you to correctly match some enzymes with the substrates on which they act. Pepsin does *not* break down sucrose — that is done by sucrase produced by intestinal glands — and, therefore, choice (B) is the correct one.

201. **(A)**   Choice (A) is correct because villi and microvilli are found in the small intestine. While villi are small, but visible, projections of the mucosa, microvilli can only be visualized with an electron microscope. Along with larger foldings of the intestine, these structures serve to greatly increase the surface area of the intenstinal lining.

202. **(C)**   The ovoid mass of food that enters the esophagus from the mouth is called a bolus, so choice (C) is correct. The term chyme refers to the semi-liquid material that enters the duodenum from the stompach; pylorus refers to the *opening* through which chyme enters the duodenum; and, the caecum is a blind pouch at the end of the small intestine where it meets the large intestine.

203. **(B)**   There are two sources of amylase — the salivary glands and the pancreas. Choice (B) correctly identifies these glands. The stomach and small intestine both produce enzymes, but neither produces amylase.

204. **(D)** This item tests your knowledge of both the respiratory and digestive tracts. Because of evolutionary adaptations that led to lung breathing in vertebrates, the back of the pharynx came to have a dual role. It allows passage of food while the organism is swallowing and also serves as the passageway for air during inhalation and exhalation. The nasal cavity and trachea are components of the respiratory tract exclusively and the esophagus only serves the digestive tract.

205. **(A)** Compound (2) is immediately identified as a carboxylic acid by the 1H peak at 12.0δ in the nmr. This limits possible answers to (A) and (D), since (B) and (C) are aldehydes. The key to distinguishing between (A) and (D) is the integration of the areas containing the aromatic protons (7.2 δ), and alkenic protons (4.7 - 5.5δ). Since the spectrum shows five aromatic and two alkenic protons, the structure must be (A), cinnamic acid.

206. **(D)** This reaction is the classic iodoform test. Methyl ketones react with I_2/ OH^- to give a yellow precipitate of iodoform. CHI_3, and a carboxylic acid. None of the other compounds would so react.

207. **(A)** Bromine in carbon tetrachloride would react with the alkene; bromine would be added across the double bond and the red Br_2/CCl_4 would be decolorized. (B), Tollen's reagent, gives a positive test (silver mirro) with aldehydes. (C), aqueous sodium bicarbonate, would react and give off CO_2 with carboxylic acids. (D), aqueous silver nitrate, would react with reactive halides to give a precipitate of silver halide.

208. **(B)** Compound (1), remember, is a ketone. Ketones are reduced by sodium borohydride to give alcohols, which absorb in the infrared at ca. 3300 cm^{-1}.

209. **(D)** This question tests your knowledge of bond hybridization. Carbons that form double bonds, whether to each other or to other atoms, are sp^2. Carbons that form single bonds to four other atoms are sp^3.

210. **(C)** A resonance form with only six electrons on electronegative oxygen is very unlikely. Nitrogen has too many electrons, also. (A) is the uncharged conventionally written form. (B) and (D) are reasonable resonance contributors.

211. **(C)** To solve synthetic problems, one usually works backwards. Comparing the product to starting material, you can see that a methyl group has been added and a tertiary alcohol formed. This can be the product of a Grignard reagent and a ketone. A ketone can result form oxidation of a secondary alcohol, which can be formed by adding H^3O^+ to an alkene. This sequence is found in c, with the fourth step being hydrolysis of the Grignard adduct. (A) is not feasible since a Grignard does not add to an alkene. The first two steps of B would lead right back to the alkene. (D) has the same limitation as (A).

212. **(D)** Multiple bonds are generally shorter than single bonds because the increased overlap of orbitals brings the nuclei closer together. Furthermore, triple bonds are shorter than double bonds, for the same reason. Therefore, the acetylene bond, d, will be the shortest bond in this molecule. c is a single bond; a and b are

actually equivalent because of electron delocalization within the aromatic ring. Their length is intermediate between single and double bonds.

213. (A) The anti-conformation has the two methyl groups, which are larger than hydrogens, farthest apart, so it will have the lowest potential energy.

214. (C) The gauche conformation has the methyl groups close to each other, but not with the direct overlap of the eclipsed forms; so it is more stable than they are, but less stable than the anti-conformation.

215. (B) The eclipsed-1 conformation has the groups in direct alignment with each other, but with the hydrogens and methyl groups interacting, rather than the direct methyl-methyl interaction of eclipsed-2.

216. (D) The direct methyl-methyl interaction makes eclipsed-2 the least stable conformation.

217. (C) The carboxylate ion, which has a negative charge, is stabilized by having that charge delocalized over the entire carboxylate group.

$$R-C \overset{O}{\underset{O^-}{}} \longleftrightarrow R-C \overset{O^-}{\underset{O}{}}$$

Phenols can delocalize the charge onto the ring, to some extent, but this is not as stabilizing as having two *equivalent* resonance forms. (D) is incorrect because it is the opposite of the correct answer. (A) and (B) have nothing to do with acid strength.

218. (A) The negative charge on a phenolate ion can be delocalized onto the ring to some extent, but the delocalization is not as effective as if it were onto two equivalent oxygen atoms, as in a carboxylate ion. Nevertheless, strongly electron-withdrawing groups on the ring can stabilize the phenolate ion to the point that it is as stable as some carboxylate ions.

$$O_2N-\underset{NO_2}{\underset{|}{\bigcirc}}-O^-$$

(B) is incorrect on two counts; the nitro groups are not electron-dontating, and they would not stabilize the negative charge if they were. (C) and (D) have nothing to do with acidity. (D) is not a true statement, in any case.

219. (B) The most basic carboxylate ion is derived from the weakest acid. Since electronegative bromines stablize the carboxylate ion and increase the acidity of the acid, they decrease the basicity of the ion. Consequently, (1) is the strongest base shown. Since the effect of electronegativity decreases with distance, (3) would be a stronger base (from a weaker acid) than (2).

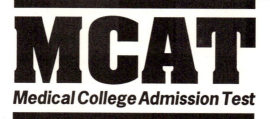

Test 6

Test 6 is also on CD-ROM in our special interactive MCAT TEST*ware®*. It is highly recommended that you take this exam on computer first. You will then have the additional study features and benefits of enforced timed conditions, individual diagnostic analysis, and instant scoring. See page 2 for guidance on how to get the most out of our MCAT book and software.

MEDICAL COLLEGE ADMISSION TEST
TEST 6
ANSWER SHEET

Section 1:
Verbal Reasoning

1. Ⓐ Ⓑ Ⓒ Ⓓ
2. Ⓐ Ⓑ Ⓒ Ⓓ
3. Ⓐ Ⓑ Ⓒ Ⓓ
4. Ⓐ Ⓑ Ⓒ Ⓓ
5. Ⓐ Ⓑ Ⓒ Ⓓ
6. Ⓐ Ⓑ Ⓒ Ⓓ
7. Ⓐ Ⓑ Ⓒ Ⓓ
8. Ⓐ Ⓑ Ⓒ Ⓓ
9. Ⓐ Ⓑ Ⓒ Ⓓ
10. Ⓐ Ⓑ Ⓒ Ⓓ
11. Ⓐ Ⓑ Ⓒ Ⓓ
12. Ⓐ Ⓑ Ⓒ Ⓓ
13. Ⓐ Ⓑ Ⓒ Ⓓ
14. Ⓐ Ⓑ Ⓒ Ⓓ
15. Ⓐ Ⓑ Ⓒ Ⓓ
16. Ⓐ Ⓑ Ⓒ Ⓓ
17. Ⓐ Ⓑ Ⓒ Ⓓ
18. Ⓐ Ⓑ Ⓒ Ⓓ
19. Ⓐ Ⓑ Ⓒ Ⓓ
20. Ⓐ Ⓑ Ⓒ Ⓓ
21. Ⓐ Ⓑ Ⓒ Ⓓ
22. Ⓐ Ⓑ Ⓒ Ⓓ
23. Ⓐ Ⓑ Ⓒ Ⓓ
24. Ⓐ Ⓑ Ⓒ Ⓓ
25. Ⓐ Ⓑ Ⓒ Ⓓ
26. Ⓐ Ⓑ Ⓒ Ⓓ
27. Ⓐ Ⓑ Ⓒ Ⓓ
28. Ⓐ Ⓑ Ⓒ Ⓓ
29. Ⓐ Ⓑ Ⓒ Ⓓ
30. Ⓐ Ⓑ Ⓒ Ⓓ
31. Ⓐ Ⓑ Ⓒ Ⓓ

32. Ⓐ Ⓑ Ⓒ Ⓓ
33. Ⓐ Ⓑ Ⓒ Ⓓ
34. Ⓐ Ⓑ Ⓒ Ⓓ
35. Ⓐ Ⓑ Ⓒ Ⓓ
36. Ⓐ Ⓑ Ⓒ Ⓓ
37. Ⓐ Ⓑ Ⓒ Ⓓ
38. Ⓐ Ⓑ Ⓒ Ⓓ
39. Ⓐ Ⓑ Ⓒ Ⓓ
40. Ⓐ Ⓑ Ⓒ Ⓓ
41. Ⓐ Ⓑ Ⓒ Ⓓ
42. Ⓐ Ⓑ Ⓒ Ⓓ
43. Ⓐ Ⓑ Ⓒ Ⓓ
44. Ⓐ Ⓑ Ⓒ Ⓓ
45. Ⓐ Ⓑ Ⓒ Ⓓ
46. Ⓐ Ⓑ Ⓒ Ⓓ
47. Ⓐ Ⓑ Ⓒ Ⓓ
48. Ⓐ Ⓑ Ⓒ Ⓓ
49. Ⓐ Ⓑ Ⓒ Ⓓ
50. Ⓐ Ⓑ Ⓒ Ⓓ
51. Ⓐ Ⓑ Ⓒ Ⓓ
52. Ⓐ Ⓑ Ⓒ Ⓓ
53. Ⓐ Ⓑ Ⓒ Ⓓ
54. Ⓐ Ⓑ Ⓒ Ⓓ
55. Ⓐ Ⓑ Ⓒ Ⓓ
56. Ⓐ Ⓑ Ⓒ Ⓓ
57. Ⓐ Ⓑ Ⓒ Ⓓ
58. Ⓐ Ⓑ Ⓒ Ⓓ
59. Ⓐ Ⓑ Ⓒ Ⓓ
60. Ⓐ Ⓑ Ⓒ Ⓓ
61. Ⓐ Ⓑ Ⓒ Ⓓ
62. Ⓐ Ⓑ Ⓒ Ⓓ
63. Ⓐ Ⓑ Ⓒ Ⓓ
64. Ⓐ Ⓑ Ⓒ Ⓓ
65. Ⓐ Ⓑ Ⓒ Ⓓ

Section 2:
Physical Sciences

66. Ⓐ Ⓑ Ⓒ Ⓓ
67. Ⓐ Ⓑ Ⓒ Ⓓ
68. Ⓐ Ⓑ Ⓒ Ⓓ
69. Ⓐ Ⓑ Ⓒ Ⓓ
70. Ⓐ Ⓑ Ⓒ Ⓓ
71. Ⓐ Ⓑ Ⓒ Ⓓ
72. Ⓐ Ⓑ Ⓒ Ⓓ
73. Ⓐ Ⓑ Ⓒ Ⓓ
74. Ⓐ Ⓑ Ⓒ Ⓓ
75. Ⓐ Ⓑ Ⓒ Ⓓ
76. Ⓐ Ⓑ Ⓒ Ⓓ
77. Ⓐ Ⓑ Ⓒ Ⓓ
78. Ⓐ Ⓑ Ⓒ Ⓓ
79. Ⓐ Ⓑ Ⓒ Ⓓ
80. Ⓐ Ⓑ Ⓒ Ⓓ
81. Ⓐ Ⓑ Ⓒ Ⓓ
82. Ⓐ Ⓑ Ⓒ Ⓓ
83. Ⓐ Ⓑ Ⓒ Ⓓ
84. Ⓐ Ⓑ Ⓒ Ⓓ
85. Ⓐ Ⓑ Ⓒ Ⓓ
86. Ⓐ Ⓑ Ⓒ Ⓓ
87. Ⓐ Ⓑ Ⓒ Ⓓ
88. Ⓐ Ⓑ Ⓒ Ⓓ
89. Ⓐ Ⓑ Ⓒ Ⓓ
90. Ⓐ Ⓑ Ⓒ Ⓓ
91. Ⓐ Ⓑ Ⓒ Ⓓ
92. Ⓐ Ⓑ Ⓒ Ⓓ
93. Ⓐ Ⓑ Ⓒ Ⓓ
94. Ⓐ Ⓑ Ⓒ Ⓓ
95. Ⓐ Ⓑ Ⓒ Ⓓ
96. Ⓐ Ⓑ Ⓒ Ⓓ

97. Ⓐ Ⓑ Ⓒ Ⓓ
98. Ⓐ Ⓑ Ⓒ Ⓓ
99. Ⓐ Ⓑ Ⓒ Ⓓ
100. Ⓐ Ⓑ Ⓒ Ⓓ
101. Ⓐ Ⓑ Ⓒ Ⓓ
102. Ⓐ Ⓑ Ⓒ Ⓓ
103. Ⓐ Ⓑ Ⓒ Ⓓ
104. Ⓐ Ⓑ Ⓒ Ⓓ
105. Ⓐ Ⓑ Ⓒ Ⓓ
106. Ⓐ Ⓑ Ⓒ Ⓓ
107. Ⓐ Ⓑ Ⓒ Ⓓ
108. Ⓐ Ⓑ Ⓒ Ⓓ
109. Ⓐ Ⓑ Ⓒ Ⓓ
110. Ⓐ Ⓑ Ⓒ Ⓓ
111. Ⓐ Ⓑ Ⓒ Ⓓ
112. Ⓐ Ⓑ Ⓒ Ⓓ
113. Ⓐ Ⓑ Ⓒ Ⓓ
114. Ⓐ Ⓑ Ⓒ Ⓓ
115. Ⓐ Ⓑ Ⓒ Ⓓ
116. Ⓐ Ⓑ Ⓒ Ⓓ
117. Ⓐ Ⓑ Ⓒ Ⓓ
118. Ⓐ Ⓑ Ⓒ Ⓓ
119. Ⓐ Ⓑ Ⓒ Ⓓ
120. Ⓐ Ⓑ Ⓒ Ⓓ
121. Ⓐ Ⓑ Ⓒ Ⓓ
122. Ⓐ Ⓑ Ⓒ Ⓓ
123. Ⓐ Ⓑ Ⓒ Ⓓ
124. Ⓐ Ⓑ Ⓒ Ⓓ
125. Ⓐ Ⓑ Ⓒ Ⓓ
126. Ⓐ Ⓑ Ⓒ Ⓓ
127. Ⓐ Ⓑ Ⓒ Ⓓ
128. Ⓐ Ⓑ Ⓒ Ⓓ
129. Ⓐ Ⓑ Ⓒ Ⓓ
130. Ⓐ Ⓑ Ⓒ Ⓓ
131. Ⓐ Ⓑ Ⓒ Ⓓ
132. Ⓐ Ⓑ Ⓒ Ⓓ
133. Ⓐ Ⓑ Ⓒ Ⓓ
134. Ⓐ Ⓑ Ⓒ Ⓓ
135. Ⓐ Ⓑ Ⓒ Ⓓ
136. Ⓐ Ⓑ Ⓒ Ⓓ
137. Ⓐ Ⓑ Ⓒ Ⓓ
138. Ⓐ Ⓑ Ⓒ Ⓓ
139. Ⓐ Ⓑ Ⓒ Ⓓ

140. Ⓐ Ⓑ Ⓒ Ⓓ
141. Ⓐ Ⓑ Ⓒ Ⓓ
142. Ⓐ Ⓑ Ⓒ Ⓓ

Section 4:
Biological Sciences

143. Ⓐ Ⓑ Ⓒ Ⓓ
144. Ⓐ Ⓑ Ⓒ Ⓓ
145. Ⓐ Ⓑ Ⓒ Ⓓ
146. Ⓐ Ⓑ Ⓒ Ⓓ
147. Ⓐ Ⓑ Ⓒ Ⓓ
148. Ⓐ Ⓑ Ⓒ Ⓓ
149. Ⓐ Ⓑ Ⓒ Ⓓ
150. Ⓐ Ⓑ Ⓒ Ⓓ
151. Ⓐ Ⓑ Ⓒ Ⓓ
152. Ⓐ Ⓑ Ⓒ Ⓓ
153. Ⓐ Ⓑ Ⓒ Ⓓ
154. Ⓐ Ⓑ Ⓒ Ⓓ
155. Ⓐ Ⓑ Ⓒ Ⓓ
156. Ⓐ Ⓑ Ⓒ Ⓓ
157. Ⓐ Ⓑ Ⓒ Ⓓ
158. Ⓐ Ⓑ Ⓒ Ⓓ
159. Ⓐ Ⓑ Ⓒ Ⓓ
160. Ⓐ Ⓑ Ⓒ Ⓓ
161. Ⓐ Ⓑ Ⓒ Ⓓ
162. Ⓐ Ⓑ Ⓒ Ⓓ
163. Ⓐ Ⓑ Ⓒ Ⓓ
164. Ⓐ Ⓑ Ⓒ Ⓓ
165. Ⓐ Ⓑ Ⓒ Ⓓ
166. Ⓐ Ⓑ Ⓒ Ⓓ
167. Ⓐ Ⓑ Ⓒ Ⓓ
168. Ⓐ Ⓑ Ⓒ Ⓓ
169. Ⓐ Ⓑ Ⓒ Ⓓ
170. Ⓐ Ⓑ Ⓒ Ⓓ
171. Ⓐ Ⓑ Ⓒ Ⓓ
172. Ⓐ Ⓑ Ⓒ Ⓓ
173. Ⓐ Ⓑ Ⓒ Ⓓ
174. Ⓐ Ⓑ Ⓒ Ⓓ
175. Ⓐ Ⓑ Ⓒ Ⓓ
176. Ⓐ Ⓑ Ⓒ Ⓓ

177. Ⓐ Ⓑ Ⓒ Ⓓ
178. Ⓐ Ⓑ Ⓒ Ⓓ
179. Ⓐ Ⓑ Ⓒ Ⓓ
180. Ⓐ Ⓑ Ⓒ Ⓓ
181. Ⓐ Ⓑ Ⓒ Ⓓ
182. Ⓐ Ⓑ Ⓒ Ⓓ
183. Ⓐ Ⓑ Ⓒ Ⓓ
184. Ⓐ Ⓑ Ⓒ Ⓓ
185. Ⓐ Ⓑ Ⓒ Ⓓ
186. Ⓐ Ⓑ Ⓒ Ⓓ
187. Ⓐ Ⓑ Ⓒ Ⓓ
188. Ⓐ Ⓑ Ⓒ Ⓓ
189. Ⓐ Ⓑ Ⓒ Ⓓ
190. Ⓐ Ⓑ Ⓒ Ⓓ
191. Ⓐ Ⓑ Ⓒ Ⓓ
192. Ⓐ Ⓑ Ⓒ Ⓓ
193. Ⓐ Ⓑ Ⓒ Ⓓ
194. Ⓐ Ⓑ Ⓒ Ⓓ
195. Ⓐ Ⓑ Ⓒ Ⓓ
196. Ⓐ Ⓑ Ⓒ Ⓓ
197. Ⓐ Ⓑ Ⓒ Ⓓ
198. Ⓐ Ⓑ Ⓒ Ⓓ
199. Ⓐ Ⓑ Ⓒ Ⓓ
200. Ⓐ Ⓑ Ⓒ Ⓓ
201. Ⓐ Ⓑ Ⓒ Ⓓ
202. Ⓐ Ⓑ Ⓒ Ⓓ
203. Ⓐ Ⓑ Ⓒ Ⓓ
204. Ⓐ Ⓑ Ⓒ Ⓓ
205. Ⓐ Ⓑ Ⓒ Ⓓ
206. Ⓐ Ⓑ Ⓒ Ⓓ
207. Ⓐ Ⓑ Ⓒ Ⓓ
208. Ⓐ Ⓑ Ⓒ Ⓓ
209. Ⓐ Ⓑ Ⓒ Ⓓ
210. Ⓐ Ⓑ Ⓒ Ⓓ
211. Ⓐ Ⓑ Ⓒ Ⓓ
212. Ⓐ Ⓑ Ⓒ Ⓓ
213. Ⓐ Ⓑ Ⓒ Ⓓ
214. Ⓐ Ⓑ Ⓒ Ⓓ
215. Ⓐ Ⓑ Ⓒ Ⓓ
216. Ⓐ Ⓑ Ⓒ Ⓓ
217. Ⓐ Ⓑ Ⓒ Ⓓ
218. Ⓐ Ⓑ Ⓒ Ⓓ
219. Ⓐ Ⓑ Ⓒ Ⓓ

TEST 6

Section 1 — Verbal Reasoning

TIME: 85 Minutes
QUESTIONS: 1-65

DIRECTIONS: The verbal reasoning section contains seven passages, each followed by a series of questions. Based on the information given in a passage, choose the one best answer to each question. If you are not sure of an answer, eliminate those choices that you know are incorrect and choose an answer from among those remaining. Fill in the corresponding circle on the answer sheet to indicate your answer.

PASSAGE I (Questions 1-9)

In his classic book *Ethics*, G. E. Moore presented an ethical theory and defended it by offering a detailed critique of a number of alternative theories.

One of the important distinctions Moore brought out was between the reasons that may lead us to think an action is right or wrong and the reasons that actually constitute an action's being right or wrong. This is a plausible distinction, but one that we are apt to overlook. The difference Moore was calling to our attention here is between the considerations that may be effective in causing us to understand or believe that an action is right and the very different matter of what makes the action right. In another context, we might see this distinction in the mechanism by which we determine or come to believe that someone is a girl and not a boy. Normally we rely on such facts as the name or the attire of the person, when in fact we know that these clues are entirely incidental to the person's actual gender. A person's being named "Mary" is a good reason for our belief that the person so named is a girl, but it is no reason at all for why the person actually is a girl.

Applying this point to the rightness of actions, Moore urged that we be careful to determine whether such things as our own or others' approval of an action is merely a reason for our belief in the rightness of an action or the sort of thing that actually makes an action right.

In challenging the idea that approval of some sort is what actually makes an action right, Moore noted that there are several difficulties with this view. For example, consider the case in which two people are disagreeing about whether or not a certain action is right. If the rightness of the act were constituted only by the individual's approval of it — if "right" simply means "approved of" — then these two people could not, in fact, disagree with one another at all. Their statements that the act in question is or is not right are not in conflict, since they are actually talking about two different things: their separate feelings of approval.

If it is said, instead, that the approval that is relevant here is general approval (the approval of most people in a society), then a moral reformer's assertion, "I know that most people approve of this action but I believe that this action is wrong," would be self-contradictory, since it means, "I know that most people approve of this action but I believe that this action is what most people do not approve of." If general approval determines rightness, then the individual moral reformer's belief would not be sufficient for reclassifying as wrong an act that is approved of by most members of the society.

Moore argued that we should not confuse our approval of an action with the reasons for it being true that the action is right. It may be true that the reason why we think an action is right is that we approve of it, but this is a very different thing from the reason why the action is, in fact, right.

1. The fundamental distinction discussed in the passage is between

    (A) reasons for our beliefs that something is right and reasons for it being right.

    (B) reasons for someone being female and reasons for our beliefs that the person is female.

    (C) reasons for something being right and reasons for it being wrong.

    (D) reasons for what we believe and reasons for what we know.

2. According to this passage, Moore considered our own or others' approval of an action to be an invalid reason for

    (A) our believing the action is right.

    (B) the action being right.

    (C) our performing the action.

    (D) None of the above.

3. The fact that someone is named "John" is a reason for

    (A) our thinking that this person is male.

    (B) why this person is male.

    (C) Both (A) and (B).

    (D) Neither (A) nor (B).

4. According to the passage, if everyone agrees that an action is right,

    (A) the action is right.

    (B) it is true that the action is right.

    (C) it is possible that the action is not right.

    (D) None of the above.

5. Which of the following would be a valid conclusion according to the passage?

    (A) Murder is wrong because everyone believes it is wrong.

    (B) Everyone believes murder is wrong because it is wrong.

    (C) Everyone should believe that murder is wrong.

    (D) None of the above.

6. Suppose someone were raised to believe that stealing is all right. Moore would accept this as an explanation for

    (A) why this person would believe that stealing is right.

    (B) why stealing would be right.

    (C) why stealing would be right for this person.

    (D) All of the above.

7. The passage implies that

    (A) we might have reasons for believing something that is in fact false.

    (B) if something is true, then we will always believe it.

    (C) if we can give reasons for believing something, then it is true.

    (D) if we cannot give reasons for believing something, then it is false.

8. In this passage, it is argued that

    (A) what is right is the same as what a person approves of.

    (B) people do not disagree about what is right.

    (C) approval is not what makes an action right.

    (D) None of the above.

9. If we were to apply Moore's principles of reasoning, we would regard the fuel gauge on an automobile as

    (A) a reason for our believing how much fuel is in the automobile.

    (B) a reason for how much fuel is in the automobile.

    (C) Both (A) and (B).

    (D) Neither (A) nor (B).

PASSAGE II (Questions 10-19)

Since life began eons ago, thousands of creatures have come and gone like the dinosaur — sometimes rendered extinct by naturally changing ecological conditions but more recently by humans and their activities.

If extinction is part of the natural order, some people ask: "Why save endangered species? What makes a relatively few animals and plants so special that effort and money should be expended to preserve them?"

Congress addressed these questions in the preamble to the Endangered Species Act of 1973, holding that endangered and threatened species of fish, wildlife, and plants "are of esthetic, ecological, educational, historical, recreational, and scientific value to the Nation and its people." In making this statement, Congress was summarizing a number of convincing arguments advanced by thoughtful scientists, conservationalists, and others who are greatly concerned by the disappearance of wildlife.

Sadly, we can no longer attribute the increasing decline in our wild animals and plants to "natural" processes. Many are declining because of exploitation, habitat alteration or destruction, pollution, or the introduction of new species of plants and animals to an area. As mandated by Congress, protecting endangered species and restoring them to the point where their existence is no longer jeopardized is the primary objective of the U.S. Fish and Wildlife Service's Endangered Species Program.

Passage of the Endangered Species Act of 1973 gave the United States one of the most far-reaching laws ever enacted by any country to prevent the extinction of imperiled animals and plants. The Act created a national program that today involves the federal government, the states, conservation organizations, individual citizens, business and industry, and foreign governments in a cooperative effort to conserve endangered wildlife throughout the world. Under the law, the Secretary of the Interior (acting through the U.S. Fish and Wildlife Service) has broad powers to protect and conserve all forms of wildlife and plants he finds in serious jeopardy. The Secretary of Commerce, acting through the National Marine Fisheries Service, has similar authority for protecting and conserving most marine life.

As of August 1984, more than 300 native mammals, birds, reptiles, crustaceans, plants, and other life forms were officially protected on the U.S. List of Endangered and Threatened Wildlife and Plants. In addition, more than 500 foreign species have been listed.

Habitat destruction is the most serious worldwide threat to wildlife and plants, followed by overexploitation for commercial, sporting, or other purposes. Disease, predation, inadequate conservation laws, and other natural or man-made factors may also contribute to a species' decline — making it a candidate for listing as endangered or threatened. The Act defines an "endangered" species as one that is in danger of extinction throughout all or a significant portion of its range. A "threatened" species is defined as one that is likely to become endangered within the foreseeable future.

The Fish and Wildlife Service follows a formal "rulemaking" procedure in determining which species should be placed on the U.S. List of Endangered and Threatened Wildlife and Plants.

A "rulemaking" is the process used by Federal agencies (and many states) to propose and later adopt regulations which have the effect of law and apply to all U.S. residents. The proposed rulemaking is published in the *Federal Register*, a daily government publication, and after a suitable period for public comment and possible revision, it is published again as a final rule. Endangered or threatened species are placed on the list, reclassified, or deleted through this process.

10. Which of the following combinations best represents the main contributing factors to the possible extinction of plants and animals?

    (A)   Habitat destruction, pollution, natural processes

    (B)   Introduction of new species into an area, disease, natural processes

    (C)   Habitat destruction, overexploitation, pollution

    (D)   Uncontrolled hunting quotas, predation, disease

11. The passage implies that it is possible for the public to influence the government's decisions regarding endangered species by

    (A)   mentioning that the rulemaking proposals become final rules only after a period of public access allowing for commentary.

(B)   indicating the need for popular vote to pass the Endangered Species Act of 1973.

(C)   citing statistics which were based on public feedback.

(D)   stating the law which requires public majority to pass the *Federal Register*.

12.   All of the following are presented as reasons for saving endangered species EXCEPT for which one?

    (A)   A variety of plants and animals offer educational value to the Nation.

    (B)   The number of diseased animals contaminating the Nation's food supply has increased dramatically over the last century.

    (C)   In general, plants and animals beautify the country.

    (D)   The study of such diverse plants and animals is of great scientific value.

13.   Which of the following best represents the main idea of the passage?

    (A)   The Endangered Species Act of 1973 was an important development in the preservation of endangered wildlife.

    (B)   The federal government's current involvement in conservation of endangered plants and animals was bolstered by public involvement in the late 1960s.

    (C)   Man-made factors have had negative effects on wildlife, forcing the intervention of the Secretaries of Commerce and Interior to work in conjunction with the public to create legitimate conservation laws for the nation.

    (D)   Modern human existence has negatively altered natural habitats, prompting the installment of the Endangered Species Act which promotes the conservation of endangered species worldwide.

14.   What is the author's purpose of mentioning dinosaurs in the beginning of the passage?

    (A)   To develop similarities between the plight of one animal to another animal described later in the passage

    (B)   To contrast ancient and modern attitudes toward wildlife

    (C)   To express the need for government control of wildlife

    (D)   To present a well-known example in order to later contrast the difference between natural and man-made extinction

15.   As opposed to "threatened" wildlife, an "endangered" species has which of the following criteria?

    I.   overexploitation for commercial purposes

    II.   danger of extinction throughout most of its life range

    III.   the likelihood of extinction in the near future

(A) II only. (B) I and II only.

(C) I and III only. (D) II and III only.

16. The U.S. government's support of wildlife conservation can be seen in which of the following examples from the passage?

(A) The passing of federal and state laws for recording wildlife in the nation

(B) The assertion that the protection and restoration of endangered species is a main objective in wildlife conservation and in the development of the laws and programs surrounding this issue

(C) The creation of federal programs to interact with national services for the protection of wildlife

(D) The accounting of public opinion and comment regarding proposals concerning endangered wildlife

17. According to the passage, all of the following apply to the "rulemaking" procedure EXCEPT for which one?

(A) The procedure is used by federal and state agencies to propose and adopt regulations.

(B) Public access to and commentary on the documented rulemaking procedure may prompt the reevaluation of the endangered species list and the proposals.

(C) The procedure produces regulations which act as laws and apply to all U.S. citizens.

(D) The proposals are only made into final rules after a period of time during which the Secretaries of Commerce and Interior approve all revisions and pass them to Congress.

18. Statistics from 1984 show which of the following results?

(A) Five-thirds more native species survived than foreign species that were endangered.

(B) There are more foreign than native endangered species which indicates that more funding is needed.

(C) The large number of endangered species listed shows the need for and continuance of conservation laws.

(D) Native creatures can survive and adapt better than foreign species to the alterations in their environment.

19. Which of the following would provide the best service to a private group's proposal to protect a certain type of mammal?

(A) Congress

(B) The city's mayor

(C) The Secretary of the Interior

(D) The Secretary of Commerce

PASSAGE III (Questions 20-29)

It is a matter for public concern that American universities begin 1989 in serious difficulty explaining what they are, what they should teach and by what right they teach.

The universities' crisis is related to a profound problem of the 20th century, a cause of war in our times, which is the problem of truth — an intellectual problem, obviously, but a political one as well. If truth doesn't exist, or cannot be determined, why do we do what we do? If it does exist and can be determined, and I possess the truth while you are in error, why should I not send you to prison or Siberia in order to eliminate error from society?

The Western civilization that produced the ferocious modern politico-ideological "truth" systems of Marxism-Leninism, mutating into Stalinism and Nazism-Fascism, is the same civilization that has most effectively resisted the ideologizing of knowledge. It has defended free thought and created, in the course of its history, the democratic political system that actually asks people to decide a nation's course. It has done this on a continuing assumption of the possibility of discovering the truth about things through reason.

The values of this civilization, "the West," are now questioned, directly or indirectly, in the course of the university controversy. First there is debate about cultural relativism, which was most publicized at Stanford University. People ask why the thought and art of the West should be taught in the American university, rather than the thought and art of China and India.

People ask why the oral literature of Africa or the preliterate cultures of the North American Indian should be shunted off onto the margins of what is considered civilization. Women note that few women are among the "great" figures taught in the university and challenge that this should be so.

A political explanation is proposed, which says European or European-descended white men have always controlled Western universities and dominated Western cultural life, imposing what suited them.

This obviously is true but it is just as obviously reductionist. To say that Western society is Eurocentric is to repeat oneself. To say that its culture has been dominated by men is to state an historical fact, not only about this civilization but all others as well. Yet self-interest, plot and power-brokerage are not satisfactory explanations. To claim that they are is to deny implicitly that values or standards exist outside the play of power, or that judgments have been or can be made which are not those of power-in-action.

Behind the cultural relativism of the controversy is the influence of "postmodernism," which says that universal principles and values, and the Western liberal, rationalist effort to discover general truths are no longer credible.

The founding assumption of the Western university is that reality is perceived through reason. Postmodern thought holds to the contrary that reason has become "pluralized" and relativized, and reality is indeterminate. Knowledge exists only as "regimes" of knowledge, which is to say political systems (an academic department or intellectual school, for example) dictate that certain things are so and use power, pain and reward to make this accepted.

The civilization we live in would be incomprehensible and unworkable if we abandoned the beliefs that reason can arbitrate the moral claims of society and that truth exists and is ascertainable. Philosopher Alastair MacIntyre argues that our moral identity and civilization are integrally related, and if we abandon a belief in truth for a cultural relativism, we are giving up all possibility of moral judgment.

From William Pfaff, "American Universities, Moral Reasoning and the Greeks." © 1989 by Los Angeles Times Syndicate.

20. According to the author, the two conflicting modes of thought in the crisis he describes are

    (A) those of preliterate and postliterate cultures.

    (B) Marxism and Nazism.

    (C) postmodernism and liberal rationalism.

    (D) Fascism and postmodernism.

21. Which of the following statements most accurately states the author's view of Western civilization's response to the problem of truth?

    (A) The West has refused to deal with the problem.

    (B) The West has abandoned rationalism in favor of repressive politico-ideological "truth" systems.

    (C) The West has used "truth" systems as an excuse for war and for exploiting non-Western cultures.

    (D) The West has produced both repressive "truth" systems and preserved free thought and open inquiry.

22. The author's discussion of the problem of truth is intended chiefly to

    (A) demonstrate the decline of moral responsibility in Western civilization.

    (B) indicate that universities are powerless to cope with large historical movements.

    (C) illustrate the harmful effects of "truth" systems.

    (D) place the current crisis in universities in a broad intellectual and political context.

23. The author believes that the threat to the values of Western civilization in the current university controversy spring from

    I.   cultural relativism

    II. postmodernism

    III. Nazism-Fascism

    (A) I only.   (B) I and II only.

    (C) II and III only.   (D) I, II, and III.

24. The author's chief objection to the explanation that says the content of university curricula results from the domination of European-descended white males is that such an explanation

(A)   reduces values and judgments to political power-plays.

(B)   does not account for the ethnic and gender variety present in modern American universities.

(C)   ignores the cultural relativism that has long dominated American thought.

(D)   is simply not true.

25.   The crisis in American universities discussed by the author involves all of the following EXCEPT

(A)   self-identity.

(B)   inadequate funding.

(C)   curriculum content.

(D)   moral basis of authority.

26.   According to the author, all of the following beliefs of Western civilization are threatened by postmodernism EXCEPT the belief that

(A)   truth can be discovered through reason.

(B)   reality is indeterminate.

(C)   reason can arbitrate society's moral claims.

(D)   general truths transcend political systems.

27.   Based on the author's discussion, it can be inferred that postmodern thought contains all of the following ideas EXCEPT

(A)   universal values do not exist.

(B)   knowledge exists only as a political system.

(C)   objective inquiry is the best means of discovering truth.

(D)   "reality" cannot be discovered through reason.

28.   Which of the following does the author regard as the worst possible consequence of the current crisis in American education?

(A)   Abandoning bases for making moral judgments

(B)   Radical change in the curriculum

(C)   The breakdown of traditional academic departments and schools

(D)   The loss of America's global influence and respect

29.   According to the author, Western civilization and American universities

(A)   necessarily find themselves in conflict from time to time.

(B)   have essentially dissimilar conceptions of truth and reality.

(C)   must join forces to resist threats from non-Western cultures.

(D)   are based on an identical assumption.

PASSAGE IV (Questions 30-37)

The relationship of a king towards his people is rightly compared to that of a father to his children, and to a head of a body composed of diverse members. For it was as fathers that the good princes and magistrates of the people of God acknowledged themselves to their subjects. And for all other well-ruled commonwealths, the style of *pater patriae* (father of his country) was ever and is commonly used with kings. The proper office of a king towards his subjects agrees very well with the office of the head towards the body and all members thereof. For from the head, being the seat of judgment, proceedeth the care and foresight of guiding and preventing all evil that may come to the body or any part thereof. The head cares for the body; so doth the king for his people. As the discourse and direction flows from the head, and the execution according thereunto belongs to the rest of the members, everyone according to their office: so is it betwixt a wise prince and his people. As the judgment coming from the head may not only employ the members, every one in its own office, as long as they are able for it; but, likewise, in case any of them affected with any infirmity must care and provide for their remedy, in case it be curable, and if otherwise has someone cut them off for fear of infecting the rest: even so is it betwixt the prince and his people. And as there is ever hope of curing any diseased member by the direction of the head, as long as it is whole; but by the contrary, if it be troubled, all the members are partakers of that pain, so is it betwixt the prince and his people.

And now to speak first of the father's part, consider what duty his children owe to him, and whether upon any pretext whatever it will not be thought monstrous and unnatural for his sons to rise up against him, to control him at their appetite, and when they think good to slay him, or to cut him off, and adopt to themselves any other they please in his room. Can any pretense of wickedness or rigor on his part be a just excuse for his children to put hand to him? In case it were true that the father hated and wronged the children never so much, will any man endowed with the least spark of reason think it lawful for them to meet him with the line? Yea, suppose the father were furiously following his sons with a drawn sword, is it lawful for them to turn and strike again, or make any resistance but by flight? I think surely if there were no more but the example of brute beasts and unreasonable creatures, it may serve well enough to qualify and prove my argument. We read often the piety that the storks have to their old and decayed parents: and generally we know that there are many sorts of beasts and fowls that with violence and many bloody strokes will beat and banish their young ones from them, how soon they perceive them to be able to fend for themselves; but we never read nor heard of any resistance on their part, except among vipers; which proves such persons as ought to be reasonable creatures, and yet unnaturally follow this example, to be endued with their viperous nature.

And for the similitude of the head and the body, it may very well fall out that the head will be forced to cut off some rotten member to keep the rest of the body in integrity: but what state the body can be in, if the head for any infirmity that can fall to it be cut off, I leave it to the reader's judgment.

To conclude, if the children may upon any pretext that can be imagined lawfully rise up against their father, cut him off, and choose any other whom they please in his room; and if the body for the well of it may for an infirmity that may be in the head strike it off, then I cannot deny that the people may rebel, control, and displace, or cut off their king, at their own pleasure, and upon respects moving them.

Adapted from James Stuart, *The True Law of Free Monarchies.* (1598)

30. Which of the following statements most accurately describes the organization of the passage?

    (A) It takes the form of a syllogism (a major premise, minor premise, and conclusion).

    (B) It takes the form of an "if X, then Y" proposition.

    (C) It takes the form of argument by analogy (two controlling metaphors).

    (D) It uses inductive logic, proceeding from particulars to a generalization.

31. The chief purpose of the passage is to

    (A) argue that kings need the consent of the governed.

    (B) demonstrate the burdens of kingship.

    (C) argue that abuse of power leads inevitably to rebellion.

    (D) argue that the king can do whatever he pleases and not be subject to criticism.

32. The author alludes to "beasts and fowls" chiefly to support his argument that

    (A) the king's subjects should not resist the king's irrational, violent behavior.

    (B) the king serves as protector for even his most unworthy subjects.

    (C) civil obedience protects man from the chaos of the natural order.

    (D) a benign monarchy is analogous to natural law.

33. Which of the following statements most accurately summarizes the relationships among the four paragraphs?

    (A) The first two present one argument and the last two present a second argument.

    (B) The first introduces two metaphors, the second and third each develop one of them, and the fourth deals with both.

    (C) Each of the first three has a different controlling metaphor, and the fourth presents a conclusion.

    (D) The first, third, and fourth draw their controlling metaphors from man, and the second derives its controlling metaphor from nature.

34. The author compares the king to all of the following EXCEPT

    (A) a father.   (B) a heart.

    (C) the head of a body.   (D) an old stork.

35. The author believes that

    (A) subjects may rebel only with ample cause.

    (B) monarchs should be replaced only when an overwhelming majority of their subjects desires change.

    (C)   violent revolution is sometimes justified.

    (D)   monarchs may never be lawfully replaced.

36.   Based on this passage, the author most likely believes in

    (A)   the divine right of kings.

    (B)   separation of church and state.

    (C)   representative government.

    (D)   the right of subjects to recall rulers.

37.   The weakest arguments in the passage result from

    (A)   a failure to define terms.

    (B)   introducing examples (such as the viper) that contradict other examples.

    (C)   the failure to provide historical background.

    (D)   taking metaphors literally, as in the head/body metaphor.

PASSAGE V (Questions 38-46)

Genius is supposed to be a power of producing excellencies which are out of the reach of rules of art; a power which no precepts can teach, and which no industry can acquire.

This opinion of the impossibility of acquiring those beauties which stamp the work with the character of Genius, supposes that it is something more fixed than in reality it is; and that we always do, and always did agree in opinion, with respect to what should be considered as the characteristic of genius. But the truth is, the degree of excellence which proclaims Genius is different, in different times and different places; and what shows it to be so is that mankind has often changed its opinion upon this matter.

When the arts were in their infancy, the power of merely drawing the likeness of any object was considered one of their greatest efforts. But when it was found that every man could be taught to do this and a great deal more merely by the observance of certain precepts, the word Genius shifted its application and was given only to him who added the peculiar character of the object he represented; to him who had invention, expression, grace, or dignity; in short, to him who possessed those qualities, or excellencies, the power of producing which could not then be taught by any known and promulgated rules.

What we now call Genius begins not where rules abstractly end, but where known vulgar and trite rules no longer hold any place. Even works of Genius, like every other effect, as they must have their cause, must likewise have their rules. It cannot be by chance that excellencies are produced with any constancy or certainty, for this is not the nature of chance. Yet the rules by which men of extraordinary parts work, are either such that they discover by their own peculiar observations, or a nice texture as not easily to admit being expressed in words; especially as artists are not very frequently skillful in that mode of communicating ideas. Unsubstantial, however, as these rules may seem and as difficult as it may be to convey them in writing, they are still seen and felt in the mind of the artist; and he works from them with as much certainty, as if they were embodied, as I may say, upon paper. It is true that these refined principles cannot always be made palpable, like the more gross rules of art. Yet it does not follow that the mind may be put in such a train that it shall perceive, by a kind of scientific sense, that propriety which words, particularly words of unpracticed writers such as we are, can but very feebly suggest.

Invention is one of the great marks of Genius, but if we consult experience, we shall find that it is by being conversant with the inventions of others that we learn to invent; as by reading the thoughts of others we learn to think.

38. Which of the following statements best describes the function of the first paragraph?

    (A)   It offers historical background for the author's topic.

    (B)   It states a position that the author will attempt to refute.

    (C)   It states the first of the author's two-part argument.

    (D)   It states the main thesis of the essay, which is developed in subsequent paragraphs.

39. "It" (line 6) refers to

    (A)   this opinion.   (B)   those beauties.

    (C)   the work.   (D)   the character of Genius.

40. Which of the following ideas is NOT contained in paragraphs two and three?

    (A)   The belief that Genius cannot be taught depends on the idea that there is a fixed, unchanging definition of Genius.

    (B)   Conceptions of Genius have changed from age to age.

    (C)   Only works that have such qualities as invention or dignity deserve to be regarded as products of Genius.

    (D)   Conceptions of Genius are related to our knowledge of the rules of art.

41. The chief idea in paragraph three is best expressed by which of the following?

    (A)   The more educated the artist, the more likely the artist is to achieve the status of Genius.

    (B)   Common people are less likely to recognize true geniuses than educated people, but this risk was greater in the past than it is in the present.

    (C)   It is more difficult to recognize Genius in the early states of an art form than when that art form is more fully developed.

    (D)   In any age, the name of Genius is applied to artists who achieve effects that could not be produced by following rules then in existence.

42. Based on the passage, with which of the following statements would the author disagree most strongly?

    (A)   Genius is innate and can never be taught.

    (B)   Standards of Genius rise as more is learned of the rules of art.

    (C)   Works of Genius follow certain rules, even if those rules are hidden from common view.

    (D)   Men of Genius may discover rules of art through their own acute observations.

43.   Which of the following ideas is contained in paragraph four?

    (A)   Works of Genius are often produced by chance.

    (B)   Works of Genius are based on artistic principles.

    (C)   Genius begins where rules end.

    (D)   Rules are seldom perceived by artists.

44.   All of the following assumptions EXCEPT which are contained in paragraph four?

    (A)   All effects have causes.

    (B)   Rules operate even when they are not consciously recognized.

    (C)   In time, all rules become vulgar and trite.

    (D)   Chance cannot consistently produce excellence.

45.   Which of the following ideas in the essay is an unsupported claim, based neither on an appeal to history nor on experience?

    I.   Artistic rules in works of Genius are seen and felt in the mind of the artist.

    II.   Artists can learn invention.

    III.   The degree of excellence that is called Genius differs in various times and locales.

    (A)   I only.   (B)   II only.

    (C)   I and III only.   (D)   I, II, and III.

46.   The primary purpose of the passage is to

    (A)   analyze the differences between genuine and supposed works of Genius.

    (B)   trace the history of different conceptions of Genius.

    (C)   distinguish between works of Genius and works of invention.

    (D)   argue that Genius is not out of the reach of the rules of art.

PASSAGE VI (Questions 47-56)

    Three months ago we wrote about the costly retreat from the humanities on all the levels of American education. It has not become apparent to us that one of the biggest problems confronting American education today is the increasing vocationalization of our colleges and universities. Schools are under pressure to become job-training centers and employment agencies.

    The pressure comes mainly from two sources. One is the growing determination of many citizens to reduce taxes which is understandable, but irresponsible when connected to the reduction of vital public services. The second source of pressure comes from parents and students who scorn courses that do not teach people how to become attractive to employers in a tightening job market.

It is absurd to believe that development of skills does not also require systematic development of the human mind. Education is being measured more by the size of the benefits the individual can extract from society than by the extent to which the individual can come into possession of his or her full powers. The result is that the life-giving juices are in danger of being drained out of education.

Instead of trying to shrink the liberal arts, Americans ought to pressure colleges and universities to increase the ratio of the humanities to the sciences.

The irony of the emphasis being placed on careers is that nothing is more valuable for anyone who has had a professional or vocational education than to be able to deal with abstractions or complexities, or to feel comfortable with subtleties of thought and language. The doctor who knows only about disease is at a disadvantage alongside the doctor who knows at least as much about people as about pathological organisms. The lawyer who argues in court from a narrow legal base is no match for the lawyer who can connect legal precedents to historical experience. The business executive whose competence in general management is bolstered by an artistic ability to deal with people is of prime value to his company. For the technologist, the engineering of consent can be as important as the engineering of moving parts. Just in terms of career preparation, therefore, a student is shortchanged by shortcutting the humanities.

But even if it could be demonstrated that the humanities contribute nothing directly to a job, they would still be an essential part of the educational equipment of any person who wants to come to terms with life. The humanities would be expendable only if human beings didn't have to make decisions that affected their lives and the lives of others; if the human past never existed or had nothing to tell us about the present; if human relations were random aspects of life; and if no special demands arose from the accident of being born a human being instead of a hen or a hog.

Finally, there would be good reason to eliminate the humanities if a free society were not absolutely dependent on a functioning citizenry. If the main purpose of a university is job training, then the underlying philosophy of our government has little meaning. The debates that went into the making of American society concerned not just institutions or governing principles but the capacity of humans to sustain those institutions. The fundamental question sensed by everyone at the American Constitutional Convention was whether the people themselves would understand what it meant to hold the ultimate power of society, and whether they had enough of a sense of history and destiny to know where they had been and where they ought to be going.

Jefferson was prouder of having been the founder of the University of Virginia than of having been President of the United States. He knew that the educated and developed mind was the best assurance that a political system could be made to work — a system based on the informed consent of the governed. If this idea fails, then all the saved tax dollars in the world will not be enough to prevent the nation from turning on itself.

Adapted from Norman Cousins, "How to Make People Smaller Than They Are" © *The Saturday Review* (December 1978).

47. The primary purpose of the passage is to

    (A) argue that the liberal arts are more vocationally useful than professional education.

    (B) lament the passing of a golden era in American higher education.

    (C) argue that the humanities are the most important part of the curriculum.

    (D) argue that too much money is being spent on vocational and professional education.

48. The author cites all of the following as sources of pressure to vocationalize American education EXCEPT

    (A) the desire for lower taxes.

    (B) measuring education in terms of benefits to be extracted from society.

    (C) the desire of individuals to develop their full powers.

    (D) parents who want their children to be competitive in the marketplace.

49. Which of the following reasons does the author offer to support his contention that Americans ought to pressure universities to increase the ratio of the humanities to the sciences?

    I.   The humanities are useful for people who have had professional or vocational educations.

    II. Free societies depend absolutely on citizens educated in the humanities.

    III. The humanities are essential in helping people understand and cope with their lives as human beings.

    (A) I only.   (B) I and II only.

    (C) II and III only.   (D) I, II, and III.

50. The author's discussion of doctors, lawyers, and business executives is designed chiefly to

    (A) provide evidence to support his claim that the humanities provide valuable job-related skills.

    (B) point out the weaknesses of vocational education.

    (C) illustrate his argument that the humanities are important for anyone wishing to come to terms with life.

    (D) argue that the "life-giving juices" are being drained out of education.

51. Judging from this passage, which of the following best expresses the author's conception of the proper primary function of education?

    (A) It ought to develop a broad range of job-related skills.

    (B) It should fulfill the emotional and psychological needs of the individual.

    (C) It ought to develop systematically the full mental capacities of the individual.

(D)   It should be tailored to the special interests and life-objectives of each individual.

52.   The evidence offered in support of the author's argument in the last paragraph can best be described as an appeal to

(A)   facts.   (B)   authority.

(C)   general beliefs.   (D)   emotion.

53.   Which of the following statements accurately describe the function and/or primary argument of paragraph seven ("Finally…")?

I.   It shifts the author's argument from private or personal concerns to societal concerns.

II.   It is an extension of his argument in paragraph five that the humanities can contribute useful job-related skills.

III.   It is the final evidence he offers to prove that the humanities are essential to anyone wishing "to come to terms with life."

(A)   I only.   (B)   I and III only.

(C)   II and III only.   (D)   I, II and III.

54.   A study showing that recent engineering graduates earn twice as much as recent humanities graduates would

(A)   force the author to revise his argument that the humanities are useful in career preparation.

(B)   undermine the author's claim that the humanities are essential for individuals in coming to terms with life.

(C)   confirm the author's statement that the underlying philosophy of our government has little meaning.

(D)   not affect the author's arguments.

55.   Paragraph six ("But even…") implicitly or explicitly affirms all of the following EXCEPT

(A)   the relevance of history.

(B)   the chaotic nature of the universe.

(C)   the necessity of moral choice.

(D)   the unique nature of human life.

56.   In context, "the engineering of consent" can best be said to refer to

(A)   technological skill.

(B)   the ability to think sequentially.

(C)   skill in dealing with human beings.

(D)   the ability to deal with abstractions.

PASSAGE VII (Questions 57-65)

The right of nature, which writers commonly call *jus naturale*, is the liberty each man has to use his own power as he wills himself for the preservation of his own nature, that is to say, of his own life; and consequently of doing anything which in his own judgment and reason he shall conceive to be the aptest means thereunto.

By Liberty is understood, according to the proper signification of the word, the absence of external impediments, which impediments may oft take away part of a man's power to do what he would, but cannot hinder him from using the power left him according as his judgment and reason shall dictate to him.

A law of nature (*lex naturalis*) is a precept or general rule found out by reason, by which a man is forbidden to do that which is destructive to his life or taketh away the means of preserving the same; and to omit that by which he thinketh it may be best preserved. Those that speak of this subject confuse *Jus* and *Lex*, Right and Law; yet these ought to be distinguished because Right consisteth in liberty to do or to forbear, whereas Law determineth and bindeth to one of them: so that Law and Right differ as much as obligation and liberty, which in one and the same matter are inconsistent.

And because the condition of man (as hath been declared in the precedent chapter) is a condition of war of everyone against everyone, in which case everyone is governed by his own reason, and there is nothing he can make of us that may not be a help unto him in preserving his life against his enemies: it followeth that in such a condition every man has a right to every thing, even to one another's body. And therefore as long as this natural right of every man to every thing endureth, there can be no security to any man (how strong or wise soever he be) of living out the time which nature ordinarily alloweth men to live. And consequently, it is a precept or general rule of reason that every man ought to endeavor peace as far as he has hope of obtaining it; and when he cannot obtain it, that he may seek and use all helps and advantages of war. The first branch of which containeth the first and fundamental law of nature, which is to seek peace and follow it. The second, the sum of the right of nature, which is to use all means we can to defend ourselves. From this fundamental law of nature, by which men are commanded to endeavor peace, is derived this second law: that a man be willing, when others are so too, insofar as for peace and defence of himself he shall think necessary, to lay down this right to all things, and be contented with so much liberty against other men as he would allow other men against himself. For as long as any man holdeth this right of doing anything he liketh, so long are all men in the condition of war. But if other men will not lay down their right, as well as he, then there is no reason for anyone to divest himself of his. For that he were to expose himself to pray (to which no man is bound) rather than dispose himself to peace. This is that law of the Gospel: Whatsoever you require that others should do to you, that do ye to them.

From Thomas Hobbes, *Leviathan.* (1651).

57. According to the author, the right of nature and a law of nature

(A) spring from the same desire for peace.

(B) are naturally compatible.

(C) have been clearly delineated by previous writers.

(D) are in conflict with one another.

58. The author derives his first law of nature from

    (A) reason. (B) observation of nature.

    (C) Biblical authority. (D) history.

59. *Lex naturalis* is based on

    I.   individual liberty

    II. obligation

    III. social contract

    (A) I only. (B) I and II only.

    (C) II and III only. (D) I, II, and III.

60. The author says that man's natural condition involves all of the following EXCEPT a state

    (A) in which considerations of self-preservation are paramount.

    (B) of constant warfare with other humans.

    (C) in which no man has a right to his neighbor's things.

    (D) in which each man is governed by his own reason.

61. One can infer from the passage that the author believes

    (A) in absolute monarchy.

    (B) that effective government depends on the consent of the governed.

    (C) that liberty is best achieved in a democratic society.

    (D) that only rugged individualists can lead satisfying lives.

62. According to the author, the first and second laws of nature spring ultimately from man's

    (A) desire for self-preservation.

    (B) need for social institutions.

    (C) desire for liberty.

    (D) essentially benign constitution.

63. The author suggests that man need not follow the second law of nature

    (A) when it conflicts with the first law of nature.

    (B) if other men refuse to relinquish their rights of nature.

    (C) when it infringes on his personal identity.

    (D) when it conflicts with Biblical teachings.

64. The author refers to the Bible chiefly to

    (A) lend authority to his argument.

(B)   further explain his second law of nature.

(C)   place his essay in the tradition of Western Christian thought.

(D)   make his argument appear less radical.

65.   Which of the following statements is most accurate?

(A)   The right of nature and the two laws of nature derive from the same impulse for self-preservation; they differ chiefly insofar as the former considers man as an individual and the latter considers man as a social being.

(B)   The right of nature deals with man's liberty whereas the two laws of nature deal with man's desire for peace and the right to defend himself.

(C)   The author believes that the laws of nature ought to take precedence over the right of nature, but that men always give priority to the right of nature when the two are in conflict.

(D)   The right of nature and the two laws of nature both derive from reason, but only the former deals with self-preservation while the latter deal only with peace and prosperity.

STOP

If time still remains, you may review work only in this section.

When the time allotted is up, you may go on to the next section.

Section 2 — Physical Sciences

TIME: 100 Minutes
QUESTIONS: 66-142

> **DIRECTIONS:** Most of the questions in this section are arranged in groups, each corresponding to a descriptive passage. Based on the information given in a passage, choose the one best answer to each question in the group. Some questions are independent of a descriptive passage and of each other. Choose the one best answer to each of these questions. If you are not sure of an answer, eliminate those choices that you know are incorrect and choose an answer from among those remaining. Fill in the corresponding circle on the answer sheet to indicate your answer. You may refer to the periodic table at any time.

PASSAGE I (Questions 66-70)

A man pulls a 25 kg crate at a constant speed of 2 m/s up a hill using a rope inclined at 25° with respect to the 30° incline. The force of friction between the crate and the slope is f = 53.33 N and is assumed to be constant over the entire 20 m long slope. The rope does not stretch as it is pulled and the tension in the rope is maintained constant. Use the value of $g = 10m/s^2$.

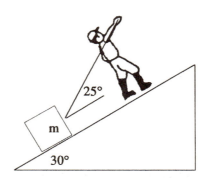

66.   How much work is done by gravity in moving the crate up the slope?

    (A)   - 5,000 J   (B)   - 4,330 J

    (C)   - 2,500 J   (D)   - 2,868 J

67.   How much work is done by the frictional force in moving the crate up the slope?

    (A)   - 1,067 J   (B)   - 4,330 J

    (C)   - 2,500 J   (D)   - 1, 570 J

68. How much work is done by the contact force (often called the NORMAL force) between the crate and the slope in moving the crate up the slope?

    (A) 0 J
    (B) 5,000 J
    (C) 2,500 J
    (D) - 1,067 J

69. How much work is done by the man in moving the crate up the slope?

    (A) 1,067 J
    (B) 4,330 J
    (C) 5,000 J
    (D) 3,567 J

70. How much power does the man output during the crate's motion?

    (A) 433 W
    (B) 500 W
    (C) 356.7 W
    (D) 106.7 W

PASSAGE II (Questions 71-75)

A 2 kg mass attached to an ideal Hookean spring is constrained to oscillate along one dimension on a horizontal frictionless surface. A mark has been placed at an arbitrary location on the table to designate the $x = 0$ position for this motion. As the mass oscillates without loss of energy it traces the path shown on the graph below.

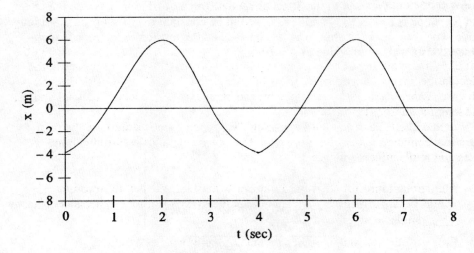

71. What is the amplitude of the motion for this oscillator?

    (A) 6 m
    (B) - 4 m
    (C) 5 m
    (D) 2 m

72. What is the period of the oscillator?

    (A) 2 s
    (B) 4 s
    (C) 6 s
    (D) 8 s

73. When is the mass moving the slowest?

    (A) 1 s   (B) 2.5 s

    (C) 5 s   (D) 6 s

74. When does the mass have its greatest acceleration?

    (A) 1 s   (B) 2.5 s

    (C) 5 s   (D) 6 s

75. What is the spring constant of the spring?

    (A) 19.74 N/m   (B) 2 N/m

    (C) 100 N/m   (D) 68.35 N/m

PASSAGE III (Questions 76–85)

Atom A located in Group V in the second row of the periodic table combines with atom B which is located in Group VII in the third row of the periodic table.

Various laboratory experiments indicate that each atom in the periodic table has a different ability to attract the electrons in a covalent bond resulting in a bond polarity. The difference in their electronegativities leads to varying degrees of ionic or covalent bonding. Measurement of the dipole moment of the molecule in the laboratory indicates the degree of polarity.

Another atom (C) whose electronic configuration is

$$1s^2 2s^2 2p^6 3s^2 3p_x^{\,1} 3p_y^{\,1} 3p_z^{\,1}$$

also combines with atom B. However, atom C forms two different compounds with atom B. When more than one compound can be formed between two elements, the molecular geometry (arrangement of atoms around the central atom) is different in each case. This difference in arrangement can be detected by measuring bond angles, bond lengths and dipole moments.

Valence Shell Electron Pair Repulsion Theory and hybridization are the two theoretical explanations offered to explain the experimentally-determined bond angles and molecular geometries.

76. The compound formed between atom A and atom B has the formula _____ , would be classified as _____, contains bonds but is a _____ because it has a _____ molecular geometry.

    (A) NCl_3 ... ionic ... polar covalent ... nonpolar ... pyramidal

    (B) NCl_3 ... covalent ... polar covalent ... polar ... pyramidal

    (C) NCl_3 ... ionic ... polar covalent ... polar ... trigonal planar

    (D) NCl_3 ... covalent ... polar covalent ... nonpolar ... trigonal planar

77. The bond angles in the molecule in question 76 are approximately _____ degrees because the repulsion between lone pair electrons and bond pair electrons _____ than the repulsion between bond pair electrons and bond pair electrons and the hybridization is _____.

    (A) 107 ... < ... sp^2 (B) 107 ... > ... sp^3

    (C) 107 ... < ... sp^3 (D) 120 ... > ... sp^2

78. The compound formed between atom C and B which is not formed by atom A and atom B has the formula _____ and exhibits _____ hybridization and a _____ molecular geometry.

    (A) PCl_3 ... sp^3 ... tetrahedral

    (B) PCl_5 ... sp^3d ... trigonal bipyramidal

    (C) PCl_5 ... sp^2d^2 ... pentagon

    (D) PCl_5 ... sp^3d ... square

79. Another molecule that would have the same number of valence shell electrons around the central atom as in question 78 but whose molecular geometry should be T-shaped might be _____. In this type of molecular geometry the lone pair (nonbinding) electrons always occupy the positions _____ because this results in _____ 90-degree repulsions.

    (A) ClF_3... above and below the triangle ... fewer

    (B) AsF_5 ... on the triangle ... fewer

    (C) ClF_3 ... on the triangle ... fewer

    (D) AsF_3 ... above and below the triangle ... more

80. Which of the following is not a valid set of quantum numbers for an electron in element C (Passage III)?

    (A) $n = 3; l = 0; m_l = 1; m_s = +^1/_2$

    (B) $n = 3; l = 1; m_l = 1; m_s = +^1/_2$

    (C) $n = 3; l = 1; m_l = 1; m_s = -^1/_2$

    (D) $n = 3; l = 1; m_l = 0; m_s = -^1/_2$

81. Which of the following molecules has only one bond between carbon atoms that exhibits sp^3-sp^2 type hybridization?

    (A) $CH_3CH_2CH = CHCH_3$

    (B) CH_3CH_2CHO

    (C) $CH_3CHOHCH_2CH_3$

    (D) $CH_3CH_2CH_2NH_2$

82. Element B contains _____ protons, _____ electrons, and _____ neutrons and will form a _____ ion whose radius will be _____ the radius of the parent atom.

    (A) 17 ... 17 ... 17 ... - 1 ... <

    (B) 17 ... 17 ... 18 ... - 1 ... <

    (C) 17 ... 17 ... 18 ... - 1 ... >

    (D) 17 ... 18 ... 18 ... +1 ... <

83. The maximum number of electrons that can be placed in the n = 3 energy level of a neutral, ground state atom of the element that would be found directly beneath element B in the periodic table is

(A)   5.   (B)   3.

(C)   8.   (D)   18.

84. The molecular orbital diagram for the molecule formed between two atoms of element A indicates that the molecule is _____, with _____ electrons in the bonding molecular orbitals and _____ electrons in the anti-bonding molecular orbitals which results in a bond order of _____ .

(A)   diamagnetic ... 8 ... 4 ... 2

(B)   paramagnetic ... 8 ... 2 ... 3

(C)   paramagnetic ... 7 ... 4 ... 2

(D)   diamagnetic ... 8 ... 2 ... 3

85. The bond formed between A and B is _____ polar than the bond formed between C and B because the electronegativity of A is _____ than that of C because electronegativities _____ from bottom to top in a family and from left to right in a row in the periodic table.

(A)   more ... > ... increase   (B)   less ... < ... decrease

(C)   more ... < ... increase   (D)   less ... < ... increase

PASSAGE IV (Questions 86-90)

A meter stick, whose center of gravity is found to be at exactly its midpoint, is pivoted at $x = 0$ cm by a frictionless pivot. It is maintained horizontal with the use of a spring balance which is attached to the stick at $x = 20$ cm. The angle (θ) between the stick and the direction of the applied force on the balance is permitted to vary between 90° and 150° while the meter stick is kept horizontal, during which time the force registered by the balance changes. A 2 N weight is hung at $x = 95$ cm on the stick so that its weight is vertically downward at that point. The table and figure below record the above information, as well as some values of the spring force vs. the angle.

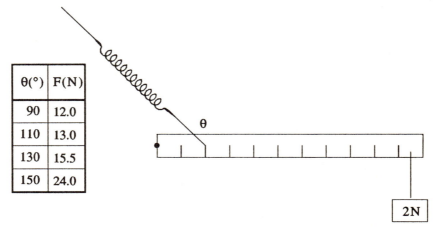

θ(°)	F(N)
90	12.0
110	13.0
130	15.5
150	24.0

86. Compute the torque on the stick about its pivot created by the 2 N mass.

    (A) 1 Nm   (B) 1.5 Nm

    (C) 2 Nm   (D) 1.9 Nm

87. Compute the torque on the stick about its pivot created by the spring balance when it is at 90°.

    (A) 0 Nm   (B) 2.4 Nm

    (C) 3.6 Nm   (D) 5 Nm

88. If the meter stick were to be held below the horizontal

    (A) the torque due to the 2 N weight would not change.

    (B) the angle between the spring balance and the stick could not be 90°.

    (C) Both (A) and (B).

    (D) the torque due to the weight of the meter stick would change.

89. Determine the weight of the meter stick by averaging the values obtained from the data.

    (A) 0.95 N   (B) 1.09 N

    (C) 2 N   (D) 1.01 N

90. Determine the horizontal force exerted by the pivot on the stick when the angle of the spring balance is 150°.

    (A) 20.8 N   (B) 24 N

    (C) 0 N   (D) 12 N

PASSAGE V (Questions 91-96)
    A thermodynamic system comprised of a non-ideal gas is taken through the cycle shown below as a P - V diagram. The process from state c to state a is adiabatic

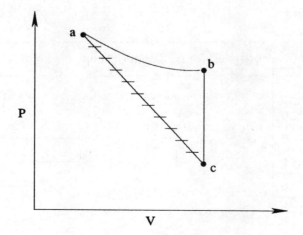

and requires that 500 J of work be done on the gas. Getting to state a from state b, however, requires that 750 J of work be done on the gas along the isothermal path shown during which time 300 J of heat flows out of the gas. The process from state b to state c takes place at constant volume.

91. How much work is done by the gas during one complete cycle traversed counterclockwise?

    (A) 0 J   (B) 250 J

    (C) - 250 J   (D) - 1, 250 J

92. What is the change in the internal energy of the gas during the process from state a to state b?

    (A) 0 J   (B) 1050 J

    (C) 450 J   (D) - 450 J

93. How much heat is absorbed by the gas during the process from state c to state a?

    (A) 500 J   (B) 250 J

    (C) 0 J   (D) - 250 J

94. What is the change in the internal energy of the gas during the process from state c to state a?

    (A) 500 J   (B) - 500 J

    (C) 0 J   (D) 750 J

95. How much heat flows out of the gas during the process from state b to state c?

    (A) 300 J   (B) 50 J

    (C) 0 J   (D) 250 J

96. What is the change in the internal energy of the gas during any complete cycle?

    (A) 0 J   (B) 250 J

    (C) - 250 J   (D) 1,250 J

QUESTIONS 97-104 are NOT based on a descriptive passage.

---

97. Consider the general thin lens problem where the object sits in medium n_0, the convex lens is made of material n_r, and the image is found in medium n_i. If the curvature radii are R_1 and R_2 as shown, then find the secondary focal length f'.

    (A) $f' = -n_0/[(n_r - n_0)/R_1 + (n_i - n_r)/R_2]$

    (B) $f' = n_i/[(n_r - n_0)/R_1 + (n_i - n_r)/R_2]$

    (C) $f' = n_i/[(n_i - n_r)/R_1 + (n_r - n_0)/R_2]$

    (D) $f' = -n_0/[(n_i - n_r)/R_1 + (n_r - n_0)/R_2]$

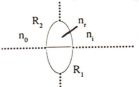

98. A block of mass m moving at speed v collides with a spring of restoring force $F = -k_1 x - k_2 x^3$ on a frictionless surface. Find the maximum compression of the spring.

(A) $k_1 / k_2 \left(\sqrt{1 + mv^2 k_2 / k_1^2} - 1 \right)$

(B) $\sqrt{k_1 / k_2} \left(\sqrt{1 + mv^2 k_2 / k_1^2} - 1 \right)^{1/2}$

(C) $k_1 / k_2 \left(\sqrt{1 + 2mv^2 k_2 / k_1^2} - 1 \right)$

(D) $\sqrt{k_1 / k_2} \left(\sqrt{1 + 2mv^2 k_2 / k_1^2} - 1 \right)^{1/2}$

99. Calculate the vector force due to a potential energy $U = kr^n$.

(A) $-knr^{n-2} \mathbf{r}$ (B) $-knr^{n-1} \mathbf{r}$

(C) $+knr^{n-2} \mathbf{r}$ (D) $+knr^{n-1} \mathbf{r}$

100. The μ-meson has the same charge as the electron, but a greater mass $m_\mu = 207 \, m_e$. Use Bohr theory to find the radius of a μ-mesonic atom with nucleus of charge Ze orbited by the μ^- as compared to the radius of the hydrogen-like atom.

(A) $r_\mu = 207 \, r_H$ (B) $r_\mu = 207^2 \, r_H$

(C) $r_\mu = r_H / 207$ (D) $r_\mu = r_H / 207^2$

101. Which of the following is a characteristic of an exothermic reaction?

(A) The potential energy of the reactants is lower than the potential energy of the products.

(B) There is a positive ΔH.

(C) There is no energy of activation.

(D) None of the above.

102. Suppose that a man jumps off a building 202 m high onto cushions having a total thickness of 2m. If the cushions are crushed to a thickness of 0.5 m, what is the man's acceleration as he slows down?

(A) 133 g

(B) 5 g

(C) 2 g

(D) 266 g

103. Tom has a mass of 70 kg and Suzy has a mass of 60 kg. They are separated by a distance of 0.5 m at a wine and cheese party. What is the gravitational potential energy of the Tom-Suzy system?

(A) 1.12×10^{-6} J   (B) -1.12×10^{-6} J

(C) 5.60×10^{-7} J   (D) -5.60×10^{-7} J

104. The principle that stated that a population remained genetically stable in succeeding generations was the

    (A) Hardy-Weinberg principle.

    (B) Darwinian principle.

    (C) Mendelian principle.

    (D) Avery, McLeod and McCarty principle.

PASSAGE VI (Questions 105-114)

Experiment 1

The following data was obtained when the reaction below was studied:

$$2A + B + 3C \longleftrightarrow Products$$

Initial Rate	[A]	[B]	[C]
3	1	1	1
6	2	1	1
27	1	1	3
3	1	4	1

Experiment 2

The concentrations of B and C were kept constant and the concentration of A was observed over time.

Time, min	[A]
0	0.400
10	0.300
20	0.200
30	0.150
40	0.100
50	0.075
60	0.500

Experiment 3

A given set of concentrations of A, B, and C was used to determine the rate of the reaction at various temperatures.

Temperature (°C)	$k(L\ mol^{-1}\ s^{-1})$
283	1.2×10^{-4}
302	3.5×10^{-4}
355	6.8×10^{-3}
393	1.8×10^{-2}
430	1.7×10^{-1}

105. The rate of disappearance of A should be _____ the rate of disappearance of B while the disappearance of C should be _____ the rate of disappearance of B.

    (A) twice ... twice

    (B) twice ... triple

    (C) one-half ... one-third

    (D) one-half ... one-half

106. What is the relationship between the concentration of A and the initial rate of the reaction?

    (A) Directly proportional   (B) Inversely proportional

    (C) No obvious relationship   (D) Linearly related

107. Tripling the concentration of C _____ the initial rate of the reaction by a factor of _____.

    (A) increases ... 3   (B) increases ... 9

    (C) increases ... 2   (D) No obvious relationship

108. Combine the answers to Questions 105 and 106 with the effect of increasing the concentration of B by a factor of 4 in order to determine the rate law for this reaction. The rate law is

    (A) rate = k[A] [B] [C]^2 (B) rate = k[A]^2 [C]

    (C) rate = k[A] [C]^2 (D) rate = k[A]^2 [B] [C]^3

109. The overall order of this reaction is

    (A) 6.   (B) 4.

    (C) 5.   (D) 3.

110. Using the order of the reaction as determined in Question 108, one of the mechanisms for the reaction might be a one-step _____ collision.

    (A) unimolecular   (B) bimolecular

    (C) termolecular   (D) six-bodied

111. What kind of graph of concentration A versus time might be used to prove that the rate law determined in Question 108 holds true for the relationship between the rate of the reaction and the concentration of A?

    (A) [A] versus time gives a straight line

    (B) [B] versus 1/time gives a straight line

    (C) 1/[A] versus time gives a straight line

    (D) ln [A] versus time gives a straight line

112. How much faster will a reaction be at 65°C compared to the same reaction at 25°C?

    (A) 4 times   (B) 8 times

    (C) 16 times   (D) 2 times

113. If the rate constant at 35°C is three times the reaction rate at 15°C, what is the activation energy in kJ for this reaction? How should the data presented in the passage be graphed to obtain the best value for the activation energy?

    (A) 9.13×10^4 ... ln 1/T versus k

    (B) 8.38×10^1 ... ln k versus $1/T$

    (C) 8.38×10^1 ... ln $1/T$ versus k

    (D) 9.13×10^4 ... ln k versus $1/T$

114. Adding a catalyst to a reaction mixture _____ the rate of the reaction because the catalyst _____ and _____ the energy of activation for the reaction.

    (A)   increases ...   changes the mechanism ... increases

    (B)   increases ... changes the mechanism ... decreases

    (C)   increases ... has no effect on the mechanism ... increases

    (D)   decreases ... changes the mechanism ... decreases

PASSAGE VII (Questions 115–119)

    A 1.5 V dry cell battery with internal resistance (r) is connected in series with an external resistor (R) and an ammeter as shown in the figure below. A current of 0.15 A is measured. A voltmeter is also attached at the terminals of the battery, as shown. With the circuit connected, it records a value of 1.40 V. When the circuit is broken, i.e., when the resistor is disconnected from the battery, the voltmeter records a value of 1.50 V.

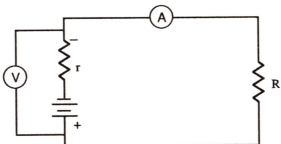

115. The voltage reading of 1.5 V recorded when the circuit is broken is called the _____ of the battery.

    (A)   energy   (B)   electromotive force

    (C)   power   (D)   equipotential

116. The value of the external resistance is

    (A) $10 \ \Omega$ (B) $8.50 \ \Omega$

    (C) $0.21 \ \Omega$ (D) $9.33 \ \Omega$

117. The value of the internal resistance of the battery is

    (A) $9.33 \ \Omega$ (B) $0.67 \ \Omega$

    (C) $1.50 \ \Omega$ (D) $10 \ \Omega$

118. The heat generated in the battery each minute is

    (A)   0.9 J   (B)   13.5 J

    (C)   0 J   (D)   2.03 J

119. When two identical dry cell batteries are placed in series with a 20Ω external resistor the resulting current in the circuit will be

    (A)   0.15 A   (B)   0.30 A

    (C)   0.14 A   (D)   0.28 A

PASSAGE VIII (Questions 120-125)

    A converging lens of focal length $f_1 = +20$ cm is located 10 cm to the left of a diverging lens of focal length $f_2 = -15$ cm. A 10 cm tall object is placed 40 cm to the left of the converging lens. The image produced by the converging lens (as if it were alone) will act as the object for the diverging lens.

120. If the diverging lens were not there, the image would be located _____ the converging lens.

    (A)   40 cm to the left of

    (B)   20 cm to the right of

    (C)   40 cm to the right of

    (D)   at infinity to the right of

121. If the diverging lens were not there, the image would be

    (A)   inverted and smaller than the object.

    (B)   inverted and the same size as the object.

    (C)   upright and larger than the object.

    (D)   not visible at all.

122. The diverging lens acts to

    (A)   confine the region for viewing the object.

    (B)   magnify the object.

    (C)   intensify the object.

    (D)   produce a virtual image of the object.

123. The object for the diverging lens is

    (A)   the same as that for the converging lens.

    (B)   real and upright.

    (C)   virtual and inverted.

    (D)   Does not exist

124. The final image produced by the combined system is located

    (A)   20 cm to the left of the converging lens.

    (B)   30 cm to the right of the diverging lens.

(C)   10 cm to the right of the diverging lens.

(D)   at infinity to the left of the diverging lens.

125.   The total magnification of the system is

(A) $-\frac{1}{3}$ (B) $+\frac{2}{3}$

(C) -1 (D) $+1$

PASSAGE IX (Questions 126-135)
Use the following data to answer the questions.

Acid Solutions:

Half Reactions					E° (volts)
Ca^{2+}	+	$2e^-$	$\longrightarrow$	Ca	- 2.9
Na^{1+}	+	$1e^-$	$\longrightarrow$	Na	- 2.7
Al^{3+}	+	$3e^-$	$\longrightarrow$	Al	- 1.7
Mn^{2+}	+	$2e^-$	$\longrightarrow$	Mn	- 1.2
Zn^{2+}	+	$2e^-$	$\longrightarrow$	Zn	- 0.8
Cu^{2+}	+	$2e^-$	$\longrightarrow$	Cu	+ 0.3
I_2 (s)	+	$2e^-$	$\longrightarrow$	$2I^-$	+ 0.5
$PtCl_4^{2-}$	+	$2e^-$	$\longrightarrow$	$Pt + 4Cl^-$	+0.7
Ag^{1+}	+	$1e^-$	$\longrightarrow$	Ag	+0.8
O_2 (g) + $4H^+$	+	$4e^-$	$\longrightarrow$	$2 H_2O$ (l)	+1.23
Cr_2O_7	+	$6e^-$	$\longrightarrow$	$2 Cr^{3+}$	+1.33
Cl_2 (g)	+	$2e^-$	$\longrightarrow$	$2 Cl^-$	+1.36
MnO_4^-	+	$5e^-$	$\longrightarrow$	Mn^{2+}	+1.51

Experiment 1
At STP, a chemist performed the following reaction:

$$Al + PtCl_4^{-2} \longrightarrow Al^{3+} + Pt + Cl^-$$

Experiment 2
The following reaction was performed at 25°C and one atmosphere:

$$Na + Mn^{+2} \longrightarrow Na^{+1} + Mn$$

Experiment 3

$$Mn \mid 0.1\ M\ Mn(NO_3)_3 \mid\mid\ 0.1\ m\ AgNO_3 \mid Ag$$

126.   Which of the following is a spontaneous reaction?

(A) $Mn^{2+} + MnO_4^-$ (B) $Zn^{2+} + Ag$

(C) $Ag^{1+} + Cl_2$ (D) $Na + I_2$

127. Consider the reaction in Experiment 1. What are the coefficients when this equation is balanced?

(A) 2, 3, 2, 3, 12

(B) 1, 1, 1, 1, 4

(C) 2, 1, 1, 1, 4

(D) 1, 2, 1, 2, 8

128. In Experiment 1, _____ is oxidized and _____ is the oxidizing agent.

(A) Al ... Al

(B) Al ... $PtCl_4^{2-}$

(C) $PtCl_4^{2-}$ ... Al

(D) $PtCl_4^{2-}$ ... Pt

129. What is the emf of the cell in Experiment 1 if all the aqueous species are at unit concentration?

(A) - 2.4

(B) 2.4

(C) 6.5

(D) - 6.5

130. Which of the following is the approximate answer for the equilibrium constant for the reaction in Experiment 2?

(A) 10^{25}

(B) 10^{51}

(C) 10^{183}

(D) 10^{-52}

131. What is the change in the Gibbs free energy ($\Delta G°$) for the reaction in Experiment 1?

(A) - 2.32 × 10^5 kJ

(B) 2.32 × 10^5 kJ

(C) - 1.39 × 10^6 kJ

(D) 1.39 × 10^6 kJ

132. How many grams of aluminum will be removed if a current of 5.0 amperes is passed through an aqueous solution of aluminum chloride for 30.0 minutes?

(A) 2.5

(B) 0.84

(C) 1.2

(D) 3.6

133. If the concentrations of $PtCl_4^{2-}$, Al^{3+}, and Cl^- are all 0.10 M, what will the emf of the cell be?

(A) 2.4

(B) 2.5

(C) 2.6

(D) 2.3

134. Consider the cell that was set up in Experiment 3: Manganese is the _____ and reduction takes place at the _____ electrode.

(A) anode ... Mn

(B) anode ... Ag

(C) cathode ... Mn

(D) cathode ... Ag

135. Which of the following substances will oxidize Zn?

(A) Na^{1+}

(B) Cu

(C) Cl^-

(D) I_2

QUESTIONS 136-142 are NOT based on a descriptive passage.

136. Hydrolysis of protein peptide bonds produces

(A) glucosides.

(B) carboxylic acids.

(C) amino acids.

(D) glucose monomers.

137. Which of the following compounds is the weakest acid?

(A) NH_3

(B) $(CH_3)_2 NH$

(C) CH_3OH

(D) CH_3CH_2ONa

138. What is the product, after hydroloysis, when methyl iodide is treated with magnesium in ether and the product reacts with ethylene oxide?

(A) $CH_3(CH_2)_3OH$

(B) $CH_3CH_2CH_2OH$

(C) $CH_3CHOHCH_3$

(D) $CH_3CH_2COCH_3$

139. Which carbohydrate, whose solubility in water increases upon addition of dilute HCl, does not have a sweet taste?

(A) Monosaccharides

(B) Disaccharides

(C) Glucose

(D) Polysaccharides

140. $H_2(g)$ reacts with $I_2(g)$ to give HI(g) at 700°K. However, when X is introduced to the system, it is observed that the reaction now occurs at the same rate at 400°K. X is a(n)

(A) substitution agent.

(B) linking agent.

(C) enzyme.

(D) catalyst.

141. The salt produced by the equimolar reaction of acetic acid with sodium hydroxide is

(A) neutral.

(B) acidic.

(C) alkaline.

(D) aprotic.

142. One mole of hemiacetal is produced by reacting

(A) a self-condensation of two moles of aldehyde.

(B) a mixed-condensation of one mole of aldehyde and one mole of ketone.

(C) two moles of alcohol with one mole of aldehyde.

(D) one mole of alcohol with one mole of aldehyde.

STOP

If time still remains, you may review work only in this section.

When the time allotted is up, you may go on to the next section.

Section 3 — Writing Sample

TIME: 60 minutes
2 Essays, separately timed
30 minutes each

DIRECTIONS: This section tests your writing skills by asking you to write two essays. You will have 30 minutes to write each one.

During the first 30 minutes, work only on the first essay. If you finish it in less than 30 minutes, you may review what you have written, but do not begin the second essay. During the second 30 minutes, work only on the second essay. If you finish it in less than 30 minutes, you may review what you have written for that essay only. Do not go back to the first essay.

Read each assigned topic carefully. Make sure your essays respond to the topics as they are assigned.

Make sure your essays are written in complete sentences and para-graphs, and are as clear as you can make them. Make any corrections or additions between the lines of your essays. Do not write in the margins.

On the day of the test, you are given three pages to write each essay. You are not required to use all of the space provided, but do not skip lines so you will not waste space. Illegible essays can not be scored.

Part 1

Consider this statement:

"Pens are most dangerous tools, more sharp by odds
Than swords, and cut more keen than whips or rods."

John Taylor (1580-1653)

Write a unified essay in which you perform the following tasks: (1) Explain what you think the above statement means (2) Describe a specific situation in which pens are *not* as powerful as swords (3) Discuss what you think determines whether or not the pen is mightier than the sword.

STOP

If time still remains, you may review work only in this section.

When the time allotted is up, you may go on to the next section.

Part 2

Consider this statement:

"Patience is the strongest of strong drinks, for it kills the giant Despair."

Douglas Jerrold (1803-1857)

Write a unified essay in which you perform the following tasks: (1) Explain what you think the above statement means (2) Describe a specific situation in which patience may *not* overcome despair (3) Discuss what you think determines whether or not patience is the best means of fighting despair.

STOP

If time still remains, you may review work only in this section.

When the time allotted is up, you may go on to the next section.

Section 4 — Biological Sciences

TIME: 100 Minutes
QUESTIONS: 143-219

DIRECTIONS: Most of the questions in this section are arranged in groups, each corresponding to a descriptive passage. Based on the information given in a passage, choose the one best answer to each question in the group. Some questions are independent of a descriptive passage and of each other. Choose the one best answer to each of these questions. If you are not sure of an answer, eliminate those choices that you know are incorrect and choose an answer from among those remaining. Fill in the corresponding circle on the answer sheet to indicate your answer. You may refer to the periodic table at any time.

PASSAGE I (Questions 143-147)

Human pedigrees are used in genetics to study inherited traits. Circles represent females, squares represent males. Parents are joined by a horizontal line between their symbols; sibling offspring are suspended below their parents from a horizontal line. The symbols of individuals affected by a specific genetic trait are darkened in as shown below.

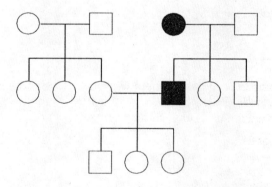

Pedigree A

143. *Could* the trait indicated in the pedigree A above be caused by a sex-linked gene?

(A)   No, this trait could not be sex-linked.

(B)   Yes, this trait could be due to a sex-linked dominant gene.

(C)   Yes, this trait could be due to a sex-linked recessive gene.

(D)   Yes, this trait appears to be due to a holandric sex-linked gene.

144. *Could* the trait indicated in the pedigree A above be caused by an autosomal gene?

    (A)   Yes, an autosomal dominant gene could cause this trait.

    (B)   Yes, an autosomal recessive gene could cause this trait.

    (C)   No, an autosomal gene could not account for this pedigree.

    (D)   Yes, (A) and (B) are true.

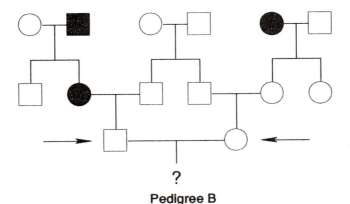

Pedigree B

145. If the trait concerned in the pedigree B above is caused by an autosomal recessive gene, what is the probability that the couple indicated by the arrows will have an affected child? (They plan to have just one child.)

    (A)   zero   (B) $1/4$

    (C) $(1/2)^3$ or $1/8$ (D) $1/4 \times 1/4$ or $1/16$

146. If the trait concerned in the pedigree B above is caused by a sex-linked dominant gene, what is the probability that the couple indicated by the arrows will have an affected child? (They will have only one child.)

    (A) $(1/2)^2$ or 14

    (B)   zero

    (C) $1/2$ for males; zero for females

    (D)   Probability cannot be determined from this pedigree.

147. If the trait concerned in pedigree C (shown on the following page) is caused by a sex-linked recessive gene, what is the change that the couple indicated by the arrows would have an affected child?

    (A) $(1/2)^2$ (B) $(1/2)^3$

    (C) $(1/2)^4$ (D) $(1/2)^5$

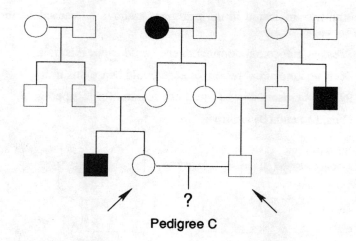

Pedigree C

PASSAGE II (Questions 148-153)

Male animals produce gametes by a process called spermatogenesis which involves two meiotic divisions and a maturation process. The overall result is the production of haploid sperm from a diploid organism. Humans have a diploid chromosomal number of 46.

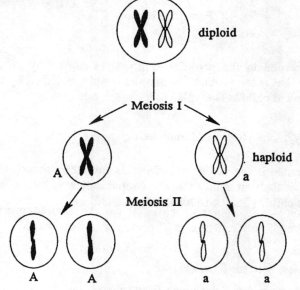

Overview of Meiosis
(Spermatogenesis in a hypothetical animal with 2N = 2)

148. In the human male, how many chromosomes would be present in a primary spermatocyte at Prophase I?

(A)   23

(B)   46

(C)   92

(D)   No chromosomes would be present, only chromatids.

149. In the human male, how many chromosomes would be present in a primary spermatocyte at Anaphase I?

    (A) 23

    (B) 46

    (C) 92

    (D) No chromosomes would be present, only chromatids.

150. In the human male, how many chromosomes would be present in a secondary spermatocyte at Anaphase II?

    (A) 23

    (B) 46

    (C) 92

    (D) No chromosomes would be present, only chromatids.

151. In the human male, how many sperm would come from four secondary spermatocytes?

    (A) 4

    (B) 8

    (C) 16

    (D) None; sperm come from primary spermatocytes.

152. In the human male, the following cells are haploid:

    (A) spermatid, sperm.

    (B) primary spermatocyte after Metaphase I.

    (C) secondary spermatocyte.

    (D) Only (A) and (C).

153. Following meoisis II, in oogenesis, one cell becomes the mature ovum. The other cells produced do not function as gametes and are known as

    (A) Barr bodies.   (B) polar bodies.

    (C) basal bodies.   (D) vitreous bodies.

PASSAGE III (Questions 154-158)

The cell membranes of living systems maintain an internal environment which is distinct from the external environment. The tubes below have selectively permeable membranes at their bottoms. The test tubes initially contain 10 ml of:

Test tube	Solution
A	distilled water
B	0.5% glucose in water
C	1.0% glucose in water

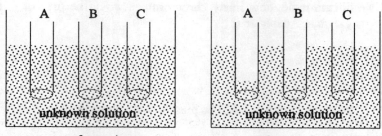

at start of experiment   after two hours

The results after two hours are shown in the above figure. Refer to these figures to answer the following questions.

154. The difference in the amount of solution in each of the tubes after two hours shows that

   (A) tube A initially had a hypotonic solution compared to the unknown solution.

   (B) tube A initially had a hypertonic solution compared to the unknown solution.

   (C) the tube C solution is isotonic to that of the unknown.

   (D) Both (A) and (C)

155. What is the concentration of the unknown solution?

   (A) 100% water

   (B) 99.5% water

   (C) 99.0% water

   (D) Cannot be determined from the information provided.

156. If a red blood cell is placed in a hypertonic solution,

   (A) the cell will shrink as water moves out.

   (B) the cell will swell as water moves inward.

   (C) the cell will maintain its shape by osmosis.

   (D) the cell will maintain its shape but its organelles will collapse inward.

157. If a cell is placed in a solution which has a concentration of solutes lower than that in the cell, the solution is said to be

   (A) hypotonic.   (B) hypertonic.

   (C) isotonic.   (D) osmotic.

158. Without expending energy, molecules can move into or out of cells by

   (A) passing though pores formed by pore proteins in the plasma membrane.

   (B) binding to a carrier protein in the plasma membrane.

(C)   diffusing though the lipid phase of the plasma membrane.

(D)   All of the above.

PASSAGE IV (Questions 159-164)

Gel electrophoresis of proteins has shown a surprising amount of diversity at the molecular level. The majority of proteins which exhibit polymorphism have only two alleles, one whose "fast" allozyme migrates rapidly compared to the other "slow" allozyme. These allozymes (variant forms of an enzyme) are often not known to confer different degrees of fitness. A population of fruit flies was examined, and "fast" and "slow" esterases were subsequently found. A representative gel electrophoretogram of six individuals' esterases is below.

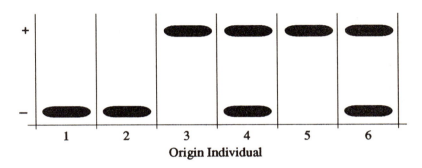

Origin Individual

159.   From the above electrophoretogram, it can be concluded that

(A)   individual #4 is heterozygous for different versions of this enzyme (allozymes).

(B)   individuals #1 and #2 only have the slow allozyme and are therefore less fit.

(C)   the most adaptive phenotype would be shown by individuals #3 and #5.

(D)   None of the above statements are correct.

160.   The relationship between different allozymes is

(A)   they are the products of different alleles.

(B)   they catalyze the same reaction.

(C)   Both (A) and (B).

(D)   None of the above.

161.   If the "slow" allozyme could only function within the lower part of the range of normal temperatures, and the "fast" allozyme functioned throughout this temperature range,

(A)   the "slow allozyme homozygote would be considered to be the most "fit" phenotype.

(B)   the "fast" allozyme homozygote would be considered to be the most "fit" phenotype.

(C)   the heterozygote would be the least fit phenotype.

(D)   the allozyme constitution of an individual would not be related to fitness.

162. The results of electrophretic studies such as described above indicate that

(A)   genotypes are not relevant to fitness.

(B)   Darwinian fitness does not apply at the molecular level.

(C)   genetic variability at the molecular level is commonly found in biological populations.

(D)   None of the above.

163. The rate at which a protein migrates in an electrical field

(A)   is related to its catalytic efficiency.

(B)   is related to its fitness.

(C)   is related to its primary structure.

(D)   Both (A) and (B).

164. If the "fast" allozyme only worked in the upper half of the normal temperature range and the "slow" allozyme only worked in the lower half of the normal temperature range,

(A)   this would be an example of heterosis.

(B)   balancing selection would work against both types of homozygotes.

(C)   the heterozygous phenotype would be most fit.

(D)   All of the above statements are correct.

QUESTIONS 165-170 are NOT based on a descriptive passage.

---

165. Following fertilization, the zygote undergoes a series of rapid mitotic divisions. The stage at which a solid ball of cells is formed is called

(A)   the morula.   (B)   the blastula.

(C)   the gastrula.   (D)   the fetus.

166. The area of the brain responsible for coordinating voluntary muscle movement is the

(A)   cerebrum.   (B)   cerebellum.

(C)   thalamus.   (D)   hypothalamus.

167. Pepsin requires _____ for proper activity.

(A)   vitamin C   (B)   enzymes

(C)   acidity   (D)   basicity

168. Enzymes

    (A)   are consumed in a reaction.

    (B)   change the final equilibrium point.

    (C)   provide heat.

    (D)   lower the activation energy required for a reaction.

169. Which of the following sequences describes the blood clotting process correctly?

    (A)   Damaged platelets + Ca⁺⁺ $\xrightarrow{enzyme}$ prothrombin $\xrightarrow{enzyme}$ fibrinogen → fibrin.

    (B)   Damaged platelets + Ca⁺⁺ → prothrombin $\xrightarrow{enzyme}$ fibrinogen → fibrin

    (C)   Damaged platelets + Ca⁺⁺ $\xrightarrow{enzyme}$ prothrombin $\xrightarrow{enzyme}$ fibrin → fibrinogen

    (D)   Damaged platelets + Na⁺ → thromboplastin → thrombin → fibrinogen → fibrin

170.   One of the simplest kinds of behavior is the knee jerk, in which a tap below the knee causes the leg to jerk up. This behavior requires as a minimum which of the following combination of structures?

    (A)   A motor neuron and a muscle

    (B)   A receptor and at least two segments of the spinal chord

    (C)   A receptor neuron, a motor neuron, and a muscle.

    (D)   An intact spinal cord and a brain

PASSAGE V (Questions 171-175)

Evolution is a central concept in biology. Understanding biology requires the study of genes in populations and the mechanisms which may result in genetic diversity, speciation, or extinction. In Hardy-Weinberg genetic equilibrium, gene and genotypic frequencies remain constant over many generations. If there were two different alleles for a particular locus, the frequency of the dominant allele "A" would be termed "p," and that of the recessive allele "a" would be called "q."

The diploid generation would be distributed with the frequencies p^2 for AA, 2pq for Aa, and q^2 for aa. These frequencies would remain the same generation after generation as long as there were no forces which disturbed this equilibrium. Disturbance could come from random events in small populations, genetic changes, assortative mating and natural selection. Evolution would never occur if populations remained in genetic equilibrium. Darwin's "Theory of Natural Selection" is the principal, unifying concept which provides the framework for ongoing biological studies today. The theory could be summarized as "differential reproduction of genetic variants results in evolutionary change."

Although many gene frequency changes may be due to genetic drift, selection is a significant factor in effecting evolutionary changes. Darwin provided the theoretical basis for the development of population genetics. Molecular biologists as well as naturalists actively study evolutionary biology today.

171. Darwin's theory of natural selection, the "survival of the fittest" as it is understood today,

    (A) is generally understood to refer to the progressive evolution of larger, stronger organisms.

    (B) refers to the relative ability of individuals with different genotypes to have different reproductive success.

    (C) has been replaced by the concept of punctuated equilibrium.

    (D) None of the above.

172. Of the following, which is NOT an assumption for Hardy-Weinberg genetic equilibrium?

    (A) No selection

    (B) Large population size

    (C) Non migration/genetic exchange with other populations

    (D) Non random mating

173. Random fluctuations in gene frequencies due to small population size is called

    (A) genetic equilibrium.   (B) heterosis.

    (C) genetic drift.   (D) natural selection.

174. Selection which acts to remove one extreme in a distribution of phenotypes is called

    (A) disruptive selection.   (B) balancing selection.

    (C) macroselection.   (D) directional selection.

175. Selection acts upon

    (A) populations.   (B) individual phenotypes.

    (C) species.   (D) genes.

PASSAGE VI (Questions 176-181)

If an organism is to grow, mature, replace injured or worn-out parts, cellular division must occur. The process of nuclear division which results in two identical daughter nuclei is called mitosis. Cytokinesis refers to the division of the cytoplasm. These complex components of cell division usually occur simultaneously, but they can occur independently. Both processes are controlled by intricate interactions between genes, their products and environmental factors. The following questions concern mitosis and cytokinesis.

176. The stage at which chromosomes condense by coiling tightly is called

    (A) prophase.   (B) metaphase.

    (C) anaphase.   (D) telophase.

177. The constricted area at which two identical chromatids are joined is called the

    (A) centriole.

    (B) centrosome.

    (C) centromere.

    (D) centrochore.

178. If the somatic chromosome number of a species is 46, how many chromosomes would be present in a cell during anaphase?

    (A) 23

    (B) 46

    (C) 92

    (D) None of the above.

179. The stage during which chromosomes replicate is

    (A) prophase.

    (B) metaphase.

    (C) anaphase.

    (D) interphase.

180. The protein structure to which spindle microtubules attach is the

    (A) centromere.

    (B) centriole.

    (C) centrosome.

    (D) kinetochore.

181. Animal cells usually undergo cytokinesis by

    (A) a contractile ring of actin filaments which cleaves one cell into two.

    (B) the phragmoplast forming a telophase furrow.

    (C) the formation of a cell plate across the equator.

    (D) binary fission.

PASSAGE VII (Questions 182-187)

Organisms have evolved mechanisms to defend themselves against foreign invaders. Vertebrates have a variety of types of white blood cells which respond to

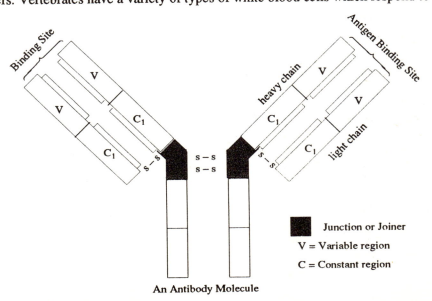

An Antibody Molecule

Junction or Joiner

V = Variable region

C = Constant region

foreign molecules. These cells come from stem cells in the bone marrow. Any specific immune cell can only make *one* kind of antibody. Mammals have immune cells which can produce antibodies which specifically react with virtually any foreign substance — the potential to form billions of different antibodies, more types of antibodies than the total number of genes in the organism. An illustration of an antibody molecule is above

182. The vertebrate immune response involves the following different types of cells which respond in a highly specific manner.

    (A)   Erythrocytes and phagocytes

    (B)   T cells and B cells

    (C)   Reticulocytes and phagocytes

    (D)   Both (A) and (B).

183. The Y-shaped antibody molecule is produced by

    (A)   infected cells.   (B)   T cells.

    (C)   B cells.   (D)   phagocytes.

184. The Y-shaped antibody molecule consists of how many different types of polypeptides?

    (A)   1   (B)   2

    (C)   3   (D)   4

185. Cell-mediated immunity is the function of

    (A)   T cells.   (B)   B cells.

    (C)   phagocytes.   (D)   reticulocytes.

186. The antibody molecule illustrated

    (A)   could bind two different kinds of antigens.

    (B)   could only bind one kind of antigen.

    (C)   is a dimer which could bind one particular type of antigen at two different sites.

    (D)   Both (B) and (C).

187. Using your knowledge of the variability of immunoglobulin structure, select the variants that are present in all members of a species.

    (A)   Allotypes   (B)   Idiotypes

    (C)   Isotypes   (D)   Phenotypes

PASSAGE VIII (Questions 188-192)
    Early microscopists discovered that every animal and plant tissue consisted of small units called cells. All living organisms are composed of one or more cells, the

basic units of biological structure and function. Various structures and organelles have evolved to support the life processes of cells. In order to understand how an organism lives and interacts with its environment, one must understand the cell.

188. There are many different kinds of cells, but all cells share the following features.

(A) mitochondria and nuclei

(B) endoplasmic reticulum and centrioles

(C) a plasma membrane and DNA genetic information

(D) All of the above.

189. The eukayotic plasma membrane basically is a bilayer of

(A) proteins.

(B) glycopeptides.

(C) phospholipids.

(D) phosphopetides.

190. The function of the nucleous is to

(A) produce ribosomal subunits.

(B) orient the cellular poles during cytokinesis.

(C) store messenger RNA before transport to the endoplasmic reticulum.

(D) process, package and store lipids and proteins for the nuclear membrane.

191. The mitochondria is the organelle which

(A) has the enzymes and cofactors for the process known as respiration.

(B) is descended from other mitochondria.

(C) breaks down organic molecules, coupling these catabolic reactions with energy-capturing reactions which store this energy in other molecules to be used for other cellular processes.

(D) All of the above.

192. The following structures are all part of a continuous network of membraneous tubes, flattened sacs, and channels found in eukaryotic cells.

(A) Golgi complex, vesicles, rough endoplasmic reticulum, perosixomes

(B) Rough endoplasmic reticulum, smooth endoplasmic reticulum, Golgi complex

(C) Endoplasmic reticulum, lysosomes, mitochondria, Golgi complex

(D) Nuclear membrane pores, vesicles, microtubules

QUESTIONS 193-197 are NOT based on a descriptive passage.

193. Which of the following molecules is thought to block the myosin (cross bridge) binding site on actin when a muscle fiber is not contracting?

(A) Calcium

(B) Troponin

(C) Tropomyosin

(D) ATP

194. To find the genetic order of three bacterial genes we do not need to know the

(A) number of wild-type cells.

(B) frequency of recombination.

(C) dominance and recessiveness of the alleles.

(D) number of double cross-over events.

195. In the kidneys, blood plasma is filtered from the capillaries into the

(A) lymphatic system.

(B) renal artery.

(C) distal convoluted tubule.

(D) Bowman's capsule.

196. During development, the stage in which there is a hollow ball of cells is called

(A) gastrulation.

(B) blastulation.

(C) morulation.

(D) the isolecithal stage.

197. A harmless animal that represents another species that is dangerous to a predator is an example of

(A) Mullerian mimicry.

(B) Batesian mimicry.

(C) cryptic appearance.

(D) mutualism.

PASSAGE IX (Questions 198-203)

In organisms that reproduce asexually, nuclear division is accomplished by mitosis and each of the daughter cells receives an exact copy of the parental genetic material. All of the offspring of asexual reproduction are essentially genetically identical, resulting in little if any genetic variability among different generations.

Sexually reproducing species, however, exhibit a high degree of genetic variability. This variability is due mainly to the process of meiosis during which gamete formation occurs. Meiosis differs from mitosis in that the daughter cells contain only half the number of chromosomes of the parental cells. This is necessary to insure that the chromosome number of a species remains constant since sexual reproduction involves the union of two gametes. The zygote formed in this manner will then have the full complement of chromosomes.

Human cells contain two copies of each chromosome type (1 maternal and 1 paternal), each of which contains slight variants of the same genes. There are 46 total chromosomes, or 23 pairs of chromosomes, in each cell. During the first meiotic division, the pairs of homologous chromosomes segregate randomly into daughter cells. Each daughter cell therefore contains some chromosomes of maternal origin and some of paternal origin. During the second meiotic division, the two chromatids that make up each chromosome separate and assort randomly into daughter cells. The number of possible chromosomal combinations which can result simply because of random assortment of chromosomes and chromatics is 2^n, where n is the number of pairs of chromosomes. In humans, the number of possible combinations is 2^{23}, or 8,388,608. The number of possible chromosomal combinations that can result when two gametes unite to form a zygote is $(2^n)^2$. Thus, it can be seen how the events which occur during meiosis increase the number of different genetic combinations and hence contribute to the potentially high genetic variability in a sexually reproducing species.

198. A clone, which is a group of genetically identical organisms derived from a single parent, is a result of which type of division?

    (A) Cytokinesis   (B) Meiosis

    (C) Reduction   (D) Mitosis

199. Which of the following statements best describes one of the major benefits of sexual reproduction?

    (A) The genetic variability associated with sexual reproduction allows a species to readily adapt to a changing environment.

    (B) The genetic variability associated with sexual reproduction is of great importance in an unchanging environment for species continuity.

    (C) Chromosome number remains constant, unlike asexual reproduction in which chromosome number doubles with each generation.

    (D) All of the progeny of sexual reproduction will be genetically identical.

200. In a cell containing 3 pairs of chromosomes, how many possible chromosomal combinations exist for each daughter cell?

    (A) 64   (B) 8

    (C) 16   (D) 3

201. In which of the following cases would asexual reproduction be more advantageous than sexual reproduction?

    (A) Gypsy moths subjected to an annual spraying using a variety of pesticides

    (B) Cabbage cultivated for its high disease resistance

    (C) Migratory birds exposed to widely varying environmental conditions

    (D) Orange trees transplanted from a native habitat to a foreign land

202. One of the important events that occurs during meiosis, but not in mitosis is

    (A) replication of the chromosomal material.

    (B) a doubling of the chromosome number.

    (C)   a reduction by half of the chromosome number.

    (D)   nuclear division.

203. During prophase of the first meiotic division, chromatids of homologous chromosomes often exchange parts, a process known as crossing over. How does this affect genetic variability?

    (A)   It increases genetic variability to a greater extent than random assortment alone.

    (B)   It decreases genetic variability by producing daughter cells that are very similar to each other.

    (C)   It does not affect genetic variability because homologous chromosomes are exactly alike.

    (D)   It decreases genetic variability by reducing the possible number of chromosomal combinations.

PASSAGE X (Questions 204-209)

    10 grams of iodine (I_2) were added to 10 grams of acetone in a 500 cc flask. 1.6 molar sodium hydroxide was added slowly to the flask with through mixing. The reaction was kept cool, and proceeded until the brown color of the iodine was gone, and all that remained was a yellow solution and a yellow precipitate.

204. The yellow precipitate is most likely

    (A)   sodium iodide.   (B)   iodoform.

    (C)   sodium acetate.   (D)   None of the above.

205. If radioactive iodine were used in the reaction, where in the products would the radioactivity be found?

    (A)   Precipitate   (B)   Supernatant

    (C)   Both (A) and (B).   (D)   It cannot be determined

206. If radioactive sodium (in the form of sodium hydroxide) were used in the reaction, where in the products would the radioactivity be found?

    (A)   Precipitate   (B)   Supernatant

    (C)   Both (A) and (B).   (D)   It cannot be determined

207. If this reaction produces 4.27 grams of the precipitate, what is the efficiency of the reaction?

    (A)   100%   (B)   95.6%

    (C)   95.2%   (D)   82.6%

208. Which of the following will react with the precipitate to produce I_2 gas?

    (A) F_2 (B) Cl_2

    (C) Br_2 (D)   All of the above.

209. If the precipitate were mixed with hexane, the result would be

    (A) $CH_3(CH_2)_4CH_2I$

    (B) $CH_3(CH_2)_3CHICH_3$

    (C) $CH_3(CH_2)_4Cl_3$

    (D) No reaction.

PASSAGE XI (Questions 210-215)

   (-) 2-bromo octane is reacted with sodium hydroxide.

210. The main product is

    (A) (-) 2-octanol.

    (B) (+) 2- octanol.

    (C) (+/-) 2-octanol.

    (D) Some optically *inactive* product.

211. This type of reaction is classified as

    (A) E1.

    (B) E2.

    (C) S_N1.

    (D) S_N2.

212. Which of the following will react in this manner faster than the 2-bromo octane?

    (A) $CH_3(CH_2)_6CH_2NBr$

    (B) $CH_3(CH_2)_4CHBrCH_2CH_3$

    (C) $CH_3(CH_2)_4CBr(CH_3)_2$

    (D) $CH_3(CH_2)_3CHBr(CH_2)_2CH_3$

213. Which of the following will react in this manner slower than the 2-bromo octane?

    (A) $CH_3(CH_2)_6CH_2NBr$

    (B) $CH_3(CH_2)_4CHBrCH_2CH_3$

    (C) $CH_3(CH_2)_4CBr(CH_3)_2$

    (D) $CH_3(CH_2)_3CHBr(CH_2)_2CH_3$

214. Which of the following is true of the above reaction?

    (A) It involves second order kinetics

    (B) It involves an elimination

    (C) Both of the above

    (D) None of the above

215. What will the major product be if (+)2-bromo octane is used?

    (A) (+) 2-bromo octanol

    (B) (-) 2-bromo octanol

    (C) (-) 2-bromo octane

    (D) (+) 2-bromo octane

QUESTIONS 216-219 are NOT based on a descriptive passage.

216. Which reagents should be used to prepare ethers by the Williamson method?

    (A) Primary alcohol, butylchloride and HCl

    (B) Primary alcohol, sodium, HCl

(C)   Sodium borohydride, butylchloride

(D)   None of the above.

217. Which of the following isomers has the lowest vapor pressure?

(A) $CH_3CH_2CH_2CH_2CH_2CH_2CH_2OH$

(B) $CH_3OCH_2CH_2CH_2CH_2CH_3$

(C) $CH_3CH_2OCH_2CH_2CH_2CH_3$

(D) $CH_3CH_2CH_{2O}CH_2CH_2CH_3$

218. What is the structural formula of the hydrogenation product of 2-methyl-2-pentene if deuterium was used as a tracer and Pt as a catalyst?

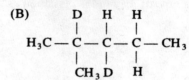

219. Which of the following bond polarity comparisons is false?

(A)   HCL > HBr   (B)   HS > HO

(C)   HF > HO   (D)   IF > BrCl

STOP

If time still remains, you may review work only in this section.

TEST 6

ANSWER KEY

1.	(A)	26.	(B)	51.	(C)	76.	(B)
2.	(B)	27.	(C)	52.	(B)	77.	(B)
3.	(A)	28.	(A)	53.	(A)	78.	(B)
4.	(C)	29.	(D)	54.	(D)	79.	(C)
5.	(D)	30.	(C)	55.	(B)	80.	(A)
6.	(A)	31.	(C)	56.	(C)	81.	(B)
7.	(A)	32.	(A)	57.	(D)	82.	(C)
8.	(C)	33.	(B)	58.	(A)	83.	(D)
9.	(A)	34.	(B)	59.	(C)	84.	(D)
10.	(C)	35.	(C)	60.	(C)	85.	(A)
11.	(A)	36.	(A)	61.	(B)	86.	(D)
12.	(B)	37.	(D)	62.	(A)	87.	(B)
13.	(D)	38.	(B)	63.	(B)	88.	(D)
14.	(D)	39.	(D)	64.	(B)	89.	(D)
15.	(B)	40.	(C)	65.	(A)	90.	(A)
16.	(B)	41.	(D)	66.	(C)	91.	(C)
17.	(D)	42.	(A)	67.	(A)	92.	(D)
18.	(C)	43.	(B)	68.	(A)	93.	(C)
19.	(C)	44.	(C)	69.	(D)	94.	(A)
20.	(C)	45.	(A)	70.	(C)	95.	(B)
21.	(D)	46.	(D)	71.	(C)	96.	(A)
22.	(D)	47.	(C)	72.	(B)	97.	(B)
23.	(B)	48.	(C)	73.	(D)	98.	(D)
24.	(A)	49.	(D)	74.	(D)	99.	(A)
25.	(B)	50.	(A)	75.	(A)	100.	(C)

101.	(D)	131.	(D)	161.	(B)	191.	(D)
102.	(A)	132.	(B)	162.	(C)	192.	(B)
103.	(D)	133.	(A)	163.	(C)	193.	(C)
104.	(A)	134.	(B)	164.	(D)	194.	(C)
105.	(B)	135.	(D)	165.	(A)	195.	(D)
106.	(A)	136.	(C)	166.	(B)	196.	(B)
107.	(B)	137.	(D)	167.	(C)	197.	(B)
108.	(C)	138.	(B)	168.	(D)	198.	(D)
109.	(D)	139.	(D)	169.	(A)	199.	(A)
110.	(C)	140.	(D)	170.	(C)	200.	(B)
111.	(D)	141.	(C)	171.	(B)	201.	(B)
112.	(C)	142.	(D)	172.	(D)	202.	(C)
113.	(B)	143.	(A)	173.	(C)	203.	(A)
114.	(B)	144.	(D)	174.	(D)	204.	(B)
115.	(B)	145.	(C)	175.	(B)	205.	(C)
116.	(D)	146.	(B)	176.	(A)	206.	(B)
117.	(B)	147.	(B)	177.	(C)	207.	(D)
118.	(A)	148.	(B)	178.	(C)	208.	(D)
119.	(C)	149.	(B)	179.	(D)	209.	(D)
120.	(C)	150.	(B)	180.	(D)	210.	(B)
121.	(B)	151.	(B)	181.	(A)	211.	(D)
122.	(D)	152.	(C)	182.	(B)	212.	(A)
123.	(C)	153.	(B)	183.	(C)	213.	(C)
124.	(A)	154.	(D)	184.	(B)	214.	(A)
125.	(D)	155.	(C)	185.	(A)	215.	(C)
126.	(D)	156.	(B)	186.	(D)	216.	(A)
127.	(A)	157.	(A)	187.	(C)	217.	(A)
128.	(B)	158.	(D)	188.	(C)	218.	(A)
129.	(B)	159.	(A)	189.	(C)	219.	(B)
130.	(B)	160.	(C)	190.	(C)		

DETAILED EXPLANATIONS
OF ANSWERS

Section 1 — Verbal Reasoning

PASSAGE I (Questions 1-9)

1.   **(A)**   is correct. While (B) is discussed in the passage, it is an analogy to the distinction being considered, not the distinction itself. The other choices are not discussed in the passage.

2.   **(B)**   is correct. The concluding paragraph of this passage makes this clear and also shows why (A) is not correct. This passage does not consider Moore's views on (C), reasons for acting.

3.   **(A)**   is correct. The second paragraph discusses the relationship between a person's name, a person's gender, and our determination of that person's gender. The name may lead us to a certain belief about the person's gender but it does not determine the person's actual gender.

4.   **(C)**   is correct. Agreement is no guarantee that an action is right, only that everyone believes it to be right. Thus, (A) and (B) are incorrect. As paragraphs 3 and 5 imply, it is possible that everyone will agree that an action is right, while the action is wrong, so (C) is the best answer.

5.   **(D)**   is correct. Referring to paragraphs two and four, it can be seen that there is no necessary connection between belief that an action is wrong and that action's being wrong, so both (A) and (B) are incorrect. Since the passage is not concerned with what people should believe, (C) is also incorrect.

6.   **(A)**   is correct. The facts of a person's upbringing would serve to explain why this person believed as he or she did, but would not explain the truth of the person's belief, so both (B) and (C) should be rejected.

7.   **(A)**   is correct. The distinction set out in the second paragraph points to a difference in factors that may cause or even justify our beliefs and factors that may cause or determine the actual status of something. Since reasons for our belief that something is true do not cause that thing to be true, neither (C) nor (D) follows from this passage. In addition, since we may believe things that are not true, (B) is not correct.

8.   **(C)**   is correct. The fourth and fifth paragraphs show that people can disagree about what is right and that their individual or collective approval does not ensure an action's rightness. Therefore, (A) and (B) should be rejected.

9.   **(A)**   is correct. The fuel gauge is the normal reason we have for holding the belief we do about how much fuel we have. The fuel gauge, however, is not cause of how much fuel we have, so (B) is false. Since (A) and only (A) is true, choices (C) and (D) can be eliminated.

PASSAGE II (Questions 10-19)

10.   **(C)**   The passage states that we can "no longer attribute the increasing decline in our wild animals and plants to "natural processes"; therefore, answers (A) and (B) which include natural processes are incorrect. The passage does not argue against any quotas, unlimited or otherwise; therefore, (D) is incorrect. By process of elimination, (C) is correct.

11.   **(A)**   The passage does not mention popular vote (B), and it offers simple statistics which require no public response (C). While the public may have a chance to comment on the *Federal Register*, it is not a document which needs to be "passed," especially by public vote (D). The passage does mention the accessibility of the *Federal Register* to the public for commentary; therefore, (A) is correct.

12.   **(B)**   While disease among animals is a given reason for the possible decline in animal number, there is no mention of disease as it relates to food supply. The educational, esthetic, and scientific values of wildlife are extolled by Congress' statement which accompanies the passing of the Endangered Species Act of 1973, making (A), (C), (D), true and therefore not the exception.

13.   **(D)**   While it is important to acknowledge the impact of the Endangered Species Act of 1973, answer (A) merely names the act and does not include an explanation of its application. (B) is incorrect because it mentions "public involvement", a topic not covered in this passage. (C) is incorrect not only because it presents again this false public interaction, but it focuses on the United States (the "Nation") and omits the connection with other countries which also honor conservation laws. (D) embodies the topics of why species are endangered, what has been done about it and by whom, making (D) the most complete answer of the four choices.

14.   **(D)**   The passage states that habitat destruction, a man-made force, is the most serious threat to wildlife and plants. To demonstrate the importance and consequence of environment, the author uses the dinosaur to show what natural extinction is as compared to man-made, habitat altering extinction of today. (A) is incorrect because the passage does not focus solely on one particular animal. (B) is incorrect because ancient attitudes are not actually presented in the passage. (C) is incorrect because the government in no way affected the life of the dinosaur.

15.   **(B)**   Option III is the definition of a "threatened" species, therefore any answer with that option is incorrect. Option I applies to both "endangered" and "threatened" species. Option II defines an "endangered" species according to the passage. (B) offers both Options I and II.

16. **(B)** The passage says that Congress made this statement in regard to the U.S. Fish and Wildlife Service's Endangered Species Program which came about as a result of the Endangered Species Act. Merely "recording" wildlife will do nothing for its preservation, so (A) is incorrect. Government programs which work above generating laws for citizens are also not worthwhile; therefore (C) is incorrect. (D) also only records the public's comments, but no action is taken, rendering the tasks useless; therefore (D) is incorrect.

17. **(D)** The Fish and Wildlife Service works with the *Federal Register*; there is no involvement of either Secretaries or Congress in the placement of a species on the published endangered list.

18. **(C)** The information the statistics offer is misinterpreted by answers (A), which distorts the numbers, and (B) which assumes too much based on the little information given, much in the same way that (D) does. (C) offers the best interpretation of the numbers of animals placed on the List of Endangered Species and Threatened Wildlife and Plants.

19. **(C)** The Secretary of Commerce has broad powers to protect and conserve forms of marine life, not mammals which is what this group is interested in; therefore, (D) is incorrect. The mayor of a city (B) does not have the specific powers that the Fish and Wildlife Service has, which works directly with the Secretary of the Interior. Congress (A) also does not have the specific power or knowledge of the Fish and Wildlife Service, a program which is also more accessible to the public.

PASSAGE III (Questions 20-29)

20. **(C)** The two modes of thought involved in the "identity crisis" discussed by the author are that of liberal rationalism, which maintains that truth can be discovered through reason, and that of postmodernism, which maintains that knowledge exists only as political systems, that reality is indeterminate, and that reason has become "pluralized." Fascism, Marxism, and Nazism are "truth" systems produced by modern Western civilization, but not the modes of thought involved in the current university crisis (hence not (D) or (B)). Both modes are those of literate cultures (hence not (A)).

21. **(D)** In paragraph three, the author asserts that Western civilization has produced such politico-ideological "truth" systems as Nazism and Marxism, but it has also been the civilization that has most effectively resisted the ideologizing of knowledge, thus preserving free thought and open inquiry. Hence it has not ignored the problem of truth (not (A)) or abandoned rationalism (not (B)). It has used "truth" systems as a basis for war, but that is only one aspect of the problem of truth in the twentieth century (hence not (C)).

22. **(D)** The author conceives of the current university crisis as part of the larger twentieth-century intellectual and political problem of truth. Hence he seeks to define that problem in paragraphs two and three before addressing the university crisis in the remainder of the passage. What the author perceives to be the possible decline of moral responsibility has not yet happened, but may if postmodern thought

prevails (hence not (A)). As the remainder of the passage makes clear, the author believes that intellectual crises in universities have far-reaching consequences (hence not (B)). The author discusses the harmful effects of "truth" systems, but that is not the primary function of his discussion of truth (hence not (C)).

23.   **(B)**   The tradition of liberal rationalism is threatened by cultural relativism (paragraph four), which is informed by the influence of postmodernism (paragraph eight). Nazism-Fascism is not involved in the current university controversy.

24.   **(A)**   The author says (paragraph seven) that self-interest, plot and power-brokerage are not satisfactory explanations because they deny that objective values or standards exist or that judgments can be anything except power-plays. He does not deny the truth of such explanations (hence not (D)), but objects to their reductionism. Historically there has not been sufficient ethnic and gender variety to deny the truth of such explanations (hence not (B)); the threat of cultural relativism is a relatively recent phenomenon (hence not (C)).

25.   **(B)**   The crisis involves self-identity (the universities' difficulty in explaining what they are), curriculum content (what they should teach), and the moral basis of their authority (by what right they teach). The author does not discuss funding problems.

26.   **(B)**   One of the beliefs of postmodern thought is that reality is indeterminate; hence that belief is not threatened by postmodernism. Other postmodern beliefs are that truth or knowledge exist only as political systems (not (D)) and that there is no such thing as universal truth and that reason has been "pluralized" (not (A)). The author says that our civilization would be unworkable if we abandon our belief that reason can arbitrate the moral claims of society; that is, if we capitulate to postmodernism, which does not share that belief (hence not (C)).

27.   **(C)**   Postmodernism asserts that the effort to discover truth through reason is no longer credible (hence not (D)), that knowledge exists only as political "regimes" (hence not (B)), and that universal values do not exist since truth is relative (hence not (A)). The tradition of liberal rationalism maintains that objective inquiry is the best means of discovering truth.

28.   **(A)** The last paragraph makes clear that the author believes the most serious consequence of the triumph of postmodern thought and capitulating to cultural relativity is that we give up all possibility of moral judgment if we give up our belief in the existence of truth (see his reference to MacIntyre in the last paragraph). Radical change in the curriculum is a likely result of the triumph of cultural relativism, but is not the author's chief worry (hence not (B)). The breakdown of traditional departments and the loss of global influence are possible results, but are not specifically addressed by the author (hence not (C) or (D)).

29.   **(D)**   The author says that Western civilization is based on the assumption of the possibility of discovering the truth about things through reason (paragraph three) and that the founding assumption of the Western university is that reality is knowable through reason (paragraph nine). Hence Western civilization and American universi-

ties have similar conceptions of truth and reality (hence not (B)). The chief threat to Western civilization is from within (hence not (C)). The author does not address the topic in (A).

PASSAGE IV (Questions 30-37)

30.   **(C)**   The passage presents its argument by means of analogy, specifically, two metaphors that are introduced at the beginning and then developed throughout the passage (the king as a father and the king as the head of a physical body). The other three choices are inaccurate.

31.   **(C)**   The primary purpose of the passage is to argue indirectly that the king may do whatever he pleases and that no one has a right to criticize him regardless of the irrationality of his behavior. The author does not believe that the king needs the consent of his subjects to rule, nor does he believe that rebellion is ever justified.

32.   **(A)**   The author uses examples drawn from the natural world to support his argument that the king's behavior, even at its most violent and irrational, ought not to be resisted by his subjects. Beasts and fowls, he says, do not resist when they are beaten and banished by their parents; by analogy, neither should subjects resist the king, their father, when he behaves in a similar fashion. The king and his subjects are analogous to the natural order, but the king depicted in this instance is not benign.

33.   **(B)**   The metaphors of the king as father and king as head are introduced in the first paragraph. The second paragraph develops the metaphor of king as father, while the third paragraph develops the king-as-head metaphor. The fourth paragraph uses both metaphors in stating the conclusion to what is a single argument throughout the passage.

34.   **(B)**   The king is compared to a father in paragraphs one, two, and four; to the head of a body in paragraphs one, three, and four; and to an old stork in paragraph two. The comparison to a stork is a part of the comparison of the king with a father; the author urges subjects to emulate storks, which regard their "old and decayed parents" with piety.

35.   **(C)**   The last paragraph makes it clear that the author believes that the king may never be lawfully replaced (they may not "choose any other whom they please in his room"). In the author's view, there is never ample cause for rebellion, and violent revolution is never justified.

36.   **(A)**   The author does not address the issue of separation of church and state, but clearly does not endorse the notion of representative government (since popular opinion has no influence on the king's behavior) or the right of recall (since rebellion is never justified). All of the author's beliefs are consistent with a belief in the divine right of kings.

37.   **(D)**   The author's metaphor comparing the king to the head of a physical body suggests that the king is the seat of wisdom and power, but the metaphor does not effectively support his argument that a king can never be replaced when the

metaphor is taken literally. Cutting the head off a physical body obviously destroys the whole, but replacing a ruler does not necessarily destroy a country. There are no key terms that the author leaves undefined (hence not (A)). The author's example of the viper is an exception that the author believes proves the "natural law" he discusses (hence not (B)).

PASSAGE V (Questions 38-46)

38.   **(B)**   The first paragraph states that it is generally believed that Genius cannot be taught through rules or acquired by hard work, a position that the author attempts to refute in the remainder of the passage. It does not offer historical background, nor is it part of the author's argument or his thesis.

39.   **(D)**   The sense of the sentence is that common opinion believes that the character of Genius ("it") is more absolute than it actually is.

40.   **(C)**   Paragraphs two and three argue that Genius has been regarded differently in different ages. As additional rules or principles of art are discovered and codified, standards of excellence that merit the name of Genius increase. As new rules governing art are discovered, those works whose qualities earlier earned them the name of Genius are understood and explained in terms of precepts that can be taught to others. Hence the idea that Genius cannot be taught presupposes that there is a fixed, unchanging definition of Genius. In fact, however, conceptions of Genius change as our knowledge of the rules of art change (hence not (A), (B), or (D)). Invention and dignity are aspects of some works of Genius, but are not necessary in all such works, nor have they been regarded as requirements in all ages.

41.   **(D)**   The author's primary point in this paragraph is that works are regarded as the product of Genius if they have qualities that cannot be produced according to rules that are known at the time they are produced. (A) may be true, but is not addressed in this paragraph. The first part of (B) is true, but it is true in all ages. The paragraph deals with changing conceptions of Genius, not with relative degrees of recognizing Genius in different ages (hence not (C)).

42.   **(A)**   The entire passage is designed to argue that Genius can be taught. The other three statements are all ones with which the author would agree (and which are in fact present in the passage in similar forms).

43.   **(B)**   The author believes that all works of Genius are based on artistic principles, even if these principles have not yet been codified. Hence works of Genius are produced by rules, not chance (hence not (A)), and Genius always operates according to rules (hence not (C)). These principles are seen and felt in the mind of the artist (hence not (D)) even if they are not easily expressed.

44.   **(C)**   Some rules become vulgar and trite, but that does not suggest that all do. All of the other choices are assumptions upon which the author's argument that all works of Genius operate in accordance with principles is based.

45.   **(A)**   I is a simple assertion, II is based on an appeal to experience, and III is based on an appeal to history.

46.   **(D)**   All of the passage is designed to refute the idea in paragraph one that Genius is beyond the reach of rules. The other choices are either mistaken ((A) and (C)) or partial explanations (B) of the passage's main purpose.

PASSAGE VI (Questions 47-56)

47.   **(C)**   The author argues that the humanities are not only neglected, but that they ought to be at the center of higher education. Although liberal arts can be vocationally useful, that is not the chief thrust of the author's argument, nor is he primarily concerned with amounts of money spent on different kinds of education or with lamenting the loss of a less vocationally-oriented past.

48.   **(C)**   (A), (B), and (D) are mentioned in paragraph two. The author believes that education in the humanities, not vocational education, develops the full powers of individuals.

49.   **(D)**   The author offers three reasons why the ratio of the humanities to the sciences should be increased: I is the chief subject of paragraph five, II of paragraphs seven and eight, and III of paragraph six.

50.   **(A)**   The author argues that doctors, lawyers, and business executives who are liberally educated have an advantage over those who are not, even when the only consideration is career preparation. (B) is a plausible answer when vocational education is compared with liberal education, but that is not the chief point of the author's discussion of doctors, lawyers, and executives in paragraph five. The author discusses (C) and (D), but not specifically in relation to these professionals.

51.   **(C)**   In paragraph three, the author suggests that the proper objective of education is to enable the individual to come into possession of his or her full powers, an idea that is repeated in the final paragraph in the author's assertion that Jefferson believed that the educated and developed mind is of paramount importance if free society is to be preserved. For the author, the primary function of education is not connected to vocational concerns (not (A)) or personal emotional needs (not (B)), nor is it to cater to the individual's special interests, which may be merely vocational.

52.   **(B)**   The author appeals to the authority of Jefferson, who knew that the educated and developed mind is the best assurance that a political system can be made to work, in support of his argument that the humanities should be given greater emphasis. His final paragraph is rhetorically effective, but is not essentially an appeal to facts, general beliefs, or emotion.

53.   **(A)**   The seventh paragraph presents the last of the author's three arguments for increased support for the humanities. The first two deal with private concerns (vocational advantages, the desire of the individual to come to terms with life), while the third focuses on the value of the humanities for the preservation and functioning of a free society.

54. **(D)** The author's argument for increasing the ratio of the humanities to the sciences in American education would not be affected because his case does not depend on potential earning power of various types of education. (A) is incorrect because his argument is that the humanities are useful in career preparation when combined with vocational or professional education in the case of doctors, lawyers, engineers, and business executives, not that education in the humanities will lead to more lucrative careers than education in the professions. "Coming to terms with life" is unrelated to annual income (hence not (B)), which is also unrelated to our government's underlying philosophy (C).

55. **(B)** Paragraph six explicitly or implicity affirms the relevance of history ("if the human past had nothing to tell us about the present"), the necessity of moral choice ("if human beings didn't have to make decisions that affect the lives of others"), and the unique nature of human life ("if no special demands arose from the accident of being born a human being"). The paragraph does not assert that the universe is chaotic; instead, it suggests that human relations are not random aspects of life.

56. **(C)** The humanities are useful in teaching people to think sequentially and to deal with abstractions, but the engineering of consent refers to the need for technologically skillful engineers to be able to deal with people, much as doctors need to know as much about people as about pathological organisms.

PASSAGE VII (Questions 57-65)

57. **(D)** The author says that law and right differ as much as obligation and liberty, which are inconsistent (paragraph three). They do spring from the same desire, but it is the desire for self-preservation (hence not (A)). They are naturally incompatible, not compatible (hence not (B)). The author's task is to define and analyze these concepts, not to rely on discussions of previous writers (hence not (C)).

58. **(A)** The first law of nature (seek peace and follow it) derives from the "general rule of reason" that "every man ought to endeavor peace as far as he has hope of obtaining it; and when he cannot obtain it, that he may seek and use all helps and advantages of war" (paragraph four). The author analyzes man's natural state, but derives his laws from a reasoning process (hence not (B)). Neither Biblical authority nor history are the sources of his laws, although they may be in agreement with both Biblical authority and human history.

59. **(C)** *Lex naturalis* (law of nature) is based on the need for social contracts to assure self-preservation for man considered as a member of society. Hence a law of nature involves obligation to others and social agreements. The right of nature is based on considerations of individual liberty (hence not I), not on considerations of man as a member of a group.

60. **(C)** In paragraph four, the author defines man's natural condition as one in which man is in a state of "war of everyone against everyone," in which each individual is therefore governed by his own reason (rather than by social contracts),

and in which man can make use of anything to preserve his life against his enemies (hence not (A), (B), or (D)).

61.   **(B)**   The author believes that man must form social contracts based on mutual obligations if man is to achieve self-preservation in society. Such contracts depend on consent if they are to work; lack of consent on either side leads to chaos and war. Hence the correct choice is (B). Absolute monarchy is not based on mutual consent. Rugged individualists probably cannot lead satisfactory lives unless they are willing to give up significant portions of personal liberty. Absolute liberty, in fact, cannot be achieved in any society, democratic or otherwise, nor does the author discuss the relative merits of democracy.

62.   **(A)**   All natural laws derive ultimately from man's desire for self-preservation. Man needs social institutions, but that need springs from his desire for self-preservation (hence not (B)). The right of nature, not the law of nature, is based on the desire for liberty (hence not (C)). The author's discussion of man's natural state makes clear it is a condition of constant warfare, not one that suggests that man's nature is essentially benign (hence not (D)).

63.   **(B)**   Toward the end of the last paragraph, the author says that man is not obligated to follow the second law of nature (to lay down his right of nature) if other men refuse to give up their right of nature. The first and second laws of nature are compatible (hence not (A)). The second law of nature is also compatible with the "law of the Gospel" (hence not (D)). The right of nature always conflicts with personal freedom, but purely personal considerations must be subordinated to social considerations if the laws of nature are to work (hence not (C)).

64.   **(B)**   The author's quotation from the Bible is essentially a restatement of his second law of nature — that man must give up his right of nature if he expects other men to do the same. His argument derives from reason, not from authority (hence not (A)), nor is he concerned with whether his argument appears radical or with his place in Western Christian thought (hence not (C) or (D)).

65.   **(A)**   The right of nature and the laws of nature do derive ultimately from the same impulse (self-preservation); the former considers the rights of man as an individual, whereas the latter seeks to establish laws that enable man to survive when interacting with other men. (B) is incorrect because the two laws of nature do not deal with man's right to defend himself; instead, they focus on man's obligation to give up certain forms of liberty in order to achieve peace. The right of nature and the law of nature do conflict, but the author does not suggest that man invariably chooses the right of nature when the two conflict (hence not (C)). The right of nature and the laws of nature both derive from reason, but they also deal with self-preservation (hence not (D)).

Section 2 — Physical Sciences

PASSAGE I (Questions 66-70)

66.   **(C)**   Work is defined through the combination of the force F on an object (mg downward) over a displacement D (along the slope) times the cosine of the angle θ between these two vectors:

$$W_g = mgD \cos \theta = (25 \text{ kg}) (10 \text{ m/s}^2) (20 \text{ m}) \cos (120°)$$

$$W_g = -2500 \text{ J}$$

Answer (A) is obtained by neglecting the relationship with the angle, answer (B) is obtained by using the angle of the slope (30°) instead of the angle between the vectors, while answer (D) is obtained by using the angle $\theta = 55°$, the sum of the two angles given.

67.   **(A)**   The frictional force f is given in the problem and thus the same relationship is to be used:

$$W_f = fD \cos \theta = (53.33 \text{ N}) (20 \text{ m}) \cos (180°)$$

$$W_f = -1067 \text{ J}$$

Answers (B) and (C) are inserted as in the previous question to imply that the work done by friction might be identical to the work done by the gravitational field.

68.   **(A)**   Once again, we rely on the same relationship to compute the work done by the contact force as:

$$W_c = ND \cos \theta = N (20 \text{ m}) \cos (90°)$$

$$W_c = 0$$

The work is zero because there is no component of the contact force along the direction of motion. Thus, it is not necessary to compute the actual force N. Answer (B) is the opposite of the simple (weight) (distance) that many believe to be the work done in opposition to gravity. Answer (C) comes from the incorrect notion that the contact force simply opposes that of gravity.

69.   **(D)**   The simplest approach here is to recognize that there is no net force on the crate (zero acceleration) and thus *no net work done*. Therefore, the sum of the works by each of the four forces is *zero*, the last force being the effort of the man through the tension in the rope. Therefore:

$$W_m = -(W_g + W_f + W_c)$$

$$W_m = -(-2500 \text{ J} - 1067 \text{ J} + 0)$$

$$W_m = +3567 \text{ J}$$

70.   **(C)**   The relationship between the power P output by any force F is:

$$P = Fv$$

where v is the speed of the object upon which the force is acting. Since we have not needed to know the actual force applied by the man we can write the power in terms of the work as:

$$P = W/t$$

where t is the time taken to perform the work, which in this case is just:

$$t = d/v \ (20 \text{ m}) / (2 \text{ m/s}) = 10 \text{ s}$$

giving:

$$P_m = W_m / t = (3567 \text{ J}) / (10 \text{ s})$$

$$P_m = 356.7 \text{ Watts}$$

PASSAGE II (Questions 71-75)

71. **(C)** The amplitude A of a simple harmonic oscillator is defined as $\frac{1}{2}$ the difference between the minimum and maximum displacement. In this case we have a maximum value of + 6 m, a minimum value of - 4m, and thus:

$$A = \frac{1}{2} ((6 \text{ m}) - (- 4 \text{ m})) = 5 \text{ m}$$

Answers (A) and (B) are both attempts to assume that the oscillator is symmetric, which it is not.

72. **(B)** The period T of the oscillator is defined as the time for one complete oscillation. Since the points at the center are deceptive, we rely on the turning points to determine this. Two consecutive maximum displacements occur at $t = 2$ and $t = 6$ seconds, thus:

$$T = 6 \text{ s} - 2 \text{ s} = 4 \text{ s}.$$

73. **(D)** The velocity of an object is found by taking the slope of the displacement vs. time graph. Thus, when the slope is *zero*, the mass has the slowest speed. This occurs at $t = 0$, $t = 2$, $t = 4$, and $t = 6$ seconds on our graph. Answers (A) and (C) are where the mass moves the fastest.

74. **(D)** As the mass reaches its minimum and maximum displacements, it experiences the greatest acceleration required to get it completely turned around and going again. This can be seen from the graph as the fastest *change* in the slope, where the slope represents the velocity of the object. Thus, at $t = 0$, $t = 2$, $t = 4$, and $t = 6$ seconds, we find our greatest acceleration. Answers (A) and (C) occur for the greatest *speed*, but the least amount of the *change* in the velocity.

75. **(A)** The relationship between the physical characteristics of the mass m, the spring of constant k, and the period T is:

$$T = 2\pi\sqrt{\frac{m}{k}}$$

$$k = \frac{4\pi^2 m}{T} = \frac{4\pi^2 (2kg)}{(4s)}$$

$$k = 19.74 \text{ N/m}$$

PASSAGE III (Questions 76-85)

The passage requires an understanding of electronic configuration, bonding, hybridization, molecular geometries and their effect on the polarity of molecules.

76. **(B)** Nitrogen is atom A and chlorine is atom B. Nitrogen will form only one compound with chlorine. No expanded octet is possible because the nitrogen atom is too small to accommodate more than 8 electrons around the central atom. The bonding is covalent because nitrogen and chlorine are both nonmetal atoms. Metals and nonmetals form ionic bonds; whereas nonmetals form polar covalent bonds with other nonmetal. A nonmetal will also form a nonpolar covalent bond with itself.

Nitrogen, the central atom, possesses 5 valence electrons. The unpaired electrons in the p subshell bond to the unpaired electron in each of 3 different chlorine atoms to give 8 valence electrons around nitrogen. Eight valence electrons form 4 pairs of electrons — 3 bonding pairs and 1 lone (non-bonding) pair of electrons. In order to minimize the repulsion between the pairs of electrons, the four pairs are arranged in a tetrahedral. However, since the lone pair of electrons occupies one of the positions in the tetrahedral the molecular geometry will no longer be a symmetrical tetrahedral but will resemble a pyramid with N at the apex.

The covalent bond between N and Cl is polar because the two atoms have different electronegativities — ability to attract the electrons in a covalent bond. The greater the difference in the electronegativity, the more polar the bond. Since the pyramidal molecule is not symmetrical, there is no way for the polarities of the bonds to cancel each other and the resulting molecule must be polar.

77. **(B)** Since repulsion between the lone pair and the bond pairs is greater than the repulsion between bond pairs, the bond angle shrinks from the normal tetrahedral angle of 109.5° to approximately 107°. The exact angle will vary with the ligand (atom around the central atom). For example, since the electron cloud between N and F in NF_3 would be more elongated (due to the greater difference in electronegativities) than the electron cloud between N and Cl in NCl_3, the bond angle in NF_3 would be expected to be less than that in NCl_3.

The hybridization is sp^3 since there must be four equivalent orbitals for the 4 pairs of electrons to occupy. The 2s and the three 2p orbitals of nitrogen are hybridized to form 4 equivalent sp^3 (since they are made from one s orbital and three p orbitals) containing one pair of electrons and three unpaired electrons that form bonds with three chlorine atoms.

78. **(B)** Phosphorus is a larger atom than nitrogen, therefore, P will form both PCl_3 and PCl_5. The bonding in PCl_3 exhibits sp^3 hybidization with the lone pair of electrons occupying one of the tetrahedrally-arranged orbitals. However, the bonding in PCl_5 is described as sp d because one of the original 3s electrons is promoted to an empty 3d orbital and hybridization results in five equivalent orbitals made from one

s, three p and one d orbital — sp^{3}d. The resulting molecule has 10 valence electrons around the central atom and is said to possess an expanded octet.

Five pairs of electrons can be arranged in two different ways — a square with one pair up or down (square pyramidal) or a triangle with one pair up and one pair down (trigonal bipyramidal). The number of 90° must be made as small as possible in order to minimize the repulsion between the electron pairs. In the square pyramidal shape there would be eight 90° repulsions; whereas in the trigonal bipyramidal there would be six 90° repulsions. Consequently, there will be 6 - 90° and 3 - 120° bond angles in the trigonal bipyramidal molecule.

All of the bonds in this molecule will be polar since the electronegativities of P and Cl are different. However, because this a symmetrical molecule, the bond polarities will cancel each other resulting in a nonpolar molecule.

79.   **(C)**   There must be 10 electrons around the central atom since P has 5 valence electrons and each chlorine shares one electron. In SF$_6$ there are 12 valence electrons. AsF$_5$ has 10 valence electrons but it would exhibit the same molecular geometry as PCl$_5$. In ClF$_3$ the Cl atom has 7 valence electrons and each F atom shares 1 electron to give 10 valence electrons or 5 pairs of electrons. However, the molecular geometry will be different because all of the valence electrons are not involved in bonds. AsF$_3$ would have 8 valence electrons around the As atom.

There are 5 pairs of electrons around the Cl. However, only 3 of these can be involved in bonds since there are 3 fluorine attached to the Cl. These must be polar covalent bonds since the electronegativities are different. The two remaining pairs of electrons are called lone pair (nonbonding pair) electrons since they occupy space but are not located between two atoms. Five pairs of electrons require a trigonal bipyramidal type molecular geometry. However, since two of the positions are occupied by the lone pair electrons, the resulting molecular geometry is called T-shaped.

Placing the lone pair electrons above and below the triangle would result in six 90° repulsions between the lone pairs and the bond pairs. Only four 90° repulsions result if the lone pairs occupy two of the positions on the triangle. Since minimizing the number of 90° repulsions is the requirement for obtaining the most stable molecular geometry, the T-shaped molecule with the lone pairs occupying the triangle positions is the most likely structure. This molecular geometry can be verified by experiments for determining the bond angles.

80.   **(A)**   The principal quantum number, n, can have an integral value excluding zero. The azimuthal quantum number, l, can be 0 to n -1. The magnetic quantum number, m_1, can have values from -l to +l. The spin quantum number, m_s, can have values of +$^1/_2$ or -$^1/_2$. Selection (A) is not a valid set because if $l = 0$, m_l must be 0, because the absolute value of m_l must not be greater than the absolute value of l.

81.   **(B)**   Draw the Lewis electron dot formulas for the compounds. If a carbon is surrounded by four sigma bonds, its hybridization will be sp^3 since the bonds must be formed from identical orbitals. A double bond consists of a sigma bond and pi bond. A carbon atom attached to 3 sigma bonds and 1 pi bond will exhibit sp^2 hybridization since only 3 equivalent oribtals were used in the bonding. The remaining electron in the 2 p orbital forms a pi bond by overlapping of the p orbitals.

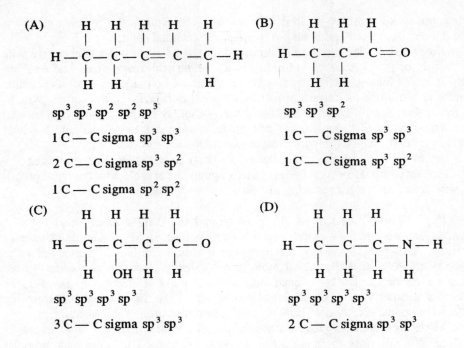

82. **(C)**   Element B is chlorine which has an atomic number of seventeen which means it has 17 protons and 17 electrons if it is a neutral atom. There are 18 neutrons in this atom if we assume that it is the atom of chlorine with a mass number of 35 (35 - 17 = 18). Chlorine forms a negative one ion since it needs only one electron to complete its outer shell of electrons. This negative one ion is larger than the parent atom because of electronic repulsion between the added electron and the other electrons in this region of space.

83. **(D)**   The element directly underneath element B (chlorine) is bromine which has a filled $n = 3$ energy level ($3s^2sp^63d^{10}$), a total of 18 electrons. The $n = 1$ energy level will hold a maximum of 2 electrons ($1s^2$), the $n = 2$ energy level will hold a maximum of 8 ($2s^22p^6$) and the $n = 4$ energy level will hold a maximum of 32 ($4s^24p^64d^{10}4f^{14}$).

84. **(D)**

Bond order = (Bonding electron - Antibonding electrons)/2

$$= (8 - 2) / 2 = 3$$

All the electrons are paired so the molecule is diamagnetic. (See figure on next page.)

85. **(A)**   The electronegativity of the atoms in the periodic table increases from bottom to top and from left to right. Therefore, N is more electronegative than P. This results in a more polar bond since the greater the difference in the electronegativity, the more polar the bond. A zero difference in electronegativity would result in a nonpolar molecule. Nitrogen, oxygen and fluorine are the most electronegative elements in the periodic table.

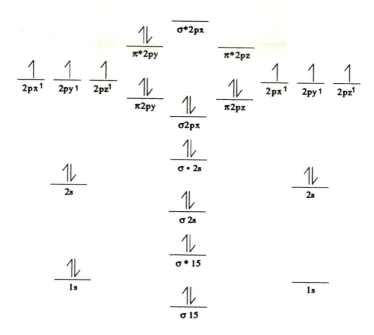

PASSAGE IV (Questions 86-90)

86. **(D)** Torque τ is determined by the product of the force *F* times the moment arm *d* from the pivot point.

$$\tau = dF = (0.95 \text{ m}) (2 \text{ N}) = 1.90 \text{ Nm}$$

87. **(B)** Torque is also found as the product of the distance *r* from the pivot times the force *F* times the sin θ ... θ being the angle between the directions of *r* and *F*. Thus:

$$\tau = rF \sin \theta = (0.2 \text{ m}) (12N) \sin (90°) = 2.4 \text{ Nm}$$

88. **(D)** Since the torque sensitively depends on the angle between the directions of *r* and *F*, any non-horizontal placement of the stick would yield a different value of the torque due to the weight of the stick which appears at the 50 cm mark and is directed vertically downward. Answer (A) is wrong, as this weight also points vertically downward under all conditions. Answer (B) is not correct, since this angle can be freely adjusted by moving the spring independent of the stick.

89. **(D)** The weight of the stick is to be determined by averaging the values obtained from each data set. The general result is:

$$\Sigma \tau_p = 0 = \tau_{sp} - (\tau_{st} + \tau_w)$$

where *p* stands for the pivot, sp for the spring, st for the stick, and *w* for the hanging weight. These separate torques are found to be:

$$0 = (0.2 \text{ m}) \, (F) \sin(\theta) - ((0.5 \text{ m}) \, (W_{st}) + (0.95 \text{ m}) \, (2 \text{ N}))$$

each of the four data sets gives a different value for W_{st} as:

$$W_{st} = ((0.2 \text{ m}) \, (F) \sin(\theta) - 1.9 \text{ Nm}) / (0.5 \text{ m})$$

From the table, these four values are 1 N, 1.09 N, 0.95 N, and 1 N. This yields the average value of:

$$W_{st} = (1 + 1.09 + 0.95 + 1) / 4 = 1.01 \text{ N}$$

90.　**(A)**　Since equilibrium prevails at any of the angles, the horizontal force exerted by the pivot must balance the horizontal force provided by the spring balance. Thus:

$$F_h = F \cos(\theta) = (24 \text{ N}) \cos(150°) = 20.8 \text{ N}$$

Answer (B) neglects the cosine dependence for this component of the force, while answer (D) is the vertical component of this spring force, not the horizontal one.

PASSAGE V (Questions 91-96)

91.　**(C)**　Since *zero* work is done during the constant volume process ($dW = PdV$), the total work is just the sum of the two given, accounting for the correct directions:

$$W_{ba} = -750 \text{ J}$$

while

$$W_{ac} = +500 \text{ J}$$

as defined by positive work being done *by* the gas. Thus, a net work of - 250 J is found. Answer (D) accounts only for magnitudes and not the different directions, while answer (B) is correct only for a *clockwise* traversal of the cycle.

92.　**(D)**　The first law of thermodynamics can be stated as

$$\Delta U = Q - W,$$

U being the internal energy of the gas and Q being the heat gained by the gas. Since the process from $a - b$ is just the reverse of the process from $b - a$, we have

$$Q_{ab} = +300 \text{ J},$$

$$W_{ab} = +750 \text{ J},$$

and therefore:

$$\Delta U_{ab} = (300 \text{ J}) - (750 \text{ J}) = -450 \text{ J}$$

93.　**(C)**　The process $c - a$ is adiabatic, and thus, by definition, no heat flows into or out of the gas during this process.

94.　**(A)**　Since this process is adiabatic, $Q_{ca} = 0$. We already know that $W_{ca} = -500$ J, therefore,

$$\Delta U_{ca} = 0 - (-500 \text{ J}) = +500 \text{ J}$$

95. **(B)** To compute the heat flow in or out of the gas we rearrange the first law as

$$Q = \Delta U + W.$$

Thus, we must know ΔU_{bc} to determine Q_{bc}. We obtain this by recognizing that the internal energy change over the entire cycle is *zero*. Thus, the sum of the answers to questions 92 and 94 must be negated in the process from b - c, pr:

$$\Delta U_{bc} = -(\Delta U_{ab} + \Delta U_{ca}) = -((-450 \text{ J}) + (500 \text{ J})) = -50 \text{ J}$$

Since no work is done during the constant volume process:

$$Q_{bc} = \Delta U_{bc} + W_{bc} = -50 \text{ J} + 0 = -50 \text{ J}$$

96. **(A)** We already relied on this information to compute the answer to Question 95, but many will think the value must be the same as the work done, thus choosing any one of the wrong answers.

INDEPENDENT QUESTIONS

97. **(B)** This is the general thin lens problem. Applying the optics equation for going from one medium to another

$$-\frac{n}{s} + \frac{n'}{s'} = \frac{n'-n}{R}$$

we get

$$-\frac{n_0}{s_0} + \frac{n_r}{s'} = \frac{n_r - n_0}{R_1}$$

and

$$-\frac{n_r}{s'} + \frac{n_i}{s'_i} = \frac{(n_i - n_r)}{R_2}$$

Add the equations to get

$$-\frac{n_0}{s_0} + \frac{n_i}{s'_i} = \frac{(n_r - n_0)}{R_1} + \frac{(n_i - n_r)}{R_2}.$$

To find the secondary focal length, set $s_0 = -\infty$

$$\frac{n_i}{f'} = \frac{n_r - n_0}{R_1} + \frac{n_i - n_r}{R_2}$$

or $\quad f' = \dfrac{n_i}{(n_r - n_0)/R_1 + (n_i - n_r)/R_2}$

98. **(D)** The given spring force is nonlinear but conservative.

$$F = -k_1 x - k_2 x^3$$

Using the work-energy theorem:

$$W = \Delta K$$

$$W = \int F \cdot dx = \tfrac{1}{2} k_1 x^2 + \tfrac{1}{4} k_2 x^4 = \tfrac{1}{2} m v^2$$

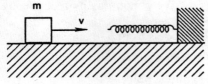

$$x^4 + 2 \frac{k_1}{k_2} x^2 = \frac{2m}{k_2} v^2$$

$$(x^2 + \frac{k_2}{k_2})^2 = 2 \frac{m}{k_2} v^2 + (\frac{k_1}{k_2})^2$$

$$x^2 = -\frac{k_1}{k_2} + \sqrt{2 \frac{m}{k_2} v^2 - \frac{k_1^2}{k_2^2}}$$

$$x = \sqrt{k_1 / k_2} \left(\sqrt{1 + \frac{2mv^2 k_2}{k_1^2}} - 1 \right)^{1/2}$$

99. **(A)** The given central potential is

$$U = k r^n$$

Hence

$$F = -\nabla U = -k \left(\hat{r} \frac{\partial}{\partial r} + \hat{\theta} \frac{1}{r} \frac{\partial}{\partial \theta} + \hat{\phi} \frac{1}{r \sin \theta} \frac{\partial}{\partial \phi} \right) r^n$$

Writing the gradient in spherical coordinates.

$$= -k \hat{r} \, n r^{n-1}$$

$$= -k n \, r^{n-2} r \hat{r} = -k n \, r^{n-2} \mathbf{r}$$

since $\dfrac{\partial r}{\partial \theta}$ and $\dfrac{\partial r}{\partial \phi}$

are zero (curvilinear orthogonal coordinates). Also

$$\mathbf{r} = x\mathbf{x} + y\mathbf{y} + z\mathbf{z}$$

in spherical coordinates.

100. **(C)** Using $F = ma$ with $a = v^2 / r$ as the centripetal acceleration and $F = kq_1 q_2 / r^2$ as the Couloumb force, we have

$$F = \frac{mv^2}{r} = \frac{kZe^2}{r^2}$$

From Bohr theory

$$L = mvr = n\hbar$$

thus $\quad v = \dfrac{n\hbar}{mr}$

$$\dfrac{m\left(\dfrac{n\hbar}{mr}\right)^2}{r} = \dfrac{kZe^2}{r^2}$$

$$r_\mu = \dfrac{n^2\hbar^2}{kZe^2 m_\mu}$$

$$r_H = \dfrac{n^2\hbar^2}{kZe^2 m_e}$$

$$r_\mu = \dfrac{m_e}{m_\mu}\, r_H = \dfrac{1}{207}\, r_H$$

where r_H is the radius of the Hydrogen-like atom in Bohr theory.

101. **(D)**   All reactions, exothermic or endothermic, that involve any type of bond breaking will have an energy of activation, though it may be very low. An exothermic reaction has a negative ΔH (change in enthalpy). Since heat is being liberated it is only logical that the potential energy of the products should be lower than the potential energy of the reactants. This is summarized in the diagram shown.

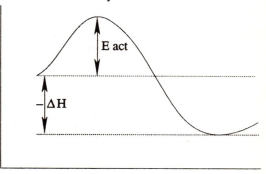

102. **(A)**   Use basic kinematics

$$v^2 - v_0 = 2a(x - x_0)$$

$$v = \sqrt{2ax}$$

$$= \sqrt{2(9.8)200}$$

$$= 62.61\ \text{m}/\text{s}$$

$$v^2 - v_0^2 = 2a(x - x_0)$$

$$0^2 - 62.61^2 = 2a(0.5 - 2)$$

$$a = 1307\ \text{m}/\text{s}^2$$

$$a = 133\ g$$

using $g = 9.8$ m/s^2

103. **(D)**   Newton's universal law of gravitation states that

$$F = -\frac{Gm_1m_2}{r^2}$$

Now integrate the force to get the potential energy.

$$U = -\int Fdr = \frac{Gm_1m_2}{R}$$

$$U = -\frac{(6.67 \times 10^{-11})(70)(60)}{0.5} = -5.60 \times 10^{-7}\,J$$

104. **(A)**   The Hardy-Weinberg principle is one of the fundamental concepts in population genetics. It states that a population remains genetically stable in succeeding generations.

PASSAGE VI (Questions 105-114)
        The passage requires an understanding of the interpretation of experimental rate data, rates of reactions, rate laws, and mathematical relationships between these.

105. **(B)**   Using the coefficients in the stoichiometric equation shows that 2 molecules of A would disappear for each B and 3 molecules of C would disappear with each molecule of B. Consequently, the rate of disappearance of A would be twice the rate of disappearance of B and the rate of disappearance of C would be three times the rate of disappearance of B. The same kind of relationships would hold for the appearance of products on the right-hand side of the equation.

106. **(A)**   Using row 1 and row 2 shows that the concentrations of B and C are constant while the concentration of A doubles (from 1 M to 1 M). The initial rate also doubles. Consequently, a direct proportion must exist between the rate and the concentration of A:

    rate = $k[A]$.

107. **(B)**   Using row 1 and row 3 shows that the concentration of A and B remains constant while the concentration of C triples (1 M to 3 M). The initial rate increases from 3 to 27 so the rate must increase by a factor of 9 (27/3 = 9).

    rate = $k[C]^2$

108. **(C)**   From the answer in 106 and 107, we already know that

    rate = $k[A]\,[C]^2$.

Using row 1 and row 4 reveals that quadrupling the concentration of B has no effect on the initial rate of the reaction. This means that B cannot be involved in the rate-determining step in the reaction and therefore, cannot be in the rate law expression.

109. **(D)**   The order of the reaction can be obtained by simply adding the superscripts in the rate equation

    $1 + 2 = 3$.

110. **(C)**   If the mechanism were to consist of a one-step process, one molecule of A and two molecules of C would have to collide simultaneously, resulting in a termolecular collision — not very likely.

111. **(D)**   Any first-order reaction will yield a straight line when the logarithm of the concentration is plotted versus the time. The natural of Naperian logarithm or the base-10 logarithm may be used in the plot. The slope of the line will give the specific rate constant k. In this case, since all the concentrations were held constant except for A, the reaction would be called a pseudo-first-order reaction. Second-order reaction yields straight lines when the reciprocal of the concentration is plotted versus time.

112. **(C)**   In general, increasing the temperature by 10° doubles the reaction rate. Since the temperature increases by 4 multiples of 10, the reaction rate will double four times — 2^4 — or 16 times. The rate will be 16 times faster at 65°C.

113. **(B)**   Using the Arrhenius equation:

$$k = Ae^{-Ea/RT}$$

a linear relationship can be derived:

$$\ln k = \ln A - E_a / RT$$

$$\ln k = - E_a / RT + \ln A$$

This equation shows that a plot of $\ln k$ versus $1/T$ would give E_a/R = slope and $\ln A$ = y-intercept. In this case, only two rate constants and two temperatures are given, so a plot is not necessary since two equations in two unknowns can be set up:

$$\ln k_1 = - E_a / RT_1 + \ln A$$

$$\ln k_2 = - E_a / RT_2 + \ln A$$

Subtracting the two equations gives

$$\ln k_1 - \ln k_2 = - e_a / R \, (1/T_1 + 1/T_2)$$

$$\ln K_1/k_2 = E_a / R \, (1/T_2 - 1/T_1)$$

The problem says $k_2 = 3k_1$. Substituting this relationship into the equation gives:

$$\ln (k_1/3k_1) = \{E_a / (8.314 \times 10^{-3} \text{ J/mol K})\} \, (1/308 - 1/298)$$

$$E_a = 8.38 \times 10^1 \text{ kJ}$$

114. **(B)**   Adding a catalyst to a reaction lowers the activation energy by providing a different pathway for the reaction — one that does not require as much energy. Since less energy is required in a collision, more collisions are effective, and therefore, the reaction rate is much faster.

PASSAGE VII (Questions 115-119)

115. **(B)**   The term Electromotive Force or EMG is historical in nature. The battery is often called a "seat of EMF." Since the EMF is actually a potential differ-

ence which drives electrical charges to higher potential, it cannot be considered an equipotential (answer (D)). Answers (A) and (C) are dimensionally incorrect.

116. **(D)**   Ohm's law gives us the relationship between the potential difference V across any resistor R and the current I through the resistor as:

$$V = IR$$

or

$$R = V/I = (1.40 \text{ V}) / (0.15 \text{ A}) = 9.33 \ \Omega.$$

Answer (A) is obtained by using the EMF of the battery instead of the terminal voltage (V_t) recorded while the resistor is connected.

117. **(B)**   We must realize that the difference between the EMF, which can be likened to the maximum possible ability for the battery to move charges, and the terminal voltage is through the internal resistance of the battery by:

$$V_t = \text{EMF} - Ir$$

$$V_t + Ir = \text{EMF}$$

$$Ir = \text{EMF} - V_t$$

$$r = (\text{EMF} - V_t) / I = ((1.5 \text{ V}) - (1.4 \text{ V})) / (0.15 \text{ A})$$

$$r = 0.67 \ \Omega$$

Note that the sum of $R + r = 10 \ \Omega$ as expected. The battery and the external resistor share the total EMF. Answer (A) is provided again for those who neglect to account for the fact that the battery is the supply of the voltage.

118. **(A)**   The heat generated within the battery is through its internal resistance and may be computed from the power generated P times the time t in 3 ways:

$$Q = Pt = IVt = I^2rt = V^2t / r$$

$$Q = (0.15 \text{ A})^2 (0.67 \ \Omega) (60 \text{ s}) = 0.9 \text{ J}$$

Answer (C) would be correct only if $r = 0$, while answer (B) incorrectly uses the full EMF to compute the heat loss ... recall that the majority of the work done by the battery is the pumping of charges into the external resistor!

119. **(C)**   Series connections of EMFs and resistors yield the simple sum as the combined effect. Thus, the total EMF will be 3.0 V, while the total internal resistance will be 1.34 Ω. Since the external resistor simply adds in series, the net resistance of this circuit will be:

$$R_{net} = 2r + R = (1.34 \ \Omega) + (20 \ \Omega) = 21.34 \ \Omega$$

Using Ohm's law we find:

$$\text{EMF}_{net} = IR_{net}$$

$$I = \text{EMF}_{net} / R_{net} = (3.0 \text{ V}) / (21.34 \ \Omega)$$

$I = 0.14$ A

Answer (A) is found by neglecting the internal resistances of the batteries, while answer (B) would be the result when the batteries are connected in parallel with the original 10Ω resistor.

PASSAGE VIII (Questions 120-125)

120. (C)   The relationship between the distance from the object to the lens o, the distance form the image to the lens i, and the focal length of the lens f is:

$$\frac{1}{o} + \frac{1}{i} = \frac{1}{f}$$

Thus, since $o = 40$ cm and $f = +20$ cm:

$$\frac{1}{i} = \frac{1}{f} - \frac{1}{o} = \frac{1}{(20 \text{ cm})} - \frac{1}{(40 \text{ cm})} = \frac{1}{40 \text{ cm}}$$

which yields the answer $i = +40$ cm. The $+$ signifies that the image is *real* and thus is located where the light actually goes — through the lens — which is to the *right* of the lens.

121. (B)   The magnification m relationships yield both the size and orientation of the image relative to the object:

$$m = -\frac{i}{o} \; ; \; |m| = \frac{h_i}{h_o}$$

where h_i and h_o are the heights of the image and object, respectively. Thus, the results for this case are:

$$m = -(40 \text{ cm}) / (40 \text{ cm}) = -1$$

$$|m| = 1$$

which say that the image is the same size as the object but *inverted* due to the *negative* result for m.

122. (D)   A diverging lens spreads light away from the optical axis, not allowing it to converge as in the formation of a real image. The image is then said to be *virtual*. Diverging lenses can only produce images smaller than the object, thus answer (B) is incorrect. The light intensity is a measure of power per unit area. Thus, answer (C) is not correct for a diverging lens which cannot intensify a beam due to its spreading effects.

123. (C)   The problem reads "The image produced by the converging lens … will act as the object for the diverging lens." Since this image is produced 40 cm to the right of the converging lens, it is found 30 cm to the right of the diverging lens. Since the light is truly traveling to the right and the lens is to the left of this "object," the object is considered *virtual* and has been *inverted* by the converging lens. Answer (A) must be incorrect simply by the statement of the problem. Answer (B) would be correct only if we considered the original object, thus ditto.

124. **(A)** Using the formula from Question 120:

$$\frac{1}{o} + \frac{1}{i} = \frac{1}{f}$$

with $o = -30$ cm *(the negative sign required for virtual)* and $f = -15$ cm

$$\frac{1}{i} = \frac{1}{f} - \frac{1}{o} = \frac{1}{(-15\,\text{cm})} - \frac{1}{(-30\,\text{cm})} = \frac{1}{-30\,\text{cm}}$$

which gives $i = -30$ cm, or 30 cm to the *left* of the diverging lens. Since the diverging lens is 10 cm to the *right* of the converging lens, this final image must be located 20 cm to the *left* of the *converging* lens. Answer (C) would be the result had the object distance been taken as *positive* instead of negative.

125. **(D)** As before, the magnification for the diverging lens is:

$$m = -\frac{i}{o} \; ; \; |m| = \frac{h_i}{h_o}$$

so that:

$$m = -(-30\,\text{cm}) / (-30\,\text{cm}) = -1$$

This says that the *inverted* object is *reinverted* but kept the same size. Therefore, the *total* magnification (m_T) is just the products of the two individual magnifications and is:

$$m_T = (-1)(-1) = +1$$

It is interesting to note that this particular optical system has simply brought a real object closer to the lens system without changing its size or orientation. Answers (A) and (B) would be correct only if demagnification occurred, which it has not. Answer (C) is the magnification of each lens separately, not the combined effect.

PASSAGE IX (Questions 126-135)

This problem set requires an understanding of oxidation–reduction reactions as well as electrochemistry. You must know the Nernst equation, the relationship between Gibbs free energy and the cell EMF, Faraday's law of electrolysis, as well as basic definitions and concepts.

126. **(D)** The half-reaction for Na is reversed and the sign of the $E°$ is changed. This oxidation half cell can then be added to the reduction half cell for I_2:

Oxidation: $\quad 2Na \longrightarrow 2Na^{1+} + 2e^- \qquad +2.7$ v

Reduction: $\quad I_2 + 2e^- \longrightarrow 2I^- \qquad +0.5$ v

Overall: $\quad 2Na + I_2 \longrightarrow 2Na^{1+} + 2I^- \;\; +3.2$ v

This is a spontaneous cell since the EMF is positive. In answer (A) both substances would have to be reduced — this is impossible. In answer (B) the EMF would be negative, indicating a nonspontaneous reaction. In answer (C) both substances would have to be reduced.

127. **(A)** In order to balance an oxidation-reduction equation, the number of electrons lost during oxidation must be equal to the number of electrons gained during the reduction process.

$$2 \, (Al \longrightarrow Al^{3+} + 3e^-)$$

$$3 \, (PtCl_2^{2-} + 2e^- \longrightarrow Pt + 4Cl^-)$$

$$2Al + 3 \, PtCl_4^{2-} \longrightarrow 2Al^{3+} + 3Pt + 12Cl^-$$

128. **(B)** Oxidation is loss (OIL) of electrons and reduction is gain (RIG) of electrons. Al loses electrons and is, therefore, oxidized. The substance that is reduced is the oxidizing agent since it takes electrons away from some other substance, therefore, $PtCl_4^{2-}$ is the oxidizing agent since it is reduced.

129. **(B)**

$$Al \longrightarrow Al^{3+} + 3e^- \qquad +1.7 \text{ v}$$

$$PtCl_4^{2-} + 2e^- \longrightarrow Pt + 4Cl^- \qquad +0.7 \text{ v}$$

$$2.4 \text{ v}$$

Although the number of electrons lost must be equal to the number of electrons gained, we do not have to multiply the EMF for each by an appropriate number to balance the electrons.

130. **(B)**

$$E° = (0.059/n) \log K$$

$$2 \, (Na \longrightarrow Na^{1+} + 1e^-) \qquad 2.7 \text{ v}$$

$$Mn^{2+} + 2e^- \longrightarrow Mn \qquad -1.2 \text{ v}$$

$$2 \, Na + Mn^{2+} \longrightarrow Na^{1+} + Mn \qquad 1.5 \text{ v}$$

$$1.5 = (0.59/2) \log K$$

$$\log K = 50.847 = \text{approximately } 51$$

$$K = 7.0 \times 10^{50} \text{ or } 10^{51}$$

Your answer requires only that you recognize that logarithms are exponents of the base 10. Therefore, you may simply use the number preceding the decimal since log K = 50.847 or log K = 51 (approximately) so $K = 10^{51}$.

131. **(D)**

$$\Delta G° = -nFE°$$

$$\Delta G° = -(6 \text{ mole e's}) (96,500 \text{ coulombs/mole e's}) \, 2.4 \text{ j/coulomb}$$

$$= -1.39 \times 10^6$$

When the Gibb's free energy is negative, the reaction is spontaneous. If the EMF for the cell is negative, the change in Gibbs free energy is negative.

132. **(B)**

$$\text{gms} = 5 \text{ amp} \times 30.0 \text{ min} \times \frac{60 \text{ min}}{1 \text{ min}} \times \frac{1 \text{ coulomb}}{1 \text{ amp sec}} \times \frac{1 \text{ F}}{96,500 \text{ c}}$$

$$\times \frac{1 \text{ mole e's}}{1 \text{ F}} \times \frac{1 \text{ mole Al}}{3 \text{ mole e's}} \times \frac{27.0 \text{ gms Al}}{1 \text{ mole Al}} = 0.84$$

The Al is the anode and it will be oxidized during any electrolysis reaction, therefore, its weight will decrease.

133. **(A)**

$$E = E° - (0.059/n) \log \{[.1]^2 [1] [.1]^{12}\} / [.1]^3$$

$$= 2.4 - (0.059/6) \log [.1]^{11}$$

$$= 2.4 - (0.059/6) (-11)$$

$$= 2.4 + 0.108$$

$$= 2.5$$

You must have a balanced equation and remember that solids are always (1) in these equations.

134. **(B)**   By convention the cell on the left is designated as the anode at which oxidation takes place. Thus silver is reduced at the silver cathode and the electrons travel through the external circuit from the Mn anode (-) to the Ag cathode (+).

135. **(D)**   In answer (A) the EMF for reducing Na^{1+} and oxidizing Zn would be negative $(- 2.7 + 0.8 = - 1.9)$. Therefore, this would be a nonspontaneous reaction and Na^{1+} will not oxidize Zn. In answer (B) both substances would have to be oxidized — this is impossible. The same situation exists in answer (C). Only answer (D) gives a positive $E°$ $(+ 0.5 + 0.8 = 1.3)$ An examination of the table reveals that any of the species on the left-hand side of the arrow that are below Zn will oxidize it. This is always true.

INDEPENDENT QUESTIONS

136. **(C)**   When proteins are boiled in dilute acids or bases they are hydrolyzed, i.e., degraded or broken down to amino acids. Amino acids are compounds whose molecules possess both the amino (- NH_2) and the carboxyl (- CO_2H) functional groups. The general formula may be written as

$$\begin{array}{c} \text{H} \\ | \\ \text{H} - \text{N} - \text{C} - \text{C} - \text{OH} , \\ | \quad | \quad \| \\ \text{H} \quad \text{Z} \quad \text{O} \end{array}$$

where Z = side group.

The union of amino acids, which results in the formation of the protein, is due to bonds that come about as a result of the elimination of a hydrogen from the -NH_2 group, and an OH from the - CO_2H group. This linkage is termed a peptide bond. It is depicted as

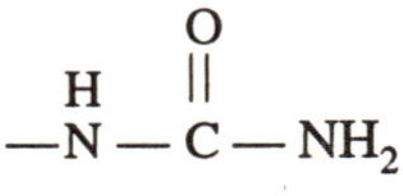

$$\overset{\displaystyle H}{-N}-\overset{\displaystyle \overset{O}{\|}}{C}-NH_2$$

peptide bond

When this substance is hydrolyzed, the following reaction occurs. In acid:

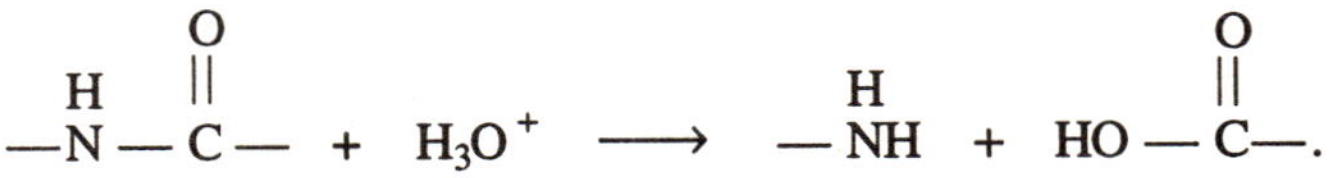

$$\overset{\displaystyle H}{-N}-\overset{\displaystyle \overset{O}{\|}}{C}- \ + \ H_3O^+ \ \longrightarrow \ \overset{\displaystyle H}{-NH} \ + \ HO-\overset{\displaystyle \overset{O}{\|}}{C}-.$$

You obtain the amino and carboxylic group.

Note: NH_2 is basic, so that in acid, you actually get - NH_3^+. Thus, you obtain a compound that possesses an amino acid and a carboxylic group, which is, as you recall, an amino acid. With base, the same result is obtained, but, you immediately obtain NH_2 and not NH_3^+. The carboxylic portion, which is acidic, reacts with the OH^- from base to yield COO^-.

137. **(D)**   Because of the presence of a pair of nonbonding electrons on nitrogen, amines are Lewis bases like alcohols and ethers. However, since nitrogen is not as electronegative as oxygen, amines have a greater tendency to react with a proton making them more basic than alcohols. Also, since alkyl groups are electron-donating, the substituted amines are more basic than ammonia. NH_4^+ is the conjugate acid of ammonia. Alkoxide ions, having a negative formal charge along with two lone pairs of electrons are more basic than amines. In order of decreasing basicity:

$$CH_3CH_2O^- > (CH_3)_2NH > NH_3 > CH_3OH > NH_4^+.$$

138. **(B)**   The reaction of Grignard reagents with ethylene oxide is an important method of preparing primary alcohols. The product contains two carbons more than the alkyl or aryl group of the Grignard reagent. The reaction may be viewed as follows:

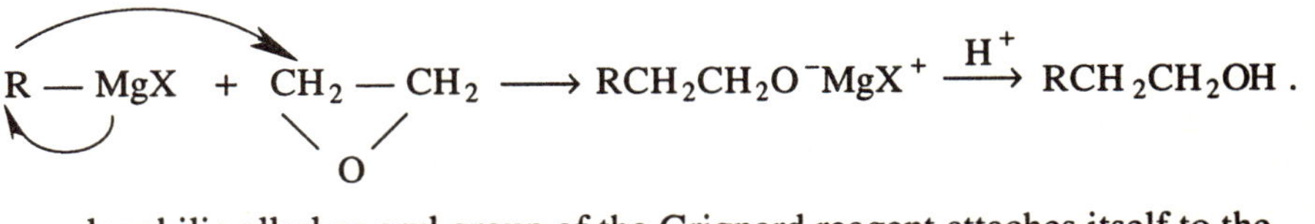

$$R-MgX \ + \ \underset{\underset{\displaystyle O}{\diagdown\diagup}}{CH_2-CH_2} \ \longrightarrow \ RCH_2CH_2O^-MgX^+ \ \overset{H^+}{\longrightarrow} \ RCH_2CH_2OH \ .$$

The nucleophilic alkyl or aryl group of the Grignard reagent attaches itself to the relatively positive carbon and the electrophilic magnesium attaches itself to the relatively negative oxygen. Here, the Grignard reagent used is methylmagnesiumiodide, which can be prepared by reacting Mg with methyl iodide in ether:

$$Mg + CH_3 - I \overset{ether}{\longrightarrow} CH_3 \, Mg \, I$$

Grignard Reagent

At this point, the ethylene oxide is added (with subsequent hydrolysis) to obtain n-propyl alcohol:

$$CH_2 - CH_2 \xrightarrow{CH_3MgI} \xrightarrow{HOH} CH_3CH_2CH_2OH.$$

with O bridging the two CH_2 groups.

139. **(D)** Carbohydrates may be defined as simple sugars and the substances that hydrolyze to yield simple sugars. Carbohydrates are placed in three classes: (1) Monosaccharides — those that do not undergo hydrolysis; (2) Disaccharides — those that may be hydrolyzed to two monosaccharide molecules; and (3) Polysaccharides — those which form many monosaccharide molecules after hydrolysis.

140. **(D)** In this reaction, X serves to reduce the temperature required for product formation to occur. This lowering of the required reaction temperature is analogous to a decrease in the activation energy of the reaction. By definition, a catalyst lowers the activation energy of a reaction. Hence, X is determined to be a catalyst. An enzyme is defined as a biochemical catalyst and thus it is inapplicable in this case since the reaction in question is not biochemical in nature.

141. **(C)**

$$HOAc + NaOH \longrightarrow NaOAc + H_2O$$

acetic acid   sodium acetate

The reaction of equimolar quantities of a weak acid and a strong base produces a basic (alkaline) salt and water.

142. **(D)** One mole of a hemiacetal is produced by reaction of one mole of aldehyde with one mole of alcohol.

$$\underset{\text{aldehyde}}{RCH} \; (=O) \quad + \quad \underset{\text{alcohol}}{R'OH} \xrightarrow[OH^-]{H^+ \text{ or}} \quad \underset{\text{hemiacetal}}{R - C(OH)(OR') - H}$$

Section 3 — Writing Sample

DEMONSTRATION ESSAY 1

John Taylor remarks upon the strength of written words by suggesting that they are even more powerful than tangible steel. No doubt, words carved by a writer's pen may do crippling harm to humans and surpass the longevity of a simple physical laceration. Taylor begins his observation regarding written words and the pens that produce them with a metaphor, likening the pens to "dangerous tools." Just as tools may be used to construct or demolish, so pens, too, may be used to enhance; but more importantly, Taylor stresses the pen's potential to destroy as implied by his choice of "painful" word pairs: sharp/swords, cut/keen, whips/rods. Like a parent cautions a young child about a knife or scissors, so Taylor reminds the reader of the harm that words can inflict.

A common response to Taylor's remark which would contradict his belief in the power of the written word can be found echoing in the playgrounds and schoolyards of all of our childhoods: "Sticks and stones may break my bones but words will never hurt me." This chant proclaims the immediate and painful results of abuse by physical objects, while attempting to combat the threat posed by words. Although visible damage will most certainly not be seen when hurling words rather than rocks, this lyric works to deny the internal psychological and emotional suffering which can be caused by disdainful words or unchecked verbal emotion. A physical wound caused by swords, whips, and rods, or sticks and stones for that matter, may soon heal; but the mental wound caused by the sharper wit of pens is often much deeper and lasting. Not only is the recorded word there for the victim to see and feel, it is there for contemporaries as well as future generations to ponder.

If one is to learn from history, one must remember that words — whether spoken or written — must be chosen carefully; for their might has been demonstrated throughout the ages. The imperishable effect of the written word as compared to the timely pain of physical abuse can be summed up when one considers the teeming amount of published accounts of modern and ancient opinion available in our libraries. Compare their accessibility to the chances of viewing the scars of a deep wound on any body. Long after the body has passed into oblivion the opinion of that person may remain among the living, but more ominously, it may be entombed on the bookshelves.

EXPLANATION OF DEMONSTRATION ESSAY 1

The essay addresses all three tasks: (1) Taylor's view of the might of power of the pen is explained and interpreted. (2) The essay contains a paragraph which contests Taylor's opinion with a childhood taunt which claims that words are unable to cause pain. (3) The essay compares the lasting effects of the written word versus the ephemeral pain of physical injury and makes a historically proven conclusion about each in relation to the other.

The grammar, spelling, and punctuation conform to suggested standards. Organization, depth of thought, control of vocabulary and variation of sentence structure are evident.

DEMONSTRATION ESSAY II

Douglas Jerrold extols the positive effects of patience as he compares it to a "strong drink," suggesting results through its usage similar to those of an alcoholic beverage. Because this metaphor seems favorable in that patience, like a drink, can slay an emotion as undesirable as despair it can be inferred that the repercussions of patience are also propitious. These characteristics are needed to overcome such a dire state of consciousness as despair. However, by using personification and by ascribing such power to Patience, the message becomes clear that if one can partake of this strongest of strong drinks, one will not be inclined to surrender to despondency and the giant Despair will be slain.

It is important to note, however, that people must be careful that they do not become complacent by relying too heavily on patience. Some literature of the past, particularly fairy tales, has presented women, for instance, with role models of overly patient females. These characters are so patient, in fact, that they become passive and do not work to better their situation. For example, some of the women passively wait or sleep, like Sleeping Beauty; or, instead of relying on their own abilities, they hope for rescue, like Cinderella as she prays for a fairy godmother, or Rapunzel as she wishes for a Prince.

Although Douglas Jerrold advocates imbibing the strong drink of Patience to conquer Despair, it seems that over-reliance on patience and passivity can induce the same ill-effects of the alcohol to which it is compared: a blurring of vision creating the inability to see what and when action must be taken. Just as it is difficult to rise from the depths of a drunken existence which is as firmly rooted in despair as it can be caused by it, it is equally laborious to stir one's own soul to action having been made dormant by the excessive patience it practiced — in moderation at one time — for its own good.

EXPLANATION OF DEMONSTRATION ESSAY II

The essay addresses all three tasks: (1) Jerrold's idea of Patience is defined and explained in relation to the metaphor and the object of Despair. (2) A conflicting view, presenting the disadvantages of patience, is presenting using examples. (3) A resolution of moderation is offered.

The essay uses relevant examples. The essay clearly, concisely, and logically presents the argument. The grammar, spelling, and punctuation conform to suggested standards. Organization, depth of thought, and control of vocabulary and sentence structure are evident.

Section 4 — Biological Sciences

PASSAGE I (Questions 143-147)

This passage requires a basic understanding of Mendelian inheritance and sex linkage, and the ability to apply the basic rules of probability of independent events.

143. **(A)**   This pedigree could not represent a sex-linked trait. A sex-linked recessive trait would have to be exhibited by all sons if exhibited by the mother. A holandric trait is carried on the Y chromosome and would not be exhibited by females. A father who showed sex-linked dominant trait would have to pass that trait on to all of his daughters.

144. **(D)**   This pedigree could represent either a dominant or recessive autosomal gene. Parents affected with a dominant autosomal trait may be heterozygotes; in this

pedigree both affected persons are heterozygotes. They may pass on the recessive trait to their offspring. Only two affected parents with normal offspring would rule out an autosomal recessive gene.

145. **(C)** The male is heterozygous since his mother exhibits the trait. The probability of his sperm carrying the recessive allele is therefore $^1/_2$. The female's mother is heterozygous because her mother exhibits the trait. The probability that the female received the recessive allele is $^1/_2$. If the female is heterozygous, $^1/_2$ of her eggs would carry the allele. Since all three events must occur in order to have a homozygous recessive child, the probability of having an affected child would be the product of these three probabilities, $^1/_2 \times ^1/_2 \times ^1/_2$.

146. **(B)** Any individual who possesses a dominant allele should show it. Since this couple does not exhibit the trait, neither of them has the allele to pass on to offspring.

147. **(B)** The female could be heterozygous for the trait in question; the chance that she is heterozygous is $^1/_2$ since her mother showed herself to be a heterozygote by having an affected son. If the female in question is heterozygous, half ($^1/_2$) of her eggs would carry the recessive gene. All daughters of this couple would receive their father's X chromosome with its dominant gene. Therefore only sons could be affected. Half ($^1/_2$) of the offspring are expected to be male: those which are fertilized by a Y-bearing sperm. All three events must occur (heterozygous female, recessive X egg, X-bearing sperm), in order to have an affected child. The chance of the occurrence is the product of the probabilities of these independent events: $^1/_2 \times ^1/_2 \times ^1/_2$.

PASSAGE II (Questions 148-153)

This passage involves meiosis, specifically spermatogenesis. In order to respond correctly to the questions in this section, one must know the stages of meiosis and the chromosomal constitution at each of these stages.

148. **(B)** The diploid number of chromosomes is present at Prophase I. These chromosomes replicate and synapse during this phase of meiosis. A replicated chromosome, two identical chromatids joined by a common centromere, is considered to be one chromosome.

149. **(B)** At Anaphase I, homologous chromosomes (each chromosome consists of identical chromatids joined at the entromere) travel to opposite poles. All of the chromosomes are present in the cell which were present before Prophase I. The chromatids will not separate until the second meiotic division.

150. **(B)** There are 46 chromosomes present in one secondary spermatocyte at Anaphase II. The centromeres replicate at the onset of Anaphase II, and the now doubled number of chromosomes travels on spindle fibers to opposite poles at Anaphase II. All of these chromosomes are present in one cell during this period. After the completion of Telophase II, each pole will result in a spermatid with 23 chromosomes.

151. **(B)** Eight sperm would result from four secondary spermatocytes after

Meiosis II. In spermatogenesis, the diploid primary spermatocyte produces two haploid secondary spermatocytes which each undergo nuclear and cytoplasmic division to produce two spermatids. Each spermatid goes through a maturation process called spermiogenesis to produce sperm. Therefore, four secondary spermatocytes would double to produce eight spermatids which would develop into eight sperm.

152. **(C)**   The two secondary spermatocytes produced after the completion of Meiosis I are haploid. They have one replicated chromosome of each type, 23 chromosomes in all. Meiosis II is similar to a mitotic division; the identical sister chromatids separate and travel to opposite poles at Anaphase II. The products of Meiosis II are haploid spermatids which develop into haploid sperm. The primary spermatocyte is diploid.

153. **(B)**   Polar bodies are small cells produced in oogenesis resulting from the divisions of primary and secondary oocytes. A Barr body is the sex chromatin mass that represents the genetically inactivated X chromosome found in the somatic cells of normal females. A basal body is a small granule usually present at the base of a flagellum or a cilium in protozoa. Vitreous bodies refer to the jelly-like substance within the eye that fills the space between the lens and the retina.

PASSAGE III (Questions 154-158)
        Understanding this passage requires a basic knowledge of osmosis, the diffusion of water across a selectively permeable membrane. The net moment of water will be from the side with a higher concentration of water to the side with a lower concentration.

154. **(D)**   Water has moved from tubes A and B but not tube C after two hours. Therefore, tube A initially had a hypotonic solution compared to the unknown, and tube C was isotonic compared to the unknown. Water moves across a selectively permeable membrane from a hypotonic solution (one with a higher water concentration) to a hypertonic solution. Tube A is 100% water; the unknown solution contains a solute and therefore has a lower water concentration. Since there is no difference in tube C's level of solution after two hours, it must have the same water concentration as the unknown solution.

155. **(C)**   Since tube C does not change fluid levels, the unknown solution must have the same concentration of water as tube C. Tube C is 1.0% glucose, therefore 99.0% water.

156. **(B)**   The red blood cell would swell as water moved inward. Water will move across a selectively permeable membrane from a hypotonic solution (less solute, more water) to a hypertonic solution (more solute, less water). The process of water moving across a semipermeable membrane is termed osmosis.

157. **(A)**   A solution which has a lower concentration of solutes is said to be hypotonic compared to the fluid in the cell. A hypertonic solution (B) has a higher concentration of solutes. Isotonic solutions (C) have the same concentration of solutes. The terms hypotonic (D) and osmotic (E) do not pertain to this question.

158. **(D)**   Molecules may move into or out of cells in several ways. Molecules such as ions and water molecules will move by diffusion through plasma membrane pores from a region of higher concentration to a region of lower concentration. Lipid-soluble molecules can diffuse directly through the lipid phase of the membrane. Carrier-facilitated diffusion involves carrier proteins, often called permeases, which interact with the molecule and ease its diffusion through the membrane.

PASSAGE IV (Questions 159-164)
Underlying this passage is an understanding of the relationship between genes and proteins. The representative electrophoretogram reveals that the enzyme in question exists in two forms which are separable by electrophoresis. Individuals may show one or both forms.

159. **(A)**   To answer this question, one must interpret the electrophoretic results and understand the meaning of the term allele. Alleles are genes which code for different versions of the same product, in this case an enzyme. Individuals 4 and 6 show both allozymes and therefore appear to be heterozygous for this gene. Individuals 1 and 2 are homozygous for the "slow" allele, but there is no evidence given concerning relative fitness of this allele. Likewise, there is no evidence that the "fast" allele in #3 and #5 is more adaptive.

160. **(C)**   This question requires the understanding that alleles code for a different molecular version of a product which serves a particular function. In this case, the alleles code for different versions of an enzyme (allozymes) whose function is to catalyze the same reaction.

161. **(B)**   This question assigns a differential range of function for the two allozymes. If one allozyme (in this case the "fast" allele product) functions throughout the normal temperature range and the other "slow" allozyme has restricted function within this range, homozygotes for the broad range allele would be most fit.

162. **(C)**   The introductory passage stated that gel electrophoresis revealed a surprising amount of diversity at the molecular level, indicating that genetic variability at the molecular level is a widespread phenomenon. The information in this section does not address fitness.

163. **(C)**   The primary structure of a protein, the specific sequence of amino acids, determines the rate at which the molecule will migrate. This electrophoretic characteristic is unrelated to catalytic efficiency and fitness.

164. **(D)**   If both allozymes could only function in half of the normal temperature range, the heterozygote which has both allozymes would have enzymes which worked throughout the range of temperatures. The superior fitness of the heterozygotes is termed heterosis, and selection for the heterozygote maintains genetic diversity and is termed balancing selection.

INDEPENDENT QUESTIONS

165. **(A)**   The mitotic divisions of the zygote lead to a solid ball of cells called

the morula. As the cells of the morula divide further, a fluid-filled cavity forms. This hollow ball of cells is the blastula. When the cells of the blastula differentiate into three layers, the mass is known as a gastrula. The developing organism is called a fetus.

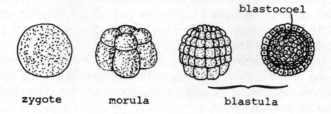

zygote   morula   blastula

166. **(B)**   The cerebellum regulates and coordinates muscle contractions. Its size in different animals corresponds roughly with the amount of muscular activity of the animal. Removal of the cerebellum results in the loss of the ability to coordinate voluntary muscle movement.

167. **(C)**   Pepsin is one of the few enzymes whose optimum pH is not 7. Pepsin requires a low pH of 1.5 to 2.5 for proper activity. The acidity of the stomach is maintained for optimal activity of the protease pepsin.

168. **(D)**   Enzymes are catalysts. Catalysts form unstable intermediates with the reactants. The complexes provide an alternate pathway for the reaction — one with a lower activation energy. This enables the reaction to proceed more readily and at a faster rate. Once the product has been formed, the enzyme is released and is free to catalyze another reaction.

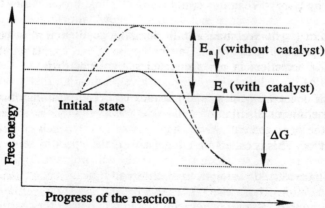

Reduction of Necessary Activation Energy by Catalysts

The activation energy (E_a) necessary to initiate the reaction is much less in the presence of a catalyst than in its absence. It is this lowering of the activation energy barrier by enzyme catalysts that makes possible most of the chemical reactions of life. Note that the free energy of reaction (ΔG) is unchanged by the catalyst; i.e., it is the same for both the catalyzed and the uncatalyzed reaction; only the activation energy is changed.

169. **(A)**   Blood clotting is initiated by damaged platelets + calcium → thrombo-plastin which acts on prothrombin → thrombin → which acts on fibrinogen molecules to produce → fibrin clot, an insoluable mass.

170. **(C)**   Highly developed animals can react extremely quickly to certain types of stimuli. This can be important when the animal comes into contact with harmful stimuli, such as fire or sharp objects piercing the skin. The faster the animal responds, the less damage is done.

These kinds of responses do not involve the brain, for conscious input is unnecessary and would slow the response. Instead, the impulse is carried from the receptor neuron directly to the spinal cord and then back out through a motor neuron to the appropriate muscle. Thus, the receptor neuron, the motor neuron, and the muscle are the only structures necessary for the reflex action to occur.

PASSAGE V (Questions 171-175)

This section involves the basic concepts of evolution and population genetics. In order to answer these questions, one must understand natural selection and the conditions under which Hardy-Weinberg genetic equilibrium prevails.

171. **(B)**   Natural selection results in a differential in reproductive success between individuals of different genotypes. In the game of evolution, the winners are genotypes which succeed in passing on more genes to the next generation than other genotypes.

172. **(D)**   Nonrandom mating would disturb Hardy-Weinberg genetic equilibrium. Nonrandom or assortive mating typically leads to an increase in homozygotes and a decrease in heterozygotes in the diploid population compared to the frequencies predicted by Hardy-Weinberg equilibrium.

173. **(C)**   For Hardy-Weinberg equilibrium, the population must be large enough for the laws of probability to prevail. In small populations, events unrelated to fitness can cause wide fluctuations in gene frequencies, or genetic drift.

174. **(D)**   If one extreme is selected against in a biological distribution, the mean of the next generation's distribution will move away from that extreme phenotype. In other words, the next generation will have fewer genes which confer the selected-against phenotype. This is called directional selection.

175. **(B)**   Individual phenotypes have different success at contributing their genes to the next generation. Those phenotypes that have relatively fewer descendants have been selected against. Selection acts on the individual phenotypes with the best adaptive traits, in order to select for survival those organisms that can respond best to certain conditions.

PASSAGE VI (Questions 176-181)

Cell and nuclear division are studied in elementary biology courses, but these cellular events are truly complex. Timing, chromosomal structure and cell structure are important to these processes. The questions in this section require an understanding of the basic structures involved and the sequence of events in mitosis and cytokinesis.

176. **(A)**   A principal prophase feature is the condensation of chromatin via coiling at several levels. Chromosomes enter metaphase in a condensed state and do not begin relaxation to a less condensed state until telophase, returning to decondensation at the following interphase.

177. **(C)**   The centromere is also called the primary construction. It is the point at which sister chromatids are joined. Because this region is relatively uncondensed, it appears to be very narrow or even undiscernable under the microscope. The spindle fibers will attach in this region on the kinetochore structures located at the centromere.

178. **(C)**   At prophase and metaphase there are 23 pairs, or 46 chromosomes, which are replicated. Each chromosomes has identical sister chromatids joined at the centromere. At anaphase, the replicated chromosomes travel to opposite poles, doubling the number of chromosomes in the cell at that time.

179. **(D)**   Replication of chromosomes occurs during the "S" stage of the cell cycle when the DNA content in the nucleus doubles. The "S" stands for synthesis, specifically, DNA synthesis. The "S" stage is in mid-interphase.

180. **(D)**   The kinetochore is the actual structure to which spindle microtubules attach. The replicated chromosome consists of two identical chromatics joined at the centromere region. Two kinetochores per chromosome develop in late prophase, one pointed toward each pole. The microtubules of the spindle attach to the kinetochores. The centriole is a self-reproducing organelle which is associated with nuclear division. The centrosome is the differentiated region of the cytoplasm which contains the centriole.

181. **(A)**   Animal cells undergo cytokinesis by means of a contractile ring of actin filaments which divide the cell into two. Pragmoplasts and cell plates are characteristic of plant cells. Binary fission is an amitotic, asexual division process of prokaryotes.

PASSAGE VII (Questions 182-187)

Although the vertebrate immune response is complex, these questions concern basic elements of that response. One needs to know the nature of cell-mediated and humoral immunity and the principal organs, cells and molecules involved.

182. **(B)**   T and B lymphocytes respond to specific invading organisms. Cells which also respond but are not listed here are Natural Killer (NK) cells which respond to viruses and non-self tissues. Erythrocytes are red blood cells which contain oxygen-transporting hemoglobin. Phagocytes are scavenger cells; they are not responsible for the immune response. Reticulocytes are young red blood cells just after loss of their nuclei. They mature into erythrocytes.

183. **(C)**   B cells or B lymphocytes produce antibodies after stimulation by a specific antigen. T cells or T lymphocytes (B) directly attack foreign cells or substances in the cell-mediated immune response. Phagocytes (D) are scavenger cells.

184. **(B)**   The Y-shaped antibody molecule consists of two identical "heavy" and two identical "light" polypeptide chains held together by disulfide bridges. There are, therefore, just two different types of polypeptides in an antibody molecule, the "heavy" chain and the "light" chain.

185. **(A)**   T cells or T lymphocytes participate in cell-mediated immunity — attacking foreign cells or substances. B cells produce specific antibodies. Reticulocytes are red blood cells which are not part of the immune process. Phagocytes are scavenger cells.

186. **(D)**   As described in the passage, antibodies are specific for one specific type of antigen. The antibody molecule illustrated has two binding sites and therefore could bind this type of antigen at both active sites.

187. **(C)**   Isotypes are variants which are present in all members of a species. Examples of isotypic variants are the different antibody classes and subclasses. Allotypes, however, are variants which are due to intraspecies genetic differences. Each individual has a specific allotype at each of its immunoglobulin gene loci, which often differ from those present in other individuals. Idiotypes are variants due to a large amount of structural heterogeneity in the immunoglobulin V regions. This is related to the production of a wide variety of different V regions to bind diverse antigens. Finally, phenotypes are the physical appearances of an individual, some phenotypes, such as blood groups, are completely determined by heredity, while others, such as statute, are readily altered by environmental agents.

PASSAGE VIII (Questions 188-192)
This section is concerned with the basics of cell architecture. The specific structure of a cell is directly related to its function. Some features are common to all cells, others vary according to the cell's origin and/or function.

188. **(C)**   All cells have a plasma membrane and DNA as genetic information. Prokaryotic cells do not have mitochondria, nuclei, endoplasmic reticulum or centrioles. Viruses are considered to be noncellular particles; they have a protein coat but no plasma membrane. RNA or DNA may serve as viral genetic information.

189. **(C)**   The plasma or cell membrane in eukaryotes consists of a phospholipid bilayer, a double layer of phospholipids with their relatively hydrophilic (polar) "heads" on the outside and their hydrophobic (nonpolar) fatty acid tails pointed inward. Different proteins and carbohydrates may or may not be present, depending on the cell type.

190. **(C)**   The nucleolus is the region of ribosomal rRNA synthesis and the assembly of ribosomal subunits. It is formed around the nucleolar organizing region on a particular chromosome, the region of DNA which codes for rRNA.

191. **(D)**   The inner membrane of the mitochondrion contains cofactors for electron transport, and the mitochondrial matrix has the enzymes of the Krebs or citric acid cycle. Thus, the process of respiration occurs within the mitochondrion. This process involves breaking down the acetyl group on acetyl coenzyme A, passing the

hydrogen atoms down electron carriers via the electron transport chain where coupled reactions form energy-rich ATP molecules from ADP. Mitochondria are descended from mitochondria; they duplicate by a binary fission process.

192. **(B)** The rough and smooth endoplasmic reticulum are continuous with the golgi complex. A vesicle is a membrane bound sac. The peroxisome is a type of vesicle which contains peroxide-forming and -destroying enzymes. Lysosomes are vesicles which contain hydrolytic enzymes. Microtubules are part of the cytoskeleton. Mitochondria are double-membraned organelles.

INDEPENDENT QUESTIONS

193. **(C)** Tropomyosin, a linear protein attaches to actin, and covers the myosin binding sites when the muscle is not contracting.

194. **(C)** Bacterial genomes are haploid. This means that they have only one copy of each gene. Thus, no recessive traits can be masked by dominant traits since the alleles are in single copies. This fact is very useful to geneticists who wish to follow traits that would be masked in diploid organisms.

195. **(D)** The blood plasma is filtered from the capillaries to the Bowman's capsule through the single-celled capillary wall and the single-celled lining of the Bowman's capsule. Therefore, the blood which originally enters the kidneys through the renal artery is filtered from the capillaries of the glomerulus into the Bowman's

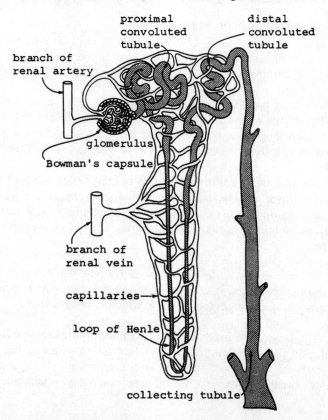

capsule. Eventually, the filtered blood leaves the kidneys after having passed through a second capillary network called the renal portal system.

196. **(B)**   A developing embryo undergoes three drastically different stages in its early development. These states are temporally continuous but have been given separate names. The single zygote divides many times and becomes a ball of cells called the morula. A fluid-filled cavity is formed in the center of the morula changing it into a hollow ball of cells called the blastula. Blastulation is followed by gastrulation where the three germ layers differentiate. The gastrula period extends until the early forms of all of the major structures are laid down in neurulation. After this, the developing organism is referred to as a fetus.

197. **(B)**   Cryptic appearance, Mullerian mimicry and Batesian mimicry are ways in which organisms can avoid becoming the victims of predators. The cryptic appearance of some organisms enables them to blend into their background, becoming invisible to their potential attackers. Mullerian mimicry involves the evolution of two or more inedible or unpleasant-tasting species to resemble one another. Batesian mimicry, however, involves the resemblance of an unprotected, harmless species to a dangerous species. This makes it difficult for the predator to distinguish between the two forms. Once the predator has tasted the noxious species, it tends to stay away from both species.

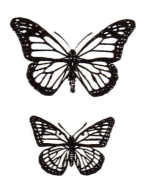

An example of Batesian mimicry.

Top: The Monarch butterfly, a distasteful species. Bottom: The Viceroy, a species that mimics the Monarch. Species in the group to which the Viceroy belongs ordinarily have a quite different appearance.

PASSAGE IX (Questions 198-203)

198. **(D)**   Mitosis gives rise to daughter cells that are identical to the parent cell and is the only type of nuclear division that could result in clone formation. Answer (A) is incorrect because cytokinesis is the division of cytoplasm which occurs in both mitosis and meiosis. Answers (B) and (C) are wrong because they refer to the same type of division which results in genetically variable daughter cells.

199. **(A)** Sexual reproduction introduces a great deal of genetic variability into a population. If the environment changes, the traits necessary to survive in the new environment may also change. When there are many variations of traits available, it is likely that some individuals will possess the traits best suited to the new environment and will be able to survive and reproduce. Answer (B) is wrong because genetic variability is not as important in an unchanging environment. Answer (C) is incorrect because chromosome number remains constant in both sexual and asexual reproduction. Answer (D) is wrong because the offspring of sexual reproduction are genetically different from each other.

200. **(B)** If a cell contains 3 pair of chromosomes, the number of possible combinations is 2^3, or 8 different combinations. For example, if a cell contains the chromosome pairs Aa, Bb, and Cc, the possible chromosome combinations are:

ABC	ABc	Abc	AbC
aBC	aBc	abC	abc

201. **(B)** Since the progeny of asexual reproduction are genetically identical, this type of reproduction is advantageous when an organism possesses certain desirable traits which would benefit future generations, such as disease resistance in plants. Answers (A), (C) and (D) are incorrect because genetic variability would be more beneficial in these cases by helping the species adapt to different environments.

202. **(C)** During meiosis, the chromosome number is reduced by half so that when two gametes unite to form a new individual, the chromosome number is once again restored to normal. Answers (A) and (D) are wrong because these events occur in both meiosis and mitosis. Answer (B) is incorrect because the chromosome number is reduced by half during meiosis.

203. **(A)** When individual chromatics exchange parts, genetic variability is increased to an even greater extent than with random assortment alone. Following crossover, each homologous chromosome contains one original chromatid and one altered chromatid. In this case, meiosis would result in four genetically different daughter cells. Answer (B) is wrong because the daughter cells will be genetically different. Answer (C) is incorrect because homologous chromosomes contain slight variations of the same genes and are not identical. Answer (D) is incorrect because the number of chromosomal combinations is not reduced.

PASSAGE X (Questions 204-219)

204. **(B)** The above reaction occurs in two steps. Iodine will react with acetone to form hydrogen iodide and triiodoactone, which is readily reversible:

$$3I_2 + CH_3COCH_3 \longleftrightarrow 3HI + CLI_3COCH_3.$$

However, the hydrogen iodide will react irreversibly with sodium hydroxide to form sodium iodide and water:

$$3NaOH + 3HI \longrightarrow 3NaI + 3H_2O.$$

The triiodoactone also reacts with the sodium hydroxide to form sodium acetate and iodoform:

$$Cl_3COCH_3 + NaOH \longrightarrow CH_3COOH + CHI_3.$$

Since iodoform is quite insoluble in water, it is the precipitate.

205. **(C)** Remember, iodine will be in the precipitate as iodoform, and in the supernatant as sodium iodide.

206 **(B)** The only compound the sodium ends up in is sodium acetate, which is quite soluble in water, and hence in the supernatant.

207. **(D)** The molecular weight of iodine is 254, hence 10 grams of I_2 will contain 0.03937 moles. Looking at the stoichiometric ratios, three moles of iodine produce one mole of the precipitate, iodoform. This gives 0.01312 moles of iodoform, which with a molecular weight of 394, gives 5.169 grams of iodoform. Since only 4.27 grams were produced, this gives $(4.27 / 5.169) \times 100 = 82.6\%$ efficiency.

208. **(D)** Remember, electronegativity *decreases* as one moves down the periodic table. This means that, since all of the listed halogens are above iodine, they can all displace it. An example using fluorine would be:

$$F_2 + 2CHI_3 \longrightarrow 2CHI_2F + I_2 \uparrow.$$

The other halogens would react the same.

209. **(D)** Remember, alkanes generally do not react.

PASSAGE XI (Questions 210-215)

210. **(B)** This is an S_N2 reaction. The OH⁻ replaces the Br, and the optical activity is reversed. See the illustration below.

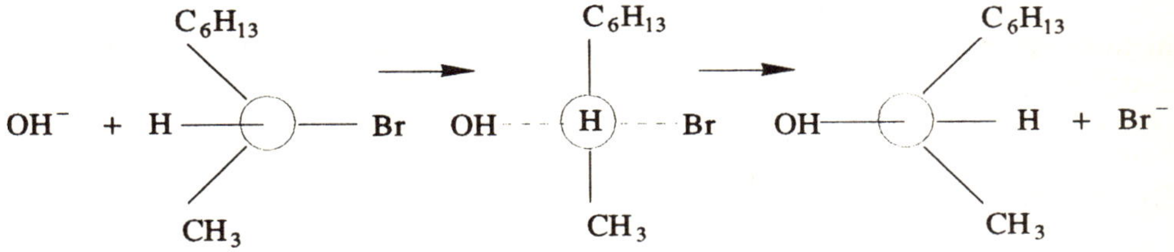

An example of an S_N2 reaction.

Note that the optical activity of the product has been reversed. Also note the intermediate form in the middle.

211. **(D)** The correct answer is (D), as was mentioned above. It involves substitution (answers (A) and (B) are elimination), and the optical activity of the product is reversed.

212. **(A)** For an S_N2 reaction with an alkyl halide, a methyl group is more reactive than a primary, which is greater than a secondary, which is greater than a tertiary. Choice (A) has the bromine on a 1° carbon, rather than a 2°, as was on the original.

213. **(C)** For the reasons cited above, the bromine in this compound is on a 3° carbon.

214. **(A)** S_N2 stands for substitution, second order kinetics. The rate law for this states:

$$\text{Rate} = k[CH_3(CH_2)_5CHBrCH_3]\,[OH^-],$$

where k is the reaction rate constant.

215. **(C)** An S_N2 reaction will still occur, and the optical activity will be reversed.

INDEPENDENT QUESTIONS

216. **(A)** The Williamson synthesis of ethers is important because of its versatility in the laboratory. This method of synthesis can be used to make asymmetrical ethers as well as symmetrical ethers. In the Williamson synthesis, an alkyl halide is allowed to react with a sodium alkoxide (or sodium phenoxide)

$$R-X \qquad + R'-O^-Na^+ \qquad \longrightarrow \qquad R-O-R' + Na^+X^-,$$

Alkyl halide   Sodium alkoxide   Ether

where R represents an alkyl group and X a halide (Cl, Br, I or F). [The yield from RX is:

$$CH_3 > 1° > 2° \,(> 3°).]$$

The sodium alkoxide is made by direct action of sodium metal on dry alcohols:

$$R-\;\;OH + Na \;\longrightarrow\; R-O^-Na^+ + {}^1/_2\,H_2 \uparrow$$

Sodium alkoxide

217. **(A)** Hydrogen bonding in alcohols serves to decrease the vapor pressure by "holding" the molecules together.

218. **(A)** Catalytic hydrogentation of an alkene is achieved by reacting the alk-

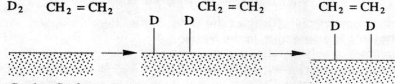

$$CH_2D - CH_2D$$

ene with H_2 (g) on the surface of an appropriate catalyst such as Pt, Pd or Ni. Using D_2 instead of H_2, the mechanism is probably described in the previous diagram.

As can be seen from the diagram, syn-addition is usually the result since only one side of the alkene is exposed to the catalyst surface.

Keeping this in mind it can be seen that the hydrogenation of 2-methyl-2-pentene occurs in the following manner:

$$
\underset{\substack{CH_3 \\ / \\ CH_3}}{C} = \underset{\substack{CH_2CH_3 \\ \backslash \\ H}}{C} \quad \xrightarrow{\hspace{2cm}} \quad CH_3\underset{CH_3}{\overset{D}{C}} - \underset{H}{\overset{D}{C}} - CH_2CH_3
$$

or in another form:

$$
H_3C - \underset{CH_3}{\overset{D}{C}} - \underset{H}{\overset{D}{C}} - \underset{H}{\overset{H}{C}} - CH_3
$$

Choice (B) is a product of anti-addition which does not occur with a platinum catalyst. Choice (C) is the catalytic hydrogenation product of 4-methyl-2-pentene. Choice (D) is also a product of anti-addition.

219. **(B)**   Polarity indicates that there is an unequal sharing of electrons between two atoms. This creates a charge distribution in the molecule where one atom is partially positive and the other is partially negative. The degree of polarity is measured by finding the difference in the ability of the two atoms to attract electrons. This tendency to attract electrons is electronegativity. The greater the electronegativity difference, the greater the degree of polarity.

In general, electronegativity increases across a period and decreases down a group of the periodic table.

When comparing the polarities of HCl and HBr, one observes that Cl is in the same group and higher than Br, thus it has greater electronegativity. Therefore, HCl is more polar than HBr. For HS and HO, O is more electronegative than S since it is higher in the same group; HO is more polar than HS. For HF and HO, F is more electronegative than O so HF is more polar than HO. F, Cl, Br and I are all in the same group. The electronegativity values vary, with F having the greatest and I the smallest. Br and Cl have intermediate values. As in all other cases, the difference between two extreme values is greater than the difference between two intermediate values, and consequently IF is more polar than BrCl. Since O is more electronegative than C, one may assume OF is more polar than CF. However, this gives the wrong answer. One must remember that we are attempting to obtain the largest electronegativity difference, not only the largest electronegativity value. Since F is the element with the greatest electronegativity value given in this choice, it is from this value that we subtract the electronegativities of C and O. Since C < O in electronegative value, Cf will give a greater electronegativity difference and hence a greater polarity value than OF.

THE PERIODIC TABLE

KEY

Atomic Number →	22
	Ti
Atomic Weight →	47.88

Group Classification → (top)
Symbol →

( ) indicates most stable or best known isotope

METALS — NONMETALS

TRANSITIONAL METALS

Alkali Metals — Alkaline Earth Metals — Halogens — Noble Gases

Group	1 IA IA	2 IIA IIA	3 IIIA IIIB	4 IVA IVB	5 VA VB	6 VIA VIB	7 VIIA VIIB	8 VIIIA VIII	9 VIIIA VIII	10 VIIIA VIII	11 IB IB	12 IIB IIB	13 IIIB IIIA	14 IVB IVA	15 VB VA	16 VIB VIA	17 VIIB VIIA	18 VIII 0
	1 H 1.008																	2 He 4.003
	3 Li 6.941	4 Be 9.012											5 B 10.811	6 C 12.011	7 N 14.007	8 O 15.999	9 F 18.998	10 Ne 20.180
	11 Na 22.990	12 Mg 24.305											13 Al 26.982	14 Si 28.086	15 P 30.974	16 S 32.066	17 Cl 35.453	18 Ar 39.948
	19 K 39.098	20 Ca 40.078	21 Sc 44.956	22 Ti 47.88	23 V 50.942	24 Cr 51.996	25 Mn 54.938	26 Fe 55.847	27 Co 58.933	28 Ni 58.693	29 Cu 63.546	30 Zn 65.39	31 Ga 69.723	32 Ge 72.61	33 As 74.922	34 Se 78.96	35 Br 79.904	36 Kr 83.8
	37 Rb 85.468	38 Sr 87.62	39 Y 88.906	40 Zr 91.224	41 Nb 92.906	42 Mo 95.94	43 Tc (97.907)	44 Ru 101.07	45 Rh 102.906	46 Pd 106.4	47 Ag 107.868	48 Cd 112.411	49 In 114.818	50 Sn 118.710	51 Sb 121.757	52 Te 127.60	53 I 126.905	54 Xe 131.29
	55 Cs 132.905	56 Ba 137.327	57 La 138.906	72 Hf 178.49	73 Ta 180.948	74 W 183.84	75 Re 186.207	76 Os 190.23	77 Ir 192.22	78 Pt 195.08	79 Au 196.967	80 Hg 200.59	81 Tl 204.383	82 Pb 207.2	83 Bi 208.980	84 Po (208.982)	85 At (209.982)	86 Rn (222.018)
	87 Fr (223.020)	88 Ra (226.025)	89 Ac (227.028)	104 Unq (261.11)	105 Unp (262.114)	106 Unh (263.118)	107 Uns (262.12)	108 Uno (265)	109 Une (266)	110 Uun (269)								

LANTHANIDE SERIES

58 Ce 140.115	59 Pr 140.908	60 Nd 144.24	61 Pm (144.913)	62 Sm 150.36	63 Eu 151.965	64 Gd 157.25	65 Tb 158.925	66 Dy 162.50	67 Ho 164.930	68 Er 167.26	69 Tm 168.934	70 Yb 173.04	71 Lu 174.967

ACTINIDE SERIES

90 Th 232.038	91 Pa 231.036	92 U 238.029	93 Np 237.048	94 Pu (244.064)	95 Am (243.061)	96 Cm (247.070)	97 Bk (247.070)	98 Cf (251.080)	99 Es (252.083)	100 Fm (257.095)	101 Md (258.1)	102 No (259.101)	103 Lr (262.11)

U.S. Medical Schools*

ALABAMA
University of Alabama School of Medicine
Office of Medical Student Services / Admissions
1670 University Blvd.
Volker Hall P-100
Birmingham, AL 35294
(205) 934-2330

University of Southern Alabama College of Medicine
Office of Admissions
Rm. 2015, Medical Sciences Bldg.
Mobile, AL 36688-0002
(334) 460-7176

ARIZONA
University of Arizona College of Medicine
Admissions Office
1501 North Campbell Ave.
Tucson, AZ 85724
(520) 626-6214

ARKANSAS
University of Arkansas College of Medicine
Office of Student Admissions, Slot 551
4301 West Markham St.
Little Rock, AR 72205
(501) 686-5354

CALIFORNIA
University of California - Davis
School of Medicine
Chair, Admissions Committee
Admissions Office
Davis, CA 95616
(530) 752-2717

University of California - Irvine
College of Medicine
Office of Admissions
Medical Sciences Bldg. 802
Irvine, CA 92697-4089
(714) 824-5388

UCLA School of Medicine
Office of Student Affairs
Division of Admissions
Center for Health Sciences
Box 957035
Rm. 12 - 105CHS
Los Angeles, CA 90024
(213) 825-6081

University of California - San Diego
Office of Admissions, 621
Medical Testing Facility
School of Medicine
La Jolla, CA 92093-0621
(619) 534-3880

University of California - San Francisco
School of Medicine, Admissions
C-200, Box 408
521 Parnassus Ave.
San Francisco, CA 94143-0408
(415) 476-4044

Loma Linda University School of Medicine
Associate Dean for Admissions
Loma Linda, CA 92350
(714) 824-4467

University of Southern California
School of Medicine
Office of Admissions
1975 Zonal Ave.
Los Angeles, CA 90033
(213) 342-2552

Stanford University School of Medicine
Office of Admissions
851 Welch Road, Rm. 154
Palo Alto, CA 94304-1677
(415) 723-6861

COLORADO
University of Colorado School of Medicine
Office of Admissions and Records
UCHSC Box C297
4200 East Ninth Ave.
Denver, CO 80262
(303) 315-7361

CONNECTICUT
University of Connecticut School of Medicine
Office of Admissions and Student Affairs
263 Farmington Ave.
Farmington, CT 06030-3906
(203) 679-4713

Yale University School of Medicine
Office of Admissions
367 Cedar Street
New Haven, CT 06510
(203) 785-2643

DISTRICT OF COLUMBIA
George Washington University School of Medicine and Health Sciences
Office of Admissions
2300 I St., N.W.
Washington, D.C. 20037
(202) 994-3506

Georgetown University School of Medicine
Office of Admissions
3900 Reservoir Road, N.W.
Washington, D.C. 20007-2195
(202) 687-1154

Howard University College of Medicine
Admissions Office
520 W Street, N.W.
Washington, D.C. 20059
(202) 806-6279

FLORIDA
University of Florida College of Medicine
Office of Student Affairs
P.O. Box 100216
Gainesville, FL 32610-0216
(352) 392-3071

University of Miami School of Medicine
Office of Admissions
R159
P.O. Box 016159
Miami, FL 33101
(305) 547-6791

University of South Florida
College of Medicine
Office of Admissions
Box 3
12901 Bruce B. Downs Blvd.
Tampa, FL 33612-4799
(813) 974-2229

GEORGIA

Emory University School of
Medicine
Medical School Admissions
1440 Clifton Road, N.E.
Atlanta, GA 30322
(404) 727-5660

Medical College of Georgia
School of Medicine
Office of Admissions
1120 15th St.
Augusta, GA 30912
(706) 721-0211

Mercer University School of
Medicine
Office of Admissions and Student
Affairs
1550 College St.
Macon, GA 31207
(912) 752-2524

Morehouse School of Medi-
cine
Admissions and Student Affairs
720 Westview Drive, S.W.
Suite 150
Atlanta, GA 30310-1495
(404) 752-1650

HAWAII

University of Hawaii
John A. Burns School of
Medicine
Office of Student Affairs
1960 East - West Road
Honolulu, HI 96822

(808) 956-8300

ILLINOIS

University of Chicago -
Pritzker School of Medicine
Office of Admissions
924 East 57th St.
Chicago, IL 60637-5416
(773) 702-1939

UHS / Chicago Medical
School
Office of Admissions
3333 Green Bay Road
North Chicago, IL 60064
(708) 578-3207

University of Illinois College
of Medicine
Office of Admissions
808 S. Wood Street
Rm. 165
Chicago, IL 60612
(312) 996-5635

Loyola University Medical
Center
Stritch School of Medicine
Office of Admissions, Rm. 200
2160 South First Ave.
Maywood, IL 60153
(708) 216-3229

Northwestern University
Medical School
Associate Dean for Admissions
303 East Chicago Ave.
Rm. 1-606
Chicago, IL 60611
(312) 908-8206

Rush Medical College of Rush
University
Office of Admissions
600 South Paulina St.
Suite 524H
Chicago, IL 60612
(312) 942-6913

Southern Illinois University
School of Medicine
Office of Student and Alumni Affairs
P.O. Box 19230
Springfield, IL 62794-1226
(217) 782-2860

INDIANA

Indiana University School of
Medicine
Medical School Admissions Office
Fesler Hall 213
1120 South Drive
Indianapolis, IN 46202-5113
(317) 274-3772

IOWA

University of Iowa College of
Medicine
Office of Student Affairs
100 Medical Administration Bldg.
Iowa City, IA 52242-1101
(319) 335-8052

KANSAS

University of Kansas School of
Medicine
Office of Admissions
3901 Rainbow Blvd.
3001 Murphy Bldg.
Kansas City, KS 66160
(913) 588-5245

KENTUCKY

University of Kentucky
College of Medicine
Admissions, Rm. MN-102
Office of Education
Chandler Medical Center
800 Rose St.
Lexington, KY 40536-0084
(606) 323-6161

University of Louisville
School of Medicine
Office of Admissions
Health Sciences Center
323 East Chestnut St.
Louisville, KY 40292
(502) 852-5193

LOUISIANA

Louisiana State University
School of Medicine
Admissions Office
1901 Perdido St.
Box P3-4
New Orleans, LA 70112
(504) 568-6262

Louisiana State University
Medical Center
School of Medicine in Shreveport
Office of Student Admissions
P.O. Box 33932
Shreveport, LA 71130-3932
(318) 675-5190

Tulane University School of
Medicine
Office of Admissions
1430 Tulane Ave., SL67
New Orleans, LA 70112
(504) 588-5187

MARYLAND
Johns Hopkins University School of Medicine
Committee on Admission
720 Rutland Ave.
Baltimore, MD 21205-2196
(410) 955-3182

University of Maryland School of Medicine
Committee on Admissions
Rm. 1-005
655 West Baltimore St.
Baltimore, MD 21201
(410) 706-7478

Uniformed Services University of the Health Sciences
F. Edward Hébert School of Medicine
Admissions Office, Rm. A-1041
4301 Jones Bridge Road
Bethesda, MD 20814-4799
(301) 295-3101

MASSACHUSETTS
Boston University School of Medicine
Admissions Office L-124
715 Albany St.
Boston, MA 02118
(617) 638-4633

Harvard Medical School
Office of Admissions
25 Shattuck St.
Boston, MA 02115
(617) 432-1550

University of Massachusetts Medical School
Office of Admissions
Rm. S1-112
55 Lake Ave., North
Worcester, MA 01655
(508) 856-2323

Tufts University School of Medicine
Committee on Admissions
136 Harrison Ave.
Boston, MA 02111
(617) 636-6571

MICHIGAN
Michigan State University
College of Human Medicine
Office of Admissions
A-239 Life Sciences
East Lansing, MI 48824
(517) 353-9620

University of Michigan Medical School
Admissions Office
M4130 Medical Science Bldg. I, C-Wing
1301 Catherine Road
Ann Arbor, MI 48109-0624
(734) 764-6317

Wayne State University School of Medicine
Director of Admissions
540 East Canfield
Detroit, MI 48201
(313) 577-1466

MINNESOTA
Mayo Medical School
Admissions Committee
200 First St., S.W.
Rochester, MN 55905
(507) 284-3671

University of Minnesota-Duluth
School of Medicine
Office of Admissions, Rm. 107
10 University Drive
Duluth, MN 55812
(218) 726-8511

University of Minnesota Medical School
Office of Admissions and Student Affairs
Box 293-UMHC
420 Delaware St., S.E.
Minneapolis, MN 55455-0310
(612) 624-1122

MISSISSIPPI
University of Mississippi School of Medicine
Chairman, Admissions Committee
2500 North State St.
Jackson, MS 39216-4505
(601) 984-5010

MISSOURI
University of Missouri-Columbia
School of Medicine
Office of Admissions
MA202 Medical Sciences Bldg.
One Hospital Drive
Columbia, MO 65212
(573) 882-2923

University of Missouri-Kansas City
School of Medicine
University Admissions Office
2411 Holmes
Kansas City, MO 64108
(816) 235-1900

Saint Louis University School of Medicine
Admissions Committee
Rm. 226
1402 South Grand Blvd.
St. Louis, MO 63104
(314) 577-8205

Washington University School of Medicine
Admissions Office
660 South Euclid Avenue
Box 8107
St. Louis, MO 63110
(314) 362-6857

NEBRASKA
Creighton University
Medical School Admissions Office
2500 California Plaza
Omaha, NB 68178
(402) 280-2798

University of Nebraska College of Medicine
Admissions Committee
600 South 42nd St.
Box 986545
Omaha, NB 68198-6585
(402) 559-6140

NEVADA
University of Nevada School of Medicine
Office of Admissions
Manville 357
Reno, NV 89557-0046
(702) 784-6001

NEW HAMPSHIRE

Dartmouth Medical School
Office of Admissions
HB 7020
306 Remsen
Hanover, NH 03755-3833
(603) 650-1505

NEW JERSEY

UMDNJ - New Jersey Medical School
Director of Admissions
185 South Orange Ave.
Newark, NJ 07103
(973) 972-4631

UMDNJ - Robert Wood Johnson Medical School
Office of Admissions
675 Hoes Lane
Piscataway, NJ 08854-5635
(732) 235-4587

NEW MEXICO

University of New Mexico School of Medicine
Office of Admissions
Basic Medical Sciences Bldg., Rm. 107
Albuquerque, NM 87131-5166
(505) 272-4766

NEW YORK

Albany Medical College
Office of Admissions
Mail Code 3
47 New Scotland Ave.
Albany, NY 12208
(518) 262-5521

Albert Einstein College of Medicine
Office of Admissions
1300 Morris Park Ave.
Rm. 211
Bronx, NY 10461
(718) 430-2106

Columbia University College of Physicians and Surgeons
630 West 168th St.
New York, NY 10032
(212) 305-3595

Cornell University Medical College
Office of Admissions
445 East 69th St., Rm. 104
New York, NY 10021
(212) 746-1067

Mount Sinai School of Medicine
Office of Admissions
Box 1002
One Gustave L. Levy Place
New York, NY 10029
(212) 241-6696

New York Medical College
Office of Admissions
Administrative Bldg.
Valhalla, NY 10595
(914) 993-4507

New York University School of Medicine
Office of Admissions
P.O. Box 1924
New York, NY 10016
(212) 263-5290

University of Rochester School of Medicine and Dentistry
Director of Admissions
Medical Center Box 601
601 Elmwood Ave.
Rochester, NY 14642
(716) 275-4539

State University of New York Health Science Center at Brooklyn
Director of Admissions
450 Clarkson Ave. - Box 60
Brooklyn, NY 11433
(718) 270-2446

State University of New York at Buffalo
Office of Medical Admissions
Farber Hall
Rm. 131
Buffalo, NY 14214-3013
(716) 829-3466

State University of New York at Stony Brook Health Sciences Center School of Medicine
Committee on Admissions
Level 4, Rm. 46
Stony Brook, NY 11794-8434
(516) 444-2113

State University of New York Health Science Center at Syracuse
College of Medicine
Admissions Committee
155 Elizabeth Blackwell Street
Syracuse, NY 13210
(315) 464-4570

NORTH CAROLINA

Bowman Gray School of Medicine of Wake Forest University
Office of Medical School Admissions
300 South Hawthorne Road
Winston-Salem, NC 27103
(336) 716-4264

Duke University School of Medicine
Committee on Admissions
Duke University Medical Center
P.O. Box 3710
Durham, NC 27710
(919) 684-2985

East Carolina University School of Medicine
Office of Admissions
Greenville, NC 27858-4354
(919) 816-2202

University of North Carolina at Chapel Hill School of Medicine
Admissions Office
130 MacNider Hall
CB #7000
Chapel Hill, NC 27599-7000
(919) 962-8331

NORTH DAKOTA

University of North Dakota School of Medicine
Secretary, Committee on Admissions
501 North Columbia Road
Grand Forks, ND 58203-9037
(701) 777-4221

OHIO

Case Western Reserve University School of Medicine
Associate Dean for Admissions and Student Affairs
10900 Euclid Ave.
Cleveland, OH 44106-4920
(216) 368-3450

University of Cincinnati
College of Medicine
Office of Admissions
P.O. Box 670552
Cincinnati, OH 45267-0552
(513) 558-7314

Medical College of Ohio
Admissions Office
3045 Arlington Ave.
Toledo, OH 43614
(419) 383-4229

Northeastern Ohio University
College of Medicine
Office of Admissions
4209 State Rt. 44
P.O. Box 95
Rootstown, OH 44272
(330) 325-2511

Ohio State University College
of Medicine
Admissions Committee
270 Meiling Hall
370 West Ninth Avenue
Columbus, OH 43210
(614) 292-7137

Wright State University
School of Medicine
Office of Student Affairs/Admissions
P.O. Box 1751
Dayton, OH 45401
(937) 873-2934

OKLAHOMA
University of Oklahoma
College of Medicine
Office of Student Admissions
BMSB 357
P.O. Box 26901
Oklahoma City, OK 73190
(405) 271-2331

OREGON
Oregon Health Sciences
University
Office of Admissions
3181 S.W. Sam Jackson Park Road
L102
Portland, OR 97201
(503) 494-8220

PENNSYLVANIA
Hahnemann University School
of Medicine
Medical School Admissions
2900 Queen Lane
Philadelphia, PA 19129
(215) 991-8202

Jefferson Medical College of
Thomas Jefferson University
Associate Dean for Admissions
1025 Walnut St.
Philadelphia, PA 19107
(215) 955-6983

Medical College of Pennsylvania
Associate Dean for Admissions
3300 Henry Avenue
Philadelphia, PA 19129
(215) 842-7009

Pennsylvania State University
College of Medicine
Admissions Office H060
P.O. Box 850
Hershey, PA 17033
(717) 531-8755

University of Pennsylvania
School of Medicine
Director of Admissions
Suite 100 - Edward J.
Stemmler Hall
3450 Hamilton Walk
Philadelphia, PA 19104-6056
(215) 898-8001

University of Pittsburgh
School of Medicine
Office of Admissions
518 Scaife Hall
Pittsburgh, PA 15261
(412) 648-9891

Temple University School of
Medicine
Admissions Office
Suite 305, Student Faculty Center
Broad and Ontario Streets
Philadelphia, PA 19140
(215) 707-3656

PUERTO RICO
Universidad Central del Caribe
School of Medicine
Office of Admissions
P.O. Box 60327

Bayamón, PR 00960-6032
(787) 740-1611

Ponce School of Medicine
Admissions Office
P.O. Box 7004
Ponce, PR 00732
(787) 840-2575

University of Puerto Rico
Central Admissions Office
School of Medicine
P.O. Box 365067
San Juan, PR 00936-5067
(787) 758-2525, Ext. 5213

RHODE ISLAND
Brown University Program in
Medicine
Office of Admission
97 Waterman St.
Box G-A212
Providence, RI 02912
(401) 863-2149

SOUTH CAROLINA
Medical University of South
Carolina
Director of Admissions
171 Ashley Avenue
Charleston, SC 29425
(803) 792-3281

University of South Carolina
School of Medicine
Senior Associate Dean for Student
Programs
Columbia, SC 29208
(803) 733-3325

SOUTH DAKOTA
University of South Dakota
School of Medicine
Office of Student Affairs, Rm. 105
414 East Clark St.
Vermillion, SD 57069-2390
(605) 677-5233

TENNESSEE
East Tennessee State University
Quillen College of Medicine
Assistant Dean for Admissions and
Records
P.O. Box 70580
Johnson City, TN 37614-0002
(423) 439-6221

Meharry Medical College
School of Medicine
Director, Admissions and Records
1005 D.B. Todd, Jr. Blvd.
Nashville, TN 37208
(615) 327-6223

University of Tennessee,
Memphis
College of Medicine
Director of Admissions
800 Madison Avenue
Memphis, TN 38163
(901) 448-5559

Vanderbilt University School
of Medicine
Office of Admissions
209 Light Hall
Nashville, TN 37232
(615) 322-2145

TEXAS

Baylor College of Medicine
Office of Admissions
One Baylor Plaza
Rm. N104
Houston, TX 77030
(713) 798-4842

Texas A&M University
College of Medicine
Associate Dean for Admissions and
Student Affairs
159 Joe H. Reynolds Medical Bldg.
College Station, TX 77843-1114
(409) 845-7744

Texas Tech University
School of Medicine
Health Sciences Center
Office of Admissions 2 B116
Lubbock, TX 79430
(806) 743-2297

University of Texas
Southwestern Medical Center
at Dallas
Office of Admissions
5323 Harry Hines Blvd.
Dallas, TX 75235-9096
(214) 688-2670

University of Texas Medical
Branch
Office of Admissions
1-212 Ashbel Smith Bldg.

Galveston, TX 77555-1305
(409) 772-1215

University of Texas College of
Medicine
Office of Admissions
6431 Fannin
Houston, TX 77225
(713) 500-5116

University of Texas
Health Sciences Center at San
Antonio
Medical School Admissions
Registrar's Office
7703 Floyd Curl Drive
San Antonio, TX 78284-7702
(512) 567-2665

UTAH

University of Utah School of
Medicine
Director, Medical School Admissions
50 North Medical Drive
Salt Lake City, UT 84132
(801) 581-7498

VERMONT

University of Vermont College
of Medicine
Admissions Office
E-109 Given Bldg.
Burlington, VT 05405
(802) 656-2154

VIRGINIA

Eastern Virginia Medical
School
Office of Admissions
721 Fairfax Ave.
Norfolk, VA 23507
(804) 446-5812

Virginia Commonwealth
University
College of Medicine
Office of Admissions
1101 East Marshall St.
Richmond, VA 23298-0565
(804) 786-9630

University of Virginia School
of Medicine
Admissions Office
Box 235
Charlottesville, VA 22908
(804) 924-5571

WASHINGTON

University of Washington
Admissions Office
1959 Northeast Pacific
Box 356340
Seattle, WA 98195
(206) 543-7212

WEST VIRGINIA

Marshall University School of
Medicine
Admissions Office
1542 Spring Valley Drive
Huntington, WV 25704
(304) 696-7312

West Virginia University
School of Medicine
Office of Admissions and Records
1170 Health Sciences Center
P.O. Box 9815
Morgantown, WV 26506-9815
(304) 293-3521

WISCONSIN

Medical College of Wisconsin
Office of Admissions and Registrar
8701 Watertown Plank Road
Milwaukee, WI 53226
(414) 257-8246

University of Wisconsin
Medical School
Admissions Committee
Medical Sciences Center, Rm. 114(
1300 University Ave.
Madison, WI 53706
(608) 265-6344

Canadian Medical Schools*

ALBERTA
University of Alberta Faculty of Medicine
Admissions Officer
245 Medical Science Bldg.
Edmonton, AB Canada T6G 2H7
(403) 492-6350

University of Calgary Faculty of Medicine
Office of Admissions
3330 Hospital Drive, N.W.
Calgary, AB Canada T2N 4N1
(403) 220-6849

BRITISH COLUMBIA
University of British Columbia
Office of the Dean, Faculty of Medicine
Admissions Office
Rm. 317-2194 Health Sciences Center Mall
Vancouver, BC Canada V6T 1Z3
(604) 822-0747

MANITOBA
University of Manitoba Faculty of Medicine
Chairman, Admissions Committee
753 McDermot Ave.
Winnipeg, MB Canada R3E 0W3
(204) 789-3568

NEWFOUNDLAND
Memorial University of Newfoundland
Office of Admissions Rm. 1751
Faculty of Medicine
St. John's, NF Canada A1B 3V6
(709) 737-6615

NOVA SCOTIA
Dalhousie University
Admissions Coordinator
Rm. C132, Lower Level
Clinical Research Center
5849 University Ave.
Halifax, NS Canada B3H 4H7
(902) 494-1874

ONTARIO
McMaster University
Admissions and Records
Rm. 187 - Health Sciences Centre
1200 Main St. West
Hamilton, ON Canada L8N 3Z5
(905) 525-9140, Ext. 2114

University of Ottawa Faculty of Medicine
Assistant to the Dean
550 Cumberland St.
P.O. Box 450, Station A
Ottawa, ON Canada K1H 6N5
(613) 562-5409

Queen's University Faculty of Medicine
Admissions Office
Rm. 224 Botterell Hall
Kingston, ON Canada K7L 3N6
(613) 545-2542

University of Toronto Faculty of Medicine
Office of Admission
One King's College Circle
Rm. 2124
Toronto, ON Canada M5S 1A8
(416) 978-2717

University of Western Ontario Faculty of Medicine - Admissions
Rm. M103
London, ON Canada N6A 5C1
(519) 661-3744

QUEBEC
Université Laval Faculty of Medicine
Faculty of Medicine, Committee for Admission
Ste-Foy, PQ Canada G1K 7P4
(418) 656-2131, Ext. 2492

McGill University Faculty of Medicine
Admissions Office
3655 Drummond St.
Rm. 633
Montreal, PQ Canada H3G 1Y6
(514) 398-3517

University of Montreal Faculty of Medicine
Committee on Admission
P.O. Box 6128, Station A
Montreal, PQ Canada H3C 3J7
(514) 343-6265

University of Sherbrooke
Faculty of Medicine
Admission Office
3001 12th Ave. North
Sherbrooke, PQ Canada J1H 5N4
(819) 564-5208

SASKATCHEWAN
University of Saskatchewan College of Medicine
Office of Admissions
Rm. B103 Health Sciences Bldg.
107 Wiggins Road
Saskatoon, SK Canada S7N 5E5
(306) 966-6896

INSTALLING REA's TEST*ware*®

System Requirements
14-inch monitor or larger; CD-ROM drive

Macintosh: Any Macintosh with a 68020 or higher processor or Power Macintosh, 4 MB of RAM minimum, System 7.1 or later. At least 5 MB of hard-disk space available.

Windows: Any PC with 4 MB of RAM minimum and at least 5 MB of hard-disk space available.

MACINTOSH INSTALLATION

1. Insert the MCAT TEST*ware*® CD-ROM into the CD-ROM drive.

2. Double-click on the REA MCAT INSTALLER icon. The installer will automatically place the program containing the MCAT TEST*ware*® into a folder entitled "REA MCAT." If the name and location are suitable, click the INSTALL button. If you want to change this, type over the existing information, and then click INSTALL.

3. Start the MCAT TEST*ware*® application by double-clicking on its icon.

WINDOWS INSTALLATION

1. Insert the MCAT TEST*ware*® CD-ROM into the CD-ROM drive.

2. From the Start Menu, choose the RUN command. When the RUN dialog box appears, type d:\setup (where D is the letter of your CD-ROM drive) at the prompt and click OK.

3. The installation process will begin. A dialog box proposing the directory "REA_MCAT" will appear. If the name and location are suitable, click OK. If you wish to specify a different name or location, type it in and click OK.

4. Start the MCAT TEST*ware*® application by double-clicking on its icon.

TECHNICAL SUPPORT

REA TEST*ware*® is backed by customer and technical support. For questions about **installation or operation of your software**, contact us at:

Research & Education Association
Phone: (732) 819-8880 (9 a.m. to 5 p.m. ET)
Fax: (732) 819-8808
Website: http://www.rea.com
E-mail: info@rea.com

USING YOUR INTERACTIVE MCAT TEST*ware*®

REA's MCAT TEST*ware*® is **EASY TO LEARN AND USE.** To achieve maximum benefits, we recommend that you take a few minutes to go through the on-screen tutorial on your computer. The "screen buttons" are also explained here to familiarize you with the program.

Program Help and Test Directions

To get help at any time during the test, choose the **Program Help** button, which reviews basic functions of the program. The **Test Directions** button allows you to review the specific exam directions during any part of the test.

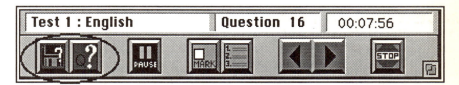

Stop Test

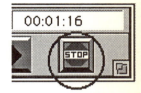

At any time during the test or when you are finished taking the test, click on the **Stop** button. The program will advance you to the next screen.

Once you leave this test, without suspending the exam, you will not be able to return to this test.

| GO TO NEXT TEST | SUSPEND EXAM | RETURN TO WHERE I WAS |

This screen allows you to go to the next test section, suspend or quit the entire test, or it can return you to the last question accessed prior to clicking the **Stop** button.

Arrow Buttons

When an answer is selected, click on the Right Arrow button or press the Return key to proceed to the next question.

Mark Questions

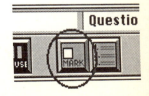

If you are unsure about an answer to a particular question, the program allows you to mark it for later review. Flag the question by clicking on the **Mark** button.

Table of Contents

To review all marked questions, review answer choices, or skip to any question within a test section, click on the **Table of Contents** button.

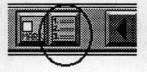

Results

Review and analyze your performance on the test by clicking on the **Results** button.

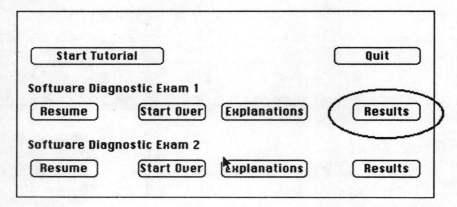

Explanations

In Explanations mode, click on the **Explanation** button to pop up a detailed explanation to any question. At the end of every explanation is a page reference to the appropriate review section in the book.

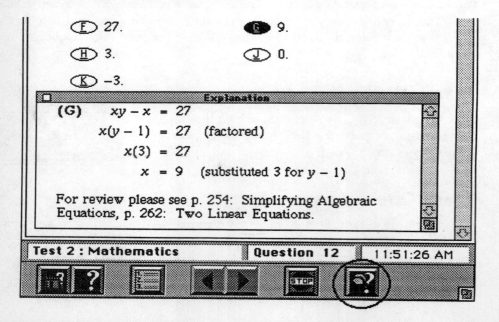